Observation Medicine

Using sample clinical protocols, order sets, and administrative policies that any hospital can use, this book gives a detailed account of how to set up and run an observation unit (OU) and reviews conditions in which observational medicine (OM) may be beneficial. In addition to clinical topics such as improving patient outcomes and avoiding readmissions, it also includes practical topics such as design, staffing, and daily operations; fiscal aspects such as coding, billing, and reimbursement; regulatory concerns such as aligning case management and utilization review with observation; nursing considerations; and more. The future of OM, and how OM can help solve the healthcare crisis from costs to access, is also discussed. Although based on U.S. practices, this book is also applicable to an international audience, and contains instructions for implementing observation in any setting or locale and in any type of hospital or other appropriate facility.

Sharon E. Mace is Professor of Medicine at the Cleveland Clinic Lerner College of Medicine of Case Western Reserve University; Director of Observation Unit, Director of Research, and previously Director of Pediatric Education/Quality Improvement at the Emergency Services Institute, Cleveland Clinic; and a member of the Faculty of MetroHealth Medical Center/Cleveland Clinic Emergency Medicine Residency in Cleveland, Ohio.

Observation Medicine

Principles and Protocols

Edited by

Sharon E. Mace
Emergency Services Institute, Cleveland Clinic, Cleveland, OH

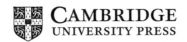

CAMBRIDGE
UNIVERSITY PRESS

CAMBRIDGE
UNIVERSITY PRESS

University Printing House, Cambridge CB2 8BS, United Kingdom

One Liberty Plaza, 20th Floor, New York, NY 10006, USA

477 Williamstown Road, Port Melbourne, VIC 3207, Australia

4843/24, 2nd Floor, Ansari Road, Daryaganj, Delhi – 110002, India

79 Anson Road, #06-04/06, Singapore 079906

Cambridge University Press is part of the University of Cambridge.

It furthers the University's mission by disseminating knowledge in the pursuit of education, learning, and research at the highest international levels of excellence.

www.cambridge.org
Information on this title: www.cambridge.org/9781107022348

First published 2017

Printed in the United Kingdom by Clays, St Ives plc

A catalog record for this publication is available from the British Library.

Library of Congress Cataloging in Publication Data
Names: Mace, Sharon E., editor.
Title: Observation medicine : principles and protocols / edited by Sharon E. Mace.
Other titles: Observation medicine (Mace)
Description: Cambridge, United Kingdom ; New York : Cambridge University Press, 2016. | Includes bibliographical references and index.
Identifiers: LCCN 2015048881 | ISBN 9781107022348 (Hardback : alk. paper)
Subjects: | MESH: Emergency Service, Hospital | Diagnostic Techniques and Procedures | Emergency Medicine–methods | Watchful Waiting–methods | Patient Admission
Classification: LCC RT48 | NLM WX 215 | DDC 616.07/5–dc23 LC record available at http://lccn.loc.gov/2015048881

ISBN 978-1-107-02234-8 Hardback

....

Contents

Advance Praise

This is a wonderful, much needed book by a wonderful, much learned author. Dr. Mace has decades of experience in observation medicine and even more in emergency medicine leadership. This book not only includes the best summary to date of what EM observation medicine has been but also provides a road map to the future. If your practice includes observation medicine, you need this book. Rock on, Dr. Mace.

Nick Jouriles, MD, FACEP Chair, EM, Cleveland Clinic Akron General: Professor & Chair, EM, Northeast Ohio Medical University; President, ED Benchmarking Alliance; Past President, American College of Emergency Physicians

"Observation Medicine: Principles and Protocols" edited by Dr. Sharon E. Mace is a relevant and timely textbook to Emergency Medicine. It has unique content as it relates to the development of both adult and pediatric observation medicine. The book is written in an easy to read format with many outstanding ideas on how to implement observation medicine in the emergency department. This is an indispensable resource!

Isabel A. Barata, MS, MD, MBA, FACP, FAAP, FACEP
Associate Professor of Pediatrics and Emergency Medicine, Hofstra Northwell School of Medicine; Pediatric Emergency Medicine Service Line Quality Director, Emergency Medicine and Pediatrics Service Line; Director of Pediatric Emergency Medicine, North Shore University Hospital

Finally! After decades, an up-to-date authority on observation units and observation medicine. If you are in any way involved in this dynamic aspect of emergency medicine, this book is for you. From the clinical to the administrative to the convoluted billing and regulatory issues, this book is a wealth of information that will help you navigate this complex area of emergency medical practice. The included clinical protocols, alone, are worth their weight in gold; they will give you an excellent basis for the wide range of problems we can safely deal with through observation medicine. I just wish we had access to the knowledge and wisdom contained in this book when we started our observation unit in 1979!

Stephen V. Cantrill, MD, FACEP
Denver Health Medical Center
University of Colorado School of Medicine

Observation medicine is the perfect tool for progressive emergency physicians to leverage improvements in cost, quality and patient satisfaction. I have seen physician groups and hospitals struggle to collect all the information necessary to build and run an observation medicine service effectively, sometimes taking years to get it right. We have needed this book for a long time, and now it's here – a single source for the best information on what, why and how to develop an observation service that lasts and adds value to your hospital partner.

James R. Blakeman
Executive Vice President
Emergency Group's Office, San Dimas, CA

Dr. Mace's Observation Medicine is a must have for all physicians and administrators who have or would like to start an observation unit. Jammed with helpful tips, useful clinical protocols and administrative guidelines, it will guarantee the success of your program!!

Ann M Dietrich, MD, FAAP, FACEP
Associate Professor Ohio University Heritage College of Medicine
Medical Director of Education Ohio ACEP

As a longstanding residency director, it is difficult to provide the training needed to keep up with the advancements in emergency care. Observation medicine is proving to be an extremely valuable addition to emergency care, and emergency medicine residents need to be exposed and trained in this facet of emergency care. Dr. Mace's textbook, Observation Medicine, provides a valuable training resource useful to all emergency medicine residencies. This textbook provides the background needed to not only work within an emergency department that has an Observation unit, but potentially to develop one. This is a great resource for training in Observation Medicine.

Michael S. Beeson, M.D., MBA
Program Director of Emergency Medicine
Professor | EM | Northeast Ohio Medical University
Director | American Board of Emergency Medicine
Cleveland Clinic Akron General

The face of health care is changing and that is a good thing. However, we are a stubborn group and change is difficult. Dr. Mace's book describes observation care in a manner that is easily understood by all healthcare providers and administrators. What we are unfamiliar with We are afraid of... Dr. Mace's book will provide the knowledge you need to embrace the change and leverage the observation services you deliver. As a nurse, we continue to care for our patients the same as we always have but in a shorter span of time, this book shares invaluable information in resource management, time management and expedited care management. This book is a MUST HAVE for success in our evolving health care environment.

Ethel Games, RN
Emergency Room Nurse
Fountain Valley Regional Hospital
Fountain Valley, California

This text will serve as the "go to" resource for health care providers managing patients in an observation unit. The book is well organized with chapters that focus on the content most relevant to contemporary observation medicine. There is no doubt it will become required reading for the observation medicine curriculum in EM residency programs.

Michael Brown, MD, MSc
Professor, Michigan State University College of Human Medicine

Chair, Department of Emergency Medicine, Michigan State University Grand Rapids, Michigan

The Textbook *Observation Medicine: Principles and Protocols* edited by Sharon E. Mace is a must have in your Emergency Medicine Library. Dr. Mace, an experienced Emergency Physician practicing Observation Medicine for Adults and Children at the Cleveland Clinic Hospital System for decades, has assembled a team of contributors representing the best and brightest of Emergency Medicine. In the ninety-six (96) Chapters of this book, the reader will learn everything you need in implementing an Observation Unit for your Emergency Department and your hospital. The breath of this book is exhaustive. The chapters are organized into multiple sections. They include: "Administration, Clinical Setting and Education, New Developments, Financial (including coding and reimbursement), Clinical Protocols, Administrative Policies, Order Sets for Adults and Pediatrics, and much more."

Economics and the desire to provide optimal care for Emergency patients who needed just a little bit more time to stabilize their care, arrive at a definitive answer, or prepare patients for safe discharge home without a hospital admission, helped to drive the development of this specialized area of Emergency Medicine.

As written, in the forward by Greg Henry, MD, FACEP, (Past President of the American College of Emergency Physicians), "Remember the goals: cost-effective care, time-efficient care, the best patient outcomes, and more compassionate human-centered care. Observation medicine can achieve these goals."

This book can help establish an Observation Unit as part of your Emergency Department through its guidance of Administration, Protocols, exploring the types of Clinical Problems that would best be served by these units. They also bring in the experts of reimbursement to help you pay for the services you provide. If you already have an Observation Unit, this book is essential to operating that unit correctly and at a higher level. If it is your responsibility, as an Emergency Department Leader (Director, Associate Director, or responsible for medical or nursing education), the protocols and educational modules will make your life easier.

Do yourself a favor and purchase this book for yourself and your department. You will be glad you made the investment.

Andrew I. Bern, MD, FACEP
Past Member, ACEP Board of Directors
Past, Chairman of the ACEP Board of Directors

We currently sit amidst one of the most transformational periods in healthcare, with a rise in consumer based value assessments that are driving care. For those with new or worsened illness or injury, observation care is a key tool after emergency department care to optimize outcomes and enhance value. This *Observation Medicine* text assembles the knowledge needed, from organization and oversight through symptom-driven approaches and disease specific care. Rather than searching through many texts or sites, Dr. Mace and her team created a singular source that uses a clear and accessible format to aid those wanting to start or improve their observation unit.

Donald M. Yealy, MD

Chair, Department of Emergency Medicine, University of Pittsburgh / University of Pittsburgh Physicians; Senior Medical Director, Health Services Division, and Vice President of Emergency and Urgent Care Services, UPMC; Professor of Emergency Medicine, Medicine, and Clinical and Translational Sciences, University of Pittsburgh School of Medicine

About the Editors

Editor

Sharon E. Mace, MD, FACEP, FAAP is board certified in emergency medicine and pediatrics. She is a Professor of Medicine at the Cleveland Clinic Lerner College of Medicine at Case Western Reserve University and is full time faculty in emergency medicine for the MetroHealth Medical Center/Cleveland Clinic Emergency Medicine Residency Program in Cleveland, Ohio. She has over 37 years of administrative and clinical experience in emergency medicine in academic and community hospital settings including nearly a decade as a Director of the Emergency Department in a Community Hospital. She is currently an attending physician in the Emergency Services Institute at the Cleveland Clinic. She is the Director of Research and has been the first and only Director of the Observation Unit at the Cleveland Clinic for the past 23 years since the inception of the "Clinical Decision Unit" in 1994, where she has been able to mentor medical students, residents and even several international fellows in observation medicine. The observation unit at the Cleveland Clinic is a 20 bed unit that places about 6,000 patients a year in the Observation Unit. She has also been Director of Pediatric Education and Quality Improvement for the Cleveland Clinic Emergency Services Institute. She has lectured nationally and internationally on emergency medicine especially observation medicine. She has served as the Chairman of the Section of Observation Medicine for the American College of Emergency Physicians and on the Observation Medicine Committee for the Society of Hospital Medicine that authored a white paper on observation medicine. She has authored over 200 articles in the medical literature, over 60 textbook chapters (excluding this textbook) and edited a previous medical textbook and now this second authoritative and comprehensive textbook on observation medicine. She has been the recipient of numerous grants and awards including a National Science Foundation Research Fellowship, Academic Residency Science Day Award, National Chapter Project Award, State Emergency Medical Services Council Award for Leadership and Excellence in Emergency Medical Services, the American Association of Women Emergency Physicians Research and Education Award, and Who's Who in America and Who's Who in the World. She has served as a course director for numerous medical courses including many national conferences on Observation Medicine and has even been a member of the Pediatric Medical Care Subcommittee for the National Presidential Commission on Children and Disasters.

Section Editors

Matthew J. Campbell, Pharm.D., BCPS obtained his Doctor of Pharmacy degree from Ohio Northern University and subsequently completed a Pharmacy Practice Residency at MetroHealth Medical Center in Cleveland, Ohio. He is a licensed pharmacist in the state of Ohio and is a Board Certified Pharmacotherapy Specialist (BCPS). He has received numerous honors and awards including the Ohio Northern University Presidential Merit Scholarship, Institutional Preceptor of the Year at the College of Pharmacy at Lake Erie College of Osteopathic Medicine, Pharmacist Mission Award at Cleveland Clinic, and the Promoting the Profession Award at Cleveland Clinic. He has had numerous presentations locally and nationally and is actively involved with pharmacy resident education at Cleveland Clinic. He practiced as a Clinical Pharmacy Specialist in the surgical ICU of a community hospital for several years and is currently the Lead Pharmacist in the Emergency Services Institute at the Cleveland Clinic in Cleveland, Ohio. He is the Section Editor for the Section IX: 1 Adult Order Sets and Section IX: 2 Pediatric Order Sets.

Karen Games, RN, has over 40 years of experience as a registered nurse and as a case manager. She received her nursing degree from South Surburban College in Illinois, and completed a Critical Care Specialty Nursing Course at Good Samaritan Hospital in Los Angeles. Her academic credentials include the following training and certifications: FHP Management Training – Quality Education System, HFMA Billing Compliance and a five year Certification Program in Case Management (CCM). She is also an InterQual Certified Trainer. She has been a consultant and a national speaker on Case Management. With her extensive nursing, case management, and administrative experience, she has had an opportunity to develop multiple programs, policies and procedures related to nursing, case management, and observation medicine. Her various administrative positions include serving as a Regional Case Management Director, a PMI Case Management Specialist, the Director of Case Management Education and Informatics for the Tenet Health System. She has also been the Director of Risk Management and Patient Safety for Desert Regional Medical Center in California and most recently, Administrative Director of Collaborative Care at Los Alamitos Medical Center, also in California. She is the Section Editor for Chapter 7: Nursing, Chapter 64: Determining the Correct Status and Chapter 65: Care Coordination.

Michael Granovsky, MD, CPC, CEDC, FACEP is board certified in emergency medicine. His certifications in coding include the American Academy of Professional Coders (AAPC) – Certified Professional Coder and AAPC – CEDC ED Specialty Certification. He has been a member of the American College of Emergency Physicians (ACEP) for 20 years, a member of the AAPC for 15 years and has served for nearly 15 years on the ACEP Physicians Coding and Nomenclature Advisory Committee (CNAC), including three years as the CNAC National Chairman. He has spoken nationally at numerous conferences and has been the author of many articles in professional publications dealing with reimbursement, practice management issues, CPT, ICD-9, CMS issues and ICD-10. He has served as the course director for the ACEP Coding and Reimbursement Conference for over a decade. He has been on the editorial board and served as the editor for ED Coding Alert. He is the Technical Editor of the AAPC ED specialized CPC–CEDC Emergency Department Coding Specialty Certification. He is the subject matter expert on the ED Specialty Exam and Study Guide for the AAPC. His service on national committees includes immediate past chairman ACEP National Coding Advisory Committee, Work Group Chair ICD-10 – ACEP Quality and Performance Committee, ACEP Expert Technical Panel for Quality Measure Development, ACEP Registry Task Force and the ACEP Reimbursement Committee – Fair Payment Work Group Chair. Dr. Granovsky is currently the Chairman of the ACEP Reimbursement Committee. As the President, Division of Coding for Logix Health; he is responsible for health policy, coding, education, and regulatory processes with oversight of seven million annual emergency department claims. He is the Section Editor for Section V: Financial Coding and Reimbursement and Chapters 1 and 2.

Contributors

Sharon E. Mace, MD, FACEP, FAAP
Professor of Medicine, Cleveland Clinic Lerner
College of Medicine at Case Western Reserve
University, Faculty, MetroHealth/Cleveland
Clinic Emergency Medicine Residency
Director, Observation Unit and Director,
Research Cleveland Clinic Cleveland, OH

Robert E. O'Connor, MD, MPH, FACEP
Chair, Physician-in-Chief, Department of
Emergency Medicine, University of Virginia
Health System, Charlottesville, Va. Chair, Board
of Directors, American College of Physicians

Louis Graff MD FACEP FACP FACC.
Professor Surgery and Emergency Medicine.
Clinical Professor Medicine.
University of Connecticut School of Medicine.
Chair Utilization Review Committee.
Hartford Healthcare Corporation Central Region
Hospitals
Farmington, CT

David Robinson, MD, MS, MMM, FACEP
Professor and Vice-Chairman of
Emergency Medicine, University of Texas
Medical School at Houston;
Chief of Emergency Services, Lyndon B. Johnson
Hospital, Harris Health System Houston, TX

Christopher W. Baugh, MD,MBA, FACEP
Medical Director of Clinical Operations and
Observation Medicine
Department of Emergency Medicine | Brigham &
Women's Hospital
Assistant Professor Harvard Medical School
Boston, MA

J. Stephen Bohan, MD, MS, FACEP, FACP
Executive Vice Chair, Emergency Medicine
Brigham and Women's Hospital
Associate Professor, Harvard Medical School
Boston, MA

Karen Games, RN
Director of Process Improvement, Los Alamitos
Medical Center

Gregory L. Henry, MD, FACEP
Clinical Professor Department of Emergency
Medicine, University of Michigan Medical School,
Ann Arbor, MI, Past President, American College
of Emergency Physicians

Elaine Thallner, MD, MS
Organizational Development and Change
Management
Staff Physician, Emergency Services Institute,
Cleveland Clinic Foundation, Cleveland, OH

Ryan Prudoff, DO, MS, FACEP
Staff Emergency Physician, Cleveland Clinic
Foundation
Clinical Associate Professor Emergency Medicine
Ohio University Heritage College of Osteopathic
Medicine
Cleveland, OH

Stephen Sayles, MD, FACEP
Director Cleveland Clinic Brunswick Emergency
Department, Cleveland Clinic Foundation,
Cleveland, OH

Robert S. Bennett, MD
Director, Observation Unit, Highland Hospital
Rochester, NY

Jonathan Glauser, MD, FACEP
Professor Emergency Medicine Case Western
Reserve University.
Faculty Emergency Medicine Residency
MetroHealth/Cleveland Clinic Cleveland, OH

David J. Paje, FACP, SFHM
Assistant Professor at University of Michigan
Medical School
Associate Director, Medical Short Stay Unit,
University of Michigan Health System

Staff Physician, Ann Arbor VA Healthcare System
Ann Arbor, MI

Peter Y. Watson, MD, FACP, SFHM
Division Head of Hospital Medicine
Henry Ford Hospital Detroit, MI

Pawan Suri, MD
Chair, Division of Observation Medicine
Program Director, Combined EM/IM Residency Program
Department of Emergency Medicine
Assistant Professor in Emergency Medicine and Internal Medicine
Virginia Commonwealth University Medical Center
Richmond, VA

Margarita Pena, MD, FACEP
Medical Director, Clinical Decision Unit
Associate Program Director, Emergency Medicine
St. John Hospital and Medical Center
Detroit, MI

L. Christine Gilmore, MD
Physician, Wake Forest Baptist Medical Center
Department of Emergency Medicine Winston-Salem, NC

Bret A. Nicks, MD, MHA, FACEP
Chief Medical Officer, Wake Forest Baptist Health - Davie Medical Center
Emergency Medicine Winston-Salem, NC

Catherine T. Puetz, MD, FACEP
Attending Physician Department of Emergency Medicine
Grand Rapids, MI

Kayur V. Patel MD, FACP, FACPE, FACHE, FACEP
Chairman, Access2MD Terre Haute, Indiana

Igor Kozunov, MBA, MHA
Chief Executive Officer, Wellness For Life Medical, LLC
Indianapolis, IN

Louella Vaughan, MBBS, MPhil, DPhil, FRACP
Consultant Physician in Acute Medicine, The Royal London Hospital
Senior Clinical Research Fellow, The Nuffield Trust,

Senior Clinical Research Fellow, Northwest London CLAHRC
London, UK

Tertius T. Tuy, MD
Singapore General Hospital, Singapore, Former Research Fellow, Cleveland Clinic Foundation, Emergency Services Institute, Cleveland, OH

W. Frank Peacock, MD, FACEP, FACC
Professor, Emergency Medicine
Associate Chair and Research Director
Baylor College of Medicine
Houston, Texas

Jieun Kim, MD
Medical Officer, Singapore General Hospital, Singapore Former Research Fellow, Cleveland Clinic Foundation, Emergency Services Institute, Cleveland, OH

T. Andrew Windsor, MD, RDMS, FAAEM
Assistant Professor, Department of Emergency Medicine
University of Maryland School of Medicine
Baltimore, MD

Amal Mattu, MD, FACEP, FAAEM
Professor and Vice-Chair, Emergency Medicine, University of Maryland, Baltimore, MD

Kami M. Hu, MD
Critical Care Medicine Fellow, University of Maryland Medical Center
Departments of Internal and Emergency Medicine
Baltimore, MD

Eric Anderson MD, MBA, FACEP, FAAEM
Faculty Cleveland Clinic – MetroHealth Emergency Medicine Residency
Faculty Emergency Medicine Cleveland Clinic Lerner College of Medicine
Cleveland, OH

Chew Yian Chai, MD, MCEM, FAMS
Consultant/ EDTU Director, National University Hospital Emergency Medicine Department, Singapore

Carol L Clark MDMBA FACEP
Professor, Oakland University William Beaumont School of Medicine
Associate Director of Research

Department of Emergency Medicine
Beaumont Health Systems- Royal Oak, MI

Michelle A. Wiener, MD, MS
Clinical Faculty, Wayne State University School
of Medicine
St. John Medical Center, Detroit , MI

Matthew Tabbut, MD, FACEP
Attending Physician, Department of Emergency
Medicine, MetroHealth Medical Center
Assistant Professor of Emergency Medicine,
Case Western Reserve University School of
Medicine
Cleveland, OH

Saurin Bhatt, MD, MBA
Faculty Cleveland Clinic – MetroHealth
Emergency Medicine Residency
Faculty Emergency Medicine Cleveland Clinic
Lerner College of Medicine, Cleveland, OH

Mark G. Moseley MD, MHA, FACEP
Vice Chairman for Clinical Affairs
The OSU Department of Emergency Medicine
Medical Director for Utilization Management
The Ohio State University Health System
Columbus, OH

Miles P. Hawley, MD, MBA
Senior Medical Director, System Hospitalist and
Observation Services
Director, Physician Advisor Services
OhioHealth Columbus, OH

Taruna Aurora, MD
Assistant Professor, Departments of Emergency &
Internal Medicine
Director, Clinical Decision Unit, Emergency
Department
Medical Director, Department of Care
Coordination and Utilization Management
Virginia Commonwealth University Health
Systems
Richmond, VA

Kimberly A. Ressler, MD, MSN
Attending Physician
Rochester General Hospital Rochester, NY

Matt Lyon, MD, FACEP
Professor and Vice Chairman
Director, Emergency Department Observation
Unit

Director, Center of Ultrasound Education and
Research
Department of Emergency Medicine and
Hospitalist Services
Medical College of Georgia, Augusta University

Leah S. Taylor, MA
Instructor, Augusta University
Augusta, GA

Robert W. Gibson, PhD, MSOTR/L FAOTA
Professor, Director of Research
Department of Emergency Medicine
Medical College of Georgia
Augusta University, Augusta, GA

Rokhsanna Sadeghi, MD, MPH
Finger Lakes Health, Attending Physician Geneva,
NY

Abhinav Chandra, MD, FACEP
Kaiser Permanente Senior Clinician Physician in
Emergency Medicine,
Director of Emergency Observation Medicine,
Kaiser Permanente South Sacramento, CA

Elizabeth A. Rees, MD
Attending Physician, Methodist Medical Center
Oak Ridge, TN. (formerly Wake Forest Baptist
Health Medical Center, Winston-Salem, NC)

Claire Pearson MD, MPH
Assistant Professor, Department of Emergency
Medicine
Division of Clinical Research, Wayne State
University School of Medicine

Robert D. Welch, MD, MS, FACEP
Professor , Wayne State University School of
Medicine
Director of Clinical Research, Department of
Emergency Medicine
Detroit Receiving Hospital, Detroit, MI

Brian Kern, MD
Attending Physician, Detroit Medical Center,
Clinical Assistant Professor, Department of
Emergency Medicine, Wayne State University
School of Medicine

Veronica Sikka MD, Phd, MHA, MPH, FACEP
Veronica Sikka, MD, PhD, MHA, MPH, FAAEM,
FACEP
Chief, Emergency Medicine

Orlando VA Medical Center
Associate Professor, Emergency Medicine
UCF School of Medicine Orlando, FL

Renee Reid, MD, FACEP
Assistant Professor, Virginia Commonwealth
University Richmond, VA

Harinder Dhindsa, MD, MBA, MPH
Associate Professor, Attending
Physician, Virginia Commonwealth University
School of Medicine, Chief of Emergency
Medicine, Richmond, VA

Aderonke Ojo, MBBS
Associate Professor of Pediatrics
Baylor College of Medicine
Attending ED Physician, Texas Children's
Hospital, Houston, TX

Fredric M. Hustey, MD, FACEP
Attending Physician Cleveland Clinic
Associate Professor, Cleveland Clinic Lerner
College of Medicine
Case Western Reserve University, Cleveland, OH

Nathaniel L. Scott, MD, FACEP
Program Director, EM / IM Combined Residency
Program
Staff Physician, Emergency Medicine and
Hospital Medicine, Hennepin County Medical
Center
Assistant Professor, University of Minnesota
Medical School Minneapolis, MN

James R. Miner, MD, FACEP
Chief of Emergency Medicine
Hennepin County Medical Center
Professor of Emergency Medicine
University of Minnesota, Minneapolis, MN

Steven J. Walsh, MD
Fellow, Carolinas Poison Center, Chapel Hill, NC

Marsha Ford, MD, FACEP
Former President, American Association Poison
Control Centers, Adjunct Professor UNC-Chapel
Hill School of Medicine, Toxicoligist/Attending
Physician Carolinas Healthcare System Charlotte,
NC

Constance J. Doyle, MD, FACEP
Clinical Instructor Emergency Medicine
University of Michigan, Attending Physician

St Joseph Mercy Hospital Emergency Medicine,
Ann Arbor, MI

Michael A. Granovsky, MD, CPC, CEDC, FACEP
President, Coding for Logix Health
Chair, ACEP Physicians Coding and
Nomenclature Advisory
Committee (CNAC)

David A. McKenzie, CAE
Reimbursement Director, American College of
Emergency Physicians Dallas, TX

Candace E. Schaeffer, RN, MBA, RHIA
Compliance Officer, Optum360

BK Kizziar, RN-BC, CCM
Member Case Management Society of America,
Owner, BK Associates Grandbury, TX

Nancy E. Skinner, RN-BC, CCM
President, Riverside HealthCare Consulting
Whitwell, TN

Robert L. Leviton, MD, MPH, CI, FACEP
Chief Medical Information Officer - Physician
Advisor
Bronx Lebanon Hospital Center, Bronx, NY

Sandra Sieck, RN, MBA
Chief Executive Officer, Sieck HealthCare
Mobile, Al

Heather Tuffin, MBChB (UCT), DipPEC (CMSA)
Improvement Advisor, Western
Cape Department of Health, Capetown,
South Africa

LA Wallis, MBChB, FRCS, DIMCRCS, Dip Sport
Med, FCEM, FIFEM
Professor and Head of Emergency Medicine,
Stellenbosch University
Head of Emergency Medicine, Western Cape
Government
President, International Federation for
Emergency Medicine
Professor and Head of Emergency Medicine,
University of Cape Town, South Africa

Malcolm Mahadevan MD, FRCS, MRCP, FAMS
Associate Professor, National University of
Singapore
Head and Senior Consultant, National University
Hospital System, Singapore

John Burke, FACEM
Deputy Director, Emergency Department
Royal Brisbane & Women's Hospital
Brisbane, Australia

Michael Ardagh, ONZM, PhD, MbChB, DCH, FACEM
Professor of Emergency Medicine, University of Otago, Christchurch, New Zealand

Said Laribi, MD, PhD
Professor of Emergency Medicine, University of Tours, France
Chair of the Emergency Medicine Department, Tours University Hospital, France

Patrick Plaisance, MD, PhD
Professor of Emergency Medicine, University Paris Diderot, France
Chair of the Emergency Room, Lariboisière University Hospital, Paris, France

Martin Mockel, MD, PhD, FESC, FAHA
Charité – Universitätsmedizin Berlin, Berlin, Germany

Julia Searle, MD, MPH
Charité – Universitätsmedizin Berlin, Berlin, Germany

Salvatore Di Somma, MD, PhD
Department of Emergency Medicine
Sant'Andrea Hospital, Rome, Italy
Department of Medical and Surgery Science and Translational Medicine
University "Sapienza", Rome, Italy

Angelo Ianni, MD
Department of Emergency Medicine
Sant'Andrea Hospital, Rome, Italy

Christina Bongiovanni , MD
Department of Emergency Medicine
Sant'Andrea Hospital, Rome, Italy

Dylan Jenkins, MBBS
Consultant, Doncaster Royal Infirmary
Doncaster, United Kingdom

Carlos-Hernan Camargo-Mila, M.D., E.A.E.S., A.C.E.P.
Professor of Surgery and Emergency Medicine
Colegio Mayor del Rosario University
Chairman of the Emergency Department
Fundación CardioInfantil - Instituto de Cardiología
Bogotá D.C. - COLOMBIA

Madeline Joseph, MD, FACEP, FAAP
Professor of Emergency Medicine and Pediatrics
Assistant Chair of Pediatric Emergency Medicine
Quality Improvement, Department of Emergency Medicine
University of Florida College of Medicine-Jacksonville, FL

Sean Bush, MD, FACEP
Professor of Emergency Medicine Brody School of Medicine East Carolina University, Attending Physician Vidant Medical Center Greenville, NC

Matthew J. Campbell, Pharm. D., BCPS
Lead Pharmacist Emergency Department,
Cleveland Clinic.
Cleveland, OH

Foreword: Onward and Upward

Science in many ways has become an international bully. It expects everyone to stop their day-to-day life as "we scientists" prod and probe the human body doing everything we can to belittle human life and reduce the patient to a soulless heart-lung preparation without value, virtue, and the essence of humanity removed. The more time the patients spend in the giant monolith known as the tertiary care hospital, the less real patient's lives become.

Enter this book and more importantly the field of observation medicine. First things first. Most books don't need a foreword! Get on with it, but in the best traditions of foreword writing I'm going to set forth a framework as to where medicine is to go if we are to have any economic viability as a profession and still meaningfully improve outcomes.

Let's draw some quick conclusions as to where medicine stands at the year 2016. What have we learned from the past? First, most things that happen in hospitals have unintended consequences, i.e. "Bad things happen; even with the best of intentions." The sooner we get you out of the hospital, the less likely you are to pick up an infection we can't cure or fall and break your hip. This is a change from my early life in medicine where we assumed that the death rate was lower inside these huge structures of science than out on the streets or at home.

Second, costs count! You can die at home for free and if we can't make a real contribution to a meaningful life, what are we doing, and why are we charging so much money for it? Human flourishing is not equivalent to having a heartbeat.

Third, Charlie Chaplin's classic film, "Modern Times" was made during the machine age when there was a wide spread fear that technology was setting the agenda for human life. "Taylorism" as the Marxist used to put it, was putting rigid unvarying thought before actions or consideration of outcomes. Substitute computer for the word machines and you have our own age.

Fourth, there is no controlled governor on the current system. Dr. John Rogers once commenting on medicine said, "They gave us an unlimited budget, and we over spent it." Will the useless CPR ever stop?

With these thoughts in mind, let's predict where medicine will be and why this book should be extremely useful. The emergency departments of America have become centers of clinical decision making. The ED is where all important decisions of inpatient v. outpatient care are now being made. Observation medicine is the new third pathway which allows a good alternative to protect inpatient populations and yet recognize that time is the only reliable test of therapy. Not all care fits into the neat four hour maximum of standard emergency department visits.

Hopefully with new opportunities to control overall costs, we will take this opportunity and seize the day. The real question is, are we going to be able to move the current system to "buy into" a healthcare product mode which addresses individual charges but can concentrate on actual costs? No economist would confuse these concepts. The bulk purchase of service will require honesty about what needs to be done for patients as opposed to what can be charged for when dealing with the government and third party payers.

Just conclude that if the days of big money and "spend at all costs" isn't over with, it shortly will be. Observation medicine should be ready to offer the cost effective alternative. If we can't do that than just burn this book and admit everyone.

Lost somewhere in ICD–10 coding, (and what isn't lost in ICD–10 coding) is the concept of making life better. Getting patients closer to their families and friends and out of rooms where the mattresses are covered in plastic and the only people who touch you wear gloves and masks.

The new world for providers looks much different than the old. It is no accident that organized medicine has not asked serious questions concerning workforce issues. 75% to 80% of the healthcare costs in America are workforce. There is almost no real research as to who should be doing just what. This is as true in urban areas as in rural outposts. It is an embarrassment that we do not have these answers which are needed if cost control is to be achieved. Even the simplest questions as to how many facilities do we need per population, hinges on the questions of utilization and cost. The number of hospital based emergency departments in the last 40 years has gone from 5,700 to slightly less than 4,000. What is the correct number of such hospitals which are needed? What is the number of free standing ERs and urgent care centers which are needed? All of these will depend on the blossoming of observation medicine. So as you proceed through this book, don't lose the forest in the ventilators. Remember the goals; cost effective care, time efficient care, the best patient outcomes, and more compassionate human centered care. Observation medicine can achieve these goals.

Ars longa vita brevis.

Greg Henry, MD

Preface

The purpose of this textbook is to provide a resource for anyone interested in observation medicine and to be a practical education for "how to" do observation in any setting or location, even internationally. Currently, there is no one source that you can reference to learn about not just the clinical aspects of observation with information including protocols and order sets; but also the administrative, business, fiscal, nursing, case management, utilization review, design, reimbursement, regulatory/governmental, and other facets of observation medicine. Monumental changes are occurring in health care not just in the United States but throughout the world and observation medicine can be on the frontlines in solving the complex issues facing healthcare now and in the future.

This text is intended to be a practicum for anyone interested in setting up or maintaining a successful Observation Unit (OU). To quote a colleague and friend, this textbook is "one stop shopping" for observation medicine. Much of the information in this textbook is not readily available elsewhere. Some of the Chapters, such as the protocols and order sets are detailed enough to serve as a "hands on' manual for observation medicine. The intent was to provide a concise, useful overview of all aspects of observation medicine starting with the clinical and expanding to the organizational and administrative aspects from set-up and staffing; to the regulatory/governmental, the business and financial, and reimbursement. This "real world" information should be applicable to any given practice setting; whether urban, suburban or rural; community-based or academic, in the United States or worldwide. In the 21st century, medicine including observation medicine is an art, a science and a business. This text is intended to address these three topics; while detailing how observation medicine operating with a patient/family centered focus can help provide the highest quality of patient care with optimal patient outcomes and be cost-effective.

I hope that everyone: clinicians, administrators, nursing, case managers, reimbursement specialists, utilization review experts, and the many others involved in any aspect of observation medicine; will find this textbook a valuable resource in their clinical practice and daily operations that can provide a useful toolkit for understanding the many complex issues with observation medicine and healthcare, and offer insights into recent developments and the future.

With any endeavor, there are many contributors. I could not have accomplished this textbook without the numerous authors and editors, as well as the individuals at Cambridge University Press. I have had the honor and pleasure of serving as the Director of the Clinical Decision Unit at the Cleveland Clinic since its beginning in 1994, more than twenty years ago. The CDU is one of the oldest OUs in existence. The 20 bed unit has averaged about 6,000 patients a year and has been in operation with the same director since its inception. Indeed, we may have the longest continuously in operation OU with the same OU director anywhere. I would like to acknowledge the numerous contributions of my colleagues and coworkers over these two decades including the many outstanding physicians, the exceptional nurses and other personal in the OU and the emergency department and the hospital staff/personnel. Thank you for allowing me to work with you and improve care for our patients. To my students, residents and fellows, thank you for allowing me to participate in your education and research. May all our patients benefit. Finally, thank you to my family and friends for their encouragement and love.

Part I

Administration: Key Concepts of Observation Medicine, and Developing and Maintaining an Observation Unit

Observation Medicine – Key Concepts: *How to Start (and Maintain) an Observation Unit: What You Need to Know*

Clinical Issues

Sharon E. Mace, MD, FACEP, FAAP

Overview and Introduction

This chapter is an introductory chapter or primer on observation medicine that answers commonly asked questions, both clinical and administrative, about observation. It gives an overview and covers the key items that are essential in setting up (and maintaining) a successful observation unit (OU). Critical items involved in creating an OU are discussed with additional information covered in later chapters.

What is Observation?

The Centers for Medicare and Medicaid Services (CMS) definition of observation status is outpatient care ordered by a physician and provided in a hospital bed to determine the need for admission:

> a well-defined set of specific, clinically appropriate services, which include ongoing short term treatment, assessment, and reassessment before a decision can be made regarding whether patients will require further treatment as hospital inpatients or if they are able to be discharged from the hospital. Observation status is commonly assigned to patients who present to the emergency department and who then require a significant period of treatment or monitoring before a decision is made concerning their admission or discharge. ... (and) in the majority of cases, the decision ... can be made in less than 48 hours, usually in less than 24 hours. In

only rare and exceptional cases do ... outpatient observation services span more than 48 hours.[1]

As noted in the CMS definition, since observation status is outpatient care, patients are not "admitted" to an OU so the terms "OU admission" or "admitted to OU" should not be used. Rather, patients are "placed in the OU" or "referred to the OU." The CMS definition also emphasizes the time-limited nature of typical observation, specifically < 24 hours in most cases.

Types of Observation Unit: Protocol Driven and Designated Unit

The types of OUs are based on whether or not they have protocols or are "protocol driven" and on whether they have a dedicated unit or dedicated space. The optimal unit is type I with both protocols and a dedicated unit. Type II is discretionary care provided in an OU. Type III, termed "a virtual OU," is protocol driven with no discrete OU, thus, the OU bed is in any location with OU beds scattered throughout the hospital. Types II and III are intermediate. The least desirable is type IV with no set protocols and no dedicated space (Table 1.1). A Type I OU is most likely to succeed and Type IV is most likely to fail. Efficiency can only be achieved with a protocol-driven OU with

Table 1.1 Types of Observation Units

Type	Protocol Driven	Dedicated Unit	Comments
Type I	Yes	Yes	Optimal, most likely to succeed
Type II	No	Yes	"Discretionary care"
Type III	Yes	No	"Virtual OU"
Type IV	No	No	Least desirable, most likely to fail

dedicated space.[2] "The strongest evidence supporting the benefits of observation care is specific to care delivered in dedicated observation units, where evidence-based evaluation and standardized protocols are used to avert inpatient admissions."[3]

This has been attributed to the fact that "ED (emergency department)-based OUs, which often provide operationally and physically distinct care to observation patients, have been touted as cost-effective alternatives to inpatient care, resulting in fewer admissions and reductions in length of stay (LOS) without a resultant increase in return ED-visits or readmissions."[4]

This was confirmed by a recent study comparing type I OUs (e.g., OUs in a dedicated space with defined protocols) versus patients receiving observation services elsewhere in the hospital. This study found type I units (versus patients receiving observation services elsewhere in the hospital) had a 23–38% shorter LOS, a 17–44% decreased probability of subsequent inpatient admission and $950 million in potential national cost savings each year. They further estimated that 11.7% of short-stay inpatients nationwide could be treated in a type I unit, with potential savings of $5.5–$8.5 billion annually.[2] As another study points out, "the operationally and physically distinct features of a designated OU may be required to realize the benefits of observation attributed to individual patients."[4]

Open and Closed Units

There are also "open" and "closed" OUs. In a closed unit, only certain designated physicians can admit to the OU. This is similar to the concept that only intensivists can admit to an intensive care unit or neurologists/neurosurgeons can admit to a neurology intensive care unit. With a closed unit, the physicians who know the OU and the operations of the unit (including the specific protocols, orders sets, and care pathways), work there on a regular basis, and, most importantly, who are held to the administrative and clinical standards for that unit are the only physicians who can treat patients in the OU. Only physicians who know the guiding principle of observation medicine – which is the rapid, efficient diagnostic evaluation and/or therapy of selected patients in less than 24 hours – and are held accountable to

these standards can refer or place patients in the OU. Historically, this has been the province of the emergency physician[4] with a majority of the OUs under ED administration.[5, 6] Observation medicine is considered to be an integral part of emergency medicine and part of the curriculum for emergency medicine residencies.[7] Recently, hospitalists have been involved with observation medicine and units.[8] (See Chapter 13 Observation Medicine and the Hospitalist .)

An administrative policy that specifically states which physicians can place patients in your OU will be useful in achieving this goal. (See Chapter 88 Administrative Policies/Guidelines.) For the rapid turnover of OU patients to occur, there must be on-site coverage, which implies coverage by ED physicians or hospitalists. Thus, a closed unit with in-house staffing 24/7, 365 days a year is ideal and helps ensure the success of the OU.

With a closed unit only one specialty can place patients in the OU, while an open unit allows any physician on the medical staff appropriately credentialed to admit patients to the hospital to place patients in the OU.[6] It is difficult, if not impossible, to make sure that the entire medical staff of the hospital knows, buys into the premise of observation, and consistently follows the administrative and clinical mandate of the OU. Moreover, the lack of availability at all times (including during office or clinic hours, during procedures or while in the operating room, and even at nights, e.g. 24/7) increases the inefficiency of the open unit and predisposes it to failure.

Hybrid Units

The term "hybrid unit" has been used to describe several variations in the OU. One definition of a hybrid unit (or combined unit) is an OU that accepts both adult and pediatric patients,[9] while another definition refers to an OU that primarily has patients placed in the OU from the ED who need further evaluation and/or treatment, but also accepts post procedure or "recovery room" type patients[10] with the premise that taking scheduled elective procedure patients may allow for "a more uniform patient census throughout the day," thereby, "improving staff utilization."[11] This is generally during the afternoon after the OU patients placed in the OU overnight from the ED have been discharged or admitted in the morning and before the busiest time of the ED, the evening shift, when most patients are placed in the OU from the ED.

Length of Stay

As per CMS guidelines, care in the OU is expected to be completed within 24 hours.[1] This has been the case as noted in multiple national surveys with a mean LOS of 15.3 hours,[5] and a median LOS of 19.5 hours in another study.[6]

Location of the Observation Unit

Cohorting observation patients in one area in a dedicated space has many advantages.[2] Diffusing observation patients in "scatter beds" throughout the hospital makes it difficult, if not impossible, for everyone throughout the hospital to identify and prioritize the observation patient.

Observation is "a process and a mindset" and not a specific location. Location may have additional logistical advantages when the OU is physically near the ED when under ED management. However, space is a major issue in hospitals, and observation care has been successfully provided in locations that are not adjacent to the ED.[5] If the OU is managed by the ED, a location adjacent to, in, or near the ED is preferable for many reasons. There is the ability for a more immediate response from ED staff if an untoward event, which although very rare, does occur;[12] if personnel have any "downtime," they may help out in the ED, but are next to the OU, which is their first and primary responsibility. This brings up the next topic of "flexible" staffing.

Staffing the Observation Unit

Flexible Staffing

In order for the OU to run at maximal efficiency, there must be the ability for an immediate response at all times: from taking the patient from the ED and placing in the OU, to responding to changes in the patient's condition, to dealing with test results and consults, and to discharging or admitting the patient. This is why there are dangers present in "flexible" or "flex" staffing. Ideally, staff covering the OU, especially nursing staffing, should be assigned only to the OU.[5] If this is not possible, then the primary responsibility of staffing should be to the OU, with other

non-OU assignments or responsibilities being secondary, and with the ability to transition quickly, easily and seamlessly, back to the OU when the OU becomes "busy" with patients being placed in the OU, being discharged, or admitted to the inpatient unit from the OU and/or with the managing of patients in the OU.

Nursing Staffing Ratios in the Observation Unit

The ebb and flow of patients in the OU mirrors that of the ED with most patients placed in the OU during the afternoon and evening hours, which is when the ED is busiest. Most patients complete their diagnostic testing and therapy by the next morning, which is the busiest time for disposition (usually discharge) of the patient. So, in reality, nursing is usually quite busy during the day shift with disposition of patients and evening shift accepting new patients in the OU. Generally, there are fewer diagnostic tests – such as stress tests, GI tests: colonoscopy or esophagoduodenoscopy, or EEG – during the night shift. Thus, for nursing staffing, the usual ratio of nurses to patients is 1:4 on days and evening shifts, and 1:5 on nights.

It is probably not a good idea to significantly increase the nurse to patient ratio at night since there is often some time lag from when the patient is seen in the ED and then placed into the OU so the early night-time hours can be busy with new patients arriving in the OU. Also, patients generally need to be transported during the night shift to stress testing and other procedures or diagnostic testing before the day shift so they can start the procedures promptly at 7 a.m. In addition, morning blood draws and other tests are usually done around 6 a.m. so they can have the results back by the time the OU day-shift physician arrives at 7 a.m. If there is any "down time" then the night shift may accomplish other tasks, such as ordering supplies or stocking for the next day. The 1 nurse to 4 OU patients (days/ evenings) and 1:5 (nights) is the recommended ratio. This is confirmed by a national survey that found the mean number of OU patients per nurse is 4.2 with 96% of nurses taking care of ≤ 4 patients,[5] (See Chapter 7 Nursing)

However, it is realized that if the OU is very "under census," nursing staffing may be temporarily assigned to another area with the provision that their first and foremost priority is the OU. If the OU is near the ED and the OU is very under census, it would be best to assign the OU nurse to ED patients that are not critically ill, since it is probably easier to pull the nurse back from the "less acute" area, such as fast track or split flow, than if he or she is caring for an intubated ICU patient with multiple intravenous (IV) medications. The premise is that it is easier to finish taking care of a low acuity patient with a sprained ankle than an acute myocardial infarction (MI) or an intubated respiratory failure patient or septic patient on multiple IV drips and return to the OU for new patients placed in the OU. Again, pulling nurses from the OU to work in other units should be avoided if possible and only done if the OU is very under census and the nurses can return to the OU as soon as they are needed.

Cross Coverage in the Observation Unit

When the OU is under the auspices of the ED, some have suggested there be "cross coverage" such that nurses work in both the ED as an ED nurse and in the OU as an OU nurse. This theory is that the nurse knows how the systems in the ED and the OU work and there is an understanding of what their colleagues do and this fosters collegiality. Conversely, it may be generally assumed that when a nurse chooses to work in a given hospital unit, they like that type of nursing care and forcing them to work elsewhere may hurt morale. One solution would be to orient the OU nurse to the ED (and OU, of course) during their orientation period so they are familiar with the processes in both the ED and the OU, but that once their orientation is over, they are scheduled primarily in the OU, but can function as an ED nurse if needed.

Nursing Staffing: Longevity and Patient Satisfaction

It is our experience that the OU nursing staff enjoys their job, are empowered in that they are expected to check all tests including laboratory and radiology reports and consult notes etc. and notify the physician of significant results, and are able to do much patient and family education. Our OU nursing staff has some of the greatest number of years of experience and most stable staffing of any unit in the hospital. The average OU nursing experience in our unit is around 15 years, of which most of the time has been in the OU. Our OU at the Cleveland Clinic, to our knowledge, may be the "oldest" continuously operating OU under the same management (e.g., since 1994 with the same OU medical director for 22 years) in the United States. Compared with the ED and other units in the hospital, the OU has one of the highest patient satisfaction scores and fewest patient complaints of any nursing unit in the hospital.[13]

Staffing the Unit: Physician

As with nursing and the advanced practice provider staffing of the OU, physician staffing is also dependent on the size of the OU. There are some parameters. The emergency physician workload time study found that the physician service time for an observation medicine patient was 55.6 minutes per patient.[14] Similarly, at a meeting of the Society of Hospital Medicine it was noted "that conventional wisdom holds that 15 patients is the optimal daily census."[15] Generally, for the physician in the OU, the busiest time is the morning shift when patient dispositions are occurring with patients being discharged or admitted. Staffing, of course, is dependent on many variables: institutional support (e.g., advanced practice providers, residents, fellows), time needed for documentation (such as scribes or dictation versus electronic medical record keeping), patient complexity, and responsibilities (e.g., is medicine reconciliation part of the physician's task or are there pharmacists who do this job).

There should always be a physician readily available on site in the area on hospital premises, even at night, who can immediately respond to the OU patients. This is a major advantage with a closed unit and points out the problem with an open unit where any physician may place patients in the OU, but they are not in house and, thereby, are unable to immediately respond, which prolongs the OU LOS and may lead to less than optimal patient care and outcomes.

Staffing the Unit: Advanced Practice Providers

The use of nurse practitioners and physician assistants in the OU has increased over the years.

There are several terms applied to these valuable and essential health care providers including Advanced Practice Providers (APP), Advanced Practice Clinicians (APC), midlevel providers and physician extenders. We have used physician assistants and more recently, advanced practice nurses, in our OU and ED to work alongside our physicians since the OU has been open over the last 23 years. We are currently evaluating and recruiting additional APPs in order to expand our OU coverage and further decrease our OU LOS.

The APP can identify patients in triage or in the ED who are likely OU candidates and evaluate them to determine whether or not they can be placed in the OU. If a patient is appropriate for the OU, they can start the history, physical evaluation, and OU orders; if not, they can begin ED diagnostic studies and treatment. This process allows patients to be quickly transitioned to the OU; if not suitable for the OU, an evaluation has already begun, which helps decrease the ED turnaround time (TAT) and ED LOS. Thus, by initially evaluating patients in triage or the ED and placing orders, the APP decreases the time to a "licensed provider," which is an important metric that EDs are evaluated on.

There are many other duties that can be assigned to the APPs that can justify the need for additional APPs in the OU. (Table 1.2) Some of the additional responsibilities that can be delegated to the APP in the OU include reviewing all reports and ancillary studies including laboratory and radiology studies that are resulted after the patient has left the ED or OU, especially "culture reports," and calling the patient and their pharmacist if any prescriptions including antibiotics are needed. When patients call in to the ED with questions or problems regarding their care in the ED or OU after they are discharged, the unit secretary pulls their ED or OU chart and gives it to the APP who can determine if the patient needs to return to the ED to be seen or needs other follow-up care. Routine "call back" programs on ED and/or OU patients have been recommended to increase patient satisfaction and Press-Ganey scores, and have identified problems with care that can be addressed, which benefits patient safety. With the emphasis on transitions of care, follow-up care, revisits to the ED and hospital readmissions; this may become more important in the future.

Table 1.2 Responsibilities of Advanced Practice Providers

- Documentation: initial history/physical examination, diagnostic studies, and treatment to occur in the OU; progress notes, discharge history, physical examination, OU course, discharge plan for continuing care
- Writes initial orders for patients placed in the OU
- Manages patients in the OU
- Discharge Planning: helps schedule follow-up testing and appointments
- Assists in seeing patients in ED who are likely candidates for the OU: does the initial history /physical examination, writes OU orders (with the caveat that OU patients are their primary responsibility)
- Reviews any follow-up ancillary ED and OU reports (laboratory, radiology, cardiac, or other studies)
- For example, reviews ED culture reports daily and if needed, writes or phones in antibiotic prescriptions
- Makes patient "call backs"
- Answers phone calls from patients discharged from the ED or OU

With the additional job responsibilities, especially in the larger OUs, there is justification for the staffing of an APP for the OU at least on the day and evening shifts. Of course, there should be onsite (in-house) physician availability 24 hours a day, 7 days a week, 365 days a year for the APP. Currently, the Medicare (and select other carriers) reimbursement for the APPs is 85% of that of the physician.

Staffing the Unit: Additional Personnel

In addition to physicians, APPs, and nursing staff, there should be consideration of additional staffing needs, again, depending on the size of the unit. Should there be unit secretaries, respiratory therapists to administer aerosols, pharmacists who perform medicine reconciliation, and technicians who assist in nursing procedures such as obtaining EKGs, drawing blood, starting IVs, etc.? What about housekeeping? Being a self-contained unit may increase efficiency and decrease LOS, particularly in larger units, so the OU does not have to rely on other hospital departments such as phlebotomy, ECG technicians, or respiratory therapy to provide services to OU patients. This eliminates the need to wait for other departments to come to the OU and perform needed services, which could increase LOS.

Administrative Staffing of the Observation Unit

There must be a physician medical director and a nursing director for the OU. It is critical to have strong leadership for the OU. The physician medical director provides both administrative and clinical leadership. The physician medical director is responsible for patient care issues such as review of patient care and appropriateness of patients placed in the OU, and OU patient quality and safety. The physician medical director in concert with the nursing director of the OU is responsible for operational issues in the OU in order to ensure the OU provides optimal patient care in an efficient and cost-effective manner. The OU medical director works with other physicians, hospital departments and personnel to set up processes for the day-to-day functioning of the OU to improve the availability and timeliness of diagnostic testing and treatment for OU patients. The physician medical director is a resource and provides oversight for the APPs. The physician medical director works with the hospital to ensure reimbursement for services provided to patients in the OU. In order to adequately provide clinical and administrative oversight for the OU, there must be some designated nonclinical administrative time for the OU physician medical director.[10]

Similarly, there must be a nursing director for the OU, who provides direction and leadership for the nursing staff in the OU. The nursing director deals with nursing and ancillary staffing of the OU, personnel issues, operations, and sets the standards for the nursing care provided in the OU. Ideally, especially with larger OUs, the physician and nursing medical directors of the OU should be separate from the ED physician and nursing directors. When there is one physician and, similarly, one nurse director for both the ED and the OU, since time is limited, the focus tends to be on the ED and not the OU. This is a mistake and sends the wrong impression that the OU is not valued enough to have its own administration. This does not imply that the OU physician and nursing directors do not provide direct patient care in addition to their administrative duties, especially in smaller OUs. Providing direct

patient care, as well as administrative direction, is desirable since it allows for the direct understanding of the processes involved and how to continually improve them and promotes credibility and respect among the OU staff.

The job descriptions in the administrative policies Chapter 88 further delineates the job responsibilities of the OU staff.

Design, Equipment, and Supplies for the Observation Unit

The design of the unit, at least partly, depends on the type of patients placed in the unit. Since the majority of patients in the OU are cardiac – especially chest pain, heart failure, or syncope – then having telemetry capability for all patients or all beds having rhythm strip and vital sign monitoring is indicated. Respiratory equipment and supplies – oxygen, aerosols, CPAP for patients with sleep apnea, etc. – should be in the design of the OU since respiratory patients also comprise a large group of OU patients. If any patients with contagious infections, such as acute gastroenteritis or pneumonia, will be placed in the OU, then the OU should not be an open ward setting or design and should have some individual cubicles that can be "enclosed" or with doors in order to meet infectious disease precautions/guidelines. Considerations for parents/families as well as other items (equipment, bed sizes/cribs, medications, etc.) need to be taken into account if pediatric patients are included in a "hybrid" unit.[7] (See Chapter 5 on Design.)

Size of the Observational Unit

How many beds should your OU have? This depends on many factors: the ED census or volume, hospital size (number of beds), the type of hospital (tertiary care or community, urban/suburban/rural), population density, financial considerations (number of 1-day stays, PEPPER report, etc.), and ED factors (LOS, TAT, % admissions). However, a rule of thumb has been that 10% of ED patients are potential OU candidates, so if your ED sees 50,000 patients a year, then about 5,000 ED patients could be placed in an OU. This applies to adult ED patients.

The percentage is lower for pediatric patients, where 5% may be a reasonable estimate. Thus, if there is an annual pediatric ED volume of 50,000 patients then about 2,500 could be placed in an OU. The percentage may differ based on whether it is a tertiary care pediatric ED or a community hospital ED that sees pediatric patients with a lower percentage of potential pediatric OU candidates in the community hospital ED, which might reflect a greater incidence of transfers/referrals to the tertiary care hospital and varying patient acuity.[7, 11]

Alternative methods for calculating the percentage of patients that could be placed in a type I OU, based on the number of short-stay inpatients, are 11.7% in one study.[2] This is similar to observation status patients comprising 10.4% of all hospital stays (of 43,853 stays in one large hospital system, inpatient was 89.6% and observation was 10.4%).[16]

Metrics, Benchmarks, Performance Improvement, and Patient Safety, Quality and Experience

Key metrics that must be reported for the OU are volume or census of OU patients, LOS for OU patients, disposition: admissions to inpatient services and discharges, and sentinel events. The benchmarks for the OU include: average LOS of 15–16 hours and about 80% of patients are discharged from the OU and conversely, only about a 15–20% are admitted to inpatient floors from the OU. Quality indicators include admissions to any of the following: intensive care unit, cardiac catheterization unit, or operating room. Sentinel events include resuscitations or codes, intubations or acute need for BiPaP, and use of vasopressors or ACLS drugs. (See Chapter 9 on Metrics and Performance Improvement, Patient Quality, Safety and Experience.)

Benefits of an Observation Unit: Clinical and Financial

The benefits of an OU are outlined in Table 1.3.

Business Plan

What are the problems facing the hospital and the ED? How can an OU help solve these issues? Is there overcrowding in the ED and a shortage of inpatient hospital beds? The opening of an OU is one of the easiest ways to add more beds to the hospital so patients are not waiting on a stretcher

Table 1.3 Benefits of an Observation Unit: Clinical and Financial*

Clinical Benefits of an Observation Unit (OU)

- Improved patient care
- Fewer missed diagnoses
- Decreased risk/malpractice liability
- Third option for emergency physician/hospital staff: admit to inpatient, discharge, or observation
- Shorter length of stay (LOS)
- Increased patient and family satisfaction
- Improved patient safety
- Improves emergency department (ED) throughput (decreased LOS, faster turn-around times)
- Expands the capacity of the ED
- Maximizes ED efficiency and profitability
- Increased sensitivity and specificity of ED diagnosis and management
- Patients who do need care as an inpatient (from the OU) have a more specific and accurate diagnosis and are more likely to be admitted to the correct inpatient service
- Decreased exposure to the dangers of inpatient hospitalization including medication errors, falls, exposure to multi-drug resistant bacteria and other pathogens, physical deconditioning, intensive care unit/hospital psychosis (observation for 15 hours versus a typical short-stay admission of 2 or more days limits the risk)
- Increased, more appropriate referrals (more specific and accurate diagnosis) with easier evaluation since preliminary studies already done
- Organizational structure and format allows for easier adoption of clinical pathways, algorithms, etc. for the standardization of care and best practices
- Better patient outcomes

Financial Benefits of Observation Medicine

- Cost savings resulting from shorter hospital stay and efficient use of resources
- Allows an inpatient bed to be filled by a patient with a more profitable diagnosis related group (DRG) payment

Table 1.3 (cont.)

- When the hospital is at capacity and at or near full census, use of OU may alleviate or help avoid cancelling elective surgeries, denying elective admissions, and refusing transfers

- Adding an OU is the easiest, fastest, and less expensive way to increase hospital capacity and add more beds

- Avoids inpatient admission that may have otherwise resulted in a loss for the hospital (several common diagnoses such as heart failure are recognized to not fully cover average inpatient hospital costs)

- Cost to manage a patient in the OU is less than in the inpatient floor (inpatient care has higher fixed costs and a longer LOS in addition to bundled payments, which generally leads to a loss for the hospital, whereas placement of the same patient in the OU would lead to a profit)

- Increased revenue if appropriate patients are placed in OU (bill for observation codes and fee-for-service basis as per ambulatory payment system) (use of current procedural terminology (CPT) billing codes after 8 hours have passed in OU) (hospital and physician billing)

- OU is currently not under the DRG system for completely bundled payments as with inpatient care but is now part of the list of Comprehensive APCs which bundle most labs and ancillary studies for the facility. The physician component is still billed separately to Medicare

- Risk of denial is lower than for inpatient unit (patients with short inpatient stays, especially 1–2 days, are targeted by payers as likely inappropriate)

- Risk of audits is lower than for inpatient unit (patients with short inpatient stays especially 1–2 days, are targeted by payers as likely inappropriate)

- Increased revenue since revenue created by the OU may be separate from or overlap with revenues resulting from patients who would have previously been sent home from the ED

* This not an all-inclusive list but gives some of the many benefits of a Type I observation unit.

in the ED for an inpatient hospital bed. Does the ED have a problem with a long LOS and slow turnaround times? An OU will increase ED efficiency, decrease ED wait times and turnaround times, and shorten the ED LOS.

Does your ED have poor patient satisfaction and low Press-Ganey scores? A less crowded, more organized ED that can off load ED patients to a more pleasant, quieter, and less chaotic location – specifically an OU – should improve patient satisfaction, Press-Ganey scores, etc.

What is highlighted in the Program for Evaluating Payment Patterns Electronic Report (PEPPER) report for your hospital? Has there been an excessive number of denials for 1-day inpatient admissions? Has your hospital been fined and had overpayments recouped? Placing patients in an OU instead of them being categorized as an inpatient admission for ≤ 24 hours should help ameliorate this problem.

There are likely other issues facing your institution and emergency department. The implementation of a well-organized and well-maintained OU should have a positive impact on the myriad of throughput challenges facing the hospital and ED.

Before opening an OU, talk with the payers in your region, discuss the advantages of observation with them, and give them time to set up their processes and information technology so they can pay you appropriately for services. Prior to opening your OU, have the systems in place, so you can identify OU patients and appropriately bill for your services with the recognition that you can bill for both physician services and hospital services. You must also be in compliance with all the local, state, and federal regulations, so meeting with your reimbursement specialists, coders, and compliance team is essential.

Hospital administration must be involved and supportive of the OU. Nursing and ancillary personnel in the OU and ED are key to the success of the OU as well as other departments in the hospital, such as stress testing, other cardiac testing (e.g., echocardiology, holter monitoring), radiology (for CT scans, MRIs, V/Q scans, etc.), gastroenterology procedure lab (if esophagogastroduodenoscopy or colonoscopies are to be done while patients are in the OU), and interventional radiology procedures. The physicians and advanced practice practitioners who will be staffing the unit must have "buy-in" for the OU to succeed. The medical staff should be apprised of the OU and how it fits into the patient care process. Presentations to the medical staff are invaluable in answering their questions or concerns and by explaining how the OU will benefit their practices. Face-to-face meetings will help attain their support and be instrumental in setting up referrals for the OU patients.

Meetings not only with internal hospital personnel/departments and physicians, but also key external "players" (such as payers), are important not only when setting up or starting an OU, but also in sustaining the efficient day-to-day operations of the OU. This organizational framework and preparation and ongoing maintenance is essential to the successful initiation and continuation of the OU.

References

1. Centers for Medicare and Medicaid Services (CMS). Medicare benefit policy manual, Chapter 6: Hospital services covered under Part B. Baltimore, MD: CMS; [revised Mar 1, 2013]. www.cms.gov/Regulations-and-Guidance/Guidance/Transmittals/downloads/R42BP.pdf and www.cms.gov/Regulations-and-Guidance/Guidance/Manuals/downloads/bp102c06.pdf (Accessed March 2016)

2. Ross MA, Hockenberry JM, Mutter R, et al. Protocol-driven emergency department observation units offer savings, shorter stays and reduced admissions. *Health Affairs* 2013; 32(12): 2149–2156.

3. Baugh CW, Venkatesh AK, Hilton JA, et al. Making greater use of dedicated hospital observation units for many short-stay patients could save $3.1 billion a year. *Health Affairs* 2012; 31(10): 2314–2323.

4. Macy ML, Hall M, Shah SS, et al. Differences in designations of observation care in US freestanding Children's Hospitals: are they virtual or real? *J Hosp Medicine* 2012; 7(4): 287–293.

5. Mace SE, Graff L, Mikhail M, et al. A national survey of observation units in the United States. *Am J Emerg Med* 2003 21:529–533.

6. Osborne A, Weston J, Wheatley M, et al. Characteristics of hospital observation services: a society of cardiovascular patient care survey. *Critical Pathways in Cardiology* 2013; 12(2): 45–48.

7. Mace SE, Shah J. Observation medicine in emergency medicine residency programs. *Acad Emerg Med* 2002; 9: 169–171.

8. Barsuk J, Casey D, Graff L, et al. The Observation Unit: an operational overview for the hospitalist. Society of Hospital Medicine White Paper. May 21, 2009. www.hospitalmedicine.org/Content/NavigationMenu/Publications/WhitePapers/White_Papers.htm (Accessed March 2015)

9. Mace SE. Pediatric observation medicine. *Emerg Med Clinics North Am* 2001: 19(1): 239–254.

10. Ross MA, Naylor S, Compton S, et al. Maximizing use of the emergency department observation unit: a novel hybrid design. *Ann Emerg Med* 2001; 37: 267–274.

11. Zebrack M, Kadish H, Nelson D. The pediatric hybrid observation unit: an analysis of 6477 consecutive patient encounters. *Pediatrics* 2005; 115 (5): e535–e542.

12. Mace SE. Resuscitations in an observation unit. *J Quality in Clinical Practice* 1999; 19 (3):155–163.

13. Mace SE. Patient complaints in an observation unit. *J Quality Clinical Practice* 1998; 18(2): 151–158.

14. Graff LG, Wolf S, Dinwoodie R, et al. Emergency physician workload: a time study. *Ann Emerg Med* 1993: 22(7): 1156–1163.

15. Maguire P. What's the ideal number of patients to see? *Today's Hospitalist*, July 2009. Available on-line at: www.todayshospitalist.com/index.php?b=articles_read&cnt +824 (Accessed March 2016)

16. Sheehy AM, Graf B, Gangireddy S, et al. Hospitalized but not admitted. Characteristics of patients with "Observation Status" at an academic medical center. *JAMA Intern Med* 2013; 173(2): 1991–1998.

2

Observation Medicine – Key Concepts: *How to Start (and Maintain) an Observation Unit: What You Need to Know*

Administrative Issues

Sharon E. Mace, MD, FACEP, FAAP

OVERVIEW

There has been a steady increase in the frequency and duration of observation encounters in recent years.[1, 2] In the United States, observation encounters for Medicare beneficiaries increased from 86.9 to 116.6 observation stay events per 1,000 inpatient admissions per month over a 2-year period during 2007–2009, while there was a decrease in inpatient admissions for the same time period. The overall result was a 34% increase in the ratio of observation stays to inpatient admissions.[2] According to the government, these trends have continued with an increase in observation, yet a decrease in inpatient hospital services again in 2010 to 2011.[3] The Medicare Payment Advisory Commission (Med-PAC) report notes a 28.5% increase in outpatient services with a concurrent 12.6% decrease in inpatient discharges for the 2006–2012 period.[3]

The volume of observation visits and the duration of observation visits are both increasing. There was nearly a 68% increase in observation visits from 28 to approximately 47 visits per 1,000 Part B beneficiaries for the period between 2006 and 2011.[4] Looking at the annual number of observation hours for Medicare beneficiaries from 2006 through 2010, there was a 70% increase from 23 million to 39 million.[1] Moreover, the number of observation stays exceeding 72 hours increased by 88% from 2007 through 2009.[2]

References: Overview

1. Medicare Payment Advisory Commission. *A Data Book: Health Care Spending and the Medicare Program.* June 2012. Section 7. www.medpac.gov/documents/Jun12dataBookEntireReport.pdf (Accessed March 2016)

2. Feng Z, Wright B, Mor V. Sharp rise in Medicare enrollees being held in hospitals for observation raises concerns about causes and consequences. *Health Aff (Millwood)* 2012; 31(6): 1251–1259.

3. MedPAC report to Congress: hospital inpatient and outpatient services. www.medpac.gov/documents/mar14_EntireReport.pdfchapters (Accessed March 2016)

4. MedPAC report to Congress: hospital inpatient and outpatient services. www.medpac.gov/chaptersMar13_Ch03.pdf (Accessed March 2016)

THE TWO-MIDNIGHT RULE

In response to this recent increase in the number and duration of observation stays, the Centers for Medicare and Medicaid Services (CMS) enacted a rules change on October 1, 2013.[5] This rules change classifies most hospital encounters of < 2 midnights as observation, while those ≥ 2 midnights are categorized as inpatients. There has been much discussion and controversy regarding what the impact of this new rule will be.[6–8]

The 2014 Medicare payment rules include an amended definition of inpatient status. In order to qualify as an inpatient the following conditions must be met: patients receive only medically necessary services ordered by a physician and their hospitalization lasts through two midnights. In the CY 2016 OPPS final rule, CMS maintains the benchmark established by the original two-midnight rule, but permits greater flexibility for determining when an admission that does not meet the benchmark should nonetheless be payable under Part A on a case-by-case basis. The CY 2016 OPPS final rule also discusses a shift in the enforcement of the two-midnight rule from Medicare Administrative Contractors (MACs) to Quality Improvement Organizations (QIOs).[9]

References: Two-Midnight Rule

5. Centers for Medicare and Medicaid Services inpatient prospective payment system 1599-F. Fiscal year 2014 Final rule. www.gpo.gov/fdsys/pkg/FR-2013-08-19/pdf/2013-18956.pdf (Accessed March 2016)

6. Sheehy AM, Caponi B, Gangireddy S, et al. Observation and inpatient status: clinical impact of the 2-midnight rule. *Journal of Hospital Medicine* 2014; 9(4): 203–209.

7. www.healthcapital.com/hcc/newsletter/01_14/2-Midnight%20Rule.pdf (Accessed March 2016)

8. Society of Hospital Medicine Public Policy Committee. The Observation Status Problem. Impact and Recommendations for Change. Society of Hospital Medicine Whitepaper, July 2014. Available at www.hospital medicine.org/advocacy (Accessed March 2016)

9. www.cms.gov/Newsroom/MediaReleaseDatabase/Fact-sheets/2015-Fact-sheets-items/2015-10-30-4.html (Accessed March 2016)

BACKGROUND

What Is Observation?

Before discussing the two-midnight rule, several caveats must be noted.[1] First, the term observation has been applied to many types of patient encounters. There is a distinction between observation medicine that is protocol driven – that has specific protocols, guidelines, and order sets; that has explicit clinical guidelines with strong administrative leadership; and that is generally applied to patients cohorted in a specific area of the hospital, most frequently in an emergency department (ED) based observation unit (OU), known as a type I OU – versus observation medicine that is non-protocol driven, without guidelines and order sets, without strong administrative organization and leadership, and with observation patients placed throughout the hospital instead of in a discrete unit or area.[2-4] This optimal construct is clearly different from observation in "scatter beds" in inpatient areas. "When observation is used as a billing status in inpatient areas without changes in care delivery, it's largely a cost-shifting exercise – relieving the hospital of the risk of adverse action by the RAC (recovery audit contractor) but increasing the patient's financial burden."[3]

The success of this format and organization (e.g., type I OU) is detailed in the evidence-based chapters in this textbook. This is what is generally referred to as "ED observation" or "simple observation." Placing patients in "observation" or "observation status" without this clinical and administrative organizational structure is generally doomed to fail and frequently exceeds the previously stated time-based goals of 24 hours. The incidence of ED OUs in the United States has grown from about 19% according to a 2003 study[5] with a higher incidence (about 36%) in academic centers in a 2002 study[6] to about one-third of all EDs in the United States having a dedicated OU.[7-9] The administration of the OUs is usually under the ED.[8, 10]

Next, although the stated target for simple observation is 24 hours, the goal is generally to discharge the patient well before 24 hours. Indeed, the mean length of stay (LOS) is 15.3 hours[5] and the median LOS is 19 hours[10] according to two different surveys with a desired minimum of 8 hours and a maximum of 24 hours.[9]

Simple versus Complex or Extended Observation

Recently, the application of these same principles of observation medicine on a more extended time frame, often ≤ 48 hours instead of ≤ 24 hours as the set goal, has been advocated for several reasons including the concern for readmissions, with the expectation that somewhat more complex patients (e.g., those with more than one chief complaint or problem and with multiple comorbidities) might be diagnosed and treated in a shorter time frame than the usual several-day inpatient hospital admission if the same principles of observation are applied. The term "complex" or "extended" observation has been applied to this patient population. (See Chapters 16 and 17 on extended or complex observation.)

This book is designed to provide the tools for achieving success with observation patients, whether "simple" versus "complex" or "extended" observation patients, with the acknowledgment that they are two different patient populations.

Historically, inappropriate labelling of patients as observation, especially adding observation status in postoperative patients, created problems and liabilities, and was one reason why in years past payment was denied for anything other than the three cardinal diagnoses of chest pain, asthma, and heart failure. These three diagnoses were singled out because of the extensive evidence-based medicine verifying the benefits of observation in the literature.[9,11] Later, as additional research documenting the advantages of observation as applied to other diagnoses and conditions was identified, payment was no longer limited to these three core diagnoses.

Misclassifying and/or reclassifying patients as observation or inpatient creates problems; the ideal is to place patients in the correct status from the beginning rather than rectifying an erroneous categorization. (See Chapter 64 on Determining the Correct Status.)

Impact of the Two-Midnight Rule

The impact of the two-midnight rule is yet to be determined.[12] As mentioned, CMS enacted the rules change on October 1, 2013 that categorized the majority of patient–hospital encounters of < 2 midnights as observation, while those ≥ 2 midnights as hospital inpatient stays.[13] However, on April 1, 2014, a bill was signed into law that directs CMS to delay enforcement of the two-midnight rule. This means that CMS has postponed postpayment audits of the two-midnight rule until after March 31, 2015. However, the rule is still in effect and hospitals have to meet its requirements. CMS has applied prepayment "probe and educate" reviews to see if hospitals are in compliance. There is also pending legislation in Congress that directs CMS to create criteria for short inpatient stays.[14, 15]

> As of October 1, 2015, MACs have completed the third round of Inpatient Probe and Educate reviews (although some provider education may continue beyond this date)... Beginning in January 2016, Recovery Auditor Contractors (RACs) may conduct patient status reviews only for those providers that have been referred by the QIO (Quality Improvement Organization) as exhibiting persistent noncompliance with medicare payment policies, including but not limited to: having high denial rates and consistently failing to adhere to the Two Midnight rule (including repeatedly submitting inappropriate inpatient claims for stays that do not span one midnight) or failing to improve their performance after QIO educational intervention.[16]

So the jury is still out and the results are yet to be determined. However, what can and should we be doing in the meantime? First and foremost, make sure documentation is complete and accurate, no matter what status the patient is in.

Table 2.1 Inpatient Admission Documentation Checklist

- Documentation is complete and accurate
- Documentation details what is happening with or to the patient
- Documentation includes an estimated length of stay
- Documentation includes a plan of care
- Documentation includes physician certification of medical necessity
- Documentation of the patient's admission must be dated, timed, and signed

(Table 2.1) Physician documentation must provide a complete picture of what is happening with or to the patient. The physician must certify medical necessity, sign, date, and time the patient's inpatient admission. The physician documentation should include an estimate of the patient's LOS and the physician's plan of care for the patient. (See Chapter 66 on Medical Necessity.)

No matter what happens with the two-midnight rule or when, we can be certain that auditors will be scrutinizing medical records and frequently employing a look back period that may be several years. It is also likely that 1- and 2-day stays will be targeted for audits regarding medical necessity and for accurate and complete documentation. Undoubtedly, case management and utilization review will be extremely busy in the near future. In addition, the billing department should be compliant with the new rules.[17–21] Ongoing information and updates may be obtained from the CMS National Provider Calls.[22]

References: Background

1. Centers for Medicaid and Medicare Services. CMS finalizes FY 2014 policy and payments changes for inpatient stays in acute-care and long-term care hospitals. www.cms.gov/Newsroom/MediaReleaseDatabase/Fact-Sheets/2013-Fact-Sheets-Items/2013-08-02-2.html (Accessed March 2016)

2. Ross MA, Hockenberry JM, Barrett M, et al. Protocol driven emergency department observation units offer savings, shorter stays and reduced admissions. *Health Affairs* 2013; 32(12): 2149–2156.

3. Baugh CW, Schur JD. Observation care – high-value care or a cost-shifting loophole? *New Engl J Med* 2013; 369(4): 302–305.

4. Baugh CW, Venkatesh AK, Hilton JA, et al. Making greater use of dedicated hospital

observation units for many short-stay patients could save $3.1 billion a year. *Health Affairs* 2012; 31(10): 2314–2322.

5. Mace SE, Graff L, Mikhail M, et al. A national survey of observation units in the United States. *Am J Emerg Med* 2003; 21: 529–533.

6. Mace SE, Shah J. Observation medicine in emergency medicine residency programs. *Acad Emerg Med* 2002; 9:169–171.

7. Graff LG. *Observation Medicine: The Healthcare System's Tincture of Time.* American College of Emergency Physicians Web site: www.acep.org/WorkArea?Download/Asset.aspx?id=45885 (Accessed March 2016)

8. Venkatesh AK, Geisler P, Gibson Chambers JJ, et al. Use of observation care in US emergency departments, 2001 to 2008. *PLos ONE* 2011; 6(9):1–10 (e24326).

9. Baugh CW, Venkatesh AK, Bohan JS. Emergency department observation units: a clinical and financial benefit for hospitals. *Health Care Manage Rev* 2011; 36(1): 28–37.

10. Osborne A, Weston J, Wheatley M, et al. Characteristics of hospital observation services: A Society of Cardiovascular Patient Care survey. *Critical Pathways in Cardiology* 2013; 12(2): 45–49.

11. Department of Health and Human Services (DHHS) Centers for Medicare and Medicaid Services (CMS). CMS Manual System Pub. 100-02 Medicare Benefit Policy. Transmittal 42. Date: December 16, 2005. Available at www.cms.gov/Regulations-and-Guidance/Transmittals/downloads/R42BP.pdf (Accessed March 2016)

12. Sheehy AM, Caponi B, Ganigreddy S, et al. Observation and inpatient status: clinical impact of the 2-midnight rule. *J Hosp Med* 2014; 9(4): 203–209.

13. Centers for Medicare and Medicaid Services Hospital inpatient prospective payment system 1599-F. Fiscal year 2014 Final rule. Federal register/Vol. 78, No.160/Monday, August 19, 2013/Rules and Regulations. www.gpo.gov/fdsys/pkg/FR-2013-18956.pdf (Accessed March 2016)

14. Don't ignore the two-midnight rule. It's still in effect. *Hosp Case Manag* 2014; 22(5): 57–66.

15. CMS announces delay in two-midnight rule enforcement. *Hosp Peer Rev* 2014; 39(4): 37–38.

16. www.cms.gov/Research-Statistics-Data-and-Systems/Monitoring-Programs/Medicare-FFS-Compliance-Programs/Medical-Review/InpatientHospitalReviews.html) (Accessed March 2016)

17. Carlson J. Auditing inpatient stays. "Two-midnight" rule may still prove costly. *Mod Healthc* 2013 September 9; 43(36):9–10.

18. Is the two-midnight rule much ado about nothing? *Hosp Case Manag* 2013 December; 21(12): 161–164.

19. Egusquiza D. 8 critical steps for 2-midnight compliance. *Healthc Financ Manage* 2014 February; 68(2): 54–57.

20. Edelberg C. A. closer look at the two-midnight rule, what it means for ED providers. *ED Manag* 2013 December; 25(12): 142–143.

21. Cesta T. Case management insider. The 2-midnight rule – a game changer for case management. *Hosp Case Manag* 2014 April; 22(4): 47–50.

22. www.cms.gov/Outreach-and-Education/Outreach/NPC/National-Provider-Calls- and-Events.html (Accessed March 2016)

PEPPER REPORT

What Is the PEPPER Report?

The Program for Evaluating Payment Patterns Electronic Report, known as the PEPPER report, is an electronic data report that contains hospital-specific information for various areas targeted by CMS. An individual hospital's PEPPER report contains hospital-specific Medicare claims data for targeted areas. Areas targeted by CMS include 1-day stays, hospital readmissions, and diagnosis-related groups (DRGs) that have historically been associated with high rates of Medicare payment errors.[1]

What Is Contained in the PEPPER Report?

The PEPPER report gives data on areas targeted by CMS where there are likely payment errors secondary to billing, MS-DRG (Medicare Severity Adjusted – DRG) coding, and/or problems with medical necessity for admissions. The information contained in the PEPPER report should assist hospitals in identifying possible overpayments as well as possible underpayments. It can assist in identifying potential problems and can be used to establish what items should be targeted for internal audits and validation analysis. It can aid in finding areas where medical necessity may be questionable, overcoding or undercoding occurs, and readmissions are too common. It can help detect areas where the hospital may be susceptible to denials from the Recovery Audit Contractors (RACs).[2]

CMS makes the PEPPER report available to fiscal intermediaries (FIs) and to the MACs. RACs have the ability to provide PEPPER data to the individual hospital. PEPPER has various target areas that have been identified as high risk for payment errors.[2]

The PEPPER report provides a spreadsheet of information unique to a given hospital, which can be compared with other hospitals in your region, state, MAC jurisdiction, and the country.[3] The worksheets in the PEPPER report show the hospital's percentiles in each target area and compares the hospital's numbers or percentiles with other acute care hospitals, as well as listing the hospital's top DRGs for 1-day stays and the statewide top DRGs for 1-day stays for the fiscal year. A high number of short stays suggests that the inpatient admission wasn't necessary or the patient should have been managed on an outpatient basis, perhaps in observation status.[2]

How Can the PEPPER Report Be Used?

The PEPPER report for any given hospital should be compared with other hospitals in the region or state, and items that stand out from other institutions that may be outliers should be evaluated to see if they indicate a problem. Generally, any time the hospital falls ≥ 80th percentile or < 20th percentile suggests an issue that should be addressed. When the hospital is uniformly low in relation to the medical necessity measures, then this may be an indicator that there is over-utilization of observation services, while hospital scores in the high range suggest coding errors or problems with regard to medical necessity.[4] Results ≥ 80th percentile or < 20th percentile imply that the hospital may be inappropriately using observation services.[3] It is also useful to determine what DRGs comprise the greatest number of 1-day stays and then review them for appropriate level of care.[1]

A PEPPER Compare Worksheet on short-term acute care hospitals shows the individual hospital findings based on the unusualness of the findings relative to other hospitals in the state or region including outlier values and the extent of the potential problem, which is the outlier value times the number of discharges. PEPPER may include a variety of tables and graphs that compare an individual hospital with others. "Having admissions in the outlier range does increase your risk of review by your Quality Improvement Organization (QIO), which could mean the hospital has to pay back money it has received because of noncompliance in reviewing cases prior to admission."[2]

Similarly, compare the 30-day readmission rate for the hospital with other acute care institutions in the state and ascertain whether or not there was incomplete care during the first admission and the second admission occurred in order to provide services that should have been rendered during the first or initial hospital stay.[1]

In the past, PEPPER reports were distributed to hospitals by their state Medicare QIO as a way to support the Hospital Payment Monitoring Program (HPMP). Currently, QIOs are no longer providing these reports. The PEPPER reports have been sent to hospitals by mail, but are now available through a secure portal from a website maintained by TMF Health Quality Institute.

The TMF Health Quality Institute is under contract from CMS to furnish comparative data reports not only to providers but also to MACs in an attempt to decrease Medicare fee-for-service improper payments. For example, if a hospital has a high number of 1-day inpatient stays for chest pain in its PEPPER report, this is an area noted to be at high risk for payment errors, which raises a red flag and may trigger a government contractor to do an audit on the hospital's 1-day inpatient chest pain stays.[5] This illustrates the importance of placing patients in the proper status initially and raises the question of how many of these 1-day inpatient chest pain stays or inpatient admissions could have been placed in observation status in an OU (which is outpatient status) instead, avoiding the high rating and misclassification of patients and the increased risk of an audit. In some instances, the use of observation status could be an alternative for an inpatient admission.

How Can One Access the PEPPER Report?

A hospital's PEPPER report is accessible at a secure website via TMF.[6] TMF Health Quality Institute is the contractor for the CMS PEPPER program, whose job is to prepare the PEPPER reports for specific institutions/facilities using claims data. Note: there are PEPPER reports not only for short-term acute care facilities, (which is relevant for observation medicine) but also for long-term acute care facilities.[7] There is also a training/resource website maintained by the TMF Health Quality Institute.[8]

What Can Happen if There Are Errors in Payment?

PEPPER reports concentrate on LOS issues, specifically 1-day stays, and on certain MS-DRGS that have been problems in the past.[9] There are significant financial consequences that can greatly impact an institution's bottom line so it is crucial that every patient is coded correctly and compliant.[10] Regarding observation, there are two types of coding errors. When patients are misclassified as outpatients instead of as inpatients, then the hospital does not receive appropriate inpatient payment. Conversely, when observation patients are misclassified as inpatients, when audited and such mistakes are detected, the hospital not only will be compelled to return inappropriate payments but also can be fined and have to pay penalties and interest on any misclassifications identified during an audit.[10]

Revision of the PEPPER Report Based on the Two-Midnight Rule

Because of the two-midnight rule for inpatient admissions, the PEPPER compliance tool has been recently revised.[11] The two-midnight rule was adopted by the Inpatient Prospective Payment System (IPPS) regulation in 2014. The two-midnight rule usually assumes that hospital stays crossing two midnights are appropriately billed as an inpatient, and conversely, shorter stays are generally not reported as an inpatient stay, with a few exceptions, excluding patients who are admitted for inpatient-only procedures. This revised PEPPER report has six new target areas: 2-day stays for medical DRGs, 2-day stays for surgical DRGs, 1-day stays for medical DRGs, 1-day stays for surgical DRGs, same-day stays for medical DRGs, and same-day stay for surgical DRGs. Observation status metrics should help recognize overpayments and underpayments. The CMS website gives information on the IPPS 2014 and other rulings.[12]

References: PEPPER Report

1. PEPPER can help you focus on likely RAC targets. *Hospital Case Management*; 2010 December; 18(12): 181–182.

2. PEPPER can identify areas where denials may occur. *Hospital Case Management*; 2005 June; 13(6): 84–86.

3. http://store.relearning.com/by-topic/pepper-1/pepper.html (Accessed March 2016)

4. Wiedemann LA. Seasoning your compliance plan with PEPPER. *How to read PEPPER data on payment errors*; 2007 January; 78(1): 44–49.

5. www.hcpro.com/print/HOM-218293–5750/What-is-PEPPER-data-and-how-can -it-help-prepare-for-a-RAC-audit? (Accessed March 2016)

6. TMF Health Quality Institute http://pepperresourcs.org/PEPPER/SecurePEPPER Access.aspx (Accessed March 2016)

7. Kulus J. PEPPER gives corporate compliance guidelines. *Provider: Long Term & Post-Acute Care*. 2013 March; www.providermagazine.com/archives/2014_Archives/Pages/0314 (Accessed March 2016)

8. TMF health Quality Institute http://hospitals.tmf.org/PEPPERResources/tabid/1115/Default.aspx (Accessed March 2016)

9. www.hcpro.com/HIM-245049–865/Use-PEPPER-reports-to-stay-on-top-of-common-coding-errors (Accessed March 2016)

10. Corrati RR. Report data identify risk areas for improper payments. *Healthcare Financial Management* 2011 October; 65(10): 88–92.

11. Report on Medicare Compliance: PEPPER compliance tool is revised for two-midnight rule in time for June release. Atlantic Information Services, Inc. 2014 May; 23(16). Available online at www.AIShealth.com (Accessed March 2016)

12. Centers for Medicare and Medicaid Services. www.cms.gov/Medicare/medicare-Fee-for-Service-Payment/AcuteInpatientPPS/FY2014-IPPS-FinalRule (Accessed March 2016)

CRITERIA FOR INPATIENT ADMISSION OR OBSERVATION

Overview

Recently, the National Government Services, and MAC, published their views on the process of clinical and reimbursement or payment decisions regarding observation.[1] In step one, the treating physician should ascertain whether the patient can be discharged home from the ED. If the answer is no, discharge is not appropriate, then the practitioner proceeds to step two and "understand[s] that the patient will need ongoing inpatient services with a high degree of certitude or assess the likelihood that care may be rendered within a 48-hour timeframe."[1] Extended or complex observation could be considered for this situation where there is "outpatient observation up to 48 hours of care (with) appropriate diagnostic and therapeutic care." However, "Physicians should use a 24-hour period as a benchmark, i.e. they should order admission for patients who are expected to need hospital care for 24 hours or more, and treat other patients on an outpatient basis."[1] This again reinforces the 24-hour time frame for observation (or "simple" observation).

Medical Necessity Screening Tools

There are several medical necessity screening tools that Medicare and its contractors may select to use in their determination of medical necessity. The Milliman care guidelines[2] or McKesson's Interqual[3,4] are two commonly used screening tools, although there are other proprietary systems.[5] The criteria used may vary from state to state or jurisdiction. Moreover, Medicare does not mandate the use of any particular screening criteria.

The key components of any criteria pertain to intensity of service (IS) and severity of illness (SI); both criteria must be met in order to substantiate the medical necessity for inpatient admission versus observation status or another service in the hospital system. There are similarities between the inpatient admission and observation criteria, however, inpatient SI and IS criteria generally indicate higher acuity. The criteria are arranged by body system, for example, general, cardiorespiratory, central nervous system, gastrointestinal, metabolic, obstetrics, and surgery/trauma. Components of the SI criteria include assessments, monitoring, medication administration, intravenous fluids, administration of blood products, and psychiatric crisis intervention.[5]

The usual process involves a hospital case manager (or care coordinator) or member of the utilization management staff reviewing the patient's record.[4,6] Ideally, this process would begin prospectively in the ED, but generally within the first 24 hours of a patient's admission to determine if the particular screening tool's criteria are met. Documentation by the treating physician is critical to establishing the IS and the SI.

There may be times where a specific patient does not meet inpatient criteria, but requires an inpatient admission. In these instances, the physician in conjunction with the case manager or utilization review staff member should consider the overall scenario to decide on the need for hospitalization. Excellent documentation of medical necessity is crucial in these cases.

There are times when the initial review of a record fails to meet screening criteria for medical necessity. Generally, a medical review, which is a second-level review, occurs in which a physician or nurse reviews the record for clinical documentation to support the hospital admission and payment. This emphasizes the critical importance of excellent documentation in order to provide proof of medical necessity. (See Chapter 66 Medical Necessity)

There are also instances where screening criteria have been met, yet the payer denies payment because documentation does not support the medical necessity of admission. Hospitals can appeal payment denials, but this involves additional time and expense so it is best to assign the correct status at the beginning. (See Chapter 67 Denials and Appeals)

Unfortunately, the criteria for determining inpatient hospital admission versus observation are not always well defined so the decision usually defers to physician judgment. Indeed, the accuracy of the various criteria in predicting the need for hospitalization for both medical and surgical patients has been questioned by some.[7–10]

Again, incorrect patient status, for example, inpatient admission versus observation, has many negative repercussions. Categorizing a patient as inpatient when he or she should have been observation leads to payment errors with the potential for denial of payment, and perhaps, more importantly, compliance issues related to overpayments. On the other hand, there is the potential for revenue loss when a patient is in observation and should have been an inpatient.

Changes in Observation Status: From Inpatient to Observation

There are very strict criteria for changing inpatient status to observation and the change must occur "*before*" the patient is discharged from the hospital.[11] Some key prerequisites for changing from inpatient to observation status are as follows: the hospital has not already submitted the inpatient claim to Medicare; the Utilization Committee makes the decision, the physician agrees with the Utilization Committee's decision, and the physician documents this concurrence in the patient's medical record; and the UB04 outpatient bill is submitted with the condition code 44, "inpatient admission changed to outpatient" in one of the Form locators 18–28.[12] Code 44 can still be used even with the two-midnight rule.[13] However, there is one caveat: Medicare anticipates that the use of this code 44 modifier is used infrequently and frequent usage may be a red flag that triggers an audit.

Changes in Observation Status: From Observation to Inpatient Admission

A patient in observation status may be admitted to inpatient status at any time for medically necessary continued care, provided inpatient medical necessity screening criteria are met at the time of the hospital inpatient admission, which should be documented. However, two important points must be mentioned. First, the inpatient medical necessity screening criteria must be determined at or from the time of the inpatient admission and *not* from the time the patient was first placed in observation. Second, the patient can never be retroactively switched from observation to inpatient, since a retroactive change would imply that the observation never happened.

References: Criteria for Inpatient Admission or Observation

1. www.ngsmedicare.com/ngs/portal/ngsmedicare (Accessed March 2016)

2. www.careguidelines.com (Accessed 2016)

3. www.mckesson.com/about-mckesson/our-company/businesses/mckesson-health-solutions/interqual-evidence-based-clinical-content (Accessed 2016)

4. Mitus AJ. The birth of interqual. *Professional Case Management* 2008; 13(4): 228–233.

5. www.acep.org/Clinical–Practice-Management/Utilization-Review-FAQ (Accessed March 2016)

6. McKendry MJ, Van Horn J. Tips, tools and techniques. *Case Management* 2004; 9(2): 61–71.

7. Wang H, Robinson RD, Coppola M, et al. The accuracy of interqual criteria in determining the need for observation versus hospitalization in emergency department patients with chronic heart failure. *Critical Pathways in Cardiology* 2013; 12(4): 192–196.

8. Irwin CB, Nigl J, Lowe RA. Accuracy of interqual criteria in determining the hospitalization need in medicare patients with gastrointestinal bleeding. *Acad Emerg Med* 2000; 7:552–553 (abstract).

9. Irvin CB, Monfette K, Lowe R. Retrospective evaluation of potential Medicare admission denials using interqual and Milliman Roberts admission criteria. *Acad Emerg Med* 2000; 7:543 (abstract).

10. Rutledge R. An analysis of 25 Milliman & Robertson guidelines for surgery: data driven versus consensus-derived clinical practice guidelines. *Ann Surg* 1998; 228(4): 579–585.

11. www.cms.gov/Regulations-and-Guidance/Guidance/Transmittals/downloads/R299CP.pdf (Accessed March 2016)

12. www.cms.gov/Outreach-and-Education/Medicare-Learning-Network-MLN/MLNMattersArticles/downloads/SE0622.pdf (Accessed 2016)

13. Confusion ahead as CMS changes inpatient criteria. *Hospital Case Management* 2013 October; 21(10): 133–136.

INPATIENT PROSPECTIVE PAYMENT SYSTEM (IPPS)

What Is IPPS?

The IPPS is "a system of payment for the operating costs of acute care hospital inpatient stays under Medicare Part A (Hospital Insurance) based on prospectively set rates."[1] Under the IPPS, each case is classified into a DRG. Each DRG has a payment weight assigned to it, based on the average resources used to treat Medicare patients in that DRG. The base payment rate is split into a labor-related and nonlabor share. The labor-related share is adjusted by the wage index according to where the hospital is located. (Note: If in Alaska or Hawaii, there is also a nonlabor cost of living adjustment factor.) The base payment is multiplied by the DRG relative weight. There is an add-on, termed the disproportionate share hospital (DSH) adjustment, for hospitals that treat a high-percentage of low-income patients. There is also an add-on adjustment, the indirect medical education (IME) adjustment, for approved teaching hospitals. For specific cases that are unusually costly, termed outlier cases, the IPPS is increased.[1]

The specific DRGs are referenced in the International Classification of Diseases (ICD). The ICD is maintained by the National Center for Health Statistics (NCHS) and the CMS. The current version is the ICD-10-CM (International Classification of Diseases 10th revision clinical modification).[2] The U.S. Department of Health and Human Services issued a final rule finalizing October 1, 2015 as the new compliance date to transition to the ICD-10 code sets.[3] There is also the Current Procedural Terminology (CPT), which is "the medical nomenclature used to report medical procedures and services under public and private health insurance programs."[4] Various manuals are available that list the ICD-9 and ICD-10 codes and the CPT codes.[5–7]

In general, Medicare Part A covers hospital care, skilled-nursing facility care, nursing home care (as long as custodial care isn't the only care needed), hospice, and home health services.[8] Medicare Part B "covers services (like lab tests, surgeries, and doctor visits) and supplies (like wheelchairs and walkers) considered medically necessary to treat a disease or condition."[9]

Inpatient Hospital Stays, IPPS, Targeting Short Inpatient Stays, Reimbursement and Observation

As noted, Medicare's payment for inpatient admissions is determined by using the ICD-10 diagnosis codes), submitted by the hospital to determine the DRG, which ultimately decides the payment for the inpatient admission. According to Medicare's inpatient prospective reimbursement system, every DRG has a known mean LOS and this mean LOS is used to determine the DRG's relative weight and, therefore, payment. Short inpatient hospital stays, for example, meaningfully less than the average LOS, raise concerns that there is potential overpayment and that the admission was "inappropriate" so Medicare and the QIOs monitor hospital discharge data and specifically target short hospital stays. Any hospital that has a high incidence of short inpatient hospital stays is very likely to be audited; if any inappropriate admissions are discovered, repayment and fines or sanctions can be onerous with tremendous financial consequences. Excellent documentation, especially focused on IS and SI, are useful in justifying an admission.[10]

However, in a number of cases, observation status (placement in observation status but not "admitted" to observation since observation is considered an outpatient service) is a viable option to an inpatient admission and, as detailed in later chapters, may even be better in terms of patient/family satisfaction, lower costs, and better patient outcomes with fewer returns to the ED and readmissions to the hospital.

References: Inpatient Prospective Payment System (IPPS)

1. www.cms.gov/Medicare/Medicare-Fee-for-Service-Payment/AcuteInpatientPPS/index.html (Accessed March 2016)

2. www.cdc.gov/nchs/icd/icd9.htm (Accessed March 2016)

3. http://cms.gov/Medicare/Coding/ICD10/index.html (Accessed March 2016)

4. www.cdc.gov/nchs/icd/icd10cm.htm (Accessed March 2016)

5. ICD-9-CM (International Classification of Diseases 9th Revision Clinical Modification). Hart AC, Stegman MS, Ford B (eds.) Optum Insight, Inc., 2012, sixth ed.

6. ICD-10-CM. Official Guidelines for Coding and Reporting –Fy 2015. Department of Health and Human Services, 2015. ,

7. Gabber W, Kachur KH, Canter KV. Current Procedural Coding Expert: CPT Codes with Medicare Essentials Enhanced for Accuracy. American Medical Association, 2011.

8. www.medicare.gov/what-medicare-covers/part-a/what-part-a-covers.html (Accessed March 2016)

9. www.medicare.gov/what-medicare-covers/part-b/what-medicare-part-b-covers.html (Accessed march 2016)

10. www.acep.org/Clinical–Practice-Management/Utilization-Review-FAQ (Accessed March 2016)

MEDICARE'S HOSPITAL PAYMENT MONITORING PROGRAM (HPMP)

The Medicare HPMP was established by CMS to measure, monitor, and decrease payment errors for hospitals (both short- and long-term acute care hospitals) that receive reimbursement via the IPPS using DRGs. The goal is to pay only for services that are "reasonable and necessary" in order to protect the Medicare trust fund. By analyzing claims, doing audits, and modifying the program, Medicare expects to improve payment accuracy.[1–4] The Comprehensive Error Rate Testing (CERT) program and HPMP were established by CMS to randomly sample and review claims submitted to Medicare.[1]

CMS contracts with various Medicare QIOs. The 53 QIOs have a dual function: to analyze and then report data back to CMS, and to provide educational outreach for Medicare providers. In the past when ICD-9 was used, the Clinical Data Abstraction Center checked for the accuracy of documentation and ICD coding, and for the medical necessity of admissions by looking at 62 hospital discharges on a monthly basis for every state and Puerto Rico, and forwards any errors to the state QIOs for review. After performing a focused audit on high-risk areas using Medicare's own inpatient hospital discharge data, HPMP sends the results to the hospital as the PEPPER report.

Targeted areas detailed in the PEPPER report include 1-day inpatient hospital stays, 7-day readmissions, 3-day nursing home qualifying stays, the coding of complications and of comorbidities, and certain primary diagnoses/DRGs that have been historically associated with high Medicare payment error rates. The 1-day inpatient hospital stays gives details on the hospital's top-10 1-day stays. The coding of complications and comorbidities has been utilized to achieve a higher-paying DRG. Primary diagnoses or DRGs that have been associated with a high error rate and with a focus by CMS include 1-day stays for chest pain, 1-day stays for gastroenteritis and other digestive disorders, 1-day stays for nutritional and metabolic disorders, back problems, simple pneumonia, complex pneumonia, septicemia, heart failure and shock, and intracranial hemorrhage and stroke with infarct. Perhaps, many of these 1-day inpatient stays could be managed as observation status.

References: Medicare's Hospital Payment Monitoring Program (HPMP)

1. www.cms.gov/apps/er_report/preview_er_report .asp?from=public&which=long&reportid=7& tab=3/ (Accessed March 2016)
2. www.pepperresources.org (Accessed March 2016)
3. www.primaris.org/sites/default/files/resources/ HPMP/hpmp%20info%20sheet.pdf (Accessed March 2016)
4. www.acep.org/Clinical–Practice-Management/ Utilization-Review-FAQ (Accessed March 2016)

OBSERVATION MEDICINE BILLING: THE CONTROVERSY

Observation services may be viewed by the patient and his or her family, and sometimes by the health care provider, "as admission."[1] Observation is considered an outpatient service by Medicare.[2–4] (Table 2.2)

Table 2.2 CMS Manual on Outpatient Observation Services*

A. Outpatient Observation Services Defined

"Observation care is a well-defined set of specific, clinically appropriate services, which include ongoing short term treatment, assessment, and reassessment before a decision can be made regarding whether patients will require further treatment as hospital inpatients or if they are able to be discharged from the hospital. Observation status is commonly assigned to patients who present to the emergency department and who then require a significant period of treatment or monitoring before a decision is made concerning their admission or discharge."

"Observation services are covered only when provided by the order of a physician ... In the majority of cases, the decision whether to discharge ... or to admit the patient as an inpatient can be made in less than 48 hours, usually in less than 24 hours. In only rare and exceptional cases do reasonable and necessary outpatient services span more than 48 hours."

B. Coverage of Outpatient Observation Services

"The purpose of observation is to determine the need for further treatment or for inpatient admission. Thus, a patient in observation may improve and be released, or be admitted as an inpatient."

C. Notification of Beneficiary

"All hospital observation services ... that are medically reasonable and necessary are covered by Medicare, ... If a hospital intends to place or retain a beneficiary in observation for a noncovered service, it must give the beneficiary proper written advance notice of noncoverage ... "

* from reference 4: *Medicare Benefit Policy Manual*, Chapter 6: Hospital Services Covered Under Part B. 20.5 – Outpatient Observation Services. www.cms.gov/ Regulations-and-Guidance/Guidance/Manuals/Downloads/ bp102c15.pdf (Accessed March 2016)

However, when a patient is placed in a hospital bed even if it is "observation status," this "hospitalization without admission" may create confusion and financial issues.[1] Since observation care is deemed an "outpatient service," Medicare Part A (the hospital billing part) will not cover care rendered in the OU. However, Medicare Part B (outpatient services billing part) and some private insurers will cover observation hospital services, but Medicare Part B does not cover inpatient pharmacy charges and has an additional 20% co-pay for each individual charge incurred.

So when patients are given their usual daily medications while in observation status, these self-administered medications are charged to the patient. It is unrealistic to ask patients who are acutely ill or injured and are undergoing a medical or surgical emergency to be required to have all their medications with them so they can give themselves their own medications for many reasons, including but not limited to: they may not be at home when stricken by the acute injury or illness or they may not have the capacity at the time of the acute presentation to be able to gather all their medications to bring with them. It also poses a safety risk for the patient and the health care givers to ascertain that these are the correct and current medications for the given patient who is now acutely ill or injured and in a different clinical situation than when at home.[5]

If a patient will be discharged to a skilled-nursing facility from observation status, then observation days do not count toward the 3-day prequalifying inpatient stay that Medicare requires for patients needing skilled-nursing facility care on discharge.[5]

Importantly, inpatient admission falling under Medicare Part A is associated with a fairly high deductible ($1,288 in 2016), which must be funded by the patient before additional insurance coverage for the visit takes place. The co-pays for an OU visit that is not excessively long (e.g., 15 hours) are likely to be less costly than a short-stay inpatient admission. Indeed for certain diagnoses, "a recent Office of the Inspector General (OIG) report suggested that observation patients may pay less out of pocket than inpatients."[6] However, the 20% co-pays coupled with medication charges associated with observation can add up for very long observation stays and in some scenarios eventually exceed the Part A deductible.

This "loophole" has been criticized by multiple individuals and institutions including a recent *New England Journal of Medicine* article that recommended the following reforms in the Medicare payment policies in order "to encourage high-value observation care and minimize cost-shifting": "CMS should reform observation payment policies" by 1. "capping the total out-of-pocket expense at the inpatient deductible amount (which would) keep observation stays from costing patients more than inpatient admissions, which are generally more resource intensive", 2. "covering self-administered medications," and 3. including time in observation "toward the 3 days of hospitalization that qualify a patient for skilled-nursing-facility benefits."[5]

Importantly, in 2016 observation was added to the growing list of Medicare comprehensive APCs. The reimbursement for the observation Medicare comprehensive APC for 2016 is $2,174. The structure of the comprehensive APC includes payment for most typical ancillary services such as diagnostic studies, infused medications, and many small procedures. As such, the patient is now more protected because their 20% co-pay for this large basket of services is $435.

There has been litigation challenging the Medicare rules. There are bills recently filed in Congress that would support this Medicare reform.[5] CMS has also authorized some pilot programs that would allow time in observation to be included toward the 3 days of hospitalization that qualify for skilled-nursing benefits.

Some institutions have an information sheet regarding observation status that they distribute to patients who are being placed in observation that explains the Medicare payment policies regarding observation, and have patients sign acknowledging receipt of this information with the appropriate personnel to contact (such as case management, utilization review, financial counselors) if they have any questions.[4] Acknowledgment of the information does not waive the patient's right to request a review of the decision to assign the patient to observation.

References: Observation Medicine Billing: The Controversy

1. Sheely AM, Graf B, Gangireddy S, et al. Characteristics of patients with "observation status" at an academic medical center. *JAMA Intern Med* 2013; 173(21): 1991–1998.

2. Centers for Medicare and Medicaid Services. Are you a hospital inpatient or outpatient? www.medicare.gov/publications/pubs/pdf/11435.pdf (Accessed March 2016)

3. Centers for Medicare Advocacy Inc. Observation status. www.medicareadvocacy.org/medicare-info/observation-status#definition (Accessed March 2016)

4. *Medicare Benefit Policy Manual.* Chapter 6: Hospital Services Covered Under Part B. 20.5 – Outpatient Observation Services. www.cms.gov/Regulations-and-Guidance/Guidance/Manuals/Downloads/bp102c15.pdf (Accessed March 2016)

5. Baugh CW, Schuur JD. Observation care – high-value care or a cost-shifting loophole? *N Engl J Med* 2013; 369(4): 302–305.

6. Society of Hospital Medicine Public Policy Committee. The Observation Status Problem. Impact and Recommendations for Change. Society of Hospital Medicine Whitepaper, July 2014. Available at www.hospital medicine.org/advocacy (Accessed March 2016)

Summary

In the past, CMS has been somewhat of a "passive" payer of claims. More recently, they have shifted to being an active participant in value-based purchasing. This has led to an increased incidence of audits and greater accountability. There has been a proliferation of various Medicare and Medicaid integrity contractors. There is every indication that this shift in perspective and focus will continue in the future.

Glossary of Terms

ACA	= Affordable Care Act
CC	= Comorbidities or Complications
CERT	= Comprehensive Error Rate Testing
CFR	= Code of Federal Regulation
CMS	= Centers for Medicare and Medicaid Services
CPT	= Current Procedural Terminology
DHHS	= Department of Health and Human Services
DRG	= Diagnosis-Related Group
DSH	= Disproportionate Share Hospital
ED	= Emergency Department
FI	= Fiscal Intermediary
FISS	= Fiscal Intermediary Standard System
HCPCS	= Healthcare Common Procedure Coding System
HICN	= Healthcare Insurance Claim Number
HIPPA	= Healthcare Insurance Portability and Accountability Act
HPMP	= Hospital Payment Monitoring Program
ICD-9-CM	= International Classification of Diseases 9th revision, Clinical Modification
ICD-10-CM	= International Classification of Diseases 10th revision, Clinical Modification
IME	= Indirect Medical Education
IPPS	= Inpatient Prospective Payment System
IS	= Intensity of Service
LCD	= Local Coverage Determination
LOS	= Length of Stay
MAC	= Medicare Administrative Contractor
MCC	= Major Comorbidities or Complications
MIC	= Medicare Integrity Contractor
MS-DRG	= Medicare Severity Adjusted - DRG
NCD	= National Coverage Determination
NPP	= Non-physician Practitioner
OIG	= Office of Inspector General
OU	= Observation Unit
PEPP	= Payment Error Prevention Program
PEPPER	= Program for Evaluating Payment Patterns Electronic Report
PHI	= Protected Health Information
QIO	= Quality Improvement Organization
RAC	= Recovery Audit Contractor
RUG	= Resource Utilization Group
SI	= Severity of Illness
ZPIC	= Zone Program Integrity Contractors

* This chapter is intended to give a synopsis of key administrative issues. Changes are occurring and updates should be done on a regular basis by providers and institutions.

Chapter

3

Observation Medicine Development Over Time

Louis Graff IV, MD, FACEP, FACP

Observation Medicine Concept: Improved Delineation of Appropriate Level of Care

Recognition of the major failings of the traditional approach to the evaluation and management of patients with acute illnesses and conditions led to the development of Observation Medicine (OM). In the traditional approach, patients were brought to emergency departments (EDs) for evaluation and management by a physician over a 3–4 hour time period. During that time a history, physical, and some rapid tests were performed and the physician would either release the patient home or admit the patient to the hospital. Prompt decision on disposition was needed and even required since agencies such as the Joint Commission and the United States Federal Government prohibited prolonged ED stays. Over time leaders in emergency medicine (EM) recognized there were many patients who needed more evaluation and management than could be provided in 3–4 hours in the ED, but inpatient admission for days was not needed.

From a quality viewpoint the traditional approach was failing because many patients were being discharged home from the ED without diagnosing their serious, dangerous disease. Acute myocardial infarction (MI) was being missed in 2–5% of patients who presented atypically with the physician inadvertently missing the diagnosis and sending them home.[1] This resulted in a doubling of the patient's risk of death and risk to the physician's career comprising 30% of malpractice payments to families who lost their loved ones.[2] Other conditions similarly were not being diagnosed because of the limitations of the 3–4 hours ED evaluation but could have been diagnosed and treated if they had more than 3–4 hours evaluation.

From a utilization viewpoint the traditional approach was failing because many patients were being admitted to inpatient hospital services who were found to have no serious dangerous disease and/or needed < 24 hours of acute therapy. The majority of patients admitted for chest pain were found to not have any serious, dangerous disease during inpatient hospitalization.[3] Four out of five patients with acute asthma attacks not completely treated in the ED could be treated successfully if the therapy continued for another 8–24 hours.[4]

OM provided a "third pathway" for disposition of patients from the ED. In the 1980s and 1990s leaders in this field had operationalized the observation concept in their observation units (OUs) and validated its worth with their research. They recognized that observation service could be provided to many patients who needed more than the 3–4 hours of ED service but did not need inpatient services provided for days. It improved quality by providing a pathway that selected patients with a low probability of serious, dangerous disease who could receive an additional 8–24 hours of evaluation. For low-probability chest pain patients this resulted in reduction of the missed MI rate (with its concomitant doubled mortality) from 2–5% to < 0.5%.[5] It improved utilization by providing a pathway that selected patients with an emergent condition who could receive an additional 8–24 hours of short-term therapy without having to be hospitalized. The observation approach for these patients as an alternative to acute inpatient hospitalization reduced costs by > 50%.[6,7]

Development of Leadership

Empowerment of excellent leadership has been crucial in the development of OM. This has been necessary at each individual hospital and necessary on a national level.

The American College of Emergency Physicians (ACEP) has taken a leadership role in supporting observation services including policy statements, guidelines, offering courses on observation services, forming a section on Short Term Observation Services, and online references on ACEP's web site.[8-12]

The Society for Academic Emergency Medicine (SAEM) also recognized the importance of ED observation services and formed an OM Committee, which created an OM bibliography and curriculum.[13-15] An edition of *Emergency Medicine Clinics of North America on Observation Medicine* and the first textbooks of OM were written by ACEP/SAEM leaders in OM.[16-18]

Evolution of Observation Unit Staff

ED OUs developed in the 1960s and 1970s were staffed with physicians available 24 hours a day, 7 days a week. These emergency physicians (EPs) were available not just during morning rounds as for inpatient services with private physicians, but at all times. Thus, they were always able to respond rapidly to changes in a patient's condition, and to respond whenever the patient's evaluation and treatment plan ended with discharge home or inpatient admission. The nurses were working side by side with the physicians throughout the day and night as a collaborative team in these ED OUs, which facilitated efficiency of communication and action whenever appropriate and not just at a selected time of the day such as morning rounds. In contrast, the nurses on the inpatient units spent most of their time following the orders written by physicians when they admit the patient or during their once-a-day rounds. The rest of the time the physicians are in their offices during the day and at their homes during the evening and night. They would be called by a nurse to come back to the hospital only in special dire circumstances.

Creation of Functional Physical Plants

This development of EDs with full time EPs created the opportunity for ED observation services. Many EDs were designed in the 1960s and 1970s with observation units. They designated an area of the ED or an area adjacent or near the ED for providing observation services.

Development of Best Practice Operations

By the 1990s there was a robust literature on the safety and effectiveness of ED observation services as an alternative to acute care hospital admission and this has continued into the next millennium. There are now randomized clinical trials (RCTs) on patients with chest pain[7,9-21], asthma[6,22], atrial fibrillation[23], syncope[24], TIA[25], and many others. (See Chapters 22 Chest Pain, 27 Asthma, 24 Atrial Fibrillation, 25 Syncope, and evidence-based Chapters 80 Diagnosis/Clinical Condition and 81 Age-Related.) All these RCTs have validated what prior, less sophisticated research trials have shown in the past. That is, *for selected patients, observation provides equivalent or superior clinical patient care compared with traditional acute care hospital inpatient services and it does that at half the cost.*

Development of Financial Viability

Reimbursement and rational cost-effective structuring is needed for the success of an observation program. The origins and development of OM have been in the ED for the last three decades with EPs negotiating most of the issues for the present reimbursement structure.

Physician reimbursement (Part B reimbursement) for observation services was not available for those who originally developed these services. The patient observed in an ED OU received more than double the physician services compared to patients admitted or discharged home at the end of their ED evaluation and management.[26] ACEP leaders went to the American Medical Association's (AMA's) Current Procedural Terminology (CPT) committee and their RVS Update Committee (RUC) where RVS = Relative Value Scale and successfully negotiated new CPT codes for physician reimbursement of observation services.

Either CPT 99218, 99219, or 99220 are used for evaluation and management of observation patients during their initial stay and CPT 99217 for disposition services the next day. ACEP leaders in 1998 returned to the AMA's committees and successfully negotiated new CPT codes for physician reimbursement of observation services for patients whose observation stay and discharge does not extend over to a second day (either CPT 99234, 99235, 99236). These are still the CPT codes used by any physician who provides observation services.

Facility reimbursement (Part A reimbursement) for observation services was simple at the start of the creation of observation services, but has become increasingly complex over time. In the original model, observation service charges for a room rate are similar to that for an inpatient room rate. In 2000 Medicare implemented prospective payment for outpatient services with APCs (ambulatory payment categories). Hospitals were paid for each outpatient service that had an assigned APC.

Unfortunately, Medicare refused to assign an APC for observation so they stopped Part A payment for observation. They had identified many hospitals were double charging Medicare for surgical procedures by charging for observation inappropriately, in addition to the appropriate charge for the surgical procedure, which included recovery after the procedure.

Advocates from Emergency Medicine, the Society of Chest Pain Centers, the American Heart Association, the American College of Cardiology, and the American College of Nuclear Cardiology met with CMS on this issue and clarified the value and cost-effectiveness of the rational use of observation (extended diagnostic or therapeutic use and not post procedure). In 2003 CMS did again agree to make Part A payments for observation with the creation of an APC for observation (APC #0339). But they only agreed to pay for observation for selected conditions: chest pain, congestive heart failure, and asthma.

In 2007, ACEP leaders were successful in advocating for CMS to remove this list and pay for any condition that was appropriate for observation. This negotiation entailed the discontinuation of APC #0339 and the creation of two new composite APCs (#8002 and #8003) that are Part A payment to the hospitals for both the ED visit (or the clinic visit if they came from a clinic) and the observation services. With this success nearly all payers recognized and agreed to pay for observation services and in many cases became aggressive advocates for the use of observation services.

References

1 Lee TH, Cook EF, Rouan GW, Weisberg MC, Goldman L. Ruling out myocardial infarction: prospective multicenter validation of a 12 hour strategy for low risk patients. *Clinical Research* 1989; 37:524A.

2 Karcz A, et al. Massachusetts emergency medicine closed malpractice claims: 1988–1990. *Ann Emerg Med* 1993; 22:553.

3 Pope JH, Aufderheide TP, Ruthazer R, et al. Missed diagnoses of acute cardiac ischemia in the emergency department. *N Engl J Med* 2000; 342:1163–70.

4 Murphy DG, Zalenskio RJ, Raucci JC et al. The utility of extended emergency department treatment of asthma. *Ann Emerg Med* 1989; 8:467.

5 Graff LG, Dallara J, Ross MA, et al. Impact on the care of the emergency department chest pain patient from the Chest Pain Evaluation Registry (CHEPER) study. *Am J Cardiol* 1997; 80:563–568.

6 Rydman RJ, Isola ML, Roberts RR, et al. Emergency Department Observation Unit versus hospital inpatient care for a chronic asthmatic population: a randomized trial of health status outcome and cost. *Med Care.* 1998; 36: 599–609.

7 Roberts R, et al. A randomized clinical trial of inpatient versus observation care in the evaluation and management of chest pain patients. *JAMA* 1997; 278:1670–1676.

8 American College Emergency Physicians. Emergency Department Observation Units. *Ann Emerg Med* 1988; 17:95–96.

9 American College Emergency Physicians Practice Management Committee. American College Emergency Physicians. Management of Observation Units. *Ann Emerg Med* 1988; 17:1348–1352.

10 Brillman J, Dunbar L, Graff L, et al. American College of Emergency Physicians Section of Observation Services: management of observation units. *Ann Emerg Med* 1995; 25:823–830.

11 Ross MA, Aorora T, Graff LG, Suri P, Ojo A, Bohan S, Clark C, O'Malley R. State of Art: Emergency Department Observation Unit. *Critical Pathways in Cardiology* 2012; 11(3):128–138.

12 Graff LG (Editor in Chief). *Observation Medicine: The Healthcare System's Tincture of Time.* Online Textbook of the American College of Emergency Physicians Observation Medicine Section at www.acep.org/acepmembership.aspx?id=30260

13 Graff LG, Dunbar L, Gibler B, Goldfrank L, Leikin J, Severance H, Schultz C, Yealy D, Watkins R, Zun L. Observation Medicine: an annotated bibliography. *Amer J Emerg Med* 1992; 10:84–93.

14 Graff LG, Dunbar L, Gibler WB, et al. Observation Committee of the Society of Academic Emergency Medicine. Observation medicine curriculum. *Ann Emerg Med* 1992; 21:963–966.

15 Graff LG, Zun L, Leiken J, Gibler WB, et al. Observation Committee of the Society for Academic Emergency Medicine. Emergency department observation beds improve patient care: Society for Academic Emergency Medicine debate. *Ann Emerg Med* 1992; 21:967–975.

16 Ross M, Graff L (eds.). Principles of observation medicine. *Emerg Med Clin North Am* 2001; 19.

17 Graff LG (ed.). *Observation Medicine*. Butterworth-Heinemann, Stoneham, MA, 1993.

18 Graff LG (ed.). *Observation Units: Implementation and Management Strategies.* American College of Emergency Physicians, Dallas, TX, 1998.

19 Gomez M. An emergency department based protocol for rapidly ruling out myocardial ischemia reduces hospital time and expense: Results of a randomized study (ROMIO). *J Am Coll Cardiol* 1996; 28:25–33.

20 Farkouh ME, Smars PA, Reeder GS, et al. A clinical trial of a chest-pain observation unit for patients with unstable angina. *N Engl J Med* 1998; 339:1882–1888.

21 Goodacre S, et al. Randomised controlled trial and economic evaluation of a chest pain observation unit compared with routine care. *Br Med J* 2004; 328:254–264.

22 McDermott, et al. Treatment of acute asthma patients as outpatients in an observation unit versus as an inpatient in the hospital. *Arch Int Med* 1997; 157:2055–2062.

23 Decker WW, et al. A prospective, randomized clinical trial of an emergency department observation unit for acute atrial fibrillation. *Ann Emerg Med* 2008; 52:322–328.

24 Shen, W, Beinborn, D. Random clinical trial of observation unit versus in patient services in evaluation and management of patients with syncope. *EP Lab Digest* May 2005.

25 Ross M, et al. An emergency department management protocol for patients with Transient Ischemic Attacks: a randomized clinical trial. *Ann Emerg Med* 2007.

26 Graff LG, Clark S. Emergency physician critical care services: a time study at an American and an English Emergency Department. *Arch Emerg Med* 1993; 10:145–154.

Observation Medicine Principles

4

Louis Graff IV, MD, FACEP, FACP

Most patients after a 2-to-4-hour emergency department (ED) evaluation are identified as being safe for outpatient treatment or severely ill requiring acute care inpatient hospitalization, but for some it is unclear what their severity of illness is and/or their intensity of service needs. These patients need a "tincture of time" of 8–24 hours of outpatient observation level of care. The physician needs to "pause" their disposition decision (outpatient vs. inpatient) and place the patient in outpatient observation level of care for limited-intensity and limited-time services. With observation 80% of patients will be found to be safe for outpatient treatment and 20% found as severely ill requiring inpatient hospitalization.[1,2]

Principles of observation medicine need to be followed to ensure optimal outcomes for these patients.[1-4] Physicians need to make a correct level-of-care determination by identifying patients with a focused patient care goal and limited duration and intensity of service need. Since these patients are judged as potentially seriously ill, they need a hospital site of service. Such services can only be provided with acute care staffing and require structure and patient care protocols for continuing care in an outpatient setting. Superior leadership providing intensive managerial review is needed to ensure adequate structure, adequate resources, continuous performance improvement, and expertise of personnel. With compliance with all these principles, the outcome will be high-quality economical service that is unique to observation services.

Observation Is the Correct Level of Care

The most difficult and most crucial task to ensure optimal observation services is for the physician to reliably identify patients for whom observation is the correct level of care. These patients must have focused patient goal needs of diagnostic evaluation and/or short-term therapy and/or management of psychosocial needs. Their therapeutic needs must have limited duration and limited intensity of service. Details on the approach to evaluate patients with respect to the threshold for observation and the threshold for inpatient admission are discussed in Chapter 19 Medical Necessity Risk Stratification.

Threshold for observation is determined by the missed diagnosis rate. For a syndrome (e.g., chest pain chief complaint) it is the rate of missed diagnosis and the rate of testing (e.g., for chest pain it is rule out myocardial infarction [MI] testing rate). There is average performance in missed diagnosis rate (e.g. 2%–5% of patients with acute MI) have their diagnosis missed at the initial ED evaluation and the rate of rule-out-MI testing.[2, 5-6] The ideal is zero missed diagnosis rate with the goal being best practice performance always on the journey toward zero. With feedback to individual physicians of their cases with a missed diagnosis and feedback to the group of lessons learned, individuals and the entire group of physicians can lower their threshold for observation (extended evaluations) rather than discharge home after the initial ED evaluation. In this example (Figure 4.1) the group diagnostic performance from 2% to < 0.5% missed MI rate as the threshold for observation decreased as the percentage of ED chest pain patients with a rule-out-MI rate increased from 35% to 50%.

Threshold for inpatient admission is determined by the observation usage rate. If patients who have moderate to high probability of disease/risk of adverse event are placed in inpatient admission and patients who have low probability of disease/risk are placed in observation, then a portion of patients with negative evaluations (final diagnosis is their presenting chief complaint) will have been in observation level of care and a portion in inpatient level of care. In the earlier example of chest pain patients and rule-out

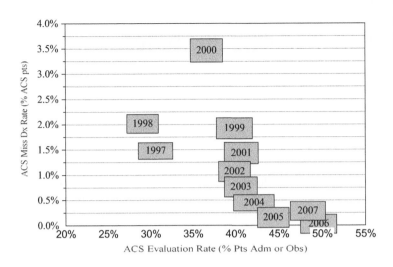

Figure 4.1 ACS Evaluation Rate vs. ACS Miss Dx Rate
National Average is 2% Miss Dx Rate

MI, the observation rate is the number of observation patients with final diagnosis of chest pain divided by the sum of the number of observation patients with final diagnosis of chest pain and the number of admitted inpatients with final diagnosis of chest pain. If the observation usage rate is very high, it indicates there is too much observation and moderate probability/risk patients are not being admitted, since if moderate probability/risk patients were being admitted, some admitted inpatients would have the final diagnosis of chest pain and not all acute MI and other serious diseases. If the observation rate is very low, it indicates there is too little observation since if moderate probability/ risk patients are being admitted, many admitted inpatients would have a final diagnosis of chest pain. Ideal is a moderate observation usage rate correlating with the ideal observation rate as identified by the missed diagnosis rate.

The OU rate has the largest n so it is the primary rate for the OU leadership to use. The observation usage rate is calculated from the many patients observed and admitted each month and can be calculated by physician each month, while the missed diagnosis rate is calculated from the few missed diagnosis cases and can only be calculated infrequently for most institutions for the whole group only once a year.

Hospital Site of Service

Hospital site of service is mandatory for observation services. The patients who are appropriate for observation level of care are those ED patients who are determined during the ED evaluation to possibly require inpatient hospitalization level of care. They are by definition patients who are possibly moderate to high risk of an adverse event and the most appropriate setting for observation services is adjacent to or inside an acute care hospital where their acute, dangerous, serious condition could be promptly and effectively treated.

Acute Care Staffing

Acute care hospital personnel are required for an OU. Observation services are a higher level of care service than the ED and personnel need to be able to respond and stabilize complications suffered by patients who are determined to have acute, dangerous, and serious conditions. These patients are then transferred to the inpatient admission level of care. Thus, staff need to be equivalent to those that provide services in the acute care hospital.

Continuing Care in Outpatient Setting

Rather than an episode of care as provided in the usual outpatient clinic or ED setting, the OU needs to provide continuing care similar to that provided to inpatient admissions. This requires order sets, protocols, rounds, and all the components of care necessary for high-quality, efficient services.

Intensive Managerial Review

The complexity of care provided in OUs requires intensive managerial review. The services are outpatient and need to be coordinated with the complexity of the acute care hospital. Physician and nursing leadership need to be empowered and responsible for continuous performance improvement, developing and implementing protocols, and ensuring the highest quality of care and utilization of resources. Operational issues such as budget, recruitment of staff, adequacy of staffing, development and education of staff need active, effective observation services leadership.

Economical Service

The nature of observation services properly structured and operated results in costs of services half of those provided as traditional acute care inpatient hospital services.[7-8] Rather than once-a-day rounds by physicians, the ideal OU has rounds every 8 hours by physicians, which results in decisions and actions taken in a much more rapid cycle than possible in a traditional acute care hospital. OU staff are trained to function with this rapid cycle (8–24 hours) care plan rather than a 4–5 day care plan. Randomized clinical trials of diagnostic evaluation of chest pain[9] and emergent therapy of acute asthma attacks[10] are two examples of many studies that have shown properly structured and operated OUs provide economical service.

References

1. Graff LG (ed.). *Observation Medicine*. Butterworth-Heinemann, Stoneham, MA, 1993.

2. Graff LG (Editor in Chief). *Observation Medicine: the Healthcare System's Tincture of Time*. Online Textbook of the American College of Emergency Physicians Observation Medicine Section at www.acep.org/acepmembership.aspx?id=30260

3. Brillman J, Dunbar L, Graff L, et al. American College of Emergency Physicians Section of Observation Services: management of observation units. *Ann Emerg Med* 1995; 25:823–830.

4. Ross MA, Aorora T, Graff LG, et al. State of art: emergency department observation unit. *Critical Pathways in Cardiology* 2012; 11(3): 128–138.

5. Graff LG, Dallara J, Ross MA, et al. Impact on the care of the emergency department chest pain patient from the Chest Pain Evaluation Registry (CHEPER) study. *Am J Cardiol* 1997; 80:563.

6. Goodacre S, Nicholl J, Dixon S, et al. Randomised controlled trial and economic evaluation of a chest pain observation unit compared with routine care. *Br Med J* 2004; 328:254.

7. Roberts RR, Zalenski RJ, Mensah EK, et al. Costs of an emergency department-based accelerated diagnostic protocol vs hospitalization in patients with chest pain: a randomized controlled trial. *JAMA* 1997; 278:1670–1676.

8. Rydman RJ, Isola ML, Roberts RR, et al. Emergency department observation unit versus hospital inpatient care for a chronic asthmatic population: a randomized trial of health status outcome and cost. *Med Care* 1998; 36:599–609.

9. Roberts RR, Zalenski RJ, Mensah EK, et al. Cost of an emergency department-based accelerated diagnostic protocol vs. hospitalization in patients with chest pain: a randomized controlled trial. *JAMA* 1997; 278:1670–1676.

10. McDermott M, Murphy D, Zalenski R, et al. A comparison between emergency department diagnostic and treatment unit and inpatient care in the management of acute asthma. *Arch Intern Med* 1997; 157:2055–2062.

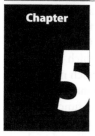

Chapter 5

Design

David Robinson, MD, MS, MMM, FACEP

Successful observation units (OUs) have several features that have changed little since the late 1980s.[1,2] Since the majority of observable patients are identified from the Emergency Department (ED), a successful OU commonly fulfills the following functions. An OU should augment the clinical capacity of the ED.[1,3,4] Next, its design and function should improve the quality of diagnostic and therapeutic care from the ED.[1,4,5] The third and most compelling function is that an OU should enhance the revenue cycle of a hospital by delivering lower cost, more efficient strategies for managing observable diagnoses.[3,5–8] If the third function cannot be achieved, then the need for an OU comes into question.[3,6,7,9]

OUs are designed to serve as a bridge for those patients requiring extended care beyond what is a reasonable time for the ED or similar outpatient setting, but not requiring the resources or intensity of services found in an inpatient service. Effective observation care is delineated in many references and is summarized by the following goals:[1,2,10,11]

1. Improve the quality of the acute care patient when a short-stay diagnostic or therapeutic workup is planned.
2. Provide a designated physician and nurse who shall be responsible for the patient's observation care.
3. Establish a dedicated location for this observable care.

4. Provide written protocols and procedures established by the hospital and medical staff that clearly delineates the type of care, the methods from which observation care will be performed, qualifying criteria to and from the unit, and criteria for discharge from the OU or admission to the hospital.
5. Provide a documented, ongoing quality review process.

Successful OUs also share several design features that follow the three 'Ps' of hospital unit design: Proximity, Personnel, and Process. The choice of hospital OU location is largely dependent on the available resources, space, training, and hospital budget. There are 4 types of OUs based on two variables (Table 5.1).[12] The first variable is whether or not the personnel are specifically trained in observation care and are familiar with the care protocols and processes. The second variable is if the unit is physically located in one location, preferably in close proximity to the ED, or if the observation patients are scattered throughout the hospital. The most effective units are those managed by trained personnel in a location where all observation patients are concentrated (type I OU).[2,4,9,12] (Note: This is similar to the Types of Observation Units in Table 1.1 in Chapter 1 where protocol driven is similar to trained personnel and dedicated unit is similar to unit in one location.)

Table 5.1 Types of Observation Units

Type	Trained Personnel Familiar with Protocols and Processes	Unit in One Location Ideally near ED	Efficiency
I	Well informed	Yes	Most efficiency
II	Well informed	No	Intermediate efficiency
III	Generally informed	Yes	Intermediate efficiency
IV	Generally informed	No	Least efficiency

The location of the OU significantly benefits the unit's operations and is a primary driver of its clinical and operational effectiveness. OUs with specific identifiable hospital locations improve long-term hospital costs by reducing redundant equipment costs, administrative workload, and transfer times from the ED.[10,12,13] There is no specific requirement for an OU to be located in a specific location although most hospital-based OUs are generally located near or adjacent to the ED[11] and nearly one-third of all hospitals now have an existing OU.[9,11] OUs located next to the ED permit seamless, integrated care pathways originating from the ED, have and can share resources such as staffing (phlebotomy and ECG technicians, nursing, clinicians) and equipment.[3,11,12] OUs located far from the ED must provide separate resources and nursing. Care protocols may be different when personnel and location varies, resulting in redundant test ordering and increased cost. Unfortunately, the creation of a new OU is often a capital budget consideration that is in direct competition with other ED expansion projects.[3,6]

Room size is a factor in many OU expansion projects. With miniaturization of telemetry systems and electronic records, and smaller computers with flat screen monitors, a modern OU room may require as little as 120 square feet per room.[14] Since a primary function of an OU is to complete a diagnostic workup, one must consider what diagnostic tools the OU will require before considering room size. For example, if a Chest Pain OU is considering performing bedside cardiac echocardiography or portable radiography, would the rooms accommodate these devices? Toilets, showers, televisions, and sleeper chairs may provide additional comfort for patients and guests. As an extended-stay room for patients, OUs deploying standard hospital inpatient beds may require rooms of 150 to 160 square feet.[14] Regulations vary from state to state, but room size and amenities such as the requirement for windows are generally more liberal for OUs than for inpatient beds, making it easier to convert inpatient beds to observation beds, rather than vice-versa.

Estimating the unit size requires three metrics: the anticipated ED volume, the expected nurse ratio for staffing, and the average time for processing the observable patient. In general, 5–10% of the ED volume might be suitable observation patients.[3,9] Most resources suggest that OU staffing is best suited for 4:1 to 6:1 nursing.[12,15] A hospital with an anticipated ED volume of 60,000, therefore, might expect to have 3,000–6,000 qualified observation patients. Using 12 hours (0.5 days) for an average protocol completion time (including transfer or discharge time), then the calculation of OU estimated size is (0.5 [bed-days/patient] × 3,000–6,000) / 365 days, or 4 to 8 beds. A 5- or 10-bed unit with 5:1 nursing would be a reasonable estimate while still anticipating further growth.[12,15]

Personnel are a considerable factor in the operational efficiency and cost of an OU.[3] A cornerstone to efficient OU operations are highly trained nurses and staff in protocol management.[16] OU-trained personnel managing an OU in a designated area (Type I OU) results in better operational efficiencies than an OU with concentrated patients but without trained personnel (Type III).[10,12,17] There is no specific policy mandating that OUs have specialized health care providers trained in observation medicine, although systems with trained OU personnel have reported better economic and noneconomic outcomes than OUs without specific provider training.[3,6,12,18]

OU systems employing nursing and ancillary staff specifically trained and knowledgeable about the clinical care pathways (e.g., chest pain protocols) can further be trained to manage the flow of patient care.[16] All nurses and ancillary staff (technicians, phlebotomists, and others) should be familiar with each care pathway. Regulatory billing guidelines outline specific documentation requirements for observation services, but have not mandated any specialty training in observation medicine as a prerequisite for establishing an OU. As a result, there may be much variability in the quality of training from the hospital's physicians, nurses, and staff.[11] Units staffed by physicians, nurses, and staff who as part of their practice, participate in observation services, and have at least some knowledge of the processes of observation medicine (e.g., risk stratification, care pathways, and billing requirements) would be considered 'generally informed' and occupy the Type III or IV units. Physicians and nurses who utilize goal-directed care pathways, are specifically trained in observation processes, and participate in the OUs quality assurance oversight, utilization review, and feedback are considered "well informed."[10,12,17] These groups of providers are found in Type I and II units. While these descriptive classifications are useful, hospitals may modify a particular observation unit type to better meet its patient care goals and needs and particular institutional goals (Table 5.1).

Resources are available for observation medicine training, design, and operations management, including sample care-directed protocols. These may be found from the American College of Emergency Medicine website (www.acep.org) or the Society of Chest Pain Centers and Providers (www.scpcp.org) and in Chapters 82–87 in this book.

References

1. American College of Emergency Physicians. Emergency department observation units. *Ann Emerg Med.* 1988; 17:95–96.

2. American College of Emergency Physicians. Management of Observation Units [policy resource and education paper]. Approved January 2008. www.acep.org (Accessed February 20, 2016)

3. Baugh CW, Venkatesh AK, Bohan JS. Emergency department observation units: A clinical and financial benefit for hospitals. *Health Care Management Review.* 2011; 36 (1):28–37

4. Ross MA, Naylor A, Compton S. Maximizing use of the emergency department observation unit: A novel hybrid design. *Ann Emerg Med.* 2001; 37(3):267–274.

5. Graff LG, Dallara J, Ross MA, et al. Impact on the care of the emergency department chest pain patient from the Chest Pain Evaluation Registry (CHEPER) study. *American J Cardiology.* 1997; 80:563–568.

6. Sieck S. Cost effectiveness of chest pain units. *Cardiol Clin.* 2005; 23:589–599.

7. Robinson D, Woods P, Snedecker C, et al. A comparison trial for stratifying intermediate risk chest pain: Benefits of emergency department observation centers. *Preventive Cardiol.* 2002; 5:23–30.

8. Roberts R, Graff L. Economic issues in observation unit medicine. *Emer Med Clinics of N America.* 2001; 19(1):19–33.

9. Graff LG. In *Observation Medicine, The Healthcare System's Tincture of Time.* Update August 2011. Retrieved March 28, 2012, from American College of Emergency Physicians website: www.acep.org/Workarea/ DownloadAsset.aspx?id=45885 (Accessed February 20, 2016)

10. American College of Emergency Physicians. Chest Pain Units in Emergency Departments. A report from the Short Term Observation Services Section. Aug. 8, 1994. www.acep.org (Accessed February 20, 2016)

11. Mace SE, Graff L, Mikhail M, et al. A national survey of observation units in the United States. *Amer J Emerg. Med* 2003; 21(7):529–533.

12. Robinson DJ. Hospital based observation unit design. In *Observation Medicine, The Healthcare System's Tincture of Time.* Update August 2011. Retrieved March 28, 2012, from American College of Emergency Physicians website: www.acep.org/Content.aspx? id=46142&terms=observation (Accessed February 20, 2016)

13. Cooke MW, Higgins J, Kidd P. Use of emergency observation and assessment wards: A systematic literature review. *Emerg Med J.* 2003; 20:138–142.

14. Huddy J. In: Huddy J, ed. *Emergency Department Design; A Practical Guide to Planning for the Future.* Dallas, TX: American College of Emergency Physicians; 2002.

15. Graff LG. Observation unit staffing. In Graff LG, ed. *Observation Medicine.* Newton, MA: Butterworth-Heinemann; 1993:89–98.

16. Emergency Nurses Association. Observation Units/Clinical Decision Units. [Position Statement]. Revised Sept 1997.

17. Brillman J, Mathers-Dunbar L. American College of Emergency Physicians: Management of observation units. *Ann Emerg Med.* June 1995; 25:823–830.

18. Rotter T, Kugler J, Koch R, et al. A systematic review and meta-analysis of clinical pathways on length of stay, hospital costs and patient outcomes. *BMC Health Services Research.* 2008; 8 (265): 1–15. www.biomedcentral.com/ 472–6963/8/265 (Accessed February 20, 2016)

Chapter

6

Staffing Considerations

Christopher W. Baugh, MD, MBA, FACEP
J. Stephen Bohan, MD, MS, FACEP, FACP

While the staff needed to operate an Emergency Department Observation Unit (ED OU) are no different than those required for the ED proper, the distribution of staff varies according to the unique aspects of the individual institution and can be modified depending on the location of the unit relative to the ED. To ensure high-quality patient care for this added service there must be adequate dedicated personnel and oversight. Customarily, ED staffing is based on a combination of visit volume, visit acuity, and the number of treatment spaces or rooms; the ED OU is no different.

Leadership

An ED OU should have clear physician and nursing leadership. This structure establishes accountability, training, oversight, and feedback. A clear leadership structure encourages communication and allows staff to elevate concerns. The most important initial task of leadership is to develop standardized management pathways and order sets. ED OU-centric staff training, which includes insights into the appropriateness of specific patients for observation care,[1–3] maximizes the potential of the unit. Clinicians need to understand patient characteristics that allow safe and expeditious care with a high likelihood of disposition to home within 24 hours. Finally, leadership should develop a policy manual that provides transparency as to the goals and available resources, update it regularly and make it easily accessible.[4]

Nurses

Observation units (OUs) are typically staffed by registered nurses, who have the clinical skills and experience to care for this patient population. Ideally the nurses should be experienced ED staff as they can carry the ED culture into the ED OU. However, other non-ED nurses, if imbued with the ED culture (e.g., rapid throughput), may be utilized. Nurses are the only staff likely to be present 24/7 in the ED OU, typically representing the highest operating cost. A survey of OUs found that one nurse cares for a mean 4.2 patients.[8] One nurse is needed per shift for every four to six patients in an OU. This varies with the institutional model, and whether Advanced Practice Providers (APPs) are present. ED OU patients tend to be more independent and less acutely ill than their counterparts on the inpatient floors or those in an extended or complex OU. Although the acuity of OU patients seems to be increasing over the years,[5,6] nurses generally care for fewer patients in the OU than is usual on the inpatient floor in order to ensure faster throughput and the "front loading" of diagnostics and therapy essential for an efficient OU to ensure shorter length of stay (LOS). The OU ratio of one nurse to four or five patients is similar to and was derived from the nurse:patient ratio for a stepdown unit. In the absence of an APP, nurses can be given more autonomy and can, for example, track down test results, thus maintaining the aggressive throughput goals of an EDU. In this model (operative at Cleveland Clinic for about 20 years, S. Mace, personal communication) nurses, with these additional responsibilities, would generally care for fewer patients, for example, a 1:4 ratio during the day and a 1:5 ratio at night. Although more recently, in order to further decrease OU LOS and for some cost saving (e.g., APPs are less expensive than emergency physicians), in the Cleveland Clinic model APPs have been added during the day and some evening hours, with the OU nurses continuing to fulfill their somewhat autonomous role on the late evening and night shift (e.g., for 12 hours a day). Thus far, national guidelines for nursing ratios have not specifically addressed the observation setting. Usually an ED OU will have a fixed number of beds, which will determine the

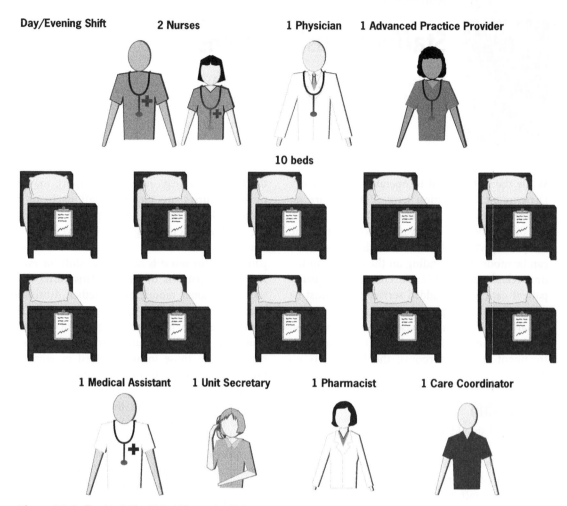

Day/Evening Shift **2 Nurses** **1 Physician** **1 Advanced Practice Provider**

10 beds

1 Medical Assistant **1 Unit Secretary** **1 Pharmacist** **1 Care Coordinator**

Figure 6.1 Staffing Model for 10-Bed Observation Unit
(Courtesy of Dr. C.W. Baugh, Dr. S.E. Mace and Center for Medical Art and Photography, Cleveland Clinic)

number of nurses needed based on the staffing ratio above. For example, a typical 10-bed observation unit will be staffed by three nurses on the day/evening shift and two nurses on nights (see Figure 6.1).

Physicians

Payer requirements and quality standards generally dictate that an attending physician personally perform both an observation admission and discharge assessment.[7] However, during the course of the observation period, the attending physician need only be immediately available, not physically present. This allows for cross coverage of other areas in the hospital, including ED acute care, but *requires additional staff* to support this model. The number of patients assigned to any

single physician must recognize the demands of both volume and complexity, taking provider capacity into account, not just at the averages, but also at peak times as well.[6] With the assistance of additional staff such as resident physicians or an APP, an uninterrupted minimum of an hour is usually needed to round on a typical 10-bed OU, but this does not include the time needed to do a thorough history, physical examination, discuss plans with the primary care physicians and consultants, with the patient and family, and the OU nursing staff, as well as write additional orders and complete the needed documentation. Local conditions such as the location of the unit and the presence of other providers affect the amount of physician coverage. Resident physicians should not be counted in any staffing model, although exposure to this growing aspect of practice is useful. (See Staffing the Unit: Physicians from Chapter 1 Clinical Issues.)

While there may be a demonstrated need for an ED OU, the available space is not always within or immediately adjacent to the ED. As a result, institutions must determine the staffing model that accounts for logistics to allow the responsible physicians to be available to the observation patients. For example, if an ED OU is created on the opposite side of a large hospital and results in long transit times, it may not be practical to expect that physician to be responsible for both locations simultaneously. However, a brief elevator ride may not impose any significant obstacle to adequate coverage.

Advanced Practice Providers

Many OUs are staffed by physician extenders, such as Nurse Practitioners or Physician Assistants. These professionals, commonly used in the United States and also called APPs, Advanced Practice Clinicians or midlevel providers, have special training to function autonomously in many clinical settings. These providers offer a less expensive alternative to a direct physician presence in the OU. Stationed in the OU, an APP is available to assess patients, respond to nursing questions or suggestions, ensure results are followed up and testing is completed. In some institutions, the APP is also expected to "help out" and adds coverage to the ED when they are not busy in the OU.

Even with the use of an APP, a supervising physician should be ultimately responsible and available for each patient in observation. Critical decisions, such as the overall management plan and endpoints for discharge, are usually made by the supervising physician and subsequently managed by the APP. If a patient decompensates or if test results are concerning, the supervising physician is reengaged to intervene. However, much of the hands-on work needed to care for observation patients can be safely handled by an APP. Some institutions do not require all observation patients to be personally seen by a physician if they rely on experienced APPs for routine observation care. However, there are implications for billing/reimbursement if this is the case, since the reimbursement may be less for an APP compared to the physician.

Ancillary Staff and Consultants

A 10-bed ED OU should be staffed by at least one medical assistant and one unit secretary. Coverage may vary overnight, when patients tend to be less active. Case management is another crucial partner essential to be engaged and present every day in an OU to assist with safe and timely dispositions of observation patients. In addition, a strong relationship with consultant services is, as is the case in the ED, essential to the success of the unit. Not surprisingly, the need for consultants tends to mirror the most frequent types of complaints managed in observation.[8] Consultations need to occur in a timely manner and recommendations for further diagnostics and treatments must consider the time frame and resources specific to the ED OU. Finally, consultations are more efficient when the consulting service has been involved in the development of clinical protocols.

References

1. Crenshaw LA, Lindsell CJ, Storrow AB, et al. An evaluation of emergency physician selection of observation unit patients. *Am J Emerg Med* 2006 May;24(3):271–279.

2. Burkhardt J, Peacock WF, Emerman CL. Predictors of emergency department observation unit outcomes. *Acad Emerg Med* 2005 Sep;12(9):869–874.

3. Ross MA, Compton S, Richardson D, et al. The use and effectiveness of an emergency department observation unit for elderly patients. *Ann Emerg Med* 2003 May;41(5):668–677.

4. Brillman J, Mathers-Dunbar L, Graff L, et al. Management of observation units. American College of Emergency Physicians. *Ann Emerg Med* 1995 Jun;25(6):823–830.

5. Greene J. Nurse groups, administrators battle over mandatory nursing ratios: California law debated on national stage. *Ann Emerg Med* 2009 September;54(3):31–33.

6. Baugh CW, Venkatesh AK, Bohan JS. Emergency department observation units: A clinical and financial benefit for hospitals. *Health Care Manage Rev* 2011 Jan–Mar;36(1):28–37.

7. Centers for Medicare & Medicaid Services (CMS). CMS Manual System: Pub 100-04 Medicare Claims Processing. 2008 February 22nd; Transmittal 1466.

8. Mace SE, Graff L, Mikhail M, et al. A national survey of observation units in the United States. *Am J Emerg Med* 2003 Nov;21(7): 529–533.

7

Nursing

Sharon E. Mace, MD, FACEP, FAAP
Karen Games, RN

Observation Unit Location: To Cohort or Not Cohort Observation Unit Patients

Whether to place observation patients scattered throughout the hospital into inpatient units is a common question. This practice should be discouraged for many reasons and is often a reason why observation status (OS) fails.

"Observation is a mindset and a process, not a location"; this quote of mine (Dr. Mace) emphasizes the importance of guidelines, protocols, policies, procedures, and other administrative and organizational mechanisms coupled with the observation unit (OU) physician and nursing mindset that is focused on the timely, efficient evaluation and/or treatment of patients and that observation can be done anywhere, even in a designated area of the emergency department (ED).

However, cohorting OU patients has many advantages. There is a precedent for grouping like patients in a hospital. This is the case for intensive care units, pediatric units, cardiology telemetry or step-down units and other specialty units, such as neurology. The advantages have been well elucidated.

The OU should be viewed in a similar manner as these other specialty units. The OU staff comprises a wide array of personnel in addition to nurses: from unit secretaries or coordinators to respiratory therapists, technicians, housekeeping, and others, depending on the setup of the OU. Having a specific unit or area for OU patients helps to develop an esprit de corps and enhance team building among the OU staff. They know the tenets of the OU, which are the efficient and cost-effective diagnostic evaluation and treatment of patients with various illnesses and injuries. Cohorting OU patients fosters this mindset and distinguishes the OU patient from other inpatients.

This also advances the OU concept throughout the hospital. Other departments – for example, cardiology, pulmonary, radiology, and laboratory – can easily and quickly recognize the OU patient. When radiology calls the unit to request it send a patient to the radiology department for a CT scan, for example, they likely will not be aware of the patient being in OS if the observation patients are scattered throughout the hospital. Even with color coding of charts, color coding patient identification bands, or signs on the patient's door, etc., the respective department, such as radiology, may not be aware of the patient's OS until he or she arrives in the department for his or her test. Being in a specific location readily lets everyone throughout the hospital know that this patient is an observation patient or a "high-priority" patient. The OU could be likened to "an express lane" at the supermarket where there is a quick turnaround.

If OU patients are randomly placed in beds throughout the hospital, then there must be a mechanism for identifying the observation patient as being unique or different from other patients on the inpatient units. Various methods have been used to distinguish the observation patient from the other inpatients on the same inpatient floor or unit. These include color coding the patient's charts, using different name bands for OU patients, and color coding the room numbers or signage on the patient's door. Unfortunately, unless other methods are used to identify the OU patient, individuals may not be aware of the patient's OS until they arrive at the patient's room or bedside. Consider phlebotomy as one example: unless their blood draw list identifies OU patients and a system is set up to prioritize the OU patients in the queue, they will not be automatically identified by the floor or area they are in, so their blood draws would be the same as anyone on a given floor and they would not be prioritized. Other instances would be how to easily and quickly identify OU patients in the daily list of radiology patients for a CT scan or inpatients having a stress test.

Not all hospitals are large enough to have a distinct OU or can afford to build a separate OU. However, OU patients can be grouped in a specific part of a given floor or consistently assigned specific beds so they can be readily identified, starting at the point of registration and throughout the entire process. Having OU patients dispersed throughout the hospital necessitates developing and maintaining various mechanisms for their identification, whether color coding, different charts, etc., which could be cumbersome and time consuming.

These techniques do identify the observation patient from other inpatients on the same floor. However, by training and by good clinical practice, if there is another patient on the same inpatient floor who is "crashing" then there is the possibility or even the likelihood that nursing personnel and resources may be, justifiably, diverted to the most seriously ill patients. When faced with more seriously ill or, even occasionally, critical patients, it is possible, even likely, that the nurse, physician or other health care provider will prioritize caring for the most seriously ill or injured patient first and the OU patient will be lower on the list.

Cohorting all observation patients in the same location, whether an designated unit or a section of a given inpatient floor, generally avoids this "ranking" of patients by acuity since, by definition, all the observation patients are at the same "low acuity" ranking and are patients who do not need intensive nursing or physician care. This grouping of patients promotes the "rapid turnaround" approach and the attitude that this is a "short-term" unit or area in which patients can only be diagnosed and treated for 24 hours or less, which also makes it more explicit to the patients and families, physicians, and other hospital personnel.

To summarize, this concept of "clustering" like patients is similar to the grouping of other types of patients, such as intensive care unit patients or cardiac step-down patients, etc., and engenders the same benefits as cohorting any patient types. Nursing and other personnel are part of a "specialized" unit that fosters an esprit de corp and anyone, including ancillary services such as laboratory or radiology, can readily identify these patients and the "short-term" rationale for their care.

Observation Unit Staffing

Once the location of the OU is determined, then another key issue in setting up an OU is personnel. One mistake that dooms an OU to failure is not to assign additional staffing hours and/or additional personnel to care for OU patients when opening an OU. This is true for physician or physician extenders, as well as for nursing and ancillary personnel. In the zeal to start an OU, sometimes, personnel especially from the ED are expected to take on the additional responsibility of OU patients in addition to the current demands of caring for ED patients. When this happens, the OU patient is second on the list after the ED patient, which defeats the premise of the OU for prompt, efficient diagnostic evaluation and treatment.

Additional nursing staff and/or nursing hours and physician coverage or hours, and perhaps, midlevel providers, will be necessary when opening an OU. There should be consideration of staffing as for additional inpatient beds. Generally, for the nursing staffing of the OU, there is a 1:4 or 1:5 nurse to patient ratio.[1] This ratio may be decreased slightly at night since some diagnostic testing, such as stress tests, are not done at night; although patients are still undergoing diagnostic testing and therapy – such as cardiac monitoring, having blood drawn and ECGs done – and receiving IV fluids, treatments, and medications at night.

Additional physician coverage or a combination of midlevel providers with physician coverage is also necessary since there is continuing care (including availability to review diagnostic testing and discuss results with consultants) and ongoing evaluation of patient response to treatment, and so on, in addition to the initial evaluation (history, physical examination, and OU plan of care) and discharge planning (with reevaluation: history, physical examination, medical course/decision making). In some institutions, the ED evaluation is transitioned into the initial OU evaluation when the same physicians are responsible for the OU. This is the case in our OU and to avoid any concerns, our practice is to waive the emergency fee and bill only for the observation fee(s) since the same physicians are caring for the patient. (This refers to the physician billing. Hospital billing is different. See Coding and Reimbursement chapters: Chapter 62 for Physicians and Chapter 63 for the Hospital.)

Depending on the number of observation patients, the physician/midlevel provider staffing may vary but additional hours and or providers must be added, otherwise the observation patients will end up waiting until the physicians or midlevel providers finish treating other patients in the ED and only then are available to reevaluate the observation patient, write additional orders and determine a disposition (discharge or inpatient admission), which defeats the purpose of observation.

Unlike nursing in which there are some suggested staffing ratios, there seems to be more variation in physician/midlevel provider staffing and the ideal physician/midlevel provider staffing has not been determined. One suggested model as used previously in our OU has one physician and midlevel provider to care for all 20 patients in our OU during the day shift, which is a 1:10 provider to patient ratio. During the evening and nights, the secondary ED coverage in the "fast track" or less acute areas may cover the OU, but again there should be additional coverage especially in the evening. (See Chapter 1 Clinical Issues.)

We are considering other staffing models, including expanding the midlevel provider coverage to 24 hours a day with physician oversight. In this model the midlevel provider and physician's first responsibility would be the OU patients, making sure the initial evaluation/orders are complete, reevaluating patients on the evening shift and documenting their findings with a progress note ideally on every shift, and doing the discharge evaluation with an updated history, physical examination, clinical course, diagnosis, and the discharge plan, which is different from and in addition to the initial evaluation conducted when the patient is placed in observation.

In addition to nursing and physician staffing, other personnel should be considered, especially if it is a large OU. The OU will need personnel similar to that needed for running an equivalent-sized inpatient unit. The question should be asked "What personnel are essential for an inpatient unit with the number of patients in your OU?" For example, a 20-bed inpatient floor would have nursing staffing and physician/midlevel providers plus a unit secretary, housekeeping, transport, "technicians" or patient care assistants who assist

the nursing staff with various tasks (from doing vital signs to transport, hygiene, nutrition, etc.). One suggestion is to use the ancillary personnel numbers for a general inpatient floor. For example, if a 25-bed floor has four patient care assistants, then a 12- bed OU should probably have two patient care assistants. Other services, such as housekeeping or transport, need to be assigned to the OU as well.

Observation Unit Design, Equipment, Supplies

The OU is unique in that it has characteristics of both an inpatient unit yet is considered an outpatient service. (See Chapter 6 Observation Unit Design.) When we started our OU over two decades ago, there were no other OUs that we could go and observe their setup, design, and staffing. Since the unit was under the auspices of the ED, our blueprints were similar to that for an ED. Mentioning some of our early issues related to design may help others avoid similar problems.

For example, rooms in the ED may have a room with a sink, but do not generally have showers in each room. Patients in observation are expected to be there for a short time but may be overnight, so in the morning patients waiting for or returning from a stress test or other procedures may want to take a shower. We did not put such bathroom facilities in our OU so our creative nurses invented "bath in a bed" to allow for morning hygiene, but shower facilities are desirable.

Initially, we did not have phone lines in every patient room, so on day one, the few phone lines assigned to the OU were overwhelmed by families phoning in and patients phoning home so that the consultants, and ancillary services calling for patients to be transported to stress testing, etc., could not get through. Needless to say, we immediately put phone lines in every patient room. A small kitchen area to heat up patient meals, etc., is also desirable.

I consider this the "4Ts" of patient amenities: telephone, television, toileting (hygiene) and, more recently, technology (internet access for patients and families). While waiting for diagnostic testing or undergoing treatment, a television and, currently, outlets and internet access for patients and their families are becoming essential in every room. This is all fundamental to improving patient and family satisfaction.

The majority of patients in an OU are cardiac patients: chest pain, heart failure, atrial fibrillation, syncope, etc., and have cardiac monitoring ordered. We made the mistake of not putting in cardiac monitoring in every room so on day one we had to find portable monitors until we could hardware additional permanent monitors (at an expense).

Another consideration is the ability to include patients with infections, such as pneumonia, bronchitis, croup, bronchiolitis, gastroenteritis, and diarrhea with dehydration, etc., in the OU. This is a large group of patients who can be cared for in an OU so consideration for these "contagious" patients or patients with communicable diseases should be included in the OU design. Ideally, individual rooms, with doors instead of curtains, etc., along with the usual standard infectious disease precautions will enable these patients to be placed in the OU. (See administrative policy on infectious diseases in Chapter 88 Administrative Policies.)

The OU needs to be stocked with the usual inpatient supplies and equipment, such as linens. Thought should be given to what medications to include in the pharmacy stock or pixis in the OU. Common medications that patients take daily may need to be included since patients will need to take their usual daily medications, in addition to various IV medications, etc., as used in the ED. The OU is designed for low-acuity, low-risk patients so the instances of resuscitations or "codes" should be infrequent, although chest pain patients sometimes do rule in for a myocardial infarction.[2] Thus, the pharmacy may need to stock both "routine floor stock" as well as emergency medications. The instances of intubations, resuscitations or codes has been rare in the OU, although when we had the first resuscitation in the OU, we had to go to the ED to get a "crash cart"; fortunately the ED was nearby, adjacent to the OU, but on review at our monthly Observation Unit Meeting, a recommendation from quality improvement was to have a "code cart" and an airway cart located in the OU unit for easier and immediate access.

Observation Unit Census: "Time Lag before the Observation Unit Is Consistently Full"

Initially, it takes time, usually about 6 months to a year, before everyone, especially the physicians

(and others including nursing), is comfortable with the OU and placing patients in the OU. This is true for the ED physicians as well as other physicians throughout the hospital. If the physicians and/or midlevel providers are familiar with the working of an OU, perhaps, having worked in another OU or acquainted with observation medicine during their training/education, this time lag before the OU is full may be shorter. But in general, there is a delay before the staff/personnel, especially the physicians, are familiar with and understand the processes and systems involved with the OU and are willing to place patients in OS and the OU is consistently full every day. This is to be expected and anticipated so staffing may need to be adjusted or "ramped up" as the OU daily census grows over time.

Observation Unit Staffing: Staffing for the Daily and Hourly Census in the Observation Unit

As mentioned, there may be a lag, usually 6–12 months, before the OU is consistently at full census. There may also be variations in the daily OU census so if there are "peaks and valleys" and if a consistent pattern is identified, nursing staffing may be adjusted appropriately. The observation census tends to follow the ED census, such that when the ED is busy, the OU tends to receive a lot of patients and be full. In our institution, the ED census and, similarly, the OU census tend to be lower on weekends so we decrease the nursing staffing on weekends in the ED and the OU. (The physician/midlevel provider staffing in the ED is also decreased on weekends.) For pediatric EDs and pediatric OUs, the ED census is likely higher on weekends (and evenings) so staffing in the pediatric ED and pediatric OU could take this into consideration. However, if there is "flex" nursing staffing, there may need to be an on-call list or other avenues for increasing the nursing staffing to meet the demand.

Generally, the highest influx of patients into the OU is during the evening shift and the greatest efflux or disposition of patients from the OU is in the late morning and early afternoon. One possible solution to this hourly variation in the OU census is to allow postprocedure recovery patients be cared for in the OU since it is anticipated that these patients will recover quickly (in 2–3 hours) and be discharged around dinner time, thereby freeing up the OU beds for the influx from the ED on the busiest ED shift, the evening shift. We have not allowed non-OU patients including postprocedure at our institution, but other institutions have tried this practice.

This practice should be clearly differentiated from the practice of putting admitted patients into the OU until a bed opens up on an inpatient floor. This is a dangerous practice and should be avoided. The OU is *not and should not become* "a holding unit." The recommendation is not to put admitted patients into the OU. This eliminates beds for the true OU patients; in addition, this creates excessive work by the OU nurses who have to do nursing intake on an admitted patient and then move the patient out to another floor where the patient again sees another nurse. This practice is also uncomfortable and unpopular with the patients and families, and gives the appearance of musical chairs or musical beds. This does not give a very flattering view of the hospital to the patient or their family. Needless to say, moving a sick patient or someone in pain multiple times from one bed to another until he or she reaches his or her final inpatient location creates much discomfort for the patient.

Assigning Observation Unit Nursing and Other Personnel to Other Areas and "Pulling Observation Unit Staff/Personnel"

The purpose of the OU is the quick turnaround of patients. If nurses are simultaneously assigned to both the ED and the OU, the problem of dealing with the most severely ill or highest acuity patients arises. By training and good clinical practice; clinicians, whether physicians or nursing or ancillary personnel, will always prioritize the sickest or most acute patients. Therefore, nursing personnel should be assigned to the OU. Pulling nurses from other units to respond when patients are placed in the OU is a dangerous practice and *is to be avoided*. It is difficult, if not impossible, for a nurse who is caring for a given patient in the ED or on an inpatient floor or other area of the hospital to abruptly stop what he or she is doing and transition to another area, the OU, to take care a new patient placed in OS.

If OU nurses are to be pulled from the OU, then they should be assigned to an area near the OU since they can relocate quickly and they should be caring for "short-term" patients. For example, it may be easier for the nurse to assist in the ED, especially in the "fast-track" area, rather than the inpatient floors or even other areas of the ED since these "fast-track" patients are usually seen, evaluated and discharged very quickly, freeing up the OU nurse to return more rapidly to the OU.

It is preferable to staff the OU first and in instances when the OU census is low, then allowing the OU nurse to assist in the ED, with the caveat that when a patient is placed in OS, any patients that nurse is caring for in the ED are immediately transitioned to another ED nurse so the OU nurse can then begin caring for and orienting the new OU patient to the OU. If the OU nurses do work in the ED, then there should be cross training so nurses from primarily the OU or primarily the ED can work in the other unit, if needed. Usually, nurses and other personnel who work in a given unit prefer the type of patient care specific to that unit so reassigning personnel to other areas may create some dissatisfaction.

Balancing the demand of the OU for the ready availability of staff to begin the patient's management in order to ensure a rapid disposition and quick turnover of OU patients with concerns over cost, especially personnel costs, can be difficult. Indeed, personnel costs, specifically nursing, are the largest item in the OU budget. However, factors that lengthen the OU stay are detrimental to the efficiency of the OU and can have major negative consequences in terms of patient outcome, quality of care, reimbursement, risk management, and patient/family satisfaction. A valid cost analysis is likely to confirm the value of the OU, and justify the personnel and other costs involved. (See Chapter 68: The Business Case for Observation Units.)

Administration of the Observation Unit: Physician Medical Director of the Observation Unit

There must be a physician medical director of the OU. The physician medical director has a dual function: clinical and administrative. The physician medical director is responsible for ensuring quality patient care in the OU with the best possible patient outcomes. He or she oversees the provision of medical care in the OU (for OS patients). He or she is also the administrative leader of the OU and works conjointly with the nurse manager of the OU to foster the efficient operation of the OU.

In order to fulfill the clinical and administrative responsibilities of the OU, the physician medical director of the OU should have protected nonclinical administrative time.[1] There are many varied complex roles performed by the medical director of the OU, who has a leadership role for the physicians and the entire OU. (See job description for the physician medical director in Chapter 88 Administrative Policies.)

Administration of the Observation Unit: Nurse Manager of the Observation Unit

No matter what the size – for example, number of beds and thus, number of patients – there must be a nursing administrator or nurse manager for the OU just as there is a physician administrator for the OU.

Whether the nurse manager is a full-time administrator or part-time and works some clinical shifts may depend on the size and other factors related to the OU as well as to the hospital. As a general rule, it is usually good practice for administrative personnel, whether nursing or physicians, to work a few shifts or hours in the OU and/or to be able to respond to clinical needs and do "hands on" care for patients when the need arises. This is a way to experience firsthand

the issues involved in caring for OU patients and become knowledgeable about the details of the day-to-day functioning of the OU, as well as to gain credibility among the OU staff and physicians.

If the OU is larger, or more specifically, a "high-volume" unit, which has a large number of patients, then there is likely more than enough for the nurse manager of the OU to do and the OU probably deserves its own nurse manager, in addition to the nurse manager of the ED, even if the OU is under the auspices of the ED.

Summary

This chapter discusses some of the commonly asked questions regarding the setup of an OU with a focus on those issues that impact nursing staffing. Based on our decades of experience, for an OU to succeed, there must be the following: personnel (clinical and administrative); resources (space or location, equipment, supplies); specific and general (clinical and administrative) guidelines, policies, procedures, order sets, and other tools; a mandatory time frame; strong leadership empowered to clinically and administratively manage the OU with administrative support from the hospital; and a multidisciplinary teamwork approach.

References

1. Mace SE, Graff L, Mikhail M, et al. A national survey of observation units in the United States. *Am J Emerg Med* 2003; 21: 529–533.

2. Mace SE. Resuscitations in an observation unit. *Journal of Quality in Clinical Practice* 1999; 19 (3):155–164.

Risk Management

Chapter 8

Gregory L. Henry, MD, FACEP

Introduction

Observation units have and will become a valuable tool for health care systems to manage both patients and risk. With such units, physicians can improve quality, and meet both patient and provider expectations. It is important to note that in most emergency departments (EDs), the principle complaints of patients have not changed over the years. "I waited too long," and "they never told me anything," are still common refrains heard around ED waiting rooms. Complaints are from frustration with unmet expectations. Such frustration leads to anger, which, in America today, leads to lawsuits. Risk management must deal with causes of unmet expectations if it is to mitigate the problems of the current medical/legal quagmire. It is only from this broader approach that better patient care and patient expectations will be realized.

Insurance companies have become in some ways the final arbiters of medical care, and they never take risk; they spread risk. Insurance rates will not go down until the actual risk goes down. This will only be accomplished through planned changes in the behavior of individuals, and more importantly through changes in the system. If the ED systems for evaluating patients leads to frustration, that is, long delays, poor service, etc., complaints and lawsuits can be expected. If the ED systems for evaluating patients lead to bad outcomes, that is, failure to diagnose serious disease, lawsuits are not just expected, but a certainty. The traditional ED system for evaluating patients fails to diagnose a considerable number of patients with acute myocardial infarctions and releases them home with false reassurance. Other serious conditions are similarly not reliably identified in the traditional ED. Observation units are a tool to address many of these risk problems in emergency medicine. More than that, they actually provide better care for less cost, which is a laudable goal of the health care system. Observation units represent the new third pathway, joining discharge and admission as outcomes from an ED visit.

What Is Risk Management?

The actual definition of risk management has varied over the years, but the traditional role of risk management has been protection of the institution, the health care workers, and the asset base on which they function. Risk management has carried a negative connotation not only for the patients, but for the doctors. People from risk management departments have been viewed as meddling, non-physicians, or at least non-practicing physicians, who have come to preach as opposed to improve. Risk management has been viewed as an office in the hospital bureaucracy rather than a way to practice. It may be that the term "risk management" has outlived its usefulness. Patient safety is and should be the more refined view of risk management.

Who Has the Real Risk?

The newer modes of risk management recognize that the only real risk is to the patient. The people who can truly be harmed by inadequate care are the people receiving that care. The only way to manage risk is to change the system and the care that is given. A quality assurance program that does not run hand and glove with a risk management program is doomed to failure. They are two sides of the same coin. The function of risk management is to make certain that every patient feels he or she has been handled in a correct and humane manner. It is not just to manage claims and complaints, but to have a continuous feedback loop into the care that is given so the problems are *anticipated*. The true effect of a risk management program should be to help modify the system. Perception is the only reality; the perception of care, as well as the care itself, is critical to the intrinsic operations of any ED.

The Quality of Risk Management Data

A tremendous problem in discussing risk management and quality assurance is that the information collected over the years has been spurious at best. Most risk management departments define their losses as failure to treat or failure to diagnose, which rarely gets at the basic problems involved. When considering an evaluation of appendicitis, for example, the recorded claim is always failure to diagnose. When in fact, with the vast majority of such claims the patient did not have the criteria on which the decision to operate could be made. The real problem was in the follow-up care, time interval for being seen again, and the way in which the patient was instructed. It is not that a diagnosis was not made, but that a definitive diagnosis at that moment in time could not be made and that further evaluation on a time-structured basis was needed. This is a question of the quality of the discharge program and the quality of system integration rather than a simple failure to diagnose.

This type of overly broad and nonspecific data collection is essentially useless when it comes to improving the system. Humans only respond to specifics. A physician and a system must know exactly what behavior requires changing if they are to act in a predictable manner. Risk management data in the future will need to be much more carefully scrutinized and collected so that we actually understand the system, decision, or specific action that requires change. Most human beings, if handled correctly, can understand that medicine is complex. Instant decisions are often impossible. Correctly constructed systems that get the patient into health care, as opposed to into the hospital, will be required in the future if costs are to be controlled and patient safety assessed.

System Thinking

Just as Deming totally changed the manufacturing world with his views of quality assurance, the current medical system, which has grown up since WWII, needs such an overhaul.[2] In the United States, since the end of WWII, there has been maximal money and minimal intelligence put into asking serious outcome questions with regard to health care outcomes. The questions of

"what do we want from a health care system?" and "what should be the services provided by that system?" have never been seriously asked in a structured format. If medicine is to be more than a glorified magic show with the patient entertained by periods of incarceration in less-than-sterile buildings with toys and gadgets, definitive outlines of where we need to go must be drawn. To this end, fundamental questions about the function of hospital versus outpatient care will need to be addressed. System thinking is defining what outcomes will drive the health care system of the future. This form of thinking must be done as a partnership with those receiving the service. The focus must not be on identifying good and bad physicians, but on identifying good and bad systems for providing defined medical service.

Ultimately, physicians alone will not determine health care. A combination of scientific input by physicians and the wants and desires of the broader society will determine what services will be given and in what settings. As resources become more limited and the population continues to age at a rate that has never before been contemplated, the need to define what actual role and outcome medicine can play is paramount. Observation units cannot become holding units for the diffident. They can't be another place to die. People can die at home for free. Risk increases when the expectations of the general society are not mirrored in its institutions. If the expectation of the general society is that everyone with abdominal pain is admitted to the hospital, whether it has anything to do with their improved health or not, failure to admit places extra risk on health care providers. That is why serious discussion needs to be undertaken. Drive-through deliveries, drive-through mastectomies, termination of life-support systems, and the like are not as much scientific questions as they are sociologic questions. Risk management has been the interface between technical and scientific knowledge that has not yet become inculcated into societal beliefs.

Improved Communications

No discussion in a textbook of this generation would be complete without genuflecting to the intellectual god of communications. What people think is greatly a function of what they are told. If it is the norm that patients die at home, as it is in many countries, there is no problem with a death at home. In the United States where death is accompanied by sirens, ventilators, and transplants, communications with families becomes critical. The decision to employ expensive inpatient, high-tech medicine to a defined end point will more and more require the input of patients, their families, and some true medical knowledge as to the likelihood that such interventions would restore meaningful life. It is often difficult to say in one brief moment in the ED to what degree family and patients understand the seriousness of their disease and the likelihood of a return to reasonable function. An often-overlooked function of observation units is not just for physicians to monitor the course of a disease so as to be better able to predict interventional outcomes, but for families to become educated on the various options and what might to be done with regard to their loved ones. The real communication of medical facts, as applied to the emotions of the ill, is a milieu devoutly to be wished. Restructuring the ED by adding a third disposition pathway, observation, to the traditional dispositions of hospital admission or discharge empowers the ED staff to have hours, rather than minutes, to spend communicating with patients and their families. But limitations are needed. The system fails when the observation units become a step in the pathway from nursing home to funeral home.

Improved Cost-Effectiveness

The EDs of the United States are increasingly becoming the arbiters of the application of science to human problems. At any hour, day or night, EDs are available throughout this country to process human misery and enter people into the health care system. This need is not decreasing. Whether the primary interests are social, such as the poor and uninsured, or a mixture of medically and financially important issues, such as in managed care, a tempest in medical care exists in EDs. The sorting out function has never been more important and has never required more skilled practitioners. It also requires wisdom. It is only in knowing what to do and to whom, that we are able to balance the three imperatives of access, quality, and cost. There is an ill-defined sense that there exists some linear relationship between the amount of money spent on health care and the health of society. Yet, some countries which spend less than one-third that of the United States (on a gross

national product basis) on health care actually produce better overall health outcomes. A third disposition pathway (transfer to observation) prevents the ED staff from hasty decisions on hospital admission and allows hours, rather than minutes, before decisions must be made on committing a patient to extensive, costly evaluation in a hospitalized setting. No one wants to talk about the fact that the larger community need is not medical observation units but psychiatric observation units. In many locations effective care to medical patients is being destroyed by overwhelmed and grossly inefficient psychiatric systems.

Legal Issues

When providers and consumers cannot agree on problems in risk management, resolution does not occur in the medical world, but in the realm of jurisprudence. The questions become of duty, breach, harm done, and the proximate cause. The relationship between these elements is the exclusive arena of the law. Medical malpractice has been present in English Common Law since at least 1290 AD. Since the case of Hill versus Chynault in 1377, we have specific case law on which to base future legal decisions. The concepts of health and specific medical abilities in diagnosis and treatments have varied tremendously since the first medical/legal cases. The concepts of physician as assuming the role of healer have not changed in the last millennium. In legal terms, the physician is the retained agent and servant of the patient. The degree to which we understand our servant role is a measure of our maturity in medicine. By the same token, physicians and the medical community are health advisors to the individual. It is the interaction between the patient's rights and the physician's duty where risk management is most challenged. Into the future, as resources diminish, the skilled physician is the one who can help the society truly choose amongst options that will provide meaningful life with the most judicious use of resources. Creating a system for selected patients to receive prolonged observation with ED staff enables emergency medicine to better meet both its moral and legal obligations.

High-Risk Situations

EDs must come to grips with the fact that high-risk situations do exist. The role of observation units should be in simultaneously increasing the quality of care, reducing the overall cost of care, and providing the least disruption to patients' lives. The options of either ED discharge or an in-hospital admission must be supplemented by the third choice of observation. The third pathway is often the most intelligent pathway with certain types of conditions such as chest pain, abdomen pain, headache, asthma, and change in mental status.

Chest pain cases still constitute approximately 30% of all monies lost in emergency medicine malpractice cases.[3] A physician who believes he knows the exact cause of chest pain of every patient after the initial history and physical is often referred to by another name: Defendant Physician. Chest pain is a constellation of diseases in which the initial history and physical may reveal nothing, while the patient actually has incredibly severe disease. Only through proper observation, retesting, and the application of certain test modalities will the question of chest pain be resolved. It is the ideal example of that intermediate condition in which decisions can be made without admission to the hospital, but often require more than an initial history and a physical. Various TIA and stroke syndromes are becoming the new norm for observation work-up.

Abdominal pain still constitutes a large percentage of money lost in emergency medicine malpractice.[4] The progression of disease may not be clear. Abdominal pain can be sensitive, but highly nonspecific. In those cases, in which time sensitive management is required, the observation unit may be ideal. Certainly many patients with abdominal pain can go home and return in specifically stated times for reevaluation. The observation unit is ideal for those patients who have difficulty in logistics, transportation, understanding their disease, or for those patients the physician has a high level of concern about the presence of serious disease.

Resolution of head pain with therapy is no indication that severe disease does not exist.[5] The performance of studies such as lumbar punctures, CT scans, and therapies with multiple drugs may require a more prolonged ED evaluation. In such cases, observation and treatment may be essential in arriving at a diagnosis without missing potentially life-threatening disease.

The vast majority of diabetics who have mild to moderate ketoacidosis can be managed with aggressive fluids, insulin, and electrolyte therapy and can be reversed without resorting to inpatient care. Such patients often understand the nature of their disease and how they got into trouble; actually admitting such patients, because it is an artificial situation, may prolong the time to stabilize and enter them back into the usual outpatient world.

Asthmatics, as a group, constitute the largest number of return visits to EDs.[6] This is frequently because they are not using their medications correctly, are going back into contact with irritants, or have not been properly stabilized before discharge. Observation/treatment units provide for proper therapy and allow systematically administered steroids and other medications to stabilize the condition of the patient prior to discharge.

The quintessential ED patient is the alcoholic with mild alteration of mental status who may or may not have hit his head. Such patients are often minimally confused and yet hospitals simply do not have the resources to admit all such patients. Observation units are where frequent repeat examinations can be performed, and where community resources and family support can be organized to facilitate the proper management of such patients. Inpatient therapy offers little to such patients who will then again return to the streets. The coordination function with regard to

Risk Management Approach

Risk Management Goals

Improve service
Improve outcome
Help manage poor outcomes

Strategy to Decrease Risk

Patient feels handled correctly & humanely
Risk management data on system

On system function
On decisions
On actions
On outcomes

Observation to Redesign System

Improve communications
Improve cost-effectiveness

Observe High-Risk Patients

Chest pain patients
Abdominal pain patients
Headache patients
Asthma patients
Mental status patients
TIA

such community and family services, which can be carried out in a rapid treatment and decision unit, are often overlooked. The availability of resources for patients with altered mental status and psychiatric disease is often tremendously constricted in nonregular work hours. It is frequently the function of the ED to not only stabilize the medical situation, but the social situation as well. This may be best accomplished through a rapid treatment and decision unit.

Conclusion

Risk management, in its older format of protecting the institution at all costs, is rapidly dying.

Risk management in the future will look at the causes of risk and provide feedback and input into the system to control such risks by improving the care. The institution, the physician, and the patient will all be at less risk if systems are broadly understood by the people they serve. Some consensus as to what services will be offered and where those services are best provided is needed in this society. A total rethinking is necessary as to the role of the in-hospital setting. The new role of risk management in providing feedback to improving the system, as well as communications with patients and their families, will be critical as we are more and more challenged to judiciously utilize resources.

References

1. Henry G. *Emergency Medicine Risk Management: A Comprehensive Review*, 2nd ed. American College of Emergency Physicians, Dallas, TX, 2001.

2. Deming, WE. *Out of Crisis.* Massachusetts Institute of Technology, Center for Advanced Engineering Study, Cambridge, MA, 1982.

3. Rogers JT. *Risk Management in Emergency Medicine.* American College of Emergency Physicians, Dallas, TX, 1985.

4. Ibid.

5. Henry G. *Headache, Emergency Medicine Concepts in Clinical Practice*, 4th ed. Rosen/Barkan et al., C.V. Mosby-Yearbook Inc., St. Louis, MO, 1998.

6. Butz AM. Outcomes of emergency room treatment of children with asthma. *J Asthma.* 1991;28(4):255.

Metrics and Performance Improvement
Patient Quality, Safety, and Experience

Sharon E. Mace, MD, FACEP, FAAP
Elaine Thallner, MD, MS, FACEP

Introduction

Quality improvement requires a method for measuring and analyzing information about a process, program, and/or system.[1] Tracking metrics can be a valuable tool for assessment of a system or benchmark.[2,3] Metrics are a first step in a comprehensive Performance Improvement (PI)[4] or Continuous Quality Improvement (CQI) program.[5] CQI has been defined as a continual process or methodology for positive change or improvement in a system or program by making system improvements or modifying the practice or procedure of how things are done.

In health care, the desired end result of any PI or CQI process is to make a positive impact on patient care, with the hope of improved patient outcomes, which may include an array of results ranging from a decreased length of stay (LOS) to improved quality of life as well as a decrease in morbidity and mortality.[6-8]

More recently, another factor, cost, has been added to this process. In addition to improving patient care, there now needs to be a component included that looks at the costs involved in providing quality care. So the equation has become value = quality/cost whereby increased quality and/or decreased cost increase value. This corresponds with the Centers for Medicare Services' focus on transitioning from volume-based care to value-based care.

Components of a comprehensive PI or CQI program include quality, patient safety, and patient experience.[9,10] Patient quality focuses on improving patient care and achieving better outcomes by modifying processes and changing and improving the system as well as monitoring individual performance. The goal of patient safety is to foster an environment that enhances the identification of problems instead of ignoring or concealing problems. The objective of a patient experience program is to create the best experience for everyone involved, especially the patient and family, but also for the health care workers, as well as including improved communication, patient-centered care initiatives and empowerment of the patient.

Examples of "tools" in the PI "toolbox" or approach include any number of forms from the Toyota production mode (Demming approach), the aviation flight team model, the plan/act/do/check method, lean initiatives, and six sigma.[11]

The Importance of Observation Medicine

Numerous studies have documented the many advantages of observation medicine in terms of lower cost, decreased missed diagnoses, improved risk management, fewer admissions, improved quality of life, shorter length of stays, greater patient satisfaction,[12] lower readmission rate, less returns to the emergency department (ED), improved efficiency of the ED, better patient care and patient outcomes with fewer complications and adverse events, and decreased morbidity and mortality. Yet little has been published on CQI, and even less on metrics for the observation unit (OU), although CQI for the OU may be an asset in identifying problems, saving money, improving efficiency, defining issues, developing new processes, or making further improvements in the system and processes.[5,13-15]

Components of a CQI Program

Critical components for the OU to function optimally include policies and procedures, protocols, standardized order sets, and clinical pathways. (See Clinical Protocols Chapters 82–87, Administrative Policies Chapter 88, Order Sets Chapters 89–96.) Benchmarking against other OUs is a useful methodology for ascertaining whether the OU is performing at its full potential. Comparison with national or even international benchmarks or standards can help determine how your specific institution/OU is performing and if there is an opportunity for improvement. Internal comparisons over a given timeframe (e.g., daily, monthly, quarterly, or yearly) at your own institution/OU can gauge whether issues are developing or if there is progress toward a given goal.

Observation Unit Database

Information essential for an OU database begins with the patients placed in observation status. Such information is required for many purposes, in addition to metrics and the CQI program. Some of the reasons mandating an OU database are communication among health care providers and transitions of care including patient care for referrals and follow-up; regulatory requirements whether local, state, or federal; meeting the standards for various organizations, such as the Joint Commission on Accreditation of Healthcare Organizations (JCAHO or the "Joint"); for reimbursement from government programs, health maintenance organizations, and other insurers/payers; in addition to training, education and research. Of course, maintaining patient confidentiality and meeting the Health Information and Portability Act (HIPPA) requirements, as with any patient information, is mandatory.

Suggested data elements for individual OU patients are listed in Table 9.1. Various components, such as mandatory patient identifiers such as name and medical record number, are needed for many reasons including follow-up on laboratory tests, procedures, and for referrals. At a minimum, the final diagnosis is essential clinical information. Times are required in order to calculate LOS. LOS for the OU does not include the time spent in the ED. Onset is from when the order to place in observation is written and then nursing acknowledges and documents the observation orders. LOS may be the most important metric for an OU.

The specific procedures and the time required for them is a requirement for the database since the time out of the OU for various diagnostic or therapeutic procedures, such as an endoscopy or stress test, should be subtracted from the OU time (e.g., time discharged from observation – time placed in observation) in order to accurately

Table 9.1 Data Set for Individual Patients in the Observation Unit (OU)*

I. Patient Identifiers
  - Medical record number
  - Name

II. Demographics
  - Age
  - Gender
  - Ethnicity

III. Time
  - Length of stay (LOS) in observation
  - Date placed in observation**
  - Time placed in observation**
  - Date discharged from observation (or admitted to an inpatient floor)
  - Time discharged from observation (or admitted to an inpatient floor)

IV. Disposition: admitted, (if yes, what floor or unit); discharged, expired, other (give detail, e.g., left against medical advice)

V. Clinical
  Chief complaint(s)
  Final diagnoses
  Comorbidities
  Procedures (list all)
  Time for the procedure(s)***
  Laboratory tests
  Radiology tests
  Consults

VI. Health Care Coverage/Insurance

* This is not an all-inclusive list, but one suggested data set that can be tailored to the needs of your individual unit. Insurance information may be in a separate data set from the clinical parameters.
* This does not include such personnel information as address, phone, emergency contact. Billing information such as the insurer(s) may be in a separate data set.
** Needed to determine or calculate length of stay.
*** Facility requirements include subtracting procedure times (time for a procedure and/or away from OU, as for a stress test as an example) from overall OU length of stay.

report the LOS for facility billing purposes. However, in some cases and depending upon the payer, an average for a specific procedure may be given. Although one should be able to determine or reiterate how this average was determined or calculated.

Suggested data elements useful for regular, such as monthly and yearly, statistics, and for designing metrics for the OU and evaluation

Table 9.2 Data Elements for Observation Unit Database*

- Number of patients placed in observation
- OU diagnoses
- OU length of stay
- Disposition from OU
  - Inpatient admissions:
    - Inpatient service: cardiology, general surgery (for example)
    - Inpatient floor: intensive care unit (ICU): medical ICU, surgical ICU, cardiology ICU, respiratory ICU, step-down, ward
  - Discharge: home, nursing home, rehabilitation
  - Transfer
  - Expired
  - Other: LAMA (left against medical advice)
- Chief complaint
- Final diagnoses
- Demographics: age, gender, ethnicity
- Health care coverage/insurance**

* This is not an all-inclusive list, but one suggested data set that can be tailored to the needs of your individual unit.
** May be in a different data set.

of the OU are given in Table 9.2. There are five to six basic or minimal overall variables needed to build a dataset for the OU, which include the number of patients placed in observation, their LOS, disposition: admit or discharge, and final diagnosis: noncardiac chest pain, unstable angina, myocardial infarction (MI), nonspecific abdominal pain, appendicitis, cholecystitis, etc. The chief complaint is also a useful data element.

Additional clinical information such as laboratory tests (e.g. cardiac enzymes), diagnostic studies (e.g. stress tests, CT scans, ultrasounds, MRI), procedures (esophagogastroduodenoscopy [EGD], colonoscopy, etc.), and consults may be valuable input for a clinical database. Provider information regarding the physicians and the advanced practice clinicians may be a useful factor to add to the OU database.

Whether or not there is an electronic medical record or a written log should not be an obstacle to a database for the OU. Even a handwritten registry for the OU can be utilized as a basis for data analysis. (See Appendix 9.1: Clinical Decision Unit or CDU log.)

Specialized or customized databases can be designed to the requirements of the particular OU or institution. If the institution is part of a chest pain registry, for example, then additional variables can be added to encompass the registry, such as type of stress test, results of stress test, number of patients who rule in for MI or those with an positive enzymes or a NSTEMI (non ST elevation MI). Trend analysis of the OU data set may be valuable for operations regarding resource utilization, staffing, use of ancillary tests, and other support services.

Documentation for the Observation Unit

Essential documentation for the OU begins with an appropriate history and physical examination of the patient and the reason(s) for placing the patient in observation status, whether this is done by the physician or the advanced level practitioner. Along with the justification for the observation care, there should be a plan outlining the diagnostic studies to be performed and/or treatment to be given, and a strategy for discharge, which enumerates the conditions for discharge and the conditions for admission. Progress notes are also an important part of the documentation.

Nursing assessments are a critical part of the OU record and generally include an admission nursing assessment and a notation in the records of the patient's discharge (or admission) including the time when discharged or admitted. Key elements of the nursing OU documentation include vital signs, and if appropriate, pain assessments, neurologic checks, and/or vascular checks. Any patient and/or family education/teaching by OU nursing staff or other personnel such as respiratory therapists, nurse educators, or nurse clinical specialists should be noted.

Any and all procedures and treatments should be documented. These include any respiratory treatments, intravenous fluids, medications administered, diagnostic studies or procedures or therapeutic interventions. Diagnostic interventions may range from an arterial blood gas to a lumbar puncture, a stress test or an EGD. Treatment commonly includes intravenous fluids and parenteral medications, especially pain medications, antiemetics and antibiotics, but can also include procedures such as an incision and drainage or wound care.

Table 9.3 Metrics for the Observation Unit (OU)

- *Length of Stay (LOS) Metrics*
  - LOS > 24 hours
  - LOS < 6–8 hours
- *Observation Unit Metrics Similar to Emergency Department Metrics*
  - Volume: number of patients placed in observation unit
  - Disposition
    - Admissions to inpatient services
    - Discharges from observation unit
    - Other: left before treatment completed (LBTC) and left against medical advice (LAMA)
  - Transfers
  - Returns to ED/OU/Hospital within 72 hours
  - Complaints
  - Incident/SERS (Safety Event Reporting System) reports (such as falls)
- *Acuity Metrics*
  - Admit to Intensive Care Unit: cardiac, respiratory, medical, surgical, pediatric
  - To operating room
  - To cardiac catheterization lab
- *Process Indicators*
  - Process (steps) involved in obtaining results for cardiac enzymes
- *Outcome Indicators*
  - Morbidity
  - Mortality
- *Rate-Based Indicators*
  - Admission rate to inpatient unit > 20%
  - Myocardial infarction rule in > 10%
- *Sentinel Event Indicators*
  - Deaths
  - Codes
  - Resuscitations
  - Airway interventions: intubations, unplanned use of mechanical ventilation (Bipap, CPAP)
  - Cardiac: use of thrombolytics, emergent cardioversion, shock, life-threatening dysrhythmias and/or use of ACLS drugs/protocols
  - Occurrence of rapid response team (RRT) or medical emergency team (MET) calls (for an in-house OU)
- *Benchmarks*
  - Overall LOS < 24 hours, average LOS < 15–16 hours (national)
  - Complaints < 2%

Again, if such therapeutic or diagnostic procedures are done, and the patient is away from the OU, perhaps, in the endoscopy suite or in interventional radiology, the total time away from the OU should be noted and then subtracted from the total time in the OU as required for reimbursement depending on the payer. Some payers may allow for an average time for a procedure such as a stress test or endoscopy to be used instead of the exact time for an individual patient.

Metrics for the Observation Unit

Length of Stay Metrics

Long Length of Stay (Greater than 24 Hours)

Many key OU metrics center on LOS. (Table 9.3) Most OUs have as their policy disposition of the patient in a specific time frame, usually 24 hours. Therefore, the number of patients in the OU with an extremely long stay in the OU, for example, greater than 24 hours, is an outlier. These cases are generally reviewed to determine the reason for the inappropriately long OU stay and potential solutions.

For example, when our OU started, we noted that patients with a LOS > 24 hours tended to be waiting for a stress test or a gastroenterology test (such as an EGD or colonoscopy), which often did not occur until late in the day or was even cancelled. We invited the administrators/physicians in charge of stress testing and endoscopy suite, respectively, to our monthly CDU meetings; the collaborative result was leaving a set number of early morning openings slotted for CDU patients, which if unfilled then went to outside referrals or inpatients.

Short Length of Stay (Less than 8 Hours)

A very short LOS, usually a LOS < 6–8 hours is another metric. Patients in the OU for < a given number of hours suggests that they were inappropriately admitted to the OU. If they were placed in the OU and then admitted quickly as inpatients, this suggests they should have been directly admitted from the ED and were too ill for the OU. Conversely, if they were placed in the OU and were discharged very quickly, this indicates that they could have been discharged from the ED and did not need an OU stay. Such extremely short OU stays have a cost: an inordinate amount of valuable nursing time and resources. OU stays, no matter how long the patient's LOS is, require a nursing OU admission assessment that costs a significant amount of nursing time. Moreover, there is an inconvenience, and perhaps, even some discomfort, to the patient and family, if the patient is transferred from one unit to another. Another reason for looking at LOS < 8 hours is reimbursement, with some payers not reimbursing for stays less than 8 hours.

It is important to have an active CQI program with metrics for reviewing data since not all outliers are inappropriate. As an example, a patient seen in the ED with chest pain with negative enzymes and a normal ECG is placed in observation status. At 4 hours, a second set of enzymes is positive, the ECG is unchanged and he is admitted to the hospital with a diagnosis of a NSTEMI. This patient would be an outlier because he ruled in for MI and had a short LOS of < 8 hours, but on review, it may have been appropriate care assuming the patient did not have unstable angina and was not on an IV drip (e.g., nitroglycerin).

Conversely, OU CQI would note the metric regarding the number of prolonged OU stays > 24 hours, compare this metric with previous months, noting whether there is an unexpected increase (or decrease). Cases > 24 hours are then flagged for review. If the increased LOS was due to inability to obtain a specific test, such as a stress test, then this should be reviewed and actions taken to make sure the required resources are available.

At the time the patient is placed in observation status, the patient and family should be informed about observation being a short stay (e.g., < 24 hour) and that discharge is anticipated within 1 day or < 24 hours.

Metrics Similar to Emergency Department Metrics

Several metrics for the OU are patterned after metrics for the ED. Volume data, for example, is analogous to that for the ED. The number of patients placed in OU status (OU volume) is analogous to the number of ED visits or ED volume. Disposition statistics are comparable to that for the ED: number of patients admitted, discharged or transferred from the OU, number of patients in the OU that left against medical advice (LAMA) or left before treatment completed (LBTC).

Complaints, LBTC including LAMA, and transfers are standard categories that are reviewed for the ED and for the OU. Incident or Safety Event Reporting System (SERS) reports, such as falls, should be evaluated, whether it occurred in the ED or the OU.

Complaints

It should be noted that the number of complaints for the OU are believed to be less than for the ED and for other nursing units in the hospital. The fast turnaround of patients with rapid access to diagnostic testing and therapy tends to result in fewer complaints. To our knowledge, there is only one report that dealt specifically with the type of complaints encountered in the OU. This study found that the majority of complaints (43%) involved staffing issues (interpersonal relations, behavior or attitude) with a 10:1 ratio for nursing to physician complaints, perhaps, at least partly related to the fact that patient time spent with nursing far outweighs that with the time spent with physicians. However, the next categories of complaints were similar to those recorded for other areas of the hospital as opposed to those received in EDs: discharge processes 25%, environmental concerns (unclean or uncomfortable rooms) 17.9%, difficulties with diagnostic investigations 10.7%, and miscellaneous issues 3.6%.[14]

Acuity Metrics

By definition, the patients placed in observation are low-risk, low-acuity patients who do not need intensive nursing or physician care (see CDU administrative policy) and are expected to have a high likelihood of being discharged home in less than 24 hours. Patients who are admitted to an intensive care unit (ICU), go to the operating room or to the cardiac catheterization laboratory are higher-acuity patients, which makes these groups an important metric to track as part of OU case review.

Types of Indicators for the Observation Unit

Indicators are a tool used to identify critical components of patient care, and can be employed for CQI activities that evaluate the quality of patient care and support activities. Types of indicators include structure, process, outcome, and sentinel.[16]

Structural Indicators

Structure or structural indicators are utilized to assess items such as equipment, supplies, physical design, staffing levels, and even organizational culture; process indicators focus on procedural issues. Structure indicators would help identify whether specific equipment has a high failure rate or supplies have an unusually short life span or significantly high rate of breakage.

Process Indicators

Process indicators center on procedures or processes, asking such questions as "Did all chest pain patients get aspirin?", or "Were the appropriate stress tests ordered?", or "What is the incidence of 'blood redraws' because of lost or mislabeled etc. specimens?" Then analyzing "What are the interrelated actions that must occur for obtaining a set of cardiac enzymes starting from the time the order was written, the blood drawn and labeled, to the result reported and the physician notified?" and ascertaining what happened when the specimen was lost or mislabeled and taking steps to prevent this from occurring in the future. "Was the clinical pathway or process followed?" If not, what was the rationale? "Was the procedure done correctly and in a timely fashion?"

Outcome Indicators

Outcome indicators measure patients' responses to treatment; these indicators include mortality and measures of morbidity such as incidence of MI, dysrhythmias, and shock.

Rate-Based Indicators

Rate-based indicators use a specified threshold or given level. For example, if the usual admission rate to the inpatient service from the OU is 20% (and conversely, the discharge rate is 80%), whenever the inpatient admission rate goes above say 20% or the discharge rate falls below 80%, then a review of admissions from the OU to the inpatient floors is warranted. In the multicenter chest pain study, the rule in MI rate for OUs was 6.9%.[17] If your OU statistics reveal a high rule in MI rate of say > 10%, then all the OU cases that ruled in for an MI for the given time period (e.g., month, quarter, or year) should be reviewed to determine if there are any CQI issues or trends.

Sentinel-Event Indicators

Sentinel-event indicators are used to screen for serious patient care events and mandate review whenever they occur. Customary CQI sentinel events for the ED and hospital should also be evaluated when they occur in the OU. Such sentinel events include deaths, codes or resuscitations, airway interventions that indicate respiratory failure as signified by intubation or the unplanned use of mechanical ventilation (e.g., Bipap or CPAP), the use of thrombolytics, and the occurrence of life-threatening dysrhythmias requiring the use of ACLS drugs/protocols or emergent cardioversion.

Benchmarks

Benchmarking is the process of measuring patient outcomes and/or patient care delivery or services

Table 9.4 Clinical Decision Unit Meeting (CDU) Agenda

1. Approval of monthly minutes
2. Monthly/Quarterly/Yearly Statistics
3. Metrics
4. Policies:
   - Revision/update of old policies
   - Adoption of new policies

   Procedures:
   - Revision/update of old procedures
   - Adoption of new procedures
5. Order Sets
   - Revision/update of previous order sets
   - Adoption of new order sets
6. Triggers for Review (LOS > 24 hours, < 6–8 hours, ICU admissions, others)
7. Chart reviews
8. Complaints
9. Discussion with invited departments/individuals
10. Old business
11. New business
12. Other

against a set standard or goal, which may be an internal or institutional standard, or external based on comparison with other health care organizations or even a national or international standard. The goal of 10 minutes from the door of the ED to the ECG is an example of an external national benchmark.

Protocols, Clinical Pathways, and Standardized Order Sets

Protocols, pathways, order sets have been shown to reduce costs, standardize care, cut LOS, lessen morbidity and mortality, and most importantly, improve patient outcomes; they are an important part of any CQI program. (See Chapters 82–96)

Observation Unit or Clinical Decision Unit Meetings

The CDU monthly meetings serve as a forum to review data regarding the OU, revise old policies/procedures/order sets, approve drafts of any new policies/procedures/order sets, analyze any metrics or statistics, review charts identified through the CQI process, set new goals or benchmarks, and invite representatives of other departments to discuss any issues of concern or areas for improvement. A CDU meeting agenda is outlined in Table 9.4.

Summary

There must be a well-organized framework and administrative support for the OU to be successful. An active, robust OU PI/CQI program is critical to a well-functioning OU and ongoing learning and improvements.

Appendix 9.1: Observation Unit Patient Log

CDU PATIENT LOG

Patient Name	Medical Record #	Diagnosis	Age	Gender	Date/Time of CDU Arrival	Date/Time of CDU Discharge	LOS	Discharge or Admit (Floor, ICU, OR or Cath Lab)

ICU = Intensive Care Unit
OR = Operating Room
Cath Lab = Catheterization Lab
LOS = Length of Stay

References

1. Batalden PB, Nelson EC, Gardent PB, et al. Leading macrosystems and mesosystems for microsystem peak performance. In: Nelson EC, Batalden PB, Godfrey MM (eds). *Quality by Design*. San Francisco, CA, Josey-Bass, 2007; ch. 4, pp. 69–105.

2. Francis RCE, Spies CD, Kerner T. Quality management and benchmarking in emergency medicine. *Curr Opin Anesthesiol*, 2008; 21: 233–239.

3. Specific Aims. In: Nelson EC, Batalden PB, Godfrey MM (eds). *Quality by Design*. San Francisco, CA, Josey-Bass, 2007; ch. 18, pp. 308–312.

4. Blumenthal D. Performance improvement in health care – seizing the moment. *N Engl J Med*, 2012; 366(21): 1953–1955.

5. Mace SE. Patient quality (continuous quality improvement), safety and experience for the observation unit. In: *Observation Medicine*. American College of Emergency Physicians, www.acep (Accessed March 20162012).

6. Glickman SW, Schulman KA, Peterson ED, et al. Evidence-based perspectives on pay for performance and quality of patient care and outcomes in emergency medicine. *Ann Emerg Med*, 2008; 51: 622–631.

7. Baker WE. Evaluation of clinical performance in emergency medicine. *Emerg Med Clin N Am*, 2009; 27: 615–626.

8. Langberg ML, Black JT. Dead souls comparing Dartmouth atlas benchmarks with CMS outcomes. *N Engl J Med*, 2009; 361(122):e109.

9. Wachter RM. The nature and frequency of medical errors and adverse events. In: Wachter RM. *Understanding Patient Safety*. New York: McGraw Hill, 2008; ch. 1, pp. 3–16.

10. Hudson S. Patient experience: How to get the journey right from start to finish. *Health Service Journal*, March 29, 2012; 122 (6300): 28–29.

11. Glasgow JM, Scott-Caziewell J, Jill R, et al. Guiding inpatient quality improvement: a systematic review of lean and six sigma. *Jt. Comm J Qual Patient Safety*, Dec 2010; 36(12): 531–532.

12. Graff L. Observation units for elimination of missed myocardial infarction errors. *Maryland Medicine*, 2001; suppl; 40–42.

13. Mace SE. Continuous quality improvement for the clinical decision unit. *Healthcare Quality*, 2004; 26(1): 29–36.

14. Mace SE. An analysis of patient complaints in an observation unit. *J Qual Clin Practice*, 1998; 18(2): 151–158.

15. Mace SE. Resuscitations in an observation unit. *J Qual Clin Practice*, 1999; 19: 155–164.

16. Donabedian A. The quality of care: How can it be measured. *JAMA*, 1988; 121(11): 1145–1150.

17. Graff LG, Dallara J, Ross MA, et al. Impact on the care of the emergency department chest pain patient evaluation registry (CHEPER) study. *Amer J Card* 1997; 80(5): 563–568.

Part II

Observation Medicine: Clinical Setting and Education

Chapter

10

The Community Hospital Perspective in a Suburban/Rural Setting

Ryan Prudoff, DO, MS, FACEP
Stephen Sayles, MD, FACEP

Observation medicine or Clinical Decision Units (CDUs) can be a valuable asset in the small-to-medium rural community setting. It is important to have a good working relationship with your hospital administration to allow for a mutually beneficial arrangement. There are a myriad of factors that contribute to a highly functioning CDU, which can improve the overall flow of the Emergency Department (ED). The CDU, however, should be regarded as a separate "service line" and should be viewed as such with careful consideration given to:

1. How the service will improve patient care and decrease physician liability
2. How ED through-put will be affected
3. Ancillary service involvement
4. Additional work required
5. ED group financials vs. hospital financial repercussions

Our community hospital functions with a four-bed CDU with a yearly ED volume of 26,700 patients. Of all hospital admissions, 5.5% were placed in observation – with the ED managing 58% of those observation patients in an ED CDU and 42% placed in observation status throughout the hospital.

Prior to implementation of the ED observation unit (OU), the average length of stay (LOS) for all hospital observation patients was 27 hours. The LOS for patients managed through the ED OU averaged 15 hours and the LOS for observation patients in the hospital (e.g., non-ED OU observation patients) remained at 27 hours. Over 12 months of operation, 848 patients were evaluated in the CDU, saving the hospital the equivalent of 424 patient days. The implementation of the CDU resulted in improvement in the back-end ED processing of patients and ED patient flow or turnaround time, as well as adding value to the hospital by increasing bed availability for higher-acuity patients.

Tantamount to our successful operation was the idea that the bed was the most valuable commodity in the flow equation. We employed 24-hour CDU management, meaning discharges occur more promptly in an attempt to improve turnaround time. Although consideration was given to the time of day discharges occurred, patients were given the option to be discharged late in the evening if their workup was complete. Also, our CDU was designated a closed unit which eliminated the dependence and delays that occur from waiting on "non-ED physicians" to evaluate or discharge patients.

We initially reviewed the information from ACEP's observation medicine section for a menu of common observation conditions (www.acep.org/Clinical–Practice-Management/Observation-Medicine) and selected those conditions that would be optimally treated with the resources available at our facility. As the comfort level of both physicians and observation nursing staff increased, we began to expand the services provided in the CDU. We selected chest pain, asthma, and COPD initially because the patients could be continually monitored and treated as if they would be on the hospital floor. We believe the proximity of the CDU to the ED adds an advantage to patients by providing access to emergency physicians for rapid response if a patient's condition deteriorates or they do not respond as desired to medical management.

Initiation of clinical care pathways was instituted for those conditions placed in the OU, which allows for consistent high-quality care and limited treatment variability. We used established care plans as the framework for those conditions selected for evaluation in the OU. Through close collaboration with the available subspecialists, we created site-specific protocols leveraging the facility's available resources. We also established inclusion and exclusion criteria for each care plan.

Conversely, we excluded patient conditions requiring a high amount of social resources, which can monopolize CDU staff and detract from the management of observation patients. For example, a patient under the influence of chemical substances or having psychiatric issues can have high demands on the CDU staff. Additionally we found that patients who could not ambulate or perform activities of daily living or with severe dementia were failures for treatment in the CDU. These failures were due to other ancillary services needed to be involved in their medical care and the additional time needed to coordinate follow-up. This is consistent with the findings of a recent study regarding the types of CDU patients that will need inpatient admission from the CDU. In this study, frailty and sociodemographic factors were the greatest predictors of inpatient admission from the CDU.[1] As a general rule, patients placed in the OU should have only a few discrete issues that can be addressed simply, and should be able to walk in and out of the CDU.

The number of observation services that EDs can potentially provide is growing and determining which services are right for your facility may be dependent on what ancillary services or diagnostic services are available. Overall, observation medicine has been a success at our facility and our CDU continues to expand services – most recently in the form of Pediatric Observation.

Pediatric Observation in the Community Setting

Observation of pediatric patients improves compliance with therapy, decreases patient bounce backs and allows for the closer monitoring of patients. Since management of both adult and pediatric patients ("hybrid unit"; see hybrid units in Chapter 1) occurred in the four-bed CDU, we found the variable experience of nursing staff and the requirements of young children/toddlers increased staff anxiety. We addressed staffing concerns by treating only school-aged children, that is, children 5 years and above. In addition, we required at least one parent to remain in the OU with the child at all times. This allows for the patient's family to be updated on any changes in condition, decreases delays in locating the guardian in the event that the patient is decompensated and requires transfer, and allows patients to be discharged in real time. (See Pediatric Observation Chapters 53 and 54, and The Evidence Basis for Age-Related Observation care Chapter 81.)

With the assistance of our local pediatricians, we limited our services to high-yield complaints such as asthma, dehydration, non-differentiated abdominal pain, cellulitis, and urinary tract infections. Aggressive treatment and frequent reevaluation allowed for faster disposition and turnaround. This is important in the rural community setting where the pediatrician is often not available 24 hours a day.

We have had success with the selected patient populations and complaints chosen for observation treatment. We have decreased the patients' overall LOS, improved hospital resource utilization, and increased hospital bed availability.

References

1. Zdradzinski MJ, Phelan MP, Mace SE. Impact of frailty and sociodemographic factors on hospital admission from an emergency department observation unit. *AJMQ* (accepted for publication 2016)

Chapter

11

The Urban Community Hospital

Robert S. Bennett, MD

A community hospital is an ideal setting for an observation unit (OU). Although many OUs have been developed at large academic institutions to deal with issues of crowding in emergency departments (EDs) and inpatient units, there are other compelling reasons to support their presence in additional settings. In surveys conducted between 2007 and 2008, approximately a third of all EDs in the United States were found to have dedicated OUs. About 56% of these are administered through the ED.[1,2] There is clearly an opportunity for expansion to the remaining facilities that do not yet have dedicated OUs.

A community hospital ED may not have the volume to fill a large OU. However, a small unit (for example, ten beds or fewer) can provide flexibility to manage short-stay hospital patients or extended-stay ED patients. The pressure on EDs to complete full evaluations, including procedures and radiology studies with limited availability (such as MRI), has resulted in longer stays. These patients can be referred to an OU to decompress the ED, with the OU functioning as a clinical decision unit (CDU). There is growing evidence that many "short-stay" patients managed on an inpatient unit are similar to OU patients.[1] A community OU may be able to provide more cost-effective and high-quality care to these patients as well.

The key to the successful operation of a community hospital OU is the cultivation of strong relationships with diverse services. The ED providers facilitate the referral of appropriate patients. Frequent interactions and feedback regarding patient outcomes is essential. In an environment that has become increasingly regulated, availability of and collegiality with utilization managers will assist with patient selection. Geriatric services, which are becoming the focus of many EDs and OUs, should follow suit. It is time-consuming to evaluate, treat, and discharge an elderly patient presenting to the ED since many of their problems are multidimensional. OUs can provide a less hectic setting where more time can be taken to evaluate the often complex set of circumstances that led to an elderly patient's arrival to the hospital. Solid support from physical therapy and social work consultants is vital in determining appropriate and safe disposition for geriatric patients. (See also Chapter 55 Geriatric Observation Medicine and Chapter 81 Age-Related Observation Care)

Most observation services include a large census of patients with cardiac problems such as chest pain, syncope or arrhythmias. Therefore, it is worthwhile to nurture a collaborative relationship with the hospital cardiology department. Many patients with low-risk chest pain require a noninvasive study. If the plan is to perform the study as part of the OU stay, then scheduling studies should be prioritized and patients should be prepared with standardized order sets (NPO, beta blockers held, and appropriate attire available). (see Chapter 89 Adult Order Sets) Availability of testing or consultation with a cardiologist early in the day can optimize operational efficiency.

The presence of an OU in a community hospital can be a great asset. Institutions value the additional revenues that can be produced with high patient satisfaction and reduced lengths of stay.[3] Patients are clearly satisfied with cost-effective and efficient care. Forging and maintaining strong relationships with the many partner services that support the OU is pivotal to the success of any OU.

References

1. Wiler JL, Ross MA, Ginde AA. National Study of Emergency Department Observation Services. *Academic Emergency Medicine* 2011; 18:959–965.

2. Venkatesh AK, Geisler BP, Gibson Chambers JJ, et al. Use of observation care in US emergency departments, 2001 to 2008. *PLoS ONE* 2011; 6(9):e24326. Doi: 10.1371/journal.pone.0024326.

3. Baugh CW, Venkatesh AK, Bohan JS. Emergency department observation units: a clinical and financial benefit for hospitals. *Health Care Manage Rev* 2011;36(1): 28–37.

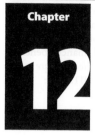

Chapter

12

The Tertiary Care Hospital and Academic Setting

Jonathan Glauser, MD, FACEP

Observation medicine started in the community setting as a way of working up certain discrete problems that were quite common in the community setting and could be resolved within 24 hours: chest pain, asthma, COPD exacerbations, and, slightly later, heart failure. These presentations were common in all emergency departments (EDs), and lent themselves to standardized workups with treatment protocols. Moreover, since patients often did not have to physically leave the location of the ED, these workups could be pursued expeditiously and more economically than on an in-patient floor, and without delays and interruptions while awaiting bed assignments, transfer of care to another service, or transport upstairs.

Tertiary care hospitals work differently from community hospitals in certain fundamental ways. Patients with solid organ transplants, for example, are seen nearly exclusively at transplant centers, so that community hospitals seldom manage transplant complications or even the routine emergency care of such patients when it is not related to the transplant itself. Similarly, tertiary referral centers treat patients with certain chronic illnesses that may not present in the community setting at all because the underlying disease is rare, or because community primary care physicians seldom are the major provider of these patients' care. Medical disorders such as primary pulmonary hypertension, inflammatory bowel disease, thrombocytopenic purpuras, leukemias, myelofibrosis, gastroparesis, postural hypotension (POTS), refractory headaches (which historically do not clear with standardized therapy for migraine), and other entities force patients to come to tertiary centers exclusively, including for their emergency care.

It should be noted that a variety of urologic, neurosurgical, colorectal and ENT procedures are performed solely within a relative handful of centers. Some patients therefore will be referred from outside emergency departments to tertiary care EDs. Many of these patients, while having possibly rare illnesses, may not require a prolonged hospitalization, but simply an evaluation by a consultant who is not available at all in a community hospital. These patients may be observed overnight pending an evaluation by a consultant with unique expertise not found elsewhere in the city or even the state, and not necessarily present overnight at the tertiary center.

Patients with common problems typically managed in the community setting may require referral for care in a tertiary hospital, even if that care can still be accomplished within 24 hours. It is one thing to manage congestive heart failure overnight with diuresis, education in diet, and evaluation for acute coronary syndrome. It may be a completely different matter in the patient with an ejection fraction of 15%, who is already on a transplant list, and with a course of therapy maxed out on a regimen including diuretics, aldosterone, beta blockers, and ACE inhibitors.

Tertiary care hospitals almost by definition are in an urban setting, or at the very least require a large catchment area to exist. A recent report noted that hospitals with ED-managed observation units are more likely to be located in an urban area and to have reported boarding in the ED.[1] It is therefore reasonable to expect that tertiary care hospitals in particular will derive the aforementioned benefits of OUs to urban hospitals in terms of patient flow and in ameliorating bed shortages upstairs. These are also medical centers that tend to be larger, have more specific admitting services, and therefore more complex bed arrangements for specific categories of problems, with ensuing difficulties arranging the proper floor and service for patients going upstairs. The Crohn's patient with a simple flare will not go to the same floor or service as the one with a collection on abdominal CT. The patient with Goodpasture's disease and hemoptysis may not go to the same pulmonary service as the lung transplant patient.

From a financial perspective, there is the threat of audits of patients who "should have" been admitted on observation stay by agencies charged with recouping dollars, especially by the nation's largest health insurer, the Centers for Medicare and Medicaid Services (CMS).[2] The incentives for tertiary care centers to have or establish OUs are self-evident, especially to any emergency physician who has ever composed a letter justifying why a hospital admission was necessary as opposed to a less expensive observation stay. It should be self-evident that a recovery audit contractor (RAC) who gets paid to extract money from hospitals will not be impressed that a patient who drove 300 miles to the ED had to be fully admitted to the hospital so that he or she could be seen by a specific consultant hematologist or urologist the next day. Given the interactions that emergency physicians have with nearly every service in a complex institution, as well as the time sensitivity inherent to the practice, emergency medicine may be uniquely situated to perform observation medicine in the setting of the tertiary care ED.[3]

The optimal size of a tertiary care hospital's OU has yet to be defined. Some may make the case that the future hospital will be comprised of intensive care beds and operating rooms, with the remainder being divided among short-stay and observation beds – in which case the future observation unit may need to be very large indeed. There is ongoing pressure to accomplish imaging more expeditiously as well. For example, keeping an elderly patient with a negative X-ray who has acute hip pain after a fall for an MRI is more unacceptable than it was 10–15 years ago. Interventional radiology may be expected to perform more interventions or tube placements immediately on patients staying in an OU when in the past it would have been unthinkable to not formally admit them to the hospital. Since tertiary care centers in general have more ready access to technology and interventional services, it is reasonable to assume that the need for diagnostic studies will enhance the value of the OU even more in the tertiary referral medical center.

It will always be unacceptable for the emergency physician to not make accurate assessments and diagnoses in any hospital setting. The enhanced knowledge content, the availability of technology at tertiary centers, and the immutable fact that certain illnesses can only declare themselves after a period of time all ensure that observation medicine will become ever more critical to the function and financial survival of these referral centers.

References

1. Wiler JL, Ross MA, Ginde AA. National study of emergency department observation services. *Acad Emerg Med* 2011; 18(9): 959–965.

2. Terra SM. Regulatory issues: recovery audit contractors and their impact on case management. *Prof Case Manag* 2009; 14: 217–23.

3. Baugh CW, Venkatesh AK, Bohan JS. Emergency department observation units: a clinical and financial benefit for hospitals. *Health Care Manage Rev* 2011; 36(1): 28–37.

Chapter

13

Observation Medicine and the Hospitalist

David G. Paje, MD, FACP, SFHM
Peter Y. Watson, MD, FACP, SFHM

The concept of observation medicine (OM) evolved from the same need for a more efficient delivery of hospital-based services that gave rise to the hospitalist movement. Whereas observation was initially defined through specific government directives, the early years of hospital medicine were shaped in part by managed care forces.[1,2] Nonetheless, both were conceived to reduce cost while improving the quality of care in the hospital setting.

Since observation can be provided anywhere on hospital premises, whether in a designated unit or in a general unit, it is essential for the hospitalist to understand this new paradigm and to recognize certain clinical and operational aspects that distinguish observation from the usual inpatient care. This distinction starts with selecting the right patients, and the key to this is properly matching patients' medical needs with the appropriate resources and level of care. Those placed in observation are generally lower risk in terms of severity of illness or likelihood for short-term adverse outcomes. However, many of them present with diagnostic uncertainties for potentially life threatening conditions, such as myocardial infarction, serious arrhythmia or cerebral ischemia. The hospitalist must apply evidence-based clinical algorithms and risk-stratification tools to safely and efficiently identify patients who are ideal candidates for observation.

When observation patients are placed in regular inpatient beds alongside admitted patients who have more complex needs, the opportunity to drive throughput may be lost in the overall unit workflow. Formulating clinical pathways that are goal-directed and clearly defining parameters for disposition allow nurse-driven care and lead to shorter lengths of stay. In addition, identifying a dedicated hospitalist to round primarily on observation patients should minimize the effect of competing priorities from admitted patients who are generally sicker. Alternatively, placing

all observation patients in a designated geographic area or unit would be ideal, and this has been shown to have the potential to improve efficiency and clinical outcomes.[3–5]

Hospitalists must also be aware that the usual routine in hospital operations, particularly with regards to laboratory, imaging, testing and consultative services, may inadvertently delay the care of observation patients. This is because staffing and scheduling for these services are based on the typical ebb and flow in demand that is mainly influenced by inpatient ordering practices and by traditional physician rounding times. Hospitalists need to collaborate with hospital leadership and other key stakeholders to design a reasonable expedited process specifically for observation patients.[6] Also, hospitalists should adopt a scheduling model that ensures around-the-clock on-site coverage, especially since observation patients can be admitted or discharged at any time of the day, and since some clinical conditions may need frequent and timely physician reassessments. Furthermore, these patients are best managed with a mind-set that evaluates their progress in terms of the hours rather than the days they have been in the hospital.

For institutions that have observation units (OUs) that are run by hospitalists, there may be a temptation to accommodate patients with higher acuity including admitted patients who are waiting for inpatient beds. This is particularly true when hospital occupancy is high and when the emergency department (ED) is busy. Nevertheless, routinely allowing this practice defeats the purpose of a designated OU, that is, to drive throughput by grouping together patients who have more predictable and shorter lengths of stay.[7] Keeping the integrity of this cohort is crucial to the success of the unit, which translates to increased bed availability and improved ED throughput.[8,9]

In conclusion, providing observation services is consistent with the hospitalist's mission of optimizing resource utilization while at the same time advancing the quality of care in the hospital setting. However, the challenges and demands of observation that differentiate it from the usual inpatient care require the hospitalist to adopt operational adjustments that are directed at improving throughput and efficiency.

References

1. Wachter RM, Goldman L. The emerging role of "hospitalists" in the American health care system. *N Engl J Med*, 1996. 335(7): 514–7.

2. *Medicare Benefit Policy Manual*, in Chapter 6 – Hospital Services Covered Under Part B. Centers for Medicare and Medicaid Services, 2011.

3. Abenhaim HA, Kahn SR, Raffoul J, et al. Program description: a hospitalist-run, medical short-stay unit in a teaching hospital. *CMAJ*, 2000. 163(11): 1477–80.

4. Daly, S, Campbell DA, Cameron PA. Short-stay units and observation medicine: a systematic review. *Med J Aust*, 2003. 178(11): 559–63.

5. Barsuk JH, Casey DE Jr, Graff LG IV, et al. *The Observation Unit: An Operational Overview for the Hospitalist*. Society of Hospital Medicine, 2007. www.hospitalmedicine.org/Content/NavigationMenu/Publications/WhitePapers/White_Papers.htm. Accessed February 12, 2016.

6. Lucas BP, Kunapley R, Mba B, et al. A hospitalist-run short-stay unit: features that predict length-of-stay and eventual admission to traditional inpatient services. *J Hosp Med*, 2009. 4(5): 276–84.

7. Cooke MW, Higgins J, Kidd P. Use of emergency observation and assessment wards: a systematic literature review. *Emerg Med J*, 2003. 20(2): 138–42.

8. Krantz MJ, Zwang O, Rowan SB, et al. A cooperative care model: cardiologists and hospitalists reduce length of stay in a chest pain observation unit. *Crit Pathw Cardiol*, 2005. 4(2): 55–8.

9. Leykum LK, Huerta V, Mortense E. Implementation of a hospitalist-run observation unit and impact on length of stay (LOS): a brief report. *J Hosp Med*, 2010. 5(9): E2–5.

Chapter

14

Training and Education – Residents

Pawan Suri, MD

Many academic and community Emergency Departments (EDs) now have observation units (OUs).[1] Emergency Medicine (EM) residents are often exposed to these units during their training and may be expected to manage patients in an OU. Graff et al., in their paper on Observation Medicine (OM) curriculum, state that managing patients in an OU is governed by extended care principles in contrast to the episodic care principles applied in the ED.[2] Thus, emergency physicians need to gain additional knowledge to provide observation services. OM can be seen as a bridge between emergency care and acute inpatient care. Following patients in an OU beyond the acute presentation in the ED may allow residents to gain a deeper appreciation of the natural history of disease and enable them to make better disposition decisions. A structured OU rotation for EM residents enhances the educational experience in all areas of Accreditation Council on Graduate Medical Education (ACGME) core competencies.[3] Other groups that may benefit from an OU rotation include medical students, midlevel providers, internal medicine and pediatric residents, and pharmacy residents.

Graff et al. divided the OU rotation curriculum into four topics: history of OM, types of services, characteristics of services, and management of the ED OU. A model curriculum should balance clinical experience with didactic teaching. A fully developed rotation would ideally introduce the first-year resident to principles of OM with incremental responsibilities under attending supervision such that by the final year of residency, the resident feels comfortable managing multiple patients in the OU. The didactic part of the rotation should include core curriculum lectures, a reading list pertaining to commonly encountered observation diagnoses and review of recent literature. Starting at the post-graduate year (PGY)-1 year, residents can be introduced

to the basic principles of OM, existing protocols and understanding the global as well as disease-specific exclusion and inclusion criteria for patient selection. (See Chapter 82 on Clinical Protocols.) As residents progresses to the PGY-2 level and beyond, they are encouraged to clinically manage multiple patients, learn the administrative aspect of OM, help develop new protocols, participate in quality assurance, (see Chapter 9) and learn the nuances of observation billing and coding (see Chapters 62 and 63). Prerequisites for setting up a successful OU rotation start with dedicated OU leadership with a commitment to teach. There has to be institutional and departmental support that allows for faculty time to develop teaching resources.

In 2008, the authors instituted a required rotation in OM for second-year EM residents at the Virginia Commonwealth University's ten-bed OU. The residents have an 8-hour workday that starts at 7 a.m. with signout from the overnight midlevel provider. The structure of the rotation mimics the ED multitasking approach. Residents participate in work rounds with contemporaneous admissions and discharges. The approach is disposition driven and yet allows for bedside teaching. The residents participate in field trips to various testing areas like nuclear medicine, ECHO lab, stress testing, electrophysiology, and endoscopy to get a behind-the-scene look and get a chance to meet with consultants face to face. Unlike in the busy ED environment, residents in the OU get the opportunity to address patients' social needs and communicate with primary care physicians to ensure a safe discharge and minimize recidivism. In addition, we encourage residents to hone their skills in ancillary testing such as bedside ultrasound to help management decisions. Residents are given reading assignments and get a daily quiz. The response to our OU rotations has been overwhelmingly positive.[3]

Our situation is somewhat unique in that we have two dedicated EM and Internal Medicine dual-boarded physicians staffing the OU. In other academic departments where it may not be possible to devote a full rotation to Observation Medicine, it may be possible to combine OU experience with an existing EM rotation, Ultrasound, Toxicology, or Procedure elective.

References

1. Wiler JL, Glinde, AA. National study of emergency department observation services. *Annals of Emergency Medicine*, September 2010;56 (3) Suppl.: S142.

2. Graft LG, Dunbar L, Gibler WB, et al. Observation medicine curriculum. *Annals of Emergency Medicine*, August 1992;21:963–966.

3. Coleman K, Aurora T, Kurz MC, et al. Evaluating the educational impact of an observation unit rotation for emergency medicine residents on ACGME core competencies. *Academic Emergency Medicine*, May 2010;17(5), Suppl.

Chapter

15

Training and Education – Medical Students/Fellows

Margarita E. Pena, MD, FACEP

Incorporating observation medicine (OM) into medical education is important. The incentives to decrease a patient's hospital length of stay and provide more outpatient services have changed the arena in which a medical student learns clinical medicine. As the number of patients placed in a dedicated observation area increases, so does the likelihood that a student physician will care for patients in this setting. This trend is expected to continue as the value and necessity of placing patients in an observation unit (OU) versus an inpatient unit increases.[1-3] Fortunately, studies suggest clinical teaching is not jeopardized in short-stay areas.[4,5]

OM education should ideally be introduced during student physicians' clinical rotations. In this way they gain a general understanding about the types of patients and conditions that they will see in an observation setting and start to learn about the factors that differentiate observation versus inpatient care.[6]

Medical students are likely to be exposed to OM during those clinical rotations where patients have the option of being placed in an OU setting such as pediatrics, internal medicine, surgery, and especially emergency medicine (EM). This is for several reasons. Currently, over half of U.S. hospitals with an OU are administratively managed by ED staff.[1] In a survey of EM residency programs, almost two-thirds of all hospitals had or were planning to open an OU.[7] Therefore, in those hospitals with EDOUs staffed by emergency physicians, medical students learn from physicians knowledgeable in OM. For example, at this author's institution, our 30-bed Clinical Decision Unit (CDU) is a closed unit that is managed and staffed by attending emergency physicians who rotate their shifts between the ED and CDU.

Observation orders for patients are entered electronically in the ED by attending and resident physicians. Our EM residents rotate in the CDU starting their second year and have a more dedicated month during their third year. Lectures on OM topics are given on a regular basis as part of the EM resident didactic lecture series, which medical students are encouraged to attend. Therefore, medical students rotating in our ED learn about the science and clinical aspects of OM firsthand by working with EM attendings and residents experienced in caring for patients in a dedicated OU setting. There is also an opportunity for fourth year medical students to do a 1-month OM elective where they receive additional didactic teaching and work directly with the attending CDU physician.

Interestingly, for medical students planning to interview for an EM residency position, the Emergency Medicine Residents Association website encourages familiarity with the practice of observation.[8]

Fellowships in OM provide an opportunity after residency training to gain expertise and prepare for a directorship. Current programs offer board certified or prepared emergency physicians 1- to 2-year EM OM Fellowships that focus on clinical, administrative, and research training and the possibility to earn a degree in business administration or public health during the fellowship.

Although there is currently no consensus curriculum for OM fellowship training, the American College of Emergency Physicians (ACEP) section of Observation Medicine and the Society of Academic Emergency Medicine (SAEM) interest group are actively working to address this need.[9]

References

1. Wiler JL, Ross MA, Ginde AA. National study of emergency department observation services. *Acad Emerg Med* 2011; 18(9):959–965.

2. Baugh CW, Venkatesh AK, Bohan JS. Emergency department observation units: A clinical and financial benefit for hospitals. *Health Care Manage Rev* 2011; 36(1): 28–37.

3. Roberts R, Graff L. Economic issues in observation unit medicine. *Emerg Med Clin N Amer* 2001; 19(1): 19–33.

4. O'Riordan DC, Ingram Clark CL. Potential availability of patients in a short stay ward for medical student teaching. *Ann R Coll Surg Eng* (suppl) 1997; 79:15–16.

5. Marks MK, Baskin MN, Lovejoy FH Jr, et al. Intern learning and education in a short stay unit. A qualitative study. *Arch Pediatr Adolesc Med* 1997; 151(2):193–198.

6. Graff LG (ed). *Observation Medicine: The Healthcare's System Tincture of Time.* www.iep.org/Our%20 Physicians/Journal%20Club/ Observation%20Medicine% 2002.03.11/Observation% 20Medicine.pdf (Accessed February 12, 2016)

7. Mace SE, Shah J. Observation medicine in emergency medicine residency programs. *Acad Emerg Med* 2002; 9 (2):169–171.

8. EMRA website: Emergency Medicine issues to know for your interview. www.emra.org/ content.aspx?id=854 (Accessed February 12, 2016)

9. SAEM website: Observational Medicine interest group objectives. www.saem.org/ observational-medicine-0 (Accessed February 12, 2016)

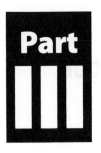

Part III

New Developments in Observation Medicine

Chapter

16

Extended and Complex Observation

L. Christine Gilmore, MD
Bret A. Nicks, MD, MHA, FACEP

Key Points:

- Limited literature on approach to extended or complex observation
- Consider combining/modifying existing protocols for increased complexity
- Patients improving but requiring additional time may benefit from extended observation
- Robust quality improvement (QI) program essential to achieve high-quality and efficient patient care

Background

Observation medicine (OM) originated over three decades ago to meet many pressing health care issues. While improved diagnostic evaluation, short-term therapy of many emergent conditions, and enhanced quality and cost containment remain at the forefront today, the expanding role of OM continues – and has become an integral component of Emergency Medicine (EM). In many parts of the world, Emergency Departments (EDs) strain to accommodate increasing patient volumes with more complex illness with the concurrent decrease in overall inpatient bed capacity.[1] At the same time, operational and quality care metrics continue to increase, reflecting the importance of healthcare delivery and transitions of care through the entire care process. With ongoing scrutiny and potential penalties for short-stay hospital admissions versus observation, hospitals are incentivized to maximize efficiency and avoid unnecessary inpatient admissions.[2] In this shifting milieu of patient care, the growth of observation services has been notable.[3] Protocols abound for successful management of increasingly diverse conditions in the single-disease-focused observation patient. However, the process of caring for complex or extended observation patients is less well defined. Resource utilization issues, however, are unlikely to abate, and observation unit

(OU) providers may be asked to extend the care opportunities for patients who do not fit the well-established protocols.

Streamlined, evidence-based protocols encourage efficiency in the Emergency Department Observation Unit (ED OU); careful patient selection is mandatory. The approach is characterized by focused care for a patient requiring 6 to 24 hours of low-intensity treatment or diagnostic interventions before definitive disposition.[4] The operational and economic value of observation has been demonstrated in these patients with a single problem, such as low-risk chest pain, asthma or pediatric croup.[5–8]

Virtually no literature describes an ED OU approach when the clinical picture cannot be similarly reduced. Realdi et al. described a "Rapid Intense Observation" unit (RIO) for management of complex patients.[9] The authors used broad admission criteria; all acutely ill patients were eligible with exceptions of marked clinical instability, immediate subspecialty needs, residential or social care issues or severe behavioral disturbances. In many ways, the Italian RIO approach is similar to American ED OUs, with clear clinical pathways and protocols employed to expedite care and optimize efficiency. Initial emphasis is on ruling out emergency conditions with subsequent diagnosis or treatment of acute maladies. Similar to ED OUs, undifferentiated chest pain, syncope, and arrhythmias were the most common admitting complaints in the RIO. (See Chapter 21 on Acute Medicine.) Key differences, however, underscore the limitations of caring for increasing complexity in an ED setting. The RIO unit was primarily managed by Internal Medicine physicians, rounding multiple times daily, and utilized operational and staffing resources commensurate with inpatient care. Additionally, the 24-to-72-hour time frame and 35% admission rate described under the RIO model exceed the popular ED OU parameter of a 20% admission rate from the ED

OU to hospital inpatient. It is not surprising that, to date, no literature describes management of a similarly broad, undifferentiated population in an ED OU.

Using existing evidence-based protocols in combination or briefly extending the period of observation does allow for consideration of more complex patients with a foundation in the current literature. While this may allow for expanding inclusion criteria, maintaining careful patient selection amenable to evidence-based, protocol-driven care logically preserves the operational efficiency of the ED OU. Further study is needed to determine the role and value of observation in complex patients. In addition to patient outcomes and operational benefits, changes in staffing, reimbursement and facility resources – including actual bed numbers – will require reevaluation as the scope of OM expands.

Pathophysiology

Pertinent pathophysiology will vary according to complaint.

Inclusion criteria

Patients with simple issues that could be successfully managed by combining existing observational protocols may be appropriate for extended or complex observation. Those with an acute medical condition in the setting of well-managed comorbidities may also be appropriate for some units if otherwise stable. Extended observation may be considered in patients who are improving but require a small amount of additional time beyond 24 hours to meet discharge criteria. These patients should have a predictable clinical course. For example, a dehydrated patient with recently resolved nausea, vomiting and diarrhea could be stable for discharge if allowed additional time for correction of electrolyte abnormalities. Social workers or psychiatric case workers may allow for ED OU management of patients with complicating psychosocial issues to be addressed before discharge.

Exclusion Criteria

Those with high acuity, complications, or high risk of severe illness are likely to need staffing and services beyond the capacity of an ED OU and should be admitted to an inpatient hospital service. A robust resource utilization/quality assurance (QA)/quality improvement (QI) program is necessary to ensure that complex patients are being appropriately differentiated from patient's with complications prior to ED OU admission. Patients who will obviously require beyond 1–2 days stabilizing medical concerns should be admitted.

Management/Intervention

Management will be similar to traditional patients with emphasis on communication, reassessment and quality assurance. Communication is especially important with extended observation patients, who may be cared for by an increased number of providers. A formal transfer of care system should be in place to ensure accurate relay of medical information through the transitions of care. Extending observation a few hours may be useful if it obviates admission, and if quality, efficiently focused care is provided regardless if the patient ultimately requires hospitalization. Although extended observation requires flexibility in length of stay (LOS) benchmarks and a clearly defined documentation process, admission criteria should still exclude patients not expected to improve in the unit. Close attention to maximum LOS and a means for addressing outliers should be incorporated into the ED OU's operating policy.[10]

A unit's need and ability to manage more complex patients will depend on the staffing model, ancillary resources, and operational demands of the institution. Patients with underlying comorbidities may be managed in the ED OU. When used in combination, protocols may require modification for the scope of care being provided, interventions needed, and medications required. Protocols may be used in combination to manage a patient with a chief complaint and ancillary issues arising from treatment. For instance, a hyperglycemia protocol may be used to treat elevated blood sugar secondary to steroids administered to a patient for a chronic obstructive pulmonary disease (COPD) exacerbation. Deconstructing aspects of the presenting complaint may also allow for management of greater complexity. Consider cellulitis with hyperglycemia. A provider might combine cellulitis and hyperglycemia protocols to address an elevated blood sugar in a patient with otherwise uncomplicated cellulitis. A retrospective analysis by Shrock suggests that cellulitis patients with history of diabetes mellitus (DM), typically associated with a poorer outcome, are not more likely to be admitted or "fail" observation than those without DM.[11] Although this was a retrospective analysis, the article demonstrates several interesting points: 1) There is a need for well-designed, prospective studies to determine clinical predictors for successful observation management. A recent prospective study suggests that frailty and sociodemographic factors significantly impact hospital admission from an ED OU.[12] 2) Clinical predictors may be useful in revising and expanding admission criteria. 3) Patients with increasing complexity – such as comorbid DM and cellulitis – may still be appropriate for OM. Regardless of the nature of complexity and approach to management, QI/QA and peer review are essential. Close attention to patient outcomes is necessary to determine the success of management involving modification or combination of existing protocols. (See patient quality in Chapter 9 on Metrics and Performance.)

An ED OU is often institution specific and reflects its needs and culture. Observation protocols, patient admissions, care pathways and staffing models require buy-in from all shareholders including hospital administration, physicians, nursing and support staff. Units with a limited number of simple, protocol-driven pathways might be effectively staffed by midlevel providers with MD oversight and rounding. Units incorporating complex pathways and conditions, however, might require more extensive physician staffing. Avoiding unnecessary admissions, freeing inpatient beds and expediting ED throughput may justify the expanded staffing model in a busy urban center – however, this may be more problematic in smaller settings with less volume. (See Chapter 10 on Community Hospital Perspective.) Similarly, some health systems or hospitals may choose to subsidize groups staffing ED OUs in exchange for operational benefits gained by expanding the OU. It is important to address goals of the ED OU as well as reimbursement with all interested parties before altering the scope of care. Nurses, pharmacists and ancillary staff should be considered in these discussions.

Finally, appropriate facilities and equipment should be available. Beds approved for 23-hour use only should be upgraded to inpatient standards if extended observation is to be considered. Dietary services should be available. Any additional pharmaceutical or medical equipment needs should also be assessed prior to expanding admission criteria.

Summary

OM is expanding towards the uncharted realm of caring for complex patients. More research into the need for, value of and outcomes in caring for these patients is needed. The low-intensity, short-term focused care provided by the ED OU may be extended to patients with greater complexity by modifying or combining protocols. In some facilities with high volumes or important resource utilization issues, units may consider increasing staffing or working with hospitalists to manage patients with acute and chronic issues. Reimbursement schemes, group and institutional buy-in and staffing needs are vital considerations.

References

1. Kellermann AL. Crisis in the emergency department. *N Engl J Med.* 2006;355 (13):1300–1303.

2. Zenner P, Mattie L, Zaharias K. Recovery audit contractor (RAC) basics. 2008; 24. Available: http:// publications.milliman.com/ research/health-rr/pdfs/ recovery-audit-contractor-basics-RR11-01–08.pdf. Accessed February 2016.

3. Venkatesh A. ED Observation Units lower health care costs. Available: www.emra.org/ emra_articles.aspx?id=42328. Accessed February 2012.

4. Graff LG. Observation medicine: The healthcare system's tincture of time. ACEP, 2009;24. Available: www .acep.org/WorkArea/Download Asset.aspx?id=45885. Accessed February 2012.

5. McDermott MF, Murphy DG, Zalenski RJ, et al. A comparison between emergency diagnostic and treatment unit and inpatient care in the management of acute asthma. *Arch Intern Med.* 1997;157:2055–2062.

6. Roberts RR, Zalenski RJ, Mensah EK, et al. Costs of an emergency department-based accelerated diagnostic protocol vs hospitalization in patients with chest pain: a randomized controlled trial. *JAMA.* 1997;278:1670–1676.

7. Goodacre S, Nicholl J, Dixon S. Randomised controlled trial and economic evaluation of a chest pain observation unit compared with routine care. *BMJ*. 2004;328:254.

8. Greenberg RA, Dudley NC, Rittichier KK. A reduction in hospitalization, length of stay, and hospital charges for croup with the institution of a pediatric observation unit. *Am J Emerg Med*. 2006;24: 818–821.

9. Realdi G, Giannini S, Fioretto P, et al. Diagnostic pathways of the complex patients: rapid intensive observation in an Acute Medical Unit. *Intern Emerg Med*. 2011;6(1):85–92.

10. ACEP Clinical and Practice Management. Emergency Department Observation Services. Revised and approved by the ACEP Board of Directors January 2008. www.acep.org/content.aspx?id=29204. Accessed February 2012.

11. Schrock J, Laskey S, Cydulka, R. Predicting observation unit treatment failures in patients with skin and soft tissue infections. *Int J Emerg Med*. June 2008; 1(2):85–90.

12. Zdradzinski MJ, Phelan MP, Mace SE. Impact of fraility and sociodemographic factors on hospital admission from an emergency department observation unit. *AJMQ* (accepted for publication 2016)

Chapter

17 Extended Observation Services

Catherine T. Puetz, MD, FACEP

The use of short-stay units for observing patients as an alternative to hospitalization dates back to 1972.[1] Observation Units (OUs) have emerged as a viable solution to hospitals facing emergency department (ED) overcrowding, lack of available inpatient beds, and the movement by the Centers for Medicare and Medicaid Services (CMS) and other third-party payers to expand the list of treatments and procedures considered as outpatient services.

OUs have allowed physicians to provide better care in a shorter time period at a decreased cost to hospitals. Observation care begins after it is determined by the ED that the patient is unsafe to go home based on his or her medical condition and requires more time to determine the need for inpatient admission or discharge. The time frame for observation services is a minimum of 8 hours to no greater than 48 hours unless there are unforeseen medical circumstances that would require this. The typical observation patient length of stay is < 23 hours. In the past, CMS limited the diagnosis list to chest pain, asthma, and congestive heart failure (CHF). However, this changed a few years ago when the payment for observation services would cover all conditions.[2] With these changes, Medicare claims data indicated a trend for more observation services extending beyond 48 hours from 3% in 2006 to 6% in 2008.[3] These statistics are concerning for two reasons: first being the fact that Medicare and private third-party payers will not reimburse hospitals after 48 hours in observation and second the financial burden an *extended* observation stay has on Medicare beneficiaries. These beneficiaries are subjected to higher co-pays and are more likely to be impacted by the CMS rules regarding self-administered medications. Being cognizant of these barriers still doesn't resolve the problem OUs face in the 48th hour: what to do with those patients still categorized as observation status and not safe for discharge.

Unfortunately, there is very little research to demonstrate that keeping patients in a dedicated OU beyond 23 hours is still more cost-effective when considering the other options such as transferring a patient categorized as observation status to an inpatient bed[4] or discharging the patient to an unsafe environment. The OU at my institution is a 25-bed unit that manages observation status patients up to 48 hours and longer if needed. Those of us intimately involved in the development of the OU for our organization were well aware of the barriers that existed and we have developed a system that provides efficient comprehensive medical care, addresses patient's needs for safe discharge, addresses financial concerns from the moment they are placed in observation, and provides 24-hour access for utilization management to readdress a patient's status as mandated by Medicare beneficiaries patient rights.

The flow of our unit begins with the decision from the ED provider that the patient is unable to be safely discharged from the ED due to his or her underlying medical issue. If the patient's condition fits the criteria of one of the preestablished observation diagnosis a "transfer to observation" order is placed, the observation care set orders for that specific condition are initiated and the patient will be moved to the separate medical OU. It has been clearly established that one of the reasons ED OUs are so successful is that clear inclusion/exclusion criteria exist and goals of observation stays are already in place for staff to follow.[5] (See Chapters 82–87.) The problem remains that there are patients that require further observation who don't fit the preexisting criteria but still only meet observation status. Most hospitals utilize the Milliman or InterQual criteria to determine patient status. These criteria are complex to understand; at my institution, we utilize our Patient Placement Department to assist the ED in assigning the correct status at the time a bed is requested. After the review is complete and the status is determined to be observation this patient subset will be transferred to the medical OU for further care. We have discovered that with the recent changes in shifting more care to outpatient services, our patient population is older and our length of stay has increased. We are currently in the midst of collecting this data and therefore it is not currently available. However, a recent study indicates that fraility and sociodemographic factors, but not age, are significant predictors of inpatient admission from the observation unit.[6]

The processes that we have set in place to help facilitate care have helped streamline care and we are very careful to educate our Medicare patients about their status and the impact it has on them financially. All patients that are transferred to the medical OU are notified of their status and what that means regarding co-pays and the self-administration of medications. We require all of our patients to read the information sheet of what it means to be in observation and we have them sign the form indicating their understanding of the process. A copy of the agreement is left with the patient and a copy is included in the medical record.

Our approach to observation care is that of a comprehensive team. Our team consists of observation specific nurses, acute care midlevel providers (PAs, NPs), physicians, care management, utilization management, environmental services, PT/OT and pharmacy. Each day begins with a checkpoint where the plan of care is discussed amongst the team. It is at these meetings, where we have utilization management review the patient to determine if the patient meets inpatient status or not. Those patients that meet inpatient criteria are admitted to the hospitalist service in an inpatient bed. For those patients who don't meet inpatient criteria, the goals of their stay are discussed as well as some of the outpatient and home needs that they may require. The care management staff meets with every patient in the OU a minimum of once but often more times to discuss financial concerns, care coordination issues, and health care access. The team works with families regarding financial concerns and Medicare-related issues. The availability of reassessing patient status is 24/7 in our organization, making it easier for us to keep our commitment to assign the correct status to the patient as his or her medical condition indicates.

Our organization accepts the fact that the aging population and their increased medical needs will result in longer observation stays due to medical necessity. The observation services provided in the dedicated OU unit of our organization are safe and efficient for our patients leading to desirable outcomes for the patient and the organization.

Hopefully, the Acute Care Organizations (ACOs) will recognize that with the ever growing elderly population and the trend towards more complex services being provided as an outpatient, the need for extended observation stays is inevitable and the use of ED OUs for the care of these patients is still more cost-effective than having these patients placed in an inpatient bed. (See Chapter 20 on ACOs.)

References

1. Gururaj VJ, Allen JE, Russo RM. Short stay in an outpatient department: An alternative to hospitalization. *Am J Dis Child* 1972; 123:128–132.

2. Hale DK. *Observation Status: A Guide to Compliant Level of Care Determination*, Second Edition. HC Pro, Inc. 2008.

3. Clark C. AHA: Observation Status Fears on the Rise. Health Leaders Media. October 29, 2010.

4. Ross MA, Compton S, Richardson D, et al. The use and effectiveness of an emergency department observation unit for elderly patients. *Ann Emerg Med* 2003; 41(5):668–677.

5. Koenig BO, Ross MA, Jackson RE. An emergency department observation unit protocol for acute-onset atrial fibrillation is feasible. *Ann Emerg Med* 2002; 39:374–381.

6. Zdradzinski MJ, Phelan MP, Mace SE. Impact of fraility and sociodemographic factors on hospital admission from an emergency department observation unit. *AJMQ* (accepted for publication 2016).

Chapter

18

Hospital Readmissions

Sharon E. Mace, MD, FACEP, FAAP

Overview

Hospital readmissions are not only common but also costly.[1] They have become a key focus in health care. In the United States, approximately 20% of Medicare beneficiaries are readmitted to the hospital within 30 days of discharge.[1] Moreover, the estimated cost of these readmissions is 17.4 billion dollars per year.[1] Therefore, it should not be a surprise that hospital readmissions are being scrutinized in an effort to decrease hospital readmissions and costs. Evidence of this intense scrutiny is demonstrated by the increasing use of hospital readmissions for public reporting and pay-for-performance.[2,3]

In the United States, the Centers for Medicare and Medicaid Services (CMS) and the Veterans Health Administration (VHA) publicly report 30-day readmission rates for three medical conditions: heart failure, pneumonia and acute myocardial infarction (MI).[4,5] CMS reduces Medicare reimbursements to hospitals that have excessive readmission rates of these three conditions.[6] The most expensive Diagnosis-Related Group (DRG) diagnosis for hospitalizations in general and the most frequent diagnosis for 30-day readmissions is heart failure with a cost of 15 billion in the United States.[7]

Moreover, CMS intends to expand its readmission program that penalizes hospitals with excessive readmission rates to include surgical procedures in addition to the three medical conditions: heart failure, pneumonia and acute MI.[6,8]

Decreasing readmission rates has become a national priority. As mentioned, CMS publicly reports these rates. The National Quality Forum (NQF) has endorsed hospital risk-standardized readmission rates (RSRRs) as performance measures, with specific endorsed measures: RSRR for heart failure, acute MI (AMI), elective primary total hip arthroplasty (THA) and total knee arthroplasty (TKA).[8] Recently, the Patient Protection

Affordable Care Act of 2010 created new financial incentives for reducing readmission rates using the publicly reported measures.[9] By 2015, hospitals with high readmission rates can lose ≤ 3% of their Medicare reimbursement.[10] This financial impetus has led to many initiatives at all levels: local, state and national, which will be discussed as potential solutions to the readmissions dilemma.

Rates of 30-Day Readmissions

Not all readmissions are preventable or avoidable.[3,11] Moreover, the incidence of 30-day of "preventable or avoidable readmissions" varies greatly.[11] Often quoted percentages of preventable admissions are in the 18% or 20% range.[1,2] However, rates up to as high as 47% or even 59% in studies that used only administrative data have been reported.[12,13] The incidence of avoidable readmission rates was as low as 9.3% to a high of 39.9% of all readmissions, according to one meta-analysis, depending at least in part on the method utilized to determine if the readmission was preventable (e.g., on the number of reviewers).[14]

Should 30-Day Readmissions Be Used as a Metric?

Some experts have questioned the use of 30-day readmissions as a metric.[11-18] A prospective multicenter study found that the methodology used to determine readmissions can greatly affect the readmission rate. They found that the readmission rates "cannot be determined accurately on the basis of administrative data alone" and "is a subjective judgment that requires detailed patient data, multiple reviewers and an analysis that accounts for differing reviewer accuracy when collating judgments." They concluded that "urgent readmissions should be used with caution to gauge the quality of hospital care."[15]

Others have also echoed these sentiments. "Readmission rates are not a reliable measure of hospital quality in cardiac surgery."[16] "Most readmissions at our public, safety net hospital were unavoidable" and "these findings suggest that readmissions do not necessarily reflect inadequate medical care, may reflect resource constraints that are unlikely to be addressable in systems caring for a large burden of uninsured patients, and merit individualized review."[17]

Several problems with using 30-day readmissions as a metric have been noted.[11] These reasons include the following: only a small percentage of readmissions at 30 days are preventable, the majority of variables that determine hospital readmission rates are "patient- and community-level factors that are well outside the hospital's control," and high admission rates could be "the result of low mortality rates or good access to hospital care." Furthermore, they cite other unforeseen consequences of using the 30-day readmission rate: in their zeal to reduce readmission rates, hospitals are bypassing other "more urgent issues, such as patient safety" and there are "better, more targeted policies" that will improve discharge planning and care coordination.[11]

Some readmissions may be "unavoidable" or "not preventable" and/or are outside the purview of the hospital.[11-18] The "socioeconomic disparities in readmission raises the question of whether CMS's readmission measures and associated financial penalties should be adjusted for the effects of factors beyond hospital influence at the individual or neighborhood level, such as poverty and lack of social support."[18] This is because all-cause readmission statistics "are only partially influenced by quality of care."[14]

International Perspective

It should be noted that this emphasis on readmissions is not unique to the United States, but is a worldwide issue with varying but somewhat similar 30-day readmission rates (16.0%, 16.7%) and similar risk factors, specifically increased illness severity as denoted by longer hospital stay, comorbidity (e.g., active malignancy, anemia), and higher Charlson scores, which are all associated with increased readmission rates.[15,19-21]

Report to Congress

In a report to Congress, "Payment Policy for Inpatient Readmissions," the recommendations

Table 18.1: Recommendations for How Hospitals Can Reduce Readmissions*

- Provide better, safer care during the inpatient stay
- Attend to patient's medication needs at discharge
- Improve communication with patients before and after discharge
- Improve communication with other providers
- Review practice patterns

* From "Payment Policy for Inpatient Readmissions" from www.medpac.gov/documents/Jun07_EntireReport.pdf.

for ways for hospitals to reduce readmissions were "provide better, safer care during the inpatient stay," "attend to patient's medication needs at discharge," "improve communication with patients before and after discharge," "improve communication with other providers" and "review practice patterns."[2] (Table 18.1) There has been literature evaluating these recommendations and suggested methods for their implementation, which will be addressed in the sections to follow.

Patient Disease/Illness/Injury Factors

The factors contributing to 30-day readmissions are just beginning to be elucidated, but some variables have been identified. (Table 18.2) Many of the factors can be correlated with the patient's disease or clinical condition, especially the severity of their disease.[22] Prior admissions,[23-26] need for medications, such as chronic steroid use,[27,28] and new need for home oxygen[29] may be markers for significant underlying chronic illnesses/diseases and have been associated with increased readmission rates. Significant comorbidity – including kidney injury, renal failure, dialysis, cardiovascular disease including heart failure, immunosuppression, bleeding disorders (including those from anticoagulant and other therapies), diabetes, anemia and AIDS – have been noted to increase the risk of readmission.[25,28-36] An increased number of comorbidities or a higher Charlson score are also associated with increased readmission rates.[24,26,29,37,38] Psychiatric illnesses/mental health comorbidities[39,40] and dementia[41] have been linked to an increased risk of 30-day readmissions.

Prolonged length of stay (LOS) and intensive care unit (ICU) admission as indicators of severity of disease have been linked to increased 30-day

Table 18.2: Factors Associated with High 30-Day Readmission Rates*

I. DISEASE/ILLNESS

   A. Severity of the Index or Primary Illness/Disease

      1. Prior hospital admissions**
      2. Prior emergency department visits**
      3. Medications: new prescription of home oxygen, chronic steroid use, immunosuppressive drugs, others**

   B. Comorbidity

      1. Specific medical comorbidities: heart failure, renal failure, dialysis, immunosuppression, bleeding disorders, anemia, AIDS
      2. Increased number of comorbidities
      3. Mental health/psychiatric illness
      4. Dementia

   C. Complexity or Problems Occurring During Index Admission**

      1. ICU admission
      2. Length of hospitalization (longer LOS): prolonged inpatient stay
      3. More extensive or complicated surgery (e.g., longer operating room time)
      4. Post-operative complications
      5. Complications of injury
      6. Complications of procedures: such as percutaneous coronary intervention (PCI)
      7. Postoperative or postprocedure dysrhythmias
      8. Laboratory abnormalities: hemoglobin (anemia), sodium (hyponatremia), hyperglycemia
      9. Discharge from hospital other than to home (e.g., skilled nursing facility, rehabilitation facility)

II. PATIENT VARIABLES

   A. Demographics***

      1. Age (especially elderly)
      2. Gender
      3. Race

   B. Ability to Do Activities of Daily Living/Need for Assistance***

      1. Activity
      2. Functional impairment
      3. Mobility
      4. Exercise

   C. Individual Risk Factors***

      1. Smoking
      2. Substance abuse
      3. Obesity

   D. Socioeconomic

      1. Lack of social supports: family/caregivers
        - Married vs. single (married has spouse for support and care giving)
      2. Homeless
      3. High poverty areas, lower household income, type of insurance coverage

III. ACCESS TO CARE***

      1. Geography (location: where you live)
      2. Regional differences (by county, whether urban/suburban/rural)
      3. Access to care
      4. Low per capita primary care
      5. Health care utilization

IV. IN-HOSPITAL VARIABLES

   A. Factors related to the care given during the index or initial stay

      1. Operative factors
      2. Procedure factors
      3. Treatment
      4. Complications

   B. Factors related to discharge process

      1. Patient and family education prior to discharge

   C. Factors related to follow-up care

      1. Transitions of care
      2. Follow-up phone calls
      3. Patient follow-up arranged prior to discharge
      4. Timely follow-up appointments
      5. Needed service(s) arranged prior to discharge: home health care, visiting nurse, etc.
      6. Home visits by a health care provider

* This is likely not an all-inclusive list but gives some of the factors associated with readmissions. Variables may be added, deleted or changed when additional research becomes available.
** These may be markers of disease complexity and/or severity of illness.
*** Noted in some studies but not others, may apply to one disease or condition but not others.

readmissions.[24,34,42,43] Factors occurring during the index admission related to the complexity of care – for example, more extensive and/or complicated surgery and/or prolonged operative time – have been associated with greater risks of 30-day readmissions.[27,37] Complications occurring from procedures – such as percutaneous coronary intervention (PCI) or surgery related to a patient's traumatic injury – during the initial or index hospital admission have been correlated with higher 30-day readmissions rates.[26,27,34,37,44–48] Although there is a wide range of complications from bleeding to dysrhythmias, wound infections seem to be the most common postoperative complication.[45,47,48]

Laboratory abnormalities during the initial or index visit are being evaluated for their effect on 30-day readmissions. Kidney injury (e.g., abnormal creatinine and blood urea nitrogen) and the degree or severity of kidney injury was associated with increased readmission rates.[30,31,47] Anemia has generally been correlated with higher 30-day readmission rates, especially for medical patients.[25,29,49] For hyperglycemia there were conflicting reports: one study found an association with readmission rates,[50] while another did not.[51] Electrolyte abnormalities, specifically hyponatremia,[52] and an elevated white blood cell count[53] were independent predictors of a greater readmission rate.

Demographic Variables

Demographic variables are also correlated with readmissions rates with older patients having higher readmission rates in most studies,[18,26,28,34,54–56] but not all studies.[43] Gender has mixed results with some studies finding that females having higher readmission rates,[32,34] while others report males having significantly higher readmission rates than females,[18,57] and others noted that gender had no effect.[43] Similarly, race has been associated with increased readmission rates in African Americans versus Caucasians according to some reports[34,43,54,58,59] but not others,[24,27] with socioeconomic factors (poverty, location of service) possibly accounting for some of the disparity for African Americans having higher readmission rates than Caucasians.[54,57]

Individual Factors

Individual factors have been looked at. Smoking,[32,48] substance abuse,[17] and "patient noncompliance"[17,60] are correlated with higher readmission rates. Most studies found that obesity or increased body mass index was associated with higher readmission rates,[27,54,61] while others did not.[48]

Functionality and ability to do activities of daily living and mobility/exercise have also been linked with 30-day readmissions. Measures of frailty and diminished or dependent functionality as indicated by lack of activity, lack of mobility, and history of falls in the preceding 6 months are predictors of increased readmissions.[26,62–64] Similarly, discharge destination, comparing discharge to a nursing home or skilled nursing facility instead of to home, has been linked to an increase in readmission rates.[26,27]

Socioeconomic Factors

Socioeconomic factors are noted to have an effect.[54,57,65] Those with a lower median income have higher 30-day readmission rates.[17,54,57] Patients from high poverty areas have been noted to have higher readmission rates.[17,18] Medicaid-enrolled patients have a higher rate of 30-day readmissions than commercially insured patients.[34,37,43,54,65–68] The homeless have higher readmission rates.[69] Lack of social supports is a negative variable. Those with a spouse for support and care giving do better with fewer 30-day readmissions than unmarried or widowed individuals in most studies.[24,43]

Access to Care, Health Care Utilization and Community Factors

Access to care has been evaluated. Health care utilization, low per capita primary care/access to care and geography/regional differences (where you live by neighborhood, county, region, or census region) may affect the readmission rates.[17,18,65,68] Whether the patient lives in an urban versus rural area has been linked with readmission rates in some studies[65,68] but not others.[45] The relationship between number of health care providers and readmissions has been evaluated and is inversely linked to the number of general practitioners (e.g., a decrease in readmissions occurred with an increased per capita number of general practitioners).[65] Proximity to a health care provider/hospital or the distance to care has been linked to readmission rates.[65,68]

Comparing emergent with elective admissions shows higher readmission rates for those admitted emergently.[54,68] As noted, the type of insurance coverage has also been associated with readmission rates with patients having "Medicaid" and "Medicare or State-financed insurance" more likely than patients with private (or commercial) insurance or health maintenance organization insurance to be readmitted.[34,37,43,54,65–68]

Hospital Factors

When hospital variables are looked at, the volume may be a factor with higher-volume institutions or high-performing hospitals having lower readmission rates.[67,70] Adherence to best practices has been advocated as a method to decrease readmission rates and improve patient outcomes. Of interest was the finding in this *New England Journal* study that "high adherence to reported surgical process measures was only marginally associated with reduced readmission rates."[67] Readmission rates are higher at teaching hospitals according to several studies.[10,67] Number of hospital beds, ownership type (for-profit, nonprofit or government) and multihospital affiliation or not had no effect on readmission rates according to one study,[10] while another study found lower readmission rates at larger (> 400 beds) hospitals and at private nonprofit hospitals (vs. for-profit or public hospitals).[67]

Hospital variables can be categorized into three groups: factors relevant to the operation or procedure or treatment for a given condition or illness, factors applicable to the discharge process and factors germane to follow-up care. Readmission rates vary with the diagnosis at the index hospitalization.[71] The specific illness/diagnosis or type of operation or procedure performed for a given condition or illness has been looked at with differences in 30-day readmission rates noted according to the types of procedures or surgery done (e.g., vascular surgery, major joint replacement, bowel procedures, coronary-artery bypass grafting, lobectomy, cardiac stent, others),[67,68] but whether a different surgical approach or technique is associated with a lower readmission rate is variable and may be somewhat dependent on the specific technical procedure. This suggests that the technical approach for each procedure or operation should be evaluated individually. For example, two reports found no difference based on the type of operation

performed (e.g., laparoscopic vs. open procedure),[72,73] while others report that certain technical aspects may make a difference in readmission rates.[74]

Regarding medical conditions, cardiac care has been examined. Giving aspirin, beta blockers, angiotensin-converting enzyme (ACE) or angiotensin receptor blocker (ARB) inhibitors at hospital discharge has been associated with a lower 30-day readmission rate.[34,75,76] The initial correct antibiotic affected hospital readmission for pneumonia.[77] Moreover, it seems likely that the results will be highly specific for a given procedure or operation or illness/condition.[68,73,74] Problems related to the discharge process and follow-up care have also been implicated as a factor in increasing the readmission rate.[10]

Potential Solutions

Various programs focusing on the patient during their admission have been suggested as a means to decrease readmissions. Such programs often involve targeting high-risk patients (e.g., frail and elderly), a team management approach, active case management, and/or units for the high-risk (often elderly) patients and a focus on discharge instructions and/or transitions of care and/or follow-up care.[10,79–93]

Achieving patient/family understanding of discharge instructions – whether by using medication reconciliation and counseling, teach-back mechanisms or other approaches – has been advocated as one approach to decreasing readmissions.[75,77,79,81,83]

Improving transitions of care has been recommended as a method for lowering 30-day readmission rates.[84,85]

Follow-up phone calls to discharged patients has been recommended.[79] Arranging timely follow-up appointments prior to the patient's discharge from the hospital has been suggested as another promising approach.[79,86]

Home visits by a health care practitioner – whether a community paramedic, a nurse, community health worker, pharmacist, nurse practitioner, physician assistant, or physician – after the patient's discharge from the hospital may be one avenue for decreasing readmissions.[86–91] Receipt of hospice or home-based palliative care postdischarge was associated with lower odds of hospital readmission.[92]

Solutions may also be related to socioeconomic variables that may be beyond the reach of an individual provider, hospital or even health care system, but depend on societal as well as individual factors.

Potential Solutions: Observation Medicine

As noted, hospital variables include factors relevant to the operation or procedure or treatment for a given condition or illness. This area of focus could be based on "Best Practices" and standardized care, including care paths, protocols, and order sets, as has been demonstrated to be effective with observation medicine when practiced in a focused unit with specific criteria and set pathways. As proven in the evidence-based chapters (both for disease-specific conditions and for age-based considerations), the correct application of observation medicine shows much promise and based on preliminary evidence could be extremely valuable in achieving the goal of decreased 30-day readmissions. Initial studies have found a decrease in returns to the emergency department (ED) and in readmissions to the hospital. For example, in the study by Peacock et al., the 90-day return visit to the ED for congestive heart failure patients treated in the ED observation unit was decreased by 64% over standard inpatient care.[93] In the article by Roberts et al., the readmission rate was 4.8% for the ED chest pain unit patients versus 6.1% for standard inpatient care.[94]

The evidence-based chapters have other articles detailing the decreased readmissions, improvement in quality-of-life measures, and decreased morbidity and mortality with the use of protocol-driven, standardized observation units. (Chapters 80 and 81)

Summary

Hospital readmissions, which are common, costly, and not unique to any one system or country, are a focus of health care and governmental agencies in an attempt to control costs and improve patient quality and outcomes. The etiology of readmissions appears to be multifactorial and complex. Factors cited as contributing to readmissions involve not only hospital variables but also demographic, individual, socioeconomic and community/geographic considerations.

The rate of 30-day preventable readmissions is highly variable depending on the methodology utilized to determine what is an avoidable or preventable admission. The use of "avoidable" readmissions as a metric for hospital payment has been questioned because of the effect of socioeconomic factors and patient/disease variables outside the control of a given hospital(s) or health care system on some readmissions.

Recommendations for ways to decrease hospital readmissions have been issued. Various solutions have been proposed in an attempt to decrease the readmission rate. Observation medicine has been effective in reducing costs, decreasing the LOS, increasing patient/family satisfaction, decreasing ED return visits, decreasing readmissions, and improving patient care and outcomes. (See evidence-based Chapters 80 and 81) It seems likely the promise of observation medicine may be able to have a positive impact on readmission rates.

References

1. Jencks SF, Williams MV, Coleman EA. Rehospitalizations among patients in the Medicare fee-for-service program. *N Engl J Med* 2009; 360(14): 1418–1428.

2. Medicare Payment Advisory Committee (MedCAP). Report to the Congress: Creating greater efficiency in Medicare. Available at: www.medpac.gov/documents/Jun07_Entire Report.pdf. Accessed February 2016.

3. Rosen AK, Chen Q, Shin MH, et al. Medical and surgical readmissions in the Veterans Health Administration. What proportions are related to the index Hospitalization? *Medical Care* 2014; 52(3):243–249.

4. Centers for Medicare and Medicaid Services (CMS). CMS Hospital Compare Web site. Available at: www.cms.gov/Medicare/Medicare-Fee-for-Service-Payment/AcuteInpatientPPS/Readmissions-Reduction-Program.html. Accessed February 2016.

5. Department of Veterans Affairs. VA Hospital Compare. Available at: www.hospitalcompare.va.gov. Accessed February 2016.

6. Department of Health and Human Services; Centers for Medicare and Medicaid Services. Medicare Program Hospital Inpatient Perspective Payment Systems for Acute Care Hospitals and the Long Term Care Hospital

Prospective Payment System and Proposed Fiscal Year 2014 Rates; Quality Reporting Requirements for Specific Providers; Hospital Conditions of Participation; Medicare program; FY 2014 Hospice Wage Index and Payment Rate Update; Hospice Quality Reporting Requirements; and Updates on Payment Reform; Proposed Rules. Federal Register 78 (May 10, 2013): 27486–27823. Available at: www.gpo.gov/fdsys/pkg/FR-2013-05-10/pdf/2013-10234.pdf. Accessed February 2016.

7. Pina IL. Trends in heart failure hospitalizations. *Curr Heart Fail Rep* 2012; 9(4):346–353.

8. National Quality forum (NQF) website. Available at: www.qualityforum.org/News_And_Resources/Press_Releases/2013/NQF_Upholds_Endorsement_of_Planned_Readmissions_Measures.aspx. Accessed February 2016.

9. Federal Register, Patient Protection Affordable Care Act. Available at: www.gpo.gov/fdsys/pkg/FR-2013-03-11/pdf/2013-04952.pdf. Accessed February 2016.

10. Bradley EH, Curry L, Horwitz LI, et al. Hospital strategies associated with 30-day readmission rates for patients with heart failure. *Circ Cardiovasc Qual Outcomes* 2013; 6:444–450.

11. Joynt KE. Thirty-day readmissions – truth and consequences. *N Engl J Med* 2012; 366(15):1366–1369.

12. Feigenbaum P, Neuwirth E, Trowbridge L, et al. Factors contributing to all-cause 30-day readmissions: a structured case series across 18 hospitals. *Med Care* 2012; 50(7):599–607.

13. Van Walraven C, Bennett C, Jennings A, et al. Proportion of hospital admissions deemed avoidable: a systematic review. *CMAJ* 2011; 183(7): E391–E402.

14. Van Walraven C, Jennings A, Forster AJ. A meta-analysis of the hospital 30-day avoidable readmission rate. *J Eval Clin Pract* 2012; 18(6):1211–1218.

15. Van Walraven C, Jennings A, Taljaard M, et al. Incidence of potentially avoidable urgent readmissions and their relation to all-cause urgent readmissions. *CMAJ* 2011; 183 (14):e1067–1072.

16. Shih T, Dimick JB. Reliability of readmission rates as a hospital quality measure in cardiac surgery. *Ann Thorac Surg* 2014; 97(4):1214–1218.

17. Shimizu E, Glaspy K, Witt MD, et al. Readmissions at a public safety net hospital. *PLoS One.* 2014 Mar 11; 9(3):e 91244.

18. Hu J, Gonsahn MD, Nerenz DR, et al. Socioeconomic status and readmissions: evidence from an urban teaching hospital. *Health Aff (Millwood)* 2014; 33(5):786–791.

19. Shu CC, Lin YF, Ko WJ. Risk factors for 30-day readmission in general medical patients admitted from the emergency department: a single center study. *Intern Med J* 2012; 42 (6):677–682.

20. Tuppin P, Cuerq A, de Peretti C, et al. First hospitalization for heart failure in France in 2009: patient characteristics and 30-day follow-up. *Arch Cardiovasc Dis* 2013; 106(11):570–585.

21. Blunt I, Bardsley M, Grove A, et al. Classifying emergency 30-day readmissions in England using routine hospital data 2004–2010: what is the scope for reduction? *Emerg Med J* 2015; 32(1):44–50.

22. Kiridly DN, Karkenny AJ, Hutzler LH, et al. The effect of severity of disease on cost burden of 30-day readmissions following total joint arthroplasty. J Arthroplasty 2014; 29(8):1545–1547.

23. Hummel SL, Katrapati P, Gillespie BW, et al. Impact of prior admissions on 30 day readmission in medicare heart failure inpatients. *Mayo Clin Proc* 2014; 89(5):623–630.

24. Garrison GM, Mansukhani MP, Bohn B. Predictors of thirty-day readmissions among hospitalized family medicine patients. *J Am Board Fam Med* 2013; 26(1):71–77.

25. Borenstein J, Aronow HU, Bolton LB, et al. Early recognition of risk factors for adverse outcomes during hospitalization among Medicare patients: a prospective cohort study. *BMC Geriatr* 2013; 13:72.

26. Moore L, Stelfox HT, Turgeon AF, et al. Rates, patterns, and determinants of unplanned admission after traumatic injury: a multicenter cohort study. *Ann Surg* 2014; 259 (2):374–380.

27. Kelly KN, Iannuzzi JC, et al. Risk factors associated with 30-day postoperative readmissions in major gastrointestinal resections. *J Gastrointest Surg* 2014; 18(1):35–43.

28. Khavanin N, Bethke KP, Lovecchio FC, et al. Risk factors for unplanned readmissions following excisional breast surgery. *Breast J* 2014; 20(3):288–294.

29. Nguyen HQ, Chu L, Liu IL, Lee JS, et al. Associations between physical activity and 30 day readmission risk in chronic obstructive pulmonary disease. *Ann Am Thor Soc* 2014; 11 (5):695–705.

30. Brown JR, Parikh CR, Ross CS, et al. Impact of perioperative acute kidney injury as a severity index for thirty-day readmission after cardiac surgery. *Ann Thor Surg* 2014; 97(1):111–117.

31. Whittaker D, Soine LA, Errico KM. Patient and process factors associated with all-cause 30-day readmission among patients with heart failure.

J Am Assoc Nurse Pract 2015; 27:105–113.

32. McPhee JT, Nguyen LL, Ho KJ, et al. Risk prediction of 30-day readmission after infrainguinal bypass for critical limb ischemia. *J Vasc Surg* 2013; 57 (6):1481–1488.

33. Ahmad R, Schmidt BH, Rattner, DW, et al. Factors influencing readmission after curative gastrectomy for gastric cancer. *J Am Coll Surg* 2014; 218:1215–1222.

34. Wasfy JH, Rosenfield K, Zelevinsky K, et al. A prediction model to identify patients at high risk for 30-day readmission after percutaneous coronary intervention. *Circ Cardiovasc Qual Outcomes* 2013; 6(4):429–435.

35. David D, Britting L, Dalton J. Cardiac acute care nurse practitioner and 30-day readmission. *J Cardiovasc Nurs* 2015; 30(3):248–255.

36. Fleishman JA, Yehia BR, Korthuis PT, et al. Thirty day readmission rate among adults living with HIV. *AIDS* 2013; 27 (13):2059–2068.

37. Wang MC, Shivakoti M, Sparapani RA, et al. Thirty day readmissions after elective spine surgery for degenerative conditions among US Medicare beneficiaries. *Spine J* 2012; 12 (10):902–911.

38. Brandao LF, Zargar H, Laydner H, et al. 30-day hospital readmission after robotic partial nephrectomy; are we prepared for Medicare Readmission Reduction Program? *J Urol* 2014; 192 (3):677–681.

39. Ketterer MW, Draus C, McCord J, et al. Behavioral factors and hospital admissions/readmissions in patients with CHF. *Psychosomatics* 2014; 55(1): 45–50.

40. Burke RE, Donze J, Schnipper JL, Contribution of psychiatric illness and substance abuse to 30-day readmission rate. *J Hosp Med* 2013; 8(8): 450–455.

41. Daiello LA, Gardener R, Epstein-Lubow G, Butterfield K. Association of dementia with early rehospitalization among Medicare beneficiaries. *Arch Gerontol Geriatr* 2014; 59:162–168.

42. Clement RC, Derman PB, Graham DS, et al. Risk factors, causes and the economic implications of unplanned readmissions following total hip arthroplasty. *J Arthroplasty* 2013; 28(8 suppl):7–10. doi 10:1016/j.

43. Dailey EA, Cizik A, Kasten J, et al. Risk factors for readmission of orthopedic surgical patients. *J Bone Joint Surg AM* 2013; 95 (11):10012–1019.

44. Glance LG, Kellerman AL, Osler TM, et al. Hospital readmission after noncardiac surgery: the role of major complications. *JAMA Surg* 2014; doi: 10.1001 [Epub ahead of print].

45. Greenblatt DY, Greenberg CC, Kind A, Havlena JA, et al. Causes and implications of readmission after abdominal aortic aneurysm repair. *Ann Surg* 2012; 256(4):596–605.

46. Vogel TR, Dombrovskiy VY, Lowry SF, et al. Impact of infectious complications after elective surgery on hospital readmission and late deaths in the U.S. Medicare population. *Surg Infect (Larchmt)* 2012; 13 (5):307–311.

47. Shehata N, Forster A, Rothwell DM. et al. Does anemia impact hospital readmission after coronary artery bypass surgery? *Transfusion* 2013; 53 (8):1688–1697.

48. Lovecchio F, Farmer R, Souza J, et al. Risk factors for 30-day readmission in patients undergoing ventral hernia repair. *Surgery* 2014; 155(4): 702–710.

49. Lin RJ, Evans AT, Chused AE, et al. Anemia in general medical inpatients prolongs length of stay and increases 30-day readmission rate. *Southern Med J* 2013; 106(5): 316–320.

50. Evans NR, Dhatariya KK. Assessing the relationship between admission glucose levels, subsequent length of hospital stay, readmission and mortality. *Clin Med* 2012; 12 (2):137–139.

51. Lee LJ, Emons MF, Martin SA, et al. Association of blood glucose levels with in-hospital mortality and 30 day readmission in patients undergoing invasive cardiovascular surgery. *Curr Medical Research & Opinion* 2012; 28(10):1657–1665.

52. Deitelzweig S, Amin A, Christian R, et al. Health care utilization, costs, and readmission rates associated with hyponatremia. *Hosp Pract* 2013; 41(1):89–95.

53. Brown JR, Landis RC, Chaisson K, et al. Preoperative white blood cell count and risk of 30-day readmission after cardiac surgery. *Int J Inflam* 2013; doi: 10.1155/2013/781024 [Epub Jul 18, 2013].

54. Li Z, Armstrong EJ, Parker JP, Danielsen B, et al. Hospital variation in readmission after bypass surgery in California. *Circ Cardiovasc Qual Outcomes* 2012; 5(5):729–737.

55. Hageman MG, Bossen JK, Smith RM, et al. Predictors of readmission in orthopedic trauma surgery. *J Orthop Trauma* 2014; 28(10): e247–e249.

56. Paquette JM, Solon P, Rafferty JF, et al. Readmission for dehydration of renal failure after ileostomy creation. *Dis Colon Rectum* 2013; 56(8): 974–979.

57. Mather JF, Fortunato GJ, Ash JL, et al. Prediction of 30 pneumonia 30-day readmissions: a single-center attempt to increase model performance. *Respir Care* 2014; 59(2):199–208.

58. Schneider EB, Haider AH, Hyder O, et al. Assessing short and long term outcomes among black vs. white Medicare patients undergoing resection of colorectal cancer. *Am J Surg* 2013; 205(4): 402–408.

59. Singh JA, Lu X, Rosenthal GE, et al. Racial disparities in knee and hip total joint arthroplasty: an 18-year analysis of national Medicare data. *Ann Rheum Dis*; Sep 18 [Epub ahead of print].

60. Vaziri S, Cox JB, Friedman WA. Readmisssions in neurosurgery: a qualitative inquiry. *World Neurosurg* 2014; S1878–8750.

61. Silber JH, Rosenbaum PR, Kelz RR, et al. Medical and financial risks associated with surgery in the elderly obese. *Ann Surg* 2012; 256(1):79–86.

62. Robinson TN, Wu DS, Pointer L, et al. Simple frailty score predicts postoperative complications across surgical specialties. *Am J Surg* 2013; 206 (4):544–550.

63. Fisher SR, Kuo VF, Sharma G, et al. Mobility after discharge as a marker for 30-day readmission. *J Gerontol A Biol Sci Med Sci* 2013; 68(7): 805–810.

64. Jones TS, Dunn CL, Wu DS, et al. Relationship between asking an older adult about falls and surgical outcomes. *JAMA Surg* 2013; 148(12): 1132–1138.

65. Herrin J, St. Andre J, Kenward K, et al. Community factors and hospital readmission rates. *Health Serv Res* 2015; 50(1): 20–39.

66. Allen LS, Smoyer Tomic KE, Smith DM. Rates and predictors of 30 day readmission among commercially insured and Medicaid-enrolled patients hospitalized with systolic heart failure. *Circ Heart Fail* 2012; 5 (6):672–679.

67. Tsai TC, Joynt KE, Orav EJ, et al. Variation in surgical-readmission rates and quality of hospital care. *N Engl J Med* 2013; 369(12):1134–1142.

68. Engelbert TL, Fernandez-Taylor S, Gupta PK, et al. Clinical characteristics associated with readmission among patients undergoing vascular surgery. *J Vasc Surg* 2014; 59(5):1349–1355.

69. Doran KM, Ragins KT, Iacomacci AL, et al. The revolving hospital door: hospital readmissions among patients who are homeless. *Med Care* 2013; 51(9):767–773.

70. Dharmarajan K, Hsieh AF, Lin Z, et al. Hospital readmission performance and patterns of readmission: retrospective cohort study of Medicare admissions. *BMJ* 2013; 347: F6571.

71. Lemieux J, Sennett C, Wang R, et al. Hospital readmission rates in Medicare advantage plans. *Am J Manag Care* 2012; 18(2): 96–104.

72. Parnaby CN, Ramsay G, Macvleod CS, et al. Complications after laparoscopic and open subtotal colectomy for inflammatory colitis: a case-matched comparison. *Colorectal Dis* 2013; 15(11):1399–1405.

73. Helgstrand F, Jorgensen LN, Kehlet H, et al. Nationwide prospective study on readmission after umbilical or epigastric hernia repair. *Hernia* 2013; 17(4):487–492.

74. Schweppe ML, Seyle TM, Swenson RD, et al. Does surgical approach in total hip arthroplasty affect rehabilitation, discharge disposition, and readmission rate? *Surg Technol Int* 2013; 23:219–227.

75. Schmeida M, Savrin R. Acute myocardial infarction rehospitalization of the Medicare fee-for-service patient: a state-level analysis exploring 30-day readmission factors. *Prof Case Manag* 2013; 18(6):295–302.

76. Brown JR, Conley SM, Niles NW. Predicting readmission or death after acute ST-elevation myocardial infarction. *Clin Cardiol* 2013; 36(10): 570–575.

77. Schmeida M, Savrin RA. Pneumonia rehospitalization of the Medicare fee-for-service patient: a state-level analysis: exploring 30-day readmission factors. *Prof Case Manag* 2012; 17(3):126–131.

78. Rosen AK, Loveland S, Shin M, et al. Examining the impact of the AHRQ Patient Safety Indicators (PSIs) on the Veterans Health Administration: the case of readmissions. *Med Care* 2013; 51910:37–44.

79. Bates OL, O'Connor N, Dunn D, et al. Applying STAAR Interventions in Incremental Bundles: Improving Post-CABG Surgical Patient Care. *Worldviews Evid Based Nurs* 2014; 11(2):89–97.

80. Segelman M, Szydlowski J, Kinosian B, et al. Hospitalization in the program of all inclusive care for the elderly. *J Am Geriatr Soc* 2014; 62(2):320–324.

81. Markley J, Andow V, Sabharwal K, et al. A project to reengineer discharges reduces 30day readmission rates, *Am J Nurs* 2013; 113(7):55–64.

82. Flood KL, McGrew l D, Green D, et al. Effects of an acute care for elders unit on costs and 30-day readmissions" *JAMA Intern Med* 2013; 173(11): 981–987.

83. Pal A, Babbott S, Wlikinson ST. Can the targeted use of a discharge pharmacist significantly decrease 30-day readmissions? *Hosp Pharm* 2013; 48(5):380–388.

84. Kirkham HS, Clark BL, Paynter J, et al. The effect of a collaborative pharmacist-hospital care transition program on the likelihood of 30 day readmission. *Am J Health Sys Pharm* 2014; 71 (9):739–745.

85. Baldwin KM, Black D, Hammond S. Developing a rural transitional care community case management program using clinical nurse specialists. *Clin Nurse Spec* 2014; 28(3):147–155.

86. Ryan J, Kang S, Dolacky S, et al. Change in readmissions and follow-up visits as part of a heart failure readmission quality improvement initiative. *Am J Med* 2013; 126(11): 989–984.

87. ED staff, paramedics work to reduce readmits. *Hosp Case Manag* 2014; 22(3):36–37.

88. New program set to intervene to prevent readmissions, repeat ED visits due to acute exacerbations of asthma. *ED Manag* 2013; 25(12): 139–141.

89. Hall MH, Esposito RA, Pekmezaris R, et al. Cardiac surgery nurse practitioner home visits prevent CABG readmissions. *Ann Thorac Surg* 2014; 97(5):1488–1895.

90. Novak CJ, Hastanan S, Moradi M, et al. Reducing unnecessary hospital readmissions: the pharmacist's role in care transitions. *Consult Pharm* 2012; 27(3):174–179.

91. Nabagiez JP, Shariff MA, Khan MA, et al. Physician assistant home visit program to reduce hospital admissions. *J Thorac Cardiovasc Surg* 2013; 145 (1):225–231.

92. Enguidanos S, Vesper E, Lorenz K, et al. 30 day readmissions among seriously ill older adults. *J Palliat Med* 2012; 15(12):1356–1361.

93. Peacock WF, Remer EE, Aponte J, et al. Effective observation unit treatment of decompensated heart failure. *Congest Heart Fail* 2002; 8(2): 68–73.

94. Roberts RR, Zalenski RJ, Mensah EK, et al. Costs of an emergency department-based accelerated diagnostic protocol vs. hospitalization in patients with chest pain: a randomized controlled trial. *JAMA* 1997; 278(20):1670–1676.

Chapter

19
Level of Care Determination
Medical Necessity Risk Stratification

Louis Graff IV, FACEP, FAAP

Medical Necessity determination is a central task of the physician evaluating patients in the emergency department (ED). Those identified as having a serious dangerous disease or as likely (moderate to high probability) of having a serious dangerous disease need admission for inpatient evaluation and treatment. Those identified as having low probability of a serious dangerous disease are appropriate for outpatient evaluation and management in observation. Those identified as unlikely (very low probability) of having a serious dangerous disease are appropriate for discharge home and scheduled outpatient evaluation and management. Accurate disposition of patients has great importance for high quality of patient care and proper utilization of resources.

Threshold to Observe: Missed Diagnosis Rate

Optimal threshold for observation is the amount of observation with the lowest possible missed diagnosis rate. The purpose of observation is to provide additional services after the ED visit to patients who might have a serious disease and might suffer adverse effects if discharged home. The missed diagnosis rate is the metric to judge whether the threshold for observation is adequate and is the percentage of a serious dangerous disease that the diagnosis missed at the initial visit. If the missed diagnosis rate is not near zero, then the physician's threshold for observation is too high and the physician will fail to place in observation low-probability-of-disease patients, some of whom have a serious disease and would be identified if observed. The rule-out evaluation rate is the percentage of chief complaint patients who are 'ruled out' for a serious disease. For example, for chest pain (CP) patients and acute myocardial infarction(MI), the rule-out evaluation rate is the percentage of ED CP patients placed in observation or inpatient admission so they can get a full rule-out evaluation for acute MI. In the example illustrated in Figure 19.1, the optimal threshold for observation is the CP evaluation rate at which the missed MI diagnosis rate is very low.

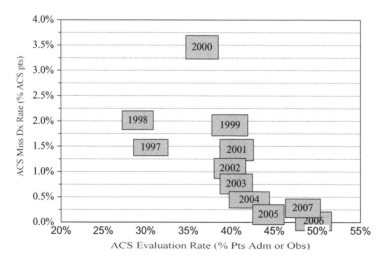

Figure 19.1 Acute Coronary Syndrome (ACS) Evaluation Rate vs Acute Coronary Syndrome (ACS) Miss Diagnosis Rate

Performance improvement efforts focus on lowering the physicians' threshold for observation so they observe all patients who might have a serious dangerous disease and lower the missed diagnosis rate to near zero. For a syndrome (e.g., CP chief complaint) it is the rate of missed diagnosis and the rate of testing (e.g., for CP, it is rule-out MI testing rate). There is an average performance with a missed diagnosis rate of 2% to 5% (e.g., 2–5% of patients with acute MI have their diagnosis missed at the initial ED evaluation). The ideal is zero-missed diagnosis rate with the goal being best practice performance always on the journey toward zero. With feedback to individual physicians of their cases with a missed diagnosis and feedback to the group of lessons learned, both individuals and the entire group of physicians can lower their threshold for observation (extended evaluations) rather than discharge home after the initial ED evaluation. In this example (Figure 19.1) the group diagnostic performance went from 2% to < 0.5% missed MI rate as the threshold for observation lowered with the percentage of ED CP patients with a rule-out MI rate increased from 35% to 50%.

Threshold for Inpatient Admission: Observation Usage Rate

Observation usage rate is the metric to judge whether the threshold to admit patients to the inpatient service is too low or too high. It is for a given chief complaint the number of observation patients with final diagnosis of the chief complaint divided by the number of observation patients with final diagnosis of the chief complaint plus the number of admitted inpatient patients with final diagnosis of the chief complaint. For example, the CP observation usage rate is calculated by dividing the number of observation CP patients with a final diagnosis of CP by the number of observation CP patients and the number of inpatient admit patients with the final diagnosis of CP. If the CP observation usage is very high (e.g., 90%), then there is a quality-of-care issue because the only patients being admitted are those with very high probability of disease. If moderate probability of disease patients were admitted as inpatients, then the CP observation usage rate would be lower because there would be patients evaluated in the inpatient service who turned out to not have a serious dangerous

disease and were given a final diagnosis of CP. If the CP observation usage is very low (e.g., 10%), then there is a utilization issue because many patients with low probability of disease were admitted. If patients with low probability of disease were observed rather than admitted as inpatients, then the CP observation usage would be higher because there would be many evaluated in the observation unit who turned out to not have a serious disease and were given a final diagnosis of CP.

The Utilization Review Process

Severity of illness (SI) and intensity of service (IS) are the yin and yang of medical necessity (see Chapter 66 Medical Necessity). There must be documentation of both to justify acute inpatient admission. Patients needing acute care hospitalization must have documentation by the clinician that shows SI to the nurse who is performing primary Utilization Review (UR) review using a UR screening system (such as Interqual) or to the physician (when there is no evidence of Medical Necessity on primary UR review) who is performing the secondary UR review. Patients needing acute care hospitalization must also have documentation by the clinician that shows IS to the nurse performing primary UR review provision or to the physician (when there is no evidence of IS on primary UR review) performing the secondary UR review.

Primary UR review is performed by a UR nurse using Interqual or other screening UR programs. The UR nurse identifies SI consistent with acute inpatient hospitalization from documentation of serious objective findings. These can be abnormal lab tests such as serum potassium less than 2.0 or they can abnormal physical findings such as low systolic blood pressure consistent with shock. The nurse identifies IS consistent with acute inpatient hospitalization from the orders for therapy documented by the clinician.

Secondary UR review is performed by a UR physician using his or her clinical judgment. The UR physician examines the clinician's documentation for what is documented in SI. This can be the clinician documentation of an admitting diagnosis that requires inpatient hospitalization evaluation and treatment (e.g., acute MI). Or this can be when the admitting clinician has concern (moderate to high probability) that the patient

Table 19.1 ABCD2 TIA Risk Stratification Score

Age ≥ 60		Yes +1
BP ≥ 140/90 initial evaluation		Yes +1
Clinical Features of the TIA:	Unilateral weakness	+2
	Speech disturbance	+1
	Other Symptoms	+0
Duration of Symptoms	< 10 minutes	+0
	10–59 minutes	+1
	≥ 60 minutes	+2
Diabetes Mellitus in Patient's History		Yes +1

Table 19.2 Cardiac Risk Score Tool for Possible ACS

Nondiagnostic EKG Changes (1 point)

EKG ST segment changes (< 1 mm ST seg change)

or T wave changes or LBBB

Age/Sex (1 point)

(Male > 45 years old; Female > 55 years old)

Past History CAD (2 points)

(Angina or PCI or Coronary surgery or MI)

Cardiac Risk Factors (up to 5 points)

Family history of CAD

Hyperlipidemia

Diabetes mellitus

History of smoking

Hypertension

Chest Pain (up to 3 points)

Substernal

Exercise related

Relieved with NTG

Chest Pain Equivalent (up to 4 points)

Syncope

SOB/dyspnea

Rapid heart beat

Unexplained weakness

ADD UP TOTAL# POINTS ABOVE:

_____

(Each Risk Factor counts as 1 point except Past History CAD = 2 points)

has a serious dangerous diagnosis or is at risk of adverse event if not provided inpatient services. In these circumstances the UR physician examines the evidence for clinician's risk stratification. Inpatient admission is medically necessary if the findings are consistent with the patient being at risk of suffering an adverse event if treated by outpatient rather than inpatient level of care.

Risk Stratification

The level of evidence for the physician's risk stratification can range from very formal risk stratification systems to those based on judgment by experts. When there is a formal, evidence-based, nationally recognized system that is the most reliable approach. An example of a formal, evidence-based, nationally recognized risk stratification system is the ABCD2 risk stratification for transient ischemic attacks (TIAs)[1] (Table 19.1). The risk of suffering a stroke within days is proportional to the score with moderate to high risk if the score is 4 or more. Less reliable evidence for risk stratification than the use of evidence based guidelines from national societies and other evidence in the literature is by appropriate physicians and leadership in the health care institution to form an institutional consensus. An example of such a consensus is the CP risk stratification in Table 19.2 derived from the American College of Cardiology guidelines and

from the TIMI score.[2] For many clinical situations there is no formal risk stratification system in existence and in such circumstances the physician makes a judgment on what is the patient's most likely disease and what is the risk to the patient. Clarity in the physician's documentation is important for those performing the UR review for evidence for medical necessity and more importantly for working to improve the accuracy of the risk stratification.

The goal of the physician's risk stratification is to accurately place the patient in the correct level of care. With many patients it is clear after their initial evaluation that they need acute care hospitalization and with others it is clear they are safe to release home. But with some it is not clear whether or not they have a serious condition and observation is a tool to clarify their diagnosis. Observation is appropriate for those whom the physician judges as having some risk/probability of disease and observation is needed to clarify their situation (threshold for observation). Observation is not appropriate for those who have moderate to high risk/probability of disease and need inpatient hospitalization (threshold for inpatient admission).

References

1) Johnston SC, Rothwell PM, Nguyen-Huynh MN, et al. Validation and refinement of scores to predict very early stroke risk after transient ischaemic attack. *Lancet* 2007;369(9558): 283–292.

2) Scott Wright R, Anderson JL, Adams CD, et al. Table 6 and Table 7 of 2011 ACCF/AHA Focused Update incorporated into the ACC/AHA 2007 Guidelines for the Management of Patients with Unstable Angina/ Non–ST-Elevation Myocardial Infarction. *J Am Coll Cardiol*, 2011; 57: 215–367.

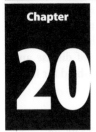

Chapter

20

Accountable Care Organizations

Kayur V. Patel, MD, FACP, FACPE, FACHE, FACEP
Igor Kozunov, MBA, MHA

Introduction

Accountable Care Organizations (ACOs) are the future of our health care landscape, and for Observation Medicine (OM), the future is very bright. The demand for efficiency and improved outcomes placed on ACOs will give rise to Observation Units (OUs) where patient–physician collaboration will be improved, acute testing will be provided timely and accurately, and care coordination and efficiency will rule the day. Hospitals of tomorrow will look drastically different to insiders from the way they do today and OM will be at the forefront of the upcoming changes.

Accountable Care Organizations Aim to Disrupt the Health Care Industry

ACOs are poised to disrupt the medical industry and change medical care as we know it. Such is the hope of those who believe that poor care coordination is at the center of our health care woes. To proponents of better care coordination, an ACO is the long-awaited panacea. ACOs are a force that will finally make health care organizations care about efficiency and outcomes. A policy that will realign financial incentives and teach providers to do better rather than doing more. One thing is certain – if these hopes come true, the coming changes will thrust OM front and center as a prominent force that will help lead many hospitals to salvation.

So What Exactly is an ACO?

Since the 1970s, one of the scariest three-letter acronyms in Medicine was HMO (Health Maintenance Organization). This failed policy invention is blamed for much modern anguish. Its legacy is a jaded medical community trained to distrust any policy innovation, however well-intentioned it may be.

Upon its first introduction, the vague concept of an ACO set off countless alarms as cynical physicians suspected ACOs of being a poorly concealed attempt at reviving the HMO formula. Even ACO's origins resembled those of HMO. Both are policy inventions, introduced by inventive policy entrepreneurs. In the case of ACO, we have Dr. Elliott Fisher to thank.

Dr. Fisher, the Director of the Center for Health Policy Research at Dartmouth Medical School, introduced the concept of an ACO in 2006 in a discussion with the Medicare Payment Advisory Commission. The new term remained out of the spotlight until it was adopted and popularized by politicians jockeying for a federal health care overhaul.

In 2010, only 4 years after its inception, the once-vague term became a reality. Signed into law as part of the Patient Protection and Affordable Care Act in 2010 by President Obama, ACOs took aim at business-as-usual in health care.

Centers for Medicare and Medicaid Services (CMS) describes ACOs as "groups of doctors, hospitals, and other health care providers, who come together voluntarily to give coordinated high quality care to their Medicare patients."[1]

CMS continues, "The goal of coordinated care is to ensure that patients, especially the chronically ill, get the right care at the right time, while avoiding unnecessary duplication of services and preventing medical errors."[1]

For skeptics, ACO's founders clearly outlined the difference between an HMO and an ACO in the latter's three core principles:

- ACOs must be provider-led organizations with a strong base of primary care that are collectively accountable for quality and total per capita costs across the full continuum of care for a population of patients;
- Payments to ACOs need to be linked to quality improvements that also reduce overall costs; and

- ACOs must use reliable and progressively more sophisticated performance measurement, to support improvement and provide confidence that savings are achieved through improvements in care.[2]

Since the signing of the Act by President Obama, the medical community waited in tense anticipation. Finally, a year after the passage, ACO guidelines were finally issued in March 2011. Another year later, the first ACOs were approved by CMS in early 2012.

What the First ACOs Look Like

As of the writing of this chapter, Medicare announced its first 27 ACOs (150 additional ACO applications are pending). These early ACOs fall somewhere between what ACO cheerleaders and naysayers have been predicting. It is now clear that the concept was not dead-on-arrival, as some naysayers believed. Hundreds of hospitals and provider organizations are putting forth the time and the effort needed to join the ranks of ACOs. Yet, most organizations are being careful and not quick to move in, in contrast with the rosy predictions painted by ACO cheerleaders.

The majority of these early ACOs are surprisingly small. Many are barely over the required 5,000-patient threshold. Of the 27 first ACOs, only 10 are hospitals. The rest are smaller, physician-led organizations.[3]

What these early ACOs demonstrate is that health care organizations are taking the aims of CMS seriously. In the process, new strategies to improve care coordination and efficiency are being evaluated. Among them is the growing field of OM.

ACOs are Poised to Fuel Growth of Observation Medicine

For the world of OM, ACOs are set to fuel an unprecedented growth of the profession. It is clear to even the most skeptical observer that only a substantial improvement in inpatient care efficiency and outcomes will separate successful ACOs from the losers. OM is one of the few specialties prepared for the upcoming evolution of inpatient care and its practitioners are already being viewed by aspiring ACOs as key drivers of ACO strategy.

The early ACOs eased many fears among the skeptics. The anticipation that ACOs were going to be largely driven by hospitals failed to materialize thus far. Most early ACOs are physician-driven. The regulators are also being serious about anticompetitive concerns. Stark laws have not been loosened and hospitals were not given an opportunity to gobble up market share under an ACO banner.

The regulators made it clear that they are serious and the bar has been set high. ACOs cannot avoid downside risk and have to be all the way in or out. For those who choose to participate, the only way to make an ACO a profitable proposition is to meet CMS's goals.

CMS put in place 33 measures to determine whether participating ACOs earn their rewards.[4] Among these measures is a strong focus on Care Coordination and Patient Safety. As new ACOs search for ways to address these measures and meet CMS's benchmarks, OM is presented with a rare opportunity for professional *intrapreneurship* – an opportunity to craft a solid value proposition for the field and to solidify its central role in the growing ranks of ACOs.

Observation Units Become Crucial Components of ACO Strategy

By now, it is evident that private insurance companies will soon join the Federal Government in supporting ACOs. Together, they are poised to create a perfect storm that will force health care organizations to shift away from the traditional "do more–bill more" culture.

Today, many hospital business models can be described simply as "keeping their beds full." However, as financial incentives shift away from care volume and toward better outcomes and efficiency, the newly formed ACOs will find that keeping patients out of the hospital has become more profitable.

Faced with this new reality, health care executives are reconsidering their assumptions about how their organizations will make money in the future. One shift that is already taking place is the slow death of a general hospital bed. Traditionally, a full bed meant revenue and a reasonable margin for most hospitals. This assumption is being undone by CMS guidelines and an ACO's ability to prevent avoidable hospitalizations will soon separate the winners from the losers under the new model. Yet, many hospitals are full of excess general beds and their mere presence can often lead to an overuse of hospital's resources, regardless of the community's true needs.[5] Enter an OU – the ACO's guard against avoidable hospitalizations and medical errors.

Designed for the strategic aims of their parent ACOs, OUs facilitate patient-physician interaction, rapid acute testing, and care coordination. The results of the growth of such units will include more efficient care, speedy testing and discharges, improved patient-physician collaboration, and focused care coordination – all gradually closing the traditional fault lines that are common in many community hospitals.

In the drive toward ACOs, OUs will change the entire landscape of a community hospital. Hospitals of tomorrow will no longer possess massive inventories of general beds. Most will consist of three main hubs: the Emergency Department, Intensive Care Units, and Observation Units. While all hospital departments will be affected by the ACO model, some of the most dramatic results will be driven mainly by Observation Medicine – the field that is no longer ahead of its time and whose practitioners will help bridge the gap between hospitals of today and our collective vision for tomorrow.

1. Centers for Medicare and Medicaid Services. Accountable Care Organizations [homepage on the Internet]. Available from www.cms.gov/Medicare/Medicare-Fee-for-Service-Payment/ACO/index.html?redirect=/aco/ (Accessed February 2016)

2. McClellan M, McKethan A, Lewis J, et al. A national strategy to put accountable care into practice. *Health Affairs*, 2010; 29(5):982–990. Available from http://content.healthaffairs.org/content/29/5/982 (Accessed February 2016)

3. Centers for Medicare and Medicaid Services. First Accountable Care Organizations under the Medicare Shared Savings Program. Fact Sheets. 2012.

4. Medicare Program; Medicare Shared Savings Program: Accountable Care Organizations, final rule. 76 Fed. Reg. 212 (2012).

5. Goodman D, Grumbach K. Does Having More Physicians Lead to Better Health System Performance? *Journal of the American Medical Association*, 2008; 299(3): 335–337.

Chapter

21

Acute Medicine in the United Kingdom

Louella Vaughan, MBBS, MPhil, DPhil, FRACP

The context of Observation Medicine in the United Kingdom is internationally unique due to the recent development of Acute Medicine as a subspeciality branch of General (Internal) Medicine. This chapter will provide a brief overview of Acute Medicine in the UK, its links with British Emergency Medicine, and its role in Observation Medicine.

Overview

Acute Medicine was developed in the UK as a response to concerns about patient safety, the increasing numbers of medical hospital admissions, and the emergence of new treatments where timeliness is crucial to success.[1] Its rapid spread and integration into the fabric of the National Health Service, however, was driven by the "four hour rule," a governmental performance target introduced in 2003/4 which mandated that 98% of patients presenting to an Emergency Department (ED) must be seen, treated, and then admitted or discharged in under 4 hours.[2] There are now over 210 Acute Medical Units (AMUs) in the UK, which manage the majority (90%) of emergency medical admissions to hospital for the first 48–72 hours of stay. (See Chapters 16 and 17 on Extended or Complex Observation.)

Due to the rapid growth of the discipline, there is a high degree of variability across AMUs.[3] However, the units essentially form an intermediate area between the ED and the downstream wards with an appropriate allocation and organization of resources to manage the medically unwell patient. As a result, AMUs share features of both EDs and general medical wards. The ideal unit, as outlined in the Royal College of Physician's Acute Medicine Guidelines,[4] comprises a separate 'trolley area' for the further assessment and immediate treatment of patients, a high-dependency area for Level One and Two care, bedded bays, a small clinic area for outpatients,

and allied health assessment facilities. Although AMUs and EDs are ideally co-located, most units accept patients only via referral from the ED or a General Practitioner, with the ED retaining the task of primary assessment and triage of unscheduled emergency patients. Staffing in the units is multidisciplinary, with dedicated support from physiotherapy, occupational therapy, pharmacy, and other allied health staff. These broadly skilled teams are capable of not only delivering appropriate care to those patients with life-threatening illnesses, but also arranging and facilitating the early supported discharge of patients with less severe illness but complex needs.

The fact that Acute Medicine is a relatively new speciality has led to a particularly strong emphasis on patient safety and operational organization. Specialist society standards for AMUs[4, 5] refer specifically to the need for the rapid assessment of patients, the use of early warning scoring systems, ready access to diagnostic services, and timely and coordinated discharge planning. The use of key performance indicators to monitor unit performance, such as mortality and morbidity data, discharge and readmission rates, and patient experience, has been strongly encouraged and will be soon be governmentally mandated.

The extent to which AMUs have taken on the task of Observation Medicine varies from hospital to hospital and is dictated by local circumstances. Many larger hospitals or those where the AMU is not co-located with the ED will often also have traditional ED-led Observation Units (OU) or Clinical Decision Units (CDU). *(See Chapter 1 [clinical] and Chapter 2 [administrative] on observation medicine.)* Some hospitals have shared observational space, to which the ED, medical and/or surgical teams can place patients. Decisions about which unit is most appropriate for any given patient are usually governed by considerations regarding potential risk, rather than being tightly defined by condition. For example, many hospitals have a single protocol for chest pain, with the stipulation that those with low risk pain are admitted to the OU, those with intermediate or high risk to the AMU and those with very high risk directly to the Cardiology service. Similarly, patients with non-life-threatening overdoses tend to be cared for by EDs where the facility exists, with only serious or life-threatening overdoses being transferred for full inpatient care.

The size and nature of AMUs means that they are able to admit a broad range of conditions for observation, such as chest pain, deep venous thrombosis, rule-out pulmonary embolism, spontaneous pneumonthorax, pleural effusion, and cellulitis. In many AMUs, the care pathways include ambulatory components. It is usual care, for example, for a patient with suspected deep vein thrombosis to be treated predominantly as an outpatient, with the patient receiving his or her initial assessment and follow-up via the AMU before transitioning to full outpatient care. Similarly, AMU pathways for cellulitis often stipulate that patients are administered intravenous antibiotics for 24–48 hours, with poorly responding, but otherwise well patients then being transferred to an ambulatory pathway for ongoing intravenous antibiotics. Some patients return daily to the units for antibiotic administration, while others have nurses give their antibiotics at home with weekly medical review on the AMU. The multidisciplinary nature of the staffing also means that elderly patients, such as those with falls, can often be seen, rapidly assessed, and then discharged with increased or interim packages of care, thus avoiding lengthy inpatient stays.

Outcome

Although AMUs are almost ubiquitous throughout the UK, only a relatively small number of units have published before-and-after studies in peer-reviewed journals and only one unit has performed any economic modelling.[6] Two studies reported significant reductions in inpatient mortality; four studies found significant reductions in length of stay between 1.5 and 2.5 days; and eight studies described improvements in various aspects of hospital functioning, such as reductions in the numbers of emergency patients awaiting inpatient beds and improved patient triage to inpatient specialties. The non-peer-reviewed literature supports these findings.

The success of the model in the UK has led to its adoption in Australia, New Zealand and the Netherlands. Eight non-peer-reviewed reports of 48 units in Australia and New Zealand confirmed almost uniform reductions in length of stay (0.4 to 3.0 days), although a number of hospitals reported small increases in readmission rates.

Conclusion

Acute Medical Units have been a highly successful innovation in the United Kingdom, with rapid diffusion of the units throughout the UK. They have been shown to reduce length of stay, promote safe patient care, and improve other aspects of hospital functioning. With regard to observation medicine, many AMUs perform the same function as ED-led OUs, with patients being admitted for up to 48 hours for observation. A key point of difference, however, is the ability of AMUs to provide ongoing ambulatory care for patients.

References

1. Federation of Medical Royal Colleges. *Acute medicine: the physician's role. Proposals for the future. A working party report of the Federation of Medical Royal Colleges.* London: Royal College of Physicians; 2000.

2. Alberti G. *Transforming Emergency Care in England.* Department of Health, London; 2004.

3. Ward D, Potter J, Ingham J, et al. Acute medical care. The right person, in the right setting–first time: how does practice match the report recommendations? *Clin Med* 2009;9(6):553–6.

4. Royal College of Physicians of London. Acute medical care: the right person, in the right setting — first time. Report of the Acute Medicine Task Force. RCPL, London; 2007.

5. Royal College of Physicians of Edinburgh. *RCPE UK Consensus Statement on Acute Medicine.* RCPE, Edinburgh; 2008.

6. Scott I, Vaughan L, Bell D. Effectiveness of acute medical units in hospitals: a systematic review. *Int J Qual Health Care* 2009;21:397–407.

Part IV

Clinical

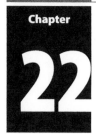

Chest Pain

Tertius T. Tuy, MD
W. Frank Peacock, MD, FACEP

Background

With 5.5 million patients per year presenting with chest pain (CP),[1] it is the second most common nontraumatic complaint to the emergency department (ED) after abdominal pain.[2] While a large proportion of patients with CP will ultimately be diagnosed with noncardiac pathology (gastrointestinal, pulmonary, psychiatric, etc.), up to 50% may have cardiac-related CP.[3] Because CP of cardiac origin can result in precipitous adverse outcomes, it is commonly the focus of prolonged evaluation. While this chapter will focus on the approach to the evaluation of CP that is potentially cardiac in origin, care should be given to consider alternative etiologies. Some of the most feared causes of acute CP are pulmonary embolus, pneumothorax, cardiac tamponade, aortic dissection, and acute coronary syndrome (ACS). Among these, ACS may be difficult to rule out in the ED setting, and may require a prolonged period of time to be effectively excluded. Thus observation units (OUs) are utilized providing an intermediate and supervised placement for patients requiring further evaluation.[4]

Since the clinical examination alone can rarely include or preclude the possibility of ACS, reperfusion therapy is heavily dependent on electrocardiograms (ECGs) and serial cardiac biomarker investigations. Without serial evaluations about 5% of patients with ACS could be misdiagnosed and potentially inappropriately sent home from the ED, which is associated with an increased mortality rate.[5,6] In order to prevent missed acute myocardial infarctions (AMIs), the American Heart Association and American College of Cardiology (AHA/ACC) have recommended that potential ACS patients should be observed for a short period of time while having serial cardiac biomarker testing, diagnostic imaging, and in some cases, provocative stress testing.[7]

OUs provide a location for patients to undergo these investigations. As reported in the Chest Pain Evaluation Registry (CHEPER), OUs have a miss rate of 0.4%, while EDs without an OU have a miss rate of 4.3%.[8] Furthermore, for patients with undifferentiated or atypical CP without diagnostic ECGs or cardiac biomarkers, the current guidelines from the American College of Cardiology and the American Heart Association suggest that these patients be evaluated in an OU.[4]

OUs have been shown to decrease missed MI rates, reduce length of stay (LOS), decrease costs, and improve patient satisfaction while maintaining equivalent or better patient outcomes. One of the earliest studies (data collected in 1993–1995) documented a decrease in the hospital admission rate, total cost, and LOS for an accelerated diagnostic protocol in a CP OU.[9] In this study, the mean total cost per patient was $1,528 for CP OU vs. $2,095 for inpatients (p < 0.01), and the mean LOS (in hours) was 33.1 for the CP OU vs. 44.8 hours (p < 0.01).[9] Likewise, other more recent analyses comparing CP OU to hospital admissions have demonstrated a decrease in both the number of admissions (54% vs. 37%) and the number of ACS patients discharged (14% vs. 6%), an increase in quality of life (at 6 months following treatment), and a decrease in costs of management[10] (all without changing the rate of cardiac events).[11] Newer technology using cardiac MRI in the OU reduced median hospitalization cost by $588 (95% CI $336 to $811) compared to inpatient strategy for patients with emergent non-low-risk CP.[12] Another study compared an ED OU with an in-hospital OU and found that fewer CP patients were converted to full inpatient admission from the ED OU: 7.9% vs. 19.2% of the in-hospital OU (p < 0.0001), and that the ED OU was more cost effective than the inpatient OU. The mean cost per patient for the ED OU was $889.87 (95% CI 862.8–916.9), while the inpatient OU totaled $1039.70 (95% CI 991.7–1087.7O).[13]

Other studies have found similar evaluation and outcome improvements. In the rule out myocardial ischemia (ROMIO) trial, a rapid ED-based rule out protocol was compared with routine hospital care. The rapid ED protocol patients had a shorter hospital stay (median 11.9 vs. 22.8 hours, p = 0.0001), lower initial ($893 vs. $1,349, p = 0.0001), and 30-day ($898 vs. $1,522, p = 0.0001) hospital charges than the patients with routine care.[14] Another study that compared patients admitted to a short stay unit with patients admitted as inpatients found similar results.[15] Patients eligible for admission to the OU were either admitted to the hospital in various units or to the OU. The median total costs at 6 months was significantly lower for the OU ($1,927) than for patients admitted to the wards ($4,712), step-down or intermediate care units ($4,031), or coronary care units ($9,201); although the cost was higher than for an ED visit ($403) (p < 0.0001). Moreover, the rate of major complications, recurrent myocardial infarction or cardiac death during the 6 months after the initial presentation was similar for those in the OU vs. those who were inpatients.[15]

These findings have not been limited to the United States. The Effectiveness and Safety of Chest Pain Assessment to Prevent Emergency Admission (ESCAPE) trial, a British study, demonstrated improved health utility at follow-up in the CP OU patients vs. inpatients. This was similar to the aforementioned studies done in the United States. The proportion of admitted patients decreased from 54% to 37% (p < 0.001), and the proportion discharged with ACS decreased from 14% to 6% (p = 0.264). Rates of cardiac events were unchanged. There was a saving of £78 per patient (p = 0.052). More importantly, there was a significant (p = 0.022) improved health utility during follow-up with 0.0137 quality-adjusted life years gained. From this analysis, the authors concluded that "Care in a chest pain observation unit can improve outcomes and may reduce costs to the health service. It seems to be more effective and more cost effective than routine care."[11]

The OU may offer improved patient satisfaction in low-risk CP patients compared to standard hospitalization.[11] The Chest Pain Evaluation in the Emergency Room (CHEER) study randomly assigned 424 patients with unstable angina to either a routine monitored bed under the care of the cardiology service (N = 212) or to the CP OU located in the ED under a strict protocol (N = 212). There was no significant difference in the rate of cardiac events between the two groups during the hospital stay (Odds Ratio [OR] 0.5 CI 0.19–1.29, p = 0.15), 30 days after discharge (OR 0.5 CI 0.2–1.24, p = 0.13), or event-free survival over 180 days (p = 0.58).[16] There were 15 primary events in the hospital admission group (13 myocardial infarction [MI], 2 congestive heart failure [CHF]) and only 7 events in the ED OU group (5 MI, 1 CHF, 1 death from cardiovascular causes). Resource use during the first 6 months was greater among the hospital admission group than among those in the ED OU group (p < 0.01).[16]

Thus the preponderance of the literature suggests that CP OUs are a safe and effective means of evaluating patients at low to intermediate risk of ACS. By providing an intermediate location for further care and evaluations, their use has alleviated an unnecessary financial burden on the patient and medical care system associated with unwarranted hospital admissions. At the same time it has similar rates of adverse events as those admitted to the hospital.[17]

Pathophysiology

CP associated with ACS is caused by myocardial ischemia from inadequate oxygen perfusion (oxygen supply relative to demand). Coronary artery disease predisposes patients to plaque rupture, and subsequent occlusion of the coronary vessels by platelet activation and thrombus formation. Ischemia and myocardial infarction leads to aberrations of the conduction system and/or the release of cellular components, which manifest as electrocardiographic or cardiac biomarker changes. The evaluation and management of patients with suspected ACS starts with the early detection of cellular injury with an electrocardiogram or cellular necrosis by cardiac biomarkers.

Risk Stratification

Classically, patients with pain consistent with ACS suffer from a substernal, crushing pain or pressure which lasts > 20 minutes. The pain may radiate to the arms, shoulders or jaw; it can be associated with diaphoresis, shortness of breath, or a sense of impending doom. However, several etiologies (esophageal spasm, gastroesophageal reflux disease, musculoskeletal pain, etc.) may mimic typical angina. Additionally, ACS may present with atypical symptoms and may be subsequently misdiagnosed. Patients with atypical symptoms tend to be female, diabetic, and elderly. Regardless of the types/natures of CP, at a minimum, patients should be adequately risk stratified for ACS. Yet with its limited sensitivity and specificity for ACS, accurate risk stratification based solely on clinical examination is not recommended.

Risk Scores

Since clinical evaluation lacks precision at identifying CP patients as high risk (c-stat 0.55), several risk scoring systems have been developed to stratify patients into low, moderate, or high risk for ACS. Patients with high risk are likely to benefit from immediate reperfusion therapy, while those of intermediate to low risk may benefit from observation. A number of validated risk scoring systems exist, and include Thrombolysis in Myocardial Infarction (TIMI), Platelet Glycoprotein IIb/IIIa in Unstable Angina Using Integrilin Therapy (PURSUIT), and the Global Registry of Acute Coronary Events (GRACE) risk scores. It is open to debate as to which risk score is superior in determining risk. A cohort study of 460 ACS patients by de Araújo et al. looked at the predictive ability of these three risk scores to predict death or MI within 1 year. It found that in terms of predictive accuracy, the GRACE score (c-stat 0.715, CI: 0.672–0.756) outperformed both the PURSUIT (c-stat 0.630, CI: 0.584–0.674) and the TIMI scores (c-stat 0.585, CI: 0.539–0.631).[18] However, Lee et al. performed an analysis on 4,743 patients presenting to the ED with potential ACS and found less variation between the scoring systems for predicting death, MI, and revascularization within 30 days. The TIMI score had the best predictive value (0.757 CI: 0.728–0.758), followed by GRACE (0.728 CI 0.701–0.755) and PURSUIT scores (0.691 CI 0.662–0.720).[19] Ultimately, regardless of which score is utilized, all have sufficient predictive value and may be used to determine patients at risk for ischemic events. Patients at low to moderate risk are good candidates for OU admission.

Criteria for the Observation Unit

Inclusion Criteria

Patients of low to intermediate risk are candidates for admission to the OU for further evaluation. Appropriate OU candidates would include:

1. CP that is potentially related to ischemic heart disease or CP that is unlikely related to ischemic heart disease but the patient has a significant history of coronary artery disease
2. Stable vital signs and hemodynamic presentation (no hypotension, hypoperfusion, or mental status change)
3. Comorbidities requiring low intensity of care
4. Negative or indeterminate ECG
5. Negative or indeterminate cardiac biomarkers

Exclusion Criteria

Patients who are at high risk for ACS are not appropriate candidates and should be admitted for hospital management. These patients may have:

1. Ischemic changes on ECG (acute ST-changes, new left bundle branch block and newly inverted T-waves believed to be ischemic in origin)
2. Cardiac marker results consistent with acute myocardial infarction (e.g., significantly elevated or rising)
3. Unlikely probability of going home within 24 hours
4. High risk by scoring system

Observation Unit Evaluation

CP has been the number one reason for admission and discharge from the OU between 2001 and 2008.[20] Although the majority of patients admitted to the CP OU will have a final diagnosis that is either musculoskeletal, gastroesophageal, or nonspecific in origin, the main focus is the rule-out of an ACS. Existing rapid rule-out protocols use a multi-marker or delta biomarkers approach, which may exclude non ST-elevated myocardial infarction (NSTEMI) in as little as 90 minutes. However, these protocols are for a certain subset of patients at low risk for ACS and if ruled out, they should not be admitted to the OU unless they require further evaluation. Several noncardiac acute etiologies of chest pain (pneumonia, pneumothorax, pulmonary embolus, etc.) may also benefit from placement in the OU (see pneumonia Chapter 29, pneumothorax Chapter 30, and abdominal pain Chapter 45).

OUs provide an intermediate location for up to 24 hours of monitoring and evaluation in individuals with low to moderate suspicion for ACS. OUs have been proven to improve outcomes, decrease LOS, reduce costs, and improve overall patient satisfaction. Evaluations revolve predominantly around serial cardiac markers, serial ECGs, and stress testing. Although telemetry is commonly available for use in the OU, a study of 248 patients in a CP OU demonstrated that telemetry did not improve detection rates of cardiac events or admissions for arrhythmias compared to patients without telemetry.[21]

Serial Electrocardiogram (ECG)

The ECG is an important part of the investigation of potential ACS. The ECG evolution of an AMI typically begins with hyperacute T waves, progresses to ST-elevation, which is then followed by Q and inverted T waves. Although the specificities for ECGs are adequate, they ultimately lack sufficient sensitivity for discharge decision making. Further, ECG changes are not specific to ACS and other diagnoses should be considered (Table 22.1). The initial ECG has a poor sensitivity (55.4%) for detecting an MI while serial ECGs modestly improve the sensitivity to 68.1%.[22] One study found nondiagnostic ECGs (secondary ST and T segment changes, < 2 mm ST elevation, previous ischemic changes, etc.) were associated with missed MI and unstable angina (UA).[23] Delayed clinical presentations may increase the difficulty to interpret ECGs and may contribute to a decreased sensitivity. In fact, after 12 hours ECGs may start to normalize and interpretations may become more difficult. To prevent misinterpretation of normalizing ECG, serial assessment may reveal evolving changes. It is recommended that a baseline ECG be obtained within 10 minutes of arrival to the ED and repeated thereafter if clinical suspicion remains. Compared to a single ECG, serial ECGs could adjudicate 16.2% more AMIs and improve diagnostic utility.[24]

Cardiac Markers

In the absence of a diagnostic ECG, cardiac markers (e.g., CK-MB, troponin) serve as a primary tool for ruling out ACS. In the setting of an anginal equivalent, elevation of cardiac markers above the 99th percentile of the upper reference limit is highly associated with cardiac necrosis from ACS. However, depending on the assay platform utilized, cardiac marker studies may take 8–12 hours from the initial ischemic event before becoming diagnostic for ACS. In

Table 22.1: ECG Differentials for STEMI

Increased T-wave Amplitude

 – Acute Myocardial Infarction

 – Benign Early Repolarization

 – Hyperkalemia

 – Left Ventricular Hypertrophy

ST-Elevation

 – Acute Myocardial Infarction

 – Benign Early Repolarization

 – Left Ventricular Hypertrophy

 – Left or Right Bundle Branch Block

 – Left Ventricular Aneurysm

 – NonSpecific Intraventricular Conduction Defect

 – Pericarditis

 – Pulmonary Embolism

 – Takotsubo Cardiomyopathy

 – J wave of Osborne

Q-waves

 – False Lead Poling

 – Hypertrophic Obstructive Cardiomyopathy

 – Left Bundle Branch Block

 – Left Ventricular Hypertrophy

 – Preexcitation in Wolf Parkinson White

T-wave Inversion

 – Acute Myocarditis

 – Long QTc

 – Pacemaker

 – Pericarditis

 – Persistent Juvenile T-Wave Pattern

 – Pulmonary Embolism

 – Stroke

 – Takotsubo Cardiomyopathy

fact, even when using newer higher sensitivity troponins, approximately 30% of patients with confirmed NSTEMI had initially negative cardiac markers.[25] Newer troponin platforms demonstrate little improvement in diagnostic accuracy when performed in serial fashion at least 3 hours after symptom onset. Therefore the 2011 European Society of Cardiology (ESC) recommendations are that a second set of cardiac markers should be repeated in as little as 6 hours from the onset of symptoms. Other professional societies (ACCF/AHA, ACEP, etc.), which have not updated their guidance, still have recommendations suggesting that serial troponin measures are required for 8–12 hours after symptom onset[4,26], or 90 min after an initially negative baseline troponin value for patients presenting within 8 hours of symptoms.[26] Because ED patients may spend hours waiting for their serial cardiac markers to return, the OU provides an alternate location for patients to be evaluated while minimizing the costs associated with ED or in-hospital room.

Troponin, CK-MB, and Myoglobin

When cardiac necrosis occurs, creatinine kinase MB isoform, myoglobin, and cardiac troponin are released into the blood stream. Although sensitivities and specificities vary with time (Table 22.2), cardiac troponins tend to have the greatest specificity and sensitivity among the three. Thus the ACC/AHA and the ESC suggests that cardiac troponins should the marker of choice for cardiac necrosis when available. Interpretation and application of cardiac biomarkers requires knowledge on their natural history following cardiac insult.[27] Cardiac troponin becomes detectable within 3–6 hours of myocardial necrosis, peaks at 12 hours and may remaining elevated for approximately 14 days. High sensitivity troponin tests are capable of detecting cardiac necrosis earlier and can identify reinfarction (using delta values). Of the other markers, myoglobin and CK-MB peak at about 4 and 12 hours, and remain elevated for 12 and 24–48 hours respectively. Therefore, CK-MB and myoglobin can also be used when there is suspicion for infarction or reinfarction.

Table 22.2: Standard Cardiac Biomarkers

	Onset	Peak	Disappearance	Advantages	Disadvantages	Sensitivity (Initial/ Serial)*	Specificity (Initial/ Serial)*
Myoglobin	2 hours	4 hours	8–12 hours	– Short half-life allows detection of reinfarction – Rapid rule-out of AMI	– Nonspecific to cardiac muscle	49%/89%	91%/87%
CKMB	4 hours	12–24 hours	2–3 days	– Short half-life allows detection of reinfarction	– Slightly nonspecific to cardiac muscle (large amount of skeletal muscle damage: rhabdomyolysis, muscular degeneration, trauma)	42%/79%	97%/96%
Troponin I/T	3–6 hours	12 hours	7–14 days	– Able to detect recent infarct – Specific to myocytes	– Difficult to detect reinfarction	39%/ 90–100%	93%/ 83–96%

* Sensitivity and specificity in detection of acute myocardial infarction

Provocative Stress Test and/or Imaging

In selected ACS patients with negative serial biomarkers and ECGs, provocative stress tests may be indicated.[28–33] However, there is some contention whether a stress test while in the OU confers a mortality benefit compared to an early outpatient stress test.[34]

Depending on the institution, a variety of stress tests may be implemented during the OU stay. Exercise stress tests (assessed by ECG or echocardiogram) are cost-efficient, easily performed, and provide insight into presence of inducible ischemia from physiologic stress. A study compared ED-initiated cardiac treadmill exercise stress testing with admitted patients.[35] The average patient charge was $467 with a LOS of 5.5 hours for the ED stress test patients, while the inpatient average patient charge was $2,340 with a 2-day LOS.[35] For individuals who cannot meet the target heart rate for a variety of reasons (inability to exercise, structural deficits, extreme pain), a pharmacological stress test may be used instead.

Although exercise stress tests are commonly implemented, there are other modalities of cardiac imaging that can be used to evaluate the likelihood of ACS. Another technique of imaging, myocardial perfusion imaging (MPI) uses technetium-99m and coronary artery vasodilators to provide information about relative blood flow to the myocardium. In detecting coronary artery disease MPI has a good sensitivity of 92% and a decent specificity of 63–71%.[33] This should be considered for women as exercise treadmill test in women has poor negative predictive value (68%) for coronary artery disease and may misrepresent the presence or absence of coronary artery disease in 36%.[36]

Computer tomography angiogram (CTA) can also provide insight into whether there is significant coronary plaque or stenosis. In fact CTA had a sensitivity of 100% and specificity of 54% for detection of a coronary plaque.[37] In the Rule-out Myocardial Infarction using Computer Assisted Tomography (ROMICAT) study, CTA was used for rapid rule-out of low risk ACS patients in the ED. ROMICAT demonstrated that low-risk CP patients with a negative CTA had 100% negative predictive value for coronary artery disease and could be discharged home immediately.[37]

Cardiac magnetic resonance (CMR) imaging can provide information about cardiac function, ischemia, viability, and coronary anatomy. In individuals with negative ECGs and cardiac markers, dobutamine stress CMR was more sensitive (86.2 vs. 74.3%) and specific (85.7 and 69.8%) for detecting 50% stenosis than a stress echo.[38] When using adenosine, perfusion CMR had a sensitivity and specificity for detecting coronary artery disease of 90% and 81% respectively.[39]

Immediate Management of Newly Confirmed ACS in the OU

During the OU stay, if patients are identified as high risk for an ACS event (positive serial biomarkers or ECGs, a clinical presentation consistent with ACS, or developing new or worsening heart failure symptoms) they should receive guideline-consistent ACS care. This includes antiplatelet and antithrombotic therapy. Oxygen, nitrates, and morphine have no demonstrated mortality benefits[40–42] and their use could be given for symptomatic treatment. Beta-blockade may be considered (except when there is evidence of heart block, hypotension, and/or acute heart failure). The physician should decide whether the patient is a candidate for either reperfusion therapy or medical management, and hospital admission to the appropriate intensive care unit should be arranged. Subsequent management of ACS should be done on an inpatient basis.

Disposition

Low-risk patients who have had an acute ACS excluded may be candidates for early discharge without a myocardial perfusion evaluation. The ASPECT study reported outcomes in patients with TIMI risk scores of zero at zero and 2-hour serial biomarker testing results and found early discharge, rather than OU stress testing, an effective strategy.[43] The decision on whether higher-risk patients require immediate evocative myocardial perfusion evaluation, or may be discharged for outpatient stress testing, is less clear. Patients discharged with elevated risk (elevated cardiac markers, ST-depressions, advanced age, or history of HF) can have up to 14-fold increase in mortality and they may benefit from earlier stress testing.[4]

Chest Pain Center Quality Improvement

While a number of professional societies (AHA, ACC, ESC) provide extensive recommendations on the management of patients with confirmed ACS, few detail specific "best practices" for the patient with suspected but unconfirmed ACS. The Society of Chest Pain Centers and Providers (SCPCP) currently accredits CP OUs on their process for evaluating patients with suspected ACS. While little objective data exists establishing improved outcomes after any quality certification process (e.g., Joint Commission Certification), using the Centers for Medicare and Medicaid Studies database, SCPCP accreditation is associated with markedly greater rates of guideline compliance than nonaccredited CP centers.[44]

Summary

In the management of CP, the observation unit serves as a location to safely determine if an ACS exists. Patients who have low to intermediate suspicion for ACS may be effectively managed during the < 24-hour placement. Observed care, serial cardiac markers and ECGs, as well as provocative stress test and imaging are the foundation for OU care. Therefore, in this selected patient population, the OU strategy can be used without incurring added risk and reduces the unnecessary cost associated with prolonged inpatient admission stay. Once ACS and other serious pathology have been ruled out, patients may be safely discharged and managed in an outpatient setting.

References

1. Bhuiya FA, Pitts SR, McCaig LF. Emergency department visits for chest pain and abdominal pain: United States, 1999–2008. *NCHS Data Brief*. 2010 Sep;(43):1–8.

2. Nawar EW, Niska RW, Xu J. National Hospital Ambulatory Medical Care Survey: 2005 emergency department summary. *Adv Data*. 2007 Jun 29;(386):1–32.

3. Eslick GD. Usefulness of chest pain character and location as diagnostic indicators of an acute coronary syndrome. *Am J Cardiol*. 2005 May 15; 95(10):1228–1231.

4. Anderson JL, Adams CD, Antman EM, et al. ACC/AHA 2007 Guidelines for the Management of Patients With Unstable Angina/Non-ST-Elevation Myocardial Infarction: A Report of the American College of Cardiology/American Heart Association Task Force on Practice Guidelines (Writing Committee to Revise the 2002 Guidelines for the Management of Patients With Unstable Angina/Non-ST-Elevation Myocardial Infarction) Developed in Collaboration with the American College of Emergency Physicians, the Society for Cardiovascular Angiography and Interventions, and the Society of Thoracic Surgeons Endorsed by the American Association of Cardiovascular and Pulmonary Rehabilitation and the Society for Academic Emergency Medicine. *J Am Coll Cardiol*. 2007 Aug 14;50 (7):e1–157.

5. Lee TH, Rouan GW, Weisberg MC, et al. Clinical characteristics and natural history of patients with acute myocardial infarction sent home from the emergency room. *Am J Cardiol*. 1987 Aug 1;60(4):219–224.

6. Body R, Carley S, Wibberley C, et al. The value of symptoms and signs in the emergent diagnosis of acute coronary syndromes. *Resuscitation*. 2010 Mar; 81(3):281–286.

7. Wright RS, Anderson JL, Adams CD, et al. 2011 ACCF/AHA focused update incorporated into the ACC/AHA 2007 Guidelines for the Management of Patients with Unstable Angina/Non-ST-Elevation Myocardial Infarction: a report of the American College of Cardiology Foundation/American Heart Association Task Force on Practice Guidelines developed in collaboration with the American Academy of Family Physicians, Society for Cardiovascular Angiography and Interventions, and the Society of Thoracic Surgeons. *J Am Coll Cardiol*. 2011 May 10;57(19):e215–367.

8. Graff LG, Dallara J, Ross MA, et al. Impact on the care of the emergency department chest pain patient from the chest pain evaluation registry (CHEPER) study. *Am J Cardiol*. 1997 Sep 1; 80(5):563–568.

9. Roberts RR, Zalenski RJ, Mensah EK, et al. Costs of an emergency department-based accelerated diagnostic protocol vs hospitalization in patients with chest pain: a randomized controlled trial. *JAMA*. 1997 Nov 26;278(20):1670–1676.

10. Goodacre S, Dixon S. Is a chest pain observation unit likely to be cost effective at my hospital? Extrapolation of data from a

randomised controlled trial. *Emerg Med J.* 2005 Jun;22(6):418–422.

11. Goodacre S, Nicholl J, Dixon S, et al. Randomised controlled trial and economic evaluation of a chest pain observation unit compared with routine care. *BMJ.* 2004 Jan 31;328(7434):254.

12. Miller CD, Hwang W, Hoekstra JW, et al. Stress cardiac magnetic resonance imaging with observation unit care reduces cost for patients with emergent chest pain: a randomized trial. *Ann Emerg Med.* 2010 Sep;56(3):209–219 e2.

13. Jagminas L, Partridge R. A comparison of emergency department versus inhospital chest pain observation units. *Am J Emerg Med.* 2005 Mar;23(2):111–113.

14. Gomez MA, Anderson JL, Karagounis LA, et al. An emergency department-based protocol for rapidly ruling out myocardial ischemia reduces hospital time and expense: results of a randomized study (ROMIO). *J Am Coll Cardiol.* 1996 Jul;28(1):25–33.

15. Gaspoz JM, Lee TH, Weinstein MC, et al. Cost-effectiveness of a new short-stay unit to "rule out" acute myocardial infarction in low risk patients. *J Am Coll Cardiol.* 1994 Nov 1;24(5):1249–1259.

16. Farkouh ME, Smars PA, Reeder GS, et al. A Clinical Trial of a Chest-Pain Observation Unit for Patients with Unstable Angina. *New England Journal of Medicine.* 1998;339(26):1882–1888.

17. Cullen MW, Reeder GS, Farkouh ME, et al. Outcomes in patients with chest pain evaluated in a chest pain unit: the chest pain evaluation in the emergency room study cohort. *Am Heart J.* 2011 May;161(5):871–877.

18. de Araújo Gonçalves P, Ferreira J, Aguiar C, et al.

TIMI, PURSUIT, and GRACE risk scores: sustained prognostic value and interaction with revascularization in NSTE-ACS. *European Heart Journal.* 2005 May;26(9):865–872.

19. Lee B, Chang AM, Matsuura AC, et al. Comparison of cardiac risk scores in ED patients with potential acute coronary syndrome. *Crit Pathw Cardiol.* 2011 Jun;10(2):64–68.

20. Venkatesh AK, Geisler BP, Gibson Chambers JJ, et al. Use of observation care in US emergency departments, 2001 to 2008. *PLoS One.* 2011;6(9):e24326.

21. Grossman SA, Shapiro NI, Mottley JL, et al. Is telemetry useful in evaluating chest pain patients in an observation unit? *Intern Emerg Med.* 2011 Dec;6(6):543–546.

22. Nable JV, Brady W. The evolution of electrocardiographic changes in ST-segment elevation myocardial infarction. *Am J Emerg Med.* 2009 Jul;27(6):734–746.

23. Pope JH, Aufderheide TP, Ruthazer R, et al. Missed diagnoses of acute cardiac ischemia in the emergency department. *N Engl J Med.* 2000 Apr 20;342(16):1163–1170.

24. Fesmire FM, Percy RF, Bardoner JB, et al. Usefulness of automated serial 12-lead ECG monitoring during the initial emergency department evaluation of patients with chest pain. *Ann Emerg Med.* 1998 Jan;31(1):3–11.

25. Meune C, Balmelli C, Twerenbold R, et al. Patients with acute coronary syndrome and normal high-sensitivity troponin. *Am J Med.* 2011 Dec;124(12):1151–1157.

26. Fesmire FM, Decker WW, Diercks DB, et al. Clinical policy: critical issues in the evaluation and management

of adult patients with non-ST-segment elevation acute coronary syndromes. *Ann Emerg Med.* 2006 Sep;48(3):270–301.

27. Wu AH, Apple FS, Gibler WB, et al. National Academy of Clinical Biochemistry Standards of Laboratory Practice: recommendations for the use of cardiac markers in coronary artery diseases. *Clin Chem.* 1999 Jul;45(7):1104–1121.

28. Pellikka PA, Nagueh SF, Elhendy AA, et al. American Society of Echocardiography recommendations for performance, interpretation, and application of stress echocardiography. *J Am Soc Echocardiogr.* 2007 Sep;20(9):1021–1041.

29. Bluemke DA, Achenbach S, Budoff M, et al. Noninvasive coronary artery imaging: magnetic resonance angiography and multidetector computed tomography angiography: a scientific statement from the american heart association committee on cardiovascular imaging and intervention of the council on cardiovascular radiology and intervention, and the councils on clinical cardiology and cardiovascular disease in the young. *Circulation.* 2008 Jul 29; 118(5):586–606.

30. Garber AM, Solomon NA. Cost-effectiveness of alternative test strategies for the diagnosis of coronary artery disease. *Ann Intern Med.* 1999 May 4; 130(9):719–728.

31. Kim C, Kwok YS, Heagerty P, et al. Pharmacologic stress testing for coronary disease diagnosis: A meta-analysis. *Am Heart J.* 2001 Dec;142(6):934–944.

32. Gianrossi R, Detrano R, Mulvihill D, et al. Exercise-induced ST depression in the diagnosis of coronary artery disease. A meta-analysis.

Circulation. 1989 Jul; 80(1):87–98.

33. Amini B, Patel CB, Lewin MR, et al. Diagnostic nuclear medicine in the ED. *Am J Emerg Med.* 2011 Jan; 29(1):91–101.

34. Rahman F, Mitra B, Cameron PA, et al. Stress testing before discharge is not required for patients with low and intermediate risk of acute coronary syndrome after emergency department short stay assessment. *Emerg Med Australas.* 2010 Oct; 22(5):449–456.

35. Kerns JR, Shaub TF, Fontanarosa PB. Emergency cardiac stress testing in the evaluation of emergency department patients with atypical chest pain. *Ann Emerg Med.* 1993 May; 22(5):794–798.

36. Curzen N, Patel D, Clarke D, et al. Women with chest pain: is exercise testing worthwhile? *Heart.* 1996 Aug;76(2):156–160.

37. Hoffmann U, Bamberg F, Chae CU, et al. Coronary computed tomography angiography for early triage of patients with acute chest pain: the ROMICAT (Rule Out Myocardial Infarction using Computer Assisted Tomography) trial. *J Am Coll Cardiol.* 2009 May 5; 53(18):1642–1650.

38. Nagel E, Lehmkuhl HB, Bocksch W, et al. Noninvasive diagnosis of ischemia-induced wall motion abnormalities with the use of high-dose dobutamine stress MRI: comparison with dobutamine stress echocardiography. *Circulation.* 1999 Feb 16; 99(6):763–770.

39. Hamon M, Fau G, Nee G, et al. Meta-analysis of the diagnostic performance of stress perfusion cardiovascular magnetic resonance for detection of coronary artery disease. *J Cardiovasc Magn Reson.* 2010;12(1):29.

40. Cabello JB, Burls A, Emparanza JI, et al. Oxygen therapy for acute myocardial infarction. *Cochrane Database Syst Rev.* 2010;(6):CD007160.

41. Yusuf S, Collins R, MacMahon S, et al. Effect of intravenous nitrates on mortality in acute myocardial infarction: an overview of the randomised trials. *Lancet.* 1988 May 14; 1(8594):1088–92.

42. Meine TJ, Roe MT, Chen AY, et al. Association of intravenous morphine use and outcomes in acute coronary syndromes: results from the CRUSADE Quality Improvement Initiative. *Am Heart J.* 2005 Jun;149(6):1043–1049.

43. Than M, Cullen L, Reid CM, et al. A 2-h diagnostic protocol to assess patients with chest pain symptoms in the Asia-Pacific region (ASPECT): a prospective observational validation study. *Lancet.* 2011 Mar 26;377 (9771):1077–1084.

44. Ross MA, Amsterdam E, Peacock WF, et al. Chest pain center accreditation is associated with better performance of centers for Medicare and Medicaid services core measures for acute myocardial infarction. *Am J Cardiol.* 2008 Jul 15; 102(2):120–124.

Chapter 23

Heart Failure

Jieun Kim, MD
W. Frank Peacock, MD, FACEP

Introduction

Heart failure (HF) has been a consistently increasing burden in both clinical management and health care spending. Annual expenditures on HF management are massive. Beyond costs, HF is becoming one of the major causes of mortality in the United States.[1] More than 4 million Medicare beneficiaries have HF and approximately half will die within 5 years.[1] In 2008, the overall prevalence of HF reached 5.7 million people, with estimated direct and indirect cost of HF alone to exceed 37.2 billion dollars.[2] The majority of the HF cost is due to inpatient hospitalization. Because the incidence of HF is expected to increase dramatically due to the aging population and improved survival from acute coronary syndrome (ACS), new strategies to decrease the clinical burden and economic costs are needed.

Based on American College of Cardiology/American Heart Association (ACC/AHA) and Agency for Healthcare Research and Quality (AHRQ) guidelines, it has been suggested that up to 50% of admitted HF patients are low-risk and may be candidates for outpatient therapy.[3] In this context, the HF observation unit (OU) can be an innovative alternative means of managing selected HF patients in an acute setting. Clinical management in the OU can provide specialized care for HF patients and is reported to shorten hospital length of stay (LOS), reduce the number of intensive care unit (ICU) admissions, and decrease the rate of 30-day hospital readmissions, thus reducing health care cost without difference in outcome.[4]

In a prospective observational study, emergency department (ED) HF patients of equivalent severity who were admitted as inpatients were compared to those treated in the ED OU. The study found no significant difference in outcome, but major benefits from ED OU management in a decrease in time from ED triage to disposition, reduced mean bed hours of inpatient 58.5 hours to 25.7 hour in ED OU, and significant cost savings from $7824 as an inpatient to $4203 from ED OU.[5] Furthermore, another study shows that during the same time period, annualized hospital costs declined by nearly $100,000, predominately the result of the 30-day readmission avoidance advantage in ED OU.[6]

Presentation of HF in the Emergency Setting

The common presentations of acute decompensated heart failure (ADHF) in the ED are shortness of breath, fatigue, and swelling of the legs. The presentation could be either an acute pump dysfunction reflecting worsening of cardiac function, or an insidious presentation as a consequence of pathologic neurohormonal and hemodynamic cascade from myocardial stress. Without a worsening of underlying circulatory function, failure to adhere to prescribed medications or dietary regimes may also lead to ADHF presentation in the ED.[4, 7]

Effective ADHF management in the ED encompasses two objectives: first, to correctly diagnose ADHF and second, to initiate an appropriate treatment in a timely manner. Both aspects of care should be equally emphasized since inability to accomplish either could have deleterious effects in ADHF patients.

Diagnosis of ADHF

The first challenge of HF management begins in the ED, where rapid and accurate identification of ADHF is necessary.[6] HF is a clinical syndrome and its diagnosis is based on signs and symptoms from the patient's initial history and physical examination, supported by radiographic findings, and laboratory results, such as biomarkers.[8]

History and Physical Examination

The most common presenting symptom of HF is dyspnea. Unfortunately, a chief complaint of dyspnea is nonspecific since it can be produced by multiple other medical conditions such as COPD, asthma, pneumonia, and myocardial ischemia.[6] Moreover, other typical physical examination findings of ADHF (e.g., rales, peripheral edema) are nondiagnostic since they are also a common presentation of other comorbidities[8] and may be missing at hospital presentation.[9] For instance, in one study, rales, edema, and elevated mean jugular venous pressure were absent in 18 of 43 patients with a documented pulmonary capillary wedge pressure (PCWP) > 22 mmHg.[10] Unfortunately, diagnostic accuracy can further decrease with other confounding factors, such as gender. Female patients can present with atypical signs and symptoms of cardiovascular disease, which can contribute to diagnostic complexity in ADHF.[11]

Radiographic Findings and Biomarkers

Similarly, radiographic features of ADHF are not always reliable. Pulmonary congestion can be minimal or absent in patients with significantly elevated pulmonary artery wedge pressure[12] and ECG and x-ray findings are either non-specific or insensitive. In one study, approximately one of every five patients admitted from the ED with ADHF had no signs of congestion on chest radiography.[13] In a large registry study (ADHERE), 26% of patients did not have evidence of pulmonary congestion on their initial chest radiograph.[14]

Consequently, biomarkers such as serum B-type natriuretic peptide (BNP) and its N-terminal prohormone (NT-proBNP) have been integrated into diagnostic decision making in suspected HF to improve accuracy and help assess the severity of potential ADHF. BNP levels are associated with New York Heart Association (NYHA) functional class, and were reported as the single most accurate predictor of the presence of HF.[6] In one study, a BNP cutoff of 100 pg/ml had a sensitivity of 90%, specificity of 76%, and an accuracy of 83% for the diagnosis of ADHF. From the PRIDE study, NTproBNP was shown to have a rule-in cutpoint of 900 pg/mL with a sensitivity of 90%, specificity of 85%, and an accuracy of 87%. NT-proBNP's rule-out cutpoint of 300 pg/mL has a sensitivity of 99%, specificity of 68%, and negative predictive value of 99%.[15] Despite its high sensitivity, BNP has several confounders that include renal failure and body mass index (BMI).[16] Therefore, BNP's role in diagnosing ADHF should be coupled with clinical impression.

Noninvasive Bioimpedance Technology

Providing a noninvasive and convenient diagnostic investigation has been evaluated using bioimpedance (BI) technology. BI measures the reactance and resistance of the body and can provide plots of a patient's volume status,[17] thus, providing real-time hydration status of the patient. Nevertheless, the precise role of BI in the ED is still undefined and large-scale studies are still needed to assess its ED utility.[6]

The Initial Treatment Goal in ED

The goal of initial treatment of ADHF is to stabilize hemodynamics, support oxygenation and ventilation, and to relieve symptoms. The primary objectives in hemodynamic stabilization are to lower the pulmonary capillary wedge pressure, reduce systemic vascular resistance, and provide a modest improvement in cardiac index.[18] In the hypertensive patient, these objectives can be achieved through a reduction in blood pressure (BP) by vasodilation and diuresis, which will also increase oxygenation of patients. Patients will benefit from maintaining a low BP, which will decrease peripheral vascular resistance and lead to an immediate clinical improvement.[17]

Simultaneously, all suspected ADHF patients should be monitored for coronary artery disease (CAD) as well as electrolyte imbalance. CAD is one of the most common causes of HF, thus, cardiac markers should be checked to detect any underlying acute myocardial infarction (AMI). Concurrently, abnormalities in potassium, sodium, magnesium, creatinine and BUN should be monitored since the patient will undergo diuresis. Significant derangement of electrolytes will need correction and will guide individualized care with supplemented electrolytes.

The Observation Unit in the Emergency Setting

The OU can be an alternative option for appropriate patients by providing optimized care to ADHF patients, thereby, reducing hospital admissions and healthcare costs. Studies have shown

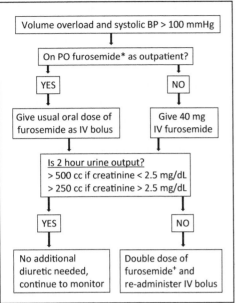

Figure 23.1 Acute Decompensated Heart Failure Patient Management Flow Chart

Volume overload and systolic BP > 100 mmHg

On PO furosemide* as outpatient?

YES — NO

Give usual oral dose of furosemide as IV bolus

Give 40 mg IV furosemide

Is 2 hour urine output?
> 500 cc if creatinine < 2.5 mg/dL
> 250 cc if creatinine > 2.5 mg/dL

YES — NO

No additional diuretic needed, continue to monitor

Double dose of furosemide+ and re-administer IV bolus

*Or furosemide equivalent

+Bolus doses > 160 mg suggest patient is not likely to succeed OU management. Inpatient hospitalization should be considered.

that safe and effective HF management strategies in the ED OU can decrease the number of ED visits, hospitalizations, and ICU admissions; thus decreasing costs and improving quality of life and mortality when compared to non-OU management programs.[11] Outcomes before and after institution of an ED OU HF protocol found ED HF revisit rates declined by 56% and the 90-day HF rehospitalization rate decreased by 64%. Furthermore, the 90-day rates of OU HF readmission decreased from 18% to 11% and the 90-day death rate decreased from 4% to 1 %.[27] ED OU management has been shown to reduce hospital LOS more than 20 hours per patient and provides a cost saving of approximately $3600 per patient.[5] Studies have suggested that up to 50% of patients could be discharged home after initial therapy.[3] These patients can be expected to greatly benefit from OU management as their clinical symptoms improve sufficiently within a few hours of ED admission.

The implementation of OU management not only decreases the overall healthcare costs, but more importantly can directly benefit patients as well. In the OU, patients can receive appropriate and intensive HF therapy without requiring several days of hospitalization. This enables patients to receive the full benefit of hospitalization in a short period of time, thus, preventing an extended inpatient admission and/or multiple outpatient visits. For instance, ejection fraction (EF)

measurement can be assessed in the OU and significant delays as may occur in the outpatient setting are prevented. Optimization of medication can be accomplished in a more controlled environment. One recommended ADHF patient management flow chart is presented in Figure 23.1.

OU Entry Criteria

In order to provide optimal care, patients should be carefully selected and transferred to the HF OU from the ED. First, patients should have a recent clinical history consistent with an acute decompensation episode such as shortness of breath, orthopnea, dyspnea upon exertion, paroxysmal nocturnal dyspnea, swollen legs or abdomen, or weight gain associated with fluid retention.[11] Physical examination should be consistent with findings of ADHF like jugular venous distinction, an audible S3 or S4 heart sound (galloping rhythms), positive abdominal jugular reflex, rales, and peripheral edema. Chest radiograph findings associated with HF include cardiomegaly, pulmonary vascular congestion, Kerley B lines, pulmonary edema, and pleural effusion.[11] Previous history of HF should be also taken as it has been shown as one of the most reliable predictors of a HF diagnosis is a history of ADHF.[19]

BNP levels are helpful for the exclusion of HF. Therefore, patient, eligibility to the HF OU includes a BNP level of > 100 pg/mL (normal

BNP levels are < 100 pg/mL). HF can be excluded from the differential for patients with BNP < 100 pg/mL as its negative predictive value is as high as 96%.[20] Clinicians should pay close attention to patients with moderately elevated levels to exclude other causes of elevated PCWP.

OU Exclusion Criteria

Severely compromised, unstable patients should not be admitted to the OU, especially, patients with a high probability of unfavorable outcomes due to acute myocardial ischemia or other critical conditions as they should be hospitalized as inpatients. Increased blood urea nitrogen (> 43 mg/dL) and low admission systolic blood pressure (≤ 115 mmHg) are two of the most significant independent predictors of acute mortality in patients with ADHF and showed a 12.9% increased mortality rate in one study.[11,21–22] Patients with an elevated BUN (43 mg/dL), low systolic BP (SBP ≤ 115 mmHg), and elevated creatinine (2.75 mg/dL) are strong predictors of acute mortality, thus, they should not be admitted to the OU.[21–22]

In addition, patients with airway instability, cardiac arrhythmias requiring continuous intravenous (IV) intervention, and inadequate systemic perfusion should not be admitted to the OU.[23] For similar reasons, patients requiring vasodilator therapy, including agents such as nitrates and nitroprusside,[6] are generally not good OU candidates. While intravenous vasodilators have potential benefits of reversing the decompensation by stabilizing hemodynamics, their need reflects a severity of illness beyond OU management.[23]

Appropriate OU Therapy

The main objectives of ADHF management in OU is to determine the type of HF (e.g., systolic or diastolic), to identify the factors that led to acute decompensation, to reduce fluid overload, to optimize ACE inhibitor therapy, to educate the patient, and to arrange patient treatment after discharge.[6]

Pharmalogical Therapy

Diuretics

Diuretics are often the first line of therapy for ADHF patients for the rapid and effective reduction of fluid thereby relieving dyspnea.[24] One recommended regimen is presented in Figure 23.1. Despite the substantial clinical utility of diuretics, clinicians must understand their potential side effects and limitations in managing ADHF.[6] Diuretics can result in decreased renal perfusion and neurohormonal activation by increasing renin and norepinephrine.[25] In addition to renal dysfunction and maladaptive neurohormonal activation, a number of studies have reported other adverse effects including hypotension and electrolyte imbalance.[6]

Despite decades of clinical usage of loop diuretics, guidelines of dosage and mode of administration have not been firmly established. The DOSE trial provides objective clinical outcome with various diuretic strategies. The study prospectively compared different strategies in mode of administration of different furosemide dosages. Overall, there was no significant difference in the patients' global assessment of symptoms or in the mean change in the creatinine level for IV bolus and continuous infusion strategies as well as high-dose or low-dose diuretics. In fact, the high-dose strategy was associated with greater diuresis and more favorable outcomes in some secondary measures, but also with transient worsening of renal function.[26]

Until the advent of new technologies, diuretics will continue to be employed as the main therapeutic agent of ADHF, but physicians should be aware of the adverse effects and employ diuretics judiciously.[6]

ACE Inhibitor

When used chronically, angiotensin-converting enzyme (ACE) inhibitors have been shown to alleviate symptoms, improve clinical status, and reduce the risk of death and the combined risk of death and hospitalization.[26] ACE inhibitors antagonize the renin-angiotensin-aldosterone system thus making them a good class of agents for chronic HF treatment. There are many studies showing the benefits of ACE inhibitors in chronic HF, but few have been conducted in the acute setting. Due to lack of large controlled studies and the potential for adverse events such as hypotension and renal dysfunction, ACE inhibitors are not currently considered as standard of care in the acute management of ADHF. Nevertheless, the limited data and anecdotal reports of successful use in the OU are encouraging and warrant further investigation to determine their utility in these patients.[6]

Ejection Fraction

EF is considered the "single most important measurement in HF"[11] by noninvasively assessing ventricular function. EF is useful in defining the etiology and HF type and is recommended to help determine treatment strategies.

Criteria for Hospital Admission from the OU

Patients should be admitted to the hospital for further management when their clinical condition fails to improve or deteriorates. Patients who exhibit sustained ventricular tachycardia, symptomatic cardiac arrhythmias, worsening renal function, unstable vital signs, ischemic chest pain, ECG changes, or develop elevated cardiac biomarkers of necrosis should be strongly considered for ICU admission.[11]

Even without clinical deterioration, failure to have sufficient urinary output or a further need for diuresis requires hospitalization. Persistent dyspnea or electrolyte imbalance also justifies the need for inpatient hospitalization.

Finally, patients who require extra care in social and medical circumstances should be considered for a long-term care plan. These patients include those with physical disabilities, mental challenges, financial troubles, or severe substance abuse problems.[11]

It is crucial that the utility of OU management is not overlooked or denied because of the further need of subsequent hospital admission after OU management. Even when patients require hospitalization after an OU admission, they will have a subsequently decreased overall LOS for more than 20 hours[5] compared to similar patients directly admitted to the hospital.[6]

Criteria for Discharge

Since every HF patient presents with unique symptoms and baseline health status, an individualized discharge evaluation should be made for each patient. Certain basic criteria must be met to insure an optimal outpatient course. Patients should report subjective improvement in symptoms, have achieved an adequate response to diuretic therapy with a total net urine output greater than 1 liter, and have normal cardiac biomarkers. The patients should also be ambulatory or at their baseline, exhibit stable electrolytes, have no new presentation of clinically significant arrhythmias, and have a normal range of vital signs with a systolic blood pressure ≥ 95 mmHg and a resting pulse rate ≤ 100 beats per minute.[11]

Although improvement in clinical congestion is a subjective assessment, objective measurements such as a reduction in jugular venous pressure, resolution of rales, edema, and orthopnea, and change in the patient's weight from presentation to discharge can be assessed, and suggest a greater probability of outpatient success. This can be also demonstrated by the patient's ambulation without dyspnea on exertion.[11]

Discharge Instruction and Patient Education

Every patient should be given clear discharge instructions with adequate follow-up prior to discharge. The optimal discharge instructions include proper diet recommendations, medication schedules, and patient education to prevent readmission and deterioration of their cardiac condition. In order to achieve this goal, appropriate consultation from cardiology, nutritional therapy, and social work may be required. ADHF patients with systolic dysfunction should be considered for beta-blockers at discharge. Studies have demonstrated that patients who have beta-blockers prescribed at hospital discharge are much more likely to be on this lifesaving medication 1 year later than those whose initiation is deferred to the outpatient environment.[21]

Finally, patient education is an important part of OU management of ADHF to prevent recurrent ED visits and or readmission. Patients should be educated on general HF knowledge, the purpose and effect of pharmacological therapies, dietary adherence, healthy lifestyle choices, early signs and symptoms of decompensation, advantages of smoking cessation, and medical assistance resources. A multidisciplinary collaboration among physicians, nursing staff, and social workers can dramatically increase the positive outcomes from patient education thus reducing hospital readmissions and the general health care burden from ADHF.

References

1. Mensah G, Brown D. An overview of cardiovascular disease burden in the United States. *Health Aff* 2007;26: 38–48.

2. American Heart Association, American Stroke Association. Heart Disease and Stroke Statistics—2011 Update. 2011. Available at: http://circ.ahajournals.org/content/123/4/e18.full.pdf. Accessed: February 2011.

3. Graff L, Orledge J, Radford MJ, et al. Correlation of the Agency for Health Care Policy and Research congestive heart failure admission guideline with mortality: peer review organization voluntary hospital association initiative to decrease events (PROVIDE) for congestive heart failure. *Ann Emerg Med.* 1999;34(4 Pt 1):429–437.

4. Silva MA, Peacock WF, Diercks DB. Optimizing treatment and outcomes in acute heart failure: beyond initial triage. *Congest Heart Fail.* May–Jun;12(3): 137–145.

5. Storrow AB, Collins SP, Lyons MS, et al. Emergency department observation of heart failure: preliminary analysis of safety and cost. *Congest Heart Fail.* 2005 Mar–Apr;11(2):68–72.

6. Albert NM, WF. Patient outcome and costs after implementation of an acute heart failure management program in an emergency department obsevation unit. *J Internat Soc Heart and Lung Transplant.* 1999;18(1):92.

7. Peacock WF, Fonarow GC, et al. Society of Chest Pain Centers recommendations for the evaluation and management of the observation stay acute heart failure patients. *Acute Cardiac Care.* 2009;11:3–42.

8. Heart Failure Society of America. Executive Summary: HFSA 2010 Comprehensive Heart Failure Practice Guideline. *J Card Fail.* 2010;16:475–539.

9. Amin A, Hospitalized patients with acute decompensated heart failure: recognition, risk stratification, and treatment review. *Jour of Hospital Medicine.* 2008;3(6):S16–24.

10. Stevensen LW, Perloff JK. The limited reliability of physical signs for estimating hemodynamics in chronic heart failure. *JAMA.* 1989; 261(6):884–888.

11. Peacock WF, Young J, Collins S, et al. Heart failure observation units: optimizing care. *Ann Emerg Med.* 2006 Jan;47(1):22–33. Epub 2005 Aug 15.

12. Mahdyoon H, Klein R, Eyler W, et al. Radiographic pulmonary congestion in end-stage congestive heart failure. *Am J Cardiol.* 1989;63(9): 625–627.

13. Collins S, Lindsell CJ, Storrow AB, et al. Prevalence of negative chest radiography in the emergency department patient with decompensated heart failure. *Ann Emerg Med.* 2005;47(1):13–18.

14. Costanzo MR, Johannes RS, Pine M, et al. The safety of intravenous diuretics alone versus diuretics plus parenteral vasoactive therapies in hospitalized patients with acutely decompensated heart failure: a propensity score and instrumental variable analysis using the Acutely Decompensated Heart Failure National Registry (ADHERE) database. *Am Heart J.* 2007; 154(2):267–277.

15. Januzzi JL, Camargo CA, Anwaruddin S, et al. The N-Terminal Pro-BNP Investigation of Dyspnea in the Emergency Department (PRIDE) Study. *Am J Cardiol.* 2005;95:948–954.

16. Silver MA, Maisel A, Yanct CW, et al. BNP Consensus Panel 2004; a clinical approach for the diagnostic, prognostic, screening, treatment monitoring, and therapeutic roles of natriuretic peptides in cardiovascular diseases. *Congest Heart Fail.* 2004;10(5 suppl 3):1–30.

17. Di Somma S, De Berardinis B, Bongiovanni C, et al. Use of BNP and bioimpedance to drive therapy in heart failure patients. *Congest Heart Fail.* 2010; 16 Suppl 1:S56–61.

18. Peacock WF. Acute emergency department management of heart failure. *Heart Fail Rev.* 2003;8:335–338.

19. Hobbs RE. Using BNP to diagnose, manage, and treat heart failure. *Cleve Clin J Med.* 2003;70:333–336.

20. Fonarow GC, Adams KF Jr, Abraham WT, et al., for the ADHERE Scientific Advisory Committee, Study Group, and Investigators. Risk stratification for in-hospital mortality in acutely decompensated heart failure: classification and regression tree analysis. *JAMA.* 2005;293:572–580.

21. Elkayam U, Tasissa Gm Binanay C, et al. Use and impact of inotropes and vasodilator therapy during heart failure hospitalization in the ESCAPE trail. *Circulation.* 2004;110(17 suppl):III–515.

22. Peacock WF. Rapid optimization: strategies for optimal care of decompensated congestive heart-failure patients in the emergency department. *Rev Cardiovasc Med.* 2002;3(suppl 4):S41–S48.

23. Nieminen MS, Böhm M, Cowie MR, et al. Executive summary of the guidelines on the diagnosis and treatment of acute heart failure: the Task Force on Acute Heart Failure

of the European Society of Cardiology. *Eur Heart J.* 2005;26:384–416.

24. Brewster UC, Setaro JF, Perazella MA. The renin-angiotension-aldosterone system: cardiorenal effects and implications for renal and cardiovascular disease states. *Am Med Sci.* 2003 Jul;326(1):15–24.

25. Felker GM, Lee KL, Bull DA, et al. Diuretic strategies in patients with acute decompensated heart failure. *N Engl J Med* 2011;364:797–805.

26. Hunt SA, Abraham W, Chin M, et al. ACC/AHA Practice Guideline: 2009 Focused Update incorporated into the ACC/AHA 2005 Guidelines for the Diagnosis and the Management of Heart Failure in Adults. *Circulation.* 2009;119:e391–e479.

27. Peacock WF, Remer E, Aponte J, et al. Effective observation unit treatment of decompensated heart failure. *Congest Heart Fail.* 2002 Mar–Apr;8(2):68–73.

Chapter

Atrial Fibrillation

Catherine T. Puetz, MD, FACEP

Background

Atrial fibrillation (AF) is a cardiovascular disease in which the upper chambers of the heart (the atria) beat in a rapid disorganized manner resulting in the presence of a fast irregular heartbeat. This arrhythmia is estimated to currently affect more than 7 million persons in the United States and Europe. It is the most common cardiac arrhythmia that exists with a prevalence that ranges from 0.1% among adults < 55 to 9% in those > 80.[1,2] With the projection of the elderly population increasing, the prevalence of AF is expected to increase 2.5-fold times the current level by the year 2050. The management and treatment costs present a significant financial burden on the health care system. The cost of treatment for AF in 2005 was approximately $6.5 billion. These costs can be attributed to increased inpatient stays and other health care services.[3]

The incidence of AF is significantly higher in men than women, regardless of age, and more common in whites than blacks. The presence of AF without associated comorbidities occurs in 10–15% of cases.[4] In developed countries, the most common comorbidities of AF include hypertension and coronary artery disease (CAD), followed by valvular heart disease (rheumatic heart disease) and thyroid disorders. Patients with hypertension have a 1.42-fold increase in developing AF. Because of the relatively high incidence of hypertension in the general population it is the most common disorder in patients with AF.[5] Ordinarily, AF is not associated with CAD unless it is complicated by an acute myocardial infarction (AMI) or heart failure (HF). AF in the setting of AMI is associated with 40% increase in mortality compared with those patients in sinus rhythm with AMI.[6]

Pathophysiology/Electrophysiology

The primary histopathologic changes in AF are progressive atrial fibrosis and loss of atrial muscle mass.[7] The normal electrical conduction system of the heart begins with an impulse fired from the sinoatrial (SA) node that propagates to the atrioventricular (AV) node resulting in contraction of the ventricle. In AF this synchronized cycle is disrupted. The electrical conduction system in patients with AF does not begin in the sinoatrial (SA) node. Rather the irregular impulses may be due to proarrhythmic atrial fibrotic areas, ectopic foci within the pulmonary vein, the heart having increased susceptibility to autonomic stimuli, circulation of antibodies against cardiac myosin heavy chains, and very rarely atrial myocarditis.[8] As a result the normal timing of the heart's pacemaker is thrown off causing the heart to beat faster or quiver. The atrial rate is generally fast (300–600 beats per minute), however, not all of these are conducted through the AV node so the ventricular rate is much slower (usually about 110–180 beats per minute).[9,10] The contraction of the two upper chambers of the heart (atria) will not be synchronized with the contractions of bottom of the heart (ventricle) causing the irregularly irregular heart beat of AF. The hemodynamic functions affected during AF are the loss of synchronous atrial activity, irregular ventricular response, rapid heart rate, and impaired coronary blood flow.

The American College of Cardiology (ACC), American Heart Association (AHA), and the European Society of Cardiology (ESC) established classifications of AF based on timing and duration of symptoms.[8] The classification of AF is separated in three patterns: paroxysmal AF, persistent AF, and permanent AF. When categorizing patients it is based on the most frequent pattern found on presentation.[8] Paroxysmal AF is categorized by episodes of AF that resolve spontaneously within 7 days, with most episodes lasting < 24 hours. Paroxysmal AF is found in younger patients and often with holter monitoring. Paroxysmal AF can progress to permanent AF, therefore, aggressive attempts to restore and maintain sinus rhythm are indicated. Persistent AF is associated with recurrent episodes that last more than 7 days.[8] Persistent AF is less likely to spontaneously convert and will require some form of cardioversion to restore sinus rhythm. The persistence of AF for a long time (e.g., a year or more) is defined as permanent AF.[8] In addition to these classifications, the ACC/AHA/ESC guidelines define additional AF categories in terms of other characteristics of the patient. Lone AF is the occurrence of AF in the absence of clinical or echocardiographic findings of cardiovascular disease in patients < 60 years of age.[8] Nonvalvular AF occurs in the absence of rheumatic mitral valve disease, a prosthetic heart valve, or mitral valve repair.[8] Secondary AF occurs in the setting of a primary condition such as AMI, cardiac surgery, pericarditis, alcohol intake "holiday heart syndrome," myocarditis, pulmonary diseases, hyperthyroidism, or metabolic syndromes.[8]

Management of AF

There are three objectives that need to be addressed when managing patients with AF: rate control, prevention of thromboembolism, and rhythm restoration. It is important to remember that 70% of patients that present acutely with AF will convert spontaneously.[11] The choice between rhythm control and rate control has been studied extensively and the conclusion was that neither treatment was inferior to the other for the outcome measures of mortality or quality of life.[12, 13] In the emergency department (ED), the initial therapy for hemodynamically stable AF patients would be ventricular rate control with subsequent consideration to some form of cardioversion (pharmacologic versus electrical) to relieve symptoms and improve cardiac output. Rate control occurs when AV nodal conduction is depressed.[14]

The agents most commonly used are beta-blockers, calcium channel blockers, digoxin and amiodarone. Beta-blockers cause prolongation of the AV refractory period by targeting the beta-adrenergic receptors. Calcium antagonists decrease heart rate by blocking the calcium channel during the plateau phase of the action potential during cardiac contraction. Digoxin's effect on the AV node is via enhancement of vagal tone.[14] In review of the evidence-based studies on rate control when monotherapy was used in the treatment of AF, both calcium antagonists and beta-blockers were more effective than digoxin in controlling heart rate at high levels of sympathetic drive. There was, however, no significant difference in terms of the effectiveness of rate control between calcium channel blockers and beta-blockers.[14,15] Beta-blocker therapy is preferred in AF patients with hypertension, AMI, and ischemic heart disease but relatively contraindicated in asthmatics.[14] Calcium antagonists should be avoided in AF patients with signs of HF. The effectiveness of AV nodal blockade on restoring sinus rhythm is no better than placebo.[14]

Cardioversion is used to restore sinus rhythm. Electrical cardioversion is the treatment of choice in the hemodynamically unstable AF patient. The stable AF patient can either be treated with pharmacological cardioversion (PC) or electrical cardioversion (EC). The restoration of sinus rhythm by either method has a higher success rate in the acute presentation of AF (< 48 hour), 80–90% (EC) versus 60–80% (PC).[14] The drawbacks of using EC include the need for procedural sedation with its associated risks. There are advantages and disadvantages of using anti-arrhythmic medication. Advantages are simplicity, convenience, and no need for procedural sedation. Disadvantages are the drug-related pro-arrhythmic effects and the lack of effect on chronic AF. The most common anti-arrhythmic medications used for PC are amiodarone, flecainide, procainamide, propafenone, sotalol, and ibutelide.[16,17]

Regardless of which treatment approach is pursued, thromboembolic prevention is essential in AF. Stroke is one of the major complications of AF. The annual risk of stroke in patients with AF is in the range of 3%–8% per year.[2] The risk of stroke increases with age as demonstrated in the Framingham Study. The annual risk of stroke attributable to AF was 1.5% in participants 50–59 years old and 23.5% in those aged 80–89 years old.[2] Thromboembolic events occur as a result of thrombus formation in the left atrium or left atrial appendage. The uncoordinated contraction of the atria in AF over time leads to dilation of the right and left atrium resulting in blood stasis and clot formation. The low peak velocities present in the left atrial appendage, as demonstrated on pulse wave Doppler echocardiography, also promotes thrombus formation.[8] Another finding on echocardiography is spontaneous echo contrast.[8] This is the presence of smoke-like images that are felt to represent increased red blood cell aggregation in the setting of low flow. The presence of this as noted on echocardiography is a predisposing factor to thrombus formation. AF also appears to activate the clotting system as evidenced by the presence of increased thrombotic and fibrinolytic markers in AF patients.[8] The risk of thrombus development increases the longer AF is present, especially when > 48 hours.

There currently are several scoring systems available to help clinicians estimate the stroke risk in patients with AF. One of the most popular risk assessment tools used is the $CHADS_2$ score. This scoring system assigns single points for the following conditions: Congestive Heart Failure (CHF), Hypertension, Age ≥ 75, and Diabetes; it assigns two points for a prior history of stroke or TIA. Patients with $CHADS_2$ score of ≥ 2 have a high risk and merit anticoagulation therapy.[18] The $CHADS_2$ score was felt to have limitations in assessing risk as it didn't incorporate a number of documented stroke risk factors.

These additional risks now addressed by the new CHA_2DS_2-VASc Score include vascular disease (prior MI, peripheral artery disease, aortic plaque), additional age category, and sex category (female gender).[19] As with the previous scoring system, the CHA_2DS_2-VASc scoring assigns one point to each risk, with the exception of age ≥ 75 and prior CVA/TIA/thromboembolic event, which are both given two points. The risk scores will determine which form of anticoagulation is recommended for AF patients. Scores ≥ 2 indicates a high risk of stroke and oral anticoagulation is recommended. Moderate risk patients (score ≥ 1) are recommended to take oral anticoagulation therapy also and those with a score of 0 have a very low risk and either no antithrombotic therapy or aspirin are recommended.[19]

Anticoagulation is one of the most important considerations to be made in the acute management of AF. (See Chapter 33 on anticoagulants.) The risk of thromboembolism in either chemical or electrical cardioversion is the same. Transesophageal echocardiography (TEE) is a good predictor of acute risk. If the presence of thrombus is not seen in the cardiac chambers or left atrial appendage and there is no evidence of spontaneous echo contrast visualized on echo, cardioversion has a low acute risk of stroke.[8] Anticoagulation is indicated for those patients in AF of suspected duration of > 48 hours that will be undergoing EC after 4–6 weeks of therapy.[8]

The goal of long-term anticoagulation in AF is to reduce risk of thromboembolism. The choice of therapy selected should be balanced between the risk of stroke and the risk of bleeding, which unfortunately both increase with age. Warfarin has long been the anticoagulation treatment of choice for AF patients with moderate to high risk for thromboembolism. The goal of therapy is maintaining an international normalized ratio (INR) in the range of 2.0–3.0, except in patients who are at significant risk for stroke (patients with artificial valves, those with rheumatic heart disease, and those with recurrent prior strokes) where the goal INR should be maintained between 2.5 and 3.5.[8]

Warfarin therapy is complex because of its narrow therapeutic window and variable pharmacodynamics and pharmacokinetics. It also interacts with many drugs and foods and requires frequent monitoring. These limitations of warfarin result in undertreatment of a considerable portion of people with AF at great risk.

Newer anticoagulation therapies have recently become available for use. They are direct Factor Xa inhibitors (e.g., rivaroxaban, edoxaban, apixaban) and direct thrombin inhibitors (e.g., dabigatran).[20] The results of the RE-LY trial found that dabigatran at a dose of 150 mg was superior to warfarin in the reduction of stroke and systemic embolism (per year: warfarin 1.69%, dabigatran 1.11%), but with a similar rate of major hemorrhage (per year: warfarin 3.36%, dabigatran 3.11%).[21] These new anticoagulants have the advantage of stable pharmacodynamics and pharmacokinetics, eliminating the need for frequent monitoring. The major disadvantages of their use include cost and that there is currently no specific way to reverse the anticoagulant effects of the drug in the event of major bleeding with the exception of idarucizumab, which is a monoclonal antibody antidote specifically for the reversal of dabigatran.[22] However, there is much research in this area and it is likely that reversal agents for all

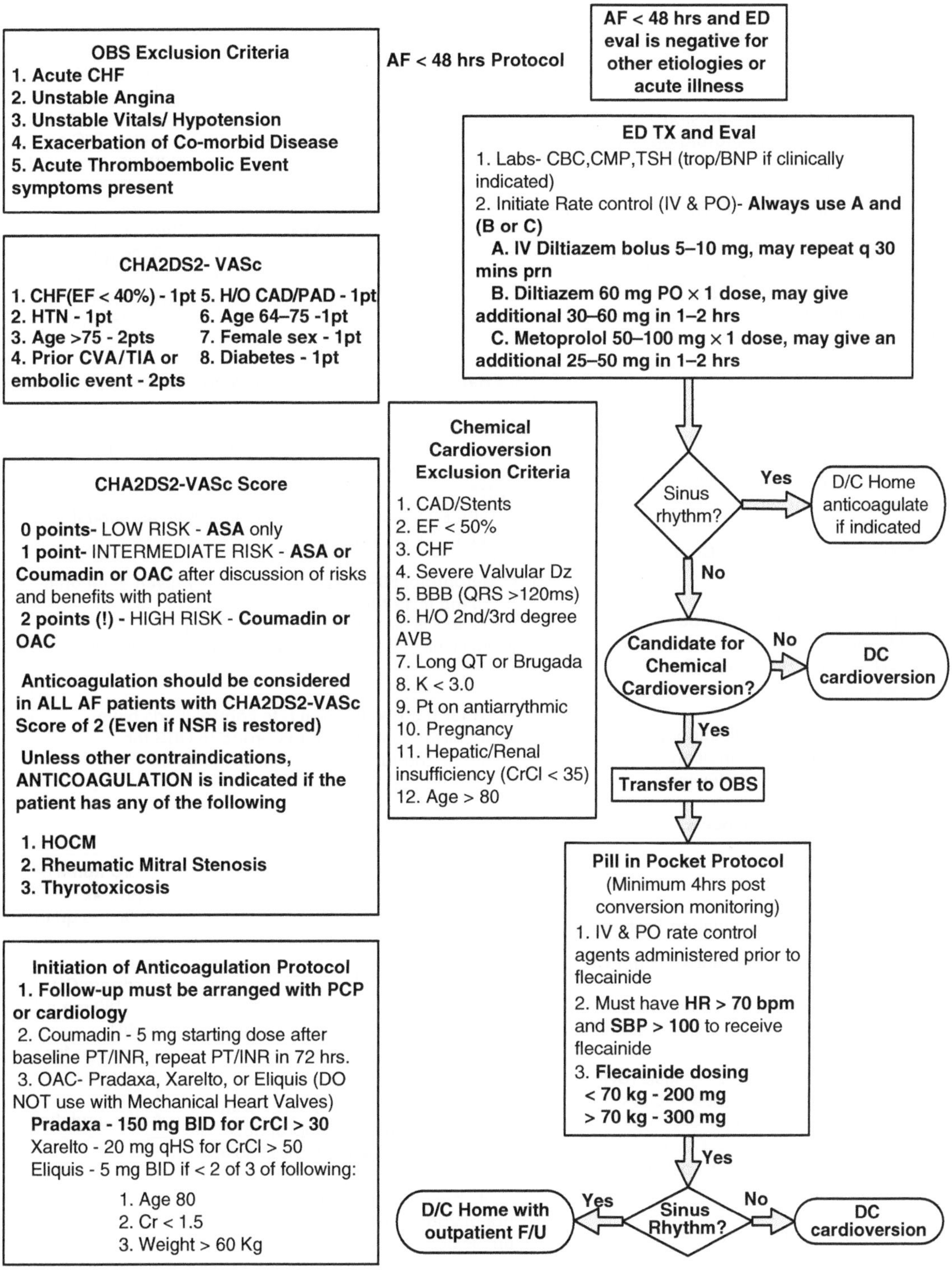

OBS Exclusion Criteria
1. Acute CHF
2. Unstable Angina
3. Unstable Vitals/ Hypotension
4. Exacerbation of Co-morbid Disease
5. Acute Thromboembolic Event symptoms present

CHA2DS2- VASc
1. CHF(EF < 40%) - 1pt   5. H/O CAD/PAD - 1pt
2. HTN - 1pt
3. Age >75 - 2pts
4. Prior CVA/TIA or embolic event - 2pts

6. Age 64–75 -1pt
7. Female sex - 1pt
8. Diabetes - 1pt

CHA2DS2-VASc Score

0 points- LOW RISK - **ASA** only
1 point- INTERMEDIATE RISK - **ASA or Coumadin or OAC** after discussion of risks and benefits with patient
2 points (!) - HIGH RISK - **Coumadin or OAC**

Anticoagulation should be considered in ALL AF patients with CHA2DS2-VASc Score of 2 (Even if NSR is restored)

Unless other contraindications, ANTICOAGULATION is indicated if the patient has any of the following

1. HOCM
2. Rheumatic Mitral Stenosis
3. Thyrotoxicosis

Initiation of Anticoagulation Protocol
1. Follow-up must be arranged with PCP or cardiology
2. Coumadin - 5 mg starting dose after baseline PT/INR, repeat PT/INR in 72 hrs.
3. OAC- Pradaxa, Xarelto, or Eliquis (DO NOT use with Mechanical Heart Valves)
Pradaxa - 150 mg BID for CrCl > 30
Xarelto - 20 mg qHS for CrCl > 50
Eliquis - 5 mg BID if < 2 of 3 of following:
　　1. Age 80
　　2. Cr < 1.5
　　3. Weight > 60 Kg

AF < 48 hrs Protocol

AF < 48 hrs and ED eval is negative for other etiologies or acute illness

ED TX and Eval
1. Labs- CBC,CMP,TSH (trop/BNP if clinically indicated)
2. Initiate Rate control (IV & PO)- **Always use A and (B or C)**
　A. IV Diltiazem bolus 5–10 mg, may repeat q 30 mins prn
　B. Diltiazem 60 mg PO × 1 dose, may give additional 30–60 mg in 1–2 hrs
　C. Metoprolol 50–100 mg × 1 dose, may give an additional 25–50 mg in 1–2 hrs

Chemical Cardioversion Exclusion Criteria
1. CAD/Stents
2. EF < 50%
3. CHF
4. Severe Valvular Dz
5. BBB (QRS >120ms)
6. H/O 2nd/3rd degree AVB
7. Long QT or Brugada
8. K < 3.0
9. Pt on antiarrythmic
10. Pregnancy
11. Hepatic/Renal insufficiency (CrCl < 35)
12. Age > 80

Sinus rhythm? — Yes → D/C Home anticoagulate if indicated

No ↓

Candidate for Chemical Cardioversion? — No → DC cardioversion

Yes ↓

Transfer to OBS

Pill in Pocket Protocol
(Minimum 4hrs post conversion monitoring)
1. IV & PO rate control agents administered prior to flecainide
2. Must have **HR > 70 bpm** and **SBP > 100** to receive flecainide
3. **Flecainide dosing**
　< 70 kg - 200 mg
　> 70 kg - 300 mg

Yes ↓

Sinus Rhythm? — Yes → D/C Home with outpatient F/U
— No → DC cardioversion

Figure 24.1 Atrial Fibrillation Clinical Algorithm: Atrial Fibrillation < 48 hours duration

of the novel or new oral anticoagulants (NOACs) or non vitamin K oral antagonists will be available in the near future. The specific NOAC reversal agent, idarucizumab, is indicated only for the reversal of the anticoagulant effects of dabigatran for emergency surgery/urgent procedures or with life-threatening or uncontrolled bleeding.

Exclusion Criteria

1. Acute CHF
2. Unstable Angina
3. Unstable Vitals/ Hypotension
4. Exacerbation of Co-morbid Disease

CHA2DS2- VASc

1. CHF(EF < 40%) - 1pt 5. H/O CAD/PAD- 1pt
2. HTN - 1pt 6. Age 64–75 -1pt
3. Age >75 - 2pts 7. Female sex - 1pt
4. Prior CVA/TIA or 8. Diabetes - 1pt
embolic event - 2pts

CHA2DS2-VASc Score

0 points - LOW RISK - **ASA** only
1 point - INTERMEDIATE RISK - **ASA or Coumadin or OAC** after discussion of risks and benefits with patient
2 points (!) - HIGH RISK - **Coumadin or OAC**

***Anticoagulation should be considered in ALL AF patients with CHA2DS2-VASc Score of 2 (Even if NSR is restored) ***

Unless other contraindications, ANTICOAGULATION is indicated if the patient has any of the following
1. HOCM
2. Rheumatic Mitral Stenosis
3. Thyrotoxicosis

Initiation of Anticoagulation Protocol

1. Follow-up must be arranged with PCP or cardiology
2. Coumadin - Starting dose 5 mg after baseline PT/INR drawn, repeat PT/INR in 72 hrs
3. OAC- Pradaxa, Xarelto, or Eliquis (DO NOT use with Mechanical Heart Valves)
   Pradaxa - 150 mg BID for CrCl > 30
   Xarelto - 20 mg qHS for CrCl > 50
   Eliquis - 5 mg BID if < 2 of 3 of following:
      1. Age 80
      2. Cr < 1.5
      3. Weight > 60 Kg

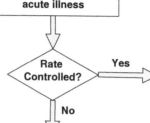

AF > 48 hours Protocol

AF present > 48 hrs & ED Eval is negative for other causes or acute illness

Rate Controlled? — **Yes** →

No ↓

ED Rate control Rx (IV & PO)- Always use 1 and (2 or 3)

1. **IV Diltiazem bolus 5–20 mg, may repeat q 30 mins prn** while waiting for oral medication to work **(Goal is patient comfort, not optimal rates initially)**
   AND
2. **Diltiazem 60 mg PO × 1 dose, may give additional 30–60 mg in 1–2 hrs**
   Or
3. **Metoprolol 50–100mg × 1 dose, may given additional 25–50 mg in 1–2 hrs**
4. If patient is already on a rate controlling medicine, give an additional dose of that medication in conjunction with IV bolus

*** After both IV and oral rate control meds have been started, consider transferring to OBS for telemetry and further rate control indicated ***

Transfer to OBS

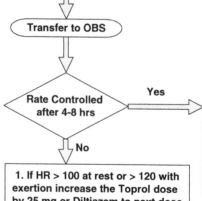

1. If rate controlled without ED therapy DO NOT start any rate control therapy
2. If ED therapy resulted in rate control, D/C on:
   Toprol XL 25–50 mg qd or BID
   or
   Cardizem CD 120–180 mg qd or BID
3. Start anticoagulation
4. D/C Home with appropriate follow up

Rate Controlled after 4-8 hrs — **Yes** →

No ↓

1. If HR > 100 at rest or > 120 with exertion increase the Toprol dose by 25 mg or Diltiazem to next dose level
2. If HR is not optimized within 4 hrs of 2nd dose - consider admission

1. **D/C home** on: **Toprol XL 25–50 mg qd or BID** or **Cardizem CD 120–180 mg qd or BID**
2. Arrange for follow up
3. Start Anticoagulation

Figure 24.2 Atrial Fibrillation Clinical Algorithm: Atrial Fibrillation > 48 hours duration

Inclusion/ Exclusion Criteria

Patients appropriate for an observation unit (OU) are those patients with symptomatic paroxysmal AF or persistent AF that require rate control and are hemodynamically stable. Patients that should be excluded from OU placement are those that are medically unstable and/or have confounding comorbid factors as the cause of their AF (e.g., secondary causes of their AF). The observation stay will evaluate the need for rate control, rhythm correction (EC vs. PC), and assessing the patient's thromboembolic risk. (Figures 24.1 and 24.2)

Observation Interventions

AF patients in OUs should be managed on an individual basis. The factors to be considered are the patient's symptoms, the known duration of the AF, and the presence of structural heart disease. There are currently many evidence-based studies published demonstrating a variety of ways to treat AF in the setting of observation.[23,24] None of these studies demonstrated a statistically significant difference in one treatment method over the other. There is evidence to suggest that the use of treatment protocols for the management of AF in observation improves patient outcomes and decreases the need for inpatient admission.[25–24,26] (Figures 24.1 and 24.2)

Conclusion

AF is becoming a serious cardiac epidemic along with CAD and CHF. The financial burden of this disease process will only increase as the population continues to age. The management of AF in OUs has been demonstrated to not only be safe but also cost-effective due to the decreased need for hospitalization of these patients.

References

1. GO AS, Hylek EM, Phillips KA, et al. Prevalence of diagnosed atrial fibrillation in adults: national implications for rhythm management and stroke prevention: the AnTicoagulation and Risk Factors in Atrial Fibrillation (ATRIA) Study. *JAMA*. 2001; 285 (18):2370–2375.

2. Lloyd-Jones DM, Wang TJ, Leip EP, et al. Lifetime risk for development of atrial fibrillation: the Framingham Hear t Study. *Circulation*. 2004; 110(9):1042–1046.

3. Coyne KS, Paramore C, Grandy S, et al. Assessing the direct costs of treating nonvalvular atrial fibrillation in the United States. *Value Health*. 2006; 9(5):348–356.

4. Krahn AD, Manfreda J, Tate RB, et al. the natural history of atrial fibrillation: incidence, risk factors, and prognosis in the Manitoba Follow-Up Study. *Am J Med*. 1995; 98 (5):476–484.

5. Cameron A, Schwartz MJ, Kronmal RA, et al. Prevalence and significance of atrial fibrillation in coronary artery disease (CASS Registry). *Am J Cardiol*. 1988; 61 (10):714–717.

6. Wong CK, White HD, Wilcox RG, et al. New atrial fibrillation after acute myocardial infarction independently predicts death: the GUSTO-III experience. *Am Heart J*. 2000; 140(6):878–885.

7. 2 Bharati S, Lev M. Histology of the normal and diseased atrium. In: Falk RH, Podrid PJ, eds. *Atrial Fibrillation: Mechanisms and Management*. New York: Raven Press, 1992.

8. Fuster V, Ryden LE, Cannom DS, et al. ACC/AHA/ASC guidelines for the management of patients with atrial fibrillation: a report to the American College of Cardiology/American Heart Association Task Force on Practice Guidelines and the European Society of Cardiology Committee for Practice Guidelines: developed in collaboration with the European Heart Rhythm Association and the Heart Rhythm and the heart Rhythm society. *Circulation*. 2006; 114 (7)e257–e354.

9. Schotten U, Verheule S, Kirchhof P, et al. Pathophysiological mechanisms of atrial fibrillation: a translational appraisal. *Physio Rev* 2011; 91:265.

10. Allessie MA, Konings K, Kirchhof CJ, et al. Electrophysiologic mechanisms of perpetuation of atrial fibrillation. *Am J Cardiol* 1996; 77:10A.

11. Danias PG, Caulfield TA, Weigner MJ, et al. Likelihood of spontaneous conversion of atrial fibrillation to sinus rhythm. *Journal of the American College of Cardiology*. 1998; 31(3):588–592.

12. Wyse DG, Waldo AL, DiMarco JP, et al. Atrial Fibrillation Follow up Investigation of Rhythm Management (AFFIRM) Investigators. A comparison of rate control and rhythm control in patients with atrial fibrillation. *NEJM*.2002; 347(23):1825–1833.

13. VanGelder IC, Hagens VE, Bosker HA, et al. A comparison of rate control and rhythm control in patients with recurrent persistent atrial fibrillation. *NEJM*. 2002; 347:1834–1840.

14. Wakai A, O'Neill JO. Emergency management of atrial fibrillation. *Postgrad Med J*. 2003; 79:313–319.

15. Levy S. Pharmacologic management of atrial fibrillation: current therapeutic strategies. *Am Heart J*. 2001; 141:S15–21.

16. Alboni P, Botto GL, Baldi N, et al. Outpatient treatment of recent-onset atrial fibrillation with the "pill in the pocket" approach. *N Engl J Med*. 2004; 351: 2384–2391.

17. Reiffel JA. Atrial fibrillation: what have recent trials taught us regarding pharmacologic management of rate and rhythm control? *PACE*. 2011; 34:247–259.

18. Gage BF, Waterman AD, Shannon W, et al. Validation of clinical classification schemes for predicting strokes: results from the National Registry of Atrial Fibrillation. *JAMA*. 2001. 285(22):2864–2870.

19. Lip GY, Niewlaat R, Pisters R, et al. Refining clinical risk stratification for predicting stroke and thromboembolism in atrial fibrillation using a novel risk factor-based approach: the euro heart survey on atrial fibrillation. *Chest*. 2010; 137(2):263–272.

20. Ahrens I, Lip GY, Pete K. New oral anticoagulant drugs in cardiovascular disease. *Thromb Haemost*. 2010; 104(1):49–60

21. Connolly SJ, et al. Dabigatran versus warfarin in patients with atrial fibrillation. *New England Journal of Medicine*. 2009; 361.

22. Pollack CV Jr, Reilly PA, Eikelboom J, et al. Idarucizumab for dabigatran reversal. *NEJM* 2015;373:511–520.

23. Decker WW, Smars PA, et al. A prospective, randomized trial of an emergency department observation unit for acute onset atrial fibrillation. *Ann Emerg Med*. 2008 Oct; 52 (4):322–328.

24. Vinson DR, Hoehn T, Graber DJ, et al. Managing emergency department patients with recent – onset atrial fibrillation. *J Emerg Med*. 2012; 42 (2):139–148.

25. Koenig BO, Ross MA, Jackson RE. An emergency department observation unit protocol for acute-onset atrial fibrillation is feasible. *Ann Emerg Med*. 2002; 39:374–381.

26. Ross MA, Comptom S, Medado P, et al. An emergency department diagnostic protocol for patients with transient ischemic attack: a randomized controlled trial. *Ann Emerg Med*. 2007; 50(2):109–119.

Chapter

25

Syncope

T. Andrew Windsor, MD, RDMS, FAAEM
Amal Mattu, MD, FACEP, FAAEM

Introduction

Syncope is a common presenting complaint in the emergency department (ED) representing 1–3% of annual ED visits and up to 6% of hospital admissions yearly.[1,2] It is defined as a transient loss of consciousness and postural tone with spontaneous full recovery and is a result of cerebral hypoperfusion. The differential diagnosis for syncope is broad, encompassing many possible etiologies from benign, self-limited events to life-threatening disease. This wide spectrum frequently prompts inpatient admissions with a mean cost of $5,400 per admission and approximately $2 billion annually.[3,4,5] Inpatient syncope evaluations are often low-yield, and serious cardiac or neurologic etiologies are only found in less than 20%.[6]

Several clinical decision rules and novel protocols have been developed to help providers determine the short-term risk of death after syncope, including Osservatorio Epidemiologico-sulla Sincopenel Lazio (OESIL; Table 25.1),[7] Syncope Evaluation in the Emergency Department Study (SEEDS),[8] San Francisco Syncope Rule (SFSR; Table 25.2),[9] Short Term Prognosis of Syncope (STePs),[10] Evaluation of Guidelines in Syncope Study (EGSYS),[11] and Risk stratification of Syncope in the Emergency Department (ROSE; Table 25.3).[12] Unfortunately there is no clear consensus on a standardized evaluation or risk profile, and the majority of these rules have not been reliably validated. As well, there is a lack of convincing evidence showing which patients benefit from short-term observation to prevent future adverse events.

The concept of syncope units (dedicated observation units [OUs]) that are equipped with the capability for common applicable diagnostic tests and ready access to specialist consultation and follow-up) has been introduced and lauded by some.[8,11] Early studies have showed that the patients who were managed in these units had significantly lower inpatient hospitalization rate and shorter length of stay (LOS) without negatively affecting the adverse outcomes or recurrence rates. Furthermore, there was an associated cost savings of approximately 20%.[11] In the SEEDS paper, there was small but significantly higher diagnostic yield in the syncope unit group when compared to standard care.[8]

Table 25.1[7] The OESIL Score:

1 point awarded for each; score ≥ 2 indicates increased risk of cardiac death:

- Age > 65 years
- History of CV disease
- Syncope without prodromes
- Abnormal ECG

Table 25.2[9] San Francisco Syncope Rule:

A patient is high risk for serious outcome if they have any of the following:

- C - History of congestive heart failure
- H - Hematocrit < 30%
- E - Abnormal ECG
- S - Shortness of breath
- S - Systolic blood pressure < 90 mmHg

Table 25.3[12] ROSE Rule:

Admit if any of the following are present:

- B - Brain natriuretic peptide (BNP) levels of 300 pg per mL or greater
  - Bradycardia of 50 beats per minute or less
- R - Rectal examination with positive fecal occult blood test (physician discretion)
- A - Anemia (hemoglobin of 9 g per dL or less)
- C - Chest pain with syncope
- E - ECG with Q waves
- S - Oxygen Saturation of 94% or less on room air

Pathophysiology

Syncope is classified as cardiac, neurally mediated (reflex), orthostatic, or neurologic. [13 Table 25.4 provides examples of each type. Neurally mediated is the most common type and is mostly seen in older adolescents and young adults.[14] The most worrisome etiologies are cardiovascular (such as acute coronary syndrome [ACS], arrhythmias, and structural or functional disease) and neurologic (preceding stroke or due to severe basilar insufficiency). Orthostatic syncope is most commonly encountered in the setting of volume depletion or a drug effect, but it is important to note that persons with underlying cardiac disease can have features similar to orthostatic intolerance.

Discussion

A primary motivator for inpatient admission should be a high concern for a risk of dysrhythmia or sudden death, and that further observation may establish a diagnosis, detect a future event, or allow intervention in a potentially life-threatening circumstance. The reality is that a large proportion of people admitted with a diagnosis of syncope are discharged without a specific etiology for their symptom. Exactly which patients benefit

from brief hospitalization is not well defined in the literature. Furthermore, hospitalization has not been shown to reduce long-term adverse events.[10] The major benefits of OUs are that they have been shown to provide high-quality and cost-effective care for many conditions, and may be appropriate for those patients who are neither high-risk nor very low-risk but need further evaluation.

Initial risk stratification can help a clinician decide which patients are at higher risk for adverse events and therefore require early workup with hospital or OU admission. Unfortunately the clinical decision rules developed for this purpose do not uniformly address length of prognosis. Some of these rules have not always performed as well as initially presented in attempts at external validation, but it is notable that there is vast heterogeneity amongst the structure of study design, endpoints and application of the individual rule criteria. The SFSR used an endpoint of 7 days and has evaluated the short-term risk of patients discharged from the ED with a reported 96% sensitivity and 62% specificity.[9,15] In a review by Serrano et al. the SFSR and OESIL have been determined to be sufficiently developed for clinical practice.[16] In another study,[17] the SFSR

Table 25.4[13]

Classification	Type	Example
Cardiovascular	Arrhythmia	AV block (2nd degree type II or 3rd degree, bradyarrhythmias, Brugada syndrome, pre-excitation QRS complex (WPW), supraventricular or ventricular tachyarrhythmias
	Functional	ACS, CHF
	Obstructive	Cardiac myxoma, hypertrophic cardiomyopathy
	Structural	Aortic dissection, aortic stenosis, pulmonary embolus, pulmonary stenosis
Neurally Mediated	Carotid hypersensitivity	Carotid massage, head rotation or shaving
	Situational	Cough, defecation, urination, visualization of blood
	Vasovagal	Stress, fear response
Neurologic	Cerebrovascular	Severe basilar artery insufficiency, subclavian steal
Psychiatric	Psychogenic	Anxiety, somatization disorders, "spells"
Orthostatic	Autonomic insufficiency	Connective tissue diseases, diabetes mellitus, spinal cord injury
	Drug effect	Alcohol, anti-hypertensives, drugs of abuse, vaso- or venodilators
Volume/Blood Deficit	Hypovolemia	Dehydration, hemorrhage

and OESIL were compared with clinical judgment and not found to be statistically different for predicting adverse events at 10 days. It is notable, however, that following each clinical rule, no discharged patient would have died, but two patients in the clinical judgment arm died. The relatively novel ROSE rule has an 87% sensitivity and a 98% negative predictive value for 1-month serious outcome in patients with syncope presenting to the ED.[12] It has been shown to perform poorly with an inadequate sensitivity for predicting adverse outcomes at 1 year, however.[18]

Evidence suggests that younger patients with an initial normal evaluation, symptoms consistent with vasovagal or orthostatic syncope, no history of heart disease, and no family history of sudden death are at low risk of an adverse event and may be safely followed as outpatients without further immediate intervention or treatment.[4,19]

Patient Criteria

Patient Selection – Inclusion

It is appropriate to admit an adult patient to an OU who presents to the ED after suffering an unexplained syncopal event for further evaluation and possible diagnostic testing with the goal of establishing a definitive cause. It may also be appropriate to admit a patient to an OU for whom a history of syncope is unclear but cannot be ruled out based on history and physical exam alone.

Patient Selection – Exclusion

Patients who are inappropriate to admit to an OU include (1) those with a clearly identified cause of syncope during the initial ED evaluation and who do not need further treatment and (2) patients with any condition that would require hospital admission independently from the syncopal event, including sustained bradycardia, type II second-degree or complete heart block, sustained supraventricular tachycardia (SVT) or ventricular tachycardia (VT), pre-excited QRS complex, Brugada syndrome, confirmed acute coronary syndrome (ACS), evidence of heart failure, stroke, subarachnoid hemorrhage, shock, coma, symptomatic anemia, major trauma, or cardiac arrest. Patients with known non-syncope syndromes, including light-headedness, dizziness, vertigo, seizure, mechanical falls, metabolic syndrome,

intoxication, etc.[8,10] may not need OU admission for syncope, but may be appropriate candidates for the OU for other reasons including patients in whom the above diagnoses are unclear and/or need further evaluation. (See on Vertigo and Dizziness Chapter 37, Geriatrics Chapter 55, Seizures Chapter 36, etc.)

Management

Patients appropriately admitted to an OU will likely benefit from continued monitoring and further diagnostic testing. All patients should have orthostatic vital signs and standard 12-lead electrocardiography[4,19], and will likely already have had these performed during the initial ED evaluation. A chest radiograph is appropriate for patients with an abnormal physical examination, chest pain, shortness of breath, or concern for pneumonia. Laboratory testing should only be ordered as clinically indicated by the history and physical examination and not as a routine broad laboratory panel. Only 2–3% of patients evaluated for syncope will have abnormal laboratory results.[20] A reasonable initial laboratory evaluation might include a fingerstick blood glucose measurement, a pregnancy test for women of childbearing age, a CBC if SFSR or ROSE are intended to be used for risk stratification, and a BNP measurement if the ROSE tool is utilized. BNP seems to rise from baseline to a peak between 18 hours and 1 week after an acute syncopal episode in many patients. The reasons for this are not clear.[21]

The American Heart Association (AHA)/American College of Cardiology Foundation (ACCF) and the American College of Emergency Physicians (ACEP) guidelines regarding the evaluation of syncope offer an algorithmic approach. If the initial evaluation (history, physical examination, electrocardiogram (ECG), appropriate labs) is nondiagnostic, echocardiography and ischemic evaluation are recommended. Those whose syncope remains unexplained at this point may require tilt-table testing, electrophysiologic studies, or continuous electrocardiographic monitoring.[4,19] A study evaluating 341 consecutive patients referred to a syncope unit showed that history and physical were more reliable in establishing a diagnosis (14%) than results from ECG (10%), Holter monitor (5%), electrophysiology (5%), or echocardiography (1%).[22]

Echocardiography

Echocardiography is a rapid, noninvasive modality that enables the provider to ascertain functional and structural information about the heart and some of the surrounding structures. It can be diagnostic in aortic stenosis or dissection, pericardial effusions/tamponade, hypertrophic cardiomyopathy, obstructive cardiac lesions, and wall motion abnormalities suggestive of ischemic disease. It has been shown to be more useful for those with an abnormal cardiac history or abnormal ECG.[23] In an observation setting, those with a normal cardiac history and normal ECG are unlikely to have an abnormal structural echocardiogram.[2]

Graded Exercise Testing

Options for exercise testing include treadmill or bicycle testing while performing an ECG or echocardiogram. Treadmill testing is the traditional form of exercise stress testing, but can be difficult for the elderly, obese, or those with orthopedic problems. Bicycle testing may be better tolerated by some while still allowing for full physical exertion. If the ECG is abnormal at baseline, or the test would be difficult to interpret alone, echocardiography allows dynamic assessment of cardiac function. Myocardial perfusion scanning exists as another option for patients unsuitable for physical exercise test. Stress testing has been shown to be more useful at confirming coronary artery disease (CAD) than excluding it.[24] (See Stress Testing Chapter 26.)

Electrocardiographic Monitoring

The purpose of continuous electrocardiographic monitoring or telemetry is to capture any potential arrhythmia events if clinically suspected. Despite being commonplace in ED and OUs, prolonged continuous telemetry monitoring is not routinely recommended by the AHA/ACCF and ACEP guidelines.[4,19] Those who have a high pre-test probability for arrhythmias or syncope recurrence, or those with ECG abnormalities should be monitored. The criteria for an abnormal ECG vary greatly among guidelines, however a generally applicable definition would be any non-sinus rhythm, or an ECG with any new changes compared to a previous ECG. In addition to evaluating the ECG for changes indicative of ischemia, the ECG should be closely inspected for dysrhythmias and AV blocks, prolonged QT, pre-excitation, ventricular hypertrophy, Brugada Syndrome, and arrhythmogenic foci. The diagnostic yield of ECG monitoring during short-stay admissions to detect dysrhythmias may be as high as 16% and increases with length of surveillance.[25]

Tilt-Table Testing

Indications for tilt-table testing include suspicion for neurally mediated syncope. However, the 2006 AHA/ACCF scientific statement does not recommend its routine use in the evaluation of syncope. The sensitivity ranges from 26% to 80%, and the specificity is approximately 90%. If the pre-test probability is high in an otherwise healthy patient, a negative test does not effectively exclude the diagnosis.[19]

Electrophysiology

Routine electrophysiologic evaluation is not recommended, but indications for electrophysiology include patients with structural heart disease, CAD with syncope, CAD with an ejection fraction < 35%, and possibly non-ischemic dilated cardiomyopathy.[19]

Computed Tomography

There is no compelling evidence to suggest that a Computed Tomography (CT) scan of the head is routinely indicated in a patient with simple history of syncope and an otherwise normal neurologic examination.[4]

Outcome

The primary outcome in an observation setting is to rule out immediately life-threatening etiologies, such as ACS, arrhythmias or neurologic causes if clinically appropriate. A possible secondary outcome is establishing an etiology for the patient's syncope. Patients who develop abnormal vital signs, ECG abnormalities, additional symptoms, or other high-risk features should have immediate specialist referral or admission. If clinical suspicion for arrhythmia is high, but observation monitoring has not revealed any further episodes, the patient may be referred for outpatient monitoring with a 48-hour Holter monitor, 30-day monitor, or implantable loop recorder. Any patient discharged from an OU should have close follow-up either with a primary care provider or a specialist within 24–48 hours.

Conclusion

The use of OUs in the evaluation of syncope is increasing, and a definitive, validated management plan for the observation setting has not yet been established. There are a number of clinical decision tools at the disposal of the treating physician to aid in determining which patients may be at higher risk for adverse events and warrant admission. These rules help the clinician with risk stratification, but they have not been well validated and are varied in short-term reliability. Common findings amongst these studies that portend poor outcomes include 1) older age, 2) ECG abnormalities, 3) history of cardiac disease, and 4) lack of typical prodrome and/or additional symptoms before syncope. Several national specialty organizations have offered their recommendations for appropriate workup of patients presenting with syncope, and some are moving towards a standardized evaluation. Further research is needed to develop and validate this standardized application. A multidisciplinary approach to the patient with syncope aids in management, and dedicated syncope units with treating physicians and ready access to cardiologists, electrophysiologists, and diagnostic testing may decrease admission length and improve diagnostic yield.

References

1. Soteriades ES, Evans JC, Larson MG, et al. Incidence and prognosis of syncope. *N Engl J Med.* 2002 Sep 19;347(12): 878–885.

2. Anderson KL, Limkakeng A, Damuth E, et al. Cardiac evaluation for structural abnormalities may not be required in patients presenting with syncope and a normal ECG result in an observation unit setting. *Ann Emerg Med.* 2012 May 24. (Epub ahead of print)

3. Sun BC, Emond JA, Camargo CA, Jr. Direct medical costs of syncope-related hospitalizations in the United States. *Am J Cardiol.* 2005; 95 (5): 668–671.

4. Huff JS, Decker WW, Quinn JV, et al. American College of Emergency Physicians. Clinical policy: critical issues in the evaluation and management of adult patients presenting to the emergency department with syncope. *Ann Emerg Med.* 2007; 49(4): 431–444.

5. Alshekhlee A, Shen WK, Mackall J, et al. Incidence and mortality rates of syncope in the United States. *Am J Med.* 2009 Feb; 122(2): 181–188.

6. Kapoor W.N., Hanusa B.H. Is syncope a risk factor for poor outcomes? Comparison of patients with and without syncope. *Am J Med.* 1996 Jun; 100(6): 646–655.

7. Colivicchi F, Ammirati F, Melina D, et al. Development and prospective validation of a risk stratification system for patients with syncope in the emergency department: the OESIL risk score. *Eur Heart J.* 2003; 24: 811–819.

8. Shen WK, Decker WW, Smars PA, et al. Syncope Evaluation in the Emergency Departments (SEEDS): a multidisciplinary approach to syncope management. *Circulation.* 2004; 110: 3636–3645.

9. Quinn JV, Stiell IG, McDermott DA, et al. Derivation of the San Francisco Syncope Rule to predict patients with short-term serious outcomes. *Ann Emerg Med.* 2004; 43: 224–232.

10. Costantino G, Perego F, Dipaola F, et al. on behalf of the STePS Investigators. Short- and long-term prognosis of syncope, risk factors, and role of hospital admission results from the STePS (Short-Term Prognosis of Syncope) study. *J Am Coll Cardiol* 2008; 51: 276–283.

11. Del Rosso A, Ungar AR, Maggi R, et al. Clinical predictors of cardiac syncope at initial evaluation in patients referred urgently to a general hospital: the EGSYS score. *Heart* 2008; 94: 1620–1626.

12. Reed MJ, Newby DE, Coull AJ, et al. The ROSE (risk stratification of syncope in the emergency department) study. *J Am Coll Cardiol.* 2010; 55(8): 713–721.

13. Gauer RL. Evaluation of syncope. *Am Fam Physician.* 2011 Sep 15;84(6): 640–650.

14. Linzer M, Yang EH, Estes NA III, et al. Diagnosing syncope. Part 1: Value of history, physical examination, and electrocardiography. Clinical Efficacy Assessment Project of the American College of Physicians. *Ann Intern Med.* 1997; 126(12): 989–996.

15. Quinn J, McDermott D, Stiell I, et al. Prospective validation of the San Francisco Syncope Rule to predict patients with serious outcomes. *Ann Emerg Med.* 2006 May; 47(5): 448–454.

16. Serrano LA, Hess EP, Bellolio MF, et al. Accuracy and quality of clinical decision rules for syncope in the emergency department: a systematic review and meta-analysis. *Ann Emerg Med.* 2010 Oct; 56(4): 362–373.e1.

17. Dipaola FCG, Perego F, Borella M, et al. San Francisco Syncope

Rule, Osservatorio Epidemiologicosulla Sincopenel Lazio risk score, and clinical judgment in the assessment of short-term outcome of syncope. *Am J Emerg Med.* 2010; 28: 432–439.

18. Reed MJ, Henderson SS, Newby DE, et al. One-year prognosis after syncope and the failure of the ROSE decision instrument to predict one-year adverse events. *Ann Emerg Med.* 2011 Sep; 58(3): 250–256.

19. Strickberger SA, Benson DW, Biaggioni I, et al. AHA/ACCF scientific statement on the evaluation of syncope: from the American Heart Association Councils on Clinical Cardiology, Cardiovascular Nursing, Cardiovascular Disease in the Young, and Stroke, and the Quality of Care and Outcomes Research Interdisciplinary Working Group; and the American College of Cardiology Foundation In Collaboration With the Heart Rhythm Society. *J Am Coll Cardiol.* 2006; 47(2): 473–484.

20. Sarasin FP, Louis-Simonet M, Carballo D, et al. Prospective evaluation of patients with syncope: a population-based study. *Am J Med.* 2001; 111(3): 177–184.

21. Reed MJ, Gibson L. The effect of syncope on brain natriuretic peptide. *Emerg Med J.* 2011 Dec; 28(12): 1066–1067.

22. Alboni P, Brignole M, Menozzi C, et al. Diagnostic value of history in patients with syncope with or without heart disease. *J Am Coll Cardiol.* 2001; 37(7): 1921–1928.

23. Sarasin FP, Junod AF, Carballo D, et al. Role of echocardiography in the evaluation of syncope: a prospective study. *Heart.* 2002; 88(4): 363–367.

24. Banerjee A, Newman DR, Van den Bruel A, et al. Diagnostic accuracy of exercise stress testing for coronary artery disease: a systematic review and meta-analysis of prospective studies. *Int J Clin Pract.* 2012 May; 66(5): 477–492.

25. Croci F, Brignole M, Alboni P, et al. The application of a standardized strategy of evaluation in patients with syncope referred to three syncope units. *Europace.* 2002;4(4): 351–355.

Chapter

26

Stress Testing

Kami M. Hu, MD
Amal Mattu, MD, FACEP, FAAEM

Introduction

Chest pain is one of the leading chief complaints in the emergency department (ED), accounting for approximately 5.2% of all visits in 2012.[1] Unfortunately only 30% of these patients are discharged with a definitive diagnosis,[2] and studies have reported a miss rate of approximately 2–5% for acute coronary syndrome (ACS) in patients discharged home from the ED.[3,4] A missed acute myocardial infarction (MI) carries a 30-day mortality rate of up to 39%,[3] and diagnostic errors in chest pain complaints and acute MI are responsible for the majority of malpractice lawsuits, the highest percentage of settled cases, and the highest payouts.[5] These facts account for why, despite a less than 20% incidence of ACS in ED patients with chest pain,[3,4] approximately half are admitted for further assessment, resulting in an estimated annual cost of over $13 billion.[6] Observation units (OUs) and "chest pain units" (CPUs) have been proven to lower these costs without worsening outcomes,[7,8] and chest pain patients are increasingly admitted to OUs for further monitoring, serial cardiac biomarkers, and frequently, cardiac stress tests. The immediate purpose of these actions is to determine whether obstructive coronary artery disease (CAD), leading to ACS, is the cause of the patient's chest pain. Which type of stress test the patient undergoes is influenced by institutional protocol, but it is important for health care providers to know about these tests and how to select them based on a patient's personal history and best interests.

Discussion

Pretest Probability

While knowledge regarding the variety of available tests is important, a discussion of test selection without a discussion on pretest probability is inappropriate. Statistically, the posttest probability of a diagnosis is dependent on the pretest probability and the diagnostic accuracy of the test in question. The reliability of a stress test result, therefore, depends on the patient's inherent likelihood of CAD, and this probability should help determine the chosen modality.

The pretest probability of CAD can be estimated based on the patient's age, sex, chest pain characteristics, and is classically categorized as very low, low, intermediate, or high risk (Table 26.1).[9] OUs are primarily utilized for patients at low or intermediate risk – patients who cannot be discharged home but do not clearly warrant inpatient care. The 2014 ACC/AHA guideline for the management of non-ST-elevation ACS offers a Class IIa recommendation for non-invasive testing for patients with "possible ACS" and negative initial work-up either prior to or within 72 hours of ED discharge.[9,10] Of note, very-low risk patients should not undergo stress testing, and high-risk patients should be referred for functional imaging or invasive coronary angiography.[11]

Pharmacologic Stress Agents

The primary pharmacologic stress agents include coronary vasodilators (adenosine, dipyridamole/persantine, regadenoson/lexiscan) and a synthetic catecholamine (dobutamine). They should be utilized in patients who cannot exercise maximally in order to achieve appropriate stress on the heart, but the agent chosen should depend on the individual patient. In nuclear stress tests, for example, vasodilators should be utilized in patients with bundle branch blocks or ventricular pacemakers in order to overcome false-positive perfusion defects that occur in these patients during exercise. Dobutamine, however, is the agent of choice

Table 26.1 Pretest Probability of Coronary Artery Disease by Age, Gender, and Symptoms

Age (y)	Gender	Character of Chest Pain/Likelihood of Angina Pectoris			
		Typical/Probable	**Atypical/Possible**	**Nonanginal**	**Asymptomatic**
30–39	Male	Intermediate	Intermediate	Low	Very low
	Female	Intermediate	Very Low	Very Low	Very low
40–49	Male	High	Intermediate	Intermediate	Low
	Female	Intermediate	Low	Very Low	Very low
50–59	Male	High	Intermediate	Intermediate	Low
	Female	Intermediate	Intermediate	Low	Very low
60–69	Male	High	Intermediate	Intermediate	Low
	Female	High	Intermediate	Intermediate	Low

Pretest probability of CAD: High > 90%, Intermediate 10–90%, Low < 10%, Very Low < 5%
Adapted from the 2002 ACC/AHA Updates for Exercise Testing.9

in patients with active bronchospastic disease (COPD, asthma), and in patients who cannot tolerate medications that will interfere with the vasodilator agents (xanthine derivatives, such as theophylline). Further information regarding the various stress agents is listed in Table 26.2.

Types of Stress Tests

Stress tests evaluate a patient's cardiac response to increased work and myocardial oxygen demand. The "stress" is provided by either exercise or pharmacologic mimics, and depending on the modality, these tests provide information about the patient's coronary integrity either by anatomic or functional assessment (or both, in some cases).

Stress Electrocardiogram (treadmill stress test, exercise tolerance test/ETT) – This test assesses for ECG changes such as ST-segment depression or elevations, elicited by patient exercise via bicycle or, most commonly, treadmill. The most standard protocol used is the Bruce protocol, in which patients are subjected to gradually increasing treadmill speed and incline. Patient heart rate and blood pressure are monitored before, during, and after the test, and the reactivity and stability of these parameters and patient's exercise capacity provide prognostic information, even if no ischemic ECG changes are noted. The Duke Treadmill Score (DTS), determined by exercise capacity, ST changes,

and anginal severity, is also used for risk stratification and has proven predictive value. A higher risk by DTS is proportional to risk of CAD and mortality; a low risk DTS is associated with a 0.25% annual mortality risk, while there is a 5% annual mortality with a high risk DTS.[12] ETT has the lowest overall sensitivity and specificity for detecting cardiac ischemia, 68% and 77%, respectively,[10] but has a high negative predictive value in low to intermediate risk patients[13] and remains the initial test of choice in patients with a normal baseline ECG who are able to exercise and are not on digoxin, in whom the accuracy approaches that of stress imaging.[14]

Nuclear Stress Test – Nuclear scanning, a form of myocardial perfusion imaging (MPI), involves the intravenous injection of radioactive isotopes such as thallium-201, technetium-99m sestamibi, or technetium-99 tetrofosmin in conjunction with gamma imaging, such as with single positron emission computed tomography (SPECT) or cardiac positron emission tomography (PET), to capture and measure the blood flow to the heart during stress and at rest. SPECT is the more commonly used imaging technique, with an average sensitivity of 88% and specificity of 74%,[15] and in addition to assessing for coronary artery stenosis, it provides information on left ventricle size and measurements of prior infarcts, if present. The

Table 26.2 Pharmacologic Stress Agents*

Drug	Side Effects	Contraindications	Additional Notes
Coronary Vasodilators			
Adenosine	Chest pain Flushing Headache Nausea Dizziness Dyspnea	• Active bronchospasm or reactive airway disease • 2nd–3rd degree AV heart block without pace maker • Sinus node disease (aka sick sinus syndrome or symptomatic bradycardia) without pace maker • Hypersensitivity to adenosine *Relative:* • Hypotension (sbp < 90 mmHg)	• Ineffective in patients who have taken xanthine derivatives (theophylline, aminophylline, caffeine) or dipyridamole in the past 24 hours • For serious side effects, discontinuation of medication is effective due to extremely short half life
Dipyridamole (Persantine)	Chest pain Hypotension Flushing Headache Nausea Dizziness Dyspnea	• Active bronchospasm or reactive airway disease • 2nd–3rd degree AV block without pacer • Hypersensitivity to dipyridamole *Relative:* • Heart failure/severe left ventricular dysfunction • Atrial tachycardias with rapid ventricular response • Hypotension (sbp < 90 mmHg)	• Ineffective in patients who have taken xanthine derivatives (theophylline, aminophylline, caffeine) in the past 24 hours • Administration of aminophylline counteracts effects
Regadenoson (Lexiscan)	Chest pain Tachycardia Arrhythmia Headache Flushing Nausea Dizziness Dyspnea	• 2nd–3rd degree AV block or sinus node dysfunction without pacer *Relative:* • Active bronchospasm or reactive airway disease • Hypotension (sbp < 90 mmHg)	• May be ineffective in patients who have taken xanthine derivatives (theophylline, aminophylline, caffeine) in the past 24 hours • Administration of aminophylline counteracts effects
Synthetic Catecholamines			
Dobutamine	Tachyarrhythmia Hypertension Chest pain Headache Tremor Palpitations Chills	• Significant aortic stenosis or obstructive cardiomyopathy • Hypersensitivity to dobutamine *Relative:* • Uncontrolled hypertension • Atrial tachyarrhythmias with rapid ventricular response • Hypovolemia	• Agent of choice in bronchospastic patients • Administration of esmolol counteracts effects

* Information collected from Lexicomp and Micromedex databases, June 2012.
AV = atrioventricular
Sbp = systolic blood pressure

ability to synchronize with the patient's ECG, or "ECG-gating," also allows assessment of systolic function. Of note, SPECT MPI currently delivers the most ionizing radiation of all the stress imaging modalities (average effective dose 16.8 mSv, depending on radionuclide and protocol used)[16] although recent studies have been successful at decreasing radiation without sacrificing test accuracy.[17] PET has been proven to be more accurate than SPECT (87% vs. 71% respectively), likely due to better pictures resulting from improved spatial resolution and better correction of soft tissue attenuation artifact.[18] Compared to MPI with SPECT, it has a higher sensitivity,[18] a lower dosimetry,[16] and is performed much more quickly, but its higher cost and lower availability limit its use. Nuclear MPIs are effective tests for risk-stratification; negative tests are associated with a 1–2% per year cardiac event (death or MI) rate if pharmacologic SPECT was used and a < 1% per year event rate if exercise SPECT was used,[19] while a negative myocardial perfusion PET scan is associated with a 0.09% per year cardiac event rate.[20]

Stress Echocardiogram – The stress "echo" uses ultrasonography to assess cardiac activity. While it does not identify specific coronary stenoses, it detects ischemia as new or worsening wall motion abnormalities, decreased wall thickening, or compensatory hyperkinesis in response to cardiac stress. It is logical then, that this test has a rather weak positive predictive value (5–53% in a recent meta-analysis).[13] Its negative predictive value is fairly high however (89–100%),[13] with a < 1% per year cardiac event rate in patients with a normal exercise echocardiogram[21] and 1.2% per year event rate for normal pharmacologic stress echo.[22] The stress echo also provides information on cardiac structure and function, and can concurrently assess for signs to indicate other etiologies of chest pain such as pulmonary embolism, or pericardial effusion. Limitations are those of standard echocardiography, including poor acoustic windows in patients who are obese or have obstructive lung disease. The use of contrast enhancement can help ameliorate these poor views, and a negative contrast-enhanced stress echo has been associated with a 0.8% per year ACS rate in recent studies.[23]

Stress Cardiovascular Magnetic Resonance Imaging – Stress Cardiovascular Magnetic Resonance Imaging (CMR) is also a type of MPI and is one of the newer imaging modalities for evaluation of chest pain and detection of CAD. Coupling pharmacologic stress via adenosine or dobutamine with gadolinium-enhanced magnetic resonance imaging, stress CMR provides a great deal of information due to its excellent spatial resolution and soft-tissue differentiation capabilities. In patients presenting with chest pain, it detects CAD with a reported sensitivity of 96% and specificity of 83%,[24] with an NPV of 100%.[25] It provides anatomic, functional, and prognostic information, and as a part of an accelerated diagnostic protocol that includes both OU admission and monitoring with stress CMR, this modality decreases medical costs without increasing adverse events, when compared to standard inpatient admission.[26]

Computed Tomography Coronary Angiography – Computed Tomography Coronary Angiography (CTCAs) are included in this chapter because they are used in OUs for CAD diagnosis. The standard CTCA is not an actual stress test, although protocols for "stress myocardial CT perfusion" are currently being developed and tested to add a functional assessment to what is now primarily anatomic.[27] CTCAs utilize multi-slice scanners and intravenous contrast to produce 3D images of the heart and coronary vessels with resolution that allows measurement of stenosis severity. CTCAs are quick and have been proven to have high sensitivity and specificity, with negative predictive values of 94–100%.[28,29] In addition to the standard negatives associated with contrasted CTs, the image quality of the CTCA is limited by elevated heart rates and the test must often be administered with beta-blockers in order to achieve slower rates for optimal images.[30] Despite its disadvantages, studies have demonstrated its utility in disposition of chest pain patients; use of CTCA is associated with decreased admission rates from the ED, shorter lengths of stay, and higher detection of CAD when compared with standard "rule-out" protocols.[31]

Testing in Women

Cardiovascular testing in women can be challenging for a variety of reasons. Women with coronary disease generally have more diffuse, less obstructive CAD than their male counterparts.[32] They often present later in life and therefore have, at baseline, decreased exercise capacities that hinder test performance.[33] They are more likely to have baseline ST-segment and T-wave anomalies that might confuse ETT interpretation, they are more subject to soft-tissue attenuation artifact in nuclear studies and poor acoustic windows during echocardiography due to breast tissue, they have smaller cardiac chambers which can affect interpretation of nuclear imaging,[33] and their chest pain is more frequently atypical, affecting pretest risk stratification and conduction of the tests themselves. It is therefore important for providers to be aware of differences in test accuracy in the female population.

The ETT remains the initial test of choice in intermediate-risk women presenting with chest pain, with an average sensitivity and specificity of 61% and 70%, respectively.[34] Occurrence of ST depressions seems to have less prognostic value in women than men,[35] but exercise capacity and chronotropic response remain helpful indicators of future risk in women.[36,37] Stress echo sensitivity is similar to that in men, but specificity is higher in women (80% vs. 56% in men).[38] For SPECT, sensitivity and specificity are both approximately 88%.[39] CTCA has been shown to have a comparable sensitivity between men and women, 96% vs. 90%, both with excellent NPVs (100% and 99%, respectively).[40] The high spatial resolution of CMR mitigates issues such as breast attenuation and small cardiac chamber size; a recent study found no difference in its prognostic value between men and women, and actually demonstrated an impressive annual major adverse cardiac event rate of only 0.3% in women who had negative stress CMR.[41]

Of note, the WOMEN trial recently found that even in females with high exercise tolerance, the mere report of more frequent chest pain was associated with a higher risk of abnormal findings on exercise testing.[42] This study has not yet been repeated, but providers should be on guard and consider frequency of chest pain when determining pretest probability.

Patient Characteristics

Patients undergoing stress testing in OUs should be patients at least 18 years of age, with negative cardiac biomarkers, a negative or non-diagnostic ECG, and no ongoing or worsening chest pain after 6–8 hours of monitoring.[10] It is important to note the absolute contraindications to stress testing: recent acute MI (within 48 hours), unstable angina not stabilized by medical therapy, uncontrolled arrhythmias causing hemodynamic instability or symptoms, severe aortic stenosis, uncontrolled heart failure, and presence or suspicion of acute pulmonary embolism, myocarditis, pericarditis, and aortic dissection. Specific contraindications to the various stress test modalities are included in Table 26.3.

Management

In preparation for stress testing, patients should be made NPO (nil per os) 4–6 hours prior to the test, should not smoke or use nicotine replacement, and should not be given anything containing caffeine during their stay (no caffeine in the prior 12–24 hours is ideal). Patient home medications should generally be continued; although nitrates, beta-blockers, and nondihydropyridine calcium channel blockers may affect exercise response and therefore test accuracy. Depending on the reason for their use, consider holding these medicines until after exercise testing. Diabetic patients should not take oral antihyperglycemics until after testing, and patients on insulin should generally take one-half of their usual dose and eat a light meal 2–4 hours prior to testing, although treatment can be tailored according to blood glucose monitoring in the unit. Patients who have taken theophylline or aminophylline in the prior 24 hours are excluded from pharmacologic stress testing with adenosine, dipyridamole, or regadenoson due to decreased efficacy of the agents in testing. If outside of that time frame, these medications should be held until after the test has been completed.

Outcome

In the setting of short-stay CPU/OUs, stress testing has one main purpose: to risk stratify patients with regards to CAD in order to determine appropriateness of discharge or guide referrals for more intense and urgent management.

Table 26.3 Stress Test Characteristics

Test	Diagnostic Performance	Advantages	Disadvantages	Prognostic Value (Annual Cardiac Event Rate After Negative Test)
Stress Electrocardiogram (ECG)	Sensitivity: 70% Specificity: 77%[10] NPV: 89–100% PPV: 0–77%[12]	• Inexpensive • Widely available • Quick (15–30 min) • Provides information about exercise capacity and prognosis • No radiation exposure	• Does not identify culprit arteries, severity of stenosis or extent of ischemia (therefore less useful after prior MI or revascularization) • Decreased accuracy in females[42] • Cannot use in patients on digoxin or with various baseline ECG abnormalities, or paced rhythms[10]	• Based on DTS risk[44] • Low risk: 0.9% • Medium risk: 1.7% • High Risk: 4.4% *Cardiac event = Cardiac death or MI*
Stress Echo cardiogram	Sensitivity: 86% Specificity: 81%[14, 20] NPV: 89–100% PPV: 5–53%[12] Accuracy: 84–87%[45, 46]	• Fairly quick (< 60 min) • No radiation exposure • Can be used in patients unable to exercise • Can be used in patients with baseline ECG abnormalities • May diagnose other etiologies of chest pain	• Diagnostic views may be limited by operator skill, patient body habitus, or tachycardia • Requires specialist interpretation • Labor intensive	• Pharmacologic stress negative: 1.2%[22] • Exercise stress negative: < 1%[21] *Cardiac event = MI, cardiac death, revascularization[21] (+anginal hospitalization)[22]*
Nuclear myocardial perfusion imaging: Single-photon emission computed tomography	Sensitivity: 82–88% Specificity: 61–74%[10] Accuracy: 71%[18]	• Can be used in patients unable to exercise • Can be used in patients with baseline ECG abnormalities	• Length of time for test (2–6 hours) • On average, the most radiation exposure of any stress test (16.8mSv)[15]	• Pharmacologic stress negative: 1–2% • Exercise stress negative: < 1%[19] *Cardiac event = MI or death*

132

	Advantages	Test characteristics	Disadvantages	Prognostic data
Nuclear myocardial perfusion imaging Positron emission tomography (PET)	• Fairly quick (< 60 min) • Higher accuracy and less radiation than SPECT[18] • Can be used in patients unable to exercise • Can be used in patients with baseline ECG abnormalities	Sensitivity: 84–96% Specificity: 81–93%[47] Accuracy: 87%[18]	• Radiation exposure (avg. 6.1mSv)[48] • Expensive, less widely available • Difficult to perform with exercise stress	• Negative 82Rb-PET: 0.09%[20] *Cardiac event = MI, cardiac death, revascularization*
Stress cardiac magnetic resonance imaging (CMR)	• Fairly quick (< 60 min) • Offers anatomic, functional, and prognostic information • No ionizing radiation	Sensitivity: 96–100% Specificity: 83–91% NPV:100%[24,25] PPV: 67%[24]	• Expensive, less widely available • Contraindicated in patients with renal failure, specific metallic devices, claustrophobia • Limited in patients who are unable to breath-hold, or with arrhythmias	• Negative stress: 1.5%[49] *Cardiac event = MI, death, revascularization, ischemic hospitalization*
Computed tomography coronary angiography (CTCA)	• Very quick (~5 min) • Offers anatomic and prognostic information • Can also assess for pulmonary embolism and aortic dissection (the "triple rule out")	Sensitivity: 96–99% Specificity:85–86% NPV:93–95% PPV: 92–96%[28,29]	• No functional assessment • Requires slow heart rate for optimal images • Radiation exposure (avg. 3.7mSv)[15] • Contraindicated in patients with contrast allergy or renal failure • Risk of contrast-induced nephropathy	• Nonobstructive CAD: 1.4% • Negative for CAD: 0.17%[50] and 99.7% survival at 2.3yrs[51] *Cardiac event: MI, revascularization, all-cause mortality*

NPV = negative predictive value, PPV = positive predictive value, DTS = Duke treadmill score, MI = myocardial infarction, mSV = milliseiverts, CAD = coronary artery disease

Conclusion

Each stress test provides a different array of information, with a different risk-benefit profile and a different overall worth that is specific to the patient being tested, depending on his or her pretest probability. A standard exercise ECG (quick, low-risk, and inexpensive) though imperfect is nevertheless very helpful at decreasing the likelihood that obstructive CAD is the etiology for a patient's chest pain. The negative predictive value of any test is diminished, however, in patients with high pretest probability. Functional testing or testing that concomitantly offers possible therapeutic intervention, such as coronary angiography, is more appropriate in this population.

Stress testing is useful for CAD diagnosis, functional assessment, and prognosis/risk-stratification. In the context of observation medicine, its utilization has been proven to lower cost burden without increasing adverse events when compared to standard inpatient admissions for ACS rule-outs. Providers should be careful, however, about adhering to protocols that subject patients to knee-jerk testing that is not tailored to their individual circumstances or needs. Evidence shows that the majority of low risk chest pain patients in OUs undergo stress tests despite very low pretest probabilities, and when abnormal test results occur, they rarely require action.[43] It is the provider's responsibility to tailor the test to the individual patient, to weigh the risks and benefits, and to withhold stress testing in patients who do not require it. This provider-directed imaging strategy has been proven to lower costs without changes in length of stay or increase in 30-day ACS[8] and is more aligned with the physician's duty to the patients in his care.

References

1. National Hospital Ambulatory Medical Care Survey: 2012 State and National Summary Tables. CDC. www.cdc.gov/nchs/data/ahcd/nhamcs_emergency/2009_ed_web_tables.pdf. [Accessed 18 February 2016]

2. Lindsell CJ, Anantharaman V, Diercks D, et al. The Internet Tracking Registry of Acute Coronary Syndromes (i*trACS): a multicenter registry of patients with suspicion of acute coronary syndromes reported using the standardized reporting guidelines for emergency department chest pain studies. *Ann Emerg Med.* 2006;48(6):666–677.

3. Pope JH, Aufderheide TP, Ruthazer R, et al. Missed diagnoses of acute cardiac ischemia in the emergency department. *N Engl J Med.* 2000;342(16):1163–1170.

4. Christensen J, Innes G, McKnight D, et al. Safety and efficiency of emergency department assessment of chest discomfort. *CMAJ.* 2004;170(12):1803–1807.

5. Brown TW, McCarthy ML, Kelen GD, et al. An epidemiologic study of closed emergency department malpractice claims in a national database of physician malpractice insurers. *Acad Emerg Med.* 2010;17:553–560

6. Wilkinson K, Severance H. Identification of chest pain patients appropriate for an emergency department observation unit. *Emerg Med Clin North Am.* 2001;19:35–66.

7. Goodacre S, Nicholl J, Dixon S, et al. Randomised controlled trial and economic evaluation of a chest pain observation unit compared with routine care. *BMJ.* 2004;328(7434):254.

8. Miller CD, Hoekstra JW, Lefebvre C, et al. Provider-directed imaging stress testing reduces health care expenditures in lower-risk chest pain patients presenting to the emergency department. *Circ Cardiovasc Imaging.* 2012;5(1):111–118.

9. Gibbons RJ, Balady GJ, Bricker JT, et al. ACC/AHA 2002 guideline update for exercise testing: summary article: a report of the American College of Cardiology/American Heart Association Task Force on Practice Guidelines (Committee to Update the 1997 Exercise Testing Guidelines). *J Am Coll Cardiol.* 2002;40:1531–1540.

10. Amsterdam EA, Wenger NK, Brindis RG, et al. 2014 AHA/ACC guideline for the management of patients with non-ST-elevation acute coronary syndromes: executive summary: a report of the American College of Cardiology/American Heart Association Task Force on Practice Guidelines. *Circulation.* 2014;130(25):2354–94.

11. Morise AP. Are the American College of Cardiology/American Heart Association guidelines for exercise testing for suspected coronary artery disease correct? *Chest.* 2000;118:535–541.

12. Mark DB, Shaw L, Harrell FE Jr, et al. Prognostic value of a treadmill exercise score in outpatients with suspected coronary artery disease. *N Engl J Med.* 1991;325:849–853.

13. Amsterdam EA, Kirk JD, Bluemke DA, et al. American Heart Association Exercise, Cardiac Rehabilitation, and Prevention Committee of the Council on Clinical Cardiology, Council on Cardiovascular Nursing, and Interdisciplinary Council on Quality of Care and Outcomes Research. Testing of low-risk patients presenting to the emergency department with chest pain: a scientific statement from the American Heart Association. *Circulation.* 2010;122(17):1756–1776.

14. Simari RD, Miller TD, Zinsmeister AR, et al. Capabilities of supine exercise electrocardiography versus exercise radionuclide angiography in predicting coronary events. *Am J Cardiol* 1991; 67:573–577.

15. Klocke FJ, Baird MG, Bateman TM, et al. ACC/AHA/ASNC guidelines for the clinical use of cardiac radionuclide imaging: a report of the American College of Cardiology/American Heart Association Task Force on Practice Guidelines (ACC/AHA/ASNC Committee to Revise the 1995 Guidelines for the Clinical Use of Cardiac Radionuclide Imaging); 2003.

16. Scott-Moncrieff A, Yang J, Levine D, et al. Real-world estimated effective radiation doses from commonly used cardiac testing and procedural modalities. *Can J Cardiol.* 2011;27(5):613–618.

17. Duvall WL, Wijetunga MN, Klein TM, et al. Stress-only Tc-99m Myocardial Perfusion Imaging in an Emergency Department Chest Pain Unit. *J Emerg Med.* 2012;42(6):642–650.

18. Bateman TM, Heller GV, McGhie AI, et al. Diagnostic accuracy of rest/stress ECG-gated Rb-82 myocardial perfusion PET: comparison with ECG-gated Tc-99m sestamibi SPECT. *J Nucl Cardiol.* 2006;13(1):24–33.

19. Navare SM, Mather JF, Shaw LJ, et al. Comparison of risk stratification with pharmacologic and exercise stress myocardial perfusion imaging: a meta-analysis. *J Nucl Cardiol.* 2004;11(5):551–561.

20. Chow BJ, Wong JW, Yoshinaga K, et al. Prognostic significance of dipyridamole-induced ST depression in patients with normal 82Rb PET myocardial perfusion imaging. *J Nucl Med.* 2005;46(7):1095–1101.

21. Pellikka PA, Nagueh SF, Elhendy AA, et al. American Society of Echocardiography recommendations for performance, interpretation, and application of stress echocardiography. *J Am Soc Echocardiogr.* 2007;20(9):1021–1041.

22. Bedetti G, Pasanisi EM, Tintori G, et al. Stress echo in chest pain unit: the SPEED trial. *Int J Cardiol.* 2005 Jul 20;102(3):461–467.

23. Gaibazzi N, Reverberi C, Badano L. Usefulness of contrast stress-echocardiography or exercise-electrocardiography to predict long-term acute coronary syndromes in patients presenting with chest pain without electrocardiographic abnormalities or 12-hour troponin elevation. *Am J Cardiol.*2011;107(2):161–167.

24. Plein S, Greenwood JP, et al. Assessment of non-ST-segment elevation acute coronary syndromes with cardiac magnetic resonance imaging. *J Am Coll Cardiol.* 2004;44:2173–2181.

25. Lerakis S, McLean DS, Anadiotis AV,et al. Prognostic value of adenosine stress cardiovascular magnetic resonance in patients with low-risk chest pain. *J Cardiovasc Magn Reson.* 2009;11:37.

26. Miller CD, Hwang W, Case D, et al. Stress CMR imaging observation unit in the emergency department reduces 1-year medical care costs in patients with acute chest pain: a randomized study for comparison with inpatient care. *JACC Cardiovasc Imaging.* 2011;4(8):862–870.

27. Blankstein R, Shturman LD, Rogers IS, et al. Adenosine-induced stress myocardial perfusion imaging using dual-source cardiac computed tomography. *J Am Coll Cardiol* 2009; 54:1072–1084.

28. Chow BJ, Abraham A, Wells GA, et al. Diagnostic accuracy and impact of computed tomographic coronary angiography on utilization of invasive coronary angiography. *Circ Cardiovasc Imaging.* 2009;2:16–23.

29. Hu XH, Zheng WL, Wang D, et al. Accuracy of high-pitch prospectively ECG-triggering CT coronary angiography for assessment of stenosis in 103 patients: Comparison with invasive coronary angiography. *Clin Radiol.* 2012; 67(11):1083–1088; Available online 2012 May 19.

30. Giesler T, Baum U, Ropers D, et al. Noninvasive visualization of coronary arteries using contrast-enhanced multidetector CT: influence of heart rate on image quality and stenosis detection.*AJR.* 2002;179:911–916.

31. Litt HI, Gatsonis C, Synder B, et al. CT angiography for safe discharge of patients with possible acute coronary syndromes. *N Engl J Med.* 2012; 366:1393–1403.

32. BaireyMerz CN, Shaw LJ, Reis SE, et al. WISE Investigators. Insights from the NHLBI-Sponsored Women's Ischemia Syndrome Evaluation (WISE) Study: Part II: gender differences in presentation, diagnosis, and outcome with regard to gender-based pathophysiology of atherosclerosis and macrovascular and microvascular coronary disease. *J Am Coll Cardiol.* 2006;47(3 Suppl):S21–29.

33. Mieres JH, Shaw LJ, Hendel RC et al. Writing Group on Perfusion Imaging in Women. American Society of Nuclear Cardiology consensus statement: Task Force on Women and Coronary Artery Disease – the role of myocardial perfusion imaging in the clinical evaluation of coronary artery disease in women [correction].*J Nucl Cardiol.* 2003;10(1):95–101.n

34. Kwok Y, Kim C, Grady D, et al. Meta-analysis of exercise testing to detect coronary artery disease in women. *Am J Cardiol.* 1999;83:660–666.

35. Gulati M, Pandey DK, Arnsdorf MF, et al. Exercise capacity and the risk of death in women: the St James Women Take Heart Project. *Circulation.* 2003;108:1554–1559.

36. Roger VL, Jacobsen SJ, Pellikka PA, et al. Prognostic value of treadmill exercise testing: a population-based study in Olmsted county, Minnesota. *Circulation.* 1998;98:2836–2841.

37. Lauer MS, Francis GS, Okin PM, et al. Impaired chronotropic response to exercise stress testing as a predictor of mortality. *JAMA.* 1999;281:524–529.

38. Marwick TH, Anderson T, Williams MJ, et al. Exercise echocardiography is an accurate and costefficienttechnique for detection of coronary artery disease in women. *J Am Coll Cardiol.* 1995;26:335–341.

39. Mieres JH, Makaryus AN, Cacciabaudo JM, et al. Value of electrocardiographically gated single-photon emission computed tomographic myocardial perfusion scintigraphy in a cohort of symptomatic postmenopausal women. *Am J Cardiol.* 2007;99:1096–1099.

40. Tsang JC, Min JK, Lin FY, et al. Sex comparison of diagnostic accuracy of 64-multidetector row coronary computed tomographic angiography: Results from the multicenter ACCURACY trial. *J Cardiovasc Comput Tomogr.* Published online 2012 June 4.

41. Coelho-Filho OR, Seabra LF, Mongeon FP, et al. Stress myocardial perfusion imaging by CMR provides strong prognostic value to cardiac events regardless of patient's sex. *JACC Cardiovasc Imaging.* 2011;4(8):850–861.

42. Mieres JH, Heller GV, Hendel RC, et al. Signs and symptoms of suspected myocardial ischemia in women: results from the What is the Optimal Method for Ischemia Evaluation in Women? trial. *J Womens Health.* 2011;20(9):1261–1268.

43. Penumetsa SC, Mallidi J, Friderici JL, et al. Outcomes of patients admitted for observation of chest pain. *Arch Intern Med.* Published online 7 May 2012. [Accessed June 12, 2012].

44. Kwok JM, Miller TD, Christian TF, et al. Prognostic value of a treadmill exercise score in symptomatic patients with nonspecific ST-T abnormalities on resting ECG. *JAMA.* 1999;282(110):1047–1053.

45. Cheitlin MD, Armstrong WF, Aurigemma GP, et al. ACC/AHA/ASE 2003 guideline update for the clinical application of echocardiography. A report of the American College of Cardiology/American Heart Association Task Force on Practice Guidelines (ACC/AHA/ASE Committee to Update the 1997 Guidelines for the Clinical Application of Echocardiography); 2003. www.accorg/clinical/guidelines/echo/index.pdf. [Accessed June 12, 2012].

46. Picano E, Molinaro S, Pasanisi E. The diagnostic accuracy of pharmacological stress echocardiography for the assessment of coronary artery disease: a meta-analysis. *Cardiovasc Ultrasound.* 2008;6:30.

47. Husmann L, Wiegand M, Valenta I, et al. Diagnostic accuracy of myocardial perfusion imaging with single photon emission computed tomography and positron emission tomography: a comparison with coronary angiography. *Int J Cardiovasc Imaging.* 2008;24(5):511–518.

48. Einstein AJ, Moser KW, Thompson RC, et al. Radiation dose to patients from cardiac diagnostic imaging. *Circulation.* 2007;116(11):1290–1305.

49. Bertaso AG, Richardson JD, Wong DT, et al. Prognostic value of adenosine stress perfusion cardiac MRI with late gadolinium enhancement in an intermediate cardiovascular risk population. *Int J Cardiol.* 2012 Jun 2. [Epub ahead of print] [Accessed June 14, 2012].

50. Hulten EA, Carbonaro S, Petrillo SP, et al. Prognostic value of cardiac computed tomography angiography: a systematic review and meta-analysis. *J Am Coll Cardiol.* 2011;57(10):1239.

51. Min JK, Dunning A, Lin FY, et al. Age- and sex-related differences in all-cause mortality risk based on coronary computed tomography angiography findings. Results from the international multicenter CONFIRM (Coronary CT Angiography Evaluation for Clinical Outcomes: An International Multicenter Registry) of 23,854 patients without known coronary artery disease. *J Am Coll Cardiol.* 2011;58(8):849–860.

52. Genders TS, Petersen SE, Pugliese F, et al. The optimal imaging strategy for patients with stable chest pain: A cost-effectiveness analysis. *Ann Intern Med.* 2015;162:474–484.

Asthma

Eric Anderson, MD, MBA, FACEP, FAAEM

Introduction

The exact definition of asthma varies by medical discipline. Generally speaking, for emergency physicians, asthma can be considered a chronic condition of recurrent hyper-responsiveness of airways characterized by inflammation and airflow obstruction.[1] Medical treatment strategies involve reducing or preventing airway inflammation and obstruction with anti-inflammatory and bronchodilator medicines. Patient education strategies involve general education about asthma, recognizing and treating exacerbations before they become severe, avoidance of known asthma triggers, and importance of medication compliance.

Asthma is a condition commonly encountered in emergency medicine. Approximately 1.8% of annual emergency department (ED) visits are due to asthma.[2] The condition affects approximately 7–10% of U.S. adults, which represents approximately 22 million Americans.[3,4] Prevalence statistics are similar in Canada.[5] There are approximately 2 million annual ED visits for asthma. There are approximately 500,000 hospital admissions annually for asthma in the United States. Asthma prevalence increased in the 1980s and 1990s, and was noted to plateau in the mid 2000s. Death rates have decreased as well, from 5637 in 1995 to 3816 in 2004.[6,7,8] Though death rates have decreased, they remain high in certain demographic groups: women 2.3 and African Americans 3.4 per 10,000 people with current asthma.[6] The death rate for the general population is less than 2 per 10,000 population.[6] Overall hospitalization rate in the United States in 2005 was 10.3 hospitalizations per 10,000 adults and 19 hospitalizations per 10,000 children.[9] Canada has similar statistics with estimated deaths in 1995 of 400–500 and a death rate in 2004 of 268, which works out to an overall death rate of about 1 per 100,000 Canadian population.[10]

Disposition of Asthma Patients Presenting to Emergency Departments

Of patients that present to the ED for evaluation of asthma, most are ddischarged home. In a study of asthma care in U.S. EDs by Tsai et al., 79% of asthma patients were discharged home, 16% were admitted to the general medical ward or to the observation unit (OU), 2% were admitted to the intensive care unit (icu), and 3% other (left against medical advice or unknown). Only 3% of asthma patients had pneumonia.[4] A Canadian study yielded a similar high discharge rate: 90% of patients were discharged and 7% were admitted.[3] Ginde et al. reviewed asthma care and found a discharge rate of 85–90%.[2]

Cost of Care for Asthma

The approximate annual cost of asthma care in the United States is 18 billion dollars.[11] This cost estimate does not include lost wages from time away from work or cost to patients for medications and follow-up care. Cost of medications was found to be an important barrier to care according to approximately 50% of patients.[12] Asthma is the main cause of missed school days for children.[13] Patients with asthma have 17 mean work days missed annually.[14] OU care of asthma has been shown to be cost-effective when compared to inpatient costs.[13]

Inclusion and Exclusion Criteria for Observation Unit

Presentations of asthma to the ED generally are broken into broad categories: mild, moderate, severe, and life threatening. Table 27.1 lists the various categories of asthma severity as well as the diagnostic criteria for each category. For the

Table 27.1 Asthma Severity

	Ability to Speak	Physical Activity	Pulse	PEFR	pCO$_2$
Mild	Speaks in sentences	Activity causes SOB	< 100	> 70% predicted	< 42
Moderate	Short phrases	Limited activity	100–120	40–69% predicted	< 42
Severe	Words	SOB at rest	> 120	< 40% predicted	> 42
Life threatening	Cannot speak due to work of breathing	Tolerates no activity	Bradycardia	< 25% predicted if patient can perform test	> 42, ABG usually not needed due to imminent respiratory arrest

SOB = shortness of breath
PEFR = peak expiratory flow rate
ABG = arterial blood gas
Adapted from References:[15,16]

purpose of this chapter, the moderate and severe categories will be discussed. Mild exacerbations are generally treated at home or the physician's office. Life-threatening asthma clearly needs to be admitted if not immediately intubated. Patients suitable for the OU are those who have shown improvement during ED treatment, however, the patient or the physician feel that the patient needs more time for medications to take effect or additional treatment. Inclusion and exclusion criteria should be developed for OUs treating patients with asthma. Table 27.2 illustrates general guidelines, inclusion criteria, and exclusion criteria for asthma patients being considered for OUs. OU patients should be discharged within the time constraints of the OU. Whatever the time constraints of your unit, patients should be expected to improve to the point of discharge within that allowed time frame. Patients who are expected to take more than the allowed time in the OU should be hospitalized from the ED. The OU should not be used to decide which patients need an ICU versus medical bed. Most OUs are not considered mini-ICUs and ICU potential patients should remain in the ED until a decision is firmly made about admission to the ICU versus the medical floor.

Treatment in Observation Unit

OU treatment consists of inhaled beta agonists at prescribed intervals, usually every 1–4 hours, inhaled anticholinergic medications, intravenous (IV) or oral steroids, and supplemental oxygen as needed. The opportunity should be taken during the OU stay for asthma education about the prevention of exacerbations and treatment by nurses or asthma educators, pamphlets or video tapes. Smoking cessation education should also occur at this time in applicable patients. Periodic assessments by nursing and/or physician staff should occur to determine response to treatment. Response to treatment should be measured by several subjective and objective criteria. Objective criteria about patient response to treatment include the following: improvement in PEFR or FEV1 to > 70% of predicted or back to patient's historical discharge values, improvement of vital signs, and improvement of pulse oxygen saturation readings. Auscultation of wheezes is not a reliable indicator of pulmonary status. However, pulmonary auscultation in combination with physician clinical judgment and the patient's opinion of their clinical status are useful guides in disposition decisions. Some patients will indicate that they are always discharged with a mild wheeze and that they feel well enough to go home. In these cases, review of the evolution of objective parameters (PEFR, FEV1, vital signs, and pulse oxygen saturation) will guide in disposition decisions.

Medications

There are several classes of therapeutic agents used in the treatment of asthma. OU treatment will be an extension and continuation of treatment initiated in the ED. Inhaled short-acting beta adrenergic agonists cause bronchodilation by stimulation of the enzyme adenyl cyclase, which changes intracellular adenosine triphosphate (ATP) to cyclic adenosine monophosphate (cAMP). This causes intracellular calcium to bind to cell membranes,

Table 27.2 Inclusion and Exclusion Criteria for Adult Asthma Patients in an Observation Unit

Inclusion	Exclusion
Improved clinical course in ED (measured PEFR or FEV1) but patient not well enough to go home	Systolic BP < 80 or > 200
Expected discharge within time parameters of the observation unit	Respiratory Rate > 40
No new symptoms suspicious for ACS, CHF	Pulse > 140
No pneumothorax	Hypoxia (or changed from patient's baseline if on home O$_2$)
Unit has capabilities to perform respiratory treatments and assessments	Unable to speak due to SOB
Unit has capability to intervene if patient decompensates	Indecision between ICU vs. medical floor
	Pulse Oximetry < 80 on room air, pH < 7.3 or > 7.5, pO$_2$ < 60, pCO$_2$ > 50
	ECG changes consistent with ACS

ED = emergency department
PEFR = peak expiratory flow rate
FEV1 = forced expiratory volume one second
ACS = acute coronary syndrome
CHF = congestive heart failure
ICU = intensive care unit
SOB = shortness of breath
ECG = electrocardiogram

The primary anticholinergic agent used for asthma is ipratropium bromide. Ipratropium bromide is a synthetic quaternary derivative of atropine. It has virtually replaced atropine, as the inhaled anticholinergic of choice, due to its improved side effect profile. Anticholinergic medications competitively antagonize acetylcholine at the post ganglionic junction of the parasympathetic nerve terminal.[15] This results in bronchodilation of the larger airways, which compliments the dilation of smaller airways caused by beta2 agonists.[15]

The combination of an inhaled beta2 agonist and an inhaled anticholinergic agent has been shown to decrease hospitalizations in patients with severe airway obstruction.[17,18]

The exact mechanism of systemic corticosteroids has not been fully elucidated, but the effect is felt to be due to increasing responsiveness to beta2 agonists and decreasing inflammation. Onset of action is 4 to 8 hours after administration. Use of systemic corticosteroids administered within an hour of admission results in a decreased need for hospitalization.[15] The usual dose is oral prednisone 40–80 mg daily or methylprednisolone 1 mg/kg.[15]

Supplemental oxygen should be administered to patients to maintain an oxygen saturation of greater than 90%. Magnesium, usually used in moderate to severe asthma is generally administered in the ED. The dose is 1–2 grams IV over 30 min.

Heliox and ketamine are used for severe asthma and, thus, are not appropriate for OU patients. Leukotriene modifiers, mast cell modifiers, and theophylline are maintenance medications and are not used during an acute asthma attack. Aminophylline has virtually disappeared from the pharmacologic armamentarium due to its side effects profile. Generally patients sick enough to require positive pressure ventilation are sick enough to be admitted to the hospital.

which reduces myocytoplasmic calcium concentration thereby causing bronchial smooth muscle relaxation.[15] Three doses, 2.5–5 mg each, administered every 20 minutes in the ED is a safe initial strategy. Sixty to seventy percent of patients will respond well enough to the initial three doses to be discharged home.[16] Further treatments for patients that have a response that is not sufficient to allow discharge home can be given in the OU if it is felt that the patient will require more than 1–2 hours more of treatment and less than the time constraints of the unit, usually < 24 hours. Patients anticipated to require more prolonged treatment should be admitted to the hospital directly from the ED.

Disposition

Patients who fail to respond or become worse during treatment should be hospitalized. Some patients may become worse to the point of requiring intubation. The OU should have staff, equipment, and expertise to manage acutely decompensating asthma patients. Certain patients are at increased risk for death during an asthma exacerbation. Those who have had repeated ED visits, repeated hospitalizations, ICU stays or prior intubations with asthma warrant close monitoring of their respiratory status. Medical conditions that complicate asthma care include congestive heart failure, pneumonia, psychiatric conditions, and substance abuse. Other risk factors that increase the risk of death in asthma are listed in Table 27.3.

Patients who respond to treatment and are deemed fit for discharge should have discharge instructions reviewed with them prior to discharge. There should be an asthma treatment plan if symptoms become worse, in the follow-up instructions. Patients with asthma severe enough to place them in an OU will generally require oral corticosteroids for 3–10 days after discharge.[15, 16] Those who have returned for the second time or whose symptoms persisted for several weeks prior to presentation may require a longer oral treatment course and a slow taper over a longer period of time. A Canadian study showed that patients at risk for relapse and return visit to the ED include those with the following characteristics: ethnicity (white), gender (female), prior ED visits and hospital admissions, and recent treatment with oral corticosteroids.[19] Discharge instructions should include with whom (person or clinic) and when the patient should follow up. The patient should have prescriptions for needed medications: oral corticosteroids, meter dose inhalers for beta adrenergic medications and anticholinergic medications. Prescriptions for maintenance meter dose inhalers for long acting beta2 adrenoreceptor agonist and inhaled steroids should be written if patient is on these medications and has run out. The patient should be educated in the use of a spacer device. If the patient does not have one, a prescription for a spacer device should be provided. The patient can use the inhaled corticosteroid while on the tapering dose of oral corticosteroids.[16]

Conclusion

Treatment of appropriate patients with asthma in an OU is an efficient and safe utilization of limited health care resources. These patients should be expected to be discharged from the OU after a period of treatment that is expected to be within the time parameters of the OU. The OU should have the capability to perform serial evaluations and treatments of asthma patients. The personnel in the OU should have the ability to intervene if the patient becomes unexpectedly worse during the treatment period. Use of an OU can free up hospital beds for sicker patients. OU treatment can be done at less cost than hospitalization.[20,21] Treatment time in the OU is less than treatment time in the hospital.[20]

Table 27.3 Risk Factors for Death in Asthma

Asthma History
Pervious ICU admit or intubation for asthma
Two or more hospitalizations with asthma in the last year
Three or more ED visits for asthma in the last year
Hospitalization or ED visit for asthma in the past month
Using > 2 canisters of SABA per month
Difficulty perceiving severity of asthma
Social History
Low socioeconomic status or inner city residence
Illicit drug use
Comorbidities
Cardiovascular disease
Other chronic lung disease
Chronic psychiatric disease
Physician Factors
Failure to evaluate severity
Failure to disposition appropriately
Failure to prescribe appropriate therapy
Failure to address comorbidities

ICU = intensive care unit
ED = emergency department
SABA = short acting beta2 agonist
Adapted from References:[13,16]

References

1. Fanta CH, Fletcher SW. An overview of asthma management. Up to date. 2012 www.uptodate.com/contents/an-overview-of-asthma-management?source=see_link

2. Ginde AA, Espinola JA, Camargo CA. Improved overall trends but persistent racial disparities in emergency department visits for acute asthma, 1993–2005. *J Aller Clin Immunol* 2008;122: 313–318.

3. Rowe BH, Voaklander DC, Wang D, et al. Asthma presentations by adults to emergency departments in Alberta Canada a large population based study. *Chest* 2009;135: 57–65.

4. Tsai CL, Sullivan AF, Gordon JA. Quality of care for acute asthma in 63 US emergency departments. *J Allergy clin Immunol* 2009;123:354–361.

5. Manfreda J, Becklake MR, Sears MR, et al. Prevalence of asthma symptoms among adults aged 20–44 yrs in Canada. *Can Med Assoc J* 2001; 164:995–1001.

6. Moorman JE, Rudd RA, Johnson CA, et al. National surveillance for asthma: United States, 1980–2004. *MMWR Surveill Summ* 2007;56:1–54.

7. Sly RM. Decreases in asthma mortality in the United States. *Ann Allergy Asthma Immunol* 2000;85:121–127.

8. Sly RM. Continuing decreases in asthma mortality in the United States. *Ann Allergy Asthma Immunol* 2004;92: 313–318.

9. Agency for healthcare research and quality, Rockville, MD HCUP statistical brief # 58. Hospital stays related to asthma for children. 2006, 2008. www.hcup-us.ahrq.gov/ reports/statbriefs/sb58.jsp

10. Hodder R, Lougheed MD, Fitzgerald JM, et al. Management of acute asthma in adults in the emergency department: assisted ventilation. *CMAJ* 2010;182(3): 265–272.

11. Akinbani L. Asthma prevalence, healthcare use and mortality: United States, 2003–5. www.cdc.gov/nchs/ product/pubs/pubd/hestats/ asthma03-05/asthma03-05.htm.

12. Crane S, Sailer D, Patch SC. Improving asthma care in emergency departments: Results of a multihospital collaborative quality initiative in rural western North Carolina. *NCMJ* 2011;72 (2):111–117.

13. Mace SE. Asthma therapy in the observation unit. *Emerg Med Clin of N America* 2001; 19(1):1–16.

14. Tapp S, Lasserson TJ, Rowe BH. Education interventions for adults who attend the emergency room for acute asthma (Review). *The Cochrane Collaboration*. The Cochrane Library 2010 issue 10. Pub John Wiley & Sons Ltd. 1–60.

15. Cydulka RK. *Acute Asthma in Adults. Emergency Medicine: A Comprehensive Study Guide.* Tintinalli JE, Ma J, Cline DM, et al. (eds.) 7th ed 2011; 504–511.

16. Camargo CA, Rachelefsky G, Schatz. Managing asthma exacerbations in the emergency department: summary of the national asthma education and prevention program expert panel report 3 guidelines for the management of asthma exacerbations. *J Em Med* 2009;37:2S:S6–S17.

17. Plotnick LH, Ducharme FM. Combined inhaled anticholinergics and beta2-agonists for initial treatment of acute asthma in children. *Cochrane Database Syst Rev* 2000; (4):CD000060.

18. Rodrigo GJ, Castro-Rodriguez JA. Anticholinergics in the treatment of children and adults with acute asthma: a systematic review with meta-analysis. *Thorax* 2005;60: 740–746.

19. Rowe BH, Villa-Roel C, Sivilotte LA, et al. Relapse after emergency department discharge for acute asthma. *SAEM* 2008;15(8):709–17.

20. Leykum LK, Huerta V, Mortensen. Implementation of a hospitalist-run observation unit and impact on length of stay (LOS): a brief report. *J of Hosp Med* 2010;5: E2–E5.

21. Rydman RJ, Isola ML, Roberts R et al. Emergency department observation unit versus hospital inpatient care for a chronic asthmatic population: a randomized trial of health status outcome and cost. *Med Care* 1998;36(4): 599–609.

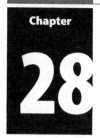

28

Acute Exacerbation of Chronic Obstructive Pulmonary Disease and Bronchitis

Eric Anderson, MD, MBA, FACEP, FAAEM

Introduction

Chronic obstructive pulmonary disease (COPD) is commonly encountered in the emergency department (ED). COPD is the term used to describe a spectrum of pulmonary disease that includes a reversible component of airway obstruction, a chronic cough with sputum component (bronchitis) and an emphysematous component where there is irreversible destruction of terminal airways. There are 1.5 million ED visits in the United States due to COPD.[1] COPD is the third most common cause for hospital admissions, with an estimated 726,000 admissions in 2000.[2] COPD is the fourth leading cause of death in the United States.[2,3] According to the World Health Organization, COPD is projected to be the third leading cause of death and the fifth leading cause of disability worldwide by the year 2020.[4] The mortality of COPD is significant with a greater than 50% mortality rate within 10 years of diagnosis.[5] The World Health Organization estimates that 80 million people worldwide suffer from moderate COPD and that there were 3 million deaths worldwide due to COPD.[4] The cost of COPD to society is significant. In 2007, the total estimated expenditure for COPD in the United States was $42.6 billion with direct medical costs accounting for 26.7 billion.[6] COPD was listed as the primary or secondary diagnosis in 8.5% of all U.S. admissions for patients > 25 years old and 11.5–15.1% of all hospitalizations in patients > 65 years old.[7]

Pathophysiology

COPD is characterized by airway obstruction and inflammation. Unlike asthma, the obstruction is not fully reversible. There is an inflammatory component and a component due to destruction of elastic recoil of the smaller airways as well as narrowing of the airways due to mucosal edema, bronchospasm and bronchoconstriction.[8] COPD has two main types, chronic bronchitis and emphysema.

Emphysema, which represents approximately 15% of patients with COPD, is characterized by a progressive destruction of lung tissue as a result of a cellular and chemotactic response to chronic irritants in the terminal airways.[9] The most common irritants are cigarette smoke and recurrent industrial exposures. A similar response is seen in alpha 1-protease deficiency where the enzyme elastase, elaborated by polymorphonucleocytes, destroys the alveolar septum, which provides support for the bronchial walls. Without the alveolar septal support, the bronchioles collapse early during expiration resulting in airway obstruction. Alpha 1-protease (and alpha 2-macroglobulin) inactivate elastase and provide protection against alveolar septal destruction.[9]

Emphysema is a pathological diagnosis based on lung tissue findings. The small airways collapse prematurely on exhalation. These patients compensate for the diminishing lung function by expanding the chest cavity to increase the available lung capacity. These patients do not ventilate well and will increase the work of breathing to compensate. The rate and depth of breathing will be increased in order to maintain adequate ventilation. This increased work of breathing causes increased metabolic energy demands. The problem is ventilation not oxygenation.[9] Clinical findings that typify the emphysematous patient include tendency to be thin, have a barrel chest, use pursed lipped breathing, and maintain oxygenation. This presentation has come to be known as the "pink puffer."

Chronic bronchitis is characterized by the hypersecretion of mucus and airway inflammation and obstruction with decreased airflow. There is a loss of surfactant and protease inhibitor producing pulmonary epithelial cells, which are replaced by mucus producing cells.[8] There is recruitment of inflammatory cells, which leads to chronic inflammation and narrowing of the airways. This results in fibrosis and narrowing resulting in chronic bronchitis.[5] These patients will have a chronic cough. Chronic hypoxia and decreased cardiac output secondary to pulmonary hypertension and cor pulmonale gives these patients the appearance of mild cyanosis and peripheral edema.[9] The underlying problem is one of poor oxygenation. The classic appearance of these patients is that they will tend to retain CO_2, appear somewhat edematous and cyanotic, the "blue bloater." Chronic Bronchitis is a diagnosis based on clinical findings: cough producing sputum for 3 months out of the year for 2 consecutive years not attributable to another cause.

Most COPD patients present with a combination of chronic bronchitis and emphysema symptoms. It is the rare patient that will be purely one or the other.[5]

A dominant risk factor for the development of COPD is cigarette smoking. Fifteen percent of chronic smokers develop COPD. Why some smokers develop COPD and others do not is not clearly understood. Five to ten percent of COPD patients have never smoked.[10] Alpha 1 antitrypsin deficiency is present in 1–2% of COPD patients.[5] Other factors that predispose for the development of COPD include indoor and outdoor air pollution from fuel burning and occupational exposures.[4,11]

The Global initiative for chronic obstructive lung disease (GOLD) has adopted a definition for COPD that recognizes airflow limitation as often being progressive and associated with an abnormal inflammatory response of the lungs to noxious particles and gases.[4,12] The GOLD classification of COPD has four stages of severity. With Stage I Mild COPD, the FEV1 is $\geq 80\%$ of predicted, with or without chronic symptoms (cough, sputum production). Stage II Moderate COPD is FEV1 between 50% and 79% of predicted and the patient may have dyspnea on exertion and cough. Stage III Severe COPD is FEV1 between 30% and 40% of predicted, and reduced exercise capacity. Stage IV very severe COPD is FEV1 $< 30\%$ predicted or $< 50\%$ predicted with chronic respiratory failure. In all stages the FEV1/FVC ratio is < 0.70. Since most EDs do not have formal pulmonary function testing, clinicians evaluate the severity of the exacerbation clinically.

The Anthonisen criteria are historical factors used to grade the acute exacerbation of COPD. Three symptoms are used to evaluate the patient. Increased sputum production, increased sputum purulence and the presence of dyspnea are used in the Anthonisen criteria. Type III patients have three symptoms, Type II patients have two of the three symptoms and Type I have one symptom.[13] Since patients presenting to the ED usually have at least dyspnea, most are Type I or II. Guidelines recommend antibiotics at discharge for Type I and II.[13] The Anthonisen criteria have a high clinical utility in the ED setting.

Clinical Presentation

The typical COPD patient will present to the ED complaining of shortness of breath (SOB) and cough productive of phlegm. There may be wheezing and minimal or no response to medications. In many cases the patient will know their diagnosis. In other cases the patient will report only a breathing problem, lung problem or frequent use of inhalers. Key elements of the history include onset and duration of symptoms, presence of SOB, fever, chest pain, cough, production of phlegm, change in phlegm amount or purulence and recent respiratory infection. Other historical keys include smoking, prior similar presentations to EDs and prior intubations or ICU stays for shortness of breath.

Differential diagnosis includes cardiovascular disease (CVD) where chest pain may or may not be a prominent complaint. CVD may present with SOB only. Differentiating COPD from CVD may be difficult on clinical grounds alone as many patients have both conditions and both conditions have symptoms and physical examination elements that overlap. Patients with CVD and COPD have more frequent COPD exacerbations and incur higher costs than patients with COPD alone.[14] Cardiac enzymes will help only if positive. Congestive heart failure (CHF) can be difficult to distinguish from chronic bronchitis as both conditions may present with SOB, edema and CO_2 retention. Patient history and B type naturetic peptide (BNP) level will help in these situations. Some patients will have both conditions. Pneumonia may be distinguished by focal infiltrates on chest radiograph, though again there is overlap in the symptoms and physical examination findings. Other conditions with similar presentations to COPD are listed in Table 28.1.

Table 28.1 Differential Diagnosis of Chronic Obstructive Pulmonary Disease (COPD) Exacerbation

Cardiac

Acute Coronary syndrome

Congestive heart failure

Pulmonary

Pneumonia

Asthma

Pulmonary embolus

Pneumothorax

Other

Carbon monoxide

Hemoglobinopathy

Severe anemia

Table 28.2 Predictors of Poor Outcome in Chronic Obstructive Pulmonary Disease (COPD) Exacerbations (Death, Prolonged Hospitalization, Mechanical Ventilation)

Patient Characteristics	Male sex
	Age > 70 years
	Continued smoking
	Poor functional performance status
Historical Characteristics	Prior hospitalizations for COPD within the last 6 months
	Maintenance corticosteroids
	Maintenance oxygen
Physical Examination Findings	Increased heart rate
	Increased respiratory rate
	Cyanosis
	Low body mass index
	Neurologic impairment
	Asterixis
	Accessory muscle use on inspiration
	Abdominal muscle use on expiration
Labs	Blood gas results: low pH, low oxygen, high pCO_2

Adapted from Roche et al. [15]

Emergency Department Management

This chapter focuses on the observation unit (OU) management of COPD exacerbations so ED management will only be covered briefly here. Patients are treated with beta adrenergic agonists, anticholinergics, corticosteroids, supplemental oxygen as needed and hydration as needed. Antibiotics will be used on most acute exacerbations of COPD. Evaluations to rule out confounding conditions include: a good history and physical examination, chest radiography, electrocardiogram, BNP, and cardiac enzymes. A decision about disposition must be made during the emergency evaluation and treatment period. Clinical factors associated with poor outcome, death or need for invasive mechanical ventilation include: advanced age, high respiratory rate, high pulse rate, low body mass index, neurologic impairment, number of previous COPD exacerbation admissions, smoking, number of Anthonisen criteria, poor performance status, SpO_2, APACHE II Score (Acute Physiology and Chronic Health Evaluation II), and blood gas values: low pH, low oxygen saturation, and high pCO_2. (See Table 28.2.)[15]

Treatment of decompensated comorbid conditions such as CHF, diabetes, hypertension and others should be initiated in the ED. As mentioned earlier, patients with comorbid conditions will tend to have more COPD exacerbations and require more resources than patients with COPD alone.[14]

A relatively high percentage of patients, up to 59% in one study, with acute exacerbation of COPD are admitted from the ED.[13] Approximately 15% of patients discharged from the ED returned within 2 weeks for readmission.[5] Patients suitable for the OU include those who demonstrated some clinical improvement of their symptoms during the ED stay. OU patients should be those where it is expected that their symptoms are expected to improve during the period in the OU. Patients who are expected to require a longer period of treatment should be admitted to the hospital from the ED.

Observation Unit Management

Treatment should be continued in the OU at intervals that facilitate clinical improvement. Therapeutic

Table 28.3 Treatment for Chronic Obstructive Pulmonary Disease (COPD)

Medication	Dosage	Therapeutic Effect	Common Side Effect
Short-acting beta adrenergic agonists Albuterol, Levalbuterol	Albuterol 2.5–5 mg neb every 2 to 4 hrs. Levalbuterol 0.63–1.25 mg neb every 4 hrs.	Bronchodilation of small airways	Tremulousness, anxiety, nausea, some decrease in serum potassium
Anticholinergics Ipratropium	0.5 mg neb every 4 hrs.	Bronchodilation of large airways	Tachycardia, palpitations, nausea
Antibiotics	First-line: amoxicillin, trimethoprim-sulfamethoxazole, doxycycline Second-line: Advanced generation quinolones, 2nd or 3rd generation cephalosporins, amoxicillin/clavulanate	Treat infections that may be contributing to the acute attack	Per the antibiotic chosen
Corticosteroids	Prednisone 40–60 mg po or Methyprednisolone 125 mg IV	Decreases inflammatory response	Hyperglycemia, fluid retention, weight gain, adrenal suppression
Oxygen	As needed to keep O_2 saturation above 92%, between 88 and 92% in known CO_2 retainers	Improve oxygenation	Respiratory depression in CO_2 retainers
Treatment of comorbid conditions			

Neb = nebulizer

modalities include: bronchodilators, anticholinergic agents, corticosteroids, supplemental oxygen, antibiotics, and stabilization and treatment of other medical conditions that may have been exacerbated. (See Table 28.3.)

Short-acting beta adrenergic agonists administered via nebulizer device or metered dose inhaler are first-line agents to treat the reversible component of COPD. Albuterol and levalbuterol are the primary short-acting beta adrenergic agents used in COPD. Salmeterol a long-acting beta adrenergic agent is used as maintenance therapy and is not used as treatment in the acute exacerbation of COPD. The pharmacology of these agents is detailed in Chapter 27 on Asthma.

The anticholinergic agent ipratropium bromide is a synthetic quaternary derivative of atropine. This agent works to competitively antagonize acetylcholine at the post ganglionic junction of the parasympathetic nerve terminal.[16] This results in dilation of the larger airways which compliments the dilation of the smaller airways caused by beta 2 agonists.[16]

Short acting beta agonists and anticholinergics are complimentary agents used to treat the bronchospasm component of COPD. Albuterol 2.5–5 mg with atrovent 0.5 mg given via nebulizer every 2–4 hours while in the OU will work to improve pulmonary function.

As described in Chapter 27 on asthma, the exact mechanism of action of corticosteroids in not fully understood. Onset of action is 4–8 hours after administration. The typical dose is prednisone 60 mg orally daily or methylprednisolone 1 mg/kg IV every 6 hours.[16]

Supplemental oxygen should be administered to patients on home oxygen therapy and others as needed to keep the saturation greater than 92%. Caution must be used in COPD patients who are chronically hypoxic and have adapted to hypoxia not to provide too much oxygen and suppress the hypoxic respiratory drive. These patients will tolerate some degree of hypoxia with saturations in the high 80s or low 90s. Review of the medical record with particular attention to prior arterial blood gas results (to determine if the patient is a

CO_2 retainer) and discussions with knowledgeable patients about their baseline respiratory status will help to determine the patient's oxygen requirement.

The bronchitis component of COPD is treated with antibiotics. Antibiotics are recommended for Anthonisen Type I and II exacerbation of COPD.[13] Typical bacteria in the sputum of COPD patients include: *Streptococcus pneumonia, Haemophilus influenzae, Moraxella catarrhalis* and *Pseudomonas aeruginosa*. Typical viruses include: rhinovirus, influenza, parainfluenza, respiratory syncytial virus, coronavirus and adenovirus.[5] *P. aeruginosa* should be considered in more severe cases and in patients who have recently been hospitalized or had several courses of antibiotics in the last year.[13] Antibacterial coverage should take into consideration the local bacterial sensitivity and prevalence patterns of the typical bacterial species listed above. Typical (first-line) antibiotics include: trimethoprim-sulfamethoxazole, ampicillin and doxycycline. However, some authors recommend amoxicillin/clavulanate, second- and third-generation cephalosporins or advanced generation quinolones (moxifloxacin, levofloxacin) as superior to the first-line antibiotics.[5] Treatment with antibiotics decreases short-term mortality, treatment failures and sputum purulence.[13]

Corticosteroids are used in the acute exacerbation of COPD to treat the inflammatory component of COPD. Corticosteroids have been shown to reduce admission rates, decrease the length of hospital stay and decrease treatment failures defined as relapse or hospitalization within 30 days.[13,17,18] Corticosteroids are effective when given orally or parenterally. Typical treatments are Prednisone 40-60 mg orally per day. There has been no benefit to taking more than 60 mg of Prednisone daily.[8] Methylprednisolone 125 mg IV may be given to patients who cannot take oral medications.[5]

Noninvasive positive pressure ventilation (NIPPV) is typically initiated in the ED when the patient is not responding to treatment or initiated on ED arrival and discontinued after the patient improves. In general, patients that require continual NIPPV should be admitted to the hospital and not to the OU while on NIPPV, as they require a higher level of monitoring and care.

Disposition

Patients who fail to respond to treatment will need to be admitted to the hospital. Some patients will unexpectedly decompensate to the point of needing NIPPV or intubation and mechanical ventilation. Personnel who staff the OU need to be able to recognize respiratory decompensation and have the skills and equipment needed to intervene. Predictors of poor outcome are listed in Table 28.2.

Patients deemed well enough to go home should have discharge instructions reviewed with them prior to discharge. Recommendation of smoking cessation should be made for those that continue to smoke. Discharge instructions should be time and person (or clinic) specific as to when and whom the patient is to follow up. Instructions about COPD, bronchitis and other comorbid conditions and medications should be provided. Warning of signs of reasons to return sooner than their scheduled follow-up time should be part of the COPD instructions. Prescriptions for prednisone, inhalers, antibiotics and refills of maintenance medications should be provided.

Conclusion

COPD is a chronic condition that has several components: inflammatory and obstructive. Chronic Bronchitis can be exacerbated by bacterial or viral infection. These conditions are worsened by cigarette smoking. Of COPD patients that seek care in EDs, 50–60% require admission to hospital from the ED and 20–30% will relapse within 4 weeks.[13] There are no specific data on relapse rates or admission rates for COPD patients seen in OUs and research can be done in this area. Treatment of appropriate COPD patients in the OU can save inpatient beds for sicker patients.

References

1. Tsai, CL, Rowe BH, Cydulka RK, et al. ED visit volume and quality of care in acute exacerbations of chronic obstructive pulmonary disease. *Am J of Emerg Med* 2009;27:1040–1049.

2. Mannino DM, Homa DM, Akimbami LJ, et al. Chronic obstructive pulmonary disease surveillance – United States. 1971–2000. *MMWR Surveil Summ* 2002;51: 1–16.

3. Mannino DM, Braman S. The epidemiology and economics of chronic obstructive pulmonary disease. *Proc Am Thorac Soc* 2007;4:502–506.

4. Arbex MA, de Souza Conceicao GM, Cendon SP, et al. Urban air pollution and chronic obstructive pulmonary disease-related emergency department visits. *J Epid Comm Health* 2009;63:777–783.

5. Howes DS, Bellazzini MA. *Chronic Obstructive Pulmonary Disease. The Clinical Practice of Emergency Medicine*, 5th ed. Wolfson AB et al. (eds.) 2010;439–443.

6. Simoni-Wastila L, Blanchette CM, Zhao L, et al. Hospital and emergency department utilization associated with treatment for chronic obstructive pulmonary disease in a managed-care medicare population. *Curr Med Research & Opin* 2009;25(11): 2729–2735.

7. Holguin F, Folch E, Redd SC, et al. Comorbidity an mortality in COPD related hospitalizations in the United States, 1979 to 2001. *Chest* 2005; 128:2005–2011.

8. Bates CG, Cydulka RK. *Chronic Obstructive Pulmonary Disease.*

Emergency Medicine: A Comprehensive Study Guide. Tintinalli et al. (eds.) ACEP 2011;511–517.

9. Anderson E. Chronic Obstructive Pulmonary Disease. Critical decisions in emergency medicine. *ACEP* 2002;16(11):15–22.

10. Barnes PJ. New therapies for Chronic Obstructive Pulmonary Disease. *Thorax* 1998;53(2):137–47.

11. Liu Y, Perez-Padilla R, Hudson NL, et al. Outdoor and indoor air pollution and COPD related diseases in high and low income countries. *Int J Tuberc Lung Dis* 2008;12:115–127.

12. Pauwels RA, Buist AS, Calverley PM, et al. Global strategy for the diagnosis management and prevention of chronic obstructive pulmonary disease. NHLBF WHO Global initiative for chronic obstructive lung disease (GOLD). Workshop summary. *Am J Resp Crit Care Med* 2001;163:1256–1276.

13. Bhutani M, Cydulka R, Rowe B, et al. Assessment and management of chronic obstructive pulmonary disease in the emergency department and beyond. *Expert Review of*

Respiratory Medicine 2011 (Aug);5.4:549–565.

14. Dalal AA, Shah M, Lunacsek O, et al. Clinical and economic burden of patients diagnosed with COPD with comorbid cardiovascular disease. *Respir Med* 2011;105: 1516–1522.

15. Roche N, Rabbat A, Zureik M, et al. Chronic obstructive pulmonary disease exacerbations in emergency departments: predictors of outcome. *Curr Opin in Pul Med* 2010;16:112–117.

16. Cydulka RK. *Acute Asthma in Adults. Emergency Medicine: A Comprehensive Study Guide.* Tintinalli JE et al. (eds.) 7th edition 2011;504–511.

17. Bullard MJ, Liaw SJ, Tsai YH, et al. Early corticosteroid use in acute exacerbations of chornic airflow obstruction. *Am J Emerg Med* 1996;14: 139–143.

18. Neiwoehner DE, Erbland ML, Deupree RH, et al. Effect of systemic glucocorticoids in exacerbations of chronic obstructive pulmonary disease. Depart of veterans affairs cooperative study group. *N Eng J Med* 1999; 340: 1941–1947.

Chapter 29

Community Acquired Pneumonia

Eric Anderson, MD, MBA, FACEP, FAAEM

Introduction

Pneumonia is a common complaint treated daily in emergency departments (EDs). There are approximately 5–6 million patients diagnosed with community acquired pneumonia (CAP) annually.[1] There are approximately 1.5 million ED visits annually due to pneumonia.[2] CAP causes approximately 4 million episodes of illness and results in more than 1 million hospital admissions in the United States each year.[3,4]

CAP is the leading cause of death due to infectious diseases in Western countries.[5] CAP is a leading cause of intensive care unit (ICU) death internationally.[5,6]

The average mortality rate for hospitalized patients is 13%, however the range is from 8% mortality in nonhospitalized to 36.5% in patients admitted to the ICU.[7,8,9] Approximately 10% of hospitalized CAP patients are admitted to the ICU.[10] In the United States, CAP is the seventh leading cause of death with an annual estimated economic cost of 9 billion dollars.[11]

Definitions[12]

1. Health care associated pneumonia (HCAP) occurs in patients who: have been hospitalized for more than 2 days within the last 90 days, reside in a nursing home or long-term care facility, are hemodialysis patients, are on immunosuppressive therapy or wound care within the last 30 days.
2. Hospital acquired pneumonia (HAP): occurs after 48 hours of hospital admission.
3. Ventilator associated pneumonia (VAP): occurs after the first 48 to 72 hours post intubation.
4. Community acquired pneumonia (CAP): occurs in patients who do not meet the criteria for HCAP, HAP, and VAP.

Presentation and Disposition of Patients Presenting to the ED with CAP

Patients will present to the ED in various states of illness ranging from nonspecific symptoms to septic. The very young and the very old may not present with respiratory symptoms at all. The elderly or very young may simply present with a fever or malaise or alteration of baseline mental status. Classic symptoms for pneumonia include: cough productive of phlegm, fever, pleuritic chest pain, and general malaise with or without shortness of breath. The patient may have all or any combination of the symptoms slowly increasing over several days. There may also be loss of appetite or unexplained general fatigue.

Risk factors for CAP include: chronic conditions such as diabetes, chronic renal failure, liver disease, congestive heart failure (CHF), chronic obstructive pulmonary disease (COPD), valvular heart disease, muscular dystrophies, nasogastric tubes, stroke, chronic alcoholism, and neoplasia. See Table 29.1.

Emergency Department

Initial ED management of CAP includes identification of the illness and initiation of treatment. Intravenous (IV) fluids and supplemental oxygen are administered as needed and antibiotic treatment is initiated (see later in chapter). The disposition is based on the patient's hemodynamic stability and the physician's impression of the likelihood that the patient will recover on oral antibiotics at home.

There are several clinical grading scales to help with this decision. confusion, urea concentration, respiratory rate, blood pressure (CURB) and pneumonia severity index (PSI) are two of the commonly used clinical tools used to assess the

Table 29.1 Risk Factors for Development of Pneumonia

Diabetes

Stroke

COPD

Congestive heart failure

End stage renal disease

Liver disease

Muscular dystrophy

Chest wall deformity

Various feeding tubes

Seizure disorder

Chronic alcoholism

Illicit drug use

Elderly

Immunosuppression

Table 29.2 Factors Associated with Subsequent Hospitalization after an Observation Unit Stay

Tuberculosis

Alcoholism

Chronic debilitation

Comorbid illness

Osteoporosis

Persistent symptoms

Persistent fever

Adapted from Chan et al.[16]

severity of pneumonia. CURB uses four clinical parameters to assess the severity of pneumonia: confusion, urea concentration greater than 7 mmol/L, respiratory rate greater than 30 breaths per minute and low blood pressure. Two or more of these criteria indicate an increased risk of death.[1] CURB 65 takes age greater than or equal to 65 years old into account as well as the other CURB criteria.[12]

The PSI uses 20 demographic, clinical, and laboratory criteria to determine the severity of pneumonia. The PSI rule was derived and validated as part of the pneumonia patient outcomes research team (PORT), which prospectively studied 14,199 adults to determine which patients were at low risk of death.[14] These criteria are used to categorize patients into five classes of increasing risk of death.[1,14]

Other indexes include the shock index (SI: pulse rate divided by the systolic blood pressure). The adjusted shock index (ASI) is the same as SI but uses a pulse rate adjusted for temperature by decreasing the pulse rate by 10 for each 1 degree C above 37 degrees C. There is the confusion, age, respiratory rate, shock index (CARSI); CARASI is the same as CARSI but uses the adjusted shock index.[13,15]

Patients deemed well enough to go home should have antibiotics initiated in the ED prior to discharge. Patients who require intubation or

pharmacologic blood pressure support should be admitted to the ICU.

Patients admitted to the medical floor are assessed as being too ill to go home or to the observation unit (OU). These patients usually may demonstrate several of the risk factors for pneumonia (Table 29.1) or medical conditions that are associated with subsequent admission to the hospital after an OU stay (Table 29.2). In some cases it will be the clinical judgment of the emergency physician that warrants admission. In other cases it will be the social environment into which the patient is being discharged that will mandate hospitalization until the social situation can be improved.

Patients admitted to the OU should be expected to be improved within 24 hours or within the time parameters of your OU. Inclusion and exclusion criteria for OU referral are listed in Table 29.3. Patients should not be placed into the OU if they require emergent intubation or pharmacologic blood pressure support, or have a markedly abnormal vital sign, new hypoxia, and/or ECG changes consistent with an acute coronary syndrome.

Observation Unit Management

Antibiotic treatment should be initiated in the ED or soon after admission to the OU. There are various treatment regimes. Generally parenteral treatment regime should be initiated in the ED and continued in the OU with transition to the outpatient regime at the time of discharge. If the patient has not improved enough for discharge, the patient will be admitted. Signs that a patient is ready for discharge include: decreased general malaise or weakness, less shortness of breath, decreased cough, decreased fever, and an overall improved sense of well-being. Signs that a patient

Table 29.3 Inclusion and Exclusion Criteria for Pneumonia Patients in an Observation Unit

Inclusion	Exclusion
Improved clinical course in ED	BP < 80 or > 200 systolic
Expected discharge within time parameters of the observation unit	RR > 40
No new symptoms suspicious for ACS	HR > 140
No pneumothorax	Hypoxia (changed from patient's baseline if on home O$_2$)
Unit has capabilities to perform respiratory assessments	Unable to speak due to shortness of breath
Unit has capability to intervene if patient decompensates	Indecision between ICU vs. medical floor
	Pulse oxygen saturation < 80 on room air, pH < 7.3 or > 7.5, pO$_2$ < 60, pCO$_2$ > 50
	ECG changes consistent with ACS
	Emergent intubation
	Pharmacologic blood pressure support

is not well enough for discharge include: worsening of the presenting symptoms or exacerbation of chronic underlying conditions (diabetes, CHF, COPD). The development of hypoxia or hypotension or worsening general weakness are signs that the patient is not yet well enough to go home. Some elderly or debilitated patients may be slightly improved but may not be well enough to go home and resume their activities of daily living (feeding, ambulation, personal hygiene, etc.). A study by Chan et al. found that certain underlying medical conditions were associated with subsequent hospitalization after an OU stay.[16] (See Table 29.2.)

Likely organisms in CAP include: *Pneumococcus, Legionella, Mycoplasma, Haemophilus influenzae, Chlamydia pneumonia, and Moraxella catarrhalis.*[16]

Antibiotic treatment in the OU continues the ceftriaxone (1 g IV q 24 h) and azithromycin (500 mg IV q 24 h) initiated in the emergency department. Patients who are penicillin allergic may be treated with levofloxacin (750 mg IV q 24 h).[17]

If community aspiration pneumonia is suspected treatment should be initiated with ampicillin/sulbactam (1.5–3 g IV q 6–8 h, decrease if impaired creatinine clearance) or clindamycin (600–900 mg q 8 h) for penicillin allergic patients.[17]

Outpatient regimes after the OU stay include: oral clarithromycin (250–500 q 12 h, decrease if impaired creatinine clearance), azithromycin (250 mg daily), and as a second-line choice doxycycline (100 mg q 12 h).[17,18] Respiratory flouroquinolones, levofloxacin (750 mg daily), may also be used, but the Centers for Disease Control recommends reserving these agents for those who cannot tolerate or have failed other therapy or have significant comorbidities without criteria for HCAP.[18]

Disposition

At the time of discharge patients should be given a prescription for the appropriate antibiotic as well as pneumonia home-going instructions. The patient should be informed as to which symptoms indicate a worsening condition and warrant a return to the ED. Antipyretics and analgesics should be prescribed as needed. Follow-up instructions should be person or clinic specific and time specific and symptom specific. Instructions regarding modification of routine medications, if any, should also be given.

Summary

Patients presenting to the ED with pneumonia and placed in the OU should be stable and have an expected clinical course that will allow discharge within the time constraints of the OU. Patients that have new hypoxia or hypotension should not be admitted to the OU. Patients who are placed on mechanical ventilation should not be placed in the OU. OU treatment should consist of antibiotics, analgesics, antipyretics, hydration, and antiemetics as needed. Treatment of stable chronic medical conditions should also be maintained in the OU. Patients who are improved and able to go home after treatment may be discharged with appropriate antibiotics and pneumonia care instructions. Patients who have not improved sufficiently to go home should be admitted. There are several pneumonia severity rating scales that will aid the physician in deciding questionable cases.

The OU admission is useful for the management of patients who are not quite ill enough to warrant a full hospital admission but the ED may have reservations about immediate discharge to home. The OU has been shown to decrease costs of care and decrease utilization of inpatient beds.[19,20]

References

1. Kontou P, Kuti JL, Nicolau DP. Validation of the infectious disease society of America/American Thoracic Society criteria to predict severe community-acquired pneumonia caused by streptococcus pneumonia. *Am J of Emerg Med* 2009;27: 968–974.

2. McCaig LF, Nawar EW. National Hospital Ambulatory Medical Care Survey: 2004 emergency department summary. *Adv Data* 2006 Jun 23;(372):1–29.

3. Aujesky, D, McCausland JB, Whittle J, et al. Reasons why emergency department providers do not rely on the pneumonia severity index to determine the initial site of treatment for patients with pneumonia. *CID* 2009;49: e100–e108.

4. DeFranco CJ, Cullen KA, Kozak LJ. National Hospital discharge survey 2005 annual summary with detailed diagnosis and procedure data. *Vital Health Stat* 2007; 13(165): 1–209.

5. Chalmers JD, Taylor JK, Mandal P, et al. Validation of the infectious diseases society of America/American thoracic society minor criteria for intensive care unit admission in community acquired pneumonia patients without major criteria for contraindications to intensive care unit care. *CID* 2011;53:503–511.

6. Trotter CL, Stuart JM, George R, et al. Increasing hospital admissions for pneumonia, England. *Emerg Inf D* 2008;14:727–733.

7. Barlett JG, Dowell SF, Mandell LA, et al. Practice guidelines for the management of community acquired pneumonia in adults. *Clin Infect Dis* 2000;31: 347–382.

8. Fine MJ, Smith MA, Carson CA, et al. Prognosis and outcomes of patients with community acquired pneumonia. A meta-analysis. *JAMA* 1996;275:134–141.

9. Marrie TJ, WU L. Factors influencing in hospital mortality in community acquired pneumonia: a prospective study of patients not initially admitted to the ICU. *Chest* 2005;127:1260–1270.

10. Infectious Disease Society of America/American Thoracic society Consensus, Guidelines on the management of adults with community acquired pneumonia. *Am J Respir Crit Care Med* 2001;163: 1730–1754.

11. Nazarian DJ, Eddy OL, Lukens TW, et al. Clinical Policy: Critical issues in the management of adult patients presenting to the emergency department with commnity acquired pneumonia. *Ann Emerg Med* 2009;54(5):704–731.

12. Slaven EM, Santanilla JI, DeBlieux PM. Healthcare associated pneumonia in the emergency department. *Sem in Respir and Critical Care Med* 2009;(30)1:46–51.

13. Musonda P, Sankaran P, Subramanian DN, et al. Prediction of mortality in community acquired pneumonia in hospitalized patients. *Am J Med Sciences.* 2011;342(6):489–93.

14. Fine MJ, Auble TE, Yealy DM, et al. A prediction rule to identify low-risk patients with community acquired pneumonia. *J Engl J Med.* 1997;336:243–250.

15. Myint PK, Bhaniani A, Bradshaw SM, et al. Usefulness of shock index and adjusted shock index in the severity assessment of community acquired pneumonia. *Respiration* 2009; 77468–77490.

16. Chan, SSW, Yuen, EHY, Kew J, et al. Community acquired pneumonia implementation of a prediction rule to guide selection of patients for outpatient treatment. *Europe J of Emerg Med* 2001;8: 279–286.

17. Rehm SJ, Sekeres JK, Neuner E, et al. Cleveland Clinic. Guidelines for infectious diseases 2012–2013. Cleveland Clinic. 2012–2013.

18. Emerman CL, Anderson E, Cline DM. Community acquired pneumonia, aspiration pneumonia and noninfectious pulmonary infiltrates. In *Emergency Medicine: A Comprehensive Study Guide.* Tintinalli J, Stapczynski JS, Ma J, et al. (eds.). McGraw-Hill Medical Pub, New York. 2011;7th ed:479–491.

19. Leykum LK, Huerta V, Mortensen. Implementation of a hospitalist-run observation unit and impact on length of stay (LOS): A brief report. *J of Hosp Med* 2010;5:E2–E5.

20. Rydman RJ, Isola ML, Roberts R, et al. Emergency department observation unit versus hospital inpatient care for a chronic asthmatic population: A randomized trial of health status outcome and cost. *Med Care* 1998;36(4): 599–609.

Chapter 30

Primary Spontaneous Pneumothorax

Chew Yian Chai, MD

Introduction

Spontaneous pneumothoraces have no preceding traumatic or iatrogenic cause. They can be further divided into two groups: primary and secondary. Primary spontaneous pneumothoraces (PSP) occur in people with no underlying parenchymal disease. Some genetic conditions, for example, Marfan's Syndrome, predispose patients to getting pneumothoraces. Secondary spontaneous pneumothoraces (SSP) tend to occur in people with underlying parenchymal disease, for example, COPD.

We discuss the management of PSP in the observation unit (OU).

Spontaneous pneumothorax occurs from the rupture of blebs and bullae. It typically occurs in tall, young people without parenchymal lung disease, and is thought to be related to increased shear forces in the apex.

Patients typically present with chest pain and mild shortness of breath. Most patients are hemodynamically stable, except for those patients with a hemopneumothorax and/or a tension pneumothorax, which are medical emergencies that require immediate decompression. *Standard erect chest radiographs (CXR) with PA and lateral views view in inspiration are recommended for the initial diagnosis of pneumothorax, rather than expiratory films (Level A).*[2] The size of the pneumothoraces does not correlate well with the clinical manifestations.[2] Therefore the management strategy is determined by clinical evaluation rather than size of the pneumothorax.

Small pneumothoraces with minimal symptoms (i.e., not tachypneic or in cardiorespiratory distress) can be observed as outpatients (Level B),[2] provided they can easily seek medical attention if there is any deterioration of their symptoms. Small pneumothoraces are defined as those with an apex to cupola distance measuring < 3 cm (American guidelines) or interpleural distance at level of hilum measuring < 2 cm (British guidelines). (See Figure 30.1) Alternatively, they can be

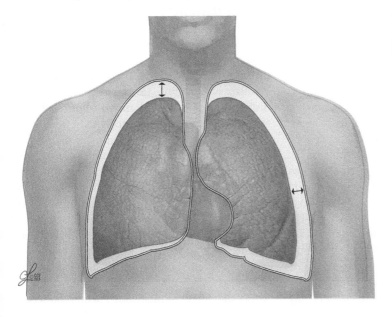

Figure 30.1 Rim of air between lung and chest wall
(Figure courtesy of Cleveland Clinic Art and Photo Department)

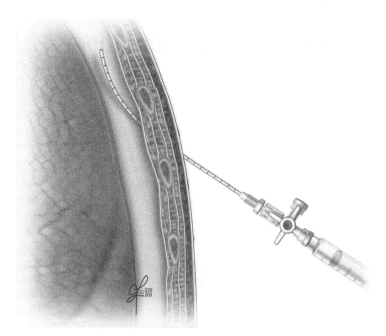

Figure 30.2 Needle aspiration of spontaneous pneumothorax
CXR = chest radiograph
COPD = chronic obstructive pulmonary disease
VATS = video assisted thoracoscopic surgery
(Figure courtesy of Cleveland Clinic Art and Photo Department)

admitted to the OU for supplemental high-flow oxygen (10 L/min), which can result in a four-fold increase in the rate of pneumothorax resolution, and a repeat CXR next day to assess interval changes. There is no evidence that active intervention improves the associated pain, which can be adequately controlled by appropriate analgesics.

For symptomatic PSP of whatever size, for example, breathlessness, active intervention – needle aspiration or chest drain insertion – should be performed (Level A).[2]

According to the American College of Chest Physicians (ACCP),[1] a pneumothorax is considered large if it measures > 3 cm from the apex to cupola. Clinical stability is defined as respiratory rate < 24 breaths/min, heart rate > 60/min or < 120/min, normal blood pressure, room air oxygen saturation > 90%, and the ability to speak in full sentences between breaths. *Patients with large PSP, but without significant breathlessness, may be managed by observation alone – though most clinicians advocate intervention in order to speed resolution (Level A).*[2]

The 2010 British Thoracic Society (BTS) Guidelines[2] recommends simple needle aspiration (NA) as the first-line treatment for all symptomatic PSP. *NA has shown equivalent success to the intervention of large-bore chest drains, plus a reduction in hospital admission and length of stay*

(LOS) (Level A).[3,4] Several meta-analyses[5,6,7] were limited by the small numbers of patients and studies, and the NA success rates range from 30–80%. NA should cease after aspiration of 2.5 liters of air, as further re-expansion is unlikely due to ongoing air leak.[2] Repeat CXR is then performed to assess resolution. *Failure of resolution will usually necessitate a second procedure such as a small bore chest drain (Level A). Further repeat NA is unlikely to be successful unless there were initial technical difficulties, for example, kinked catheter (Level B).*[2]

The ease of Seldinger (catheter over guide wire) chest drains has gained widespread usage and may be regarded as a simpler option to NA. Mini chest drains have been shown to have a similar success rate to larger chest drains,[8–13] but there are no randomized controlled trials (RCTs) to compare them to NA. In addition, it is less invasive and greatly improves the patient's comfort and cosmetic outcome. Our Center modifies this technique further, by connecting the Seldinger chest drain to a three-way adaptor and underwater seal, hence permitting a "stepwise" approach to the management of PSP. It allows repeat aspiration via the three-way adaptor connected to the chest drain, and continuous drainage to the underwater seal. (Figure 30.2) (See also Chapter 83 Specialized Clinical Protocols/Guidelines: Spontaneous Pneumothorax)

Inclusion Criteria

Patients who are haemodynamically stable, with a systolic blood pressure > 90 mmHg, and with SpO2 > 92%[2] will be included.

Exclusion Criteria

Patients with hemodynamic instability, SSP or a past history of video-assisted thoracoscopic surgery (VATS) will be admitted to the inpatient unit. Pneumothoraces secondary to trauma or complicated by hemothoraces should also be admitted to the inpatient unit. If there is a clinical suspicion of persistent air leak, they should not be admitted to the OU. Tension pneumothorax and bilateral pneumothorax are excluded. Pneumothorax with large pleural effusion (hemo/hydropneumothorax) should also be excluded. Patients with recurrence on the ipsilateral side or contralateral side will benefit from VATS as the recurrence rates have been reported to be as high as 15–40%, and are, therefore, admitted to an inpatient service.

Management/Intervention

Apical Pneumothoraces

For patients with apical pneumothoraces, they will be administered supplemental oxygen. If the apex cupola distance is > 2 cm, they will undergo needle aspiration at the second intercostal space and have a CXR repeated post aspiration. These patients will be kept in the OU and have a repeat CXR at the 14th hour. Following successful resolution, the patient can then be discharged with early review. (Figure 30.1)

Rim Pneumothoraces

For patients with rim pneumothoraces (presence of rim of air between lung and chest wall) (Figure 30.1), a 12F Seldinger chest drain will be inserted. This is connected to a three-way adaptor and underwater seal, to allow aspiration(s) and continuous passive drainage respectively. They will then be admitted to the OU and placed on supplemental oxygen. The chest drain will be clamped at the 12th hour, and a repeat CXR will be obtained at the 14th hour. For rim pneumothoraces that do not improve after clamping of the tube, repeat aspiration and underwater drainage will be continued for a further 6 hours.

The CXR will then be repeated 2 hours post clamping of the chest tube. (Figure 30.2)

Potential Complications

All patients placed in the OU under a pneumothorax protocol will have their vital signs monitored closely to detect any deterioration or complications such as hemothorax, *tension pneumothorax* (secondary to kinked or blocked catheter), re-expansion pulmonary edema, or surgical emphysema.

Hemothorax can occur due to bleeding from the bleb after chest drainage, and can be potentially life-threatening if not detected early. This will warrant immediate surgical referral for VATS to arrest the bleeding.

Re-expansion pulmonary edema (RPE) can potentially happen after a rapid expansion of lung parenchyma following a chest drain insertion for a especially large PSP that may have been present for more than a few days.[2] This is thought to be due to mechanical stress applied to the "injured" capillaries that are already "leaky." The patient typically presents with acute breathlessness and desaturation, and may cough out frothy sputum. Clinical examination of patients with RPE may reveal coarse rales in the affected lung, or less commonly in the contralateral lung. Management for RPE is largely supportive with oxygen (consider intubation if indicated) and fluids (NOT diuresis). The incidence of RPE may be up to 14% (higher in younger patients with large PSP). Fatalities have been reported, as high as 20% in one case series report.[19] Thus, one must be able to recognize RPE, and institute supportive treatment early.

Surgical emphysema is a well-recognized complication of chest drains. This is usually self-limiting, and treatment is conservative. It is usually seen with a kinked/blocked chest drain, or in patients with large air leak on a relatively small bore chest drain. Very rarely does airway obstruction or thoracic obstruction happen, in which case one will need to intervene with intubation/tracheostomy, skin incision decompression or large-bore chest drain.

Discharge Advice and Follow-Up

Patients with stable apical pneumothoraces will be discharged the next day. Patients whose pneumothoraces do not show improvement will subsequently be admitted to the respiratory unit. For rim pneumothoraces, if the lung shows good expansion, the chest tube will be removed before discharge. All patients will be discharged with pneumothorax advice and followed up by our respiratory medicine physicians within 2 weeks, with a CXR on arrival to assess resolution.

Patients who are suspected to have Marfan's syndrome will also be referred to the Cardiology Marfan's clinic for further workup.

All patients discharged after intervention or otherwise will be given written advice to return to the Emergency Department if they develop acute breathlessness or giddiness/syncope. We also reinforce lifestyle advice on issues such as smoking, air travel, and diving. Smoking increases the recurrence risk, and cessation should be encouraged. *Air travel should be avoided until full resolution (Level C).*[2] The BTS guidelines on air travel emphasize that the recurrence risk only falls significantly 1 year after the index pneumothorax, hence, in the absence of definitive surgical procedure, patients may want to defer air travel, as the consequences of a recurrence during air travel can be serious. *Diving should be permanently avoided, unless the patient has undergone bilateral surgical pleurectomy (Level C).*[2]

Summary

The goal of admitting patients with simple PSP to the OU is to treat the pneumothorax, monitor for potential complications and facilitate early discharge. Both needle aspiration and small bore chest drains compare favorably with large bore chest drains. With the use of small bore Seldinger chest drains, chest tube insertion has become minimally invasive and a much less painful procedure. This has also greatly reduced the length of stay and improved patient satisfaction.

References

1. Michael H Baumann, Charlie Strange, John E Heffner, Richard Light, Thomas J Kirby, Jeffrey Klein, James D Luketich, Edward A Panacek, Steven A Sahn. Management of spontaneous pneumothorax: an American College of Chest Physicians Delphi concensus statement. *Chest* 2012, March 9.

2. Andrew MacDuff, Anthony Arnold, John Harvey, on behalf of BTS Pleural Disease Guideline group. Management of spontaneous pneumothorax: British Thoracic Society pleural disease guideline 2010. *BMJ* 2012, March 23.

3. Win Sen Kuan, Kanwar Sudhir Lather, Malcolm Mahadevan. Primary spontaneous pneumothorax – the role of the emergency observation unit. *American Journal of Emergency Medicine* (2011) 29, 293–298.

4. Noppen M, Alexander P, Driesen P, et al. Manual aspiration versus chest tube drainage in first episodes of primary spontaneous pneumothorax. *Am J Respir Crit Care Med* 2002; 165: 1240–1244.

5. Ayed AK, Chandrasekaran C, Sukumar M, et al. Aspiration versus tube drainage in primary spontaneous pneumothorax: a randomized study. *Eur Resp J* 2006; 27:477–482.

6. Devanand A, Koh MS, Ong TH, et al. Simple aspiration versus chest-tube insertion in the management of primary spontaneous pneumothorax: a systemic review. *Respir Med* 2004; 98:579–590.

7. Zehtabchi S, Rios CL. Management of emergency department patients with primary spontaneous pneumothorax: needle aspiration or tube thoracostomy? *Ann Emerg Med* 2008; 51:91–100.

8. Wakai A, O' Sullivan RG, McCabe G. Simple aspiration versus intercostal tube drainage for primary spontaneous pneumothorax in adults. *Cochrane Database of Syst Rev* 2007; (1):CD 004479

9. Lai SM, Tee AK. Outpatient treatment of Primary Spontaneous Pneumothorax using a small-bore chest drain with a Heimlich valve: the experience of a Singapore emergency department. *Eur J Emerg Med* 2012: 19(6): 400–404.

10. Contou D, Razaki K, Katsahian S, Maitre B, Meknotso-Dessap A, Brun-Buisson C, Thille AW. Small-bore catheter versus Chest tube drainage for pneumothorax. *Am J Emerg Med* 2012 Jan 2.

11. Fysh ET, Smith NA, Lee YC. Optimal chest drain size: the rise of the small-bore pleural catheter. *Semin Respir Crit Care Med* 2010 Dec; 31(6): 760–768.

12. Horsley A, Jones L, White J, et al. Efficacy and complications of small-bore, wire-guided chest drains. *Chest* 2006; 130 (6):1857–1863.

13. Dernevik L, Roberts D, Hamraz B, et al. Management of pneumothorax with a mini-drain in ambulatory and hospitalized patients. *Scan Cardiovasc J* 2003; 37:172–176.

14. Vedam H, Barnes DJ. Comparison of large- and

small-bore intercostal catheters in the management of spontaneous pneumothorax. *Int Med J* 2003; 33: 495–499.

15. Baumann, MH. Management of spontaneous pneumothorax. *Clin Chest Med* 2006; 27: 369–381.

16. Valle P, Sullivan M, Richardson H, Bivins B, Tomlanovich M. Sequential treatment of a simple pnuemothorax. *Ann Emerg Med* 1988; 17: 936–947.

17. Matsuura Y, Nomimura T, Nurikami H, et al. Clinical evidence of re-expansion pulmonary oedema. *Chest* 1991; 100:1562–1566.

18. Pavlin DJ, Nessly MC, Cheney FW. Increased pulmonary vascular permeability as a cause of re-expansion edema in rabbits. *Am Rev Respir Dis* 1981; 124:422–427.

19. Mahfood S, Hix WR, Aaron BL, et al. Re-expansion pulmonary oedema. *Ann Thorac Surg* 1988; 45: 340–345.

20. Maunder RJ, Pierson DJ, Hudson LD. Subcutaneous and mediastinal emphysema. Pathophysiology, diagnosis and management. *Arch Intern Med* 1984; 144:1447–1453.

21. Conetta R, Barman AA, Lakovou C, et al. Acute ventilator failure from massive subcutaneous emphysema. *Chest* 1993; 104:978–980.

22. British Thoracic Society Standards of Care Committee. Managing passengers with respiratory disease planning air travel: British Thoracic Society recommendations. *Thorax* 2002; 57: 289–304.

23. British Thoracic Society Fitness to Dive Group. BTS guidelines on respiratory aspects of fitness for diving. *Thorax* 2003; 58:3–11.

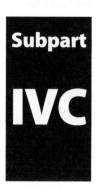

Subpart

IVC

Clinical – Vascular

Editor's Comments: Venous Thromboembolic Disease: Deep Vein Thrombosis and Pulmonary Emboli

With the trend toward outpatient care and a concern for cost-effectiveness, the possibility of using the observation unit for disorders that previously were treated only as an inpatient over several days has evolved. Patients with pulmonary emboli have generally not been considered appropriate patients for the observation unit and have previously only been treated on the hospital inpatient unit. Recently, however, the concept of risk stratification of pulmonary emboli patients, similar to the risk stratification of chest pain patients, and the management of low-risk (e.g., hemodynamically stable, non-hypoxic) pulmonary emboli patients in a non-inpatient setting, specifically the observation unit, or even as an outpatient, has emerged. Use of clinical parameters including vital signs with pulse oximetry, and laboratory/ancillary tests such as troponin, BNP, CT scan, echocardiography or other studies to document normal right ventricular function and no acute myocardial dysfunction, may allow us to risk stratify these patients, initiate treatment, and begin patient/family education in the observation unit, thereby avoiding an inpatient hospital admission.

The next several chapters – 31 Deep Vein Thrombosis, 32 Acute Pulmonary Embolism, and 33 Anticoagulants – discuss the value of observation medicine for patients with venous thromboembolic disease, specifically deep vein thrombosis and pulmonary emboli, including the management of these diseases. There has been a great deal of research recently with these disorders including the development of newer anticoagulation therapies. These agents are referred to as NOACs for novel (or newer) oral anticoagulants, or "non-vitamin K antagonist oral anticoagulants" or DOACs for direct oral anticoagulants or TSOACs for "target specific oral anticoagulants." There has also been the introduction of a reversal agent, idarucizumab, which is a monoclonal antibody antidote specifically for the reversal of the anticoagulant effects of dabigatran. It is likely that additional agents, both anticoagulants and reversal agents for other anticoagulants, will be introduced in the near future.

Anticoagulants are agents that inhibit one or more steps in the coagulation cascade. They have various mechanisms of action. The anticoagulants include unfractionated heparin, low molecular weight heparins, fondaparinux, vitamin K antagonists, direct thrombin inhibitors, and direct factor Xa inhibitors; and there are other agents that are in various stages of development. The oral direct factor Xa inhibitors, which all have an "X" in their name and all end in "Xa-ban," include rivaroxaban, apixaban, edoxaban, and betrixaban. The oral direct thrombin inhibitors (DTIs) include dabigatran.

Deep Vein Thrombosis (DVT)

Carol Lynn Clark, MD MBA FACEP
Michelle A. Wiener, MD MS

Introduction

Pulmonary embolism (PE) and deep vein thrombosis (DVT) are collectively encompassed by the term venous thromboembolism (VTE), and occur at an incidence of approximately 0.1% of persons per year.[1] VTE should be thought of as a continuum. DVT alone is a major cause of preventable morbidity and mortality worldwide, accounting for up to 600,000 U.S. hospitalizations per year.[2] Economically speaking, this translates into a substantial proportion of health care claims with an estimated total cost of 2–10 billion dollars per year in the United States alone, for the period from 1998 to 2004.[3] The incidence of primary DVT increases markedly with age, immobility, and surgery. For cases such as major orthopedic procedures (joint arthroplasty or hip fracture surgery) the risk can be as high as 40–60% without prophylaxis.[4] Several other lesser risk factors have been identified as well, including pregnancy, obesity, fracture, contraceptives, hematologic disorders, stroke, and lower extremity trauma. The most common underlying conditions associated with higher recurrence rates of DVT are increasing age (> 65 years), body mass index, cancer, limb paralysis, and an idiopathic first thrombus.[5, 6] Due to these factors, despite attempts to decrease the incidence by utilizing evidence based DVT prophylaxis, the disease burden of DVT has unfortunately remained constant due to an aging population, increasing obesity rates, and improved access to surgical care.[7]

Discussion

Early diagnosis and treatment of VTE is essential in order to reduce the risk of serious complications that are associated with this condition. While a fatal PE is the most severe and acute progression of the disease, chronic DVTs may progress to a potentially debilitating post thrombotic syndrome in as many as 50% of patients.[8,9,10] In these cases chronic pain, edema, and skin discoloration/ulceration are a common result of long-term inflammation and venous hypertension.[11] These symptoms may be severe and disabling.

The most common presenting symptoms of DVT are a combination of lower extremity pain, tenderness, erythema, and lower calf swelling.[12] However, patients will present to the Emergency Department (ED) with a wide range of clinical symptoms, which can make diagnosis difficult. The presenting symptoms may be as subtle and nonspecific as calf cramps or swelling. In a study of 87 patients with negative venograms for suspected DVT, the most common mimicking disorders were identified as muscle strain/tear (30%), twisting injury to the leg (10%), leg swelling in a paralyzed limb (9%), lymphangitis/lymph obstruction (7%), and venous insufficiency (7%).[13] In severe cases such as phlegmasia cerulea dolens, defined as a massive proximal thrombotic venous occlusion, symptoms can include sudden and severe leg pain, swelling, cyanosis, late stage compartment syndrome, or systemic circulatory collapse.

Diagnosis often begins with a standardized clinical model that combines risk factors with presenting signs and symptoms to subsequently stratify patients with a suspected DVT into high- or low-risk categories. There are many clinical prediction tools used, but the most commonly accepted model is the Wells score, which assigns point values to ten significant clinical variables in order to create a pre-test probability of DVT.[14] The pre-test probability will then guide the choice of diagnostic modality including D-dimer assays, proximal compression ultrasounds (CUS), whole leg ultrasounds and less frequently used tests such as, contrast venography, Computer Tomography scan, and Magnetic Resonance Imaging. While choosing a test modality will depend on cost, availability, and pre-morbid

Table 31.1 Half Lives of Factor X A and Direct Thrombin Inhibitors

- Apixaban: 12–15 hours

- Edoxaban: 9–14 hours

- Rivaroxaban: 5–9 hours, longer in > 60 y.o.: 11–13 hours

- Dabigatran: 12–17 hours, increases to 27.2 hours with severe renal dysfunction

conditions that might falsely elevate D-dimer levels, according to the diagnosis guidelines created by the American College of Chest Physicians (ACCP), patients with low pre-test probability should undergo initial testing with a moderately or highly sensitive D-dimer or proximal CUS. If these tests are negative, no further testing is required. However, if a D-dimer is positive further confirmation should be done with a whole leg ultrasound. For patients with a high pre-test probability whole leg US should be the preferred initial diagnostic modality.[15]

In recent years treatment of DVT has become increasingly aggressive, with initiation of anticoagulation in the ED considered paramount in halting thrombus progression. The standard treatment regimen for DVT in patients who are not at a high risk of bleeding has changed over the last several years as a new class of medications, the non-vitamin K oral anticoagulants (NOACs), have made their way onto the market. Currently available medications in the United States include apixaban (Eliquis®) dabigatran (Pradaxa®), rivaroxaban (Xarelto®) and edoxaban (Savaysa®), with others on the horizon.

These medications have revolutionized the treatment of VTE. Apixaban, edoxaban and rivaroxaban are orally absorbed direct Factor Xa inhibitors with rapid onset and relatively short half-lives. Dabigatran is a direct Thrombin inhibitor that also exhibits a short half-life. (See Table 31.1.) The benefits of these medications over other treatment regimens are that they do not require significant anticoagulation monitoring, are taken orally, and are associated with similar efficacy and a lower risk of major bleeding and intracranial hemorrhage when compared to treatment with enoxaparin plus a vitamin K antagonist (VKA) such as warfarin.[16,17]

Drawbacks to the use of the Factor Xa inhibitors are that there is currently no reversal agent,

other than time, and they are not currently recommended for pregnant women, breastfeeding women, and patients on strong CYP3A inhibitors or inducers. They are currently contraindicated if a patient has hepatic disease associated with coagulopathy, clinically relevant bleeding or if they have significant renal disease.

Reversal agents are expected to be available soon for the Factor Xa inhibitors. A reversal agent for dabigatran was recently approved in the United States. Due to the lower risk of major bleeding and in particular intracranial bleeding, the NOACs are quickly becoming the therapy of choice for VTE. Eliminating the need for frequent blood draws and the NOAC's ability to be taken orally make them significant options for treatment of these conditions. Renal function should be monitored in these medications as their bleeding risk can change if creatinine clearance decreases. The nuances of each of these medications are beyond the scope of this chapter but are important information for prescribing physicians to be aware of.[18,19,20,21]

Another treatment option available consists of administration of a "bridging" anticoagulant (intravenous unfractionated heparin), or a low-molecular-weight heparin (LMWH such as enoxaparin) with a continued course of warfarin. The advantages of LMWH over unfractionated heparin include once or twice daily injections without the need for monitoring, a long half-life, and a lower risk of major hemorrhage.[22] This again allows the patient to be treated as an outpatient without the need for hospitalization.

With both forms of acceptable outpatient treatment, enoxaparin/warfarin or the NOACs, the duration will depend on the risk of thrombus recurrence. Three months is the initial recommended time of therapy followed by reassessment of future risk. In some cases of increased risk such as recurrent VTE, significant thrombophilia or cancer, lifelong therapy may be recommended. Treatment of VTE using NOACs has become common and acceptable practice since their emergence on the market. With either drug regimen (enoxaparin/warfarin or NOACs), the patient has the benefit of being treated at home, which has been shown in studies to not only be cost-effective, but these patients also exhibit greater activity levels, higher levels of social functioning, and better treatment satisfaction scores.[23]

Chapter

32

Acute Pulmonary Embolism (PE)

David G. Paje, MD, FACP, SFHM

Introduction

Acute pulmonary embolism (PE) is a common cardiovascular emergency that affects hundreds of thousands of patients every year with a reported annual incidence of nearly 1 per 1,000 in the United States.[1,2] It is a clinical manifestation of venous thromboembolism (VTE), which is the same disease process that results in deep vein thrombosis (DVT). In general, PE is a natural sequela of DVT. Studies show that as much as 70% of patients with PE are found to have a concomitant DVT in the lower extremities, specifically in the proximal veins in two-thirds of cases. Also, among patients with symptomatic proximal DVT without symptoms of PE, 40–50% have ventilation-perfusion lung scan findings that are consistent with a high probability of PE.[3]

The occlusion of the pulmonary arterial bed that occurs in PE may lead to impairment in oxygenation as a result of ventilation-perfusion mismatch, and to more serious hemodynamic complications arising from an abrupt increase in pulmonary vascular resistance, including shock from acute right ventricular failure and sudden death from electromechanical dissociation. It is estimated that 11% of patients with acute PE die within 1 hour of onset,[4] usually even before it is recognized. However among those who do not die acutely, the case fatality rates vary depending on the clinical severity of the thromboembolic episode.

Patients with severe PE have a high risk of mortality and are best managed in a critical care environment. On the other hand, those with non-high-risk PE are usually admitted to a general medical unit and they typically stay for several days. However, various studies evaluating prognostic models have identified a group of patients with PE that are appropriate candidates for initial outpatient therapy; these patients have a low risk of fatal and nonfatal adverse outcomes.[5–11] Hence, current published guidelines recommend outpatient care for highly selected patients with PE.[12,13]

A recent administrative database review found that the median length of stay (LOS) for patients hospitalized with PE was 6 days, and the post-discharge mortality rate was 3.3%. But the adjusted risk of death after discharge was significantly higher for patients with an LOS of 4 days or less (OR, 1.55; 95% CI, 1.21–2.00) compared to those with a LOS of 5 to 6 days,[14] suggesting that patients with increased risk of complications may have been inappropriately selected for early discharge. This highlights the need to apply prognostic models and to develop explicit decision-support tools that properly identify patients who may be discharged early or treated in the outpatient setting. Providing *observation services* for further risk stratification and short-term monitoring is a reasonable alternative for non-high-risk PE patients to identify those who may need further inpatient care as well as those who may be discharged safely without the need for hospitalization.[15]

Diagnosis

Acute PE is often difficult to recognize and the diagnosis is sometimes delayed or missed. Its clinical manifestations may include dyspnea, chest pain, cough, hemoptysis, syncope, tachypnea, and tachycardia. These signs and symptoms are nonspecific and unreliable when appraised separately. However, when these findings are evaluated together with predisposing factors, the likelihood of PE can be determined.

Several *clinical decision rules* (CDR) have been developed to estimate the probability of PE, which guides the selection of the appropriate diagnostic strategy and the subsequent interpretation of test results. The most commonly used and extensively validated CDR, the *Wells rule* (Table 32.1), looks at both clinical findings and risk factors in

Table 32.1 Wells Rule and Revised Geneva Score

Clinical Decision Rule	Clinical Variable	Points
Wells Rule	Clinical signs and symptoms of DVT (minimum of leg swelling and pain with palpation of the deep vein)	3
	An alternative diagnosis is less likely than PE	3
	Heart rate greater than 100	1.5
	Immobilization or surgery in the previous 4 week	1.5
	Previous DVT/PE	1.5
	Hemoptysis	1
	Malignancy (on treatment, treated in the last 6 months or palliative)	1
	Clinical Probability	
	PE unlikely	≤ 4
	PE likely	> 4
Revised Geneva Score	Age > 65	1
	Previous DVT/PE	3
	Surgery (under general anesthesia) or fracture (of the lower limbs) within 1 month	2
	Active malignant condition (solid or hematologic malignant condition, currently active or considered cured < 1 year)	2
	Unilateral lower limb pain	3
	Hemoptysis	2
	Heart rate 75–94 beats per minute	3
	Heart rate $\geq$ 95 beats per minute	5
	Pain on lower limb deep venous palpation and unilateral edema	4
	Clinical Probability	
	PE unlikely	≤ 5
	PE likely	> 5

DVT deep vein thrombosis, *PE* pulmonary embolism

predicting the presence of PE. It includes one subjective criterion, the physician's judgment of whether an alternative diagnosis is less likely than PE. Other decision tools, such as the *revised Geneva score*, consider only objective variables. Nevertheless, both Wells and revised Geneva rules showed similar accuracy in assessing the clinical probability of PE.[16,17]

D-dimer is a product of fibrin degradation and is a highly sensitive laboratory marker for thrombosis. When the clinical probability is low, a negative D-dimer test reliably excludes PE. However, when the likelihood of PE is high, further diagnostic evaluation is required regardless of the D-dimer level. There is a wide variety of clinical conditions aside from PE that results in an elevated D-dimer, including advanced age, inflammation, trauma, recent surgery, malignancy, necrosis, autoimmune disease, or liver disease. Therefore, a positive D-dimer result is not specific for PE and it is not useful as a sole basis for its diagnosis.[18]

Imaging studies are essential in the diagnostic evaluation of PE and they are particularly indicated if the clinical suspicion is high or if the D-dimer is elevated.[19] Multidetector *computed tomography angiogram* (CTA) is currently the most readily available option. It has excellent test characteristics; its estimated sensitivity and specificity for the diagnosis of PE are at least 90% and 95%, respectively.[20] It also has the advantage of providing an alternative or a concomitant diagnosis that may account for the patient's clinical presentation. The usual limitation of CTA is the use of intravenous iodinated contrast, which is an important concern for patients at high risk for contrast-induced nephropathy especially those with underlying renal impairment. Also, in cases when the CTA is negative but the clinical probability high, further testing is necessary.

Ventilation-perfusion scintigraphy (V/Q scan) is usually the preferred alternative for patients who cannot undergo a CTA because of either renal dysfunction or allergy to iodinated contrast. V/Q scan results are reported based on criteria established in the PIOPED[21] trial using four categories: normal or near-normal, low, intermediate (nondiagnostic), and high probability of PE. A normal perfusion scan safely rules out PE in most cases, with a likelihood ratio of 0.10. A high probability V/Q scan confirms the diagnosis of PE with a high degree of certainty, especially in a

Table 32.2 European Society of Cardiology Risk Stratification of Pulmonary Embolism[13]

PE-related Early Mortality Rate			Risk Markers			Potential Treatment Implications
			Clinical (shock or hypotension)	RV-dysfunction	Myocardial injury	
High		> 15 %	+	(+)[a]	(+)[a]	Thrombolysis or embolectomy
Non-high	Intermediate	3–15 %	−	+	+	Hospital admission
				+	−	
				−	+	
	Low	< 1%	−	−	−	Early discharge or home treatment

[a] In the presence of shock or hypotension, it is not necessary to confirm RV-dysfunction or myocardial injury to classify as high risk of PE-related early mortality.
PE pulmonary embolism, RV right ventricle
Torbicki, A., et al. Guidelines on the diagnosis and management of acute pulmonary embolism: the Task Force for the Diagnosis and Management of Acute Pulmonary Embolism of the European Society of Cardiology (ESC). *Eur Heart J*, 2008; 29(18): p. 2281, by permission of Oxford University Press.

patient with a high clinical probability. Any other combination of V/Q scan result and clinical probability is not useful in excluding or establishing PE, and requires further evaluation.[13]

Direct pulmonary angiography has been the gold standard for the diagnosis of PE. It is an invasive procedure that involves direct injection of contrast dye into the pulmonary arteries. With technological advances in noninvasive alternatives, such as refinement of CT imaging, conventional direct pulmonary angiography is now rarely performed as an isolated diagnostic procedure. It is best reserved for cases where CT findings are equivocal.

Finally, *compression ultrasonography* (CUS) is another option that may be useful in evaluating patients with suspected PE. The presence of DVT in the proximal lower limb, even when asymptomatic, establishes the diagnosis of PE in patients with high clinical probability and in those with non-high clinical probability but with positive D-dimer tests (specificity of 99% and likelihood ratio of 42.2). However, the absence of DVT does not rule out PE (sensitivity of 39%).[22]

Risk Stratification

Once PE is suspected and even while diagnostic evaluation is still in progress, it is important to concurrently assess its clinical severity so that high-risk patients are identified promptly. These patients are generally hemodynamically unstable and they require more intensive management, including more aggressive interventions such as immediate thrombolysis or surgical embolectomy.[13,23] The European Society of Cardiology (ESC) guidelines, which recommend a risk-stratification approach based on the expected PE-related early mortality rate (Table 32.2), define high-risk PE by the presence of shock or systemic hypotension. It is a distinct clinical entity with an expected short-term PE-related mortality risk of more than 15%.[13]

Aside from defining high-risk PE, the ESC guidelines further classify non-high-risk PE patients as either at intermediate risk (3–15%) or at low risk (< 1%) of PE-related early mortality. Those with intermediate risk have findings consistent with the presence of right ventricular dysfunction (RVD) and/or myocardial injury.[13] Although there are no universally accepted criteria to determine the presence of RVD in patients with acute PE, widely available diagnostic tools include echocardiography, computed tomography, and brain natriuretic peptide (BNP). On the other hand, myocardial injury in patients with PE can be detected by elevations in levels of cardiac troponin T or I.[24]

However, these markers of RVD and myocardial injury are actually most useful when identifying low-risk patients. Normal echocardiographic findings, absence of right ventricular dilatation on CT or low levels of BNP or NT-proBNP are all reliable indicators of an excellent outcome, with a low risk of short-term mortality or complicated clinical course. Also, a normal cardiac troponin makes PE-related early mortality very unlikely (negative predictive value, 99–100%), irrespective of method or cutoff value applied.[13]

Nevertheless, to appropriately identify patients who may safely undergo outpatient treatment, an ideal prognostic model should not only consider PE-related early mortality but should also predict recurrent VTE, major bleeding and all-cause mortality that occur within a short period of time after PE is diagnosed. These adverse outcomes were measured as end points in several derivation and validation studies on clinical models to assess prognosis in patients diagnosed with acute PE.[25–30] Among these models are the *Pulmonary Embolism Severity Index* (PESI) and the Geneva risk score (Table 32.3).

The PESI was developed to stratify patients treated for PE into five severity classes of increasing risk of mortality within 30 days of hospitalization. The original PESI model includes 11 clinical variables that are routinely available at the time of presentation. In the derivation cohort, 59% of patients were classified as intermediate to very high risk (Class III–V) with a 14% mortality risk, while 41% were thought to be very low to low risk (Class I and II) with a 2% risk of death within 30 days.[31] A subsequent prospective validation study identified 47% of patients as low-risk (Class I and II) with an overall mortality of only 1.2% and a PE-specific mortality of 0.7%.[7] In another validation study, the 90-day mortality in low-risk patients was 1%, and there were no recurrent thromboembolic or major bleeding events.[29] A simplified version of PESI was later developed to make it easier to calculate, but a recent comparative analysis showed that the original PESI classified a higher proportion of patients as low-risk and it had a greater discriminatory power.[32]

The Geneva risk score includes six independent predictors of an adverse outcome (i.e., recurrent VTE, major bleeding and death) in patients with acute PE. In the derivation cohort, 67.2%

Table 32.3 Pulmonary Embolism Severity Index and Geneva Risk Score[25,31]

Prognostic Model	Clinical Variable	Points
Pulmonary Embolism Severity Index (PESI)	Age	Age in years
	Male sex	10
	History of cancer	30
	History of heart failure	10
	History of chronic lung disease	10
	Pulse $\geq$ 110 beats per minute	20
	Systolic blood pressure < 100 mmHg	30
	Respiratory rate $\geq$ 30 breaths per minute	20
	Temperature < 36 °C	20
	Altered mental status	60
	Arterial oxyhemoglobin saturation (SaO_2) < 90%	20
	The five risk classes based on the total point score: class I (< 65 points), class II (66–85 points), class III (86–105 points), class IV (106–125 points), and class V (> 125 points)	
Geneva Risk Score	History of cancer	2
	History of heart failure	1
	Previous DVT	1
	Concomitant DVT on ultrasound	1
	Systolic blood pressure < 100 mmHg	2
	PaO_2 < 60 mmHg (or 8 kPa)	1
	The two risk classes based on the total point score: low-risk ($\leq$ 2) and high-risk ($\geq$ 3)	

DVT deep vein thrombosis

were classified as low-risk and 32.8% were high-risk, with rates of adverse outcomes at 90 days of 2.2% and 26.1%, respectively.[25]

In summary, an appropriate risk stratification to identify low-risk patients with PE starts

Table 32.4 Initial Anticoagulation Options in Observation

Parenteral Anticoagulant		Subcutaneous Dose	Comments
Low-molecular-weight Heparin (LMWH)	Enoxaparin	1 mg/kg BID or 1.5 mg/kg daily	If CrCl < 30 ml/min, reduce dose to 1 mg/kg daily or consider UFH as an alternative
	Dalteparin	100 IU/kg BID or 200 IU/kg daily	Adjust if CrCl < 30 ml/min
	Tinzaparin	175 IU/kg daily	If CrCl < 30 ml/min, consider UFH as an alternative
Oral Anticoagulant		**Oral Dose**	**Comments**
Rivaroxaban		15 mg BID for the first 21 days, then 20 mg daily	Should be taken with food Avoid if CrCl < 30 ml/min
Apixaban		10 mg BID for 7 days, then 5 mg BID	Avoid if CrCl < 15 ml/min

CrCl creatinine clearance, *aPTT* activated partial thromboplastin time, *BID* twice daily, *BW* body weight

with excluding those who are hemodynamically unstable. Afterwards, predictive models that incorporate relevant and readily available clinical data at presentation, such as PESI and Geneva risk score, can be applied. Patients categorized as PESI Class I and II may be discharged early or be treated completely in the outpatient setting.[33] Those patients with intermediate to very high risk clinical features (PESI Class III and V) require further evaluation in the inpatient setting.

Patient Selection

Patients diagnosed with acute pulmonary embolism who are hemodynamically stable may be considered for observation services for short-term monitoring and further risk stratification to determine whether they need inpatient care or if they can be discharged to follow-up for outpatient treatment. The appropriate patients should be classified as low-risk based on a validated clinical prognostic tool, such as PESI.

Another important factor in selecting patients for observation care is their suitability for the optimal outpatient treatment regimen. Currently, the options for immediate anticoagulation for the initial treatment of VTE include rivaroxaban, apixaban and low-molecular-weight heparin (LMWH) (Table 32.4). Patients who cannot receive any of these regimens because of severe renal dysfunction or other nonspecific patient-related risk factors should be admitted for intravenous unfractionated heparin (UFH) therapy.

Observation Care

The goals of observation care for carefully selected patients with acute PE who are determined to be low-risk for adverse outcomes include initiation of anticoagulation, short-term monitoring, and further risk stratification. As soon as PE is suspected, immediate anticoagulation with an oral or a parenteral agent must be considered.[34] The appropriate choices for initial anticoagulant therapy in an observation setting are rivaroxaban, apixaban, and subcutaneous LMWH (Table 32.4). Patients should be monitored for the development of any complication related to treatment or to PE itself, including allergic reaction, thrombocytopenia, bleeding, and worsening hypoxemia. While most of the clinical variables used in risk stratification of acute PE are readily obtainable at presentation, imaging modalities, such as echocardiography and CUS, may have limited availability at some institutions. A reasonable observation stay should allow for completion of these tests when indicated.

Low-risk PE patients may be discharged after an uneventful observation stay if proper outpatient care and anticoagulant therapy can be provided. For long-term (first 3 months) treatment of PE, current guidelines prefer rivaroxaban, apixaban, edoxaban or dabigatran over a vitamin K antagonist (VKA), such as warfarin.[35] Rivaroxaban[36,37] and apixaban[38] can be initiated without the need for a parenteral anticoagulant. Edoxaban[39] and Dabigatran[40] require 5 to 10 days of initial therapy with a parenteral anticoagulant (e.g. LMWH) prior to the first dose.

If a VKA is chosen, it should be initiated on the same day as parenteral therapy is started, and the parenteral anticoagulant must be continued for a minimum of 5 days and until the international normalized ratio (INR) is 2.0 or above for at least 24 hours.[41] Because of this critical requirement and the need to monitor therapy, PE patients discharged on a VKA will need very close follow-up with their outpatient physician or with an anticoagulation clinic within 2–3 days.

For patients with PE and active cancer, extended therapy for at least the first 3 months of treatment with LMWH is preferred over VKA, rivaroxaban, apixaban, edoxaban or dabigatran.[35]

The advent of the direct-acting oral anticoagulants (DOACs) rivaroxaban, apixaban, edoxaban, and dabigatran has markedly expanded the therapeutic choices for acute PE beyond LMWH and VKA. Generally, the DOACs have comparable efficacy to VKAs in terms of preventing recurrent VTE, fatal PE and overall mortality, but with significantly lower risk of bleeding complications.[42] However, using DOACs does not eliminate the need for observation stay since some patients with low-risk PE may still require completion of their diagnostic evaluation and risk stratification. Also, devoting resources on effective patient education and ensuring access to medications prior to disposition are just as important with these newer agents.

References

1. Silverstein MD, Heit JA, Mohr DN, et al. Trends in the incidence of deep vein thrombosis and pulmonary embolism: a 25-year population-based study. *Arch Intern Med* 1998; 158(6): 585–593.

2. White RH. The epidemiology of venous thromboembolism. *Circulation* 2003; 107(23 Suppl 1): I4–8.

3. Kearon C. Natural history of venous thromboembolism. *Circulation* 2003; 107(23 Suppl 1): I22–30.

4. Dalen JE, Pulmonary embolism: what have we learned since Virchow? Natural history, pathophysiology, and diagnosis. *Chest* 2002; 122(4): 1440–1456.

5. Jakobsson C, Jimenez D, Gomez V, et al. Validation of a clinical algorithm to identify low-risk patients with pulmonary embolism. *J Thromb Haemost* 2010; 8(6): 1242–1247.

6. Jimenez D, Yusen RD, Otero R, et al. Prognostic models for selecting patients with acute pulmonary embolism for initial outpatient therapy. *Chest* 2007; 132(1): 24–30.

7. Aujesky D, Perrier A, Roy PM, et al. Validation of a clinical prognostic model to identify low-risk patients with pulmonary embolism. *J Intern Med* 2007; 261(6): 597–604.

8. Janjua M, Badshah A, Matta F, et al. Treatment of acute pulmonary embolism as outpatients or following early discharge. A systematic review. *Thromb Haemost* 2008; 100(5): 756–761.

9. Agterof MJ, Schutgens RE, Snijder RJ, et al. Out of hospital treatment of acute pulmonary embolism in patients with a low NT-proBNP level. *J Thromb Haemost* 2010; 8(6): 1235–1241.

10. Zondag W, Mos IC, Creemers-Schild D, et al. Outpatient treatment in patients with acute pulmonary embolism: the Hestia Study. *J Thromb Haemost* 2011; 9(8): 1500–1507.

11. Agterof MJ, Schutgens RE, Moumli N, et al. A prognostic model for short term adverse events in normotensive patients with pulmonary embolism. *Am J Hematol* 2011; 86(8): 646–649.

12. Snow V, Quseem A, Barry P, et al. Management of venous thromboembolism: a clinical practice guideline from the American College of Physicians and the American Academy of Family Physicians. *Ann Intern Med* 2007; 146(3): 204–210.

13. Torbicki A, Perrier A, Konstantinides S, et al. Guidelines on the diagnosis and management of acute pulmonary embolism: the Task Force for the Diagnosis and Management of Acute Pulmonary Embolism of the European Society of Cardiology (ESC). *Eur Heart J* 2008; 29(18): 2276–2315.

14. Aujesky D, Stone RA, Kim S, et al. Length of hospital stay and postdischarge mortality in patients with pulmonary embolism: a statewide perspective. *Arch Intern Med* 2008; 168(7): 706–712.

15. Bledsoe J, Hamilton D, Bess E, et al. Treatment of low-risk pulmonary embolism patients in a chest pain unit. *Crit Pathw Cardiol* 2010; 9(4): 212–215.

16. Ceriani E, Combescure C, Le Gal G, et al. Clinical prediction rules for pulmonary embolism: a systematic review and meta-analysis. *J Thromb Haemost* 2010; 8(5): 957–970.

17. Douma RA, Mos IC, Erkens PM, et al. Performance of 4 clinical decision rules in the diagnostic management of acute pulmonary embolism:

a prospective cohort study. *Ann Intern Med* 2011; 154(11): 709–718.

18. Righini M, Perrier A, DeMoerloose P, et al. D-Dimer for venous thromboembolism diagnosis: 20 years later. *J Thromb Haemost* 2008; 6(7): 1059–1071.

19. van Belle A, Buller HR, Huisman MV, et al. Effectiveness of managing suspected pulmonary embolism using an algorithm combining clinical probability, D-dimer testing, and computed tomography. *JAMA* 2006; 295(2): 172–179.

20. Qaseem A, Snow V, Barry P, et al. Current diagnosis of venous thromboembolism in primary care: a clinical practice guideline from the American Academy of Family Physicians and the American College of Physicians. *Ann Intern Med* 2007; 146(6): 454–458.

21. The PIOPED Investigators. Value of the ventilation/ perfusion scan in acute pulmonary embolism. Results of the prospective investigation of pulmonary embolism diagnosis (PIOPED). *JAMA* 1990; 263(20): 2753–2759.

22. Le Gal G, Righini M, Boehlen F, et al. A positive compression ultrasonography of the lower limb veins is highly predictive of pulmonary embolism on computed tomography in suspected patients. *Thromb Haemost* 2006; 95(6): 963–966.

23. Lankeit M, Konstantinides S. Mortality risk assessment and the role of thrombolysis in pulmonary embolism. *Clin Chest Med* 2010; 31(4): 759–769.

24. Becattini C, Vedovati MC, Agnelli G. Prognostic value of troponins in acute pulmonary embolism: a meta-analysis. *Circulation* 2007; 116(4): 427–433.

25. Wicki J, Perrier A, Pemeger TV, et al. Predicting adverse outcome in patients with acute pulmonary embolism: a risk score. *Thromb Haemost* 2000; 84(4): 548–552.

26. Uresandi F, Otero R, Cayuela A, et al. A clinical prediction rule for identifying short-term risk of adverse events in patients with pulmonary thromboembolism. *Arch Bronconeumol* 2007; 43(11): 617–622.

27. Murugappan M, Johnson JA, Gage BF, et al. Home Management Exclusion (HOME) criteria for initial treatment of acute pulmonary embolism. *Am J Respir Crit Care Med* 2008; 177: A182.

28. Nendaz MR, Bandelier P, Aujesky D, et al. Validation of a risk score identifying patients with acute pulmonary embolism, who are at low risk of clinical adverse outcome. *Thromb Haemost* 2004; 91(6): 1232–1236.

29. Aujesky D, LeManach CD, et al. Validation of a model to predict adverse outcomes in patients with pulmonary embolism. *Eur Heart J* 2006; 27(4): 476–481.

30. Otero R, Jimenez D. Pulmonary embolism at home. *Eur Respir J* 2008; 31(3): 686–687; author reply 687.

31. Aujesky D, Obrosky DS, Stone RA, et al. Derivation and validation of a prognostic model for pulmonary embolism. *Am J Respir Crit Care Med* 2005; 172(8): 1041–1046.

32. Venetz C, Jimenez D, Mean M, et al. A comparison of the original and simplified Pulmonary Embolism Severity Index. *Thromb Haemost* 2011; 106(3): 423–428.

33. Konstantinides S, Torkicki A, Agnelli G, et al. 2014 ESC Guidelines on the diagnosis and management of acute pulmonary embolism. *European Heart Journal* 2014; 35(43): 3033–3069.

34. Kearon C, Akl EA, Comerota AJ, et al. Antithrombotic Therapy for VTE Disease: Antithrombotic Therapy and Prevention of Thrombosis, 9th ed: American College of Chest Physicians Evidence-Based Clinical Practice Guidelines. *Chest* 2012; 141(2 Suppl): e419S–94S.

35. Kearon C, Akl EA, Ornelas J, et al. Antithrombotic Therapy for VTE Disease: CHEST Guideline and Expert Panel Report. *Chest* 2016; 149.

36. *FDA expands use of Xarelto to treat, reduce recurrence of blood clots.* November 8, 2012; Available from: www.fda.gov/ NewsEvents/Newsroom/ PressAnnouncements/ ucm326654.htm. (Accessed March 2016)

37. Einstein PE Investigators: Buller HR, Prins MH, Lensin AW, et al. Oral rivaroxaban for the treatment of Symptomatic Pulmonary Embolism. *N Engl J Med* 2012; 366(14): 1287–1297.

38. Agnelli G, Buller HR, Cohen A, et al. Oral Apixaban for the treatment of Acute Venous Thromboembolism. *NEJM* 2013; 369(9): 799–808.

39. Hokusai-VTE Investigators: Buller HR, Decousus H, Gross MA, et al. Edoxaban versus Warfarin for the treatment of Symptomatic Venous Thromboembolism. *NEJM* 2013; 369: 1406–1415.

40. Schulman S, Kearon C, Kakkar AK, et al. Re-Cover Study Group. Dabigatran versus warfarin in the treatment of acute venous thromboembolism. *N Engl J Med* 2009; 361(24): 2342–2352.

41. Kearon C, Akl EA, Comerota AJ, et al. Antithrombotic Therapy for VTE Disease: Antithrombotic Therapy and

Prevention of Thrombosis, 9th ed: American College of Chest Physicians Evidence-Based Clinical Practice Guidelines. *Chest* 2012; 141(2 Suppl): e419S–94S.

42. Van Der Hulle T, Kooiman J, den Exter PL, et al. Effectiveness and safety of novel oral anticoagulants as compared with vitamin K antagonists in the treatment of acute symptomatic venous thromboembolism: a systematic review and meta-analysis. *Journal of Thrombosis and Haemostasis* 2014; 12: 320–328.

Chapter

33

Anticoagulants

David G. Paje, MD, FACP, SFHM

Introduction

Since its discovery in the mid-1900s, warfarin has been the predominant anticoagulant used for the prevention and treatment of thromboembolism in patients with atrial fibrillation, venous thromboembolic disease (VTE), mechanical heart valves and other hypercoagulable states. It has a narrow therapeutic window and highly variable dosing requirements. Thus, patients must be monitored closely with regular blood work and dose adjustments to ensure that the international normalized ratio (INR) of the prothrombin time (PT) is in the desired range. However, because the optimal INR range for warfarin is not the same for all indications, rigorous investigations were performed to establish the most appropriate INR target that effectively reduces thromboembolic events for each condition while at the same time minimizing the risk of clinically significant bleeding. For the most common indications, nonvalvular atrial fibrillation (NVAF) and VTE, the target INR is from 2.0 to 3.0.

Bleeding is the most feared complication of oral anticoagulant therapy and it is directly related to the intensity of treatment.[1] Clinical studies show that warfarin increases the risk of major bleeding by 0.3–0.5% per year and the risk of intracranial hemorrhage (ICH) by 0.2%.[2] Moreover, the rate of bleeding rises sharply as the INR increases greater than 4.5,[3,4] a level that is commonly seen in patients undergoing routine outpatient monitoring of their anticoagulation.[5]

In the emergency department (ED), among patients whose INR values were obtained during their visit, almost 1 in 10 (11%) had an INR above 5.0.[6] Many of these patients present with gross bleeding.[6,7] Thus, patients with a supratherapeutic INR are frequently admitted to the hospital and are treated as inpatients.[7] However, this practice may not always be necessary in the light of current evidence particularly on the efficacy and outcomes of anticoagulation reversal strategies using vitamin K.[8,9] In the absence of clinically significant bleeding, patients with excessive anticoagulation due to warfarin may be managed safely and effectively in the observation or outpatient setting.

Pharmacology of Warfarin

Warfarin is the most commonly used vitamin K antagonist (VKA), particularly in the United States. It interferes with the final step in the hepatic synthesis of biologically active coagulation proteins, the γ-carboxylation of glutamate residues on the N-terminal regions of vitamin K-dependent factors II, VII, IX, and X. This step is necessary for the conformational change in the clotting proteins that allows binding to cofactors on phospholipid surfaces. The carboxylation process requires the reduced form of vitamin K, which results from an oxidation-reduction reaction that involves either vitamin K epoxide reductase or vitamin K reductase; both of which are directly inhibited by warfarin, the former more so than the latter.

Commercially distributed warfarin is a racemic mixture of two optically active isomers, the more potent S-enantiomer and the less potent R-enantiomer. It is highly water soluble and is rapidly absorbed from the stomach and small intestines, with a bioavailability of almost 100%. Its maximal blood concentration is reached about 90 minutes after oral administration. Warfarin is extensively protein-bound, mainly to albumin; the free fraction that is pharmacologically active varies among individuals and is independent of the total serum concentration. The two isomers of warfarin are processed in the liver through different pathways; the S-enantiomer is mostly metabolized by the p450 cytochrome enzyme CYP2C9, while the R-enantiomer is primarily oxidized by two cytochrome enzymes, CYP1A2 and CYP3A4.

The racemic mixture of warfarin has a half-life of 36–42 hours.[10]

The onset of warfarin's anticoagulant effect is based on the time it takes to sufficiently deplete the levels of circulating clotting factors, particularly factors II and X. Although the INR may increase during the first few days after starting warfarin, this merely reflects a reduction in the levels of factor VII, which has a shorter half-life of about 6 hours. Since prothrombin (factor II) has a longer half-life of about 60–72 hours, effective anticoagulation may not be achieved until after at least 5 days of treatment.[10] If higher doses were used for initiating treatment with warfarin, the INR may rise more rapidly because of a greater reduction of factor VII but this will not alter the time required to reach steady state.[11]

The relationship between the dose of warfarin and its anticoagulant effect is influenced by genetic and environmental factors that affect its absorption from the gastrointestinal tract, its metabolism in the liver and the sensitivity of its pharmacologic target, vitamin K oxide reductase (VKOR), to its inhibitory action. Thus, warfarin dosing must be individualized and periodic adjustments may be required to keep the INR in the target range. Among patients who are on long-term treatment with warfarin, several factors may lead to fluctuations in the INR, including inaccuracies in INR testing, variable dietary intake of vitamin K, changes in vitamin K or warfarin absorption, changes in warfarin metabolism, changes in vitamin K-dependent coagulation factor synthesis or metabolism, effects of concomitant medications, and patient noncompliance.[12] Because of these, maintaining optimal anticoagulation with warfarin may oftentimes be quite challenging. Even in the ideal setting of a clinical trial, the time-in-therapeutic range (TTR) achieved ranged from 29% to 75%.[13]

Excessive Anticoagulation and Bleeding Risk

For most clinical indications, the target INR is either 2.5 or 3.0, with acceptable ranges of 2.0–3.0 or 2.5–3.5, respectively.[14–16] Although the annual incidence of major bleeding associated with warfarin is estimated to be only about 1% to 3%,[2] the rate of significant bleeding events rises steeply when the INR exceeds 4.5.[3,4] In a case-control analysis of adults who suffered ICH while on warfarin, the rate of ICH was found to double for every 1-point increase in INR.[17]

In addition to the intensity of anticoagulation, other factors may contribute to the bleeding risk, including the concomitant use of other drugs that may interfere with hemostasis, prior bleeding events and advanced age. Several clinical prediction rules have been developed to predict bleeding while taking warfarin for any indication.[18] One of these, the Modified Outpatient Bleeding Risk Index (mOBRI), has been independently validated and was found to perform better than physicians' estimates of the probability of major bleeding.[19] The mOBRI includes four independent patient risk factors for major bleeding: age $\geq$ 65 years, history of gastrointestinal bleeding in the preceding 2 weeks, history of stroke, and at least one of the following comorbid conditions: recent myocardial infarction, hematocrit $<$ 30%, creatinine $>$ 1.5 mg/dL, or diabetes mellitus. One point is counted for every risk factor category and high-risk is defined as $\geq$ 3 points. For patients on anticoagulation specifically for NVAF, the HAS-BLED (Hypertension, Abnormal Renal/Liver Function, Stroke, Bleeding History or Predisposition, Labile INR, Elderly, Drugs/Alcohol Concomitantly) score is a well-validated and widely used tool to assess the risk of major bleeding.[20,21]

Most authors classify bleeding events as either major or minor (non-major). **Major bleeding** in non-surgical patients is defined by the International Society of Thrombosis and Haemostasis (ISTH) as fatal bleeding, and/or symptomatic bleeding in a critical area or organ (e.g., intracranial, intraspinal, intraocular, retroperitoneal, intraarticular, pericardial, intramuscular with compartment syndrome), and/or bleeding resulting in a drop in hemoglobin level of 2 g/dL or more or requiring the transfusion of 2 or more units of red blood cells.[22] The most prevalent site of anticoagulant-related major bleeding is the gastrointestinal tract, followed by urinary tract, intracerebral, genital tract, and retroperitoneal.[23] Based on a retrospective study, the mortality rate from major bleeding associated with warfarin was 9.5%.[23] Elderly patients (75 years and older) who generally have a higher risk of fatal thrombotic events were also found to have a higher rate of fatal bleeding, almost exclusively from ICH.[24] Also, the risk of fatal ICH may be related to the indication for anticoagulation; it is significantly more frequent in those taking warfarin for atrial fibrillation than in those who had VTE.[25–27]

Anticoagulation Reversal Strategies with Vitamin K

The anticoagulant effect of warfarin results from its inhibition of the oxidation-reduction reaction that produces the reduced vitamin-K, which is necessary for the carboxylation of the clotting factors. This involves a pair of enzymes: **vitamin K epoxide reductase**, which is sensitive to warfarin, and **vitamin K reductase**, which is less sensitive. Low doses of vitamin K (phytonadione) can overcome warfarin's inhibition of vitamin K epoxide reductase and offset its anticoagulant effect. Larger doses of vitamin K may in fact lead to warfarin resistance that may last for 1 week or more because the vitamin K that accumulates in the liver becomes available to the warfarin-insensitive reductase.

When anticoagulation becomes excessive, the goal is to promptly reduce the risk of bleeding by using strategies that will bring the INR down to safe levels while at the same time avoiding overcorrection, which may lead to thromboembolic complications. Simply withholding warfarin and allowing the INR to fall into the desired range is the most widely used approach and results in low (0.8%) incidence of major bleeding among patients with a moderate elevation of INR (6.0–10.0).[28] On the other hand, administration of either oral or intravenous vitamin K is more likely to reverse excessive anticoagulation at 24 hours compared to simply withholding warfarin.[29] However, when four randomized controlled trials (RCT) compared vitamin K to placebo for patients with INR of 4.5–10.0, the rates of major bleeding (0.8% vs. 2.0%) and thromboembolism (1.2% vs. 0.9%) were similar in both groups.[30–33] Therefore, for patients with an INR of 4.5–10.0 who are not bleeding, administration of vitamin K may lead to a more rapid correction of the INR but there is no evidence of benefit in terms of bleeding and thromboembolic outcomes.

When patients with INR values above 9.0 were studied separately, the 30-day risk of major bleeding was high (9.6%) when vitamin K was not given routinely.[34] But when 2.5 mg of oral vitamin K was given to 107 warfarin-treated patients

with INR > 10 but without evidence of bleeding, the rate of major bleeding by 90 days was low (3.7%).[9] Also, patients who are administered oral vitamin K are more likely to have an INR < 5 by day 3 compared to those who only withheld warfarin.[35] Thus, while there are no RCTs to guide the management of patients with INR > 10.0 without bleeding, using vitamin K may be a prudent option considering the substantial risk of bleeding.

Oral administration is the most preferred route of giving vitamin K to reverse anticoagulation in patients who are not bleeding. Although intravenous administration resulted in a more rapid decline in INR at 6 hours and at 12 hours, the INR values achieved at 24 hours were similar for both oral and intravenous routes.[36] Oral vitamin K at doses of 1–2.5 mg reliably corrects excessive anticoagulation without causing warfarin resistance, or anaphylactoid or skin reactions.[31,37]

Intravenous vitamin K is often used in patients who are bleeding and who need urgent reversal of anticoagulation. The suggested dose for serious or life threatening bleeding is 5–10 mg, diluted in a minimum of 50 mL of intravenous fluid and administered over a minimum of 20 minutes.[10,38] This may be repeated if necessary at 12–24 hour intervals because of the long half-life of warfarin. Anaphylactoid reactions to intravenous vitamin K have been described but are rare, and are associated with large doses, administered rapidly and with little dilution.[39]

Subcutaneous administration of vitamin K is less effective when compared to either the oral or intravenous routes; its absorption is variable and its effect on INR is unpredictable.[40,41]

Finally, the management of excessive anticoagulation in patients with mechanical heart valves who are not bleeding may be quite challenging. These patients have a high thromboembolic risk, particularly with prosthetic valves in the mitral position or with older valves in either the mitral or aortic positions. It may be prudent to adopt an approach that will minimize the likelihood of overcorrection and of warfarin resistance.

Direct Oral Anticoagulants

After about half a century of vitamin-K antagonists as the only available oral anticoagulants, two new classes of effective alternative oral medications

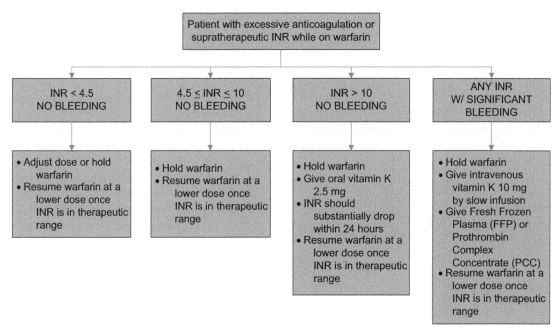

Figure 33.1 Algorithm for Managing Excessive Anticoagulation

have emerged. Collectively known as direct oral anticoagulants (DOACs), these new agents are rapidly acting, target-specific and have predictable anticoagulant effects, thus eliminating the need for routine monitoring. Dabigatran is a direct prothrombin inhibitor and has been approved to reduce the risk of stroke and systemic embolism in NVAF, to treat and prevent recurrence of VTE, and to prevent VTE after hip arthroplasty. Rivaroxaban, apixaban, and edoxaban are direct Factor Xa (FXa) inhibitors and are all indicated in patients with NVAF and VTE. In addition, both rivaroxaban and apixaban are approved for VTE prevention after hip or knee arthroplasty.

The DOACs are now the preferred anticoagulant of choice for most patients. Compared to warfarin, DOACs showed significant reductions in the risk of stroke, ICH and mortality in patients with NVAF, with similar risk of major bleeding and increased risk of gastrointestinal bleeding.[42] Among those with VTE, DOACs are at least as effective as VKAs in preventing recurrent VTE, fatal PE and overall mortality but with significantly lower rates of bleeding complications.[43]

When bleeding occurs in patients taking DOACs, the severity of bleeding and the timing of the last dose taken are the key considerations in initial management. If the bleeding is non-major

and is adequately controlled without using reversal agents, the patient may be placed in observation for continued monitoring. The DOACs have relatively short half-lives and with normal renal function, their anticoagulant effect should resolve 24–48 hours after the last dose.[44]

Patient Selection

Most warfarin-treated patients with excessive anticoagulation who are not bleeding may be managed in the outpatient setting (Figure 33.1) with either dose adjustments alone (for INR < 4.5), simply withholding warfarin (for INR 4.5–10.0), or administering low-dose oral vitamin K (for INR > 10.0). Observation care may be a reasonable alternative for those who have an unacceptably high bleeding risk from a combination of a high INR > 10.0 and the presence of other independent risk factors for major bleeding. Although clinical prediction tools have been developed to estimate bleeding risk in patients receiving anticoagulants, none has been proposed to predict bleeding specifically in patients with excessive anticoagulation.

Patients on DOACs who experience non-major bleeding that is adequately controlled without using reversal agents are also appropriate candidates for observation care. On the other hand, DOAC patients who present with major bleeding or who require the use of reversal agents should be managed in the inpatient setting.

Observation Care

Patients on warfarin treatment with an INR > 10 and without evidence of bleeding should have their dose withheld until after their INR is back in the therapeutic range. Also, they should be given oral vitamin K at a dose of 2.5 mg preferably while in the ED. Because there is a delay in clotting factor synthesis following oral vitamin K replacement, those patients who have other risk factors for major bleeding in addition to the elevated INR may be monitored closely so that more aggressive reversal measures can be instituted promptly when signs and symptoms of significant bleeding develop. Their INR may be repeated at 24 hours, at which time it is expected to fall to safer levels if hepatic function is normal, but not necessarily to the ideal therapeutic range. After discharge from observation care, patients should be followed very closely within a couple of days by their anticoagulation physician, particularly those with challenging issues such as mechanical heart valves.

A non-major bleeding episode in a patient taking a DOAC should be controlled promptly without the need for any reversal agent. Initial observation management includes holding or discontinuing succeeding doses of the anticoagulant, reviewing concomitant medications that may also affect hemostasis, evaluating renal function and managing hydration status. There is currently no readily available laboratory test that can specifically measure the anticoagulant activity of DOACs. However, common coagulation assays may be used to roughly gauge the anticoagulant effect of DOACs. The activated partial thromboplastin time (aPTT) is prolonged when there is an anticoagulant effect of dabigatran, but the aPTT may be normal even when the plasma level of dabigatran is elevated. Similarly, the PT is prolonged when there is an anticoagulant effect of FXa inhibitors, but a normal PT does not rule out elevated levels of FXa inhibitors.[45]

Since all the DOACs are at least partially eliminated through the kidneys, assessing the renal function (using Cockcroft-Gault method) is necessary in approximating the resolution of their anticoagulant effect. In patients with normal renal function, dabigatran and FXa inhibitors should be eliminated 2–3 days and 1–2 days, respectively, after the last dose. Thus, patients may be discharged from observation care if they remain clinically stable after 24–48 hours of monitoring.

Finally, patients who are seen in observation for complications related to anticoagulation should have an individualized reassessment of the benefits of continued treatment versus the risk of bleeding. This is also a good time to reconsider their options for anticoagulant therapy. Collaborating with the primary care provider or the physician responsible for managing their anticoagulation may be necessary when discussing these issues with the patient.

References

1. Oden A, Fahlen M. Oral anticoagulation and risk of death: a medical record linkage study. *BMJ*, 2002. 325(7372): 1073–1075.

2. Schulman S, Beyth RJ, Kearon C, et al. Hemorrhagic complications of anticoagulant and thrombolytic treatment: American College of Chest Physicians Evidence-Based Clinical Practice Guidelines (8th Edition). *Chest*, 2008. 133(6 Suppl): 257S–298S.

3. Hylek EM, Chang YC, Skates SJ, et al. Prospective study of the outcomes of ambulatory patients with excessive warfarin anticoagulation. *Arch Intern Med*, 2000. 160(11): 1612–1617.

4. Cannegieter SC, Rosendaal FR, Wintzen AD, et al. Optimal oral anticoagulant therapy in patients with mechanical heart valves. *N Engl J Med*, 1995. 333(1): 11–7.

5. Chiquette E, Amato MG, Bussey HI. Comparison of an anticoagulation clinic with usual medical care: anticoagulation control, patient outcomes, and health care costs. *Arch Intern Med*, 1998. 158(15): 1641–1647.

6. Newman DH, Zhitomirsky I. The prevalence of nontherapeutic and dangerous international normalized ratios among patients receiving warfarin in the emergency department. *Ann Emerg Med*, 2006. 48(2): 182–189, 189 e1.

7. Atreja A, El-Sameed YA, Jneid H, et al. Elevated international normalized ratio in the ED: clinical course and physician adherence to the published recommendations. *Am J Emerg Med*, 2005. 23(1): 40–44.

8. Denas G, Marzot F, Offellie R, et al. Effectiveness and safety of a management protocol to correct over-anticoagulation with oral vitamin K: a retrospective study of 1,043 cases. *J Thromb Thrombolysis*, 2009. 27(3): 340–347.

9. Crowther MA, Garcia D, Ageno W, et al. Oral vitamin K effectively treats international normalised ratio (INR) values in excess of 10. Results of a prospective cohort study. *Thromb Haemost*, 2010. 104(1): 118–121.

10. Ageno W, Gallus G, Wittkowsky A, et al. Oral anticoagulant therapy: Antithrombotic Therapy and Prevention of Thrombosis, 9th ed: American College of Chest Physicians Evidence-Based Clinical Practice Guidelines. *Chest*, 2012. 141(2 Suppl): e44S–88S.

11. Harrison L, Johnston M, Massicotte MP, et al. Comparison of 5-mg and 10-mg loading doses in initiation of warfarin therapy. *Ann Intern Med*, 1997. 126(2): 133–136.

12. Ansell J, Hirsh J, Hylek E, et al. Pharmacology and Management of the Vitamin K Antagonists, 8th ed: American College of Chest Physicians Evidence-Based Clinical Practice Guidelines. *Chest*, 2008. 133(6 Suppl): 160S–198S.

13. Wan Y, Heneghan C, Perera R, et al. Anticoagulation control and prediction of adverse events in patients with atrial fibrillation: a systematic review. *Circ Cardiovasc Qual Outcomes*, 2008. 1(2): 84–91.

14. You JJ, Singer DE, Howard PA, et al. Antithrombotic therapy for atrial fibrillation: Antithrombotic Therapy and Prevention of Thrombosis, 9th ed: American College of Chest Physicians Evidence-Based Clinical Practice Guidelines.

Chest, 2012. 141(2 Suppl): e531S–575S.

15. Kearon C, Akl EA, Comerota AJ, et al. Antithrombotic therapy for VTE Disease: Antithrombotic Therapy and Prevention of Thrombosis, 9th ed: American College of Chest Physicians Evidence-Based Clinical Practice Guidelines. *Chest*, 2012. 141(2 Suppl): e419S–494S.

16. Whitlock RP, Sun JC, Fremes SE, et al. Antithrombotic and thrombolytic therapy for valvular disease: Antithrombotic Therapy and Prevention of Thrombosis, 9th ed: American College of Chest Physicians Evidence-Based Clinical Practice Guidelines. *Chest*, 2012. 141(2 Suppl): e576S–600S.

17. Hylek EM, Singer DE. Risk factors for intracranial hemorrhage in outpatients taking warfarin. *Ann Intern Med*, 1994. 120(11): 897–902.

18. Dahr, K, Loewen P. The risk of bleeding with warfarin: a systematic review and performance analysis of clinical prediction rules. Thromb Haemost, 2007. 98(5): 980–987.

19. Beyth RJ, Quinn LM, Landefeld CS. Prospective evaluation of an index for predicting the risk of major bleeding in outpatients treated with warfarin. *Am J Med*, 1998. 105(2): 91–99.

20. Pisters R, Lane DA, Nieuwlaat R, et al. A novel user-friendly score (HAS-BLED) to assess 1-year risk of major bleeding in patients with atrial fibrillation. *Chest*, 2010; 138: 1093–1100.

21. Lip GY, Frison L, Halpern JL, et al. Comparative validation of a novel risk score for predicting bleeding risk in anticoagulated patients with atrial fibrillation. *Journal of the American College of Cardiology*, 2011; 57: 173–180.

22. Schulman S, Kearon C. Definition of major bleeding in clinical investigations of antihemostatic medicinal products in non-surgical patients. *Journal of Thrombosis and Haemostasis*, 2005; 3:692–694.

23. Guerrouij M, Uppal CS, Alklabi A, et al. The clinical impact of bleeding during oral anticoagulant therapy: assessment of morbidity, mortality and post-bleed anticoagulant management. *J Thromb Thrombolysis*, 2011. 31(4): 419–423.

24. Palareti G, Hirsh J, Legnani C, et al. Oral anticoagulation treatment in the elderly: a nested, prospective, case-control study. *Arch Intern Med*, 2000. 160(4): 470–478.

25. Landefeld CS, Beyth RJ. Anticoagulant-related bleeding: clinical epidemiology, prediction, and prevention. *Am J Med*, 1993. 95(3): 315–328.

26. Palareti G, Leali N, Coccheri S, et al. Bleeding complications of oral anticoagulant treatment: an inception-cohort, prospective collaborative study (ISCOAT). Italian Study on Complications of Oral Anticoagulant Therapy. *Lancet*, 1996. 348(9025): 423–428.

27. Linkins LA, Choi PT, Douketis JD. Clinical impact of bleeding in patients taking oral anticoagulant therapy for venous thromboembolism: a meta-analysis. *Ann Intern Med*, 2003. 139(11): 893–900.

28. Lousberg TR, Witt DM, Beall DG, et al. Evaluation of excessive anticoagulation in a group model health maintenance organization. *Arch Intern Med*, 1998. 158(5): 528–534.

29. Dezee KJ, Shimeall WT, Douglas KM, et al. Treatment of excessive anticoagulation with phytonadione (vitamin K):

a meta-analysis. *Arch Intern Med*, 2006. 166(4): 391–397.

30. Crowther MA, Ageno W, Garcia D, et al. Oral vitamin K versus placebo to correct excessive anticoagulation in patients receiving warfarin: a randomized trial. *Ann Intern Med*, 2009. 150(5): 293–300.

31. Crowther MA, Julian J, McCarty D, et al. Treatment of warfarin-associated coagulopathy with oral vitamin K: a randomised controlled trial. *Lancet*, 2000. 356(9241): 1551–1553.

32. Ageno W, Crowther M, Steidl L, et al. Low dose oral vitamin K to reverse acenocoumarol-induced coagulopathy: a randomized controlled trial. *Thromb Haemost*, 2002. 88(1): 48–51.

33. Ageno W, Garcia D, Silingardi M, et al. A randomized trial comparing 1 mg of oral vitamin K with no treatment in the management of warfarin-associated coagulopathy in patients with mechanical heart valves. *J Am Coll Cardiol*, 2005. 46(4): 732–733.

34. Garcia DA, Regan S, Crowther M, et al. The risk of hemorrhage among patients with warfarin-associated coagulopathy. *J Am Coll Cardiol*, 2006. 47(4): 804–808.

35. Gunther KE, Conway G, Leibach L, et al. Low-dose oral vitamin K is safe and effective for outpatient management of patients with an INR>10. *Thromb Res*, 2004. 113(3–4): 205–209.

36. Lubetsky A, Yonath H, Olchovsky D, et al. Comparison of oral vs intravenous phytonadione (vitamin K1) in patients with excessive anticoagulation: a prospective randomized controlled study. *Arch Intern Med*, 2003. 163(20): 2469–2473.

37. Crowther MA, Donovan D, Harrison L, et al. Low-dose oral vitamin K reliably reverses over-anticoagulation due to warfarin. *Thromb Haemost*, 1998. 79(6): 1116–1118.

38. Guyatt GH, Akl EA, Crowther M, et al. Executive summary: Antithrombotic Therapy and Prevention of Thrombosis, 9th ed: American College of Chest Physicians Evidence-Based Clinical Practice Guidelines. *Chest*, 2012. 141(2 Suppl): 7S–47S.

39. Fiore LD, Scola MA, Cantillon CE, et al. Anaphylactoid reactions to vitamin K. *J Thromb Thrombolysis*, 2001. 11(2): 175–183.

40. Crowther MA, Douketis JD, Schnurr T, et al. Oral vitamin K lowers the international normalized ratio more rapidly than subcutaneous vitamin K in the treatment of warfarin-associated coagulopathy. A randomized, controlled trial. *Ann Intern Med*, 2002. 137(4): 251–254.

41. Raj G, Kumar R, McKinney WP. Time course of reversal of anticoagulant effect of warfarin by intravenous and subcutaneous phytonadione. *Arch Intern Med*, 1999. 159(22): 2721–2724.

42. Ruff CT, Giugliano RP, Braunwald E, et al. Comparison of the efficacy and safety of new oral anticoagulants with warfarin in patients with atrial fibrillation: a meta-analysis of randomized trials. *Lancet*, 2014; 383: 955–962.

43. Van Der Hulle T, Kooiman J, den Exter PL, et al. Effectiveness and safety of novel oral anticoagulants as compared with vitamin K antagonists in the treatment of acute symptomatic venous thromboembolism: a systematic review and meta-analysis. *Journal of Thrombosis and Haemostasis*, 2014; 12: 320–328.

44. Jackson LR, Becker RC. Novel oral anticoagulants: pharmacology, coagulation measures, and consideration for reversal. *J Thromb Thrombolysis*, 2014; 37: 380–391.

45. Kovacs RJ, Flaker GC, Saxonhouse SJ, et al. Practical management of anticoagulation in patients with atrial fibrillation. *Journal of the American College of Cardiology*, 2015; 65: 1340–1360.

Chapter

34

Transient Ischemic Attack (TIA)

Matthew Tabbut, MD
Jonathan Glauser, MD, FACEP

TIA Definition

Every year in the United States nearly 800,000 people are affected by a new or recurrent stroke.[1] It has historically been the third leading cause of death and a leading cause of long-term disability.[2] Statistically, 15–30% of all strokes are preceded by a transient ischemic attack (TIA).[3] In the emergency department (ED), TIA accounts for approximately 300,000 patient visits annually though this may be an underestimate of the true prevalence of TIA as many do not present to a health care provider.[1,2,4]

Traditionally, TIA has been defined as an "Acute neurologic deficit caused by focal brain ischemia (attributable to a specific arterial territory) that completely resolves in 24 hours."[2,5] The differentiation between TIA and stroke historically was made when advanced brain imaging was not available and recovery was judged based on clinical symptoms. With the advent of CT and MRI, radiographic evidence of infarction can be seen in many who would have been previously classified as having a TIA.[5,6]

A new definition has been proposed that considers TIA a brief episode of neurologic dysfunction caused by focal brain or retinal ischemia without evidence of acute infarction. Some authors include a time window of less than 1 hour, since 75% of TIAs by the old definition resolve within 60 minutes.[1,3,5,6]

Recently there has been an enhanced sense of urgency regarding the workup of TIA in order to prevent subsequently debilitating strokes. The time window of greatest concern for the emergency physician is the first 48 hours to 7 days. Approximately half of all strokes that occur during the first 7 days will occur within the first 24 hours.[7]

Risk Stratification

Stroke risk is believed to be 3–5% in 2 days, 5–7% in 7 days, 8.0% in 30 days, and 9.2% in 90 days following a TIA,[8,9,10,11] although higher risk using a different methodology has also been reported: 9.9% at 2 days, 13.4% at 30 days, and 17.3% at 90 days.[9] Several scoring rules have been developed in order to risk stratify patients who are at increased risk of stroke following a TIA.

The California rule, ABCD rule, and ABCD2 rule have been used to risk stratify patients into high and low risk of subsequent stroke. The most widely used rule is the ABCD score (Table 34.1). It was derived to determine the risk of stroke following TIA at 7 days. More recently the ABCD2 score was developed by adding a history of diabetes to the ABCD score (Table 34.2).

Though the ABCD and ABCD2 rule was derived to help determine if patients are safe for

Table 34.1 ABCD Rule[2]

Factors	Score
Age ≥60 yrs	1
Elevated BP Systolic > 140 mmHg Diastolic > 90 mmHg	1
Unilateral weakness	2
Speech impairment without unilateral weakness	1
Duration ≥ 60 min	2
Duration 10 to 59 min	1
Duration < 10 min	0
Total possible points	**6**

Table 34.2 ABCD2 Rule[2]

Factors	Score
Age ≥ 60 yrs	1
Elevated BP Systolic > 140 mmHg Diastolic > 90 mmHg	1
Unilateral weakness	2
Speech impairment without unilateral weakness	1
Duration ≥ 60 min	2
Duration 10 to 50 min	1
Duration < 10 min	1
Diabetes	1
Total possible points	**7**

discharge, it has not been used specifically as entrance or exclusion criteria for ED observation units (OUs).

Role of Observation

There are no clear guidelines that establish a standard of care for the disposition of TIA patients.[12] The final decision to admit or discharge is often left to the individual institution and to physician risk tolerance. Some institutions admit all patients diagnosed with a TIA. Others who have well-established follow-up in specialized TIA clinics may discharge patients who are deemed appropriate for outpatient management to obtain their studies within the next 48 hours.[2, 13] As ED OUs have gained popularity, it is increasingly clear that patients diagnosed with TIA can be safely and efficiently managed in the observation setting as an alternative to inpatient admission.[14] In particular, OU use results in reduced risk for subsequent stroke, greater compliance with diagnostic evaluation, shorter length of stay, lower cost, and decreased hospital overcrowding and ambulance diversion.[14]

Because the risk of stroke following a TIA is highest in the first 48 hours, hospitalization has been justified in order to identify particular pathologies that may predispose to stroke. Conditions such as atrial fibrillation, carotid artery stenosis, extracranial dissections, cardiac thrombus, and cardiac arrhythmia all have been known to be causes of stroke that are potentially modifiable in the acute phase. The initial evaluation of TIA should be aimed at identifying treatable conditions to prevent stroke through a variety of imaging studies and laboratory assessments.[14]

The short-term risk of stroke in the acute phase after TIA is typically due to unstable vascular pathology, including critical carotid stenosis, cardiac thrombus, and arrhythmia.[14,15] Accelerated diagnostic protocols in the ED observation setting are aimed at uncovering these pathologies and consist of neuroimaging, telemetry monitoring, cardiac echocardiography, and carotid imaging.[16]

The evaluation of TIA in the ED observation setting provides an efficient and accurate patient assessment. Additionally it has been found to reduce unnecessary hospitalization. Rapid evaluation of TIA has been shown to reduce subsequent stroke risk. The EXPRESS trial evaluating the use of urgent, specialized clinics in the evaluation and initial treatment of TIA found an 80% reduction in risk of early recurrent stroke.[17]

From an economic standpoint, the use of accelerated diagnostic protocols in the ED OU compared to inpatient admission showed cost savings and resulted in shorter length of stay. In one report, the average cost for inpatient admission was $1,547 versus $890 for ED observation. The average length of stay for inpatient admission was 61.2 hours versus 25.6 hours for ED observation.[16]

Some categories of patients are inappropriate for admission to an OU. Patients with crescendo TIA symptoms or repeated TIA symptoms present a high risk for subsequent stroke and should be admitted to an inpatient unit. Patients with a stroke or with persistent neurologic deficits require full inpatient admission.[16]

Patients identified in the ED as having a cause for their TIA should be admitted to an inpatient unit rather than the ED OU. Thus, any head CT positive for intracranial hemorrhage, infarct or mass requires admission to the appropriate neurology or neurosurgery service. Patients with known embolic sources should be admitted to the appropriate cardiology or medical service for management of their underlying process. Any patient with known carotid stenosis > 50% should be evaluated by vascular surgery for urgent carotid endarterectomy (CEA).[16]

A certain percentage of patients will rule in for stroke even with transient symptoms that clinically appear to be a TIA.[6] Patients in the ED OU

Table 34.3 Differential Diagnosis for TIA[2,16]

Stroke
Complex migraine
Focal seizure
Todd's paralysis
Hypertensive encephalopathy
Intracranial hemorrhage
Syncope
Labyrinthine disorders
Vasospasm
Hypoglycemia
Hypernatremia
Hydrocephalus
Intracranial mass
Arteritis
Focal neuropathy

Table 34.4 ED Evaluation[2]

Glucose check	Evaluate for hypoglycemia
EKG	Evaluate for precipitating arrhythmias (i.e., atrial fibrillation)
Brain imaging (CT scan)	Differentiate between hemorrhagic lesion, mass lesion or ischemic lesion
Laboratory assessment – Complete blood count – Basic metabolic panel – Coagulation studies – Lipid profile	Evaluate for metabolic causes of symptoms and guide for medical management

Table 34.5 Observation Unit Protocol[16]

Diffusion weighted MRI	Differentiates TIA from ischemic stroke
Carotid imaging	Evaluates for stenosis that would require carotid revascularization (MRA vs CTA vs Doppler Ultrasound)
Cardiac imaging (e.g., echocardiogram)	Evaluates for cardioembolic source of TIA and for patent foramen ovale (PFO) allowing for embolism from venous circulation
Continuous telemetry monitoring	Evaluates for paroxysmal arrhythmia contributing to ischemic symptoms or differential diagnosis
Frequent neurologic assessments	Monitors for changing or evolving symptoms
Patient education	Education on stroke risk following transient ischemic attack, risk factor modification (blood pressure control, lipid control, antiplatelet agents) and smoking cessation counseling

who are found to have evidence of ischemia on their MRI should be admitted for further management and care of their stroke.

Other neurologic and vascular conditions can mimic TIA (Table 34.3). Patients with these conditions or patients who have significant comorbidities requiring > 24-hour stay should be evaluated in the ED with appropriate disposition.[16]

TIA Workup

The evaluation of TIA is time sensitive. The goal of the ED observation evaluation of TIA is to identify reversible causes of subsequent stroke. The initial ED evaluation should evaluate TIA mimics (Table 34.3), differentiate TIA from stroke and detect high-risk pathologies that require immediate intervention and admission (Table 34.4).

Purposes of an accelerated diagnostic protocol for TIA in the ED OU include confirmation of the diagnosis of TIA, evaluation for reversible causes of TIA, and determination of the need for additional therapeutic intervention to prevent subsequent stroke. Standardized protocols may consist of continuous monitoring (neurologic assessment and telemetry monitoring), brain imaging, carotid imaging, cardiac imaging, and neurology consultation (Table 34.5).

Brain Imaging
Non-Contrast CT Brain

The primary utility of CT brain imaging is to differentiate ischemic lesions versus non-ischemic lesions (i.e., tumor, aneurysm, intracranial hemorrhage) as the source of a patient's neurologic deficits.[5] CT should be performed in the ED prior to admission to the ED OU as the results have a direct impact on the need for admission and consultation.

MRI

Diffusion weighted magnetic resonance imaging (DW-MRI) serves two purposes in the ED OU. It primarily aids in the diagnostic differentiation between TIA and stroke. This technique has identified approximately 30% to 67% of patients who were clinically classified as TIA as having evidence of acute ischemia suggestive of stroke.[3, 18] Additionally DW-MRI can assist in the risk stratification of patients with TIA. While the exact results have been somewhat variable it has been consistently shown that patients with a negative DW-MRI are at less than 1% risk for stroke at 48 hours and 7 days.[18] As DW-MRI is often not readily available initially in the ED, patients can be evaluated by MRI as part of the ED observation protocol.

Vascular Imaging

Intracranial and extracranial arterial stenosis are risk factors for TIA and stroke. For those with intracranial artery stenosis the 90-day risk of stroke is 32.6% for those who also have evidence of ischemia on DW-MRI and 10.8% for those without evidence of ischemia on DW-MRI.[3] All patients evaluated in the ED OU should undergo imaging to determine the presence or absence of carotid artery stenosis with a goal of detecting carotid artery stenosis of > 50%. For patients with carotid artery stenosis < 50% there is no benefit to surgical management over medical management in reduction of stroke risk.[1] Carotid artery ultrasonography, CT angiography or MR angiography can be used to evaluate vascular caliber.

Carotid Artery Duplex Ultrasound

Carotid artery duplex ultrasonography has been considered the standard imaging modality for evaluation of carotid artery stenosis. Its major benefits include lack of radiation and its ability to evaluate the stiffness of the carotid vasculature. It is believed that increased stiffness predisposes to plaque rupture secondary to pulsatile stress from increased pulse pressure.[2] Carotid artery duplex ultrasonography has been shown to perform well in the evaluation of 70–99% stenosis

with sensitivities and specificities ranging from 86–89% and 84–87% respectively.[19, 20]

Computed Tomography Angiography

CT angiography (CTA) has become a fast, accurate, and noninvasive method of evaluating the intracranial and extracranial vasculature. It can be paired with the CT scan that patients receive in the routine workup of TIA and stroke, and is widely available.[3] Unlike duplex ultrasonography, it can provide an evaluation of the anterior and posterior carotid and cerebral vasculature. The use of CTA involves additional radiation exposure and risk for contrast induced nephropathy.[3] However, when compared to ultrasonography, CTA compared favorably with a reported sensitivity of 76% and specificity of 94% for 70–99% carotid artery stenosis.[19]

Magnetic Resonance Angiography

Magnetic resonance angiography (MRA) and contrast enhanced MRA (CE-MRA) are becoming increasingly available in the evaluation of TIA. Like CTA, it is able to provide visualization of the carotid, posterior, and intracranial vasculature. The added benefit to MRA over CTA is the avoidance of ionizing radiation.[2] The use of MRA is limited by patient tolerance, previously implanted metal devices, length of evaluation, and cost.[3] Various studies have evaluated the performance of MRA compared with gold standard arteriography and other carotid imaging modalities in the evaluation of 70–99% stenosis. Of all the noninvasive modalities evaluated, contrast enhanced MRA had the highest sensitivity and specificity of 94–95% and 90–93%.[19,20] One study reported a sensitivity of 98% and specificity of 100% for complete arterial occlusion.[20] This data suggests that MRA (particularly CE-MRA) is the most effective noninvasive imaging modality in detecting high-grade carotid artery stenosis.

Cardiac Imaging

It is believed that 20–40% of ischemic strokes are from a cardiogenic embolism.[2] Various conditions that predispose to thrombus formation or embolization include atrial fibrillation, ventricular aneurysm, heart failure with reduced ejection fraction, valvular heart disease including endocarditis, regurgitation and stenosis, and persistent foramen ovale (PFO).[3]

Echocardiography is the primary means of evaluation for potential cardiogenic processes. It is able to provide not only a structural evaluation of the heart but a functional evaluation as well. Transthoracic echocardiography (TTE) is generally considered adequate in the initial evaluation of TIA in the ED OU for the detection of intracardiac thrombus.[3,5] ED OU protocol should at minimum include TTE. If concern exists for cardiac thrombus in patients with a normal TTE, a trans-esophageal echo can be obtained. This modality has been shown to be more sensitive for detection of thrombus particularly in the left atrial appendage, aortic arch plaque, PFO or atrial septal aneurysm.[2,3,5]

Prevention of Stroke

Medical Management

Antiplatelet agents are considered the mainstay preventative treatment for atherosclerotic, ischemic cardiovascular disease. They reduce the risk for subsequent myocardial infarction, ischemic stroke, and vascular death.[21] For patients who have experienced a TIA or stroke there are currently four antiplatelet medications that are approved by the FDA. These include aspirin, aspirin/dipyridamole, clopidogrel, or ticlopidine.[1]

Aspirin

Aspirin has long been used in the secondary prevention of stroke after TIA or stroke. This cyclooxygenase (COX1) inhibitor of platelet aggregation has been shown to provide a 15% relative risk reduction for any type of subsequent stroke.[1,21] As with any anticoagulant or antiplatelet agent, there is a risk of major and minor bleeding events while taking aspirin; however this risk is smaller than that of recurrent ischemic stroke.[1] Current guidelines recommend 50–325 mg daily.[1] There is no additional benefit for doses exceeding 325 mg. Higher doses are associated with a greater risk of bleeding complications.[22] Even for patients who experience cerebral ischemic events, increasing the dosage of aspirin is not recommended.[21] Other agents have been found to be as effective or more effective than aspirin. However, aspirin is by far the least expensive of the antiplatelet agents.[1]

Aspirin/Dipyridamole

Dipyridamole is a phosphodiesterase type 5 inhibitor that decreases platelet aggregation and adhesiveness.[1,22] There have been several studies performed looking at the effectiveness of dipyridamole alone and in combination with aspirin or clopidogrel in the secondary prevention of stroke. They found the risk of stroke was reduced more with a combination of aspirin and dipyridamole than with either agent alone.[23,24] Studies indicate that there is no benefit to using dipyridamole alone; however, when used in combination with aspirin there is a significant benefit in preventing subsequent stroke.[2,5,23,24] There was no statistically different rate in major and minor bleeding complications when both medications were used.[23,24] The benefit of the aspirin plus dipyridamole is limited by side effects, particularly headache, with the combination.[23,24] Current guidelines indicate that the combination of aspirin plus extended release dipyridamole is at least as effective in preventing subsequent stroke and is an acceptable alternative to aspirin.[1] Given the side effect profile, it is not necessarily considered the first-line agent.[5]

Clopidogrel

Clopidogrel irreversibly inhibits a major adenosine diphosphate receptor on the platelet surface. It has been used both individually and in combination with aspirin in the prevention of cardiovascular disease.

There have been several major studies comparing the combination of clopidogrel and aspirin with either aspirin alone or clopidogrel alone. Taken in aggregate, studies demonstrate that the combination of aspirin and clopidogrel has not been shown to be superior to either agent alone.[21]

Clopidogrel has been shown to be equally as effective as aspirin and aspirin plus extended release dipyridamole, but has not been shown to be more effective than either option. Current guidelines recommend the use of clopidogrel 75 mg daily as monotherapy as an alternative to aspirin or aspirin plus dipyrimadole, but recommends against the use of clopidogrel plus aspirin.[1]

Ticlopidine

Ticlopidine is thienopyridine similar to clopidogrel. The use of ticlopidine has been limited by the increased rate of side effects, especially skin reactions, neutropenia, and thrombotic thrombocytopenia.[1] Ticlopidine is recommended as a second-line agent for secondary prevention of stroke and has largely been replaced by clopidogrel.[22]

Observation Recommendations

Patients who are being evaluated in the ED OU for non-cardioembolic ischemic stroke and not already taking daily antiplatelet agents should be started on an antiplatelet agent. Options listed in the AHA guidelines include aspirin 50–325 mg daily, clopidogrel 75 mg daily or aspirin/extended release dipyridamole 25/200 mg twice daily. Aspirin is typically the first-line agent given its affordable cost and safety profile. For those who fail aspirin therapy, there is no need to increase the dosage beyond 325 mg daily. Changing to a different agent can be done in consultation with a neurologist.[2]

Anticoagulation

Cardioembolism accounts for approximately 20% of ischemic strokes.[1] Anticoagulation has been shown to be effective in reducing risk of subsequent stroke in patients at risk for cardioembolic disease. Warfarin has been found to provide a 68% relative risk reduction for subsequent stroke in patients with atrial fibrillation. This exceeds the risk of major hemorrhage.[1,2]

For patients with previously diagnosed atrial fibrillation and already on anticoagulation, there is no evidence that changing levels of anticoagulation, if therapeutic (INR 2–3), will provide any additional protection against future TIA or stroke.[1]

For patients with non-cardioembolic ischemic disease there is no benefit to anticoagulation compared to antiplatelet agents. Since there is increased risk of major bleeding for patients being treated with anticoagulation, AHA guidelines recommend antiplatelet agents rather than anticoagulation for patients with non-cardioembolic ischemic stroke or TIA.[1]

Surgical Management

Carotid artery stenosis is a risk factor for cerebral ischemic symptoms. Traditionally, stenosis has been divided into < 30%, 30–49%, 50–69%, 70–99% and total occlusion where 50–69% is considered moderate stenosis and 70–99% is considered high-grade stenosis.[2,25] Symptomatic carotid artery stenosis has been shown to benefit from revascularization procedures. Traditionally CEA has been that procedure of choice. Recently carotid angioplasty and stenting have become alternatives to CEA with similar success rates.[1] The exact procedure to be performed is best determined in consultation with vascular surgery. A 2011 Cochrane review found that there was no benefit for surgical intervention over medical management for patients with carotid artery stenosis < 50%.[1,25]

One study found that patients with high-grade stenosis had a 30% reduction in their 5-year stroke risk if they had surgery within 2 weeks of their TIA.[2] The AHA guidelines recommend CEA within 2 weeks for patients who have no contra-indications to carotid revascularization.[1] Patients found to have moderate or high-grade carotid artery stenosis during workup in the ED observation setting benefit from urgent carotid revascularization procedures.

Risk Factor Modification

Hypertension

Hypertension is a risk factor for TIA and stroke. A decrease in blood pressure is associated with a lower incidence of recurrent stroke. AHA guidelines recommend an average 10/5 mmHg decrease in blood pressure.[1]

In addition to lifestyle modification (low salt diet, weight loss, exercise), diuretics with or without angiotensin converting enzyme (ACE) inhibition provide benefit.[1] There is little evidence for the utility of blood pressure management in the acute phase. Unless a patient is experiencing a hypertensive emergency, the optimization of blood pressure may be accomplished as an outpatient.[1] However if patients are in need of blood pressure control, a diuretic and ACE inhibitor can be started prior to discharge from the OU.

Diabetes

Diabetes mellitus is a risk factor for TIA and stroke. Several studies have been done comparing standard glycemic control (A1C ≤ 7–7.9%) to intensive glycemic control (A1C ≤ 6–6.5%) and have not shown benefit in reducing recurrent stroke. The AHA guidelines recommend standard glycemic control.[1]

Hyperlipidemia

Cholesterol lowering has been shown to provide benefit in long-term risk mitigation for patients who experience a TIA.[2] The AHA guidelines recommend statin therapy with a goal LDL reduction of at least 50% or absolute level < 70 mg/dL for patients who experience ischemic stroke or TIA and have evidence of atherosclerosis, LDL ≥100 mg/dL, and no coronary heart disease (CHD).[1] LDL goals should be based on the National Cholesterol Education Program (NCEP) goal of LDL < 100 mg/dL. Statin therapy may be initiated upon discharge from the ED OU.[2]

Additional Risk Factors

Other risk factors for stroke include tobacco smoking, significant alcohol consumption, obesity, and physical inactivity. The AHA guidelines recommend counseling for smoking cessation, reducing consumption of alcohol, weight loss, and 30 minutes of moderate intensity physical activity as ways of preventing stroke.[1] Patient education either verbally or video during the observation stay or written on discharge instructions may help encourage compliance.[2]

Disposition

Admission to the OU is predicated on the basis that patients will be discharged within 24 hours.[14]

Consultation

During admission to the ED OU, all patients should be evaluated by the neurology consult service. Additionally, patients found to have reversible causes of TIA and stroke (i.e., carotid artery stenosis) should be seen by the appropriate service to expedite further care.

Admission

Approximately 15% of patients will be found to have high-risk factors discovered that will require inpatient admission.[16] Factors that require inpatient admission include recurrent neurologic symptoms, evidence of acute ischemia on imaging, evidence of thromboembolism requiring anticoagulation, evidence of carotid stenosis requiring urgent revascularization or recommendation of the neurologist.[16]

Discharge

Upon presentation to the ED, patients have a 5% risk (9.9% using a different methodology) of stroke in 48 hours and 7% risk in 7 days.[8] Physicians will undoubtedly have varying levels of risk tolerance, but it is fairly universally held that patients who can be classified as having < 1% risk

Table 34.6 Risk Factor Modification[1]

Antiplatelet Agent	*If patients are not already on an agent, one should be started prior to discharge* – *Aspirin (recommended first line)* – *Additional options* • *Aspirin/dipyridamole* • *Clopidogrel* • *Ticlopidine (reserved for intolerance of other agents)* – *Changing agents based on failure of one agent can be done at the recommendation of neurology*
Hypertension	*Consider starting blood pressure control if BP > 140/90 mmHg* – *Encourage lifestyle modification* – *First-line therapy: Diuretic* – *Additional Coverage: Diuretic + ACEI (angiotensin-converting enzyme inhibitor)* – *Goal: reduction of 10/5 mmHg*
Glycemic Control	Manage diabetes according to existing guidelines – Lifestyle modification – Oral agents – Insulin
Hyperlipidemia	Consider starting statins if LDL≥100 mg/dL – Target 50% decrease LDL-C or – LDL-C < 70 mg/dL
Smoking	Patients should be counseled in smoking cessation
Lifestyle Modifications	Patients should be counseled about lifestyle modification – 30 minutes of moderate-intensity physical activity daily – weight loss

of adverse events are safe for discharge and follow-up for further outpatient management.[8] For patients who are found to have an unremarkable evaluation in the ED OU the risk of stroke was found to be 0.96% at 2 days and 1.2% at 7 days.[14]

For those who have undergone DW-MRI and found to have no evidence of ischemia, stroke risk is < 1%.[18] Patients who complete the observation protocol for TIA who have no recurrent deficits, a negative workup and normal serial exams can be discharged after neurology consultation. If patients are not already on an antiplatelet agent prior to admission, they should be started on an appropriate agent.[1] For a summary of the discharge management see Table 34.6.

Follow-Up

Patients discharged from the ED OU are still in need of urgent follow-up for long-term risk factor modification as the ongoing risk of stroke beyond the acute phase is related to vascular risk factors.[15] Patients with carotid artery stenosis not requiring immediate admission should be given urgent follow-up with vascular surgery. When discharged, patients should be given appropriate return instructions that include warning symptoms for recurrent ischemic symptoms.

Summary

The evaluation and management of TIA in the ED observation setting is primarily concerned with mitigation of future stroke risk as disability from stroke places a major burden on patients, families, and the health care system. In the ED, patients should be evaluated for TIA mimics and factors that require immediate inpatient admission. The workup prior to ED OU admission should at minimum consist of glucose check, electrocardiogram (EKG), head CT, and a basic laboratory assessment. Patients on discharge should be started on an appropriate antiplatelet or anticoagulation therapy and be educated about risk factor mitigation.

Cerebral ischemia is a time-sensitive disease. Emergency physicians will play an increasing role in TIA care and prevention of disability from subsequent stroke.

References

1. Furie KL, Kasner SE, Adams RJ, et al. Guidelines for the prevention of stroke in patients with stroke or transient ischemic attack. *Stroke*. 2011; 42:227–276.

2. Edlow JA, Metz H. Transient ischemic attack. *Emergency Medicine Practice*. 2008;10(10).

3. Ross M, Nahab F. Management of transient ischemic attacks in the twenty-first century. *Emerg Med Clin N Am*. 2009;27:51–69.

4. Kleindorfer D, Panagos P, Pancioli A, et al. Incidence and short-term prognosis of transient ischemic attack in a population-based study. *Stroke*. 2005;36:720–723.

5. Shah KH, Edlow JA. Transient ischemic attack: Review for the emergency physician. *Ann Em Med*. 2004;43:592–604.

6. Albers GW, Caplan LR, Easton JD. Transient ischemic attack – proposal for a new definition. *N Engl J Med* 2002;347: 1713–1716.

7. Chandratheva A, Mehta Z, Geraghty OC, et al. Population-based study of risk and predictors in the first few hours after TIA. *Neurology*. 2009;72:1941–1947.

8. Shah KH, Kleckner K, Edlow JA. Short-term prognosis of stroke among patients diagnosed in the emergency department with transient ischemic attack. *Ann of Emerg Med*. 2008;52:316–323.

9. Wu CM, McLaughlin K, Lorenzetti DL, et al. Early risk of stroke after transient ischemic attack: a systematic review and meta-analysis. 2007;167:2417–2422.

10. Shah KH, Metz HA, Edlow JA. Clinical Prediction Rules to stratify short-term risk of stroke among patients diagnosed in the emergency department with a transient ischemic attack. *Ann of Emerg Med*. 2009;53:662–673.

11. Giles MF, Rothwell PM. Risk of stroke after transient ischemic attack: a systematic review and meta-analysis. *Lancet Neurol*. 2007;6:1063–1072.

12. Brown MD, Reeves MJ, Glynn T, et al. Implementation of an emergency department-based transient ischemic attack clinical pathway: a pilot study in knowledge translation. *Acad Emerg Med*. 2007; 14:1114–1119.

13. Joshi JK, Ouyang B, Prabhakaran S. Should TIA patients be hospitalized or referred to a same day clinic? *Neurology*. 2011;77:2082–2088.

14. Stead LG, Bellolio MF, Suravaram S, et al. Evaluation of transient ischemic attack in an emergency department observation unit. *Neurocrit Care*. 2009; 10:204–208.

15. Giles MF, Rothwell PM. Systematic review and pooled analysis of published and unpublished validations of ABCD and ABCD2 transient ischemic attack risk scores. *Stroke*. 2010;41:667–673.

16. Ross MA, Compton S, Madado P, et al. An emergency

department diagnostic protocol for patients with transient ischemic attack: a randomized controlled trial. *Ann of Emerg Med.* 2007;50:109–119.

17. Rothwell PM, Giles MF, Chandralheva A, et al. Effect of urgent treatment of trainsient ischemic attack and minor stroke on early recurrent stroke (EXPRESS study): a prospective population-based sequential comparison. *Lancet.* 2007; 370:1432–1442.

18. Oostema JA, Brown MD, DeLano M, et al. Does diffusion-weighted imaging predict short-term risk of stroke in emergency department patients with transient ischemic attack? *Ann of Emerg Med.* 2013; 61: 62–71.

19. Wardlaw JM, Chappell FM, Best JJK, et al. Non-invasive imaging compared with intra-arterial angiography in the diagnosis of symptomatic carotid stenosis: a metaanalysis. *Lancet.* 2006; 367:1503–1512.

20. Nederkoorn PJ, Van der Graaf Y, Hunink M. Duplex ultrasonography and magnetic resonance angiography compared with digital subtraction angiography in carotid artery stenosis: a systematic review. *Stroke.* 2003;34:1324–1331.

21. Callison RC, Adams HP. Use of antiplatelet agents for prevention of ischemic stroke. *Neurol Clin.* 2008; 26:1047–1077.

22. Kral M, Herzig R, Sanal D, et al. Oral antiplatelet therapy in stroke prevention: minireview. *Biomed Pap Med Fac Univ Palacky Olomouc Czezh Repub.* 2010; 154:203–210.

23. Diener HC, Cunha L, Forbes C, et al. European Stroke Prevention Study. 2. Dipyridamole and acetylsalicylic acid in the secondary prevention of stroke. *J Neurol Sci.* 1996;143:1–13.

24. ESPRIT Study Group. Aspirin plus dipyridamole versus aspirin alone after cerebral ischemia of arterial origin (ESPRIT): randomized controlled trial. *Lancet.* 2006;367:1665–73.

25. Rerkasem K, Rothwell PM. Carotid endarterectomy for symptomatic carotid stenosis. *Cochrane Database for Systematic Reviews.* 2011;4:CD001081.

Chapter 35

Headaches

Sharon E. Mace, MD, FACEP, FAAP

Introduction

Headaches are extremely common. During a given year, nine out of ten people (90%) suffer from headaches.[1] Headache is the chief complaint in 1–4% of emergency department (ED) patients,[2–4] which accounts for approximately 5 million ED visits each year.[4,5] More than 45 million Americans suffer from chronic, recurring headaches.[6] Of the two most common headaches,[7] tension headaches have an annual prevalence of 11% with 78% of adults suffering from a tension headache at some point in time,[2] while migraine headaches affect 18% of American women and 7% of American men with an estimated 28 million individuals with migraines in the United States.[8] One-third of the US population will suffer from a migraine headache in their lifetime.[8] Approximately 70% of all headache sufferers are women.[6]

Headaches are the most common neurologic disorder, followed by stroke, Alzheimer's disease and seizures.[9,10] Headache is the ninth most common cause of physician visits.[8] Headache is the most frequent complaint in children and adolescents.[11] About 20% of the pediatric population has a significant headache.[6] Headaches are the number one reason for absenteeism from work and school. Migraine sufferers alone miss more than 157 million work and school days every year because of headaches.[6]

Headache, or cephalgia, is defined as a pain anywhere in the region of the head or neck. There are a multitude of conditions that can lead to a headache. Most of the causes of headache are benign and self-limited; although the pathology responsible for some headaches, such as meningitis, subarachnoid hemorrhage (SAH) or increased intracranial pressure from a tumor or other causes, can lead to major complications and even death if undiagnosed and untreated. It is estimated that 3.8% of ED patients with a headache have a serious or life-threatening etiology for their headache,[4] although an older study noted 17% of patients had significant lesions.[3]

The key is to differentiate the benign headache from the headache due to a significant or serious pathology, which can be quite difficult,[2,3] as evidenced by studies of SAH as an example.[12,13] Of patients with SAH, 23% were not diagnosed on their initial presentation to the ED.[12] In another study of SAH, one-third of patients died before reaching the ED and another 25% of patients died after having seen a physician for their headache.[13]

The purpose of an observation stay is to identify those with a life-threatening etiology for their headache, while concurrently managing the patient's headache pain and, if possible, begin specific treatment for the underlying etiology of the headache.[3,14]

Primary and Secondary Headaches

Headaches are categorized into primary and secondary headaches.[4] Primary headaches account for more than 90% of all headaches. Tension headaches and migraines are the most common primary headaches, while the other primary headaches, cluster headaches and trigeminal autonomic neuralgias, are much less common.

Secondary headaches are caused by an underlying condition or disease, which range from headaches due to any injury or painful condition of the head, neck or facial structures including the temporomandibular joints (TMJ), jaws, teeth, ears/nose/throat (ENT) structures (e.g., sinuses. ears, nasopharynx), head or neck musculature, to major intracranial disease or injury such as an intracranial bleed, malignancy, increased intracranial pressure, inflammatory disease (central nervous system [CNS] sarcoid, Behcet's disease, as examples) or infection (e.g., meningitis, encephalitis).

Secondary headaches also include headaches due to medications (from use, ingestion, or

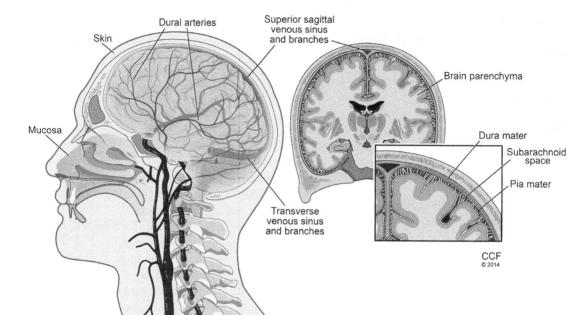

Figure 35.1 Structures Capable of Producing Pain and Non-pain Producing Structures
courtesy of Dr. Sharon E. Mace, Mr. Dave Schumick and the Medical Art and Photography Department at the Cleveland Clinic, Cleveland, Ohio.

withdrawal of prescribed or over the counter medications or drugs of abuse) or toxins (e.g., heavy metal poisoning, carbon monoxide), metabolic/endocrine causes (e.g., hypertension, dialysis, hypothyroidism, fasting, hypo/hyperglycemia) and resulting from psychiatric disorders.

Classifications of Headache

The most recent classification of headaches by the International Headache Society is the International Classification of Headache Disorders-3 (ICHD-3), published in 2013, which uses numeric codes.[7] Primary headaches are part 1 (groups 1–4). Secondary headaches are part 2 (groups 5–12). Part 3 (groups 13–14) includes the cranial neuralgias, and central and primary facial pain. The primary headaches are migraines, tension-type, cluster and trigeminal autonomic cephalgias.

The National Institute of Neurological Disorders and Stroke (NINDS) of the National Institute of Health (NIH) classification of headaches designates four categories of headaches: vascular, muscle contraction (tension), traction and inflammatory.[15]

Pathophysiology of Headaches

There are only a few structures in the cranium that are capable of generating painful stimuli including the dura at the base of the skull (basal dura), vessels (major arteries at the base of the brain, dural arteries, venous sinuses and their branches, extracranial blood vessels) and extracranial structures (skin, mucosa, muscles, fascial planes, blood vessels, nerves). Structures incapable of producing pain are the brain parenchyma, subarachnoid, pia mater and most of the dura.[2] (Figure 35.1)

Pathophysiologic mechanisms responsible for headache pain effect are (1) intra- or extra-cranial arteries undergoing distention, traction, or dilatation; (2) dura or large intracranial veins undergoing traction or displacement, (3) cranial or spinal nerves undergoing compression, traction or inflammation; (4) head and neck undergoing muscle spasm, inflammation or traction; (5) meningeal irritation; (6) increased intracranial pressure; and (7) disturbance of intracerebral serotonergic projections[2,16] Tension, presumed to be the key factor causing tension headaches, pertains to the muscle contraction of the head and/or neck. Traction results from the stretching of intracranial structures from a mass effect – as caused by a hematoma, tumor, abscess or other intracranial mass – and is typically a constant pain of variable severity. Inflammation arising from the basal dura, the head/neck soft tissues or the nerves is the pathologic process accounting for the pain from sinusitis, mastoiditis, meningitis (initial pain), and SAH (initial pain). Dilatation or distention of vessels has been suggested as the pathophysiologic mechanism behind vascular headache pain, which characteristically causes a throbbing pain, and is presumed responsible for the headache from severe hypertension and migraines,[2] although more recent data suggests other additional mechanisms. Moreover, any given headache may involve one or any permutation of these various mechanisms.

Pathophysiology of Migraines

Theories on the Pathogenesis of Migraine Headaches

The vascular or vasogenic theory, an early hypothesis, ascribed the aura of the migraine to intracranial vasoconstriction, followed by rebound dilatation of the blood vessels, which activates the perivascular nociceptive neurons and causes the headache.[17] More recently, the central neural or neurovascular hypothesis is that neural dysfunction occurs first and is followed by the vascular changes. Neural events triggered by various stimuli occurring in a genetically susceptible individual precipitate a migraine.[18]

Cortical Spreading Depression

The aberrant firing of neurons with ionic changes and the release of neurotransmitters cause abnormal activation of the trigeminal/cervical afferents. This likely involves the phenomenon of cortical spreading depression, a short-lasting depolarization wave that moves across the cerebral cortex with a brief excitation phase followed by prolonged depression of the nerve cells that occurs concurrently with a failure of brain ion homeostasis and release of neurotransmitters and metabolites from the neurons.[2]

Increased interstitial potassium and increased glutamate levels with activation of the NMDA receptor leading to an influx of calcium ions and triggering nitrogen oxide synthetase (NOS) activity is believed to precipitate the abnormal neuronal excitability that results in the cortical spreading depression with depressed electrical activity extending to adjacent areas of the cerebral cortex.[19] Both sodium and calcium enter the cells, while potassium and hydrogen ions enter the extracellular space. (Figure 35.2) The initial increasing interstitial potassium decreases the

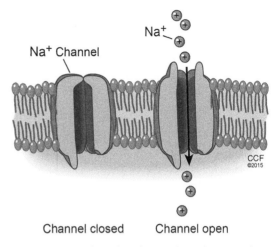

Figure 35.2 Ion channels in the neural membrane may be involved. Blocking sodium channels, for example, inhibits nerve impulse propagation
courtesy of Dr. Sharon E. Mace, Mr. Dave Schumick and the Medical Art and Photography Department at the Cleveland Clinic, Cleveland, Ohio.

resting membrane potential and could eliminate the voltage-sensitive Mg2+ block of the NMDA receptor, thus, sensitizing it to glutamate.[19]

Cortical spreading depression, thought to be the basis for the aura of migraine headaches, may lead to activation of the trigeminal nerve afferents (trigeminal nocioception) and changes the permeability of the blood-brain barrier via up-regulation and activation of matrix metalloproteinases (MMPs).[16]

Anatomy

The hallmark of migraines is the activation of the trigeminocervical pain system. Migraine pain is mediated by the trigeminal nerve (cranial nerve V), especially the ophthalmic (V1) branch, and by the upper cervical spinal cord levels (C1 and C2) via the greater occipital nerve.[20] (Figure 35.3)

Activation of the sensory afferents from the trigeminal nerve and the upper cervical spinal cord roots that innervate the dura and facial structures occurs. This input is sent via the trigeminal ganglion to the trigeminocervical complex (TCC) in the dorsal horn of the spinal cord. The first-order sensory afferents of the trigeminal nerve and the upper cervical spinal nerves synapse on second-order neurons within the TCC in the spinal cord, then these second-order neurons ascend to the third-order neurons within the thalamus and other nuclei. (Figure 35.4)

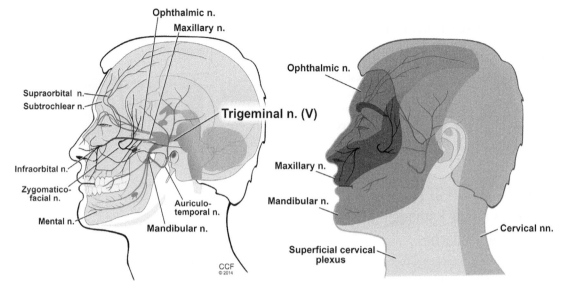

Figure 35.3 Trigeminal Nerve (Cranial Nerve V)
courtesy of Dr. Sharon E. Mace, Mr. Dave Schumick and the Medical Art and Photography Department at the Cleveland Clinic, Cleveland, Ohio.

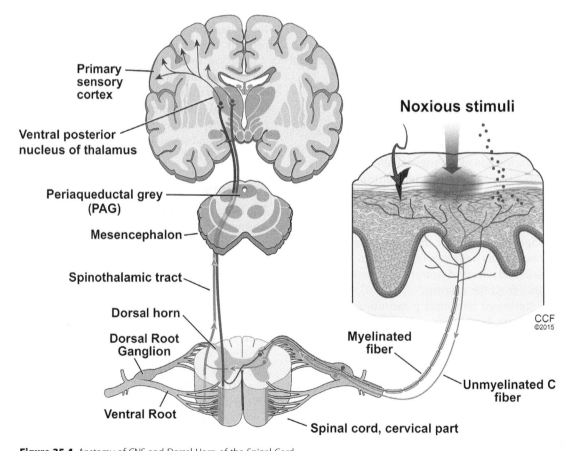

Figure 35.4 Anatomy of CNS and Dorsal Horn of the Spinal Cord
courtesy of Dr. Sharon E. Mace, Mr. Dave Schumick and the Medical Art and Photography Department at the Cleveland Clinic, Cleveland, Ohio.

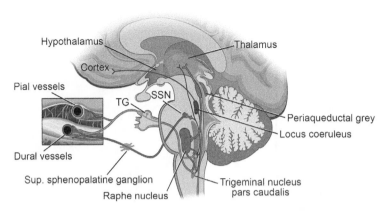

Figure 35.5 Anatomy of CNS and Trigeminocervical Complex courtesy of Dr. Sharon E. Mace, Mr. Dave Schumick and the Medical Art and Photography Department at the Cleveland Clinic, Cleveland, Ohio.

The TCC serves as the critical relay center for the transmission of nociceptive input to the higher cortical centers where pain is perceived. The TCC extends from the trigeminal nucleus caudalis in the rostral pons to the upper cervical spinal cord levels (C1 and C2). The trigeminothalamic tract consists of second-order neurons from the TCC projecting to the thalamus. The ventral posteromedial thalamic nucleus (VPM) is the key thalamic relay sending nociceptive information to the cortical pain matrix. Transmission from the spinal cord goes to the thalamus, at the upper end of the brainstem, via the spinothalamic tract, and from the spinal cord to the sensory cortex via the spinoreticular tract. (Figure 35.4 and Figure 35.5)

The CNS can alter or even abolish pain. Both inhibitory and facilitatory mechanisms can occur with upward and downward modulation.[21] Modulation of this nociceptive information occurs by projections from the periaqueductal grey (PAG), dorsal raphe nucleus (DRG), nucleus raphe magnus (NRM), locus coeruleus (LC) and the hypothalamus. Indeed, lesions in the periaqueductal grey (PAG) or the diencephalic nuclei in the rostral brainstem can precipitate a migraine headache. Multiple other second-order neurons from the TCC project to various subcortical sites suggesting that this nociceptive information is transmitted to other regions of the brain.[20] (Figure 35.4 and Figure 35.5)

Cellular and Biochemical Basis

It has been proposed that a sterile neurogenically initiated inflammation of the dura mater, characterized by vasodilatation and plasma protein extravasation, could be the cause of migraine pain. (Figure 35.6) Neurogenic plasma extravasation does occur with electrical stimulation of the trigeminal ganglion and can be blocked by various drugs, such as sumatriptan, the ergot alkaloids and indomethacin.[19] Structural alterations in the dura occur after stimulation of the trigeminal ganglion including mast cell degranulation and platelet aggregation in postcapillary venules.[22]

Neurons contain a variety of neuropeptides and neurotransmitters. Calcitonin gene-related peptide (CGRP), substance P and neurokinin A are among the substances released when trigeminal neurons are stimulated.[18,21] Release of these neuropeptides has been linked with sterile neurogenic induced inflammation. (Figure 35.6) Elevated levels of CGRP have been found in migraine patients and a CGRP antagonist has been mentioned as a treatment for migraines.[18] Nitric oxide (NO) has been shown to trigger headaches and blockade of NO synthetase (NOS) has been suggested as an abortive treatment for migraine headaches.[21] Drugs that affect the various ion channels, thereby, blocking neuronal transmission may be effective in treating headache pain.

Nociceptive fibers consist of A-δ fiber neurons and C-fiber neurons. A-δ fibers conduct sharp pain, while C-fiber neurons take longer to respond and are responsible for the dull, aching or throbbing pain.[21,22] Sodium channels are responsible for the neural transmission of most alpha-beta fibers. Sodium channel blockers, for example, the tricyclic antidepressants, are used to treat pain. Calcium channels regulate C-fiber and spinal cord neural transmission. Calcium

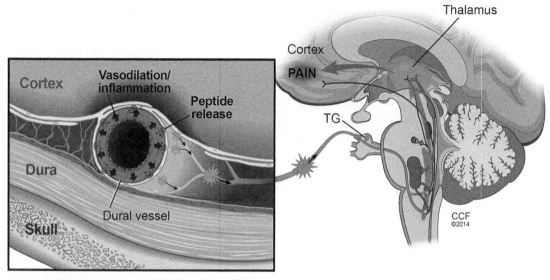

Figure 35.6 Migraine Pathophysiology with Sterile Inflammation, Vasodilatation and Release of Various Substances
courtesy of Dr. Sharon E. Mace, Mr. Dave Schumick and the Medical Art and Photography Department at the Cleveland Clinic, Cleveland, Ohio.

channel blockers, for example, gabapentin, may be used for pain therapy.[21]

Sensitization

Sensitization is the painful perception of an otherwise non-noxious stimuli. Multiple changes are present when sensitization occurs including a decreased response threshold, an increased size or magnitude of response, an expansion of receptive fields, and the development of spontaneous neural activity.[23] Migraine symptoms attributed to sensitization include the throbbing quality of the pain; the worsening of the pain with bending, coughing, or sudden movements of the head; hyperalgesia and allodynia. Hyperalgesia is the increased sensitivity to painful stimuli, while allodynia refers to the condition in which pain is produced by stimuli that are normally not painful or not noxious. Sensitization may be peripheral or central.

Peripheral sensitization refers to the increased excitability of primary afferent neurons to stimulation (usually mechanical). There is the release of proinflammatory vasoactive substances from the peripheral neurons. These proinflammatory substances – such as substance P, neurokinin A, nitric oxide (NO) and CGRP – interact with the blood vessel wall to cause vasodilatation, protein extravasation and sterile inflammation with mast cell activation and membrane disruption.[21]

Stimulation of the trigeminal ganglion leads to release of CGRP, a substance found in increased amounts in patients with acute migraines. Second-order neurons are then barraged with an increased number of stronger impulses form the primary afferent neurons. Peripheral sensitization may involve changes in ion channels, release of neuropeptides and neurotransmitters, and increased peripheral nociceptor receptivity.[22,23]

Central sensitization refers to the increased sensitivity or responsiveness of second order neurons in the TCC and higher order neurons in the CNS to mild stimuli that previously did not activate them. This may occur by increased sensitivity of higher order neurons or via disinhibition of descending modulatory pathways. There is evidence that windup or sensitization is present with migraines and that therapy may affect this hypersensitivity as with the ß adrenergic antagonists or beta blockers, propanolol and atenolol, which inhibit the firing of third-order thalmocortical neurons to dural stimulation and to glutamate injection.[17,21] Central sensitization may be related to abnormal neuronal activity in specific aminergic brainstem nuclei with prostaglandin and proinflammatory cytokines (such as interleukins [IL] and tumor necrosis factor [TNF] and cyclooxygenase enzymes) initiating and maintaining the central stimulation or a form of disinhibitory sensitization with dysfunction of descending modulatory pathways.[2,17, 22–25]

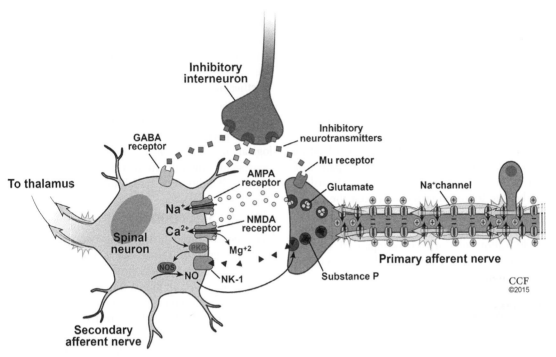

Figure 35.7 Neurotransmitters, neuropeptides, ions and receptors involved in the response to pain
courtesy of Dr. Sharon E. Mace, Mr. Dave Schumick and the Medical Art and Photography Department at the Cleveland Clinic, Cleveland, Ohio.

Pathophysiology of Pain

Periphery

When nociceptive nerve fibers in the periphery (with migraines: the trigeminal nerve, C1 and/or C2) are stimulated, local tissue damage occurs, which includes the release of chemical mediators (histamine, bradykinan, and prostaglandins) and activation of mast cells, which produces an "inflammatory soup."[21] This causes capillary leakage with plasma protein extravasation, platelet aggregation and the release of serotonin. Mast cell leukotrienes produce superoxides, which stimulate additional inflammatory cells. This inflammatory milieu initiates neuronal activity. In addition to these mediators, the cells release ions (e.g., potassium and hydrogen), cytokines and growth factors. The cations and adenosine triphosphate (ATP) are direct stimulants of the nerve. These substances (e.g., bradykinin, prostaglandin E_2, nerve growth factor) sensitize the neuron so that lower levels of input, previously subthreshold, now cause activation of the peripheral neuron with the result being peripheral sensitization. Activation of the nociceptive fibers releases neuropeptides (e.g., CGRP) that foster additional vasodilatation,

edema, and inflammation (see also pathohysiology section in seizure chapter on ion channels and on action potentials).[21–25] (Figure 35.6)

Spinal Cord and Dorsal Root Ganglion

When depolarization and conduction along the pain fibers occurs, excitatory amino acids (e.g., glutamate and aspartate) and neuropeptides (e.g., substance P) are released at the synaptic junction in the dorsal root ganglion (DRG). When the action potential reaches the DRG, glutamate (an excitatory neurotransmitter) and substance P (a neuropeptide) are released. Glutamate stimulates the AMPA receptors. Activation of the N-methyl-D-aspartate (NMDA) receptor occurs via removal of the magnesium from the NMDA receptor by glutamate and substance P. Intracellular calcium release occurs as a result of NMDA activation, which in turn, stimulates nitric oxide (NO) and protein kinase C. The inhibitory neurotransmitters, gamma-aminobutyric acid (GABA) and glycine, block the excitatory neurotransmitters, glutamate and AMPA. NMDA antagonists, such as ketamine, may decrease the pain response by blocking the NMDA receptor. NMDA receptors are widespread throughout the CNS. (Figure 35.7)

Central Nervous System

Facilitation of pain sensation is induced by glutamate, serotonin and norepinephrine; inhibition of pain occurs with GABA, glycine, and endorphins. There are mu receptors throughout the CNS: in the cortex, thalamus, spinal cord, and in the DRG. Mu receptors are generally quiescent until stimulated by painful input.[21] It may be that these mu receptors are involved in headache pain. The maladaptive pain of migraine and other primary headache disorders may be due to an imbalance between the facilitory and inhibitory systems, whereby the facilitory system dominates the inhibitory system, thereby, allowing normally nonpainful stimuli from the trigeminal nerve, C1 and/or C2 to cause pain.[21] (Figure 35.5)

Other Research

Decreased GABA levels in the brain may be a factor in the neuronal hyperexcitability or lack of inhibitory control.[24] Increased levels of CGRP, a potent vasodilator released from trigeminal ganglia neurons, are found in migrainers and are normalized when sumatriptan is administered, which may be a mechanism of action of this drug.

The tricyclic antidepressants, which block serotonin (5-hydroxytryptamine or 5-HT) reuptake, are efficacious prophylactic drugs for migraines. Serotonin is released from brainstem serotonergic nuclei. This suggests that serotonin may be involved.[21] Possible mechanisms include low serotonin levels causing a lessening of the serotonin descending pain inhibitory system, an effect on cranial vessels or on central pain pathways or by an effect on the brainstem nuclei.

Nitric oxide as a proinflammatory mediator could lead to sensitization. cGMP, a second messenger of NO, is increased in the platelets of migrainers.[24] Abnormal iron homeostasis with increased iron deposits in the PAG has been found in migrainers and those with chronic daily headaches.[24] Investigations into the genetics of migraine headaches suggests that some migraine headaches, or at least the aura, may be secondary to a channelopathy with a mutation in a voltage gated calcium channel causing an abnormal electrochemical gradient for Na+ with a build-up of the excitatory transmitter glutamate or a mutation in the sodium channel gene.[18] (Figure 35.2)

Pathophysiology Summary

Some of the possible pathophysiologic mechanisms responsible for migraine headaches are the activation of the trigeminovascular system, whether by cortical spreading depression or other mechanisms; brain stem (particularly, thalamus) activation, windup or sensitization (whether central or peripheral, or both); the electrophysiological and ion changes in the brain; and the neurogenic inflammation leading to neuronal hyperexcitability or a dyshabituation.

Patient Selection

Patients who need further diagnostic evaluation with the goal of ruling out a serious or life-threatening basis for their headache are appropriate candidates for an observation stay. Individuals who need additional pain management of their headache can be successfully treated in an observation unit (OU). Since most headache patients have tried oral and/or subcutaneous medications prior to their arrival in the ED, parenteral medications are generally warranted.[2] Additionally, if the headache diagnosis is known, the specific drugs or therapy of choice may be administered, such as oxygen for cluster headaches.

Patients inappropriate for an observation stay include those with a serious or dangerous cause of their headache. Thus, patient exclusion criteria include: increased intracranial pressure from any cause (tumor, hydrocephalus, etc.), intracranial bleed (e.g., subdural hematoma, epidural hematoma, intracerebral bleed, subarachnoid hemorrhage), acute/subacute stroke and acute CNS infection (e.g., acute encephalitis, brain abscess, epidural abscess). Bacterial meningitis is not appropriate for an OU. However, some observation protocols might allow inclusion of a patient with an uncomplicated viral meningitis patient, who has no acute focal neurologic deficits, a normal mental status and stable vital signs.

Exclusion criteria include an abnormal CT scan with a lesion needing immediate surgical intervention, hypertensive crisis (although hypertensive urgency is acceptable for observation) and patients with characteristics of high-risk headaches. Attributes of a high-risk headache include an acute alteration in mental status, co-existing seizures and headache (in a patient without a history of epilepsy), nuchal rigidity, acute visual loss (may be acute glaucoma or a stroke), new focal neurologic deficit, abnormal pupils (unequal [if not congenital] and/or sluggishly reactive), apnea or abnormal respiratory pattern, significantly abnormal vital signs (bradycardia and hypertension suggestive of Cushing's reflex), and other significant comorbidity, such as AIDS.

Patients with unstable vital signs, an altered mental status or acute psychiatric issues also should not be placed into observation. Patients unlikely to improve and be ready for discharge within < 24 hours should be considered for inpatient admission.

Observation Unit Management

The history is the most critical part of the assessment of a patient with a headache. Important data to obtain include the onset (acute "thunderclap" or gradual), duration, location, type or quality (dull throbbing, sharp lancinating, band-like, etc.) of the pain; precipitating and/or relieving factors; headache pattern; associated symptoms (nausea, vomiting, cough, myalgias, rashes, fever, chills, altered mental status, photophobia) and any history of trauma. Medications (whether prescribed, over-the-counter or illicit) and the pattern of use (initiation, discontinuation/withdrawal, tapering) should be noted since drug-related headaches are common. Allergies should be asked in view of medications for treatment and possible allergic reactions. Social history should include drug, alcohol and tobacco use, and diet (caffeine use, fasting).

Features of the physical examination that should be assessed are: vital signs; mental status; neurologic examination; head/neck/ENT examination including whether a supple or stiff neck; presence of tenderness over the temporal artery, sinuses, mastoid or temporomandibular joint; the skin for rashes or petechiae; the lungs, cardiovascular and abdominal examination.

Laboratory and radiologic studies depend on the results of the focused history and physical examination. If temporal arteritis is suspected, an erythrocyte sedimentation rate (ESR) should be drawn. A complete blood count may be useful if infection is a possibility. In women of childbearing age, a pregnancy test is generally indicated, and may be useful when deciding on drug therapy. Moreover, the differential of headache in the pregnant and peripartum woman includes additional unusual etiologies including pre-eclampsia/eclampsia and cavernous sinus thrombosis. A lumbar puncture (LP) may be diagnostic if SAH, meningitis or pseudotumor cerebri is present. Cerebrospinal fluid (CSF) analysis is warranted in order to diagnosis meningitis and perhaps, SAH. Radiology studies are based on the history and physical examination and may include CT scan, CT angiography, ultrasound and MRI/MRA.

Specific Therapy

Specific treatment for the underlying cause may begin in the OU. For hypertensive urgency, control of the blood pressure should lessen or even eliminate the headache. Steroids, specifically oral prednisone, along with scheduling a temporal artery biopsy are the treatment of choice for temporal arteritis. A LP is both diagnostic and therapeutic with removal of cerebrospinal fluid (CSF) for pseudo tumor cerebri. Intravenous (IV) caffeine and, sometimes, a blood patch are the suggested therapy for a spinal headache. Headache secondary to ophthalmologic disorders, such as acute angle glaucoma or iritis, need appropriate urgent treatment. Headache due to a non-life-threatening infection should improve with treatment of the underlying infection. The most common cause of headaches is reported to be systemic infection.[3] According to one study, systemic infection was the etiology of headache in up to 40% of patients presenting to the ED.[25] For trigeminal neuralgia, carbamazepine is the drug of choice. Oxygen is effective in about 70% of patients with a cluster headache. One medication, meperidine, should probably be avoided since it is less effective with a higher incidence of side effects than other drugs.[2] A decision on the need for preventive treatment of migraines and if so, what medications, often in conjunction with the neurologist or primary care physician, can be made while the patient is in the OU.

Pharmacologic Management

Given the myriad etiologies of headache, there is no one panacea or approach. However, several drugs have efficacy for the common primary headaches: tension-type and migraines. Since patients with migraines frequently have nausea and/or vomiting and poor po intake prior to their arrival in the ED, management generally includes IV anti-emetics to treat the nausea/vomiting and

IV rehydration for treatment of dehydration and for maintenance fluids.

Opioids are still used occasionally to treat acute episodic headaches in the ED and apprehension regarding addiction has not proven to be a valid concern in those with an acute headache.[2] However, because of their minimal success rate and the high headache reoccurrence rate, the indications for their use have declined and experts are now recommending that they be used for acute therapy of headaches only when other medications have failed or are contraindicated.[2] Indeed, in conjunction with the headache/neurology specialists, some OU protocols have eliminated opioids as standard therapy in their headache protocols (as we have in our headache treatment protocol for primary headaches). (See Headache, in the clinical protocol Chapter 82.) Similarly, for chronic headache pain, opioids are not warranted because daily opioid use can cause rebound headaches and there is a risk of narcotic abuse in this patient population.[2] (Specific drugs are discussed in the headache protocol in the protocol Chapter 82.)

Summary

Headaches represent the most common neurologic disorder. Headaches are usually benign, but may have a serious, life-threatening etiology. Patients with headaches often seek care in EDs and outpatient facilities. Their management may involve a diagnostic workup to exclude life-threatening disorders and multiple drug therapies. The OU can provide cost-effective care with an opportunity for both evaluation and treatment.

References

1. Mattu A, Goyal D, Barrett JW, et al. In: *Emergency Medicine: Avoiding the Pitfalls and Improving the Outcomes.* Malden, MA: Blackwell Publishers/BMJ Books, 2007; p. 39.

2. Kelly AM. Headache. In: Mace SE, Ducharme J, Murphy MF (eds.) *Pain Management and Sedation: Emergency Department Management.* New York: McGraw-Hill Companies, Inc., 2006; ch. 38, pp. 279–286.

3. Graff LG. Headache. In: Graff LG (ed.) *Observation Medicine.* Boston: Andover Medical Publishers, Inc., 1993; ch. 16, pp. 193–202.

4. Denny CJ, Schull MJ. Headache/Facial Pain. In: *Tintintalli's Emergency Medicine: a Comprehensive Study Guide.* 7th ed. New York, NY: McGraw-Hill; 2011; ch. 159, pp. 1113–1118.

5. Bournes V, Edlow JA. Migraine: diagnosis and pharmacologic treatment in emergency department. *Eur Rev Med Pharmacol Sci*, 2011; 15: 2156–221.

6. http://clevelandclinic.org/disorders/Headaches/hic_Overview_of_Headaches in_Adults.aspx (last accessed July 27, 2012)

7. Headache Classification Committee of the International Headache Society (2013). The International Classification of Headache Disorders (ICHD). *Cephalgia* 2013 : 33(9):629–808.

8. Headache. In: Henry GL, Jagoda A, Little NE, et al. (eds.) *Neurologic Emergencies a Symptom Oriented Approach.* New York, NY: McGraw-Hill Companies, Inc., 2003; ch. 7, pp. 157–177.

9. www.epilepsyfoundation.org/aboutepilepsy (last accessed August 5, 2012)

10. Hirtz D, Thurman DJ, Gwinn-Hardy K, et al. How common are the "common" neurologic disorders? *Neurology* 2007; 68:326–337.

11. Termine C, Ozge A, Antonaci F, et al. Overview of diagnosis and management of pediatric headache: part II: therapeutic management. *J Headache Pain* 2011; 12: 25–34.

12. Adams HP, Jergenson DD, Kassell NF, et al. Pitfalls in the recognition of subarachnoid hemorrhage. *JAMA*, 1980; 244: 794–796.

13. Kassell NF, Torner JC. Aneursymal rebleed: a preliminary report from the Cooperative Aneurysm. *Neurosurgery*, 1983; 13: 479–481.

14. Mace SE, Tan C. Headache. In: Graff LG (ed.). *Observation Medicine: The Healthcare System's Tincture of Time.* https://webapps.acep.org/WorkArea/DownloadAsset.aspx?id=45885 (last accessed July 27, 2012)

15. www.ninds.nih.gov/disorders/headache/headache.htm

16. Edlow JA, Panagos PD, Godwin SA, et al. Clinical policy: critical issues in the evaluation and management of adult patients presenting to the emergency department with an acute headache. *Ann Emerg Med*, 2008; 52(4): 407–43617.

17. Cutrer FM. Pathophysiology of migraine. *Semin Neurol* 2006; 26:171–180.

18. Goadsby PJ, Oshinsky ML. Pathophysiology of headache. In: Silberstein SD, Lipton RB, Dodick DW (eds.). *Wolff's*

Headache and Other Head Pain. New York: Oxford University Press, 2008; ch. 7, pp. 105–119.

19. Lauritzen M, King RP. Spreading depression. In: Olesen J, Goadsby PJ, Ramadan NM, et al. (eds.). *The Headaches*. Philadelphia: Lippincott Williams & Wilkins, 2006; ch. 28, pp. 269–280.

20. Andreou AP, Summ O, Charbit AR, et al. Animal models of headache: from bedside to bench and back to bedside. *Expert Rev Neurother* 2010; 10(3): 389–411.

21. Ducharme J. Neurobiology of pain. In: Mace SE, Ducharme J, Murphy MF (eds.). *Pain Management and Sedation: Emergency Department Management*. New York: McGraw-Hill Companies, Inc., 2006; ch. 30, pp. 223–227.

22. Goadsby PJ. Pathophysiology of migraine. *Neurol Clin* 2009; 27:335–360.

23. Messlinger K, Strassman AM, Burstein R. Anatomy and physiology of pain-sensitive cranial structures. In: Silberstein SD, Lipton RB, Dodick DW (eds.). *Wolff's*

Headache and Other Head Pain. New York: Oxford University Press, 2008; ch. 6, pp. 95–119.

24. Burstein R, Levy D, Jakubowski M, et al. In: Olesen J, Goadsby PJ, Ramadan NM, et al. (eds.). *The Headaches*. Philadelphia: Lippincott Williams & Wilkins, 2006, ch. 12, pp. 121–129.

25. Dhopesh V, Anwar R, Herring C. A retrospective assessment of emergency department patients with complaint of headache. *Headache* 1979; 19:37–42.

Chapter

Seizures

Sharon E. Mace, MD, FACEP, FAAP

Introduction

Approximately 5–10% of the population will experience at least one non-febrile seizure during their lifetime.[1,2] Seizures account for about 1–2% of all emergency department (ED) visits.[3] Excluding those patients with a known seizure disorder, another 300,000 individuals are diagnosed with a seizure annually, with the diagnosis generally made in the ED.[2,4] Of these, there are 200,000 new cases of seizures and epilepsy annually.[2]

These numbers do not include febrile seizures. Worldwide, febrile seizures are noted in 2–4% of children[5] and are the most common seizure in children < 5 years old, with an approximate incidence of febrile seizures at 75,000–100,000 in the United States.[6]

Excluding headaches/migraines, epilepsy is the third most common neurological disorder in the United States after stroke and Alzheimer's disease,[7] with "a prevalence greater than cerebral palsy, multiple sclerosis and Parkinson's disease combined."[2] Nearly 3 million individuals or 1% of the general population in the United States are diagnosed with epilepsy.[8] Worldwide, epilepsy affects some 50 million individuals.[9]

The number of individuals with epilepsy is expected to increase for several reasons, including the growing geriatric population and the number of returning veterans. This is because there is an increased incidence of epilepsy in the elderly and an increased risk of developing epilepsy in individuals with a traumatic brain injury.[2]

On a yearly basis in the United States, about 28% of all epilepsy patients need treatment in EDs.[10] This is not surprising, considering that up to 30% of patients treated for epilepsy continue to experience seizures ("breakthrough" seizures).[6,11]

Not only are patients with seizures common in the ED, they are "labor-intensive" in that they make considerable demands on EMS and ED resources.[12] In one ED study of patients with seizures, "advanced care, including intravenous access, laboratory work, cardiac monitoring, or oxygen administration" was required in 84% of patients and over half of the patients (55%) were administered antiepileptic drugs (AEDs).[12] Over one-fourth of patients (27%) were admitted to the hospital.[12] The annual costs (direct and indirect) each year in the United States for epilepsy and seizures is $17.6 billion.[12]

One-third of individuals who have had a single unprovoked seizure will go on to develop epilepsy. One-fourth of children with mental retardation, one in eight children with cerebral palsy, and 50% of children with both mental retardation and cerebral palsy will develop epilepsy.[2] In adults, 10% of Alzheimer patients and 22% of stroke patients can be expected to develop epilepsy. Individuals with a family member who has epilepsy are also at an increased risk of developing epilepsy, which suggests a genetic component to the disorder.[2] In children, the estimated risk of developing epilepsy is 8.7% if their mother has epilepsy and 2.4% if their father has epilepsy.[2]

Considering that the observation unit (OU), in general, is a more cost-effective alternative to inpatient care, then placing some of these patients in the OU should result in a shorter length of stay and at a lower cost than inpatient admission,[13] although a future study regarding the OU treatment of seizures is warranted to verify this conclusion.

Definitions

A seizure is the clinical manifestation(s) of an episode of an abnormal, excessive, hypersynchronous electrical discharge of a group of cortical neurons that results in a temporary disruption of brain dysfunction.[14] A seizure is a discrete, time-limited alteration in brain function that may include changes in the level of consciousness, motor activity, sensation, and/or autonomic function. Convulsions refer to a specific type of seizure with involuntary muscular contractions as its fundamental manifestation.

Seizures are classified into primary or secondary.[15] Primary or idiopathic seizures are seizures in which no identifiable cause is recognized. Secondary or symptomatic seizures are seizures that are caused by a recognizable neurological condition, for example, central nervous system infection, brain tumor, stroke, head injury, or intracranial bleed. A reactive seizure is a generally self-limited seizure in an otherwise "normal" individual due to a specific etiology, such as a drug/toxin or metabolic disorder (i.e., hypoglycemia), and is not designated as epilepsy or a seizure disorder.[14] Provoked seizures, also referred to as acute symptomatic seizures,[16] are seizures that have an obvious and immediate preceding cause (e.g., hypoglycemia, an electrolyte abnormality, exposure to a toxin/adverse event from a drug) or are due to recent acute CNS injury (such as head trauma, stroke, or CNS infection). The usage of this terminology when due to an acute metabolic abnormality or drug/toxin exposure may be acceptable since treatment of the underlying etiology should prevent recurrence of the seizure. When used following acute CNS injury the term can be misleading since the underlying cause is irreversible and there is a strong predilection toward seizure reoccurrence.[17]

Epilepsy is a clinical condition characterized by recurrent (two or more), unprovoked seizures, generally attributed to genetic susceptibility or a chronic acquired CNS pathology (such as head trauma, hypoxic encepahalopathy or a stroke), and has no immediate identifiable cause.[14] Epilepsy, by definition, does not include seizures caused by reversible etiologies, such as hypoglycemia, electrolyte or metabolic abnormalities, toxins/poisonings, drugs (illicit, prescribed or over the counter), or alcohol withdrawal seizures. The highest incidence of newly diagnosed seizures is in the extremes of age: the elderly (> 65 years old) and children (< 5 years old).[2] Seizure incidence is highest during the first decade of life, particularly during the first year of life.[12] There are many physiological reasons responsible for an increased susceptibility of the developing brain to seizure.[12]

Seizure Classifications

Seizures are categorized into generalized or partial seizures, although if there is insufficient information to classify the seizure, it is designated as "unclassified."[15,16]

A generalized seizure consists of an initial involvement of both cerebral hemispheres[18] and is characterized by a loss of consciousness (LOC). Generalized seizures are further subdivided according to the presence or absence of specific motor activity. Generalized seizures include *generalized* or *tonic-clonic (grand mal)*: muscle rigidity followed by clonic movements of the head and extremities, *absence (petit mal)*: staring with impaired awareness and responsiveness, *atypical absence*: like absence but may have incomplete and/or gradual loss of responsiveness with tonic, clonic or atonic movements, *atonic (drop attack)*: sudden total loss of muscle tone ± LOC, *myoclonic*: jerking of a muscle or group of muscles, and *tonic*: bilateral stiffening seizures.[18]

Partial (focal) seizures are seizures with an initial onset arising from a localized area of the brain (e.g., limited to part of one cerebral hemisphere).[18] Partial seizures are frequently due to a structural lesion or localized injury to the brain. Therefore, they require a diagnostic evaluation for a focal lesion such as a tumor, arteriovenous malformation (AVM), cerebrovascular accident (CVA) or intracerebral bleed; although, most individuals with partial seizures will have no etiology identified and have idiopathic (unknown) partial seizures. Partial seizures are subgrouped based on whether or not there is LOC. With simple partial seizures, consciousness is maintained; the patient with complex partial seizures may appear conscious, but is unaware and unable to interact or respond to their environment and has impaired consciousness.

In addition to these classifications of seizures, there are various epileptic syndromes that are delineated by a constellation of features.[19] Some of the more common are febrile seizures, infantile spasms, Lennox-Gastaut syndrome, benign Rolandic epilepsy, and juvenile myoclonic epilepsy.[19]

Pathophysiology of Seizures

Epileptogenesis is the series of events that changes a normal neuronal network into a hyperexcitable network.[20] A discussion of the pathophysiology of seizures can facilitate an understanding of the mechanisms underlying the occurrence of seizures and how AEDs work.

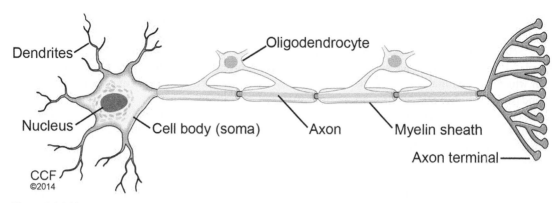

Dendrites

Oligodendrocyte

Nucleus

Cell body (soma)

Axon

Myelin sheath

Axon terminal

CCF
©2014

Figure 36.1 Neuron
The dendrites receive incoming signals from other neurons. The cell body directs the activities of the neuron (acts as a "control center") and synthesizes, breaks down, and reuses (recycles) neuronal proteins. The outgoing signal to other neurons flows along the axon. The axon terminal contains neurotransmitters.
Figures courtesy of Dr. Sharon E. Mace of the Cleveland Clinic Emergency Services, Mr. Dave Schumick of the Medical Art and Photography Department, and the Medical Art and Photography Department of the Cleveland Clinic, Cleveland, Ohio.

Neuronal circuits are composed of axonal conduction and synaptic transmission. Axonal conduction refers to the propagation of action potentials along the neuronal axon. (Figures 36.1 and 36.2) A synapse is the membrane-to-membrane contact of a nerve cell with another cell. The function of a synapse is to transmit nerve impulses, usually via a chemical transmitter substance. Key neurotransmitters in the brain include gamma (γ) aminobutyric acid (GABA), glutamate, acetylcholine, dopamine, serotonin, norepinephrine, and histamine. Synaptic transmission is the transmission or spread of nerve impulses, generally from axon terminal (presynaptic) to the postsynaptic membrane. Most commonly, synaptic transmission occurs via release of the chemical transmitters into the synaptic cleft, which then binds to a receptor for that neurotransmitter. In some instances, synaptic transmission occurs by direct propagation of the bioelectrical potential from the presynaptic to the postsynaptic membrane via a "gap junction" in which the synaptic cleft is extremely small, usually < 2 mm wide. (Figure 36.3) Both axonal conduction and synaptic transmission utilize ion channels. (Figures 36.4 and 36.5)

Cellular Physiology: Action Potential

The action potential is the fundamental mechanism of neuronal excitability. An action potential occurs in an all-or-none manner due to ion fluxes that result in a lowering of the resting membrane potential to a threshold membrane potential, which then causes depolarization to occur. (Figures 36.4 and 36.5)

Cellular Physiology: Ion Channels

Ion channels are a macromolecular protein pathway or passageway for the movement of ions into and out of the cell. Ion channels consist of proteins located in a cell's plasma membrane that have a "pore" or opening for the movement (influx or efflux) of inorganic ions (e.g., Na+, K+, Cl-, Ca^{2+}) in order to maintain or modulate the electrical potential of the cell. Thus, ion channels play a key role in the propagation of the action potential in neurons. These ion channels span the cell's membrane, thereby, transversing the lipid bilayer of a cell's plasma membrane. (Figures 36.4 and 36.5)

Movement of ions across the neuronal membrane determines the electrical membrane potential and generates the action potential. Sodium (Na +) is maintained in relatively high concentration outside the cell, while potassium (K+) is maintained in a relatively high concentration inside the cell. This electrochemical gradient is maintained by the ATP-dependent sodium-potassium pump that maintains the resting membrane potential in a polarized state at about −70 mV. (Figure 36.5) When an ion channel is opened, the ion moves passively into or out of the cell along its electrochemical gradient. (Figures 36.4 and 36.5)

There are two types of ion channels that can alter membrane potential and are accountable for excitatory and inhibitory activity: ligand-gated and voltage-gated. Conductance of ligand-gated channels is affected by a signal molecule or ligand (e.g., neurotransmitters), while the conductance of voltage-gated channels is affected by altering the transmembrane potential. Changes in intracellular

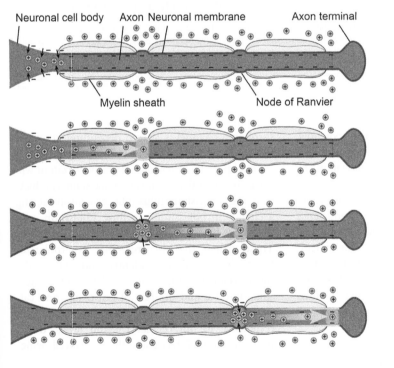

Unmyelinated Neuron

Neuronal cell body   Axon   Neuronal membrane   Axon terminal

Action potential

Myelinated Neuron

Neuronal cell body   Axon Neuronal membrane   Axon terminal

Myelin sheath   Node of Ranvier

Figure 36.2 Transmission of Impulse down Action Potential

Movement of the action potential from the neuronal cell body to the neuronal axon terminal along the axon, which allows conduction to occur. Conduction is the mechanism whereby intracellular signaling or communication within the neuron occurs, which allows the neuronal cell body to communicate with the neuronal axon terminal. Conduction involves movement of an action potential, which is generated in the cell body near the axon, down the axon to the axon terminal. The action potential occurs due to the movement of the electrically charged ions across the neuronal membrane.

Figures courtesy of Dr. Sharon E. Mace of the Cleveland Clinic Emergency Services, Mr. Dave Schumick of the Medical Art and Photography Department, and the Medical Art and Photography Department of the Cleveland Clinic, Cleveland, Ohio.

ion compartmentalization can also affect the membrane potential.[21] Sodium and calcium voltage gated ion channels act to depolarize the cell membrane toward the action potential threshold and are, therefore, excitatory.[21] Potassium voltage-gated channels cause hyperpolarization of the cell membrane away from the action potential and thus, are inhibitory. Ion channels are composed of an aggregation of polypeptide subunits. The types of subunits in the ion channels that are present in an individual neuron control the shape of the action potential and can modify the kinetic properties of the ion channel.

Ion Flows: Depolarization

Inward sodium conductance with an influx of sodium leads to a decrease in the resting membrane

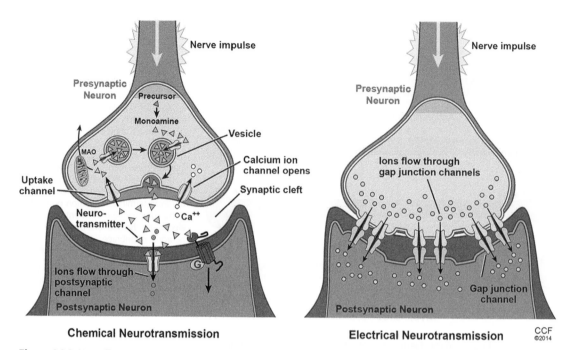

Chemical Neurotransmission   **Electrical Neurotransmission**

Figure 36.3 Neuro Transmission via Chemical Neurotransmission (Neurotransmitters) or Electrical Neurotransmission
With chemical neurotransmission, neurotransmitters are synthesized in the presynaptic neuron and then released into the synaptic cleft and travel to the postsynaptic neuron. Chemical transmission occurs via signal molecules or ligands, for example, neurotransmitters.
Electrical neurotransmission involves the use of voltage gated ion channels, including ions such as potassium, sodium or calcium.
Figures courtesy of Dr. Sharon E. Mace of the Cleveland Clinic Emergency Services, Mr. Dave Schumick of the Medical Art and Photography Department, and the Medical Art and Photography Department of the Cleveland Clinic, Cleveland, Ohio.

potential until it reaches the threshold potential, which triggers depolarization. (Figures 36.4 and 36.5) Sodium current fosters depolarization by lowering the resting membrane potential to a sub-threshold level and may foster burst firing of neurons. Increased inward calcium conductance causing an influx of calcium ions via voltage-gated channels also creates a drop in the resting membrane potential that leads to depolarization. Calcium influx also contributes to neurotransmitter release, thereby, influencing ligand-gated channels as well as affecting the firing pattern of neurons and gene expression.

Ion Flows: Hyperpolarization

The conductance of hyperpolarizing currents is predominately mediated by potassium channels, and works to diminish or inhibit excitation. Potassium conductance has many actions, including leak conductance and rectification. Leak conductance is a major influence on the resting membrane potential. Rectification pertains to the circumstance in which the direction of ion flow

through a channel is altered depending upon the voltage, which could be due to blocking of the ion channel pore by other ions. Hyperpolarization will turn on a rectifier of inward potassium conductance with potassium influx into the neuron causing a change in potassium ion flow. Potassium conductances have a multitude of effects on neurons. These include the M-current that hyperpolarizes the resting membrane potential and reduces the rate of cell firing; the A-current that sets the inter-spike interval and the rate of cell firing; and calcium activated potassium conductances that are responsive to intracellular calcium levels, determine interburst interval and the rate of cell firing.

Synaptic Transmission: Excitatory Neuurotransmitters – Glutamate

The amino acid glutamate is the primary excitatory neurotransmitter, while GABA is the major inhibitory neurotransmitter in the CNS. Glutamate receptors have been found postsynaptically on excitatory principal cells, inhibitory interneurons and some glial cells.

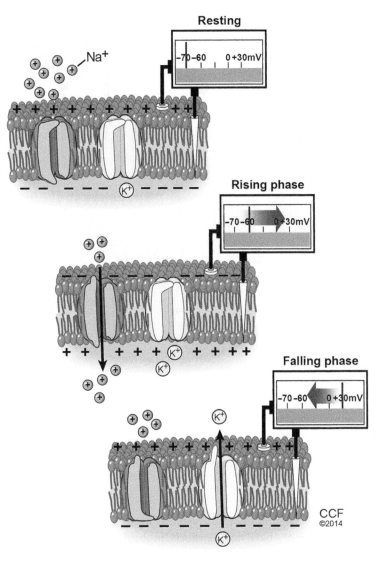

Figure 36.4 Action Potential
Action potential with resting membrane potential at around −70 millivolts.
Figures courtesy of Dr. Sharon E. Mace of the Cleveland Clinic Emergency Services, Mr. Dave Schumick of the Medical Art and Photography Department, and the Medical Art and Photography Department of the Cleveland Clinic, Cleveland, Ohio.

There are multiple subtypes of inotropic (fast synaptic transmission) glutamate receptors: α-amino-3-hydroxyl-5-methyl-4-isoxazole-proprionic acid (AMPA), kainate, and N-methyl-D-asparate (NDMA). All of these receptors open ion channels when coupled with glutamate.

Synaptic Transmission: Inhibitory Neurotransmitters – GABA Gamma-aminobutyric Acid

GABA is the main inhibitory neurotransmitter in the central nervous system (CNS).

GABA receptors have been found on almost all cortical neurons and on some glia. There are at least two types of GABA receptors: GABA-A and GABA-B. GABA-A receptors are located postsynaptically, are permeable to Cl- ions, and when activated the Cl- influx hyperpolarizes the neuronal cell membrane, thereby, inhibiting an action potential. GABA-B receptors are located presynaptically, act via second messenger systems, usually open K+ channels and have a hyperpolarizing current. This causes a decrease in transmitter release because of their presynaptic location.

Pathophysiology and Types of Epilepsy

Genetic modifications in the structure of sodium channels has been linked to various types of epilepsy from generalized epilepsy and febrile seizures to infantile myoclonic epilepsy and temporal lobe

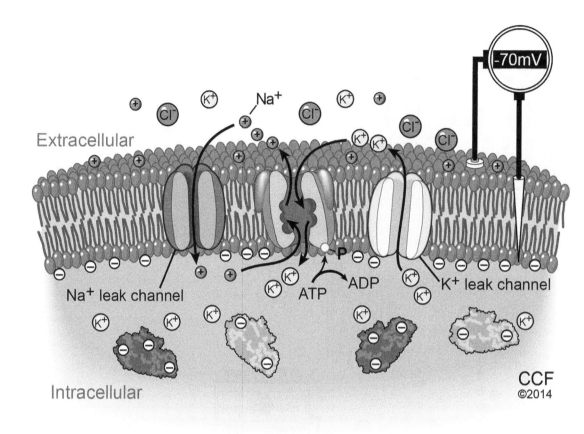

Figure 36.5 Action Potential Changes from Ion Flow Leading to Depolarization or Hyperpolarization
Figures courtesy of Dr. Sharon E. Mace of the Cleveland Clinic Emergency Services, Mr. Dave Schumick of the Medical Art and Photography Department, and the Medical Art and Photography Department of the Cleveland Clinic, Cleveland, Ohio.

epilepsy, while changes in the calcium channels have been associated with childhood absence epilepsy.[22] Genetic mutations affecting the M-current regulated by potassium ion channels are thought to be responsible for several types of epilepsy: idiopathic generalized epilepsy, benign partial epilepsy, and benign familial neonatal convulsions.

Pathophysiology and Antiepileptic Drugs

The pharmacology of most AEDs can be related to the pathophysiology. Numerous AEDs including phenytoin and carbamazepine interact with the voltage-dependent sodium channels. The AEDs levetiracetam and topiramate act partly through effects on the voltage-gated potassium channels.

In animal studies, ionotropic agonists of the excitatory glutamate receptors (AMPA, NDMA, and kainate) precipitate seizures, while antagonists of these receptors prevent seizures.

Metabotropic agonists of the glutamate receptors have varying effects, probably due to their diverse mechanisms of signal transduction and their different locations.[19]

GABA-A receptor agonists, which include the benzodiazepines and barbiturates, decrease or eliminate seizure activity. Some GABA-B agonists, for example, baclofen, cause hyperexcitability and precipitate seizures.

Summary: Neuronal Excitability

Many variables can affect neuronal hyperexcitability leading to an increased susceptibility to seizures. This has been referred to as "neuronal" or intrinsic if inside the neuron/cell or "extraneuronal" or extrinsic if in the extracellular space.[21]

Intrinsic or neuronal variables include intracellular ion concentrations, intracellular neurotransmitters (amount, available substrate, synthesis, or breakdown), voltage-gated or ligand-gated channels (number, type, location or distribution), receptors (number, type, location or distribution), modification of receptors, activation of second-messenger systems, and alteration of gene expression.

Extra-neuronal (extrinsic) factors include extracellular ion concentration, extracellular neurotransmitters (amount, available substrate, synthesis or breakdown), uptake of neurotransmitters, synapses, neuronal networks or anatomical regions of the brain.[18] The sprouting of new axons or the destruction of neurons leading to an imbalance of the excitatory/inhibitory neurons, changes in connections between the neurons with new or loss of connections are examples of how neuronal networks could affect hyperexcitability and the propensity for seizures. Current and future AEDs will likely target these molecular, cellular, and anatomic factors that lead to neuronal hyperexcitability and seizures.

Patient Evaluation

The first step is to determine whether the event was actually a seizure. The differential diagnosis is extensive and includes syncope, hyperventilation, transient ischemic attack, migraines, pseudoseizures, sleep phenomena (e.g., narcolepsy/cataplexy), drug toxicity, movement disorders (such as chorea, dystonia, myoclonic jerks, tremors, tics), and additionally in children/infants: breath holding spells and behavioral events. In an adult study, 30–40% of those seen in a first seizure clinic had experienced an earlier unrecognized seizure.[23] Similarly, a pediatric study noted "a high rate of diagnostic inaccuracy, with one quarter of patients incorrectly diagnosed as having a seizure rather than a nonepileptic event" and the diagnosis of epilepsy "missed in over one-third of children."[24] In this clinic, the diagnosis was epilepsy in 74%, nonepilepsy in 24%, and unclassifiable in 2%.

A detailed history of the event is crucial and should include: prodrome/aura if any, onset (abrupt or gradual), activity (if any): type/progression/localized or generalized/symmetric or asymmetric, consciousness, bladder/bowel incontinence, duration, postictal confusion/lethargy/headache, precipitating factors, associated symptoms (severe, persistent headache may indicate intracranial pathology), and any injuries sustained during the event.

In a patient with known seizures, determine the patient's baseline seizure pattern and whether this episode is similar to previous seizures and ascertain any precipitating factors: missed doses of seizure medications, new or changes in medications including over the counter drugs or a change from brand name to generic, alcohol/substance abuse or withdrawal, emotional stress, strenuous exercise, sleep deprivation, and any intercurrent infections or illnesses.

A prior history of unexplained injuries, tongue biting, enuresis or "passing out" may indicate unrecognized seizure activity. An important question to ask is whether there are any previous head injuries. The history should include medications including anticoagulants, allergies, social history especially alcohol/substance abuse, and family history (including seizures, other neurologic, congenital, and/or genetic disorders). Past medical history should include systemic illnesses (particularly HIV, cancer, CVA, other neurologic disorders, coagulopathy, endocrine or metabolic disorders, liver/kidney disease, previous trauma) and any recent illnesses/injuries.[6]

The physical examination should include vital signs with a temperature and pulse oxygen saturation, level of consciousness, brief mental status examination, screening for injuries (especially the head and spine), neurologic/cardiac/respiratory examination, as well as checking the neck/spine (e.g., supple or stiff, any injuries) and skin for rashes, petechiae, stigmata of inherited/congenital disorders, bruising, infections, malignancies, etc.

A dextrostix/accucheck or blood glucose is generally indicated even in known seizure patients to rule out hypoglycemia. If the patient is on an anticonvulsant that can be measured, usually an anticonvulsant level is obtained. In those with a known seizure disorder and a single unprovoked seizure similar to their previous seizure pattern, the glucose and anticonvulsant level may be the only tests that are warranted.[14]

However, if this is a first-time seizure, or there are complicating factors, or the diagnosis is uncertain, then further evaluation is usually indicated. Laboratory studies to consider are glucose, electrolytes including calcium and magnesium, renal function tests (BUN creatinine), toxicology studies, and in women of childbearing age, a pregnancy test. A seizure can cause a wide anion gap metabolic (lactic) acidosis and an elevated prolactin level immediately after the seizure, which generally resolves within 15–30 minutes. This may be useful in distinguishing a true seizure from a pseudoseizure, but must be obtained immediately after the seizure before they normalize.

Depending on the clinical circumstances, other tests may be useful. If an infection is being considered, a CBC may be warranted. If meningitis or a subarachnoid hemorrhage is in the differential, then a lumbar puncture with cerebrospinal fluid analysis is indicated. If this is a new onset partial seizure, there are focal findings or any concern for intracranial process, then a CT scan is indicated. A chest radiograph may detect an aspiration pneumonia, a tumor or other abnormality. If syncope is a possibility, an ECG is a simple, easily obtained noninvasive test. An EEG may reveal valuable information.

An EEG is infrequently obtained in the ED except for usual circumstances, such as evaluation for nonconvulsive status epilepticus in a comatose or paralyzed patient,[15] but may be part of the OU evaluation.

Patient Selection

Patients in whom any history or a valid history could not be obtained in the ED may be placed in observation until a confirmatory history and a reliable friend/family member are available to take responsibility for the patient so the patient can be safely discharged home. Repeat physical examination can be done, looking for any injuries that may have occurred during the episode and for clues to the etiology of the event, and to ascertain that the patient has fully recovered from their postictal state.

Patients who need further evaluation to determine the etiology of their "seizure-like" episode, whether to confirm a true seizure or an alternative diagnosis, are appropriate candidates for an OU. Additional testing – whether laboratory, neuroimaging, an EEG, monitoring or other specialized diagnostic studies – can be completed in the OU. If syncope is a possibility, then monitoring for dysrhythmias and a diagnostic workup can be done in the OU. (See Chapter 25 on syncope.)

Patients who need time to recover from a postictal or intoxicated state can be safely monitored in the OU. Patients for whom there is a concern for recurrent seizure activity can undergo repeat neurologic checks along with vital signs and be monitored in the OU. Patients with a known seizure

disorder, awaiting their laboratory tests including an anticonvulsant level, may have their "loading dose" of anticonvulsant medication administered in the OU. Management of any conditions that precipitated the seizure, such as an infection, should be done in order to help prevent seizure recurrence.

Since 90% of patients with alcohol withdrawal seizures will have additional seizures within a 6-hour time frame, it has been recommended that these patients be "admitted for observation and further investigation."[15]

Exclusion

Patients with unstable vital signs, acute psychiatric problems, status epilepticus, any intracranial lesion needing emergent surgical intervention, bacterial meningitis or new significant intracranial pathology (such as acute stroke or intracranial bleed) should not be admitted to an OU.

Certain patient populations are not appropriate patients for an OU admission. Human immunodeficiency virus (HIV) positive patients are a high-risk population; tend to have more serious, life-threatening etiologies for their seizures than the general population with mass lesions, meningitis, and HIV encephalopathy occurring more frequently; and usually need a more extensive diagnostic evaluation, which is unlikely to be completed in < 24 hours.[12] Although most seizures in pregnancy are not first-time seizures, the management of the pregnant patient with known or new-onset seizures is more complicated than usual and requires a multidisciplinary approach with the involvement of consultants. Initiation of treatment for first-time seizure in a pregnant patient should incorporate consultations from an obstetrician and a neurologist. Concern over risk to the fetus from AEDs adds another layer of complexity. Seizures beyond 20 weeks of gestation raise the possibility of eclampsia. It is best not to place complicated patients with seizures, such as HIV patients or pregnant patients, in the OU.

Observation Unit Management

The history is of fundamental importance after an episode, yet it may be difficult or impossible to obtain a valid history in the ED, especially in a patient with an altered mental status or who is postictal, particularly if the patient is unaccompanied and there are no family members or others from whom to obtain a history. In the OU, there is time for family or friends to come in and provide information, time to make phone calls and reach those who were present during the event, and time for the postictal or the intoxicated patient to recover and give information.

Repeat vital signs and neurologic checks can be done in the OU, with observation for any recurrent seizures or monitoring if syncope and dysrhythmias are a consideration. It has been suggested that those with alcohol withdrawal seizures be admitted for observation and additional evaluation.[15]

A diagnostic workup can be done in the OU in order to determine the etiology of the event. Was this episode a seizure or syncope or another disorder? If this was a seizure, evaluation can be done, which may involve additional laboratory tests, a neurology consult, neuroimaging (CT or MRI), lumbar puncture, EEG or other specialized testing. In patients with a known seizure disorder, once their anticonvulsant level is available, then a loading dose of anticonvulsant may be administered, although the necessity of loading anticonvulsant medications has been questioned recently.

One caveat to remember is that patients with epilepsy may have a non-epileptic seizure event or syncope or other problems/pathology. Moreover, distinguishing between a seizure and a seizure-like event can be difficult, especially in a busy ED. Additional time in the OU may be needed for determination of the etiology of the event.

Precipitating factors known to lower the seizure threshold and that trigger breakthrough seizures can be treated in the OU. Patients with a mild blood glucose and/or electrolyte abnormality, or vitamin deficiency, can have intravenous fluids with supplemental electrolytes, vitamins, glucose, and others administered to correct their deficit. Conversely, fluids and insulin can be given to lower an elevated blood sugar. Patients with a non-life-threatening infection (e.g., uncomplicated cellulitis or pharyngitis) may have treatment including antibiotics started in the OU. However, patients with seizures and serious life-threatening

or other significant infections, such as meningitis or encephalitis, are not candidates for the OU. If the patient needs adjustment in their seizure medications, then neurology consultation can be obtained in the OU.

Inclusion criteria include stable patients, who are not critically ill, who do not need emergent surgical intervention, and who are anticipated to be ready for discharge in < 24 hours. Seizure patients appropriate for observation include stable patients with new onset seizures, alcohol withdrawal seizures, uncomplicated febrile seizures, posttraumatic seizures following isolated blunt head trauma with a negative CT scan, and normal or baseline neurologic examination.[13]

Patients with precipitating conditions for their seizures that can be easily treated and are expected to improve within a 1-day (24-hour) timeframe can be placed in observation. Thus, patients with less severe infections – such as a urinary tract infection but not urosepsis, or pneumonia without hypoxia or respiratory distress, and/or electrolyte or glucose abnormalities but not diabetic ketoacidosis – may have management of their underlying illness that brought on their seizures as well as evaluation or therapy for seizure disorder in the OU.

Summary

Patients with seizures are commonly encountered in clinical practice. The OU allows a brief period of time, < 24 hours, that allows for obtaining further history and testing in order to determine the etiology of a given episode, whether a seizure or syncope or another cause. The OU affords time to complete a diagnostic evaluation and to administer therapy for the seizure including administering antiepileptics, and allows for the postictal and/or intoxicated patient to recover. The OU also provides an opportunity to repeat evaluation of the postictal patient to determine if he or she is stable for discharge and to treat any precipitating causes of the seizure.

References

1. Forsgren L, Bucht G, Eriksson S, et al. Incidence and clinical characterization of unprovoked seizures in adults; a prospective population-based study. *Epilepsia*, 1996; 37(3): 224–229.

2. www.epilepsyfoundation.org/aboutepilepsy/whatisepilepsy/statistics.cfm (last accessed July 24, 2012).

3. ACEP Clinical Policy: Critical issues in the evaluation and management of adult patients presenting to the emergency department with seizures. *Ann Emerg Med*, 2004; 43: 605–625.

4. Bagley CE, Annegers JF, Lairson Dr, et al. Cost of epilepsy in the United States: a model based on incidence and prognosis. *Epilepsia*, 1994; 35: 1230–1243.

5. Verity CM, Goldin J. Risk of epilepsy convulsions: a national cohort study. *BMJ*, 1991; 303(6814): 1373–1376.

6. Warden CR, Zibulewsky J, Mace SE, et al. Evaluation and management of seizures in the out-of-hospital and emergency department settings. *Ann Emerg Med*, 2003; 41(2): 215–224.

7. Hirtz D, Thurman DJ, Gwinn-Hardy K, et al. How common are the "common" neurologic disorders? *Neurology* 2007; 68:326–337.

8. Montouris GD, Jagoda AS. Management of breakthrough seizures in the emergency department: continuity of patient care. *Curr Med Research and Opinions*, 2007; 23(7): 1583–1592.

9. Devi PU, Manocha A, Vohora D. Seizures, antiepileptics, antioxidants and oxidative stress: an insight for researchers. *Expert Opin Pharmacother*, 2008; 9(18): 3169–3177.

10. Pashko S, McCord A, Sena MM. The cost of epilepsy and seizures in a cohort of Pennsylvania Medicaid patients. *Medical Interface*, 1993; November: 79–84.

11. Lozsadi DA, VonOertzen J, Cock HR. Epilepsy: recent advances. *Neurol*, 2010; 257: 1846–1951.

12. Huff JS, Morris DL, Kothari RU, et al. Emergency Medicine Seizure Study Group. Emergency department management of patients with seizures: a multicenter study. *Acad Emerg Med*, 2001; 8(6): 622–628.

13. Mace SE, Bent ST. Seizures. In: Graff LG (ed.). *Observation Medicine: The Healthcare System's Tincture of Time.* https://webapps.acep.org/ WorkArea/Download Assett.aspx?id=45885 (last accessed July 27, 2012)

14. Stafstrom CE. Pathophysiological mechanisms of seizures and epilepsy: a primer. In: Rho JM, Sankar R, Stafstrom CE (eds.). *Epilepsy. Mechanisms, Models, and Translational Perspective.* Boca Raton, FL, CRC Press, 2010; ch. 1: pp. 3–19.

15. Lung DD, Catlett CL, Tintinalli JE. Seizures and status epilepticus in adults. In: Tintinalli J, Stapczynski JS, Cline DM, et al. (eds.). New York; McGraw-Hill Co., 2011, ch. 165: pp. 1153–1159.

16. Huff JS, Fountain NB. Pathophysiology and definitions of seizures and status epilepticus. *Emerg Med Clin N Am*, 2011; 29: 1–13.

17. Shorvon S. The clinical forms and causes of epilepsy. In: *Handbook of Epilepsy Treatment.* Malden, MA: Blackwell Publishing, 2005; ch. 1: pp. 1–59.

18. Kellinghaus C, Luders HO. Classification of seizures. In: Wyllie E, Cascino GD, Gidal BE, Gookin HP (ed.). *Wyllie's Treatment of Epilepsy: Principles and Practice.* Philadelphia, PA: Wolters Kluwer, 2011, ch. 10: pp. 134–143.

19. Loddenkemper T. Classification of the epilepsies. In: Wyllie E, Cascino GD, Gidal BE, Goodkin HP (eds.). *Wyllie's Treatment of Epilepsy: Principles and Practice.* Philadelphia, PA: Wolter Kluwer, 2011; ch.18: pp. 229–242.

20. Dichter MA. Overview: the neurobiology of epilepsy. In: Engel J. Jr., Pedley TA, Aicardi J, et al. (eds.). *Epilepsy: a Comprehensive Textbook.* Philadelphia, PA: Wolters Kluwer/Lippincott Williams & Wilkins, 2nd ed., 2008, ch. 20: pp. 217–218.

21. www.ncbi.nlm.nih.gov/books/ NBK2510 (last accessed July 25, 2012)

22. Heinemann U, Mody I, Yaari Y. Control of neuronal excitability. In: Engel J. Jr., Pedley TA, Aicardi J, et al. (eds.). *Epilepsy: a Comprehensive Textbook.* Philadelphia, PA: Wolters Kluwer/Lippincott Williams & Wilkins, 2nd ed., 2008, ch. 21: pp. 219–231.

23. King MA, Newton MR, Jackson GD, et al. Epileptology of the first-seizure presentation: a clinical, electroencephalographic, and magnetic resonance imaging study of 300 consecutive patients. *Lancet* 352(9133): 1007–1011.

24. Hamiwka LD, Singh N, Niosi J, et al. Diagnostic inaccuracy in children with "first seizure": role for a first seizure clinic. *Epilepsia* 2007; p 48(6): 1062–1066.

Dizziness and Vertigo

Saurin Bhatt, MD

Dizziness is a common medical complaint encountered in the outpatient setting. It is estimated that up to 18% of aggregate ambulatory care visits are for the complaint of dizziness, with an increasing prevalence toward older ages.[1,2] Inadvertently, dizziness results in billions of dollars of health care costs and time lost from work. Additionally, the duration of symptoms may vary in time, potentially representing long periods of morbidity. Dizziness, often a vague complaint in itself, can represent a range of conditions from those easily treated disorders when identified to several etiologies that represent significant morbidity and mortality. It is for this reason that physicians have been looking for clinical decision strategies to help them determine the severity of this patient complaint and then initiate appropriate treatment. The goal of this chapter is not only to help the clinician to determine the correct diagnosis and treatment, but also aid in the recognition of the significant disease processes that require intervention and referral.

The emergency department (ED) and subsequently the observation unit (OU) turn out to be a common triaging area for these patients, primarily due to the amount of resources available to narrow down the complaint to a functional diagnosis. Depending on the patient, there may be a variable workup, which can be extensive. A well-functioning OU will be able to coordinate patient examination, testing, and specialist consultation in an efficient manner to remain cost and time effective for the hospital and patient. Due to the extensive differential diagnosis of dizziness, additional evaluation may require many specialties, including neurology, neurosurgery, otolaryngology, cardiology, psychiatry, geriatrics, toxicology, and social work. The role of the physician in the OU is to assimilate the information collected thus far, add tests as needed, and properly disposition the patient.

Many times, the first step in caring for the patient involves elucidating the complaint itself. This may include having the patient describe the sensations he or she is feeling without using the term "dizzy." Particular caution needs to be exercised with women and geriatric populations, as these populations may have atypical presentations of disease. Elderly patients additionally may have multiple concerning comorbidities, declining general health, polypharmacy concerns, or even socioeconomic factors that can complicate evaluation, treatment, and disposition.

Classification and Differential of Dizziness

The neurology literature has partitioned complaints of dizziness into four subtypes: presyncope, vertigo, disequilibrium, and lightheadedness. Please refer to Table 37.1 for a brief overview of these four categories. Based upon the characterization of dizziness, further workup and evaluation can proceed. This chapter will primarily focus on vertiginous-based complaints, due to the significant morbidity and mortality associated with vertiginous complaints. Additionally, cardiac and vasomotor evaluation and treatment that may be associated with presyncope dizziness complaints are discussed elsewhere. A large number of dizziness differentials require fairly basic treatment once identified and will not be the focus of this chapter.

History and Physical Examination

History

To help narrow a list of differential diagnoses, a proper history and physical examination need to be performed. History will help differentiate the dizziness subtype.

Table 37.1 Differential Diagnosis of Dizziness

Information included from reference sources[3–7,13]			
Differentials of Dizziness			
Dizziness Subtype	Type of Sensation	Temporal Characteristics	Selected Differentials
Vertigo	Spinning or motion sensation	Episodic or continuous	Benign paroxysmal positional vertigo Meniere's disease Labyrinthitis Vertebrobasilar ischemia Cerebellar infarction or hemorrhage
Presyncope	Feeling faint, or about to pass out	Episodic, may last for seconds, may be alleviated by lying down	Dehydration Anemia Cardiac ischemia Infection Hypo/Hyperglycemia
Disequilibrium	Unsteady feeling in the lower extremities	Continuous, but may vary in intensity	Multiple sensory deficits Peripheral neuropathy, Vision loss
Lightheadedness	Vague complaints, nonspecific		Medication Related Psychiatric disorders including anxiety, depression, panic attacks hyperventilation

There are specific historical factors that may be helpful to the clinician in determining the cause of the dizziness. For example, if the patient states that there have been several episodes within the past 6 months, consider that the patient may have been experiencing transient ischemic attacks (TIAs). If the patient offers a history of chiropractic manipulation, headache, or neck trauma, vertebral artery dissection should be considered. A coexistent history of any other neurological symptoms should prompt the clinician to consider a central cause of the dizziness.

If the patient by history by falls into the vertigo category, it is often helpful to determine if the complaint is suggestive of a peripheral or central lesion. As is suggested by Table 37.2, certain historical and physical examination characteristics are suggestive of a peripheral or central lesion. These are causation predictors and not determinants of the patient's symptoms. It is prudent for the examiner to not exclude a central cause solely due to the presence of one or two weak peripheral characteristics. In fact, recent literature suggests that many of these characteristics that are classically taught as strongly predictive of peripheral or central causation are not as definitive as previously thought.[24] More so, some aspects of vertiginous complaints, such as vomiting, can be found in both peripheral and central causes and therefore is an unreliable distinguishing characteristic.

For vertiginous complaints, asking about timing, triggers, progression of symptoms, and associated symptoms may be helpful. The evidence-based literature describes acute vestibular syndrome as a patient presentation lasting more than 24 hours with accompanying symptoms that include gait instability, nausea, vomiting, intolerance to head motion, and no focal neurological findings. While this represents a specific subset of dizzy patients, it also represents a specific set of patients that have been researched and from which treatment decisions have been made.

Physical Examination

Physical examination should be guided by history, but almost always include the entire neurological examination, in addition to the cardiovascular

Table 37.2 Differentiation of Peripheral Versus Central Vertigo

Information included from reference sources:[2,4,7,13,16,20]

Peripheral vs. Central Characteristics		
Characteristic	Peripheral	Central
Onset	Sudden	Gradual
Frequency	Episodic, recurrent	Constant, progressive
Duration	Seconds, minutes	Weeks, months
Nystagmus	Horizontal	Vertical
Triggered by Movement?	Yes	Symptoms may worsen, but generally are not triggered with movement.
Isolated Hearing Loss?	Yes	Other neurologic findings are usually present.
Fatigable	Yes	No
Associated Symptoms	Tinnitus, N/V	Neurologic/visual Symptoms
Postural Instability	No (may lean towards lesion)	Yes

examination. Cranial nerves should be thoroughly assessed as subtle neurological findings might be present. An assessment of gait and the presence of truncal ataxia (inability to sit upright in bed with arms crossed) may help to distinguish between a peripheral and central lesion. Cerebellar tests are also important for vertigo assessments, as cerebellar strokes may present with vertigo as the only physical manifestation of the stroke. Patients that complain of hearing abnormalities should have a complete otologic exam, including external, internal, Rinne and Weber tests. (Figure 37.1, 37.2, 37.3) Concerns regarding cardiac disease should include bruit examination and murmur assessments.

Another high yield physical examination is the complete eye examination. Nystagmus evaluation should always be performed in vertigo complaints, as its presence can provide significant information regarding the etiology of the patient's vertigo complaint. An assessment should be made in the patient's full visual fields with the eyes moved in all directions to fully assess all types of nystagmus. Refer to Table 37.3 for nystagmus characteristics, pattern type, and cause. The proper description of nystagmus is in the fast direction of movement. It is also important to note that the lack of any nystagmus or a particular type nystagmus does not rule out a stroke or particular central cause. With the exception of bidirectional nystagmus (further discussed later),

Figure 37.1 Normal Ear Anatomy

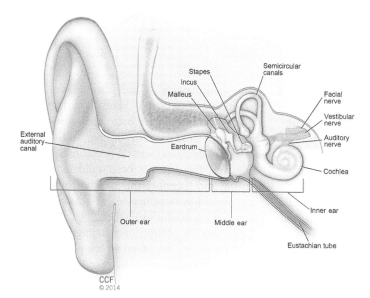

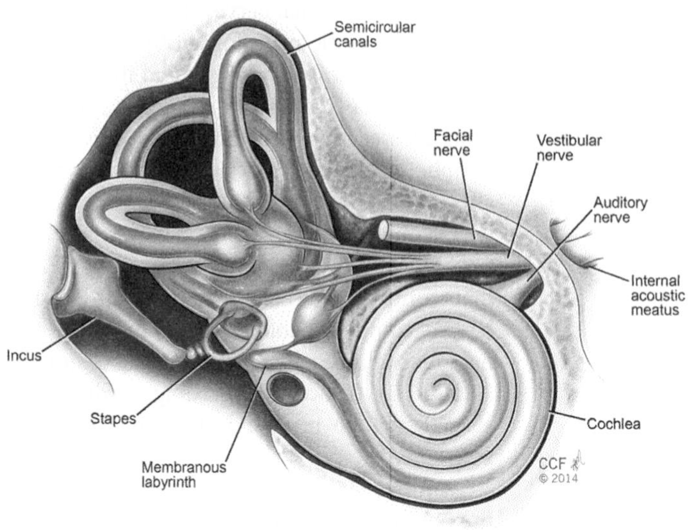

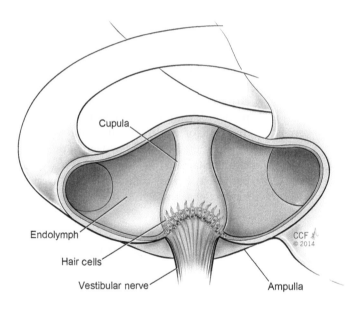

Figure 37.2 Normal Inner Ear Anatomy

Semicircular canals

Facial nerve

Vestibular nerve

Auditory nerve

Internal acoustic meatus

Incus

Stapes

Cochlea

Membranous labyrinth

CCF
© 2014

Figure 37.3 Normal Semicircular Canal

Cupula

Endolymph

Hair cells

Vestibular nerve

Ampulla

CCF
© 2014

no clinical decisions should be made exclusively on this physical examination finding. Even then, bidirectional nystagmus should be used in conjunction with other findings to come to a clinical conclusion of stroke.

Based upon recent literature, if there is a concern that there is a central cause of the patient's vertigo, two additional physical examination tests can be performed to help assess for a central cause. According to Kattah et al.,[25] a three-step examination is more sensitive than MRI within the first 24 hours in determining stroke in patients presenting with acute vertiginous symptoms. The three components of this examination include assessment of direction-changing nystagmus (also called gaze evoking or bidirectional nystagmus), horizontal head impulse testing, and assessment for skew deviation (vertical ocular misalignment). However, this has not been validated as of this writing and therefore the presence of these findings should prompt urgent CT scan or MRI and neurology specialist evaluation.

Testing for bidirectional nystagmus is an easy test to perform. A patient with a positive test will have nystagmus when looking to the left as well as the right, suggesting a dysfunction of the gaze

Table 37.3 Nystagmus

	Information included from reference sources:[17]	
	Nystagmus Evaluation	
Pattern Type	Nystagmus Characteristic	Cause
Peripheral	Upbeat torsional nystagmus with Dix-Hallpike maneuver	Benign paroxysmal Positional Vertigo
Peripheral	Unidirectional spontaneous nystagmus	Vestibular neuritis
Central	Vertical nystagmus	Strokes, Chiari malformation, multiple sclerosis
Central	Direction dependent changes	Medications (antiepileptic), stroke, multiple sclerosis
Central	Downbeating with Dix-Hallpike	Chiari malformation or cerebellar space occupying lesion
Central	Intranuclear ophthalmoplegia	Multiple sclerosis, stroke
Physiologic	Unsustained gaze dependent nystagmus	

stabilizing mechanisms of the cerebellum and brainstem.

Head impulse testing is a method for checking an intact vestibular-ocular reflex. A head thrust maneuver is performed by moving the head side to side no more than 30 degrees in either side from midline while the patient focuses on a fixed object such as the examiner's nose. The examiner alters the pace of head thrusts to ensure that the brainstem does not adapt to the movements. A positive test is when the patient is able to focus on the fixed object while the head thrusting is performed in the presence of dizziness. Avoid this maneuver in patients with known or suspected cervical spine issues. The patient's ability to fixate on an object while having a vertiginous complaint strongly suggests a central cause of symptoms.

The last test is for skew deviation. Once again the patient is asked to focus on a fixed object. One eye is covered and the covering is alternated between eyes over a short time interval (several seconds). If upon alternating the covered eye there is a vertical misalignment, it is considered a positive test for skew deviation.

Differential Diagnosis of Vertigo

The patient data after interview and examination may point to a peripheral cause of the vertiginous dizziness. Peripheral causes can be further differentiated by elucidating certain facts. The first is to determine if the patient has any migraine type symptoms. If so, the patient may have a variant of migraines known as migrainous vertigo, in which the treatment is standard migraine treatment protocols (noted in Chapter 35, Headaches).

If no migraine type symptoms are present, then the next step is to determine if the patient has any hearing loss or tinnitus present (subjectively or objectively). If none is present, then episodic events of dizziness may be considered as benign paroxysmal positional vertigo (BPPV) (Figure 37.4), whereas continuous dizziness is termed vestibular neuritis. If the patient does have hearing loss, episodic episodes likely represent Meniere's disease (Figure 37.5), whereas continuous episodes represent labrynthitis. (Table 37.4)

BPPV (Figure 37.4) can be confirmed as well as subsequently treated at the bedside by using the Dix-Hallpike maneuver (Figure 37.6). With this maneuver, the patient is instructed to keep his or her eyes open while being lowered from a sitting to a lying position with the head positioned at 45° degrees to the left or right. The head is brought to an extension to about 20° and the eyes are observed. The patient with BPPV will have an upbeating, torisonal nystagmus in the direction of that the head is turned. If this fails to elicit the nystagmus (usually delayed up to 30 seconds), an attempt can be made in the opposite direction after the patient's symptoms have subsided.

Since the etiology of BPPV is due to debris in the semicircular canals (Figure 37.4), the Epley maneuver (repositioning maneuver) can be used to remove the debris (Figure 37.7). The Epley

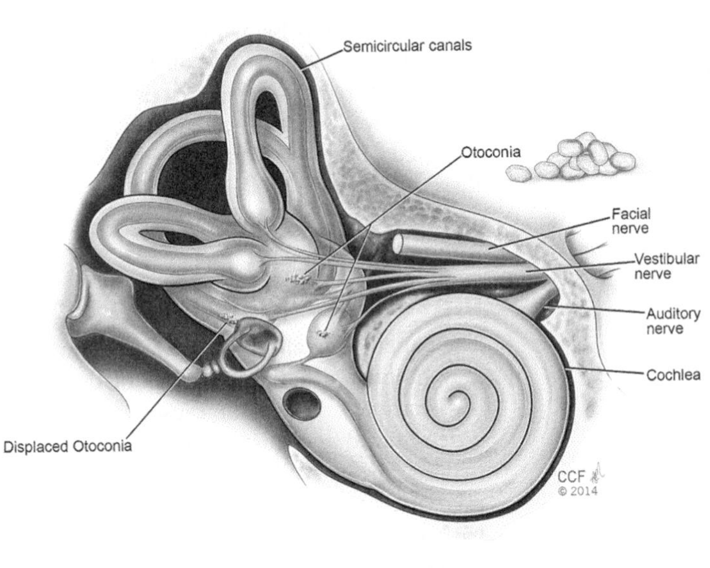

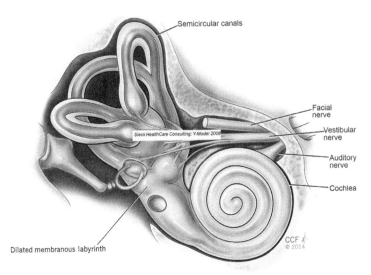

Figure 37.4 Benign Paroxysmal Positional Vertigo (BPPV)

Semicircular canals

Otoconia

Facial nerve

Vestibular nerve

Auditory nerve

Cochlea

Displaced Otoconia

CCF
© 2014

Figure 37.5 Meniere's Disease
Figures are courtesy of the Dr. Sharon E. Mace of the Emergency Services Institute of the Cleveland Clinic, the Art and Photo Department of the Cleveland Clinic and Amanda Mendelsohn (Figures 37.1–37.3) and Bill Garriott (Figures 37.4–37.7)

Semicircular canals

Sieck HealthCare Consulting: Y-Model 2008

Facial nerve

Vestibular nerve

Auditory nerve

Cochlea

Dilated membranous labyrinth

CCF
© 2014

maneuver starts with the Dix-Hallpike maneuver on the nystagmus elicited side. The patient's head is moved 90° in the opposite direction and held in that position for up to 1 minute to allow the patient to accommodate. The patient will now be looking 45° in the opposite direction. Once the patient has accommodated, the patient is rolled further in the same direction onto his or her shoulder, such that he or she is looking straight into the ground. Finally, the patient is brought back into a sitting position at the side of the bed. This maneuver may be repeated, as needed, and generally will alleviate the patient symptoms. Follow up with otolaryngology (ENT) should

be provided for further treatment as needed. Recurrence can occur, and the patient may need specialized testing and treatment not possible in the OU.

Labrynthitis and vestibular neuritis are diagnoses that usually will need ENT follow up for vestibular rehabilitation exercises. (Table 37.4) ENT consultation may be helpful to determine if antibiotics or antivirals may be necessary based upon the suspicion of symptom etiology as well as for suppressant medication recommendations. Of note, evidence-based literature suggests that patients with vestibular dysfunction will in fact learn to compensate over time, so that

Table 37.4 Vestibular Causes of Vertigo

	Benign Paroxysmal Positional Vertigo	Labrynthitis	Meniere's Disease	Vestibular Neuritis
Dizzy Episodes	Episodic	Continuous	Episodic	Continuous
Hearing Loss	No	Yes	Yes	No
Tinnitus	No	Can be present	Yes	No
Treatment	Epley maneuver Antihistamines (diphenhydramine) Anticholinergics (meclizine) Symptomatic: antiemetics or vestibular suppressant including benzodiazepines	Vestibular rehabilitation exercises Treatment if known source: can include steroids, antivirals, and antibiotics (suspected otitis media) Symptomatic treatment with antiemetics or vestibular suppressants	Diuretics, low salt diet, benzodiazepines, anticholingerics	Vestibular rehabilitation exercises Treatment if known source: can include steroids, antivirals Symptomatic treatment with antiemetics or vestibular suppressants
ENT Follow-up	Yes	Yes	Yes	Yes
Cause	Otoconia ("ear rocks"), crystals detach from otolithic membrane and collect in semicircular canal (usually posterior)	Inflammation of the labyrinth of the inner ear	Idiopathic; symptoms are due to excess fluid from the labyrinth into other areas of the inner ear	Unknown, associated with preceding or concurrent infection in ~ half of patients
Associated symptoms	Nausea, vomiting	Nausea, vomiting	Nausea, vomiting	Nausea, vomiting
Comment	May reoccur Most common vestibular disorder About 50% of dizziness in elderly is due to BPPV	Recovery can be extended to several months or years depending on the amount of damage	Triad: vertigo, hearing loss, tinnitus Surgery for cases resistant to medical management	Usually without any auditory symptoms and no neurologic symptoms other than dizziness
Typical Setting	> 50 yrs idiopathic, due to age-related dgeneration of otolithic membrane < 50 yrs trauma	Can be associated with a viral or bacterial upper respiratory infection	Young to middle-aged adults; many times after a viral infection	Sudden onset; previously well young or middle-aged adult

suppression of this compensation via medication for more than several days is not advised. If the patient is unable to perform activities of daily living (ADLs) or has a social situation that prevents discharge home, appropriate inpatient preparations should be made.

Meniere's disease has a genetic predisposition. It is treated acutely with diuretics, low salt diet, and occasionally benzodiazepines, as the causation of this disease is thought to be a fluid imbalance within the inner ear. (Figure 37.3) Again, ENT follow up would be recommended, as persistent symptoms are managed differently.

History and physical examination often are complemented with laboratory and radiographic studies. Proper testing should be guided by the patient's presentation. For vertiginous complaints, there often is little utility in obtaining laboratory

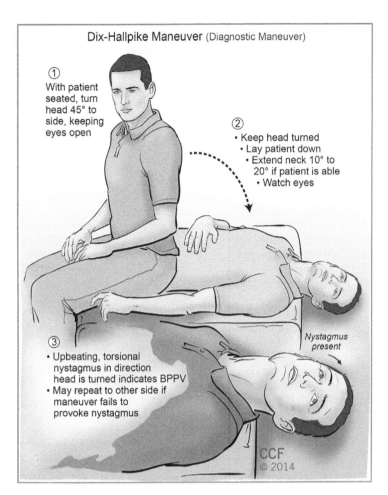

Figure 37.6 Dix-Hallpike Maneuver

Dix-Hallpike Maneuver (Diagnostic Maneuver)

① With patient seated, turn head 45° to side, keeping eyes open

② • Keep head turned
• Lay patient down
• Extend neck 10° to 20° if patient is able
• Watch eyes

③ • Upbeating, torsional nystagmus in direction head is turned indicates BPPV
• May repeat to other side if maneuver fails to provoke nystagmus

Nystagmus present

CCF
© 2014

data. Patients that fall into the dizziness categories of presyncope, disequilibrium, and lightheadedness may benefit though from additional laboratory work, especially as it may help specialists rule in other etiologies. For example, a geriatrician or psychiatrist may request medical clearance via ancillary testing for further care of the patient. Other times, ambiguous histories supplemented with laboratory data may demonstrate an easily correctable diagnosis. Laboratory tests ordered in the OU can also be obtained for trending purposes and may provide assistance for later patient care.

Radiographic studies in vertigo type complaints are almost always ordered and can be helpful in diagnosis and patient disposition. In terms of radiographic studies a chest x-ray may be helpful if there is a concern of an infectious cause of the patient's dizziness. Often CT is ordered to evaluate for intracranial pathology. A common misconception, though, is to order a CT scan and to only use

those results to rule out stroke. Noncontrast head CT is a very poor test to identify acute ischemic cerebrovascular accident (CVA) in general, and is even worse in identification of posterior fossa strokes. MRI with Diffusion Weight Imaging (DWI) is currently considered the gold standard for identification of acute ischemic stroke. As discussed previously, since there is a small percentage of posterior fossa strokes that may be missed using this test, other aspects of the patient's history, physical examination, and specialist consultation may need to be incorporated into the patient's care. Neurology admission and repeat imaging may be necessary if clinical suspicion is still high for a central process.

Central Causes of Vertigo

In an effort to aid the clinician in determining if the presenting symptoms are of a stroke, characteristics of lesions along vascular distributions

Figure 37.7 Epley Maneuver

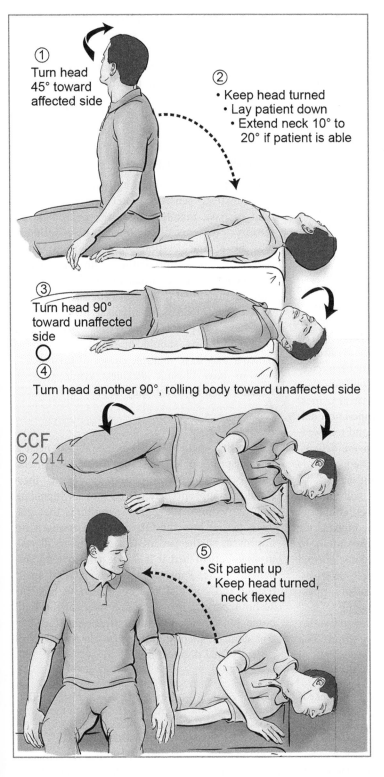

① Turn head 45° toward affected side

② • Keep head turned
• Lay patient down
• Extend neck 10° to 20° if patient is able

③ Turn head 90° toward unaffected side

④ Turn head another 90°, rolling body toward unaffected side

CCF © 2014

⑤ • Sit patient up
• Keep head turned, neck flexed

with dizziness presentations will be discussed here. As previously discussed, truncal ataxia is a good predictor of a central lesion. Generally patients may have difficulty ambulating with a peripheral lesion, but should be able to do so. With a central lesion, patients are too uncomfortable to walk and generally will fall if not properly aided. Cerebellar strokes represent only 3% of total strokes, but unfortunately will often have nonspecific findings (nausea, vomiting, unsteady gait, or headache) or subtle neurological findings (ataxia, dysarthria, and nystagmus). Usually superior cerebellar artery ischemia minimally involves the brainstem and may present with any of the aforementioned findings.

Ischemia of the anterior inferior cerebellar artery (AICA) can result in tinnitus, hearing loss, Horner Syndrome or facial weakness. Hence, care must be taken to ensure that a misdiagnosis of Meniere's disease is not given for AICA ischemia.

Posterior inferior cerebellar artery (PICA) ischemia is termed lateral medullary syndrome, also known as Wallenberg syndrome. Characteristic findings of lateral medullary syndrome are fairly extensive and include contralateral truncal and extremity sensory, pain, and temperature deficits, ipsilateral facial sensory, pain, and temperature deficits, and ipsilateral cranial nerve deficits. This, along with vertebrobasilar ischemia, tends to have very notable neurological findings.

Vertebrobasilar ischemia often will include symptoms of pupillary abnormalities, abnormal ocular movements, facial palsy, hemiplegia or quadriplegia. Other intracranial differentials to consider include space occupying lesions, normal pressure hydrocephalus, and multiple sclerosis. These can usually be identified by history, physical examination, and the proper imaging.

Integration of data is important for determination of patient diagnosis and disposition. The clinician should seek out specialist consultation in cases of increased complexity, special interventions, diagnostic help, or suspected further inpatient evaluation and treatment. Patients with dizziness complaints are frequently placed in the OU to rule out cardiac ischemia or to rule out strokes, so frequently cardiac and neurological workups are initiated within the OU. These workups are discussed elsewhere in this text.

Causes of Dizziness

Patients presenting with the disequilibrium subtype (unsteady sensation) after complete workup tend to have mainly orthopedic, neurologic or sensory problems. Additionally, polypharmacy may be a consideration and may need to be checked. Patients presenting with presyncope subtype tend to have cardiac or vasomotor conditions as their final diagnosis. Patients presenting with lightheadedness or atypical dizziness also may have polypharmacy as a cause, but psychiatric conditions should be considered. Some patients may have multiple causes of their dizziness or have chronic dizziness syndromes, of which a team approach may help.

Summary

Ultimately, a patient placed in the OU will need a final disposition within 24 hours. If the patient requires further workup and treatment, they should be appropriately placed into an inpatient bed. Sometimes, the patient symptoms that got them placed into the OU have not resolved or improved, so the patient will need to be placed in an inpatient bed if it is not safe to send the patient home. Patients may also have all their testing and consultations completed within the 24-hour period, in which case they can be sent home for further outpatient treatment. Overall, the clinical picture will help determine the patient's final disposition.

Bibliography

1. Newman-Toker DE, Hsieh YH, Carmargo CA Jr, et al. Spectrum of dizziness visits to US emergency departments: cross-sectional analysis from a nationally representative sample. *Mayo Clin Proc* 2008; 83:765–775.

2. Kroenke K, Lucas CA, Rosenberg ML, et al. Causes of persistent dizziness. *Ann Intern Med* 1992;117(11): 898–904.

3. Dros J, Maarshingh O, et al. Tests used to evaluate dizziness in primary care. *CMAJ Sept* 2010; 182 (13):E621–31.

4. Herr RD, Zun L, Mathews JJ. A directed approach to the dizzy patient. *Ann Emerg Med* 1989; 18(6):664–672.

5. Hoffman RM, Einstadter D, Kroenke K. Evaluating dizziness. *Am J Med* 1999; 107(5):468–478.

6. Kentala E, Rauch SD. A practical assessment algorithm for diagnosis of dizziness. *Otolaryngol Head Neck Surg* 2003;128(1):54–59.

7. White J. Benign paroxysmal positional vertigo: How to diagnose and quickly treat it. *Cleveland Clinic Journal of Medicine Sept* 2004; 71(9): 722–728.

8. Bronstein AM, Lempert T, Seemungal BM. Chronic dizziness: a practical approach. *Pract Neurol* 2010; 10:129–139.

9. Dizziness in the elderly. *British Journal of Hospital Medicine* Jan 2011, 72(1):M4–7.

10. Barin K, Dodson E, Dizziness in the elderly. *Otolaryngol Clin N Am* 2011; 44 437–454.

11. Thabet E, Evaluation of patients with acute vestibular syndrome. *Eur Arch Otorhinolaryngol* 2008; 265:341–349.

12. Wetmore S, Eibling D, Goebel J, et al. Challenges and opportunities in managing the dizzy older adult. *Otolaryngology–Head and Neck Surgery* 2011 144(5) 651–656.

13. Labuguen, Ronald H. Initial evaluation of vertigo. *Am Fam Physician.* 2006 Jan 15; 73(2):244–251.

14. Rubin D, Cheshire W. Evaluation of "dizziness" in the neurology office. *Semin Neurol* 2011;31:29–41.

15. Kerber K. Vertigo presentations in the emergency department. *Semin Neurol* 2009;29:482–490.

16. Kulstad C, Hannafin B. Dizzy and confused: A step-by-step evaluation of the clinician's favorite chief complaint. *Emerg Med Clin N Am* 2010;28: 453–469.

17. Kerber K, Morgenstern L, Meurer William. Nystagmus assessments documented by emergency physicians in acute dizziness presentations: A target for decision support? *Academic Emergency Medicine* 2011;18:619–626.

18. Post R, Dickerson L. Dizziness: A diagnostic approach. *Amer Fam Phys* 2010;82(4): 361–368.

19. Drachman DA, Hart CW. An approach to the dizzy patient. *Neurology* 1972;22(4): 323–334.

20. Kerber KA, Fendrick AM. The evidence base for the evaluation and management of dizziness. *J of Eval in Clin Prac* 2010;16: 186–191.

21. Kentala E, Rauch S. A practical assessment algorithm for diagnosis of dizziness. *Otolaryngology: Head and Neck Surgery* 2010;128(1): 54–59.

22. Swartz R, Longwell P. Treatment of Vertigo. *Amer Fam Physician*; Mar 15, 2005; 71(6):1115–1122.

23. Bhattacharyya N, Baugh RF, Orvidas L, et al. Clinical practice guideline: Benign paroxysmal positional vertigo *Otolaryngology–Head and Neck Surgery* 2008;139: S47–S81.

24. Tarnutzer AA, Berkowitz AL, Robinson KA, et al. Does my dizzy patient have a stroke? A systematic review of bedside diagnosis in acute vestibular syndrome. *CMAJ*, June 14, 2011;183(9):E571–E592.

25. Kattah JC, Talkad AV, Wang DZ, et al. Three-step bedside oculomotor examination more sensitive than MRI diffusion-weighted imaging. *Stroke*, 2009; 40:3504–3510.

26. Savitz SI, Caplan LR, Edlow JA. Pitfalls in the diagnosis of cerebellar Infarction. *Academic Emergency Medicine* 2007; 14:63–68.

27. Chan Y. Differential diagnosis of dizziness. *Curr Opin Otolaryngol Head Neck Surg.* 2009 Jun;17(3):200–203.

Chapter

38

Central Nervous System (CNS) Shunts

Mark G. Moseley, MD, MHA, FACEP
Miles P. Hawley, MD, MBA

Introduction

Intracranial hypertension has many different causes including brain mass, infection, hydrocephalus, cerebral venous thrombosis and idiopathic intracranial hypertension, or pseudotumor cerebri. Patients with intracranial hypertension are frequently treated with shunt placement. Shunt placement is often done to improve symptoms including headache and vision changes.[1] Shunt placement is usually performed by a neurosurgeon after medical treatment has failed. The most common types of shunts placed to relieve intracranial pressure include ventriculoperitoneal shunts and lumboperitoneal shunts.

The complication rate from shunting is high. In addition, shunts do not often completely alleviate symptoms.[2] For these reasons, patients with intracranial hypertension and ventriculoperitoneal or lumboperitoneal shunts frequently present to the emergency department (ED) with symptoms. Symptoms commonly include headache and vision changes. It can be difficult to determine on initial evaluation if the symptoms are related to shunt malfunction, underlying intracranial hypertension or another process. These patients can often complete an evaluation in the observation unit (OU).

Discussion

There is very little evidence to guide the evaluation of patients with potential shunt malfunction. Shunt failure is the most common complication of shunt placement. Shunt failure in patients with lumboperitoneal shunts occurs in 48 to 86% of patients.[2–8] Some patients will require multiple revisions. Other shunt complications include shunt infection, abdominal pain, back pain and CSF leak. Shunt infection occurs in approximately 10% of patients.[9] Rare complications include subdural and subarachnoid hemorrhage, cerebellar tonsillar herniation and syringomyelia.[10–13]

In addition to the known complications of ventriculoperitoneal or lumboperitoneal shunts, these patients often have symptoms from their underlying disease process. Patients with idiopathic intracranial hypertension often have persistent headache and vision changes despite shunting.[2]

The goal of evaluating these patients when they present to the ED is to exclude life-threatening causes of their symptoms, provide symptom relief and set up an appropriate treatment plan. For these patients this often includes excluding infection, shunt malfunction and elevated intracranial pressure.

Patient Criteria

Inclusion criteria

- Ventriculoperitoneal or lumboperitoneal shunt placed for elevated intracranial hypertension.
- Presenting complaint that may be related to shunt malfunction or elevated intracranial pressure.
- Expectation that diagnostic work-up can be completed in under 24 hours.

Exclusion criteria

- High likelihood of shunt infection or meningitis.
- New abnormality on head CT or MRI.
- Other medical conditions that make discharge in under 24 hours unlikely such as severe dehydration, uncontrolled diabetes, and uncontrolled hypertension.

Management

Patients with ventriculoperitoneal or lumboperitoneal shunts who present with symptoms such as headache or blurred vision need a complex diagnostic workup and often therapeutic treatment as well. The goal of the diagnostic workup is to exclude shunt malfunction, shunt infection and elevated intracranial pressure. Initial testing should be a noncontrast head CT scan. This is often performed in the ED prior to placing the patient in the OU. The purpose of this test is to rule out new brain mass, bleeding and significant hydrocephalus. Following a head CT, a shunt series can be obtained to look for any kinking or discontinuity in the shunt. If any abnormalities are found on the shunt series then neurosurgery should be contacted immediately to determine if urgent surgery should be performed. These patients will normally require a lumbar puncture to obtain an opening CSF pressure and CSF fluid for analysis. This often will need to be done by radiology under fluoroscopy. An opening pressure will help determine if the shunt is functioning appropriately and if the patient's symptoms are likely to be related to elevated intracranial pressure. CSF is often sent for cell count, protein, glucose, culture and gram stain. Infection can usually be ruled out based on CSF studies. Ophthalmology consultation may be necessary to evaluate for papilledema. Neurosurgical consultation is often required to assist in evaluation and adjustment of the shunt.

In addition to diagnostic evaluation, these patients also present with headache, dehydration and hypertension. Many of the principles for treating general headache apply to this patient population – quiet, hydration, darkness, rest, and anti-emetics. These patients may require opioid pain medications initially to control their symptoms. Caution should be used when using opioids, given analgesic rebound headaches and the possibility of narcotic abuse. These patients often present dehydrated due to nausea and vomiting. They will benefit from hydration with IV fluids and treatment with anti-emetics. This patient population often has comorbid hypertension. They frequently present with elevated blood pressure. This can occasionally be treated by prescribing home medications or giving oral medications. However, given that these patients frequently have nausea as a presenting symptom they often require treatment with IV medications. Blood pressure should be monitored closely during their evaluation, as uncontrolled hypertension may be contributing to their symptoms.

Outcome

There are two primary end points in this patient population: ruling out life-threatening pathology and controlling symptoms. When life-threatening pathology has been adequately ruled out then the patient needs to be evaluated for discharge. This evaluation includes ensuring that symptoms are manageable, the patient is able to tolerate PO and the patient has good follow-up. When all of these goals have been met then the patient is appropriate for discharge from observation status.

Conclusion

Management of patients with ventriculoperitoneal or lumboperitoneal shunts can be complicated. These patients often present with symptoms that could be related to shunt malfunction, infection or underlying disease process. These patients require an extended workup to rule out life-threatening pathology. In addition, these patients also require significant symptom control. With appropriate planning, this patient population can be safely managed in an OU.

References

1. Corbett JJ, Thompson HS. The rational management of idiopathic intracranial hypertension. *Arch Neurol* 1989; 46:1049.

2. McGirt MJ, Woodworth G, Thomas G, et al. Cerebrospinal fluid shunt placement for pseudotumor cerebri-associated intractable headache: predictors of treatment response and an analysis of long-term outcomes. *J Neurosurg* 2004; 101:627.

3. Burgett RA, Purvin VA, Kawasaki A. Lumboperitoneal shunting for pseudotumor cerebri. *Neurology* 1997; 49:734.

4. Eggenberger ER, Miller NR, Vitale S. Lumboperitoneal shunt for the treatment of pseudotumor cerebri. *Neurology* 1996; 46:1524.

5. Johnston I, Besser M, Morgan MK. Cerebrospinal fluid diversion in the treatment of benign intracranial hypertension. *J Neurosurg* 1988; 69:195.

6. Chumas PD, Kulkarni AV, Drake JM, et al. Lumboperitoneal shunting: a retrospective study in the pediatric population. *Neurosurgery* 1993; 32:376.

7. Rosenberg ML, Corbett JJ, Smith C, et al. Cerebrospinal

fluid diversion procedures in pseudotumor cerebri. *Neurology* 1993; 43:1071.

8. Lundar T, Nornes H. Pseudotumour cerebri-neurosurgical considerations. *Acta Neurochir Suppl (Wien)* 1990; 51:366.

9. Mayhall CG, Archer NH, Lamb VA, et al. Ventriculostomy-related infections. A prospective epidemiologic study. *N Engl J Med* 1984; 310:553.

10. Chumas PD, Armstrong DC, Drake JM, et al. Tonsillar herniation: the rule rather than the exception after lumboperitoneal shunting in the pediatric population. *J Neurosurg* 1993; 78:568.

11. Sell JJ, Rupp FW, Orrison WW Jr. Iatrogenically induced intracranial hypotension syndrome. *AJR Am J Roentgenol* 1995; 165:1513.

12. Padmanabhan R, Crompton D, Burn D, Birchall D. Acquired Chiari 1 malformation and syringomyelia following lumboperitoneal shunting for pseudotumour cerebri. *J Neurol Neurosurg Psychiatry* 2005; 76:298.

13. Suri A, Pandey P, Mehta VS. Subarachnoid hemorrhage and intracereebral hematoma following lumboperitoneal shunt for pseudotumor cerebri: a rare complication. *Neurol India* 2002; 50:508.

Chapter

39

Hyperglycemia

Pawan Suri, MD
Taruna Aurora, MD

Introduction

The clinical presentation of hyperglycemia in the emergency department (ED) varies greatly and can range from nonketotic hyperglycemia on the one end of the spectrum to diabetic ketoacidosis (DKA) on the other extreme. While some patients present with new-onset diabetes, most patients with hyperglycemia will have a prior history of Type I or Type II diabetes. Nonketotic hyperglycemia is also known as hyperosmolar hyperglycemic state (HHS) and differs from DKA due to the absence of ketoacidosis and the degree of hyperglycemia.[1] Approximately 33% of patients with hyperglycemia will have features of both DKA and HHS.[2] Regardless of the type of clinical presentation, the basic principles of hyperglycemia management are very similar.

While milder forms of DKA and HHS can be managed in an observation unit (OU), serious presentations carry significant morbidity and mortality and require inpatient admission and occasionally intensive care unit admission. New-onset diabetics who do not have a primary care physician or health insurance coverage pose a unique disposition dilemma for the treating emergency physician. While these patients often do not meet acute inpatient admission criteria, it is unsafe to discharge them without proper diabetic teaching and resources to manage their disease. We find the OU especially useful for this cohort of hyperglycemia patients.

Clinical Presentation

Significant hyperglycemia classically presents with polydipsia, polyuria, and polyphagia, with or without weight loss. DKA tends to develop rapidly over the course of a few hours to a day. The cardinal feature of DKA is the presence of an anion gap metabolic acidosis and ketonemia, both of which are absent in HHS.[1] Due to the metabolic acidosis, patients with DKA will often present with hyperventilation, abdominal pain and vomiting.[3] The abdominal pain seen in DKA is thought to be due to delayed gastric emptying and ileus associated with metabolic acidosis and electrolyte abnormalities. It is rare to see abdominal pain in the absence of acidosis.

In contrast, patients with HHS are not acidotic as evidenced by a pH of > 7.30, negative urine and serum ketones and serum bicarbonate of > 20 meq/dl. While serum glucose concentration can exceed 1000 mg/dl in HHS, it is usually less than 800 mg/dl in DKA.[1,5-6] Patients with HHS are much more likely to exhibit neurologic symptoms like lethargy, confusion and obtundation because of higher plasma osmolality.[2,5,6] These symptoms do not develop until plasma osmolality exceeds 320–330 mosmol/kg. Therefore the presence of neurological deficits in diabetic patient with plasma osmolality below 320 mosmol/kg should prompt the search for alternate causes. Some patients with HHS can even have focal neurologic signs like seizures or hemiparesis.[7]

When evaluating a patient with hyperglycemia for a possible admission to the OU, it is helpful to consider potential precipitating causes. The two most common reasons for hyperglycemia in the ED are noncompliance with antidiabetic regimen and infections.[2,5,6] Other causes include cerebrovascular accident (CVA), pancreatitis, acute myocardial infarction (MI), drugs like glucocorticoids, atypical antipsychotics, and thiazide diuretics and insulin pump malfunction. Psychological problems associated with eating disorders that lead to poor compliance with insulin regimens and cocaine use may require additional resources such as psychiatric consultation and substance abuse counseling.[8]

The serum osmolality can be calculated using the formula:

$$\text{Effective Plasma Osmolality} = [2 \times Na\ (mEq/L)] \\ + [glucose\ (mg/dL) \div 18] \\ + [BUN\ (mg/dL) \div 2.8]$$

There are two main reasons for the increased plasma osmolality seen in DKA and HHS. The first is a rise in serum glucose and the second, more important reason is the loss of free water due to glucose osmotic diuresis.[4] Anuric end-stage renal disease patients with severe hyperglycemia do not exhibit the rise in plasma osmolality and rarely develop neurologic symptoms.[9]

On physical exam, patients with DKA may have the classic Kussmaul respirations (rapid, deep breathing) and a "fruity breath" due to ketone production. The extent of dehydration in both DKA and HHS can be gauged from the physical examination, specifically looking for dry mucous membranes, decrease in skin turgor, dry axillae, and hypotension.

In DKA, there are three ketone bodies produced: acetone, acetoacetic acid, and beta-hydroxybutyric acid. In severe DKA, beta-hydroxybutyric acid is the predominant ketone. The commonly used nitorprusside test detects only acetone and acetoacetic acid and in rare circumstances it is possible to have a negative nitorprusside test in the presence of severe ketosis.[2] Some hospital labs offer beta-hydroxybutyric acid testing, but it is not widely available.

Serum sodium tends to decrease with rising serum glucose due to dilution from osmotic water movement out of the cells. Serum sodium concentration falls by approximately 1.6 meq/L for every 100 mg/dL rise in serum glucose.[10] There is an overall total body potassium deficit due to gastrointestinal losses, loss of potassium from cells due to glycogenolysis, urinary losses from glucose osmotic diuresis as well as hypovolemia-induced hyperaldosteronism. Despite a potassium deficit, the serum potassium concentration is either normal or may even be elevated[4] due to solvent drag from water movement out of the cell as well as insulin deficiency that impedes potassium uptake by cells. Further, acidemia plays a small role through a transcellular exchange of potassium with hydrogen ions resulting in a rise in serum potassium. Similarly, serum phosphate concentration is usually normal or high because of metabolic acidosis and insulin deficiency despite a total body phosphate deficit from osmotic diuresis and decreased phosphate intake.[11] Insulin therapy can unmask this low phosphate that is usually asymptomatic. Clinically evident hemolysis as well as rhabdomyolysis with myoglobinuria are rare complications of hypophosphatemia.[12,13]

There may be unexplained elevation of serum amylase and lipase in DKA without evidence of acute pancreatitis, therefore a diagnosis of pancreatitis in patients with DKA has to be made by clinical findings consistent with acute pancreatitis and abdominal CT scan.[14] Leukocytosis unrelated to infection often occurs in hyperglycemic patients but the exact etiology of this nonspecific leukocytosis is not known. Increase in white cell count corresponds to the degree of ketosis,[15] though WBCs > 25,000/microL or greater than 10% bands may favor an infectious etiology.[16]

The combination of insulin deficiency and increase in ACTH, glucagon, growth hormone and catecholamines in DKA and HHS leads to lipolysis and marked hypertriglyceridemia and hypercholesterolemia.[17] These abnormalities start to resolve within 24 hours of insulin therapy.

Patient Selection

Hyperglycemic patients presenting to the ED with blood glucose level < 600 and a pH > 7.2 can be successfully managed in an ED OU provided they do not have new onset DKA, acute mental status changes, end-stage renal disease, sepsis, acute CVA, acute MI, or infections, or significant complications. (Both glucose and ph levels for the indication for ICU admission are an arbitrary cut off with no support in literature, in general.) Patients who do not meet the blood glucose and pH criteria upon ED presentation and have treatment initiated with fluid replacement and insulin are often able to meet these criteria upon reevaluation if they remain in the ED.

Observation Unit Management

Patients with hyperglycemia who are admitted to an OU are carefully selected to exclude seriously ill patients who may require inpatient or ICU management. However, it is imperative to closely monitor and follow these patients in the OU. This may include reevaluation in order to identify and treat any underlying events that may have precipitated the hyperglycemia and to recognize any complications, as well as to assess the progress of therapy.

The primary goals of treatment of both DKA and HHS are frequent monitoring, administration of IV fluids and insulin therapy to correct hypovolemia, hyperglycemia, hyperosmolality, electrolyte abnormalities, and in the case of DKA, correct the metabolic acidosis.

All patients with hyperglycemia should have a complete blood count, serum electrolytes including serum glucose, blood urea nitrogen (BUN) and creatinine, urinalysis and an EKG done. If there is an anion gap or the presence of ketones in the urine, patients should have arterial (or venous) blood gas (ABG)(VBG) and serum ketones drawn. Optional tests may include a chest x-ray, blood and urine cultures, cardiac enzymes, amylase and lipase. For patients with new-onset hyperglycemia obtain a baseline weight and consider sending HbA1C, liver function tests (for Type II diabetics), c-peptide and insulin antibodies. Even though these test results may not be available prior to discharge, they will help follow-up care.

Most patients will have an elevated BUN and creatinine. DKA presents with a high anion gap metabolic acidosis and low serum bicarbonate. Sometimes DKA can present with serum glucose that may be only slightly elevated or even in the normal range. This occurs in patients with poor oral intake or pregnancy.[18]

Check the serum glucose every hour while the patient is on an intravenous insulin infusion. Serum electrolytes, blood urea nitrogen, creatinine should be measured every 4 hours.[19] We do not repeat ABGs during treatment and elect to rely on serial bicarbonate measurements and the anion gap to determine the extent of acidosis. If needed, the venous pH can be checked instead, which is about 0.03 units lower than arterial pH and is less painful for the patient.[20]

Fluid Replacement – The osmotic diuresis seen in DKA and HHS leads to significant volume depletion that can average up to 6 L in DKA and 10 L in HHS.[1] In addition, for each liter of fluid lost, there is concomitant loss of approximately 70 meq of sodium and potassium. Hence, one of the most important goals of therapy is to replace the intravascular volume and electrolytes.

If this is done too rapidly, it can lead to precipitous lowering of plasma osmolality and cause cerebral edema. Isotonic saline (0.9% sodium chloride) is the fluid of choice and is given at a rate of 10–15 mL/Kg per hour, not to exceed 50 mL/Kg in the first 4 hours[19] with a goal of replacing estimated deficits within the first 24 hours. Response to fluid replacement can be judged by hemodynamic monitoring and urine output. As renal perfusion increases, serum glucose is further reduced by increasing urinary loss of glucose.[21] While isotonic saline is the appropriate fluid for initial hydration, one-half isotonic saline can be used if the corrected serum sodium is normal or elevated and if concurrent potassium replacement is needed.[19]

The serum creatinine is initially elevated out of proportion to the fall in glomerular filtration rate, because acetoacetate artifactually raises measured creatinine in the standard colorimetric assay.[22] With fluid replacement, as the glomerular filtration rate rises, BUN and creatinine fall to normal levels.

Insulin Therapy – Insulin remains the cornerstone of therapy for treating hyperglycemia. For treating DKA a continuous IV regular insulin drip can be started at 0.14 U/kg per hour. Alternately, the patient can be given a bolus of 0.1 U/kg followed by a continuous infusion at 0.1 U/kg per hour.[23] Both the approaches are equally effective. Contrary to popular belief, insulin lowers serum glucose primarily by decreasing hepatic glucose production rather than enhancing peripheral utilization.[24] Insulin, in relatively low doses, exerts a potent antilipolytic effect. Insulin infusion is started after ensuring that serum potassium is above 3.3 meq/L since insulin will worsen the hypokalemia and may lead to possible arrhythmias, cardiac arrest, and respiratory muscle weakness.[19]

Initial fluid repletion will reduce serum glucose by 35–70 mg/dL per hour by increasing urinary losses and hemodilution. Addition of insulin will further reduce serum glucose. If the serum glucose does not fall by 50–70 mg/dL in the first hour, the insulin infusion should be doubled every hour until a steady decline in serum glucose is achieved. Higher doses of insulin will not produce greater than 50–70 mg/dL fall because the insulin receptors are already saturated.[25]

When the serum glucose reaches 200 mg/dL in DKA or 250–300 mg/dL in HHS, the insulin infusion rate can be reduced by half to 0.05 U/Kg per hour and the intravenous saline solution is switched to dextrose in saline.[2] Any further reduction in the serum glucose at this time below 200 mg/dL in DKA or 250–300 mg/dL in HHS may promote the development of cerebral edema. Newer insulin analogs like glulisine insulin are equally effective in treating hypoglycemia. Another alternative for treating uncomplicated, mild DKA is the use of subcutaneous insulin analogs (insulin lispro and aspart).[26]

Insulin infusion causes a rapid reversal of potassium distribution from extracellular to the intracellular space and it is very important to carefully monitor serum potassium. If the serum potassium is initially elevated despite substantial total body potassium deficit, repletion is not begun until the serum potassium concentration falls below 5.3. The use of one-half isotonic saline is preferred when adding potassium (20–40 meq/L) since it is osmotically active and if added to isotonic saline, it will yield a hypertonic solution that will be unable to correct the hyperosmolality. The goal is to maintain serum potassium between 4.0 and 5.0 meq/L. Reversing the hyperglycemia with insulin will lower the plasma osmolality, which will cause water to move from the extracellular fluid into the cells, thereby raising the serum sodium concentration.[5,10,19,27]

Bicarbonate therapy is usually not needed in the stable hyperglycemic patients admitted to an OU, though it may be indicated in severe cases with a serum pH < 6.9 or severe hyperkalemia. Side effects of bicarbonate therapy include reduced respiratory drive, increase in $pCO2$ and paradoxical CNS acidosis.[28] Bicarbonate administration can also slow down the rate of recovery of the ketosis[29] and lead to a post-treatment metabolic alkalosis.

Despite the hypophosphatemia accompanying insulin therapy, routine use of phosphate replacement is not recommended because of potential side effects like hypocalcemia and hypomagnesaemia. Phosphate replacement in the form of 20–30 meq/L of potassium phosphate added to replacement fluids is reserved for patients with a serum phosphate of < 1.0 mg/dl or patients who show signs of cardiac dysfunction, hemolytic anemia, or respiratory depression.

Cerebral edema and noncardiogenic pulmonary edema are rare complications of the treatment of DKA and HHS. Most cases of cerebral edema are seen below the age of 20.[30] OU management should include looking for symptoms like headache that may develop within 12 hours of therapy. Once developed, cerebral edema can progress rapidly to obtundation, seizures and death, with an overall mortality between 20% and 40%.[19] Ensuring that initial fluid replacement does not exceed 50 mL/Kg in the first 4 hours and not letting the blood glucose fall below 200 by switching replacement fluids to dextrose (see earlier) are two strategies used to prevent cerebral edema. Both mannitol and hypertonic saline have been used to treat cerebral edema.[30]

New-onset Diabetics – All the new-onset diabetics in our OU get a literacy test. We use REALM-R (Rapid Estimate of Adult Literacy in Medicine, Revised) available at adultmeducation. com to gauge the ability of English-speaking patients to understand diabetes teaching packet instructions. Low Literacy instruction pamphlets are available. Patients also get a visual acuity to determine if they are able to measure insulin accurately. Insulin pens are preferred for visually impaired patients. If available, a diabetes educator (usually a nurse or a midlevel provider) are excellent resources and should be involved in patient management.

For all Type I diabetics, who are usually thinner and insulin sensitive, we start insulin at a total daily dose of 0.3 units/kg/day[31] and recommend an endocrinology consult. We use a single daily subcutaneous injection of the long-acting Glargine insulin (Lantus) along with 4 units of Humalog at the largest meal. If the patient is unable to afford the Lantus, we start NPH insulin twice a day in divided doses of 0.15 units/kg/day. We ensure the patient can perform self-glucose-monitoring and is able to self-administer insulin and provide the patient with a blood glucose meter or a prescription to get one.

For Type II diabetics, who are typically obese and insulin resistant, we use oral antidiabetic medications and insulin, either alone or in combination. For patients with blood glucose < 200, start monotherapy with metformin 500 mg twice a day unless there is a contraindication (serum creatinine > 1.5, congestive heart faillure [CHF], elevated liver enzymes, alcohol abuse or IV contrast within 48 hours). Patients with blood glucose > 200 can start once daily Lantus at 0.4 units/kg/day and metformin 500 mg twice a day. Another option is to start NPH insulin 0.2 units/kg twice a day along with metformin 500 mg twice a day.[32] All patients must have access to a glucose meter and be able to use it.

Observation Unit Outcome

Tokarski et al. conducted a retrospective observational study of 101 pediatric and adult patients admitted to an OU with mild to moderate DKA over the course of a year. OU patients had a mean arterial pH of 7.3 and a mean blood glucose of 489 mg/dl. Sixty percent of patients were discharged from the OU after a mean total ED OU stay of 22.8 hours. Complications included hypoglycemia (6%) and recurrent hyperglycemia or ketosis requiring reinstitution of the insulin infusion (22%).[33] Patients with uncomplicated DKA or HHS respond well to OU management with fluid replacement and insulin and can be safely discharged. The OU also provides an opportunity for diabetic teaching that includes self-monitoring of blood glucose and insulin administration. There could be potential cost saving for the hospital if the OU can demonstrate earlier disposition as opposed to inpatient admission.

References

1. Kitabchi AE, Umpierrez GE, Murohy MB, et al. Hyperglycemic crises in adult patients with diabetes: a consensus statement from the American Diabetes Association. *Diabetes Care*, 2006. 29(12): 2739–2748.

2. Kitabchi AE, Umpierrez GE, Murphy MB, et al. Management of hyperglycemic crises in patients with diabetes. *Diabetes Care*, 2001. 24(1): 131–153.

3. Malone ML, Gennis V, Goodwin JS. Characteristics of diabetic ketoacidosis in older versus younger adults. *J Am Geriatr Soc*, 1992. 40(11): 1100–1104.

4. Arieff AI, Carroll HJ. Nonketotic hyperosmolar coma with hyperglycemia: clinical features, pathophysiology, renal function, acid-base balance, plasma-cerebrospinal fluid equilibria and the effects of therapy in 37 cases. *Medicine (Baltimore)*, 1972. 51(2): 73–94.

5. Fulop MH, Tannenbaum H, Dreyer N. Ketotic hyperosmolar coma. *Lancet*, 1973. 2(7830): 635–639.

6. Daugirdas JT, Kronfol NO, Tzamaloukas AH, et al. Hyperosmolar coma: cellular dehydration and the serum sodium concentration. *Ann Intern Med*, 1989. 110(11): 855–857.

7. Lavin PJ. Hyperglycemic hemianopia: a reversible complication of non-ketotic hyperglycemia. *Neurology*, 2005. 65(4): 616–619.

8. Nyenwe EA, Loganathan RS, Blum S, et al. Active use of cocaine: an independent risk factor for recurrent diabetic ketoacidosis in a city hospital. *Endocr Pract*, 2007. 13(1): 22–29.

9. Al-Kudsi RR, Daugindas JT, Ing TS, et al. Extreme hyperglycemia in dialysis patients. *Clin Nephrol*, 1982. 17(5): 228–231.

10. Katz MA. Hyperglycemia-induced hyponatremia – calculation of expected serum sodium depression. *N Engl J Med*, 1973. 289(16): 843–844.

11. Kebler R, McDonald, Cadnapaphornchai P. Dynamic changes in serum phosphorus levels in diabetic ketoacidosis. *Am J Med*, 1985. 79(5): 571–576.

12. Casteels K, Beckers D, Wouters C, et al. Rhabdomyolysis in diabetic ketoacidosis. *Pediatr Diabetes*, 2003. 4(1): 29–31.

13. Shilo SD, Werner D, Hershko C. Acute hemolytic anemia caused by severe hypophosphatemia in diabetic ketoacidosis. *Acta Haematol*, 1985. 73(1): 55–57.

14. Yadav D, Nair S, Norkus ED, et al. Nonspecific hyperamylasemia and hyperlipasemia in diabetic ketoacidosis: incidence and correlation with biochemical abnormalities. *Am J Gastroenterol*, 2000. 95(11): 3123–3128.

15. Stentz FB, Umpierrez GE, Cuervo R, et al. Proinflammatory cytokines, markers of cardiovascular risks, oxidative stress, and lipid peroxidation in patients with hyperglycemic crises. *Diabetes*, 2004. 53(8): 2079–2086.

16. Slovis CM, Monk VG, Slovis RG, et al. Diabetic ketoacidosis and infection: leukocyte count and differential as early predictors of serious infection. *Am J Emerg Med*, 1987. 5(1): 1–5.

17. Weidman SW, Ragland JB, Fisher JN Jr, et al. Effects of insulin on plasma lipoproteins in diabetic ketoacidosis: evidence for a change in high density lipoprotein composition during treatment. *J Lipid Res*, 1982. 23(1): 171–182.

18. Burge MR, Hardy KJ, Schade DS. Short-term fasting is a mechanism for the development of euglycemic ketoacidosis during periods of insulin deficiency. *J Clin Endocrinol Metab*, 1993. 76(5): 1192–1198.

19. Kitabchi AE, Umpierrez GE, Miles JM, et al. Hyperglycemic crises in adult patients with diabetes. *Diabetes Care*, 2009. 32(7): 1335–1343.

20. Middleton P, Kelly AM, Brown J, et al. Agreement between arterial and central venous values for pH, bicarbonate, base excess, and lactate. *Emerg Med J*, 2006. 23(8): 622–624.

21. Hillman K. Fluid resuscitation in diabetic emergencies–a reappraisal. *Intensive Care Med*, 1987. 13(1): 4–8.

22. Molitch ME, Rodman E, Hirsch CA, et al. Spurious serum creatinine elevations in ketoacidosis. *Ann Intern Med*, 1980. 93(2): 280–281.

23. Kitabchi AE, Murphy MB, Spencer J, et al. Is a priming dose of insulin necessary in a low-dose insulin protocol for the treatment of diabetic ketoacidosis? *Diabetes Care*, 2008. 31(11): 2081–2085.

24. Luzi L, Barrett EJ, Groop LC, et al. Metabolic effects of low-dose insulin therapy on glucose metabolism in diabetic ketoacidosis. *Diabetes*, 1988. 37 (11): 1470–1477.

25. Brown PM, Tompkins CV, Juul S, et al. Mechanism of action of insulin in diabetic patients: a dose-related effect on glucose production and utilisation. *Br Med J*, 1978. 1(6122): 1239–1242.

26. Umpierrez GE, Cuervo R, Karabell A, et al. Treatment of diabetic ketoacidosis with subcutaneous insulin aspart. *Diabetes Care*, 2004. 27(8): 1873–1878.

27. Hillier TA, Abbott RD, Barrett EJ. Hyponatremia: evaluating the correction factor for hyperglycemia. *Am J Med*, 1999. 106(4): 399–403.

28. Narins RG, Cohen JJ. Bicarbonate therapy for organic acidosis: the case for its continued use. *Ann Intern Med*, 1987. 106(4): 615–618.

29. Okuda Y, Adrogue HJ, Field JB, et al. Counterproductive effects of sodium bicarbonate in diabetic ketoacidosis. *J Clin Endocrinol Metab*, 1996. 81(1): 314–320.

30. Wolfsdorf J, Glaser N, Sperling MA. Diabetic ketoacidosis in infants, children, and adolescents: A consensus statement from the American Diabetes Association. *Diabetes Care*, 2006. 29(5): 1150–1159.

31. *Medical Managment of Type I Diabetes*. American Diabetes Association, 2004. Alexandria, VA.

32. Nathan DM, Buse JB, Davidson MB, et al. Medical management of hyperglycemia in type 2 diabetes: a consensus algorithm for the initiation and adjustment of therapy: a consensus statement of the American Diabetes Association and the European Association for the Study of Diabetes. *Diabetes Care*, 2009. 32(1): 193–203.

33. Tokarski GF, Kahler JK. Diabetic ketoacidosis in the emergency department and clinical decision unit. *Ann Emerg Med*, 1998. 32(3): S15.

Chapter

40

Hypoglycemia

Pawan Suri, MD
Taruna Aurora, MD

Introduction

Severe hypoglycemia is defined as an episode that is undetected by the patient or is detected so late that intervention by someone else is required to inject glucagon or take the patient to the hospital to receive intravenous (IV) glucose.[1] Varying degrees of hypoglycemia are seen in both type I and type II diabetics. Type I diabetic patients on intensive insulin therapy have a greater than threefold increased risk of severe hypoglycemia.[2] Less commonly, severe hypoglycemia may also affect patients with type II diabetes who take either oral antidiabetic medications or insulin. In the Diabetes Control and Complications Trial (DCCT), type I diabetics had a 65% incidence of severe hypoglycemia when followed over 6.5 years.[2] In contrast, the cumulative incidence of hypoglycemia in type II diabetics who were followed over a period of 6 years was 3.3% in patients taking sulfonylureas and 11.2% in patients taking insulin.[3] Thus, hypoglycemia becomes a progressively more frequent clinical problem in type II diabetics as they approach the insulin deficient end of the disease spectrum.

Risk factors for hypoglycemia include patients over age 65, those taking multiple medications and those who are frequently hospitalized.[4,5] Commonly, patients have inadvertently taken excessive or ill-timed dose of their insulin or oral hypoglycemic agent. Decrease in exogenous glucose delivery – as seen with missed meals, delayed gastric emptying or an overnight state – is another frequent cause of hypoglycemic episodes. Long-acting agents such as chlorpropamide and glyburide are more likely to cause hypoglycemia.[4,6] Renal insufficiency is associated with a fourfold increased risk for hypoglycemia in patients taking sulfonylureas. Interaction of gatifloxacin with sulfonylureas can also cause hypoglycemia.[7] This is unique to gatifloxacin and not a quinolone class effect. ACE inhibitors increase insulin sensitivity and glucose disposal, increasing the risk of hypoglycemia. Nonselective ß-blockers can impair early warning symptoms and can lead to severe hypoglycemia.[8,9] One of the best predictors for developing severe hypoglycemia is a previous episode of severe hypoglycemia. The risk is also increased in patients with high initial HbA1c levels that decreased quickly after intensive insulin therapy was begun. Other minor risk factors include male sex, higher insulin doses and adolescents.

Pathophysiology

In normal subjects the extracellular supply of glucose is carefully regulated by insulin and glucagon.[5] Insulin acts to restore normoglycemia in three ways: (a) It decreases hepatic glucose production by inhibiting both glycogenolysis and gluconeogenesis, (b) Increased glucose uptake by skeletal muscle and adipose tissue by translocating glucose transporters from an intracellular pool to the cell surface, and (c) It reduces the delivery of gluconeogenetic precursors alanine and glycerol to the liver via its antiproteolytic and antilipolytic actions. Insulin also inhibits glucagon secretion by direct inhibition of the glucagon gene in the pancreatic alpha cells,[10] which further diminishes hepatic glucose production.

The ability to suppress insulin release is an important component of the normal response to hypoglycemia. Another defense against hypoglycemia is the increased release of counter-regulatory hormones, which raise plasma glucose concentration by stimulating glucose production and by antagonizing insulin induced increase in glucose utilization. In diabetics, since insulin is supplied exogenously and cannot be suppressed, the release of conterregulatory hormones becomes the primary defense against hypoglycemia.

These hormones are, in order of importance, glucagon, epinephrine, cortisol, and growth hormone.[5,11] Glucagon acts only on the liver, increasing glucose production by stimulating both glycogenolysis and gluconeogenesis from amino acids, glycerol, and pyruvate. Epinephrine, acting via ß-adrenergic receptors has similar hepatic effects. It also increases the delivery of gluconeogenic substrates from the periphery, inhibits glucose utilization and via alpha-2 receptors inhibits insulin secretion. In addition, epinephrine induces early warning symptoms of hypoglycemia including anxiety and sweating. If the hypoglycemia is severe and persists for several hours, there is increased secretion of cortisol and growth hormone, which limit glucose utilization and enhance hepatic glucose production. It is important to understand that the actions of insulin and glucagon are interdependent. In the pancreatic islets of Langerhans, the insulin producing ß-cells form the core, surrounded by glucagon producing alpha cells. Arterial blood enters the core of each islet, delivering substrates and information first to the beta cells and then to alpha and delta cells.[12] The alpha cells rely heavily on the presence of functioning beta cells in order to function,[13] a situation that is disturbed in diabetes.

Glycemic thresholds in normal subjects

– 80 mg/dl – Insulin secretion falls to very low levels
– 65–70 mg/dl – Release of glucagon and epinephrine, early protective response: sweating, anxiety, palpitations and tremors
– < 60 mg/dl – Early cognitive dysfunction and release of cortisol and growth hormone
– 45–50 mg/dl – Lethargy and obtundation
– < 30 mg/dl – Coma and convulsions

Response to Hypoglycemia in Diabetic Patients

The protective response to hypoglycemia is impaired in many diabetic patients.[14] This is particularly true when hypoglycemia is induced either directly from exogenous insulin injection or indirectly from sulfonylurea stimulation. In these patients insulin release cannot be turned off and therefore glucose utilization and inhibition of hepatic glucose production continues. Further, both glucagon and epinephrine response to hypoglycemia are impaired in many diabetic patients. Diabetic patients who are well controlled (HbA1c levels < 8%) may have few warning symptoms when their plasma glucose concentration falls below 60 mg/dl. The absence of epinephrine induced early warning symptoms can often lead to dangerously low blood glucose levels. The concept of hypoglycemia associated autonomic failure (HAAF) in type I diabetes mellitus (DM),[15–17] posits that recent antecedent hypoglycemia causes both defective glucose counterregulation and hypoglycemia unawareness, setting up a vicious cycle. Hypoglycemic episodes may lead to up regulation of glucose transport in the brain resulting in the maintenance of glucose uptake and therefore the prevention of warning symptoms of hypoglycemia. The compensatory increase in cortisol production during the first hypoglycemia episode may also play a critical role in minimizing the protective hormonal response during a subsequent episode.[18,19] As few as 2–3 weeks of scrupulous avoidance of hypoglycemia reverses hypoglycemia unawareness and improves the reduced epinephrine component of defective glucose counter regulation.

Hypoglycemia is less common in type II DM because deficits in glucagon and epinephrine are much less prominent[20] and strict glycemic control is much more difficult to achieve.[21] However, when hypoglycemia does occur in older patients, the glucose threshold for the onset of cognitive dysfunction may overlap with the onset of symptoms, thus limiting the time to initiate self treatment and increasing the risk of severe neurological events.[22]

Patient Selection

Hypoglycemic patients on long-acting insulin or oral hypoglycemic agents who fail to respond to oral or parenteral glucose or show recurrence of hypoglycemia in the emergency department (ED) are often hospitalized for further management. While most of these patients can be successfully managed in an ED observation unit (ED OU), some may require inpatient admission. These include patients with intentional insulin or oral antidiabetic medication overdose, patients with acute or chronic renal or hepatic insufficiency, persistent mental status changes despite glucose administration or those with an acute precipitating illness like sepsis, chronic heart failure, and others.

Observation Unit Management

A thorough history is essential in determining the cause of hypoglycemia. The amount, timing and reason for any ingestion, what drug was taken, and coingestants including other diabetic medications must be noted. Laboratory tests should include a basic metabolic panel and renal function with further testing as deemed necessary.

Hypoglycemia will respond rapidly to IV Dextrose (D-glucose) 0.5–1 gm/kg available in 50 ml ampoules containing 25 g glucose in a 50% solution (D50). If thiamine deficiency from alcoholism or other forms of malnutrition is suspected, parenteral thiamine, 100 mg IV is given in conjunction with glucose.

Glucagon 5 mg, given IM raises serum glucose levels slightly and is often used in pre-hospital setting as a temporizing measure[23] when IV access has not been established. The efficacy of glucagon is dependent upon hepatic glycogen stores, which may be depleted in the setting of prolonged hypoglycemia.[24] Once the initial hypoglycemia is corrected, blood glucose should be measured twice more at 30-minute intervals and if patient remains euglycemic, serum glucose can be checked every 4–6 hours thereafter. If the patients respond to initial therapy with IV glucose based on clinical symptoms and serum glucose of more than 60 mg/dl, they should be fed a calorie rich meal.

If the hypoglycemia is due to an oral hypoglycemic medication, then holding the medication, feeding calorie rich meal and observation will suffice for the majority of patients. The role of octreotide in the observation setting is less clear. If the patient develops a second episode of hypoglycemia, the authors have on occasion safely administered octreotide, which is a somatostatin analog that inhibits insulin release from pancreatic beta islet cells.[25] The drug is rapidly and completely absorbed when given subcutaneously, reaching 100% bioavailability within 30 minutes.[26] In adults, the dose of octreotide is 50–150 mcg administered by IM or SQ injection every 6 hours. It may also be given as an IV bolus over several minutes or by continuous infusion.

When discharging a diabetic patient with hypoglycemia from the OU, consider consulting with the patient's primary care provider or endocrinologist to determine the need for modification to the current antidiabetic regimen. Since the patient is at risk for recurrence of severe hypoglycemia following the initial episode, it is important to avoid tight blood sugar control for 1–2 subsequent weeks. Consider insulin regimens that minimize the risk of hypoglycemia.[15] In a split mixed insulin regimen, moving the dose of NPH insulin to bedtime has been reported to decrease the incidence of nocturnal hypoglycemia. Another alternative is the use of basal-bolus insulin regimen that involves the use of a long-acting basal insulin analog once a day with rapid acting insulin analog with meals.

Observation Unit Outcome

Goh et al. performed a prospective observational study of consecutive patients with diabetes admitted to the ED OU for severe hypoglycemia. Out of 203 patients admitted, 170 were discharged and 33 transferred to an inpatient team for a longer period of treatment. The median length of stay for discharged patients was 23 hours. Of the 170 patients discharged, 151 were contacted at 7 and 28 days after discharge. Six patients had symptoms of recurrent hypoglycemia of which two returned to the ED and were admitted. This study showed that selected patients with hypoglycemia and be effectively and safely treated in an observation unit.[27] In our experience, carefully selected patients are ideally suited to observation management and can be safely discharged from an ED OU. The controlled environment of the ED OU also provides an excellent opportunity to further educate the patients on their disease process as well as tips to avoid future hypoglycemic episodes. There could be potential cost saving for the hospital if the ED OU can demonstrate earlier disposition as opposed to inpatient admission.

References

1. Workgroup on Hypoglycemia, American Diabetic Association (A.D.A.), Defining and reporting hypoglycemia in diabetes: a report from the American Diabetes Association Workgroup on Hypoglycemia. *Diabetes Care*, 2005. 28(5): 1245–1249.

2. Lasker RD. The diabetes control and complications trial. Implications for policy and practice. *N Engl J Med*, 1993. 329(14): 1035–1036.

3. *U.K. prospective diabetes study 16.* Overview of 6 years' therapy of type II diabetes: a progressive disease. U.K. Prospective Diabetes Study Group. *Diabetes*, 1995. 44(11): 1249–1258.

4. Krentz AJ, Ferner RE, Bailey CJ. Comparative tolerability profiles of oral antidiabetic agents. *Drug Saf*, 1994. 11(4): 223–241.

5. Shorr RI, Ray WA, Daugherty JR, et al. Incidence and risk factors for serious hypoglycemia in older persons using insulin or sulfonylureas. *Arch Intern Med*, 1997. 157(15): 1681–1686.

6. Stahl M, Berger W. Higher incidence of severe hypoglycaemia leading to hospital admission in Type 2 diabetic patients treated with long-acting versus short-acting sulphonylureas. *Diabet Med*, 1999. 16(7): 586–590.

7. Menzies DJ, Dorsainvil PA, Cunha BA, et al. Severe and persistent hypoglycemia due to gatifloxacin interaction with oral hypoglycemic agents. *Am J Med*, 2002. 113(3): 232–234.

8. ter Braak EW, Appleman AM, van de Laak M, et al. Clinical characteristics of type 1 diabetic patients with and without severe hypoglycemia. *Diabetes Care*, 2000. 23(10): 1467–1471.

9. Pedersen-Bjergaard U, Reubsaet JL, Nielsen SL, et al. Psychoactive drugs, alcohol, and severe hypoglycemia in insulin-treated diabetes: analysis of 141 cases. *Am J Med*, 2005. 118(3): 307–310.

10. Gerich JE. Oral hypoglycemic agents. *N Engl J Med*, 1989. 321(18): 1231–1245.

11. Eliasson L, Renstrom E, Ammala C, et al. PKC-dependent stimulation of exocytosis by sulfonylureas in pancreatic beta cells. *Science*, 1996. 271(5250): 813–815.

12. Spiller HA, Management of sulfonylurea ingestions. *Pediatr Emerg Care*, 1999. 15(3): 227–230.

13. Dizon AM, Kowalyk S, Hoogwerf BJ. Neuroglycopenic and other symptoms in patients with insulinomas. *Am J Med*, 1999. 106(3): 307–310.

14. Hepburn DA, Deary IJ, Frier BM, et al. Symptoms of acute insulin-induced hypoglycemia in humans with and without IDDM. *Factor-analysis approach*. *Diabetes Care*, 1991. 14(11): 949–957.

15. Cryer PE. Hypoglycaemia: the limiting factor in the glycaemic management of Type I and Type II diabetes. *Diabetologia*, 2002. 45(7): 937–948.

16. Cryer PE, Davis SN, Shamoon H. Hypoglycemia in diabetes. *Diabetes Care*, 2003. 26(6): 1902–1912.

17. Dagogo-Jack SE, Craft S, Cryer PE. Hypoglycemia-associated autonomic failure in insulin-dependent diabetes mellitus. Recent antecedent hypoglycemia reduces autonomic responses to, symptoms of, and defense against subsequent hypoglycemia. *J Clin Invest*, 1993. 91(3): 819–828.

18. Davis SN, Shavers C, Davis B, et al. Prevention of an increase in plasma cortisol during hypoglycemia preserves subsequent counterregulatory responses. *J Clin Invest*, 1997. 100(2): 429–438.

19. Davis SN, Shavers C, Costa F, et al. Role of cortisol in the pathogenesis of deficient counterregulation after antecedent hypoglycemia in normal humans. *J Clin Invest*, 1996. 98(3): 680–691.

20. MacLeod KM, Hepburn DA, Frier BM. Frequency and morbidity of severe hypoglycaemia in insulin-treated diabetic patients. *Diabet Med*, 1993. 10(3): 238–245.

21. Abraira C, Colwell JA J, Nuttall FQ, et al., Veterans Affairs Cooperative Study on glycemic control and complications in type II diabetes (VA CSDM). Results of the feasibility trial. Veterans Affairs Cooperative Study in Type II Diabetes. *Diabetes Care*, 1995. 18(8): 1113–1123.

22. Saudek CD, Duckworth WC, Giobbie-Hurder A, et al. Implantable insulin pump vs multiple-dose insulin for non-insulin-dependent diabetes mellitus: a randomized clinical trial. Department of Veterans Affairs Implantable Insulin Pump Study Group. *JAMA*, 1996. 276(16): 1322–1327.

23. Schwartz NS, Clutter WE, Shah SD, et al. Glycemic thresholds for activation of glucose counterregulatory systems are higher than the threshold for symptoms. *J Clin Invest*, 1987. 79(3): 777–781.

24. Brelje TC, Scharp DW, Sorenson RL. Three-dimensional imaging of intact isolated islets of Langerhans with confocal microscopy. *Diabetes*, 1989. 38(6): 808–814.

25. Weir GC, Bonner-Weir S. Islets of Langerhans: the puzzle of intraislet interactions and their relevance to diabetes. *J Clin Invest*, 1990. 85(4): 983–987.

26. White NH, Skor DA, Cryer PE, et al. Identification of type I diabetic patients at increased risk for hypoglycemia during intensive therapy. *N Engl J Med*, 1983. 308(9): 485–491.

27. Goh HK, Chew DE, Miranda IG, et al. 24-Hour observational ward management of diabetic patients presenting with hypoglycaemia: a prospective observational study. *Emerg Med J*, 2009. 26(10): 719–723.

Electrolyte Abnormalities

Kimberly A. Ressler, MD, MSN
Jonathan Glauser, MD, FACEP

Introduction

Patients with electrolyte abnormalities may be appropriate for the observation unit (OU) depending on the severity of the disturbance, the patient's comorbidities, and the suspected etiology of the imbalance. Optimal management of specific electrolyte problems must take into account acid-base status, patient-volume status, underlying disorders, and measurements of other electrolytes. Especially as regards the intracellular cations: potassium and magnesium, serum levels may not be an accurate indicator of total body stores. Patients with the potential for requiring lifesaving interventions or prolonged treatments are better suited for admission to higher levels of care.

Potassium

Potassium is responsible for the resting membrane potential for electrical impulses and is critical in the body's acid-base homeostasis. Buffering an acute acidosis or alkalosis entails the exchange of K^+ and H^+ across the cell membrane. A general rule is that for a change of 0.1 pH unit there is an inverse change of 0.5 mEq/L in the serum K^+.[1] Hypokalemic patients who are acidotic may require vigorous repletion.

Hypokalemia

Hypokalemia, a serum level < 3.5 mmol/L, most frequently follows potassium (K^+) losses or intracellular shifts. Diuretic therapy, both loop and thiazide, is the commonest cause. The most frequently seen extra-renal cause of hypokalemia is severe or chronic diarrhea from both volume depletion and direct K^+ losses in the stool.[2] In the presence of metabolic alkalosis, K^+ ions shift into the cells in exchange for hydrogen ions to maintain normal pH of the extracellular fluid. Respiratory acid-base abnormalities do not have this same effect on potassium.[3] Low serum magnesium may contribute to hypokalemia through renal wasting. Typically patients have no symptoms with mild hypokalemia at serum levels of 3.0–3.5 mmol/L, but patients with underlying heart disease have an increased risk of dysrhythmia even within this range.[4]

Patients appropriate for the OU include those with serum K^+ > 2.0, without severe symptoms such as ileus, rhabdomyolysis, respiratory muscle weakness, or ascending paralysis, not on digitalis and without ventricular dysrthymias. Typically, these will be patients taking a thiazide or loop diuretic, or have an acute GI fluid loss. Classic EKG changes of hypokalemia with U waves, T wave flattening, and ST segment changes should not preclude an OU stay. ECG monitoring for ventricular dysrhythmia is required during intravenous (IV) potassium replacement.[5]

Treatment

For mild and asymptomatic hypokalemia, oral replacement is preferred over IV supplementation. If oral medication is tolerated, K^+ supplements can be given as an oral dose of 20 mEq KCl every 30–60 minutes or 40–60 mEq every 4–6 hours until the goal level is reached.[3] Liquid solutions are more absorbable but tablets are better tolerated.

If hypokalemia is symptomatic or causes ECG changes, patients should be treated with IV KCl and continuous ECG monitoring. KCl is generally given as 10–20 mEq mixed in 50–100 ml saline infused over 1 hour through a large bore peripheral IV. A dose of 20 mEq should increase the serum K^+ by approximately 0.25 mEq/L.[3] After IV dosing of K^+, a maintenance IV can be given that should contain no more than KCl 40 mEq per liter bag. If the solution causes burning, it should be diluted with saline preferentially to slowing the rate of potassium repletion. Potassium phosphate can be used instead of KCl in

Table 41.1 Hypokalemia Management in the Observation Unit

Oral supplementation (if possible): 10–120 mEq/day or 40–60 mEq of KCl every 4–6 hours in divided doses. High potassium foods give more gradual increase than oral K$^+$ concentrates

Intravenous KCl 10–20 mEq in 50–100 ml over 1 hour infused through large bore IV. If burning from the infusion, may need to dilute the solution rather than slow the repletion rate

If needed, a maintenance IV can contain up to KCl 40 mEq per liter bag

Check and replete magnesium as needed

Monitor K$^+$ closely during replacement. Continuous ECG monitoring if administering IV

those patients thought to have hypophosphatemia such as those in diabetic ketoacidosis (DKA).[1] In this specific population, insulin administration should be delayed if serum K$^+$ is < 3.5. Decreased magnesium levels should be addressed simultaneously; combined deficiency with hypokalemia can increase the risk for cardiac dysrhythmias.[5] Laboratory monitoring should be done every 2–4 hours to determine the response to the potassium replacement. Consideration for causes of hypokalemia should be given while the patient is in the OU. For example, measures may include adding or substituting a potassium sparing diuretic for a current loop or thiazide diuretic in consultation with the patient's primary care provider. (Table 41.1)

Hyperkalemia

Hyperkalemia, a serum potassium (K$^+$) > 5.5 mEq/L, mandates that hemolysis during phlebotomy, extreme elevations of platelets or of white blood count first be ruled out. Acidosis, β-blockade, and digitalis toxicity can cause hyperkalemia by shifting K$^+$ from inside the cells to the extracellular space.[1] Tissue injury or necrosis from rhabdomyolysis, tumor lysis or severe burns can cause life-threatening hyperkalemia from release of intracellular K$^+$.[6] Medications including potassium sparing diuretics, angiotensin converting enzyme (ACE) inhibitors, and angiotensin receptor blockers (ARBs) can precipitate increased K$^+$ in those with renal insufficiency (RI). A history of β-blocker or nonsteroidal anti-inflammatory drug (NSAID) use should be noted. Patients with

chronic renal insufficiency (CRI) are generally able to excrete K$^+$ normally unless their kidney disease is severe (GFR < 15–20 ml/min).[6]

While there are classic ECG findings associated with hyperkalemia, some patients will have a relatively normal EKG even with severe hyperkalemia yet develop potentially fatal ventricular arrhythmias without warning.[7] The rate of the rise in serum K$^+$ may be more important than the absolute value. There is much inter-patient variability in clinical presentation and response to treatment.[8] A patient with a serum K$^+$ > 6.5 mEq/L, on digoxin, with acid-base abnormalities, wide QRS complex or absence of P waves may be inappropriate for the OU. A stable chronic renal failure (CRF) patient without ECG changes and a K$^+$ < 7 mEq/L without those ECG abnormalities may be appropriate for stabilization in the OU as a bridge to hemodialysis within the next 12 hours.

Treatment

Initial management of the hyperkalemic patient occurs in the ED prior to the OU. A repeat potassium level should be drawn to verify the level and an ECG performed. Treatment should be initiated immediately if hyperkalemia is suspected without waiting for laboratory confirmation, and continuous ECG monitoring performed. There are three treatment strategies: stabilization of cell membranes, shifting extracellular potassium into the intracellular space, and promoting loss of potassium through renal and gastrointestinal systems.[4]

The initial treatment of hyperkalemia is 10–20 ml of 10% calcium gluconate IV over 2–5 minutes, which can be repeated in 5–10 minutes.[4] Calcium antagonizes the toxic effects of hyperkalemia on the myocardium, but its protective effects last only 60 minutes and other interventions must be started simultaneously.[9] Regular insulin 10 units IV with 50 ml of 50% dextrose will shift potassium into the cell for an expected fall in plasma K$^+$ of 0.5 to 1.5 mEq/L with peak effect within 30–60 minutes.[4] If the glucose is above 250, insulin can be given without dextrose.[1] High-dose nebulized albuterol 10–20 mg results in a shift of extracellular potassium into cells within 1–2 minutes with peak effect lasting 90–120 minutes.[10] Up to 40% of renal dialysis patients may not respond to β-agonists even if not on β-blockers.[4] There is an additive decrease in serum K$^+$ if both insulin/glucose and nebulized albuterol are given together, decreasing serum

K^+ by an average of 1.21 mEq/L.[8] Research has not supported the role of bicarbonate in routine treatment for hyperkalemia, and its use may be limited to those with hyperkalemia and metabolic acidosis.

Potassium levels should be rechecked at regular intervals. In the presence of intact renal function, a potent loop diuretic such as furosemide 40–80 mg IV or ethacrynic acid 50–100 mg IV can be used to remove potassium from the body.[4] Sodium polystyrene sulfonate (SPS, Kayexalate®) as oral dose or enema exchanges Na^+ for K^+ across the intestinal wall but has not been shown to increase K^+ excretion in the stool any more than expected in diarrhea induced by laxatives.[5] A recent review does not support the use of SPS for hyperkalemia due to lack of evidence and potential risks.[10] Hemodialysis is the most effective way to remove potassium from the body. Prevention should be addressed. Medication lists should be reviewed along with diet discussion including the use of salt substitutes. Medications that slow progression of kidney disease such as ACE-inhibitors and ARBs may need to have dose adjustment or other agents prescribed.[6] Medication adjustments may have to be made in patients with heart failure and hypertension.[5] Changes should be made in collaboration with the patient's primary physician, as ACE inhibitors, beta blockers, ARBs, and potassium-sparing diuretics may be lifesaving in heart failure patients, with plans for close outpatient follow-up. See Table 41.2.

Calcium

Calcium is involved in nerve conduction, muscle contraction and blood coagulation. Only 1% of the calcium in the body is in the ECF compartment. Measured serum calcium includes that which is bound and unbound to albumin, and should be corrected for low albumin states:

Corrected Ca^{+2} (mg/dl) = measured

Ca^{+2} (mg/dl) + [0.8 × (4-albumin (gm/dl)].

Alkalosis increases binding of calcium to albumin so that for each 0.1 rise in pH the ionized Ca^{+2} is lowered by about 3–8%.[3] Respiratory alkalosis or hyperventilation can increase protein binding, decreasing ionized calcium. Correction of calcium disorders in the OU mandates measurement of serum magnesium, albumin, creatinine,

Table 41.2 Hyperkalemia Management in the Observation Unit

Treatment	Onset and Duration of Action
Calcium gluconate 10 ml of 10% solution IV over 2–5 minutes. Calcium chloride as alternative. Repeat dose in 5–10 minutes if no effect.	Effects within 1–3 minutes, duration 30–60 minutes. Start other treatment simultaneously.
10 U regular insulin with 50 ml 50% dextrose (hold the glucose if BS > 250).	Effects within 15–30 minutes, lasts 4–6 hours. Produces fall in K^+ of 0.5–1.5 mmol/L.
Beta-2 agonists: albuterol high-dose 10–20 mg via high flow nebulizer which may be repeated in 2 hours.	Onset within several minutes, lasting 1–2 hours. Lowers K^+ 0.6-1 mmol/L.
Furosemide 40–80 mg IV or ethacrynic acid 50–100 mg IV if renal function intact. Sodium polystyrene sulfonate: 20–50 grams with 100 ml of 20% sorbitol every 4–6 hours. May give 50 g as enema with 50 ml of 70% sorbitol and 100–150 ml water, retained for 1–2 hours.	
Consider need for dialysis. Address access and consult nephrology.	Immediate effect but may have rebound hyperkalemia from intracellular K^+ shifts.

Monitor K^+ closely during interventions. Address potential causes including medications that increase serum potassium: ACE inhibitors, NSAIDs, K^+-sparing diuretics, ARBs, β-blockers.

and phosphate. Tests such as serum parathormone (PTH) levels, 25-OH D3, and 1,25-$(OH)_2$ D3 levels may be helpful in tracking the etiology, but are of little relevance in the observation medicine setting.

Hypocalcemia

Hypocalcemia, ionized calcium < 2.1 mEq/L (or < 1.05 mmol/L) in the ambulatory population, is seen in patients with hypoparathyroidism (primary or iatrogenic) or CRF due to hyperphosphatemia and decreased activated vitamin D. Hypomagnesemia may exist in conjunction with low serum calcium in patients with alcoholism, diuretic use, epilepsy, and renal failure, and induces PTH resistance and decreased secretion of PTH.[3] Symptoms of hypocalcemia due to the neuromuscular excitability depend on the absolute level of serum calcium and how rapidly the decline occurred. Chvostek's or Trousseau's signs, myalgia, cramps, and paresthesias should not preclude observation care.[11] Patients with symptoms such as hypotension, psychosis, confusion, or ventricular dysrhythmias are inappropriate candidates for observation care. The differential diagnosis of hypocalcemia is broad, and often impractical to accomplish in a 24-hour stay. Following thyroid or parathyroid surgery, the cause may be obvious.

Treatment

Correction of hypocalcemia is dictated by symptoms and underlying etiology. ED OU workup should include renal function, electrolytes including magnesium, ionized calcium level, and albumin. PTH and vitamin D levels may be obtained to guide further workup as an outpatient. IV calcium replacement should be used if symptoms are present or the hypocalcemia is severe (ionized $Ca^{+2} < 1.3$ or 0.65 mmol/L).[3]

Calcium is given as chloride (360 mg of elemental calcium in 10 ml) or gluconate (93 mg of elemental calcium in 10 ml over 2–5 minutes) for an initial adult dose of 100–300 mg of calcium diluted with 5% dextrose.[1] Calcium gluconate is preferred over calcium chloride because of less local tissue irritation and lower risk of tissue necrosis with extravasation. A continuous infusion may be needed to prevent further episodes and is achieved by mixing ten 10 ml ampules of 10% calcium gluconate in one liter of 5% dextrose or 0.9% saline infused at 50 ml/hr and titrated to level of calcium.[11]

Patients receiving IV calcium should have continuous ECG monitoring to evaluate for bradycardia or heart block. Oral supplementation should be started in the OU with 1000–2600 mg of calcium carbonate or calcium citrate daily in divided doses between meals.[4] If the patient is on digitalis, calcium administration should be done cautiously and more slowly. Hypomagnesemia if present should be addressed. See Table 41.3.

Hypercalcemia

The two most common causes of hypercalcemia are hyperparathyroidism and malignancy, notably

Table 41.3 Hypocalcemia Management in the Observation Unit

Calcium gluconate 10 ml, 10% (93 mg elemental Ca) diluted in 50 ml of D5 or NS, over 5 minutes. Slow rate of infusion by half; use with caution if patient is on digitalis.	As alternative, may give calcium chloride, but it has increased risk of tissue irritation and tissue necrosis with extravasation.
If needed, can use continuous infusion of Calcium Gluconate: 10 ampules (930 mg) in 1000 ml bag of 5% dextrose or 0.9% NS given over 24 hours. Consider administration of parenteral calcium until serum calcium reaches 7–7.5 mg/dL.	
Continuous ECG monitoring while giving IV Ca^{++}. Evaluate and treat for hypomagnesemia.	
Oral calcium supplements 1000–1500 mg/day in divided doses 2–4 times daily with calcium carbonate or citrate between meals.	
Consider Vitamin D supplementation if replacement: Calcitriol 1,25 $(OH)_2D$ 0.25-2 mcg/day.	

myeloma, breast, renal, and non-small cell lung cancer. Hypercalcemia from malignancy is a poor prognostic sign.[12] Medications such as thiazide diuretics, lithium, and calcium-based antacids can contribute to hypercalcemia, especially in the dehydrated patient. Granulomatous disorders including sarcoidosis and tuberculosis cause hypercalcemia related to excessive 1,25-$(OH)_2$ Vitamin D production.[1] Patients appropriate for the OU include those with trouble concentrating, personality changes, fatigue, weakness, and nausea. Symptoms may relate to the time frame of elevation as much as to the actual calcium level. Patients with altered mentation, stupor, or coma, or requiring an extensive diagnostic workup are inappropriate for observation stay. Prior to the OU, the cause for hypercalcemia such as malignancy, sarcoid, or hyper PTH should be evident.

Treatment

The goals of treatment include identifying the cause and reducing serum calcium, especially via rehydration. Laboratory workup should include calcium, albumin, ionized calcium, renal function tests, magnesium, and potassium. Isotonic saline IV should be started with 1–2 liters over the first hour followed by 4–6 liters in the next 24 hours.[4]

Table 41.4 Hypercalcemia Management in the Observation Unit

Treatment	Comments
Saline fluid bolus by giving 1–2 L of 0.9% saline IV over first hour followed by 4–6 L of saline over 24 hours at rate of 200–300 ml/hour. Keep urine at 100–150 ml/hour.	Monitor for fluid status with hydration especially in the elderly. Use furosemide only if volume overload present.
Bisphosphonates: Zoledronic acid 4 mg IV over 30 minutes (at least 15 minutes) or Pamidronate 60–90 mg IV over 2–4 hours.	Effects within 1–3 days. Usually well-tolerated, may cause arthralgias, fever, myalgia, fatigue. Slow rate or decrease dose in renal failure.
Salmon calcitonin 4 IU/kg subcutaneously, may be repeated in 6–12 hours for Ca^{+2} > 14.	Lowers Ca^{+2} in 12–48 hours, short-term use only due to tachyphylaxis.
Steroids: prednisone 40–60 mg/day for 3–7 days or hydrocortisone 100–300 mg daily.	Use if 1, 25-$(OH)_2$ Vitamin D mediated (lymphoma, sarcoid, myeloma). Effective within 2–5 days.

Rates should be adjusted to degree of hypercalcemia, fluid status, and ability to tolerate volume expansion.[1] The role of loop diuretics in the management of hypercalcemia should be limited to management of volume overload, which generally is not present.[13]

After saline hydration, bisphosphonate therapy is the pharmacologic treatment of choice.[14] Bisphosphonates are given as a single IV infusion over 15 minutes to 4 hours, with an expected ensuing reduction in Ca^{++} after 24–72 hours. Recommended doses are pamidronate 90 mg or zoledronate 4 mg as a single infusion.[13]

For severe symptoms, subcutaneous calcitonin (4 U/kg) can be given every 12 hours, which should decrease the calcium level within 12–48 hours, and as quickly as 2 hours.[14] Calcitonin can be given simultaneously with the bisphosphonates.[13] If hypercalcemia is due to excessive Vitamin D production, as in patients with granulomatous diseases such as sarcoid or lymphoma, glucocorticoids should be administered.[1] (Table 41.4)

Magnesium

Magnesium is mostly intracellular with only 1% present in the serum for a normal value of 0.74–0.95 mmol/L (1.7–2.2 mg/dL).[4] It is a cofactor in cell metabolism, protein synthesis, and neuromuscular activity.[3] It plays a role in the body's regulation of potassium and calcium, and a low serum magnesium may not accurately reflect total body deficit.

Hypomagnesemia

Magnesium depletion typically is due to renal wasting (alcohol, diuretics) or GI losses (diarrhea, malabsorption, fistula) and is frequently seen in patients with alcoholism, poor nutrition, cirrhosis, pancreatitis, or chronic diarrhea.[3] It is the most common electrolyte abnormality in the ambulatory diabetic patient and is frequently seen in DKA.[1] Proton pump inhibitors may contribute to hypomagnesemia by increasing GI losses of magnesium.[2] Correction of low magnesium may be necessary to treat refractory hypokalemia and hypocalcemia. With the exception of those with life-threatening dysrhythmias, tetany, and seizures, patients with hypomagnesemia are often good candidates for correction in the OU. For diagnostic purposes, the fractional excretion of magnesium can distinguish renal wasting from GI loss:

$$FEMg^{+2} = \{(Urine\ Mg^{+2}\ times\ plasma\ creatinine)/0.7\ times\ (plasma\ Mg^{+2}\ times\ urine\ Cr)\}\ times\ 100$$

If $FEMg^{+2} > 2\%$, one can generally assume renal magnesium wasting.[4]

Treatment

Clinical signs and symptoms usually do not occur unless magnesium is below 1.2 mg/dL (0.49 mmol/L), at which point the patient should be treated with IV magnesium.[15] Adequate renal function should be confirmed prior to replacement of magnesium (Mg^{2+}), with dose reductions of 50–75% for RI.[16]

The initial dose is 2–4 grams of 50% magnesium sulfate in saline or dextrose given over 30–60 minutes.[1] Consensus statements recommend 6–12 grams of magnesium sulfate IV over the first 24 hours.[16] During treatment, the

Table 41.5 Hypomagnesemia Management in the Observation Unit

Establish adequate renal function

2–4 grams Magnesium sulfate IV over 10–20 minutes as emergency therapy, then up to 6–12 grams $MgSO_4$ over 8–24 hours.

Discharge home on 4–6 grams per day for 3–4 days orally: Magnesium chloride or Mag-Tab SR magnesium lactate 2–4 tablets/day if mild, 6–8 tablets if severe.

Consider diuretic adjustment (potassium sparing): amiloride or triamterene instead of a loop diuretic or a thiazide.

Monitor for decreased deep tendon reflexes (may lead to bradycardia, prolonged intervals on ECG, heart block, paralysis or apnea). Recheck serum Mg^{++} periodically.

patient should be checked for decreased deep tendon reflexes, hypotension, somnolence and heart block; Mg^{+2} levels should be re-checked. Serum K^+ and Ca^{++} abnormalities should be addressed.

Oral magnesium is limited by the common side effect of diarrhea; magnesium chloride as an enteric coated tablet is best tolerated.[1] Doses are dependent on degree of deficit but are generally 4–6 grams daily.[3] Consideration may be given toward substituting a potassium-sparing diuretic such as amiloride or triamterene for furosemide or a thiazide.[16] (Table 41.5)

Hypermagnesemia

Hypermagnesemia is relatively rare in the ED. Prominent causes include RI and excessive magnesium intake IV iatrogenically or through use of antacids and laxatives which contain magnesium, particularly in the elderly patient. The kidneys are able to adequately excrete magnesium until glomerular filtration falls below 20 ml/min.[17] Symptoms generally occur above levels of 4–6 mg/dl (1.74–2.61 mmol/L) and include nausea, vomiting, hypotension, hyporeflexia, and respiratory depression.[17] The patient without severe symptoms such as significant bradycardia or complete AV block, paralysis, or depressed level of consciousness is an appropriate candidate for the OU. Those requiring consideration of IV calcium salts or with renal failure requiring hemodialysis are not appropriate candidates.

Treatment

Workup includes testing for renal function, potassium, and calcium and obtaining a 12-lead ECG. All exogenous magnesium should be discontinued. After giving IV normal saline, a loop diuretic such as furosemide (40–80 mg IV) can be administered to enhance urinary excretion of magnesium.[3]

Sodium

Sodium is normally tightly maintained in a range of 135–145 mmol/L.[4] Water balance is regulated through the actions of antidiuretic hormone (ADH) and requires an intact thirst mechanism, as well as access to water.[18] Subtle clinical changes or life-threatening consequences depend not only on the sodium value but also how acutely the abnormality occurred. Laboratory testing may include urine and serum electrolytes, renal function, plasma and urine osmolality to determine etiology.[19]

Hyponatremia

Acute onset of hyponatremia is more likely to present with encephalopathy including visual changes, focal neurologic deficits, mental status changes, and seizures.[20] If the decline in Na^+ is more gradual, milder or no symptoms may present.[21] Patients with altered neurologic status, hemodynamic instability, or seizures are not candidates for observation care. In the hyperglycemic patient, correction should be made for osmolarity: each 100 mg/dL rise in glucose results in a 1.6 mEq/L decline in serum sodium.[1] Isotonic hyponatremia or "pseudohyponatremia" is caused by hyperlipidemia or hyperproteinemia.[3]

Hyponatremia is categorized by whether the patient is hypovolemic, euvolemic, or hypervolemic. With hypovolemic hyponatremia due to renal losses, urine $[Na^+]$ should be > 20 mEq/L. If fluid losses are predominantly extrarenal with normal renal function, urine $[Na^+]$ should be < 20 mEq/L.[3] A potential candidate for the OU is the patient with exercise-associated hyponatremia as seen in long-distance runners who drink excessive water during a race.[20] A reasonable cutoff for observation care is a serum $[Na^+]$ of approximately 120–125 mEq/L and no neurologic symptoms. Those requiring hypertonic saline for any reason should be managed in an intensive care setting.

Treatment

Unless it is completely clear that the patient's symptoms developed acutely, it is unsafe to correct sodium rapidly due to risk of osmotic demyelination syndrome (ODS), which may be irreversible. Neurologic examinations for fluctuating consciousness, dysarthria, convulsions, and disturbed consciousness should be performed.[22]

It is recommended that [Na^+] be increased by no more than 10 to 12 mEq/L during a 24-hour period, aiming for a discharge sodium in the 125–130 mEq/L range.[20] Diuresis of dilute urine can increase [Na^+] more rapidly than anticipated, and overcorrection of serum [Na^+] > 125–130 mEq/L should be avoided.[20] Patients at higher risk for ODS include alcoholics with malnutrition, hypokalemic patients, and elderly women on thiazide diuretics.[4]

Patients with hypovolemia and clinical signs of dehydration should have an initial infusion of 500–1000 cc/hr of isotonic 0.9% saline to restore volume.[20] After correction of dehydration, a hypotonic fluid (such as 0.45% saline) may be given to avoid a too rapid elevation of [Na^+], as in the patient with diuretic-induced hyponatremia.[21] Patients with euvolemic hyponatremia such as SIADH will generally respond to fluid restriction but may require long-term salt tablets to help excrete water.[21] The patient with hypervolemic hyponatremia requires both fluid restriction and diuretics and is better suited to inpatient management.

Hypernatremia

Hypernatremia, defined as serum sodium [Na^+] > 145 mEq/L, usually results from impaired water intake (dementia, mental illness, hepatic encephalopathy, or critically ill patient) or massive sodium load.[18] Initial symptoms may be nonspecific and may be masked by concomitant disease.[22] While many patients will have acute symptoms with serum [Na^+] > 158 mEq/L, the rate of change of sodium and water balance is important.[3] Correction of free water deficits should take place over at least a 48-hour period to prevent rapid fluid shifts and cerebral edema.[1] Patients with hypernatremia are generally not appropriate for care in the OU. A possible exception is the acutely dehydrated patient who is otherwise neurologically intact, with access to free water in his or her living environment.

Treatment

If hypovolemia is present, isotonic 0.9% saline should be given until hemodynamically stable and tissue perfusion restored. At that time IVF may be changed to hypotonic 0.45% saline solution.[22] The goal is to decrease serum [Na^+] by no more than 0.5 mEq/L each hour until the patient's sodium is 145 mEq/L.[4] Oral or enteral hydration with free water is generally safest.[23]

Phosphate

Phosphate is the most abundant intracellular anion. Less than 1% of total body phosphate is found in plasma. Normal levels are generally cited as 2.5–4.5 mg/dl. It is regulated by PTH and vitamin D.[1] Phosphate is essential for every intracellular reaction through the body's energy source of adenosine triphosphate.[24] Phosphate should be checked in patients if an abnormal serum potassium, magnesium, or calcium is found.[25]

Hypophosphatemia

Hypophosphatemia is relatively rare except in specific populations: DKA, chronic obstructive pulmonary disease (COPD), asthma, malignancy, long-term total parenteral nutrition, inflammatory bowel disease, anorexia nervosa, and alcoholism.[25] The most common cause of renal phosphate loss is diuretic therapy including thiazides, loop diuretics, and acetazolamide.[1] Hypophosphatemia is classified as mild 2.5–2.8 mg/dL, moderate 1.0–2.5 mg/dL, and severe < 1.0 mg/dL.[1] Patients unsuitable for the OU include those with mental obtundation, seizures, coma, respiratory failure, encephalopathy, or ileus. Phosphate disorders will seldom be the primary cause for an OU stay.

Treatment

For mild or moderate hypophosphatemia, oral replacement with potassium phosphate is 1200–1500 mg/daily given in divided doses.[3] If severe total body deficit, one may need to dose as high as 3000 mg/daily with the oral form.[25] The parenteral form of potassium phosphate IV is administered using a weight based regimen with 0.08–0.16 mmol/kg over 6 hours. Except for DKA, it is unlikely that IV phosphate will be used in the observation setting.

Hyperphosphatemia

Hyperphosphatemia, serum phosphate > 5.0 mg/dL, is most commonly seen in RF but also occurs with rhabdomyolysis, tumor lysis syndrome, or hemolysis.[1] Tetany and ventricular dysrhythmias should preclude observation stay.[25]

Treatment

Hyperphosphatemia can initially be treated with isotonic saline infusion if renal function is intact, which can enhance excretion of phosphate but may further decrease calcium.[4] For the CRF patient, hyperphosphatemia is managed with dietary restrictions and phosphate-binding salts of aluminum, magnesium, or calcium.[25] Patients deemed to require acetazolamide or dextrose/insulin are better managed in another setting.

Summary

Patients with a variety of electrolyte abnormalities are suitable for 24-hour admission into an OU. Treatment considerations include the underlying diagnosis and the patient's comorbidities. Whether a patient is appropriate for observation care should be considered on an individual basis taking into account severity and possible etiology of the electrolyte abnormality.

Bibliography

1. Gibbs MA, Tayal VS. Electrolyte disturbances. In: Marx JA, Hockerberger RS, Walls RM, editors. *Rosen's Emergency Medicine Concepts and Clinical Practice*. 6th ed. Philadelphia: Mosby Elsevier; 2010. pp. 1615–1632.

2. Unwin RJ, Luft FC, Shirley DG. Pathophysiology and management of hypokalemia: a clinical perspective. *Nat Rev Nephrol*. 2011;7:75–84.

3. Kelen GD, Hsu E. Fluids and electrolytes. In: Tintinalli JE, Stapczynski JS, Ma OJ, Cline DM, Cydulka RK, Meckles, editors. *Tintinalli's Emergency Medicine a Comprehensive Study guide*. 7th ed. New York: The McGraw-Hill Companies, Inc; 2011. pp. 117–129.

4. Weiss-Guillet EM, Takala J, Jakob SM. Diagnosis and management of electrolyte emergencies. *Best Pract Res Clin Endocrinol Metab*. 2003;17(4):623–651.

5. Alfonzo AV, Isles C, Geddes C, et al. Potassium disorders–clinical spectrum and emergency management. *Resuscitation*. 2006;70(1):10–25.

6. Nyirenda MJ, Tang JI, Padfield PL, et al. Hyperkalemia. *BMJ*. 2009;339:b4114:1019–1024.

7. Weisberg, LS. Management of severe hyperkalemia. *Crit Care Med*. 2008;36:3246–3251.

8. Elliott MJ, Ronksley PE, Clase CM, et al. Management of patients with acute hyperkalemia. *CMAJ*. 2010;182(15):1631–1635.

9. Khanna A, White WB. Management of hyperkalemia in patients with cardiovascular disease. *Am J Med*. 2009;122:215–221.

10. Pepin J, Shields C. Advances in diagnosis and management of hypokalemia and hyperkalemic emergencies. *Emerg Med Pract*. 2012;14(2):1–17.

11. Cooper MS, Gittoes NJ. Diagnosis and management of hypocalcaemia. *BMJ*. 2008;336:1298–1302.

12. Shepard MM, Smith JW. Hypercalcemia. *Am J Med Sci*. 2007;334(5):381–385.

13. Makras P, Papapoulos SE. Medical treatment of hypercalcaemia. *Hormones*. 2009;8(2)83–95.

14. LeGrand SB, Leskuski D, Zama I. Narrative Review: Furosemide for Hypercalcemia: An unproven yet common practice. *Ann Intern Med*. 2008:149:259–263.

15. Assadi F. Hypomagnesemia: An evidence-based approach to clinical cases. *Iran J Kidney Dis*. 2010;4(1):13–19.

16. Topf JM, Murray PT. Hypomagnesemia and hypermagnesemia. *Rev Endocr Metab Disord*. 2003;4:195–206.

17. Musso CG. Magnesium metabolism in health and disease. *Int Urol Nephrol*. 2009;41:357–362.

18. Archinger SG, Mortiz ML, Ayus JC. Dynatremias: Why are patients still dying? *South Med J*. 2006;99(4)353–362.

19. Adrogue HJ, Madias NE. Hypernatremia. *N Engl J Med* 2000;342(20):1493–1499.

20. Verbalis JG, Goldsmith SR, Greenberg A, et al. Hyponatremia treatment guidelines 2007: Expert panel recommendations. *Am J Med*. 2007;120(11A):S1–S21.

21. Vaidya C, Ho W, Freda BJ. Management of hyponatremia: Providing treatment and avoiding harm. *Cleve Clin J Med*. 2010;77(10):715–726.

22. Lin M, Liu SJ, Lim IT. Disorders of water imbalance. *Emerg Med Clin N Am*. 2005;23:749–770.

23. Wakil A, Atkin SL. Serum sodium disorders: Safe management. *Clin Med.* 2010;10(1): 79–82.

24. Assadi F. Hypophosphatemia: An evidence-based problem-solving approach to clinical cases. *Iran J Kidney Dis.* 2010;4 (3)195–201.

25. Shiber JR, Mattu A. Serum phosphate: Abnormalities in the emergency department. *J Emerg Med.* 2002;23(4): 395–400.

Sickle Cell Disease

42

Matt Lyon, MD FACEP
Leah Taylor, MA
Robert W. Gibson PhD, MSOTR/L

Introduction

Vaso-occlusive crisis (VOC) is the most common complication resulting from sickle cell disease (SCD) in adults.[1] VOC is caused by ischemic tissue injury as a result of occlusion of microvascular beds from abnormal, sickle-shaped red blood cells. SCD patients display a host of complications associated with micro- and occasionally macrovascular occlusion, including stroke, leg ulcers, spontaneous miscarriage, and renal insufficiency. However, the acute pain crisis is the most common reason sickle cell patients seek medical care in emergency departments (EDs).[2] Due to the recurrent nature of the acute pain crisis, possible inadequate knowledge by health care providers of this disease and the intensity of treatment needed, patients with VOC may be undermedicated in the ED.[3] This leads to low patient satisfaction, low provider satisfaction and increased costs of care. Through the use of an ED observation unit (ED OU) clinical pathway, patients suffering from VOC can be effectively managed to improve outcomes, improve satisfaction and decrease cost of care.[4]

Pathology and Clinical Presentation

SCD is a genetic disorder, which results in abnormal hemoglobin synthesis and abnormally shaped red blood cells (sickle-shaped red blood cells) when the red blood cell becomes deoxygenated. SCD is inherited in an autosomal recessive manner with heterozygous patients only rarely expressing clinical symptoms (sickle cell trait) under extreme conditions. In homozygous patients (SS) both hemoglobin genes are abnormal and express the sickle cell mutated hemoglobin. This results in the clinical syndrome of sickle cell anemia. Other sickling disorders, which are clinically similar in presentation, though milder in severity, include hemoglobin SC and hemoglobin Sβ-thalassemia disease.[5]

The hallmark of SCD is the VOC (aka Sickle Cell Crisis or pain crisis) in which there are recurrent episodes of severe pain affecting most commonly the back, legs, knees, arms, chest, and abdomen. Commonly the pain is bilateral, symmetric and usually affects the same body areas or regional distribution in subsequent attacks. VOC is the most common reason for hospitalization in patients with SCD.[6]

Factors associated with the onset of VOC include any activity that increases the requirement for oxygen, such as illness, physical stress, psychological stress and/or locations with decreased oxygen tension such as high altitude locations. However, in half of all episodes the precipitating factors are unknown. The typical VOC lasts from 3 to 14 days with a crescendo/decrescendo type pattern. Typically, the pain crisis of SCD often has an abrupt onset.[7,8] Despite oral medication treatment regimens that may begin at home, many patients require parenteral opioids for relief, and many consider the pain associated with VOC to be similar to the pain associated with bone metastasis from cancer.

Many patients with SCD experience chronic pain. VOC pain is distinctly different and occurs independently of this baseline chronic pain. How each patient is affected by his or her chronic pain as well as the VOC episodes is quite variable.[6,9] This variation is due to differences in the type of SC disease and its genetic expression, how the patient expresses or internalizes pain, his or her prior interaction with the health care system, his or her opioid tolerance, and his or her prior experience with VOC and chronic pain. Generally, patients with SCD can resume a relatively normal life in between crisis, although the chronic pain can lead to disability in some cases.[6]

Other complications from SCD may occur besides VOC. Since vaso-occlusion results in splenic infarction at a young age, the majority of patients with SCD do not have the protection from encapsulated bacteria resulting in a suppressed immune system. Thus SCD patients are susceptible to overwhelming sepsis. VOC may also occur in the lungs resulting in Acute Chest Syndrome, which includes hypoxia and dyspnea, and may progress to death if not recognized and treated appropriately. As a result of the sickle-shaped red blood cells, the red blood cells have a shortened life span, leading to a chronic anemia. During a VOC, the rate of destruction of red blood cells may increase, leading to a rapid decline in the hemoglobin (hyperhemolysis) and the possibility of severe complications.[5]

Current Management

Many patients with SCD have a relationship with a primary care physician or a hematologist who can manage the VOC with oral home medications or through infusion therapy in specialized sickle cell centers. However, many patients are remote from these centers and do not have access to specialized care, particularly when experiencing a VOC. The sudden onset of pain combined with an elevated opioid tolerance often leads to treatment in an ED setting.[10]

While the vast majority of sickle cell patients seek care in an ED on a limited or infrequent basis, a small subset of SCD patients utilize the ED on a frequent basis. The use of the ED on a frequent basis by this small subset of patients is usually due to poor social support, limited specialist or primary care, patients who have developed a more chronic form of the disease and those with a true addiction. While the proportion of sickle cell patients with an opioid addiction is similar to the general population,[11,12,13] many of these frequent users of EDs are often grouped together as exhibiting a drug-seeking behavior.[1] This perception, combined with a lack of objective measurement of the severity of the vaso-occlusion, may lead to skepticism from health care providers as to the amount or severity of pain that is associated with VOC.[3,14,15] Combined with the typical duration of a VOC of up to 2 weeks, under-treatment of pain in many cases leads to multiple ED visits during a single VOC episode, further reinforcing the stereotype of drug-seeking behavior.[16] Consequently, sickle cell patients are often distrustful of emergency physicians and may appear hostile, demanding and disruptive in the ED.[17]

Current ED management in most hospitals involves a trial of parenteral opioids and then a disposition decision. In some hospitals this involves a set number of parenteral injections, and in other hospitals this involves a specified total dose of opioids.[18] In either case, this type of treatment is labor intensive on both the nursing staff as well as the physician staff. Further, the opioid delivery is not only limited in amount and customization to the individual patient, there are usually long delays in both the initiation as well as the subsequent opioid treatments, decreasing the efficacy of treatment. As a result, undertreatment of VOC is common, leading to frequent ED visits, higher admission rates to the hospital and a high cost of care.[3]

Management Goals

Guidelines for the management of VOC in SCD have been available since 1999.[19] However, most physicians are not familiar with the treatment guidelines, and some physicians do not believe in the need for opioid therapy or the dose necessary to control the pain associated with VOC.[20] There are four essential features outlined by the pain management guideline for VOC: 1) rapid initiation of opioid therapy within 15 to 30 minutes of arrival in the ED, 2) use of adequate opioid starting dose, 3) frequent repeated doses of opioids (every 15–30 minutes) until pain is significantly improved, and 4) the need to select treatment regimens based on an individual's prior opioid-response history. Evidence to support this approach was described in the recently published Evidence-Based Management of Sickle Cell Disease: Expert Panel Report, 2014.[13,21] While these goals may be difficult to achieve in the typical ED setting, they are easily accomplished in the OU setting. By utilizing a setting that allows for extended treatment and evaluation and a clinical care pathway, all of the management goals can be met in addition to limiting many of the biases of the patient and the physician from prior ED experiences.[20] This allows the health system to realize several advantages, including decreased variability in treatment for this group of patients, increased patient satisfaction, decreased admission, improved pain control, a decrease in repeat patient ED visits during the same VOC episode, and decreased discharge of SCD patients having a life-threatening complication.[4,22]

Meeting Analgesia Guidelines

Clinical Pathway

To meet the analgesia guidelines, a clinical pathway for the evaluation and management of VOC is imperative.[23] Since patients with VOC have a similar clinical course, a pathway is a method of standardizing treatment for this disease, while also decreasing and possibly eliminating any bias or disparity on behalf of the health care provider. The use of an observation pathway allows for rapid initiation of therapy as well as decreased ED resource utilization. By using a Patient Controlled Anesthesia (PCA) delivered opioid, the patient is in control of his or her therapy, removing the bias as well as delays associated with bolus infusions of opioid. Because PCA delivery of medication is gradual, use of a PCA rarely results in the opioid high, consistent with rapid bolus infusions of narcotics. By eliminating the bolus opioid infusions, patients with opioid abuse behavior are readily identified due to resistance in use of the PCA and can be identified for alternative treatment, such as drug addiction intervention. Specific information regarding how to implement the clinical pathway while meeting the analgesia guidelines follows.

I. Rapid Initiation of Opioid Therapy

To meet the rapid initiation of opioid therapy goal, patients can be identified and initiated into the treatment protocol from the ED triage. Patients presenting to triage are initially evaluated for the presence of SCD and VOC. Many of the complicating factors of SCD can be discovered at triage, including hypoxia and hypotension. If any of these factors are discovered at triage, the patient should be treated in the ED with an appropriate triage level. However, when a patient presents with the usual VOC pain crisis, the patient can be placed directly into the ED or OU, eliminating a long wait. Once in the OU, oral or possibly parenteral opioid regimens can be started via a nurse-initiated treatment protocol. In our OU, time to triage of SC VOC averages less than 15 minutes, and time to treatment with opioids averages less than 30 minutes.[24]

II. Adequate and Repeated Opioid Until Pain Control

Utilization of opioids via a PCA protocol delivers medication on demand to the patient. This has several advantages: 1) the patient is in control of his or her opioid usage as well as the delivery rate; 2) the nursing staff is freed from rapid reassessments and intensive opioid injection schedules; and 3) the delivery of the opioid is gradual and dose-sustaining leading to a more rapid, even (less peaks and troughs) arrival at an opioid steady state. Patients are also treated with oral opioids and consideration should be given to the use of oral or parenteral nonsteroidal anti-inflammatory pain medications such as ibuprofen and ketorolac. The use of these oral medications helps to transition the patient to outpatient treatment of his or her pain crisis. Further, these medications decrease the parenteral opioid requirements. Other medications such as transdermal fentanyl should also be considered as this may be continued once discharged from the hospital.

The observation pathway for VOC is a patient-directed pathway. The patient is questioned on an hourly basis for changes in pain scale as well as the perception that he or she can manage his or her pain at home. Typically, the length of stay in our observation unit for SC VOC is 14 hours or less (depending on the time of year) with less than 16% of patients requiring admission at 24 hours of observation time.[19]

III. Individualized Treatment Regimens

Because of the variable presentation and variable opioid tolerance of each individualized patient, utilizing an individual treatment regimen improves the efficiency of the pathway. We developed an observation-specific, individualized, treatment-compliant database for monitoring the individual PCA dosages and adjunct medications for each of the sickle cell patients that utilize our hospital. This consists of the preferred opioid type, optimal initial PCA settings, preferred antiemetic and antihistamine, and adjunct medications such as long-acting transdermal or oral opioid. The database results in more consistency in treatment of individual patients regardless of who is caring for the patient in the ED. Outcome results from this intervention are not available currently, however the trend has been a lower admission rate and shorter length of stay, presumably because the opioid steady state is reached in less time due to a higher starting PCA dosage.

IV. Sickle Cell Consults and Admission Criteria

Utilizing a standard protocol with regards to admission criteria and consults, such as hematology or internal medicine, also improved the care of SC patients. Admission criteria are similar to exclusion criteria for use of the pathway: 1) development of fever or signs of infection, 2) development of hypoxia or hypotension, and 3) lack of adequate pain control after 24 hours of treatment. If any of these conditions develop, the patient should be evaluated for admission to the hospital. In our institution, the observation nurse notifies the physician if any of these conditions are met. The physician should be consulted when the patient's pain scale has not changed within 6 hours. Some physicians may be reluctant to utilize higher opioid doses during treatment as many of these patients are on large doses from initiation. Hematologists/oncologists are often more comfortable with larger doses of opioids as they often use them in oncology settings. By involving the consultant when the pain is not improving, the consultant may be able to make recommendations that may eliminate the need for admission. Pathway coordination between the admitting service and the OU assures that the patient's care is not adversely affected due to the change in physicians providing care.

Observation Protocol Implementation and Maintenance

Implementation of an observation protocol for VOC can be challenging as the goal of this pathway is to standardize care and limit variability in the patient's care. Initially, some physicians may be resistant to protocol-directed patient care. However, once established, care of the SC patient is nearly automated, yielding less physician interaction time and improving the efficiency of the ED. As with most OUs, the protocols are nurse-driven. Thus, nurse training with regards to SCD and VOC is imperative. The nursing staff of the OU is typically limited in number, so familiarity between the nurse and the sickle cell patients utilizing the OU for VOC is common.

Measures of efficacy of this pathway are determined using SC VOC metrics. Suggested metric goals are listed below in Table 42.1. These metrics are based on sickle cell analgesia guidelines and have been modified to observation medicine practice.[19,20]

Meetings between the hematology or other appropriate consultants, the observation staff,

Table 42.1 Suggested Sickle Cell Pathway Metrics and Goals

Metric	Goal
Time to ED or ED OU from Triage	15 minutes
Time to physician evaluation	30 minutes
Length of stay	12 hours
Consult rate	< 30%
Admission rate	< 15%

and the observation director on a regular basis to review the metrics is useful in meeting the metric goals. Sharing of information between the ED staff and the consultant staff helps identify problems with individual patients. Often patients, who have an increased frequency of use of the pathway, have a social, psychiatric, or non-sickle-cell-related medical problem, which increases their use of the ED. These problems can be identified and addressed through using this multidisciplinary approach.

Adjunctive Therapy

IV hydration is another area of potential controversy. Risk factors for the onset of a VOC include dehydration. However, there is little evidence that IV fluids decrease severity of VOC, length of stay, intensity of the pain, or improve outcomes. Some patients with SCD can develop pulmonary edema due to aggressive fluid intake. For example, patients with severe cardiomyopathy due to iron overload from chronic transfusion may not be able to tolerate bolus fluid orders associated with the pathway. However, many patients are dehydrated on presentation because of decreased oral intake prior to presenting to the ED. These patients should be hydrated to euvolemia shortly after admission to the OU. Continuous IV fluids at a maintenance rate are also suggested. Because patients on a PCA opioid infusion may be sleepy due to the side effects of the opioids, they may not be able to maintain adequate fluid intake while on the pathway. Further, nonsteroidal inflammatory medications (NSAIDS) may lead to decreased renal perfusion through their prostaglandin inhibitory effects, leading to renal damage when given to patients who are already dehydrated.

NSAID medications are also a useful adjunct to the opioid PCA. The effect of NSAIDS has been shown to be additive and when an oral formulation is used, patients can continue the medication after discharge to maintain the pain relief achieved on the pathway.

The goal of the pathway is to achieve a level of pain relief that can be maintained on oral medications at home. For this reason, oral oxycodone, hydrocodone, or hydromorphone should be part of the observation pathway. The pathway must be designed as not to exceed the maximum dose of acetaminophen in a 24-hour period. The strategy we utilize is one oxycodone (5 mg)-acetaminophen (325 mg) every 2 hours while on the pathway. This adjunct to the pathway should not be utilized with patients who have liver disease in order to avoid possible liver toxicity.

Home medications, particularly oral or transdermal long acting opioids, should be continued while the patient is on the observation pathway. This will help with the transition from inpatient care to home care as well as aid in achieving an opioid steady state. If the patient's long acting opioids are not continued while on the pathway, the dosage of the PCA opioids will need to be increased to account for this overall decrease in opioid delivery.

Pitfalls in Observation Management in SC VOC

As with all observation pathways, some situations may arise that lead to poor outcomes.

Populations that may not be appropriate for the sickle cell observation pathway include sickle cell patients who are pregnant or have other serious medical conditions such as cancer, severe cardiomyopathy, liver disease, or lung disease. With each of these conditions, variability in how the patient will react at each presentation to the treatment protocol can be variable, leading to uncertain outcomes from the pathway.

A multidisciplinary team consisting of the observation staff (nurse), the observation director, and consultant staff, such as hematology/oncology or internal medicine, should be considered to discuss variations in pathway design and to monitor for efficacy. This team can develop contingencies for patients who exhibit opioid abuse behavior or other psychosocial behavior detrimental to the observation pathway. Occasionally including a pain management specialist or a behavioral therapist for individual patients can help solve even some of the most challenging cases.

Conclusion

The individual with sickle cell VOC is an ideal candidate for an observation clinical pathway. Factors such as provider bias and individual patient variation to the disease can lead to variable outcome. The pathway provides for uniform treatment that leads to better outcomes, cost savings, and better patient outcomes.

References

1. Shapiro B. Benjamin LJ, Payne R, Heidrich G. Sickle cell-related pain: Perceptions of medical practitioners. *J Pain Symptom Manage* 1997;14(3):168–174.

2. Conran N, Franco-Penteado CF, Costa FF. Newer aspects of the pathophysiology of sickle cell disease vaso-occlusion. *Hemoglobin*. 2009;33(1):1–16.

3. Rupp T, Delaney K. Inadequate analgesia in emergency medicine. *Annals of Emergency Medicine*. 2004;43(4):494–503.

4. Brookoff D, Polomano R. Treating sickle cell pain like cancer pain. *Annals of Internal Medicine*. 1992;116(5):364–368.

5. Roseff SD, Sickle cell disease: a review. *Immunohematology/ American Red Cross*. 2009;25 (2):67–74.

6. McClish D, Smith WR, Dahman BA, et al. Pain site frequency and location in sickle cell disease: the PiSCES project. *Pain*. 2009;145(1–2):246–251.

7. Platt O, Thorington BD, Brambilla DJ, et al. Pain in sickle cell disease – rates and risk factors. *NEJM*. 1991;325:11–16.

8. Ballas SK, Gupta K, Adams-Graves P. Sickle cell pain: A critical reappraisal. *Blood*. 2012;120(18):3647–3656.

9. Taylor LEV, Scotts NA, Jumphreys J, et al. A review of the literature on multiple

dimensions of chronic pain in adults with sickle cell disease. *Journal of Pain and Symptom Management*. 2010;40(3): 416–435.

10. Drookoff D, Polomano R. Treating sickle cell pain like cancer pain. *Annals of Internal Medicine*. 1992;116(5): 364–368.

11. Waldrop R, Mandry C. Health professional perceptions of opioid dependence among patients with pain. *American Journal of Emergency Medicine*. 1995;13(5):529–531.

12. Smith WR, Jordan LB, Hassel KL. Frequently asked questions by hospitalist managing pain in adults with sickle cell disease.

Journal of Hospital Medicine. 2011; 6:297–303.

13. Yawn BP, Buchanan GR, Afenyi-Annan AN, et al. Management of sickle cell disease: Summary of the 2014 evidence-based report by expert panel members. JAMA. 2014;312(10):1033–1048.

14. Ballas SK. The sickle cell painful crisis in adults: phases and objective signs. *Hemoglobin.* 1995;19(6) 323–333.

15. Haywood C, Beach MC, Lanzkron S, et al. A systematic review of barriers and interventions to improve appropriate use of therapies for sickle cell disease. *Journal of the National Medical Association.* 2009;101(10):1022–1033.

16. Labbe E, Herbert D, Haynes J. Physician's attitude and practices in sickle cell disease pain management. *J Palliative Care.* 2005;21:246–251.

17. Friedman EW, Webber AB, Osborn HH, et al. Oral analgesia for treatment of painful crisis in sickle cell anemia. *Ann Emergency Medicine.* 1986;15:783–791.

18. Silbergleit R, Jancis MO, McNamara RM. Mangement of sickle cell pain crisis in the emergency department at teaching hospitals. *Journal of Emergency Medicine.* 1999;17 (4):625–630.

19. Benjamin LJ, Dampier CD, Jacox AK, et al. Guidelines for the management of acute and chronic pain in sickle-cell disease. APS Clinical Practice Guideline Series, No. 1, 1999.

20. Solomon LR. Treatment and prevention of pain due to vaso-occlusive crises in adults with sickle cell disease: an educational void. *Blood* 2008; 111:997–1003.

21. *Evidence-Based Management of Sickle Cell Disease: Expert Panel Report.* 2014; Available from: https://www.nhlbi.nih.gov/health-pro/guidelines/sickle-cell-disease-guidelines.

22. Melzer-Lange MD, Walsh-Kelly C, Lea G, et al. Patient-controlled analgesia for sickle cell pain crisis in a pediatric emergency department. 2004;20(2):2–4.

23. Rees DC, Olujohungbe AD, Parker NE, et al. Guidelines for the management of the acute painful crisis in sickle cell disease. *British Journal of Hematology.* 2003;120(5): 744–752.

24. Lyon M, Sinclair D, Renwick E. Comparison of outcomes before and after implementation of an observation unit clinical pathway for sickle cell vaso-occlusive crisis. *Florida Journal of Sickle Cell Disease and Hemoglobinopahty.* 2010. 4(1):19.

Chapter 43

Transfusions

Rokhsanna Sadeghi, MD
Jonathan Glauser, MD, FACEP

Introduction

There is a wealth of clinical situations in which patients presenting to an Emergency Department (ED) require a blood product transfusion in order to treat their condition. Many of these patients are optimal candidates for transfusion in an observation unit (OU), with correction of their presenting condition within 24 hours. The objective of this chapter is to provide an overview and guide to blood product transfusions in an OU. The products that will be covered include packed RBC, fresh frozen plasma, common plasma derivatives, and platelets. Finally, identifying and managing transfusion reactions will be discussed. Exchange transfusions, as for acute chest syndrome in sickle cell disease, and transfusions for trauma are best managed in a setting other than the OU.

Red Blood Cell Transfusion

RBC transfusion is the most common blood product transfused in clinical practice. There are approximately 85 million units of RBC transfused annually, worldwide.[1] There is a wide variation in transfusion practices among clinicians, thus multiple guidelines have been developed in order to standardize which patients would benefit from RBC transfusion in order to prevent over- and under-transfusion.

Despite multiple studies and expert panels, there is no single hemoglobin concentration threshold or "transfusion" trigger that can be applied universally. Each patient's medical condition must be taken into consideration and a clinician must fully weigh the risk of the transfusion to the benefit of having the anemia corrected.

For many decades, a transfusion trigger of hemoglobin 10 g/dL was used in clinical practice. Multiple organizations, including the AABB (formerly, American Association of Blood Banks), Australian and New Zealand Society of Blood

Transfusion, and British Committee for Standards in Hematology, have adopted the restrictive transfusion strategy as opposed to a liberal transfusion strategy.[1,2,3] Restrictive blood transfusion strategy has been found to decrease hospital length of stay and all-cause mortality.[2] Through extensive review of existing studies, these organizations have found that there is no clinical benefit to transfusing patients to maintain a hemoglobin concentration above 10 g/dL. Furthermore, a hemoglobin concentration of 5 g/dL in healthy individuals does not demonstrate inadequate oxygenation.[2]

A reason for the lack of a commonly used transfusion trigger is the absence of a reliable way to measure oxygen delivery to critical organs. Given that the objective of a blood transfusion is to increase the oxygen carrying capacity of blood, it is essential to identify patients in whom there is end-organ hypoxia, and therefore those patients who would benefit from a RBC transfusion. Making the determination of whom the benefit of transfusion outweighs the risk is a complex decision in which multiple factors need to be taken into consideration, such as age, patient's ability to compensate, coexisting cardiovascular, cerebrovascular, respiratory disease, cause of anemia, severity, and chronicity.[2] There is no consensus as to which subjective or objective findings are reliable indicators of symptomatic anemia, but fatigue, shortness of breath, increased respiratory rate and pulse are common parameters.[3] Furthermore, the cause of anemia should be identified and treated before transfusion is initiated, such as iron deficiency anemia or megaloblastic anemia. It is expected that long-term management of chronic asymptomatic anemia may involve therapy with iron, B12, folate or recombinant erythropoietin as indicated. One study involving Jehovah's Witnesses indicated that no one died with a hemoglobin in the 5–8 g/dL range because of their anemia.[4]

Once the decision has been made to transfuse RBC, a treatment end point must be defined, such

Table 43.1 Summary of Recommendations of Transfusion for Packed Red Blood Cells

Hemoglobin Concentration	Transfusion Recommendations
> 10 g/dL	Transfusion likely not necessary unless there are specific indications.*
7–10 g/dL	Transfusion may be beneficial if patient is symptomatic** or has cardiovascular or respiratory disease limiting ability to compensate.
< 7 g/dL	Transfusion appropriate, especially if known coronary artery disease and/or symptomatic. If patient is asymptomatic or other specific treatment is available, lower Hgb threshold may be used.

* Severely ill, advanced coronary artery disease, cerebrovascular, or pulmonary disease
** Symptoms include chest pain, orthostatic hypotension or tachycardia unresponsive to fluid resuscitation, or congestive heart failure

as a goal hemoglobin concentration or change in symptoms. For a 50 kg individual, one unit of RBC should increase the hemoglobin concentration by 1 g/dL or hematocrit by 3%. Likewise, if an individual is 100 kg, the hemoglobin concentration may only be raised 0.5 g/dL or the hematocrit increased 1.5% for each unit of packed RBCs transfused.[5] For the most accurate post-transfusion evaluation of hemoglobin level of increase, a blood sample should be drawn within 10–60 minutes. During this window of time, the transfusion is less affected by concurrent physiologic processes such as splenic sequestration, sepsis, and consumption.[6]

Some comments specifically related to sickle cell (SS) disease are in order. It should be noted that leukocyte-poor antigen-matched blood should be used to reduce the development of antibodies and frequency of future transfusion reactions. Exchange transfusion may prevent iron accumulation and reverse iron overload in chronically transfused patients, but is not suitable for observation care. Transfusion indications in SS disease, after discussion with the patient's hematologist, may include severe anemia, transient red cell aplasia, or acute splenic sequestration.[7] Acute

chest syndrome, stroke, and stroke prevention for those at risk by transcranial doppler are best managed in a setting other than the OU.

For OU transfusions, a set protocol for monitoring patients during and post-transfusion must be developed by each institution. Minimum level of monitoring includes frequent visual observation throughout transfusion, complete vital signs within 60 minutes prior to transfusion, complete set of vital signs 15 minutes after each transfusion initiation, and a complete set of vital signs within 60 minutes of the end of the transfusion. If there is evidence for a possible transfusion reaction, vital signs should be recorded and appropriate steps taken to address the reaction.[3] When the patient is discharged from the OU, signs of delayed transfusion reactions should be reviewed with the patient and provided in the discharge instructions. In addition, patients should be provided with a 24-hour clinical advice line.

Plasma Products and Warfarin Reversal
Fresh Frozen Plasma

Fresh frozen plasma (FFP) transfusions are used to replace plasma proteins that are deficient or defective. These may be secondary to congenital or acquired processes.[1] As with red blood cell transfusions, there are specific indications in which a patient's emergent condition can be treated with FFP transfusion in an OU. Some indications for FFP are unsuitable for management in the OU: multi-factor deficiencies or disseminated intravascular coagulation (DIC) plus bleeding, or the preoperative bleeding patient who requires multiple plasma coagulation factors. Patients with thrombotic thrombocytopenic purpura (TTP) may require plasma exchange over 2 days, and are therefore unsuitable for OU care. Massively transfused patients with clinically significant coagulation deficiencies, as with multiple trauma, will be managed elsewhere. FFP should be ABO compatible. The risk for infection transmission is not negligible, as FFP is not considered viral attenuated. This section will outline indications and guidelines on when and how to transfuse FFP.

In the OU, inherited coagulation factor deficiencies can be treated with FFP if there are no other virus safe fractionated products available, such as Factor V Leiden or Factor XI deficiencies.[2,8,9] If a patient with these deficiencies has moderate to severe bleeding or requires an

Table 43.2 Management Guidelines for Supratherapeutic INR Secondary to Warfarin[10]

INR	Recommended Management
INR higher than therapeutic range but < 5 and bleeding absent	Omit the next dose, consider lowering subsequent doses
INR 5–9, bleeding absent	Hold warfarin; If bleeding risk is high*, give vitamin K 1–2 mg PO, recheck INR in 24 hours and resume therapy at lower dose
INR > 9, bleeding absent	If low bleeding risk, hold warfarin, give vitamin K 2.5–5 mg PO or 1 mg IV, and resume warfarin at lower dose once INR < 5 If high bleeding risk*, hold warfarin, give vitamin K, consider FFP, resume warfarin at lower dose when INR < 5
Clinically significant bleeding where warfarin-induced coagulopathy is a contributing factor	Hold warfarin, give vitamin K IV up to 10 mg and FFP; assess patient until INR < 5 and bleeding stops

* High risk for bleeding: active GI conditions (PUD or IBD), concomitant antiplatelet therapy, major surgical procedure within the preceding 2 weeks, and low platelet count

to prevent unnecessary transfusions and to ensure that patients are managed in the appropriate setting.

Warfarin is a vitamin K antagonist that results in coagulopathy, which can lead to bleeding, especially if levels are supratherapeutic or if trauma occurs. This coagulopathy can lead to excessive bleeding with invasive procedures. FFP transfusion is indicated if the patient needs to undergo an emergent invasive procedure in which vitamin K could not reverse coagulopathy rapidly enough. The effect of vitamin K can be expected within 6 to 12 hours of administration, but its full effect typically only occurs after 24 hours.[10] One must keep in mind that Prothrombin Complex Concentrates (PCC) given 25–50 U/kg work more quickly than does FFP, and that for warfarin reversal 15 ml/kg of FFP must be administered – a significant volume load in many patients.[2] Generally, FFP should not be given for warfarin reversal unless there is severe bleeding.[1, 2, 8, 10]

For patients on warfarin, if the International Normalized Ratio (INR) is supratherapeutic, but less than 5 and there is no bleeding, the dose of warfarin can be decreased or next dose should be held. The risk of bleeding increases exponentially between an INR of 5–9 (Australian Consensus for Warfarin Reversal, ACWR)[11]. Patients considered to have high risk for bleeding include active peptic ulcer disease (PUD) or inflammatory bowel disease (IBD), current antiplatelet use, major surgical procedure in the past 2 weeks, and thrombocytopenia. If there is no bleeding with an INR between 5 to 9 the warfarin dose should be held, and in the presence of a high bleeding risk, vitamin K should be given. The INR should be rechecked in 24 hours, and if the level has decreased, the patient should resume warfarin at a lower dose. With an INR > 9 and no active bleeding, warfarin should be held and vitamin K administered. If the patient is at high risk for bleeding, an FFP transfusion should be considered. Once the INR is below 5, warfarin may be resumed at a lower dose. If there is clinically significant bleeding in the setting of an elevated INR, warfarin should be withheld, and vitamin K given intravenously, with FFP administered. The patient should be monitored until bleeding has stopped. Do not restart warfarin until the INR is < 5.[10]

In general, FFP will be effective when prothrombin time (PT) and activated partial thromboplastin

invasive procedure, transfusion of FFP must be considered. If a congenital bleeding disorder is suspected but unknown, it may be reasonable to administer FFP 15 ml/kg pending results, as the deficiencies will most likely be in factors VIII, IX, and XI. Rarely, patients with C1 inhibitor deficiencies presenting with angioedema may require FFP if no recombinant product is available. For patients with liver disease, FFP may also be beneficial if they are bleeding or must undergo a high-risk procedure, such as a liver biopsy. There are some recommendations that prior to liver biopsy the PT should be within 4 seconds of the normal range.[8] The severity of patients' disease and the characteristics of the planned procedure (i.e., esophagogastroduodenoscopy) or amount and location of active bleeding must be taken into consideration on an individual basis in order time (aPTT) are both 1.5 times greater than the upper limit of normal.[9] FFP will not be beneficial for patient with only minimal elevated INR. The INR of FFP has been noted to be as high as 1.3,[1] and therefore FFP cannot completely normalize the INR. The goal of an FFP transfusion is to increase plasma factor concentration to at least 30%. Typical doses for FFP are between 10–30 ml/kg. Since each unit is approximately 250 ml, volume overload may be a consideration.[9] Repeat PT and aPTT levels should be drawn after transfusion to guide treatment. FFP transfusion may need to be repeated within 6 hours if rapid reversal of coagulopathy is needed.[12] FFP should not be used for volume replacement, and its use has often been supplanted by specific recombinant viral-attenuated products.

Other Plasma Products

Cryoprecipitate

Cryoprecipitate is the cold-insoluble precipitate protein fraction derived from FFP. Cryoprecipitate contains factor VIII 60–100 units/bag, fibrinogen (factor I), von Willebrand factor (vWF), and factor XIII. Cryoprecipitate transfusions are indicated in the setting of fibrinogen deficiency with bleeding, prior to invasive procedures, trauma, or DIC.[2] When the fibrinogen level is less than 100–120 mg/dL, cryoprecipitate transfusion will elevate fibrinogen levels by approximately 50 mg/dL for every unit/10 kg body weight transfused.[8,9] There is no set guideline regarding a level at which cryoprecipitate should be transfused in presence of clinically significant hypofibrinogenemia.[8] It is cell-free, so the patient should not need Rh typing, but it is not viral-attenuated, so there is risk of infection transmission. Cryoprecipitate is second-line therapy for factor VIII deficiency (Hemophilia A disease) and for von Willebrand Disease.

Cryoprecipitate transfusions are also indicated for clinically significant bleeding or pre-procedure for patients with single factor deficiencies in which no other factor concentrates are available. Factor XIII deficiency is an example, although factor XIII concentrate is preferred, since cryoprecipitate has not undergone viral attenuation steps.[1,9] Cryoprecipitate is only recommended for patients with hemophilia A or von Willebrand disease (vWD) if isolated factor VIII concentrates or factor VIII: vWF concentrates are not available.[9] In addition, cryoprecipitate may be used for patients who are uremic and bleeding, if other treatment options have been unsuccessful.[9]

The following calculation from the American Red Cross (ARC) can be used to estimate how many cryoprecipitate units to transfuse in a patient with fibrinogen deficiency:

- $Weight\ (Kg) \times 70mL/Kg = blood\ volume\ (mL)$
- $Blood\ volume\ (mL) \times (1.0 - hematocrit)$
$$= plasma\ volume\ (mL)$$

- $fibrinogen\ required\ (mg) = (desired$
$$fibrinogen\ level(mg/dL) - initial$$
$$fibrinogen\ level\ (mg/dL)) \times$$
$$\left(plasma\ volume\ (mL) \div 100\right)$$

- $Bags\ of\ cryoprecipitate\ required$
$$= mg\ fibrinogen\ required \div 250\ mg$$
$$fibrinogen\ per\ bag\ of\ cryoprecipitate$$

For clinical bleeding, the number of bags should approximate 0.2 times the patient's body weight in kilograms. Without ongoing factor consumption or large volume blood loss, one unit of cryoprecipitate per 10 kg (of body weight) will increase fibrinogen levels by 50 mg/dL unless there is bleeding or product consumption.[9]

Quantitative and Qualitative Factor Deficiencies

The three most common inherited factor disorders are hemophilia A (factor VIII deficiency), hemophilia B (factor IX deficiency), and von Willebrand disease. In specific clinical situations, these conditions may be treated with single factor transfusions. For patients with hemophilia A and B, bleeding episodes should be urgently treated by factor replacement, within 2 hours of onset of symptoms, if possible. Ideally, treatment should commence prior to the onset of physical symptoms. Furthermore, communication with a hematologist, ideally the patient's physician, is recommended in order to achieve the highest quality of care.[13]

Hemophilia A (Factor VIII Deficiency) Recombinant factor VIII is the first line treatment for hemophilia A. It is recommended over plasma-derived factor VIII, since plasma derived transfusions carry the risk of transmission of a viral illness, while there has been no documented viral transmission with recombinant transfusion. Cryoprecipitate can be used, but overall is not recommended if factor VIII is available.[13,14] Desmopressin (DDAVP) 0.3 mcg/kg IV over 30 minutes in 50–100 ml saline or as 300 mcg nasal spray) administration should be considered for every patient, especially if they phenotypically have a mild form of hemophilia A ($\geq$ 5% factor VIII activity), since it can raise factor VIII levels to 3–6 times baseline.[14] One unit of factor VIII per kilogram of body weight will increase the plasma factor VIII level by approximately 2%.[13] Therefore, the dose of factor VIII equals weight in kg times percentage required of factor VIII times 0.5; with severe factor VIII deficiency, one should assume that the patient is starting at a factor VIII level of zero.[15]

Hemophilia B (Christmas Disease) (Factor IX Deficiency) Recombinant factor IX is the first line treatment for hemophilia B. As for factor VIII, plasma derived factor IX poses risk of transmission of viral illness.[14] One unit of factor IX per kilogram of body weight will increase the plasma factor IX level by approximately 1%. FFP use is only recommended if factor IX derivatives are not available.[13]

von Willebrand Disease von Willebrand disease (vWD) has multiple phenotypes which are associated with various clinical courses and treatment.[15] Type 1 is the mildest form and can be treated with desmopressin (DDAVP). Types 2A, 2B, 2M, and 2N can be treated with factor VIII–von Willebrand factor concentrate. Type 3 can also be treated with factor VIII–von Willebrand factor concentrate, but if there are alloantibodies present, then it is recommended to use recombinant factor VIII for treatment. Approximately 10–15% of patients with type 3 vWD develop alloantibodies that bind and inactivate vWF.[16] Platelet transfusions should also be considered as an adjunct to treatment, specifically in type 3, platelet low, or platelet-type vWD, since human platelets contain 10–15% of total blood vWF.[17] Guidelines for prophylaxis against bleeding from minor surgery recommend vWF:RCo (von Willebrand Factor: Ristocetin factor activity) and factor VIII activity levels > 30 IU/dL, and ideally > 50 IU/dL.[18]

Platelets

Platelet transfusions are essential in order to achieve hemostasis during active bleeding in a patient with thrombocytopenia. As with all blood

Table 43.3 Recommended Platelet Threshold Achieved Prior to Various Interventions[9]

Procedure	Platelet Count ($\times 10^3$/mm^3)
Spinal epidural anesthesia	80
Major invasive procedures*	40–50
Fiberoptic bronchoscopy without biopsy	20
GI endoscopy without biopsy	20

* Major invasive procedures includes central venous catheter placement, paracentesis, thoracentesis, respiratory tract biopsy, GI tract biopsies, closed liver biopsy, lumbar puncture, sinus aspiration, epidural anesthesia, and dental extraction

product transfusions, a restrictive strategy is used in order to decrease the amount of unnecessary transfusions and adverse reactions, including alloimmunization with may result in platelet refractoriness.[9] This strategy also applies to platelet transfusions. By using current guidelines in conjunction with thorough evaluation of the patient's medical condition, a safe and appropriate decision for transfusion of platelets can be made.[2]

Prophylactic platelet transfusion is recommended at platelet levels of ≤10,000/mm^3 in the absence of risk factors such as sepsis, active antibiotic use, or other abnormalities of coagulopathy.[1,2,9,19,20] If the thrombocytopenia is chronic as in bone marrow failure / myelodysplasia, the patient is asymptomatic, and has no risk factors, an even lower platelet threshold is thought to be appropriate, possibly as low as 5,000/mm^3.[9,19] It is recommended to consider platelet transfusion when platelets are ≤ 20,000/mm^3 and patients are medically unstable, but not bleeding.[9] Platelet transfusions are appropriate in massive hemorrhage if the platelet count is ≤ 50,000/mm^3, and in the presence of diffuse microvascular bleeding ≤ 100,000/mm^3.[2] Additional platelet thresholds are noted in Table 43.3.

In order to decrease the frequency of adverse reactions such as fever, non-hemolytic transfusion reactions, HLA alloimmunization, and transmitted CMV infections, platelet leukocytes reduced or apheresis platelets leukocytes reduced may be used. One unit of platelets typically increases the platelet count by 5,000–10,000/mm^3 for a 70 kg adult.[1] Platelet counts should be collected approximately

10–180 minutes after the platelet transfusion has been completed. During this time period, the transfused platelets are most vulnerable to immune platelet destruction. Additional platelet counts should be drawn at 24-hour post-transfusion, which would help identify how many of the transfused platelets are being destroyed by non-immune processes.[1]

For the majority of patients with thrombocytopenia secondary to platelet destruction, such as idiopathic thrombocytopenia purpura (ITP), thrombotic thrombocytopenia purpura (TTP), and hemolytic uremic syndrome (HUS), platelet transfusions are not indicated and are unlikely to be beneficial. If a patient is actively bleeding with thrombocytopenia in these conditions, transfusion of platelets may be required to aid in hemostasis while adjunct medications begin to work. When the platelet count is $< 30,000/mm^3$ in ITP, consider a long course of steroids and IVIG/anti-D immunoglobulin for treatment.[20,22]

Transfusion Reactions

There is a wide spectrum of transfusion reactions from mild pruritus to respiratory failure and shock. Blood product transfusions are associated with a risk of transmission of infections. The AABB, formerly American Association of Blood Banks, noted that the risks of human immunodeficiency virus (HIV) and hepatitis C virus (HCV) transmission from PRBCs from 2007–2008 were approximately 1 in 1,467,000 and 1 in 1,149,000, respectively. The risk of hepatitis B virus (HBV) transmission from 2006 to 2008 for PRBCs was approximately 1 in 300,000.[1] Bacterial (Yersinia, syphilis), parasitic (malaria, Chagas), and prion (Jakob-Creutzfeldt) transmission have also been reported. For these reasons, risks of transfusions must be weighed against the benefits, and ultimately health care providers should strive to decrease the frequency of unnecessary blood product transfusions.

Acute adverse reactions can occur within minutes to hours from onset of transfusion. The reactions include acute hemolytic transfusion reaction (AHTR), febrile non-hemolytic transfusion reactions (FNHTR), allergic transfusion reactions, transfusion-related acute lung injury (TRALI), transfusion-associated circulatory overload (TACO), and transfusion related sepsis.[23] FFP is most commonly implicated in TRALI.[24] When an acute transfusion reaction is suspected, the transfusion should be immediately held. The patient should be closely monitored and evaluated for indications of the type of reactions. Symptoms may include fevers, chills, pruritus, urticaria, tachycardia, hypotension (rarely hypertension), tachypnea, shortness of breath, bronchospasm, stridor, angioedema, chest tightness, pain in chest, back, and abdomen, congestive heart failure, pulmonary edema, generalized edema, and shock.[23] These reactions must be immediately medically managed and laboratory studies sent to further identify the cause.

Delayed reactions to blood product transfusions typically occur from 24 hours post-transfusion up to several weeks. Delayed reactions include delayed hemolytic transfusion reactions (DHTRs), post-transfusion purpura (PTP), iron overload, transfusion-associated graft-versus-host-disease (TA-GVHD), and transfusion-associated thrombosis and immunomodulation/inflammation.[23] It is imperative that patients be given information regarding warning signs of these reactions and instructions for follow-up once discharged from the OU.

References

1. Carson JL, Grossman BJ, Kleinman S, et al. Red Blood cell transfusion: a clinical practice guideline from the AABB. Ann Int Med 2012; 157 (1):49–58.

2. National Health and Medical Research Council and the Australasian Society of Blood Transfusion. Clinical practice guidelines on blood product utilization [online text]. 2001. Available at: www.nhmrc .gov.au/_files_nhmrc/ publications/attachments/ cp78.pdf?q=publications/ synopses/_files/cp78.pdf. Accessed February 20, 2016.

3. Guidelines for the clinical use of red cell transfusions. British J Haematol, 2001;113: 24–31.

4. Viele MK, Weiskopf RB. What can we learn about the need for transfusion from patients who refuse blood? The experience with Jehovah's Witnesses. Transfusion 1994; 43: 396–401.

5. Liumbruno G, Bennardello F, Lattanzio A, et al. Recommendations for the transfusion of red blood cells. Blood Transfus 2009, 7:49–64.

6. Choo Y. The HLA system in transfusion medicine. In: McCullough J, ed. Transfusion

Medicine. New York, NY: McGraw–Hill Book Co;1998:401.

7. Castro O. Management of sickle-cell disease: recent advances and controversies. *Br J Haematology.* 1999; 107: 2–11.

8. British Committee for Standards in Haematology. Guidelines for the use of fresh-frozen plasma, cryoprecipitate and cryosupernatant. *The British Society for Haematology,* 2004; 126: 11–28.

9. American Red Cross. Practice Guidelines for Blood Transfusions [online text]. 2nd ed. 2007. Available at: www.redcross.org/ www-files/Documents/ WorkingWiththeRed Cross/practiceguideline sforbloodtrans.pdf. Accessed January 5, 2012.

10. Baker RI, Coughlin PB, Gallus AS, et al. Warfarin reversal: consensus guidelines, on behalf of the Australasian Society of Thrombosis and Haemostasis. *MJA* 2004; 181: 492–497.

11. Baker RI, Coughlin PB, Gallus AS, et al. Warfarin reversal: consensus guidelines, on behalf of the Australasian Society of Thrombosis andHaemostasis. *MJA* 2004; 181: 492–497.

12. Cushman M, Lim W, Zakai N. American Society of Hematology: Clinical Practice Guide on Anticoagulant Dosing and Management of Anticoagulant-Associated Bleeding Complications in Adults [online text]. 2011. Available at: www.hematology .org/Practice/Guidelines/ 7243.aspx. Accessed February 20, 2016.

13. World Federation of Hemophilia. Guidelines for the Management of Hemophilia [online text]. 2013. Available at: www.wfh.org/2/docs/ Publications/Diagnosis_and_ Treatment/Guidelines_Mng_ Hemophilia.pdf. Accessed February 20, 2016.

14. National Hemophilia Foundation. Medical and Scientific Advisory Council Recommendations Concerning Products Licensed for the Treatment of Hemophilia and Other Bleeding Disorders [online text]. 2015. Available at: www.hemophilia.org/ NHFWeb/MainPgs/Main NHF.aspx?menuid=57& contentid=693. Accessed February 20, 2016.

15. Ansell JE. 9th National Conference on Anticoagulant Therapy. *Preface. J Thromb Thrombolysis* 2008; 25:1.

16. Mannucci, PM. Treatment of von Willebrand's Disease. *N Engl J Med* 2004;351: 683–694.

17. National Heart, Lung, and Blood Institute The-Diagnosis-Evaluation-and-Management-of-von-Willebrand-Disease-[online text]. 2008. Available at: http://catalog.nhlbi.nih.gov/ catalog/product/The-Diagnosis-Evaluation-and-Management-of-von-Willebrand-Disease-Full-Report-/08-5832. Accessed February 20, 2016.

18. American Society of Hematology: Clinical Practice Guideline on the Evaluation and Management of von Willebrand Disease [online text]. 2012. Available at: www.hematology.org/practice/ guidelines/426.aspx. Accessed February 20, 2016.

19. British Committee for Standards in Haematology. Guidelines for the use of platelet transfusions. *The British Society for Haematology,* 2003; 122: 10–23.

20. Slichter SJ. Evidence-based platelet transfusion guidelines. *American Society of Hematology Education Book.* 2007;1:172–178.

21. American Society of Hematology: Clinical Practice Guideline on the Evaluation and Management of Immune Thrombocytopenia [online text]. 2011. Available at: www.hematology.org/Practice/ Guidelines/6584.aspx. Accessed February 20, 2016.

22. Cines DB, Blanchette VS. Immune Thrombocytopenic Purpura. *N Engl J Med* 2002; 346:995–1008.

23. McCullough J, Refaai MA, Cohn CS. Blood Procurement and Red Cell Transfusion. In: Kaushansky K, Lichtman MA, Prchal JT, et al. eds. Williams Hematology. 9th ed. New York: McGraw-Hill; 2016, chapter 138. www.accessmedicine. com.library.ccf.org/content .aspx?aID=6236286. Accessed February 20, 2016.

24. Vigue B. Bench-to-bedside review: Optimizing emergency reversal of Vitamin K antagonists in severe haemorrhage – from theory to practice. *Crit Care* 2009; 13: 209.

Subpart IVG   Clinical – Infections

Chapter

Skin and Soft Tissue Infections (SSTI)

Robert S. Bennett, MD

Introduction

A growing number of patients present to emergency departments (EDs) with skin and soft tissue infections (SSTIs). Between 1993 and 2005, the number of visits to US EDs for SSTIs nearly tripled increasing from 1.2 to 3.4 million.[1] Hospital admissions for SSTIs increased by 29% from 2000 to 2004.[2] Many of these patients are ideal candidates for initial management in an observation unit (OU). Patients with SSTIs make up about 2% of all patients cared for in OUs in the United States.[3] (It is the fourth most common diagnosis, if cardiovascular conditions are grouped together.)[3] Within the broad spectrum of illness severity for SSTIs, there is a group of patients who could be appropriately cared for in an OU.

The overwhelming majority of SSTIs are caused by Staphylococcal and Streptococcal species of bacteria. More severe SSTIs, including necrotizing fasciitis or extensive cellulitis with septicemia, will require inpatient management. Patients who appear to have only mild disease can be discharged home directly from the ED with close follow-up. OU care can be an effective management choice for patients who require only a day or two of intravenous antibiotics to assure sufficient response while monitoring for clinical progression to more serious conditions.

This chapter will review the basic pathophysiology and etiology of common SSTIs, and discuss how to identify patients who can be ideally managed in an OU. Management of SSTIs will be reviewed with reference to the 2011 IDSA (Infectious Diseases Society of America) guidelines.[4] Potential challenges and pitfalls of caring for SSTI patients will be identified.

Discussion

Patients with cellulitis are the most common SSTI that should be considered as a candidate for OU care. Most uncomplicated SSTIs are caused by Streptococcal or Staphylococcal organisms. The dramatic rise in the incidence of community acquired methicillin resistant Staphylococcal (MRSA) infections has led to changes in the approach to antibiotic choice and management of abscesses. Prior to the rise in MRSA, uncomplicated cellulitis patients could be discharged home on a single antibiotic such as cephalexin.

Although most "non-suppurative" SSTIs are caused by Streptococcal species, studies have demonstrated the inability of clinicians to accurately judge the likelihood of MRSA infection.[5] Therefore, there is increased risk of failure with treatment using traditional antibiotics for cellulitis. It often makes sense, therefore, to initiate antibiotic treatment in an observation setting to assure sufficient response to the chosen regimen. The previously established practice of incision and drainage (I and D) of abscesses followed by discharge home without antibiotic coverage is being reexamined. New guidelines from the IDSA recommend antibiotic coverage after I and D under numerous conditions.[4] Some of these patients may require intravenous antibiotics and inpatient or OU care.

Clinical Presentation

The clinical manifestations of SSTIs are widely variable, but generally include presentations of skin erythema, warmth, swelling, and pain in the affected area. Patients may complain of a "spider bite," which more likely represents infection rather than any kind of bite.[6] Abscesses are sometimes obvious, but can also present more insidiously with edema and no apparent collection. An underlying abscess should be suspected in patients with presumed cellulitis who have failed to respond to initial antibiotic therapy.[7]

In the era prior to the rise in community-acquired MRSA infections, most abscesses presenting to the ED could be reliably managed by I and D without antibiotic coverage. If antibiotics were used, most patients would be treated as outpatients with oral medications. The dramatically increased prevalence of MRSA has resulted in the recognition that many patients with abscesses may now require oral or intravenous antibiotics. Thus, a number of patients who previously would be discharged home after I and D have become candidates for referral to the OU. Studies of this situation have produced conflicting results and there is general disagreement about the appropriate course of action. A 2008 *New England Journal* article[8,9] polled over 10,000 physicians regarding three different management choices for a patient presenting with a simple 5 cm abscess. Three different experts discussed rationale for selecting either I and D alone (31% of votes), I and D with anti-MRSA coverage (41% of votes) or I and D with anti-methicillin sensitive Staphylococcal aureus coverage (28% of votes).

The 2011 IDSA guidelines[4] recommend antibiotic coverage following I and D of abscesses associated with the following conditions: multiple sites of infection, rapid progression, signs and symptoms of systemic illness, associated comorbidities (such as diabetes) or immunosuppression, extremes of age, areas difficult to drain (face, hand, genitals) or lack of response to I and D. Other studies have recommended antibiotic coverage for abscesses greater than 5 cm in diameter.[10]

Laboratory Evaluation and Imaging

Patients with simple cellulitis, normal vital signs, and no underlying conditions should not require extensive laboratory evaluation. A white blood cell count (WBC) may be useful in identifying patients at risk for extended hospitalization.[11] However, most patients with SSTIs in the ED will not be triaged based upon laboratory data. Prior to the rise in prevalence of MRSA, pus from uncomplicated abscesses generally did not require culture. However, due to the change in the epidemiology of SSTIs, purulent material from an abscess or wound should be cultured if the patient is to be started on antibiotics (2011 IDSA recommendation).[4] It is widely recognized that blood cultures are not useful for the majority of patients with SSTIs.[7,12] This is especially true in patients with purulent material readily available. However, patients with extensive disease or signs of sepsis

should have blood cultures performed. This would usually preclude OU placement. It is also widely accepted that needle aspiration or biopsy of inflamed skin (or "leading edge") is not useful.[12]

Other ancillary laboratory tests for patients with SSTIs have been proposed as useful in detecting patients at risk for necrotizing infections. The Laboratory Risk Indicator for Necrotizing Fasciitis (LRINEC) score has been studied to identify patients with SSTIs who are evolving into a life-threatening infection.[13] The score is based upon laboratory values including C-reactive protein (CRP), total WBC count, serum sodium, creatinine, glucose, and hemoglobin. However, most patients with an elevated score have other signs indicating serious disease. The utility of the score in identifying early cases of necrotizing infections has not been validated. Therefore, ordering tests such as CRP in patients with SSTIs need not be routine. It has also been proposed that an elevated creatine phosphokinase level should increase suspicion of a necrotizing infection, but this has not been well studied.[7]

Under certain conditions, radiologic studies such as plain radiographs, computed tomography, or magnetic resonance imaging can provide useful information. Circumstances include concerns about osteomyelitis or foreign body retention. Duplex venograms should be considered in patients with extremity swelling more consistent with deep venous thrombosis. Bedside ultrasound has become more prevalent in many EDs and can provide assistance with diagnosing occult cutaneous abscesses. Ultrasound has been found to provide greater sensitivity and specificity in detecting deep abscesses than clinical examination alone.[14,15] Detection of abscesses with ultrasound can be readily learned by novice sonographers.[16]

Patient Selection Criteria

The selection process of appropriate patients with SSTIs for an OU has several dimensions. One dimension is the identification of patients who appear likely to fail outpatient treatment with oral antibiotics and prevent subsequent return visits to the hospital. Another is the selection of patients who clearly need intravenous antibiotics, but are likely to improve sufficiently for discharge home in less than 24 hours. Finally, patients who are at risk for deterioration or who are likely to require an extended stay should be directed to an inpatient unit.

There have been no prospectively validated selection criteria or guidelines to assist in the selection of appropriate patients with SSTIs for an OU. A retrospective cohort study identified the presence of fever in patients presenting to an ED with SSTIs to be a predictor of need for greater than 24 hours of care in the hospital.[17] However, many patients with fever could, at least initially, be managed in an OU. Conversely, there are many patients without fever presenting with complex SSTIs who are clearly not appropriate for observation care. Another retrospective cohort study attempted to predict treatment failures in OU patients treated with SSTIs. Among the variables evaluated (intravenous drug use, positive MRSA culture, abscess drainage), only female gender and white blood cell count > 15,000 were significantly associated with failure to discharge.[11]

Guidelines submitted by the Infectious Diseases Society of America (IDSA) propose hospital admission for patients presenting with SSTIs who are hypotensive or have elevated creatinine, creatine phosphokinase, or C-reactive protein levels, low serum bicarbonate level or left shift of the white blood cell differential.[12] These guidelines are not useful for identifying appropriate OU patients and would likely indicate patients at risk for more serious conditions such as septicemia or necrotizing fasciitis. Most candidates for OU care should not require the extensive laboratory evaluation proposed by the IDSA.

A classification system of illness severity has been proposed to assist in the triage of patients with SSTIs.[18] (Table 44.1). Most patients with Class 1 criteria (afebrile and healthy) could be considered for discharge home on oral antibiotics. Some of these patients should be considered as observation candidates based upon circumstances such as lack of follow-up care or predicted noncompliance. Many Class 2 patients (febrile or ill-appearing with stable comorbidity) should be considered for OU management. It would be expected that a certain proportion of these patients may require transfer to an inpatient unit for failure to improve. About 30% of patients with SSTIs required inpatient conversion in a national survey.[3] Few Class 3 patients (toxic appearance or unstable comorbidity) should be routinely considered for referral to an OU.

Table 44.1 Disposition According to Classification System for Patients with SSTIs*

Class	Patient Criteria	Disposition/ Suitability for Observation Unit Care
1	Afebrile, healthy (aside from SSTI)	Home or observation if risk features present (see text)
2	Febrile, appear ill, or stable comorbidity	Observation unit management appropriate
3	Toxic appearance, or unstable comorbidity, threatened limb	Unlikely to be safely managed in observation unit
4	Septicemia, life-threatening infection (necrotizing fasciitis)	Inpatient or intensive care unit most appropriate

SSTIs = skin and soft tissue infections
*One proposed classification system for SSTIs adapted and modified from[18]

Table 44.2 Features of Patients with SSTIs Suggesting Benefit from Observation Unit Placement

Failure of outpatient treatment
Inability to tolerate oral antibiotic
Multiple antibiotic allergies
Pain management issues but not chronic pain
Risk of noncompliance due to social circumstances
Abscess with indications for antibiotic coverage
Multiple sites of involvement
Fever (without Systemic Inflammatory Response Syndrome [SIRS])
Diabetes mellitus

SSTIs = skin and soft tissue infections

Certain features of patients with SSTIs presenting to the ED can be used to identify who would likely benefit from a stay in an OU (Table 44.2). These include failure of outpatient treatment, inability to tolerate oral antibiotic or risk of noncompliance due to social circumstances. Conversely, there are features of patients with SSTIs that would identify those who are at greater risk of complications or a prolonged stay and would be better served by disposition to an inpatient unit (Table 44.3). These include patients

Table 44.3 Features of Patients with SSTIs to Consider Exclusion from Observation Unit Placement

Features of SIRS (systemic inflammatory response syndrome)
White blood cell count > 15,000[18]
Wounds (e.g. animal or human bite) with extensive tissue damage
High-risk locations (face, neck, hand, genitals)
Pain out of proportion to clinical findings

SSTIs = skin and soft tissue infections

Table 44.4 Common Conditions that Mimic SSTIs

Venous thrombotic disease (superficial or deep)
Herpes zoster
Contact dermatitis
Septic bursitis or arthritis, gout
Insect envenomation
Fixed drug eruption

SSTIs = skin and soft tissue infections

with a white blood cell count > 15,000, high-risk SSTI locations (face or hand) and bite wounds. There is a clear need for controlled trials to determine which of these characteristics are reliable and useful.

Care should also be taken to be alert for conditions that could mimic or masquerade as an SSTI, as many of these conditions should not be managed in an OU or would require treatment other than antibiotics.[19] (Table 44.4)

Management

Antibiotic choice is the primary treatment decision for OU patients with SSTIs. Recent recommendations have led to a new terminology regarding types of cellulitis, which leads to logical selection of antibiotics. Cellulitis can usually be categorized as "purulent" or "non-purulent." Patients with obvious purulence (such as an abscess) should be treated with antibiotics effective for MRSA (clindamycin or vancomycin). If culture data becomes available, then antibiotic choice can be adjusted. Patients without obvious purulence who are not in a high-risk group for MRSA may be treated with a beta-lactam antibiotic such as cefazolin or clindamycin. Bite wounds should receive coverage with antibiotics such as ampicillin/sulbactam to cover Pasturella species.

Vancomycin has generally been the drug of choice for hospitalized patients with SSTIs. However, in the OU, there are numerous reasons to avoid using vancomycin and consider other antibiotics such as clindamycin or cefazolin. Although clindamycin has not been well studied in the treatment of MRSA infections, it is a logical choice for patients in the setting of an OU. Clindamycin doesn't require monitoring of levels as does vancomycin. It can readily be converted to an oral dose at the time of discharge. It will also cover beta-hemolytic Streptococci, making it an ideal choice

for patients with cellulitis that may not appear purulent, but have other risk factors for MRSA. The D-zone test for inducible resistance to clindamycin is performed on MRSA isolates that are resistant to erythromycin, but sensitive to clindamycin. Some patients with mild infections may still respond to clindamycin in spite of inducible resistance. However, patients with more serious infections or with slow response should be switched to other antibiotics such as vancomycin or linezolid. Cefazolin can be used for patients without evidence of purulence or obvious risk factors for MRSA. If there is lack of response or progression, then the antibiotic can be changed. Trimethoprim-sulfmethoxazole (TMP-SMZ) is mostly of use for patients who are being discharged home on oral antibiotics. It should be used for patients with purulent cellulitis or MRSA proven by culture, since it is not sufficiently active against Streptococci.[4] Other antibiotics noted to be useful in the treatment of hospitalized patients with SSTIs include linezolid, daptomycin, telavancin, and ceftaroline. Tigecycline (a tetracycline derivative) was found to be associated with higher mortality rates in clinical trials and was not included in the IDSA 2011 guidelines.[4] One might argue that management of patients with SSTIs that require less commonly used antibiotics should not take place in an OU (at least, not without consultation with an infectious disease specialist).

Discharge or Transfer Criteria

Patients who fail to respond to 24–48 hours of antibiotic treatment or develop signs of more serious illness such as necrotizing fasciitis should be transferred to an inpatient unit. Lack of response to antibiotics could also indicate the presence of a condition other than an SSTI or development of an abscess that was not identified at admission. Discharge home generally coincides with the ability to transition to oral antibiotic therapy. Although studies have shown that patients with SSTIs on intravenous antibiotics can be safely switched to oral agents after 3 to 4 days, there have been no studies of the population of patients likely to be cared for in an OU who may be able to go home in less than 24 hours.

Signs that indicate a patient can be switched to oral antibiotics and discharged home include decrease in extent and degree of erythema and edema, decrease in white blood cell count with differential shift, absence of fever, and the patient's ability to take oral medications. It may be helpful to draw an outline around the extent of erythema when a patient presents with an SSTI. On the other hand, there is some evidence that the inflammatory response to infection causing fever and erythema increases during the first 24 hours of treatment and may not necessarily indicate treatment failure.[20] There isn't any evidence to support a delay in discharge while awaiting confirmation of continued clinical improvement after switching from intravenous to oral antibiotics.[20]

At discharge from the OU, a decision will need to be made regarding total duration of therapy for treatment. There is little evidence to guide duration of antibiotic treatment after discharge from the OU. A study of outpatients receiving 5 days versus 10 days of oral antibiotic therapy with levofloxacin (not generally a good choice for the treatment of SSTIs) found no differences in outcome.[21] The IDSA guidelines recommend 7 to 14 days of therapy, with individualization based upon clinical response.[4]

Considerations regarding follow-up care should be addressed as well. If a hospital outpatient pharmacy is available, an attempt should be made to discharge patients with antibiotics in hand to enhance compliance. Patients with a primary care physician should follow-up at some point during their home treatment to assure progress towards resolution. Patients without physicians should return for a "skin check" if feasible or receive a phone call to assess their status.

Prevention of Recurrent MSRA Infections

Some patients managed in the OU may present with recurrent SSTIs presumed to be caused by MRSA. There is no evidence that decolonization strategies are useful in the reduction of recurrent MRSA SSTIs. However, the IDSA recommends consideration of intranasal mupirocin or bleach baths for patients with recurrent SSTIs in spite of optimal wound care and personal hygiene measures.[4] Of note, this recommendation is based on poor evidence and no clinical trials. It is recognized that mupirocin use could result in the selection of more resistant strains. It is also apparent that decolonization of the nares fails to address multiple other sites that are commonly colonized (axilla and groin).

Conclusion

The rise of community-acquired MRSA has resulted in a precipitous increase in patients presenting to EDs with SSTIs. These patients have produced a potential growth industry for OUs where it is feasible and practical to initiate treatment, assess response, and safely discharge. There are many unanswered questions that deserve evidence-based study, such as patient selection, optimal duration of therapy (intravenous in the hospital and oral after discharge home), objective measurements of clinical response, and appropriate management of abscesses. It is likely that patients with SSTIs can be managed more cost-effectively in an observation unit than an inpatient unit, but this too needs further study.

References

1. Pallin DJ, Egan DJ, Pelletier AJ, et al. Increased US emergency department visits for skin and soft tissue infections, and changes in antibiotic choices, during the emergence of community-associated methicillin-resistant Staphylococcus aureus. *Ann Emerg Med.* 2008;51:291–298.

2. Edelsberg J. Trends in US hospital admissions for skin and soft tissue infection. *Emerg Infect Dis.* 2009;15(9): 1516–1518.

3. Venkatesh AK, Geisler BP, Gibson Chambers JJ, et al. Use of observation care in US emergency departments, 2001 to 2008. *PLoS ONE* 2011;6(9):e24326.

Doi:10.1371/journal. pone.0024326.

4. Liu C, Bayer A, Cosgrove SE, et al. Clinical practice guidelines by the Infectious Diseases Society of America for the treatment of methicillin-resistant Staphylococcus aureus infections in adults and children. *Clinical Infectious Diseases* 2011;52(3):e18–e55.

5. Miller LG, Perdreau-Remington F, Bayer AS, et al. Clinical and epidemiologic characteristics cannot distinguish community-associated methicillin-resistant Staphylococcus aureus infection from methicillin-susceptible S. aureus infection: a prospective investigation. *Clin Infect Dis.* 2007 Feb 15; 44(4):471–482.

6. Suchard JR. "Spider bite" lesions are usually diagnosed as skin and soft-tissue infections. *J Emerg Med* Nov 2011;41(5): 473–481.

7. Abrahamian FM, Talan DA, Moran GJ. Management of skin and soft-tissue infections in the emergency department. *Infect Dis Clin N Am* 2008;22: 89–116.

8. Chambers HF, Moellering RC Jr, Kamitsuka P. Management of skin and soft-tissue infection. *N Engl J Med* 2008;359:1063–1067.

9. Hammond SP, Baden LR. Management of skin and soft-tissue infection-polling results. *N Engl J Med* 2008;359:e20.

10. Lee MC, Rios AM, Aten MF, et al. Management and outcome of children with skin and soft tissue abscesses caused by community-acquired methicillin-resistant Staphylococcus aureus. *Pediatr Infect Dis J* 2004;23: 123–127.

11. Schrock JW, Laskey S, Cydulka RK. Predicting observation unit treatment failures in patients with skin and soft tissue infections. *Int J Emerg Med* 2008;1:85–90.

12. Stevens KL, Bisno AL, Chambers HF, et al. Practice guidelines for the diagnosis and management of skin and soft-tissue infections. *Clinical Infectious Diseases* 2005;41:1373–1406.

13. Wong CH, Khin LW, Heng KS, et al. The LRINEC (laboratory risk indicator for necrotizing fasciitis) score: a tool for distinguishing necrotizing fasciitis from other soft tissue infections. *Crit Care Med* 2004;32(7):1535.

14. Tayal VS, Hasan N, Norton J, et al. The effect of soft-tissue ultrasound on the management of cellulitis in the emergency department. *Academic Emergency Medicine* 2006; 13:384–388.

15. Iverson K, Haritos D, Thomas R, et al. The effect of bedside ultrasound on diagnosis and management of soft tissue infections in a pediatric ED. *Am J Emerg Med* 2012; 30(8):1347–1351.

16. Berger T, Garrido F, Green J, et al. Bedside ultrasound performed by novices for the detection of abscess in ED patients with soft tissue infections. *Am J Emerg Med* 2012; 30(8):1569–1573.

17. Sabbaj A, Jensen B, Browning MA, et al. Soft tissue infections and emergency department disposition: predicting the need for inpatient admission. *Academic Emergency Medicine* 2009;16:1290–1297.

18. Eron LJ, Lipsky BA, Low DE, et al. Managing skin and soft tissue infections: expert panel recommendations on key decision points. *Journal of Antimicrobial Chemotherapy* 2003;52(Suppl. S1): i3–i17.

19. Falagas ME, Vergidis PI. Narrative review: diseases that masquerade as infectious cellulitis. *Ann Intern Med* 2005;142:47–55.

20. Boyter AC, Stephen J, Fegan PG, et al. Why do patients with infection remain in hospital once changed to oral antibiotics? *J Antimicrob Chemother* 1997; 39: 286–288.

21. Hepburn MJ, Dooley DP, Skidmore PJ, et al. Comparison of short-course (5 days) and standard (10 days) treatment for uncomplicated cellulitis. *Arch Intern Med* 2004;164:1669–1674.

Chapter

45

Abdominal Pain

Louis Graff IV, MD, FACEP, FACP

Abdominal pain is the most common chief complaint in the emergency department (ED) comprising 8% of patients[1] and it is one of the most difficult to diagnose with a very large differential diagnosis of serious, dangerous diseases. An organized approach of evaluation and testing is needed to have high performance in identifying these diseases in a timely manner.

Formulating a Diagnostic Approach

Initially the clinician needs to formulate a diagnostic approach by reviewing the patient's signs and symptoms considering what possible serious, dangerous diseases may be affecting the patient. The location of the pain can aid the clinician in his or her diagnostic approach. Right lower quadrant (RLQ) suggests appendicitis, renal colic, or in women ovarian disease (ovarian cyst, ovarian torsion, tubular abscess or pregnancy). Right upper quadrant (RUQ) suggests cholecystitis/lithiasis, localized bowel disease, or renal disease. Flank pain suggests most commonly renal colic, but other conditions must be considered such as aortic dissection. Left lower quadrant (LLQ) suggests diverticulitis or in women ovarian disease (ovarian cyst, ovarian torsion, tubular abscess or pregnancy). The associated symptoms can help focus the diagnostic approach. The time frame of presentation can aid the clinician in formulating his or her initial differential diagnosis for that patient.

Initial Diagnostic Approach

Once an initial differential diagnosis is formulated the physician can decide which initial tests are appropriate. The testing needs to be selective with a focus on the most likely diagnoses. There are tests available that can confirm the diagnosis if the clinician considers the diagnosis and tests to rule it out. For most patients with more than minor abdominal pain, the common tests are indicated: urinanalysis, cbc, and electrolytes. Urine pregnancy testing is indicated on all women of childbearing age unless they have had a hysterectomy, are menopausal, or are known pregnant. For patients with upper abdominal pain and clinical factors that suggest atherosclerotic disease is possible (patient age, cardiac risk factors, clinical presentation), myocardial ischemia needs to be considered with initial testing with EKG, cardiac biomarkers (troponin, CKMB, bnp) and then completion of the rule out evaluation during observation. Liver function tests and amylase/lipase are indicated for patients with upper abdominal pain as well. For patients who may be at risk of ischemic bowel disease, a lactate should be ordered. For many conditions the diagnosis is made by imaging. Pelvic ultrasound is used to diagnose women with lower abdominal pain who might have ovarian torsion, ovarian cyst, or ectopic pregnancy. Abdominal ultrasound is the best test for patients with upper abdominal pain who might have cholecystitis/lithiasis. Abdominal CT scan imaging is the definitive test for many serious dangerous conditions: appendicitis, abdominal aortic aneurysm, ischemic bowel, bowel obstruction, and volvulus.

Threshold for Testing for High Reliability

High reliability is dependent upon the clinician having high-enough suspicion and low-enough threshold for testing to identify those patients who have a serious dangerous disease. Abdominal CT scan imaging is an example of testing in abdominal pain patients that is crucial for high-quality care, but must be limited to selected patients because of risk to the patient from radiation exposure, increased service time when ordered, and cost to the patient. The threshold

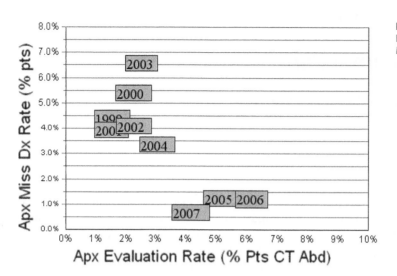

Figure 45.1 Institution's Appendicitis Evaluation Rate versus Appendicitis Missed Diagnosis Rate

for ordering this test needs to be addressed for institutions that seek to provide best practice care.

Obtaining the optimal threshold for CT scan imaging of abdominal pain patients is dependent upon measuring individual and group performance accuracy in diagnosing serious, dangerous diseases that present with abdominal pain. The goal is to identify those patients with acute appendicitis (the most common abdominal surgical emergency) who present atypically and in whom the diagnosis of appendicitis would not be evident without CT scan imaging. Patients who have risk factors for an atypical presentation of appendicitis (very young, very old, female, very early presentation, immunosuppressed) are prime candidates for abdominal CT scan imaging. Keep in mind that for young females the preferred initial imaging is ultrasound because of their increased risk from radiation exposure from CT scan imaging.

The threshold for CT scan imaging is clinically set to obtain as low a missed diagnosis rate as possible, while having as low a utilization of the CT scan imaging as possible. The method to achieve this is feedback of performance to the individual and the group. When the missed diagnosis rate is at a best practice low rate, then that sets the rate for ordering the test as measured by CT scan imaging per patients who present with a chief complaint of abdominal pain. This approach is only possible with significant performance improvement resources including an electronic database and analytic and reporting support.

Figure 45.1 shows the graph over time of the rate of CT scan imaging in abdominal pain patients versus the rate of failure to diagnose acute appendicitis. The national average for the missed diagnosis of appendicitis is approximately 8% for emergency physicians, which results in a doubling of the perforation rate and the accompanying complications.[2] Performance is improved by two components of performance feedback. First is feedback to individual practitioners of their individual missed diagnosed cases as they occur and sharing the story of lessons learned with the group. Second is periodic feedback to individual practitioners of their performance on the rate of abdominal CT scan imaging in abdominal pain patients versus their rate of missed diagnosis of appendicitis. Yearly feedback may be all that is practical, but abdominal CT scan imaging rates may be possible monthly if there is sufficient technologic and staff support.

Efforts to improve performance need to focus on the group as well as the individual. All clinicians follow their own individual performance as well as the group as a whole. It is a never-ending quest to reach zero missed diagnoses with satisfaction, when performance reaches best practice level. The challenge is particularly difficult for those patients who often present atypically with their condition and who are often not diagnosed by even the most astute physician (the very elderly, the very young, and the immunosuppressed).[2]

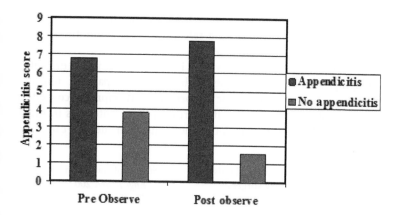

Figure 45.2 Appendicitis Score Before and After Observation (from Graff LG, et al. *Ann Emerg Med* 1991; 20: 503–507).

Role of Observation

Many patients with abdominal pain benefit from observation rather than disposition after the initial evaluation and testing. A period of observation can clarify the patient's clinical findings and improve the physician's estimate of the patient's probability of disease/risk of adverse event. A period of observation can improve the performance of the diagnostic test. Or a period of observation can make available a definitive test on an outpatient basis that is not available 24 hours a day, 7 days a week.

Clarity of the patient's clinical findings may occur with observation with signs and symptoms improving or worsening during observation, thereby, helping the physician in their formulation of the patient's probability of diagnosis. For abdominal pain patients with the diagnosis of possible appendicitis, it is often difficult upon presentation to make the diagnosis.

The appendicitis score is a 10-point system of clinical symptoms and findings with the higher the score, the more likely the patient has appendicitis. At time of presentation, patients whose diagnosis is made have a score on average of 6 points but 20% of patients who are taken to surgery have false positive surgery (normal appendix at surgery) and they have a score of 6 points as well.[1] That is, they initially have a very similar clinical picture. Patients whose diagnosis is missed have on average 2 points.[2] This is very similar to what the findings are in patients with abdominal pain who do not have appendicitis and are not taken to surgery.

Observation helps the clinician better discriminate which patients with abdominal pain have disease. For example, when considering appendicitis

the clinical findings and probability of diagnosis changes dramatically with 12 hours of observation (Figure 45.2).[3] Patients who do not have appendicitis improve and their appendicitis score drops on average 3 points,[3] while those with appendicitis on average increase their score 1 point.[3] This makes it less likely that 1 out of 5 patients will be taken to unnecessary surgery. This makes it less likely that 1 out of 10 patients will have their diagnosis missed, which doubles the risk of perforation and the concomitant complications. Even more important, many patients will be able to avoid abdominal CT scan imaging and ionizing radiation exposure and the long-term risks from radiation.[4] Thus, for many abdominal pain patients the best initial decision for the patient is to delay the decision on disposition to allow tincture of time to aid the physician in his or her decision.

Improvement in the performance of the diagnostic testing can improve during observation. For example, in abdominal pain patients with possible ACS, only one-half of those with injury (acute MI) have a positive cardiac biomarker test upon presentation.[5] The cardiac muscle has been damaged yet the cardiac biomarker is not significantly increased in the blood. But after 8 to 10 hours nearly 100% of those with injury will have a positive cardiac biomarker test identifying their acute myocardial infarction.

Observation can also make it possible for the patient to receive definitive tests safely as outpatients. For many conditions, the definitive test needed to clarify a patient's condition is only available during selected time periods of the day. For patients with possible ACS, those with unstable angina cannot be identified by cardiac biomarker testing (by definition positive cardiac biomarker test means myocardial injury [infarction]). The tests that identify unstable angina are an exercise stress test or cardiac imaging, which are only available during limited time periods during the day. With the evaluation of patients in observation over 8 to 24 hours it is possible to perform these tests, identify those with unstable angina, and safely discharge home those with a negative test.

Observation is, thus, crucial in the evaluation of patients with abdominal pain. It improves diagnostic performance.[3] It improves cost effectiveness.[1] It improves patient outcomes including patient satisfaction with their medical care. [1]

References

1. American College of Emergency Physicians Practice Management Committee: Management of observation units. *Ann Emery Med* 1988;17:1348–1352.

2. Graff L, Russell J, Seashore J, et al. False-negative and false-positive errors in abdominal pain evaluation: failure to diagnose acute appendicitis and unnecessary surgery. *Acad Emerg Med* 2000; 7: 1244–1255.

3. Graff L, Radford M, Werne C. Probability of appendicitis before and after observation. *Ann Emerg Med* 1991; 20: 503–507.

4. Brenner DJ, Hall EJ. Computed Tomography—An Increasing Source of Radiation Exposure. *N Engl J Med* 2007; 357: 2277–2284.

5. Hedges JR, Young GP, Henkel GF, et al. Serial ECGs are less accurate than serial CK-MB results for emergency department diagnosis of myocardial infarction. *Ann Emerg Med.* 1992 Dec; 21(12):1445–1450.

Chapter

46

Upper Gastrointestinal (GI) Bleeding

Abhinav Chandra, MD, FACEP

Introduction

Upper gastrointestinal bleeding (UGIB) is a common emergency with an annual incidence of 50 to 150 per 100,000 of the population. Mortality from UGIB is around 10%, and may reach 35% in patients hospitalized with other concomitant medical conditions. It results in 250,000 to 300,000 hospitalizations per year, costing $2.5 billion dollars.[1] Patients with UGIB may present in shock and require fluid resuscitation and admission. However, most episodes are self-limited, and 70–80% of patients experience only a single episode. Failure to accurately identify those at high risk for rebleed may result in significant morbidity and mortality. As a result, many patients are admitted to the hospital at a significant cost.[2]

Patient Criteria

Inclusion criteria – UGIB, hemodynamically stable after emergency department (ED) evaluation and treatment, normal mentation (or at baseline), no significant comorbidities, age < 70 years.

Exclusion criteria – Variceal Bleeding, age ≥ 70, pulse rate > 100 beats per minute, systolic blood pressure < 100 mmHg, hemoglobin ≤ 10 g/dL, use of anticoagulants, abnormal mental status, bright red blood per rectum, comorbidities (coronary artery disease, renal disease, hepatic disease, malignancy, or congestive heart failure).

Discussion

Patients with UGIB may be appropriate for observation. After ED evaluation and resuscitation, those who require extended care and are considered low risk by one of two validated scoring systems are ideal candidates. Although four risk stratification scoring systems are commonly mentioned (Rockall score, the Baylor bleeding score, the Cedars-Sinai Medical Centre Predictive Index, and the Blatchford score),[3] the Blatchford and Rockall scoring systems are the two validated tools most commonly used to risk stratify patients.

The objective of the Blatchford[4] system is to identify those patients who need endoscopy to control the bleeding. It is derived from the initial triage history, physical examination, and laboratory data, without endoscopy data. The following variables are used to determine the Blatchford score: blood urea nitrogen, hemoglobin, systolic blood pressure, heart rate, syncope, melena, heart disease, and liver disease. This system was derived from 1,748 patients presenting with UGIB at 1 of 19 hospitals in western Scotland. The logistic regression model was built by stepwise selection of explanatory variables – clinical and laboratory data obtained at the time of admission.[4] Next, they prospectively validated this derivation on a group of 197 consecutive adult patients admitted with upper gastrointestinal hemorrhage during a subsequent 3-month period in three hospitals in western Scotland. The receiver operating characteristic (ROC) curve in the validation set was 0.92 ($CI_{95\%}$ 0.88–0.95). A score of 5 or less was associated with a < 2% chance for need for intervention.[4]

The Rockall score[5] was first reported in 1995 and is one of the best known. The data presented was prospectively collected as part of a national audit of the management and outcome of acute upper gastrointestinal hemorrhage at four health regions in England. Seventy-four hospitals participated in the initial audit, which lasted from June to October 1993. A total of 4,185 cases of acute upper gastrointestinal hemorrhage identified over 4 months in 1993 and an additional 1,625 cases identified over a 3-month period in 1994 were included in the study. This study identified five independent variables that were predictive of rebleeding or death {age (points

0–2), presence of shock (points 0–2), comorbidity (points 0–3), diagnosis (points 0–2), and endoscopic stigmata of recent hemorrhage (points 0–2)}. The maximum possible score was 11, and a low-risk score was determined as a score of 0 to 2.[6] This was prospectively validated by Hay et al.[7] in 299 patients and demonstrated only 0.6% of patients had subsequent complications. This was also validated by Tham et al.[8] in 102 patients. The low-risk group of patients had no adverse outcomes.

In summary, these two risk stratification systems may be utilized to identify patients at low risk and potentially able to be discharged after early endoscopy. Patients with portal hypertension, with varicosities, taking anticoagulants, and with unstable vital signs are not ideal candidates for a clinical decision unit. The ideal patients are < 60 years old, without significant comorbidities, and felt to be reliable and compliant.

Management

Nonvariceal UGIB patients can be optimally managed initially in an ED-based Clinical Decision Unit (CDU) for up to 24 hours with hydration, proton pump inhibitors, serial hemoglobin/hematocrit measurements, serial orthostatics, and gastroenterology consult for early endoscopy, defined as within 24 hours of presentation.

The use of proton pump inhibitors (PPI) has been debated and evaluated in several trials. One study by Dr. Alan Barkum[9] analyzed data from the Canadian Registry on nonvariceal UGIB. This trial analyzed 1,869 patients with UGIB. Decreased rebleeding was significantly and independently associated with PPI use (85% of patients, mean daily dose 56 ± 53 mg) regardless of endoscopic stigmata, (odds ratio [OR]:0.53, 95% confidence interval, 95% CI:0.37–0.77). PPI use (OR:0.18, 95% CI:0.04–0.80) was independently associated with decreased mortality in patients.[9] Based on this and other trials, a Consensus Panel[10] recommended that PPIs should be provided, in the form of a bolus and then followed by an infusion, to patients with UGIB.

Outcome

Though some clinical trials have been performed in the care and treatment of nonvariceal UGIB, none have been in an ED-based CDU. Thus, the evidence about the success of observation care has been extrapolated from clinical trials performed around the world by gastroenterologists and other nonemergency medicine specialists and from one ED study.[11]

Trials have validated scoring systems, demonstrated decreased length of stay, decreased readmissions for bleeding, and decreased cost. Dr. Wrenn[11] and his team demonstrated the safety of rapid ED evaluation. Wrenn et al. studied a cohort of 96 patients presenting with UGIB who were followed in the ED for 6 hours. Thirty-eight of these patients were considered low risk as defined by lack of orthostatics, lack of underlying significant comorbid disease, hemoglobin concentration > 10 gm/dL, age < 60 years old, and felt to be reliable and compliant. Of the 38, 33 were discharged and 31 followed-up. None required readmission or transfusion.[11]

A trial by Rockall et al.[6] evaluated the safety of early discharge after endoscopy. They concluded that approximately 33% of low-risk UGIB patients are eligible for discharge after endoscopic evaluation. The rebleed rate was less than 5% and a mortality rate in this group was 0.1%.[6]

In a trial by Longstretch et al.[12], the investigators prospectively identified low-risk upper gastrointestinal hemorrhage patients using Rockall's criteria. Only one patient in 34 was readmitted for rebleed and there were no deaths. He calculated that approximately $1000 dollars was saved in hospital costs per outpatient treated.[12]

The key to the care of a patient with UGIB is appropriate risk stratification and endoscopic evaluation. The identification of low-risk findings on endoscopy in the alimentary tract allows for discharge, while the findings of high-risk features support further care. These findings have been reported in prior publications.

In an analysis of data from 37 prospective trials in which patients did not receive endoscopic therapy, Laine and Peterson[13] found that the rate of further bleeding was less than 5% in patients with a clean ulcer base and increased to 10% in patients with a flat spot. These patients would be appropriate for outpatient care after completion of observation.

A consensus statement by Barkun et al.[10] summarized high-risk endoscopic features and their rebleed rates. The bleeding risks were 22% in those with an adherent clot, 43% in those with a nonbleeding visible vessel, and 55% in those with active bleeding (oozing and spurting). Other such endoscopic features at high risk for rebleeding include ulcer size ($>$ 1 or 2 cm) and the site of bleeding (the posterior lesser gastric curvature and posterior duodenal wall).[10]

In low-risk patients, Longstretch et al.,[12] Cipolletta et al.[14], and Lee et al.[15] demonstrated cost reductions of 43–91% with the use of early endoscopy in randomized controlled studies. As mentioned, in the Longstretch et al. study, there was only one admission for rebleeding in 34 patients, no deaths and about $1,000 savings in hospital costs per outpatient treated.[12] In the Cipolletta et al. study, 95 consecutive patients at low risk for recurrent bleeding were randomized for either early discharge and outpatient care (N = 48) or hospital care (N = 47) and then followed up at 30 days for morbidity and mortality. In their trial, all patients underwent endoscopy within 12 hours of the onset of hemorrhage, which should be easily accomplished from a clinical decision unit. No patient underwent surgery or died. Rates of recurrent bleeding were 2.1% in the early discharge group and 2.2% in the hospital-treated group (one patient in each group). Median costs were $340 for the outpatient group and $3940 for the hospital group ($p = 0.001$).[14]

Lee's trial showed similar results. In his trial, all eligible patients with UGIB were randomized after admission to undergo endoscopy in 1 to 2 days (control) or early endoscopy in the ED. Patients with low-risk findings on early endoscopy were discharged directly from the ED and followed up at 30 days. In 110 consecutive patients with nonvariceal UGIB, discharge from the ED occurred in 26 of 56 (46%) patients. No patient discharged from the ED suffered an adverse outcome. The hospital stay (median of 1 day [interquartile range of 0 to 3 days] versus 2 days [interquartile range of 2 to 3 days], $p = 0.0001$) and the cost of care ($2068 [interquartile range of $928 to $3960] versus $3662 [interquartile range of $2473 to $7280], $p = 0.00006$) were significantly less for the early endoscopy group.[15]

Our understanding of gastrointestinal hemorrhage is in its infancy. The potential for increasing the CDU's role in managing gastrointestinal bleeding is exponential. Future investigations need to be done in the clinical decision unit in order to validate the results of prior studies. Information is needed to develop scoring systems for identifying low-risk patients and to identify lesions at high risk for recurrence of lower gastrointestinal bleeding. Finally, trials need to be conducted to demonstrate the impact on cost as a result of observation care under the direction of Emergency Medicine.

Conclusion

Patients may be placed in an OU for nonvariceal upper gastrointestinal hemorrhage. These patients can be safely stratified to discharge versus admission based on a validated, prognostic scoring system, and can have an early endoscopic procedure within 24 hours of observation care in a clinical decision unit.

References

1. Hay A, Maldonado L, Weingarten SR, et al. Prospective evaluation of a clinical guideline recommending hospital length of stay in upper gastrointestinal tract hemorrhage. *JAMA.* 1997; 278: 2151–2156.

2. Ferguson CB, Mitchell RM. Nonvariceal Upper Gastrointestinal Bleeding: Standard and New Treatment. *Gastroenterol Clin N Am.* 2005; 34:607

3. Das A, Wong RCK. Prediction of outcome of acute GI hemorrhage: a review of risk scores and predictive models.

Gastrointest Endosc. 2004; 60: 85–93.

4. Blatchford O, Murray WR, Blatchford MA. A risk score to predict need for treatment for upper-gastrointestinal hemorrhage. *Lancet.* 2000; 356:1318–1321.

5. Rockall TA, Logan RFA, Devlin HB, et al. Variation in outcome after acute upper gastrointestinal hemorrhage. *Lancet.* 1995; 346:346–350.

6. Rockall TA, Logan RF, Devlin HB, et al. Risk assessment after acute upper gastrointestinal hemorrhage. *Gut.* 1996; 38: 316–321.

7. Hay JA, Maldonado L, Weingarten SR, et al. Prospective evaluation of a clinical guideline recommending hospital length of stay in upper gastrointestinal tract hemorrhage. *JAMA.* 1997; 278:2151–2156.

8. Tham TCK, James C, Kelly M. Predicting outcome of acute nonvariceal upper gastrointestinal hemorrhage without endoscopy using the clinical Rockall Score. *Postgrad Med J.* 2006; 82: 757–759.

9. Barkun A, C.M., Sabbah S, Enns R, et al. The Canadian Registry on Nonvariceal Upper Gastrointestinal Bleeding and

Endoscopy (RUGBE): Endoscopic Hemostasis and Proton Pump Inhibition are Associated with Improved Outcomes in a Real-Life Setting. *Am J Gastroenterol.* 2004; 99:1238–1246.

10. Barkun A, Bardou M, Marshall JK, for the Nonvariceal Upper GI Bleeding Consensus Conference Group. Consensus recommendations for managing patients with nonvariceal upper gastrointestinal bleeding. *Ann Intern Med.* 2003; 139:843–857.

11. Wrenn KD, Thompson LB. Hemodynamically stable upper gastrointestinal bleeding. *Am J Emerg Med.* 1991 Jul; 9: 309–312.

12. Longstreth GF, Feitelberg SP. Successful outpatient management of acute upper gastrointestinal hemorrhage: use of practice guidelines in a large patient series. *Gastrointest Endosc* 1998; 47:219–222.

13. Laine L, Peterson WL. Bleeding peptic ulcer. *N Engl J Med.* 1994; 331:717–727.

14. Cipolletta L, Bianco MA, Rotondano G, et al. Outpatient management for low-risk nonvariceal upper GI bleeding: a randomized controlled trial. *Gastrointest Endosc.* 2002; 55:1–5.

15. Lee JG, Turnipseed S, Romano PS, et al. Endoscopy-based triage significantly reduces hospitalization rates and costs of treating upper GI bleeding: a randomized controlled trial. *Gastrointest Endosc.* 1999; 50:755–761.

Chapter

47

Dehydration, Gastroenteritis, and Vomiting

Elizabeth A. Rees, MD
Bret A. Nicks, MD, MHA, FACEP

Background

Many patients, from newborns to the elderly, present to the emergency department (ED) every year with a chief complaint related to dehydration. Presenting symptoms can be as varied as the potential sources of dehydration. The challenge of the emergency physician is piecing together from the history and physical examination the potentially life threatening and treatable sources of dehydration as well as correcting the dehydration and associated electrolyte abnormalities. The management of the dehydrated patient can vary widely from simple encouragement of increased oral intake to aggressive intravenous (IV) fluid and electrolyte replacement. Hospital admission rates related to dehydration have a bimodal distribution, with peaks in the very young and very old.[1] The cost of caring for dehydrated patients is spread among ambulatory care services, EDs, observation units (OUs), and inpatient hospitalizations. As it relates to observation, dehydration, often from gastroenteritis, accounts for 2% to 11.7% of the adult ED observation unit (ED OU) population.[2] The Agency for Healthcare Research and Quality considers dehydration to be a frequent, potentially preventable, acute cause of hospital admission. This is supported by a small retrospective single center observational study in which the diagnosis of dehydration was identified as the highest risk diagnosis for early return visit to the ED and subsequent admission to the hospital on early return.[3] In the elderly alone the cost of dehydration management in the inpatient setting is greater than one billion dollars a year.[4] Early and successful management of acute dehydration is an area of potential savings of limited health care dollars – and ED OU management is essential in this process.

Pathophysiology

Dehydration is the end result of total body water loss. It can be due to a multitude of causes that result from decreased intake, excessive losses, or fluid shifts from extracellular spaces. The average healthy adult requires approximately 1 to 1.5 liters of water per day. Water losses occur from urine, feces, sweating, and respiration. These losses increase with renal concentrating problems, medication effects, diarrhea, vomiting, environmental exposure, and fever. Fluid losses with vomiting, diarrhea, etc. and/or decreased fluid intake – and even the fluid shifts that can occur with ascites, effusions, and sepsis – can result in effective volume depletion and clinical dehydration.

Patients at increased risk for dehydration are those with comorbid illness as well as those with dependence on others for access to nourishment such as the very young and the debilitated elderly. Young children have an increased risk of dehydration related to their relative increase in total body water and their increased body surface area when compared to adults, as well as their dependence on others for hydration. As we age we have a relative decrease in total body water due to an increase in fat and decrease in skeletal muscle, but the risk of dehydration increases due to multiple other factors.[5]

Evaluation

A careful history and physical examination is required in patients presenting with dehydration. Historical features that are important to identify include the underlying health status of the patient, medications, and health problems, and the ability to access fluids. The physical examination when assessing for dehydration should focus on identifying potential critical, life-threatening conditions that exist. Vital signs should be performed, noting in particular the presence of fever, tachycardia, or hypotension. The physical examination should include the patient's general appearance, skin turgor, mucous membrane hydration, and capillary refill to evaluate the extent of dehydration.[5] An abdominal examination should be performed to evaluate for acute emergencies, such as evidence of appendicitis, cholecystitis, or incarcerated hernias.

Radiographic and laboratory studies should be performed at the evaluating physician's discretion to determine the extent of disease process as well to identify and rule out potentially life-threatening and treatable conditions. When indicated, studies to consider include ultrasonography and abdominal CT to evaluate for surgical pathology, and serum electrolytes or liver function tests to evaluate for complications related to dehydration itself or the precipitating cause of dehydration. Urinalysis should be considered in those patients prone to recurrent urinary tract infections or those with symptomatic dysuria. Urine output and urinalysis parameters have been used by some to assess the degree of dehydration.[6] Various dehydration scales have been suggested for assessing the degree of dehydration, but these scales have only been used in pediatric patients, particularly infants and young children.[6,7] Urine pregnancy testing should be performed in all women of childbearing age to assess for hyperemesis as a cause of their dehydration.[8]

ED OU Patient Selection – Inclusion Criteria

Careful patient selection is key to successful management in the OU setting. Appropriate patients should be hemodynamically stable with anticipation of discharge within the next 24 hours. Only mild to moderate dehydration stemming from treatable or self-limiting causes should be enrolled in the OU. Examples of appropriate presentations for OU admission are dehydration related to acute gastroenteritis, pharyngitis, or hyperemesis gravidarum, but not dehydration from an acute abdomen or diabetic ketoacidosis. If laboratory studies are performed during the initial patient evaluation, only mild electrolyte abnormalities should be present.

ED OU Patient Selection – Exclusion Criteria

Certain patients require complex care or prolonged management for treatment of dehydration and are considered poor candidates for observation dehydration protocols. In general, high-risk patients (such as those with renal failure, congestive heart failure, or liver failure) and those with hemodynamic instability should be excluded from the ED OU. Severe dehydration and marked electrolyte abnormalities are indications for hospital admission given the high likelihood of prolonged course to recovery. Conditions resulting in dehydration that require specific, focused treatment such as bowel obstruction, diabetic ketoacidosis, appendicitis, and sepsis are not amenable to ED OU care.

Management/Intervention

Observation management of dehydration allows for multiple different treatment options and interventions. IV hydration can be provided if indicated for those unable to tolerate oral fluids. Serial examinations and vital signs can be performed to evaluate response to treatment. A variety of anti-emetics can be provided to help decrease the rate of fluid loss as well as improve tolerance of oral rehydration. Most importantly, patients can be monitored for tolerance of oral fluids and ability to keep down essential medications that may factor greatly in coordinating care disposition – whether home or to an inpatient service.

As with most ED OU patients, factors related to care disposition are multifactorial. In the dehydrated patient, consideration of the underlying cause concurrent with any comorbid etiology, age, and available outpatient resources greatly impact the decision making. General guidelines for admission from the unit include unstable vital signs, cause of dehydration identified during observation requiring admission (i.e., bowel obstruction), or persistent inability to tolerate oral fluids. Patients are often safe for further management at home if their vital signs are within appropriate hemodynamic ranges, symptoms improve and the patient tolerates oral fluids, and electrolyte abnormalities resolve (if these were initially assessed). Studies of the efficacy of ED OU treatment of adults with this common condition are needed.

References

1. Agency for Healthcare Research and Quality. Preventable Hospitalizations. Part II. Detailed Statistics by Health Condition. http://archive.ahrq.gov/data/hcup/factbk5/factbk5c.htm (Accessed March 1, 2012)

2. Zalenski RJ, Rydman RJ, McCarren M, et al. Feasibility of a rapid diagnostic protocol for an emergency department chest pain unit. *Ann Emerg Med* 1997;29:99–108.

3. Gordon JA, An LC, Hayward RA, Williams BC. Initial emergency department diagnosis and return visits: risk versus perception. *Ann Emerg Med* 1998;32:569–573.

4. Xiao, et al. Economic burden of dehydration among hospitalized elderly patients; *Am J Health Sys Pharm* 2004; Dec 1; 61(23):2534–2540.

5. Armstrong J. Assessing hydration status: The elusive gold standard. *AmJ Clin Nutr* Oct 2007; 26(5):575s–584s.

6. Gorelick MH, Shaw KN, Murphy KO. Validity and reliability of clinical signs in the diagnosis of dehydration. *Pediatrics* 1997; 99(5). Available at: www.pediatrics.org/cgi/content/full/99/5/e6

7. Goldman RD, Friedman JN, Parkin PC. Validation of the clinical dehydration scale for children with acute gastroeneteritis. *Pediatrics* 2008; 122(3):545–549.

8. Cheuvront SN, Ely BR, Kenefick RW, Sawka MN. Biological variation and diagnostic accuracy of dehydration assessment markers. *Am J Clin Nutr* 2010 Sep;92(3):565–573.

Urolithiasis

Claire Pearson, MD, MPH
Robert D. Welch, MD, MS

Introduction

Urolithiasis ("urinary" or "kidney" stones) is a common medical problem for which patients often seek medical care for the symptoms of acute pain, nausea, and vomiting. The incidence of urolithiasis is over 5% of the U.S. population with a lifetime risk of 10–15% for developing a stone.[1] The majority, 70%, occur between the third and sixth decade of life, with males more commonly affected than females (7% and 3% respectively).[2] The prevalence of kidney stones has been on the rise for the past several decades.[3] Individuals that have a history of kidney stones are more likely to have a second stone with a 50% reoccurrence within 5 years and 80% within the next 20 years.[1] The costs associated with management of urolithiasis in the United States is estimated to be over $2.1 billion dollars.[4] Outpatient visits predominate but roughly 600,000 emergency department (ED) visits occur and a portion of these cases will require observation or admission.[4]

The frequency of occurrence, the need for treatment of symptoms, and, since many procedures can be done on an outpatient basis, the general lack of need for long-term hospitalization make this condition suitable for observation services. Although this section includes information on the initial diagnosis, much of the focus for observation services is on the patient in which the diagnosis has been established. Patient selection and short-term management issues are the important factors.

Discussion

Risk factors for the development of kidney stones include family history, male gender, dehydration, hot, arid climates, and history of kidney stones.[2] Metabolic diseases may also predispose to kidney stones including Crohn's disease, primary hyperparathyroidism, recurrent urinary tract infections (UTI), renal tubular acidosis, and gout.[2] Diabetes and obesity are considered to be major risk factors.[3]

Pathophysiology

Kidney stones are composed from a variety of materials, the most common being calcium oxalate, calcium phosphate, cystine, struvite, and uric acid. The majority of stones (75%) are composed of calcium oxalate with or without calcium phosphate.[2] Hyperexcretion of calcium contributes to stone formation and high-quantity dairy intake may contribute to the formation of calcium-based stones.[2] Recurrent UTI with urea-splitting bacteria such as Proteus, Klebsiella, Pseudomonas, and Staphylococcus contribute to struvite stone formation. Medications such as protease inhibitors, antibiotics, and some diuretics increase the risk of some kidney stones.[5]

The size of the stone plays a role in the ability for it to pass out of the genitourinary system. Roughly 90% of stones less than 5 mm width pass spontaneously within 4 weeks. Only 15% of stones 5mm to 8mm width pass spontaneously and only 5% greater than 8 mm will pass.[2] The location of the stone from the kidney to the bladder determines the chance of it becoming impacted along with the size of the stone. A stone may lodge in the calyx of the kidney or renal pelvis. The junction of the ureter and the renal pelvis is only 2–3 mm in diameter and impaction may occur at this site. The location in which the ureter crosses the iliac vessels is another area in which stone passage may be obstructed but the most common area for impaction is at the ureterovesicular junction. Approximately 75% of stones are located in the distal third of the ureter at the time of diagnosis. The final place a stone may be impacted is at the bladder outlet.[2]

History

Renal colic is classically acute in onset frequently with nausea and at times with vomiting. However, at times the patient may be relatively asymptomatic. Past medical problems, family history, and dietary information should be assessed during the history. Additionally, one should probe into factors that may indicate alternative causes of flank or groin pain.

Colic or spasmodic, severe intermittent pain from the flank to the groin is common for kidney stone pain. Pain in the proximal ureter or renal pelvis causes posterior flank pain and pain in the distal ureter may cause radiation of pain to the ipsilateral testicle and labia. In the ureter lower and anterior flank pain predominates and at the ureterovesical junction lower flank pain with accompanying scrotal or vulvar pain is common. Urinary symptoms may also exist including frequency and urgency.

Physical Examination

The physical examination is best used to evaluate for other causes of flank and groin pain. The classic finding of a patient with renal colic is that of someone in severe pain, but some patients can have minimal symptoms. Any important abdominal tenderness should lead one to consider and search for other causes of the pain, but the absence of major tenderness does not exclude other causes such as abdominal aortic aneurysm.

Laboratory Tests

The standard evaluation will often include a basic metabolic panel, renal function tests (blood urea nitrogen and creatinine), and urinalysis and analysis of a stone's composition.[3] Urinalysis is performed looking for red blood cells (RBCs), white blood cells (WBCs), proteins, and crystals. A urinary tract stone may be present in the absence of RBCs as about 15% will not have hematuria and RBCs may occur from other conditions such as infection, menses, appendicitis, and diverticulitis. Electrolytes should be obtained for all first-time patients presenting with a history concerning for stones, but may not be needed in all cases of patients with recurrent disease.[3]

The collection of a 24-hour urine and evaluation of urinary pH can impart information regarding stone formation.[3,5] It is not clear if a 12-hour collection (a more realistic goal for observation patients) would suffice since daily variations in fluid intake, diurnal metabolism, and other variations would not be captured.[6] Determining the type of stone can aid in the outpatient treatment and prevention for individuals with stones. Metabolic stone tests are used to help identify the underlying causes of stone formation; this typically involves a 24-hour urine collection. Knowing the stone composition can aid in identifying underlying medical conditions and certain medical conditions can aid in predicting stone composition.[7]

Imaging

Computerized tomography (CT) has become the first choice in emergency imaging with 92–100% sensitivity for the evaluation of urinary and non-urinary flank pain.[8] Data from the National Hospital Ambulatory Care Survey described a change in the use of CT for emergency evaluation of flank pain increasing from 19.6% of cases in 2000 to 45.5% in 2008 with no change in the proportion of patients (about 20%) diagnosed as having a stone.[9] The increased use is in part due to the added benefit of potentially providing a diagnosis of other sources of abdominal or flank pain, and CT is widely available in the United States. Duel energy CT utilizing advanced post-acquired processing can identify the composition of various types of stones and potentially could help guide long-term management.[10]

More recent research has evaluated the ability of CT to provide accurate diagnostic images using reduced radiation doses (low-dose CT) thereby limiting exposure. It has been shown to be an effective diagnostic modality for most patients but image quality may not be ideal for patients with a very low or high body-mass index.[11–13] For patients with a body-mass index under 30, low-dose CT imaging had 95% sensitivity and 97% specificity for ureteral stones and was 100% sensitive for those with ureteral stones larger than 3 mm.[11] This area requires more information to help determine if low-dose CT differs in the ability to identify stones in the kidney compared to the ureter[11,14,15] and to determine ideal radiation dosing parameters.[16] Some suggest that this technique may be utilized as a first-line diagnostic study if the clinician understands its limitations, but it may best be used for patients with known

(a)

(b)

(c)

(d)

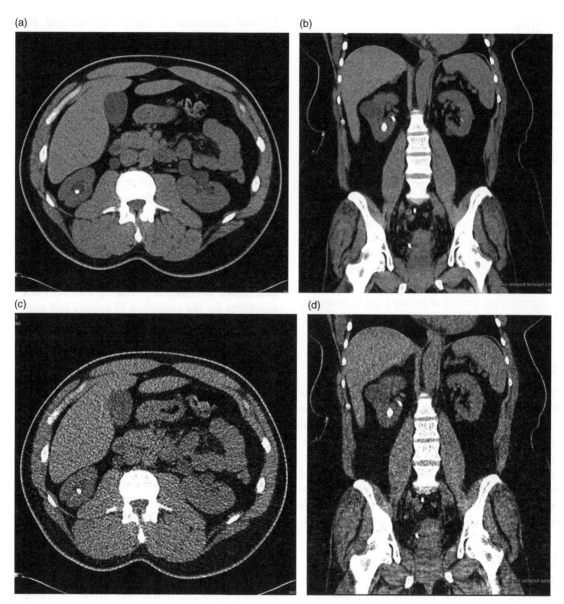

Figure 48.1 Low-Dose CT Images Compared to Full-Dose CT Images, (a) axial image using a standard-dose radiation protocol, (b) coronal image using a standard-dose radiation protocol, (c) axial image using a low-dose radiation protocol, and (d) coronal image using a low-dose radiation protocol. Both sets of images demonstrate densities in the right kidney. Two stones are seen on the coronal cuts and the incidental finding of a large right renal cyst is noted.
(Images are courtesy of Jason B. Wynberg, MD; Director, Detroit Medical Center, Kidney Stone Center)

disease to follow progress or diagnose recurrent disease.[12] Figure 48.1(a)–(d) shows images of a low- and normal-dose CT of the same patient.

Ultrasound is useful in the diagnosis of kidney stones. Advantages of ultrasound include there are no known important side effects, no radiation exposure, availability for rapid assessment, repeatability, it can detect the majority of calculi, and it is associated with low cost.[17,18] Additionally

useful information can be obtained regarding the anatomy of the kidney and ureters. For patients with the clinical finding of hematuria and flank pain, emergency limited ultrasound was found to have reasonably good sensitivity and specificity[19] and another study suggested that emergency ultrasound can be utilized to diagnose obstructive uropathy and is easily learned by physicians training in ultrasound.[20] A more recent study found that bedside ultrasonography had only moderate sensitivity and specificity for the detection of ureteral stones and had minimal impact on physicians' clinical impression of patients with possible stones.[21] Other disadvantages of ultrasound include false positives, which are secondary to surrounding anatomy, and inability to detect small stones. Additionally this diagnostic study is dependent on sonographer ability and technical quality.[17,18]

Kidney/Ureter/Bladder (KUB) radiography used to be a popular imaging modality but sensitivity was low, often around 45% to 59%.[22] Plain radiography (KUB technique) use has significantly decreased from 2000 to 2008 while ultrasound use has remained stable.[9] Advantages of using radiography include the minimal exposure to radiation and the utility for following stone passage after procedures such as extracorporeal shock wave lithotripsy (ESWL).

Studies have found that ultrasound combined with plain radiography (KUB) is more cost-effective and utilizes considerably less radiation than CT for discovering clinically significant stones.[23,24] Further studies are needed to determine if combined ultrasound and plain KUB could replace CT scan as the primary diagnostic imaging study and if these can be adequately performed at the bedside and interpreted by ED physicians.

Prior to CT, intravenous pyelography had been used for years and may still be used in places without readily available CT. One study found the sensitivity to be 94.2% and a specificity of 90.4%.[25] It is likely that many institutions have all but abandoned this diagnostic study for diagnosis among ED or observation unit (OU) patients.

Differential Diagnosis

Among the most immediately life-threatening mimics of renal colic are abdominal aortic aneurysm rupture and aortic dissection; these conditions must not be overlooked. Additional considerations include appendicitis, ectopic pregnancy, cholecystitis, pancreatitis, bowel obstruction, pyelonephritis, varicella-zoster, and musculoskeletal pain.

Patient Criteria

Most patients in whom the diagnosis of a urinary tract stone is made in the ED can be treated as an outpatient. Admission for short-term observation

and treatment is indicated when adequate pain control cannot be achieved or for intractable nausea and vomiting.[2] Additionally, severely dehydrated patients may also require observation. Patients with renal failure or patients with signs of sepsis from a urinary tract infection with tachycardia, fever, hypotension, and shock will typically need inpatient admission.[2]

Surgical intervention may be required for those with persistent obstruction, halting of stone progress, or unrelenting renal colic.[26] Those with complete obstruction require urology consultation and will need to be admitted.[2]

Management

Since the cost of kidney stone diagnosis and treatment is high and reoccurrence rates are sizeable, evaluation of the underlying cause is important.[3]

Medical Therapy

Initial medical management includes the use of nonsteroidal anti-inflammatory drugs (NSAIDS) and/or opioids for acute renal colic. NSAIDs are preferred as opioids tend to have more adverse effects.[27] In a 2006 prospective trial of acute renal colic treatment, the combination of morphine and ketorolac had greater pain relief then either analgesic drug singularly.[28] Fluid management has not been shown to have significant improvement in pain or to facilitate acute management; diuretics and high-dose fluids can cause damage.[29] However, adequate fluid hydration can help prevent reoccurrences.

Stable patients are started on oral pain management as tolerated. Adjuvant therapy includes alpha agonists (tamsulosin, terazosin, and doxazosin) or calcium channel blocker (nifedipine) to enhance stone passage. The pharmacology behind these two drug classes is the ability to inhibit smooth muscle contraction. Singh et al. performed a systematic review of trials using alpha agonist and calcium channel blockers and found that both offer significant benefit for stone expulsion.[4]

Special Considerations

Pregnant women may develop kidney stones and the risks of imaging with radiation exposure must outweigh the potential delay in diagnosis or infection, renal pathology, or premature labor. Physiologic changes of pregnancy including dilation of the renal calices, pelvis, and ureter may occur and mimic renal colic. Ultrasound has low sensitivity during pregnancy and ureteroscopy may be the study of choice for pregnant women who require interventional therapy.[30]

For patients with recurrent kidney stones the use or potential overuse of CT imaging should be evaluated. CT radiation exposure acts cumulatively, which may put individuals at increased risk for later malignancy. Although the threshold for radiation exposure is unknown, a study by Manohar et al. evaluated patients treated for kidney stones and found what was felt to be excessive exposure to radiation.[31] Since the increased use of CT scans has not lead to an increase in the portion of patients presenting with flank pain who are diagnosed with a renal stone, overuse of radiation should be a concern

for the clinician.[9] Alternative imaging or diagnostic studies previously mentioned should be strongly considered for patients with recurrent urolithiasis and prior CT imaging.

Outcome

For patients in observation the goals are progression to oral pain management and ability to tolerate oral dietary intake. Adequate hydration should be assured.

Conclusion

Kidney stones are a common emergency condition that account for significant health care dollars. Some patients will require observation and this is generally for symptom management.

References

1. Emmett M, Fenves AZ, Schwartz JC, editors. *Approach to Patient with Kidney Disease.* 9th ed. St. Louis: Elsevier; 2011.

2. Ban KM, Easter JS, editors. *Emergency Medicine, Concepts and Clinical Practice.* 7th ed. Philadelphia: Mosby; 2009.

3. Lipkin ME, Preminger GM. Demystifying the medical management of nephrolithiasis. *Rev Urol.* 2011;13(1):34–38. PubMed PMID: 21826126. Pubmed Central PMCID: 3151585. Epub 2011/08/10. eng.

4. Singh A, Alter HJ, Littlepage A. A systematic review of medical therapy to facilitate passage of ureteral calculi. *Ann Emerg Med.* 2007 Nov;50(5):552–563. PubMed PMID: 17681643. Epub 2007/08/08. eng.

5. Frassetto L, Kohlstadt I. Treatment and prevention of kidney stones: an update. *Am Fam Physician.* 2011 Dec 1; 84(11):1234–1242. PubMed PMID: 22150656. Epub 2011/ 12/14. eng.

6. Cameron M, Maalouf NM, Poindexter J, Adams-Huet B, Sakhaee K, Moe OW. The diurnal variation in urine acidification differs between normal individuals and uric acid stone formers. *Kidney international.* 2012 Jun; 81(11):1123–1130. PubMed PMID: 22297671. Pubmed Central PMCID: 3352978. Epub 2012/02/ 03. eng.

7. Pak CY, Poindexter JR, Adams-Huet B, Pearle MS. Predictive value of kidney stone composition in the detection of metabolic abnormalities. *Am J Med.* 2003 Jul;115(1): 26–32. PubMed PMID: 12867231. Epub 2003/07/18. eng.

8. Tamm EP, Silverman PM, Shuman WP. Evaluation of the patient with flank pain and possible ureteral calculus. *Radiology.* 2003 Aug;228(2): 319–329. PubMed PMID: 12819343. Epub 2003/06/ 24. eng.

9. Hyams ES, Korley FK, Pham JC, Matlaga BR. Trends in imaging use during the emergency department evaluation of flank pain. *J Urol.* 2011 Dec;186(6):2270–2274. PubMed PMID: 22014815. Epub 2011/10/22. eng.

10. Zilberman DE, Ferrandino MN, Preminger GM, Paulson EK, Lipkin ME, Boll DT. In vivo determination of urinary stone composition using dual energy computerized tomography with advanced post-acquisition processing. *Journal of Urology.* 2010 Dec;184(6):2354–2359. PubMed PMID: ISI:000284037900050. eng.

11. Poletti PA, Platon A, Rutschmann OT, Schmidlin FR, Iselin CE, Becker CD. Low-dose versus standard-dose CT protocol in patients with clinically suspected renal colic. *AJR Am J Roentgenol.* 2007 Apr;188(4):927–933. PubMed PMID: 17377025. Epub 2007/ 03/23. eng.

12. Niemann T, Kollmann T, Bongartz G. Diagnostic performance of low-dose CT for the detection of urolithiasis: a meta-analysis. *AJR Am J Roentgenol.* 2008 Aug;191(2): 396–401. PubMed PMID: 18647908. Epub 2008/07/ 24. eng.

13. Heldt JP, Smith JC, Anderson KM, Richards GD, Agarwal G, Smith DL, et al. Ureteral calculi detection using low dose computerized tomography protocols is compromised in overweight and underweight patients. *J Urol.* 2012 Jul;

188(1):124–129. PubMed PMID: 22578728. Epub 2012/05/15. eng.

14. Paulson EK, Weaver C, Ho LM, Martin L, Li J, Darsie J, et al. Conventional and reduced radiation dose of 16-MDCT for detection of nephrolithiasis and ureterolithiasis. *AJR Am J Roentgenol.* 2008 Jan;190(1):151–157. PubMed PMID: 18094305. Epub 2007/12/21. eng.

15. Heneghan JP, McGuire KA, Leder RA, DeLong DM, Yoshizumi T, Nelson RC. Helical CT for nephrolithiasis and ureterolithiasis: comparison of conventional and reduced radiation-dose techniques. *Radiology.* 2003 Nov;229(2):575–580. PubMed PMID: 14526095. Epub 2003/10/04. eng.

16. Sung MK, Singh S, Kalra MK. Current status of low dose multi-detector CT in the urinary tract. *World Journal of Radiology.* 2011 Nov 28;3(11):256–265. PubMed PMID: 22132296. Pubmed Central PMCID: 3226959. Epub 2011/12/02. eng.

17. Rao PN. Imaging for kidney stones. *World Journal of Urology.* 2004 Nov;22(5):323–7. PubMed PMID: 15290203. Epub 2004/08/04. eng.

18. Hyams ES, Shah O. Evaluation and follow-up of patients with urinary lithiasis: minimizing radiation exposure. *Current Urology Reports.* 2010 Mar;11(2):80–86. PubMed PMID: 20425094. Epub 2010/04/29. eng.

19. Gaspari RJ, Horst K. Emergency ultrasound and urinalysis in the evaluation of flank pain. *Acad Emerg Med.* 2005 Dec;12(12):1180–1184.

PubMed PMID: 16282510. Epub 2005/11/12. eng.

20. Jang TB, Casey RJ, Dyne P, Kaji A. The learning curve of resident physicians using emergency ultrasonography for obstructive uropathy. *Acad Emerg Med.* 2010 Sep;17(9):1024–1027. PubMed PMID: 20836789. Epub 2010/09/15. eng.

21. Moak JH, Lyons MS, Lindsell CJ. Bedside renal ultrasound in the evaluation of suspected ureterolithiasis. *Am J Emerg Med.* 2012 Jan;30(1):218–221. PubMed PMID: 21185667. Epub 2010/12/28. eng.

22. Levine JA, Neitlich J, Verga M, Dalrymple N, Smith RC. Ureteral calculi in patients with flank pain: correlation of plain radiography with unenhanced helical CT. *Radiology.* 1997 Jul;204(1):27–31. PubMed PMID: 9205218. Epub 1997/07/01. eng.

23. Ekici S, Sinanoglu O. Comparison of conventional radiography combined with ultrasonography versus nonenhanced helical computed tomography in evaluation of patients with renal colic. *Urol Res.* 2012 Mar 14. PubMed PMID: 22415439. Epub 2012/03/15. eng.

24. Catalano O, Nunziata A, Altei F, Siani A. Suspected ureteral colic: primary helical CT versus selective helical CT after unenhanced radiography and sonography. *AJR Am J Roentgenol.* 2002 Feb;178(2):379–387. PubMed PMID: 11804898. Epub 2002/01/24. eng.

25. Pfister SA, Deckart A, Laschke S, Dellas S, Otto U, Buitrago C, et al. Unenhanced helical computed tomography vs intravenous urography in patients with acute flank pain:

accuracy and economic impact in a randomized prospective trial. *Eur Radiol.* 2003 Nov;13(11):2513–2520. PubMed PMID: 12898174. Epub 2003/08/05. eng.

26. Preminger G, Tiselius H, Assimos D. 2007 Guideline for the management of ureteral calculi. *J Urol.* 2007;178(6):2418–2434.

27. Holdgate A, Oh CM. Is there a role for antimuscarinics in renal colic? A randomized controlled trial. *J Urol.* 2005 Aug;174(2):572–575; discussion 5. PubMed PMID: 16006900. Epub 2005/07/12. eng.

28. Safdar B, Degutis LC, Landry K, Vedere SR, Moscovitz HC, D'Onofrio G. Intravenous morphine plus ketorolac is superior to either drug alone for treatment of acute renal colic. *Ann Emerg Med.* 2006 Aug;48(2):173–181, 81 e1. PubMed PMID: 16953530. Epub 2006/09/06. eng.

29. Worster A, Richards C. Fluids and diuretics for acute ureteric colic. *Cochrane Database Syst Rev.* 2005 (3):CD004926. PubMed PMID: 16034958. Epub 2005/07/22. eng.

30. Lifshitz DA, Lingeman JE. Ureteroscopy as a first-line intervention for ureteral calculi in pregnancy. *J Endourol.* 2002 Feb;16(1):19–22. PubMed PMID: 11890444. Epub 2002/03/14. eng.

31. Manohar P, McCahy P. Repeated radiological radiation exposure in patients undergoing surgery for urinary tract stone disease in Victoria, Australia. *BJU Int.* 2011 Nov;108 Suppl 2:34–37. PubMed PMID: 22085124. Epub 2011/12/07. eng.

Chapter

49

Pyelonephritis and Urinary Tract Infections

Brian Kern, MD
Robert D. Welch, MD, MS, FACEP

Background

Urinary tract infection (UTI) may be the most frequently occurring of all bacterial infections. It is estimated that nearly 8 million patient visits and 1 million hospitalizations are accounted for by this disease. However, since UTI is not a reportable disease in the United States it is difficult to accurately determine the annual incidence of UTI. This difficulty is complicated by the common practice of not obtaining cultures in the outpatient setting and treating UTI on a presumptive basis. Ultimately, it has not been possible to accurately delineate the number of truly affected individuals.[1]

UTI affects all age groups. It is more common in females except during the neonatal period, when males are more frequently affected. The incidence of bacteriuria increases with age in women, and therefore so does the prevalence of UTI. Young women experience rates of UTI at approximately 4%, which increases to 10% at 70 years of age. In men, infection is uncommon without a predisposing source of infection such as catheterization or cystoscopy. Prevalence in men is as low as < 1% up through middle age, and then gradually increases to 10% by age 80. Rates are significantly increased in both sexes within institutionalized populations, running as high as 25% in men and 40% in women.[1–3] Although it is possible to consider the pediatric patient with pyelonephritis eligible for observation unit (OU) therapy,[4,5] the focus of this chapter is the adult patient with pyelonephritis and the information provided does not necessarily apply to the pediatric population.

Pathophysiology

The urinary tract is typically sterile and prevents the introduction of bacteria through a number of mechanisms. Complete emptying of the bladder is essential in that it prevents areas of stagnation that are predisposed to bacterial colonization. Reflux of urine is therefore a significant etiology of infection, whether in the form of congenital abnormality or from bladder overdistension. Unobstructed flow is also important in order to thoroughly wash away bacteria. Foreign bodies, such as calculi and indwelling catheters, or abnormal anatomy provide a nidus of infection. As men age, prostatic hypertrophy becomes a source of urinary obstruction as well, which can lead to UTI.[3]

Typically, bacteria invade the genitourinary system by ascent through the urethra and then into the bladder. Hematogenous and lymphatic spread of bacteria rarely provides a source for UTIs. Enteric flora are the predominant bacteria that cause UTIs. *Escherichia coli* is responsible in over 80% of infections for all populations. *Staph saprophyticus* is the next most common causative agent. Complicated UTIs are often caused by gram-positive cocci such as enterococci.[6] *Proteus, Klebsiella, Enterobacter,* and *Pseudomonas* are unusual organisms that may also cause complicated infections.[1,2,7]

Symptom presentation and the severity of illness are dependent on the extent of infection. This begins with asymptomatic bacteriuria, which is an individual with no symptoms but with greater than 10^5 colony forming units of bacteria/mL of urine. Inflammation of the bladder endothelium is known as cystitis. This results in dysuria, supra-pubic pain, and increased urinary frequency. Infection higher in the urinary tract results in inflammation of the renal parenchyma and collecting system, which is known as acute pyelonephritis. In addition to the symptoms of cystitis, pyelonephritis manifests as fever, chills, flank pain, back pain, and often nausea and vomiting. History and physical examination are the most useful tools in making the diagnosis of acute pyelonephritis.[2] Untreated acute pyelonephritis may result in renal abscess formation and ultimately renal suppuration. An infection of a normal urinary tract is uncomplicated, whereas association with structural problems or comorbid conditions results in a complicated infection. There is a higher risk of progression to a complication such as abscess formation or emphysematous pyelonephritis in complicated infections.[1,2]

Signs and symptoms of cystitis and pyelonephritis may mimic other diagnoses. For example, the differential includes pelvic inflammatory disease, ovarian torsion, appendicitis, and nephrolithiasis, all of which may present in a similar fashion. Abnormal pelvic examination and the absence of pyuria suggest a diagnosis other than pyelonephritis. Therefore a pelvic examination is indicated in all female patients. A thorough abdominal examination is also indicated in all patients in order to help identify any other pathology as well.

Most patients with uncomplicated cystitis or pyelonephritis can be managed effectively as outpatients on oral antibiotics.[6] However, patients that appear more ill may have a severe infection that warrants initial intravenous management. This would include patients that meet SIRS criteria, such as high white blood cell count or fever, or who have symptoms that otherwise preclude them from being discharged home, such as intractable nausea and vomiting. Evidence of significant dehydration is another indication for initial intravenous therapy.[8] There are no specific biomarkers yet available that can predict whether or not a patient will do well as an outpatient or if they need to be admitted. Levels of CRP, procalcitonin, and pro-atrial natriuretic peptide have all failed in predicting outcome.[9,10] Currently, the decision to discharge patients home, place them in OUs, or admit for hospitalization is based on the physician's overall clinical impression and current hospital admission criteria. However, it is unclear if emergency physicians consistently and accurately assess a patient's need for OU services. It has been found that in the past, physicians both underutilize observation services among patients who were admitted and overutilized services for patients who could be discharged directly and were not in need of short-term observation.[11] Since there are no clearly defined criteria, local protocols and practices should guide the decision-making process regarding the need for observation services. It is suggested that payment and admission criteria have and will continue to drive OU placement.

Patient Selection – Inclusions

Appropriate patients for admission to an emergency department OU (ED OU) include individuals with a clinical diagnosis of acute pyelonephritis by history of symptoms as well as by initial laboratory studies indicating pyuria and bacteriuria. Included patients should have stable vital signs who are mildly to moderately ill and who are immune-competent.[12]

Patient Selection – Exclusions

Individuals who should not be admitted to the OU include those who can clinically be discharged home primarily, are immunocompromised or have autoimmune disorders. Additional exclusions include elderly age or residing in long-term care facility, diabetes mellitus, acute renal failure, known ureteral stones, abnormal anatomy, abscess formation, single kidney or kidney transplant. Patients with severe sepsis or septic shock should also be excluded. A detailed physical examination, including pelvic examination, should be utilized to exclude patients with additional pathology.[8]

Management/Interventions

The goal of the OU is to treat the patient with intravenous antibiotics, in addition to antiemetics and fluids.[2] Patients should be adequately rehydrated and then kept on maintenance fluids. Fever and pain should also be appropriately treated.[13,14]

Initial urinalysis and gram stain along with consideration of hospital antibiogram and patterns of local sensitivity should be utilized in the selection of antibiotics. Several antibiotic regimens can be used for intravenous therapy including fluoroquinolones, aminoglycosides, and cephalosporins. Ciprofloxacin is frequently utilized in the initial empirical management.[6] All patients admitted to the OU should have a urine culture in order to guide ongoing antibiotic therapy. Blood cultures are not typically necessary or recommended. Serial examination of patients should be used to document clinical improvement or to recognize worsening clinical status.[14,15]

Imaging may also be indicated for certain individuals. Patients who fail to respond to treatment should be investigated for the presence of an abscess. Patients with recurrent infections should be investigated for obstruction or abnormal anatomy. Options for imaging include ultrasound and computed tomography. Ultrasound is useful in evaluating for intra-renal and perinephric abscess formation, as well as for the presence of hydronephrosis and hydroureter. Computed tomography has the highest sensitivity in detecting abscess or obstruction, but has the disadvantage of radiation and contrast exposure.[16,17]

Subspecialty consultation may assist in the initial management of acute pyelonephritis when certain complications do develop. For example, an infectious disease consult should be obtained in the case of a multiple-drug-resistant organism. Urology or interventional radiology consultation should also be sought in cases with abscess formation or with evidence of urinary obstruction.[2,7,14] If these or other such problems or complications arise, a review of the OU placement should be instituted and it is likely most cases would require full hospital admission.

Outcome

Most patients admitted to the OU for acute cystitis or pyelonephritis will be able to be discharged home. The primary goal is to adequately control the patient's symptoms of fever, pain, and nausea/vomiting. In this manner a patient will be able to continue therapy as an outpatient with oral antibiotics and fluids.[14]

If, however, patients develop any signs of worsening infection, or if they fail to improve with initial observation, they may need full admission to the hospital. Reasons for admission include intractable pain, nausea, or vomiting, which would preclude the individual from a successful outpatient recovery. Success or failure of OU treatment is not predicted by patient history. In addition, any patients that undergo imaging and are diagnosed with a significant complication will also likely need to be admitted for additional workup and management. Ultimately, however, most patients do rapidly improve and are able to continue therapy on an outpatient basis.[2,12,18]

Conclusion

Acute cystitis and pyelonephritis includes a spectrum of illness depending on the extent of infection. Patients may be mildly symptomatic or can be severely toxic. The diagnosis can be straightforward but other pathologies can present in similar fashion. Additionally, pyelonephritis can result in severe complications. This provides the physician with several obstacles in the successful management of this disease. However, initial management of patients in the ED OU provides an alternative to hospitalization for carefully selected patients. This allows the clinician to assess patient response to therapy, as well as to detect any other hidden pathology, prior to discharge. Patients with an adequate clinical response can be discharged on oral therapy with appropriate follow-up. By reducing the number of admissions for acute cystitis and pyelonephritis through the use of the ED OU there can be significant cost savings.[8,12,19,20]

References

1. Foxman B. Epidemiology of urinary tract infections: incidence, morbidity, and economic costs. *The American Journal of Medicine.* 2002;113 Suppl 1A:5S–13S. Epub 2002/07/13.

2. Colgan R, Williams M, Johnson JR. Diagnosis and treatment of acute pyelonephritis in women. *American Family Physician.* 2011;84(5):519–526. Epub 2011/09/06.

3. Boam WD, Miser WF. Acute focal bacterial pyelonephritis. *American Family Physician.*

1995;52(3):919–924. Epub 1995/09/01.

4. Mace SE. Pediatric observation medicine. *Emergency Medicine Clinics of North America.* 2001; 19(1):239–254. Epub 2001/02/24.

5. Macy ML, Kim CS, Sasson C, et al. Pediatric observation units in the United States: a systematic review. *Journal of Hospital Medicine: An Official Publication of the Society of Hospital Medicine.* 2010;5(3): 172–182. Epub 2010/03/18.

6. Mombelli G, Pezzoli R, Pinoja-Lutz G, et al. Oral vs intravenous ciprofloxacin in

the initial empirical management of severe pyelonephritis or complicated urinary tract infections: a prospective randomized clinical trial. *Archives of Internal Medicine.* 1999;159(1):53–58. Epub 1999/01/19.

7. Efstathiou SP, Pefanis AV, Tsioulos DI, et al. Acute pyelonephritis in adults: prediction of mortality and failure of treatment. *Archives of Internal Medicine.* 2003;163(10): 1206–1212. Epub 2003/05/28.

8. Kim K, Lee CC, Rhee JE, et al. The effects of an institutional

care map on the admission rates and medical costs in women with acute pyelonephritis. *Academic Emergency Medicine: Official Journal of the Society for Academic Emergency Medicine.* 2008;15(4):319–323. Epub 2008/03/29.

9. Claessens YE, Schmidt J, Batard E, et al. Can C-reactive protein, procalcitonin and mid-regional pro-atrial natriuretic peptide measurements guide choice of in-patient or out-patient care in acute pyelonephritis? Biomarkers In Sepsis (BIS) multicentre study. *Clinical Microbiology and Infection: The Official Publication of the European Society of Clinical Microbiology and Infectious Diseases.* 2010;16(6):753–760. Epub 2009/09/15.

10. Guinard-Barbier S, Grabar S, Chenevier-Gobeaux C, et al. Is mid-regional pro-atrial natriuretic peptide (MRproANP) an accurate marker of bacteremia in pyelonephritis? *Biomarkers: Biochemical Indicators of Exposure, Response, and Susceptibility to Chemicals.* 2011;16(4):355–363. Epub 2011/05/21.

11. Crenshaw LA, Lindsell CJ, Storrow AB, Lyons MS.

An evaluation of emergency physician selection of observation unit patients. *The American Journal of Emergency Medicine.* 2006;24(3):271–279. Epub 2006/04/26.

12. Schrock JW, Reznikova S, Weller S. The effect of an observation unit on the rate of ED admission and discharge for pyelonephritis. *The American Journal of Emergency Medicine.* 2010;28(6):682–688. Epub 2010/07/20.

13. Israel RS, Lowenstein SR, Marx JA, et al. Management of acute pyelonephritis in an emergency department observation unit. *Annals of Emergency Medicine.* 1991;20(3):253–257. Epub 1991/03/01.

14. Ward G, Jorden RC, Severance HW. Treatment of pyelonephritis in an observation unit. *Annals of Emergency Medicine.* 1991;20(3): 258–261. Epub 1991/03/01.

15. Gonzalez CM, Schaeffer AJ. Treatment of urinary tract infection: what's old, what's new, and what works. *World Journal of Urology.* 1999;17(6): 372–382. Epub 2000/02/02.

16. Chen KC, Hung SW, Seow VK, et al. The role of emergency ultrasound for evaluating acute pyelonephritis in the ED. *The*

American Journal of Emergency Medicine. 2011;29(7):721–724. Epub 2010/09/10.

17. Carnell J, Fischer J, Nagdev A. Ultrasound detection of obstructive pyelonephritis due to urolithiasis in the ED. *The American Journal of Emergency Medicine.* 2011;29(7):843 e1–3. Epub 2010/10/12.

18. Roberts R. Management of patients with infectious diseases in an emergency department observation unit. *Emergency Medicine Clinics of North America.* 2001;19(1):187–207. Epub 2001/02/24.

19. Ross MA, Compton S, Richardson D, et al. The use and effectiveness of an emergency department observation unit for elderly patients. *Annals of Emergency Medicine.* 2003;41(5):668–677. Epub 2003/04/25.

20. Gonnah R, Hegazi MO, Hmdy I, Shenoda MM. Can a change in policy reduce emergency hospital admissions? Effect of admission avoidance team, guideline implementation and maximising the observation unit. *Emergency Medicine Journal.* 2008;25 (9):575–578. Epub 2008/08/30.

Chapter 50
Pelvic Inflammatory Disease (PID)

Veronica Sikka, MD, PhD, MHA, MPH
Renee Reid, MD

Introduction

Pelvic inflammatory disease (PID) is defined by the Centers for Disease Control and Prevention (CDC) as "a spectrum of inflammatory disorders of the upper female genital tract, including any combination of endometritis, salpingitis, tubo-ovarian abscess, and pelvic peritonitis."[1] In many of these cases, sexually transmitted organisms are implicated: the most common being *N. gonorrhoeae* and *C. trachomatis*. In addition, cytomegalovirus (CMV), *M. hominis*, *U. urealyticum*, and *M. genitalium* may be associated with some cases of PID. All women who have acute PID should be tested for *N. gonorrhoeae* and *C. trachomatis* and should be screened for HIV infection.[1]

Each year, 750,000 cases of PID are diagnosed, mainly in women 15 to 29 years of age.[2] This number, unfortunately, has remained constant since the early 1990s.[3] The cost of PID is approximately $2,000 per patient, which totals to almost $1.5 billion annually.[4]

Diagnosis

It is estimated that 80 to 90% of women with a genital chlamydial infection and 10% with gonorrheal infection are asymptomatic.[1] In 2010, the CDC updated its PID guidelines, which are the basis for this section.[5]

The diagnosis of PID is based primarily on clinical evaluation. There is no one symptom, physical finding, or laboratory test that is sensitive or specific enough to definitively diagnose PID. Clinical diagnosis alone is 87% sensitive and 50% specific.[6] When compared with laparoscopy, the clinical diagnosis of PID in symptomatic patients has a positive predictive value of 65 to 90%.[6]

Table 50.1 summarizes the diagnostic criteria of PID according to the CDC.

Because of the potential for significant consequences if treatment is delayed, treatment should be based on clinical judgment without waiting for confirmation from laboratory or imaging tests. Complications of PID include infertility, ectopic pregnancy, perihepatitis (Fitz-Hugh Curtis Syndrome), tubo-ovarian abscesses, and Reiter's syndrome.

However, not all lower abdominal pain in young women is PID so other diagnoses should

Table 50.1 Clinical Diagnostic Criteria for PID (1)

One or more of the following minimum criteria must be present on pelvic examination to diagnose PID:
Cervical motion tenderness
Uterine tenderness
Adnexal tenderness

The following criteria can improve the specificity of the diagnosis:
Oral temperature > 101°F (> 38.3°C)
Abnormal cervical or vaginal mucopurulent discharge
Presence of abundant numbers of white blood cells on saline microscopy of vaginal fluid
Elevated C-reactive protein level
Laboratory documentation of cervical infection with gonorrhea or chlamydia

The following test results are the most specific criteria for diagnosing PID:
Endometrial biopsy with histopathologic evidence of endometritis
Transvaginal sonography or magnetic resonance imaging techniques showing thickened, fluid-filled tubes with or without free pelvic fluid or tubo-ovarian complex, or Doppler studies suggesting pelvic infection (e.g., tubal hyperemia)
Laparoscopic abnormalities consistent with PID

PID = pelvic inflammatory disease.
information from reference 1.

Table 50.2 Oral Treatment Regimens for Pelvic inflammatory Disease

Drug	Dosage
Option 1	
Ceftriaxone (Rocephin) plus	250 mg IM in a single dose
Doxycycline with or without	100 mg orally twice per day for 14 days
Metronidazole (Flagyl)	500 mg in a orally twice per day for 14 days
Option 2	
Cefoxitin plus	2 g IM in a single dose administered concurrently with probenecid (1 g orally)
Doxycycline with or without	100 mg orally twice per day for 14 days
Metronidazole	500 mg orally twice per day for 14 days
Option 3	
Other parenteral third generation cephalosporin (e.g., ceftizoxime [Cefizox], cefotaxime [Claforan]) plus	
Doxycycline with or without	100 mg orally twice per day for 14 days
Metronidazole	500 mg orally twice per day for 14 days

IM = intramuscularly.
Adapted from Workowski KA, Berman S; Centers for Disease Control and Prevention (CDC). Sexually transmitted diseases treatment guidelines, 2010 [published correction appears in MMWR Morb Mortal Wkly Rep. 2011;60(1):18]. MMWR Recomm Rep. 2010;59(RR-12):66.

Table 50.3 Parenteral Treatment Regimens for Pelvic Inflammatory Disease

Drug	Dosage
Regimen A	
Cefotetan (Cefotan)	2 g IV every 12 hours
or	
Cefoxitin	2 g IV every 6 hours
plus	
Doxycycline	100 mg orally or IV every 12 hours
Regimen B	
Clindamycin	900 mg IV every 8 hours
plus	
Gentamicin	Loading dose IV or IM (2 mg per kg), followed by a maintenance dose (1.5 mg per kg) every 8 hours; a single daily dose (3 to 5 mg per kg) can be substituted
Alternative regimen	
Ampicillin/sulbctam (Unasyn) plus	3 g IV every 6 hours
Doxycycline	100 mg orally or IV every 12 hours

IM = intramuscularly; IV = intravenously.
Adapted from Workowski KA, Berman S; Centers for Disease Control and Prevention (CDC). Sexually transmitted diseases treatment guidelines, 2010 [published correction appears in MMWR Morb Mortal Wkly Rep. 2011;60(1):18]. MMWR Recomm Rep. 2010;59(RR-12):65.

be considered in women 15 to 44 years of age who present with lower abdominal or pelvic pain and cervical motion or pelvic tenderness, even if these symptoms are mild.

Patient Criteria

Most women with PID are treated in the outpatient setting. Patients appropriate for the observation unit (OU) would have the presumptive diagnosis of PID and meet any of the following criteria:

1) Unable to tolerate oral antibiotics
2) Dehydrated secondary to high fever or vomiting, requiring intravenous fluids
3) Require serial abdominal examinations to rule out other pathology such as ovarian torsion or appendicitis

Evidence suggests that inpatient and outpatient antibiotic therapies are equivalent for women with mild to moderate PID.[6] Women in both groups (inpatient and outpatient antibiotic therapy) demonstrated similar clinical improvement in the short-term as well as in equivalent incidence of long-term sequelae (i.e., time to pregnancy or in the proportion of women with PID disease recurrence, chronic pelvic pain, or ectopic pregnancy).

Management

Management in the OU is a two-prong approach. The first is supportive therapy with intravenous fluids, antipyretics, and pain control. The second is antibiotics.

Tables 50.2 and 50.3 summarize the treatment guidelines for PID according to the 2010 CDC guidelines.

In patients with penicillin and cephalosporin allergies, alternative regimens include:[6]

- **Erythromycin** base 500 mg orally four times a day for 7 days

- **Erythromycin ethylsuccinate** 800 mg orally four times a day for 7 days
- **Levofloxacin** 500 mg orally once daily for 7 days
- **Ofloxacin** 300 mg orally twice a day for 7 days

Conclusion

In patients who are vomiting or unable to tolerate oral medications, the OU is an excellent option for patients with PID since they usually get better with IV fluids and medications and can usually be discharged home in < 24 hours.

References

1. Centers for Disease Control and Prevention. (2011). Diseases Characterized by Urethritis and Cervicitis. URL: www.cdc.gov/std/treatment/2010/urethritis-and-cervicitis.htm.

2. Chesson HW, Collins D, Koski K. Formulas for estimating the costs averted by sexually transmitted infection (STI) prevention programs in the United States. *Cost Effectiveness and Resource Allocation.* 2008; 6:10.

3. Sutton MY, Sternberg M, Zaidi A, et al. Trends in pelvic inflammatory disease hospital discharges and ambulatory visits, United States, 1985–2001. *Sex Transmitted Disease.* 2005; 32(12): 778–784.

4. Gradison M. Pelvic inflammatory disease. *American Family Physician.* 2012; 85(8): 791–796.

5. Workowski KA, Berman S; Centers for Disease Control and Prevention (CDC). Sexually transmitted diseases treatment guidelines, 2010 [published correction appears in *MMWR Morb Mortal Wkly Rep.* 2011; 60(1):18].*MMWR Recomm Rep.* 2010; 59(RR-12): 1–110.

6. Ness RB, Soper DE, Holley RL, et al. Effectiveness of inpatient and outpatient treatment strategies for women with pelvic inflammatory disease: Results from the Pelvic Inflammatory Disease Evaluation and Clinical Health (PEACH) Randomized Trial. *American Journal of Obstetrics and Gynecology.* 2002; 186: 929–937.5).

Chapter

51

Vaginal Bleeding

Veronica Sikka, MD, PhD, MHA, MPH
Renee Reid, MD

Introduction

Vaginal bleeding can be a cause of significant morbidity and mortality in nonpregnant patients. The average menstrual cycle lasts 28 days with normal cycles varying from 21 to 35 days. Each cycle lasts anywhere from 2 to 6 days. Oligomenorrhea refers to a decreased menstrual frequency. Polymenorrhea is increased menstrual cycles. Blood loss exceeding 80 mL per day or for more than 6 consecutive days is referred to as menorrhagia. Abnormal bleeding at irregular intervals is called metrorrhagia. Menometrorrhagia is heavy or prolonged bleeding at irregular intervals.

Diagnosis

Studies have shown that patients' estimates of vaginal bleeding correspond poorly with measured volumes.[1,2] Menstrual blood normally does not clot but a history of clotting indicates bleeding is heavy.[3]

A complete blood cell count should be obtained for all patients with significant vaginal bleeding. Hemoglobin and hematocrit (H&H), along with the patient's clinical status (e.g., symptoms and signs) may indicate the need for a blood transfusion. However, it is important to note that a patient's low H&H may be late signs of an unstable hemodynamic status, although a patient may be in shock with a normal H&H. Vital signs may be a better indicator of hemodynamic status. Thrombocytopenia may also indicate the need to also administer platelet concentrates.[4] (See Chapter 43 on Transfusions.)

For women of childbearing age, a pregnancy test (urine or blood) should be obtained to rule out pregnancy, whether an intrauterine pregnancy or an abnormal pregnancy, such as an ectopic pregnancy. Type and screen should be ordered along with coagulation studies. If the pregnant woman has vaginal bleeding and is Rh negative, then administration of Rho (D) Immune Globulin (RhoGAM) should be considered.

If the patient is symptomatic and/or the hemoglobin/hematocrit is low warranting a blood transfusion/volume repletion, the observation unit (OU) should be considered for transfusion and further workup. (See Chapter 43 on transfusions.) The evaluation in the OU can be used to determine other causes of dysfunctional uterine bleeding, including an underlying thyroid condition, coagulopathy or bleeding disorder, anticoagulant use, or liver function abnormality. A pelvic ultrasound should be performed to evaluate the endometrial cavity and the uterine corpus for thickening or the presence of fibroids. In the postmenopausal woman, endometrial thickness can be concerning for hyperplasia or carcinoma.

Patient Criteria and Management

Patients appropriate for the OU include those who are not ready to be discharged home with gynecology follow-up but are not in shock, hemodynamically unstable or will presumptively require a prolonged inpatient stay. Patients who need fluid and/or blood product administration with further evaluation of the cause of the vaginal bleeding are ideal candidates for the OU. A pelvic ultrasound can be performed while the patient is in the OU. If medical management of the bleeding is indicated, then medications can be started in the OU and continued after discharge, if needed. If a gynecology consult is warranted, it can be also be done while the patient is in the OU and follow-up arranged.

Outcome

Once the patient is hemodynamically stable and no longer symptomatic or with a significant decrease in symptoms from the dysfunctional uterine bleeding, discharge with appropriate follow-up can be considered. Causes of vaginal bleeding that require investigation can be evaluated in the OU and patients can be discharged with follow-up with either gynecology and/or hematology depending on the cause. Ultimately, patients discharged from the OU should have hemoglobins and platelet counts that are significantly improved or within normal ranges and should be hemodynamically and symptomatically stable.

References

1. Daniels RV, McCuskey C. (2003). Abnormal vaginal bleeding in the nonpregnant patient. *Emergency Medicine Clinics of North America*, 21: 751–772.

2. Morrison L, Spence J. (2000). Vaginal bleeding and pelvic pain in the nonpregnant patient. In: *Emergency Medicine: A Comprehensive Guide*. 5th edition. St. Louis, MO: McGraw-Hill: 669–680.

3. Munro MG. (2001). Dysfunctional uterine bleeding: advances in diagnosis and treatment. *Current Opinion in Obstetrics and Gynecology*, 13: 475–489.

4. Buckingham K, Fawdry A Fothergill D. (1999). Management of vaginal bleeding presenting to the accident and emergency department. *Journal of Accident and Emergency Medicine*, 16(2): 130–135.

Chapter

52

Hyperemesis Gravidarum

Veronica Sikka, MD, PhD, MHA, MPH
Harinder Dhindsa, MD, MBA, MPH

Introduction

Nausea and vomiting in pregnancy can occur in anywhere from 50 to 90% of pregnancies.[1] However, the most severe form of nausea and vomiting in pregnancy is hyperemesis gravidarum (HG), which can require aggressive management. The nausea and vomiting associated with pregnancy usually begins by 9–10 weeks of gestation, peaks at 11–13 weeks, and resolves by 12–14 weeks.[2] In a rare percentage (1–10%) of pregnancies, symptoms may continue beyond 20–22 weeks.[3]

Discussion

Hyperemesis gravidarum is characterized by persistent nausea and vomiting that can result in weight loss (> 5% of pre-pregnancy weight) and ketosis. The significant volume depletion associated with HG can result in electrolyte and acid-base imbalances, nutritional deficiencies, and threat of mortality to the mother and fetus. Severe HG requires hospitalization in 0.3–2% of pregnancies.[4]

The defining symptoms of HG include nausea and vomiting. Other symptoms include fatigue, weakness, dizziness, near-syncope, and syncope. The diagnosis of HG is primarily clinical and in many cases is nonspecific, and characterized by signs and symptoms of dehydration. Physical examination and vital signs that are suggestive of HG, include orthostatic blood pressure changes, dry mucous membranes, poor skin turgor, and weight loss.

A review of over 1,000 cases of HG found that medical complications of hyperthyroid disorders, psychiatric illness, previous molar disease, gastrointestinal disorders, pregestational diabetes, and asthma were significantly independent risk factors for HG, whereas maternal smoking and maternal age older than 30 years decreased the risk.[5] Pregnancies with female fetuses and multiple fetuses were also at increased risk.[6]

Other factors that have been proposed include ethnicity, occupational status, fetal anomalies, increased body weight, nausea and vomiting in a prior pregnancy, history of infertility, interpregnancy interval, corpus luteum in the ovary, and prior intolerance to oral contraceptives.[5]

Patient Criteria

Patients appropriate for the observation unit (OU) would have nausea and vomiting, but are hemodynamically stable, and meet any of the following criteria:

1) Unable to tolerate liquids or oral medications
2) Dehydrated, requiring intravenous fluids
3) Require serial abdominal exams and/or diagnostic testing (such as ultrasound) to rule out other pathology such as ovarian torsion or appendicitis

Signs of dehydration that can confirm the need for an observation stay include:

- Urinalysis with high ketones and specific gravity
- Electrolytes significant for low potassium or sodium and/or hyperchloremic metabolic alkalosis or acidosis
- Elevated transaminase levels, which may occur in as many as 50% of patients with hyperemesis gravidarum
- Elevated amylase levels, which are elevated in approximately 10% of patients with hyperemesis gravidarum (HG is associated with a transient hyperthyroidism and suppressed TSH levels in 50–60% of cases. The OU can be used to further work-up the potential for overt hyperthyroidism.)[6]
- Urine cultures may reveal a UTI, which can be the cause of nausea and vomiting. Intravenous antibiotics may be required.
- Hematocrit may be high from volume depletion

Management

The treatment of HG is primarily supportive with intravenous fluids and antiemetics.[7,8,9] A proposed regimen for patients who are admitted to the OU with HG includes:

1) Vitamin B-6 (pyridoxine) IV 10–25 mg daily
2) Metoclopramide 10 mg IV, IM or orally q 6 h (pregnancy class B)
3) Promethazine 12.5–25 mg IV, q 4–6 h (pregnancy class C)
4) Ondansetron 4–8 mg IV or orally q 6 h (pregnancy class B)

Steroids may be used in patients refractory to standard therapy.[9,10] It is important to use steroids cautiously and only in extremely refractory cases as they can increase the risk for oral clefts in the first 10 weeks of gestation.[10] However, if using methylprednisolone, the patient will most likely require inpatient stay and not OU admission. Thus, the use of methylprednisolone should be reserved for the inpatient setting (not the OU) with administration as ordered by the obstetrician.

Vitamin B6 has been found to reduce nausea and vomiting when compared with placebo.[1] Ondansetron, a serotonin-receptor antagonist, showed no benefit over promethazine, except for being more expensive.[1] Promethazine was compared with methylprednisolone in a randomized, double-blind, controlled trial. Methylprednisolone appeared to decrease the rate of readmission for HG. However, patients randomized to promethazine had a significantly longer duration of symptoms prior to treatment.[10]

If electrolyte abnormalities occur, these can be treated in the OU. If persistent dehydration, electrolyte loss, and/or weight loss occur despite aggressive therapy, then inpatient admission is indicated.

Conclusion

Hyperemesis gravidarum is generally self-limited and, in most cases, improves by the end of the first trimester. The majority of these patients can be successfully managed in the OU setting.

References

1. ACOG. American College of Obstetrics and Gynecology Practice Bulletin: nausea and vomiting of pregnancy. *Obstet Gynecol.* 2004;103(4):803–814.

2. Lacroix R, Eason E, Melzack R. Nausea and vomiting during pregnancy: a prospective study of its frequency, intensity, and patterns of change. *Am J Obstet Gynecol.* 2000; 182 (4):931–937.

3. Bailit JL. Hyperemesis gravidarium: epidemiologic findings from a large cohort. *Am J Obstet Gynecol.* 2005; 193 (3 Pt 1):811–814.

4. Fell DB, Dodds L, Joseph KS, et al. Risk factors for hyperemesis gravidarum requiring hospital admission during pregnancy. *Obstet Gynecol.* 2006; 107(2 Pt 1): 277–284.

5. Dodds L, Fell DB, Joseph KS, et al. Outcomes of pregnancies complicated by hyperemesis gravidarum. *Obstet Gynecol.* 2006; 107(2 Pt 1):285–292.

6. Holmgren C, Aagaard-Tillery KM, Silver RM, et al. Hyperemesis in pregnancy: an evaluation of treatment strategies with maternal and neonatal outcomes. *Am J Obstet Gynecol* 2008; 198 (1):56.e1–4.

7. Tan JY, Loh KC, Yeo GS, et al. Transient hyperthyroidism of hyperemesis gravidarum. *BJOG* 2002; 109(6): 683–688.

8. Goodwin TM. Hyperemesis gravidarum. *Obstet Gynecol Clin North Am.* 2008; 35 (3):401–417, viii.

9. Matok I, Gorodischer R, Koren G, et al. The safety of metoclopramide use in the first trimester of pregnancy. *N Engl J Med.* 2009; 2528–2535.

10. Safari HR, Alsulyman OM, Gherman RB, et al. Experience with oral methylprednisolone in the treatment of refractory hyperemesis gravidarum. *Am J Obstet Gynecol.* 1998; 178 (5):1054–1058.

Chapter

53

Pediatric Observation Medicine

Sharon E. Mace, MD, FACEP, FAAP

Introduction

Pediatric patients comprise about 27% of all emergency department (ED) visits.[1] There has been a 60.4% increase in ED visits from 1991, in which only 85 million patients were seen, to 2011, when approximately 136.3 million patients were evaluated in EDs, of which an estimated 36.8 million (27%) were infants and children.[2] There is every indication that this exponential growth in ED visits will continue. This growth along with the increased acuity and complexity of patients,[3] and expanded ED evaluation are critical factors leading to overcrowding in EDs, which has major negative consequences including detrimental effects on patient care and worse patient outcomes.[4] Moreover, overcrowding is not unique to the United States, but is a worldwide problem.[5]

Over the past few years, ED visits for pediatric patients has also been increasing.[6] Infants under 12 months of age are the age group with the highest annual per capita ED visit rate.[7] Pediatric patients, like adults, also suffer from the harmful impact of overcrowding.[8]

Observation medicine (OM) has been suggested as a potential solution to this crisis and has been successful has been in improving the quality of patient care, increasing patient/family satisfaction, decreasing missed diagnoses, creating better risk management, decreasing inappropriate hospital admissions, reducing length of stay (LOS), and creating better patient outcomes, while lowering costs.[9] This is true for pediatric patients as well as adults.[10–12]

Pathophysiology

Pediatric patients are, generally, more difficult and complex to evaluate than adults and at a higher risk.[12,13] Infants and children often have a nonspecific complaint and subtle physical examination findings. Preverbal children and infants may be unable to communicate their symptoms. Infants and children have an increased susceptibility to infection, limited physiologic reserve, and developmental and/or age considerations. Diagnostic testing and therapeutic measures can have unique considerations and challenges, ranging from concerns over radiation exposure to the difficulties in obtaining an intravenous line and/or blood work or the need to perform sedation for procedures, even simple radiology tests.

Although most pediatric patients evaluated in the ED have a minor injury or mild illness or a benign condition, the possibility of a serious limb- or life- threatening illness/injury exists and could be easily overlooked. Indeed, analysis of malpractice awards confirms the fact that failure to diagnose or a delay in diagnosis does happen, often with disastrous consequences. Common pediatric diagnoses including gastroenteritis and appendicitis are repeatedly mentioned in malpractice lawsuits. Indeed, gastroenteritis is the most frequent diagnosis in malpractice claims and 15% of all malpractice dollars paid are for missed appendicitis. Looking at cost per claim, missed meningitis tops the list and at number one accounts for 17% of all malpractice dollars paid.[13]

Physiologic, anatomic, and developmental factors add to the complexity and risk in evaluating infants and children. Patients at the extremes of age, including the very young, are known to have an increased risk of infection, including both a higher incidence and increased severity of infection, due to their lesser ability to fight infection. Pediatric patients have a limited physiologic reserve. For example, their greater body surface area and lesser renal capacity to conserve water and electrolytes increases their risk for dehydration, their proportionately greater head size predisposes them to head injury, their liver has a reduced ability to detoxify substances, and they rely on heart rate rather than stroke volume to maintain their cardiac output.

There has also been an increase in individuals with Special Health Care Needs (SHCN) and many other high-risk pediatric patients (vulnerable population).[14] Such patients range from survivors of the intensive care units (whether the Pediatric, Surgical, or Neonatal ICUs), oncology patients (on chemotherapy, radiation therapy, s/p bone marrow transplant), immunosuppressed individuals (from medications, from disease such as HIV, rheumatologic disorders, etc.) to the transplant patients (kidney, liver, pancreas, lung, heart) and those with chronic diseases (e.g., cystic fibrosis and diabetes).

Such conditions add to the complexity and risk of evaluating and managing pediatric patients, especially infants and children.

The advantages of additional time for evaluation and treatment, with further diagnostic testing and therapy, in these complex and high-risk infants and children are obvious. Moreover, an observation stay may have another benefit in pediatric patients. It has been suggested that the observation of infants and children with repeat examination may be preferred or at least equivalent to advanced diagnostic testing in some cases. For example, serial examination of the stable pediatric patient with right lower quadrant pain and a nondiagnostic or poor quality ultrasound in an observation unit (OU) may be preferable to doing an abdominal CT scan, at least in terms of avoiding radiation exposure with increased lifetime risks of malignancy.[15]

Background

The first OUs evolved in the 1960s and included adults, while the first pediatric OUs or "Short Stay Units" (SSUs) came into use in the 1970s. Since then, there has been much literature regarding the use of an observation stay for adults, with diagnoses ranging from heart failure, asthma, transient ischemic attacks (TIAs) to syncope, and especially chest pain with the rapid growth of chest pain units and even a Society of Chest Pain Centers.[9]

In spite of this early history, there has been a relative paucity of information regarding pediatric OM, along with the recognition that "there are not many pediatric observation units, which in itself is surprising considering their usefulness."[16] The first textbook of Observation Medicine by Graff had 33 chapters, not one of which dealt with pediatrics.[17] Moreover, of the limited literature regarding pediatric OM, it almost exclusively comes from tertiary care centers. This is in spite of the fact that 81% of the infants and children evaluated in EDs are seen in smaller community hospitals[18] with combined adult and pediatric EDs, which is likely an area for future growth and research. (See pediatric OU patients in Chapter 10 Observation Medicine in Community Hospitals.)

The Principles of Pediatric Observation Medicine

No matter what the age of the patient, the definition and key principles of OM are the same. OM allows patients to undergo diagnostic evaluation and/or treatment for a limited time frame, generally < 24 hours. An organizational framework that provides for administrative oversight with designated staffing and coverage, design, patient accommodations, documentation requirements, policies, procedures, protocols, order sets, care paths, and performance improvement (PI) /continuous quality improvement (CQI)/metrics is required for any OU.[9–12] (See Performance Improvement, Chapter 9.)

Patients placed in observation status, whether adult or pediatric, have the following inclusion criteria: low risk, stable, low acuity, and/or low severity, low-intensity nursing care, low-intensity physician care, and non-intensive care. Criteria for exclusion include critically ill, unstable, need intensive nursing care, need intensive physician care, and have an anticipated LOS > 24 hours. (See Protocol Chapter 82.)

Differences between Pediatric and Adult Observation Medicine: Design, Supplies, Equipment, Medications

There are some differences between the adult and pediatric OU. The supplies, equipment, and medications may differ. The primary diagnoses in the adult OU are cardiac: chest pain, heart failure, syncope etc., while the top diagnoses in the pediatric OU are respiratory (asthma, bronchiolitis, croup) and gastrointestinal (dehydration,

Table 53.1 Most Common Diagnoses in an Observation Unit*

Pediatric**	Adult***
1. Asthma	1. Chest pain
2. Dehydration	2. Abdominal pain
3. Gastroenteritis	3. Asthma: acute
4. Pneumonia	exacerbation
5. Abdominal pain	4. Congestive heart
6. Seizures	failure (CHF)
7. Fever	5. Chronic obstructive
8. Bronchiolitis	pulmonary disease: acute
9. Croup	exacerbation
10. Poisonings	6. Syncope
11. Trauma	7. Transient ischemic
	attack (TIA)
	8. Ureterolithiasis
	9. Pyelonephritis
	10. Cellulitis/Uncomplicated
	Soft Tissue Infections
	11. Gastrointestinal bleeding
	12. Acute atrial fibrillation
	13. Other non TIA, non CVA
	neurologic disorders
	14. Acute back pain
	15. Deep vein thrombosis
	16. Trauma
	17. Toxicology/overdose

* Represents the common diagnoses seen in our observation unit from 1994 to 2015.

** Pediatric diagnoses are listed in order of prevalence. Our prevalence is consistent with other units.

*** In adults, chest pain is undoubtedly the most common diagnosis in our unit and in other observation units, with about 80% estimated prevalence.[9] Depending on the individual observation unit, the prevalence of other diagnoses varies greatly depending on many factors including inclusion/exclusion criteria, age of the patient population seen in the ED; such as high percentage of elderly, hospital specialty (subspecialty availability and referral patterns), trauma vs. nontrauma, designated stroke center, etc. However, generally, abdominal pain and asthma are the next most common diagnoses, with syncope, TIA, CHF, COPD exacerbation, genitourinary complaints (kidney stones, pyelonephritis) and uncomplicated skin infections in the top ten adult diagnoses.

gastroenteritis, vomiting, diarrhea, etc.)[12,19–21] (Table 53.1), which has implications for the need for monitoring, equipment, procedures, and medications.

The focus for the adult OU is repeat ECGs and blood draws with cardiac monitoring, whereas respiratory treatments, steroids, intravenous fluids, and anti-emetics are prime considerations for the pediatric OU. Thus, there may be greater utilization of an ECG technician or a phlebotomist in the adult OU, while the respiratory therapist is more needed in the pediatric OU. Because of the higher frequency of dehydration/other gastrointestinal complaints, respiratory diagnoses, and infections encountered in the pediatric OU versus chest pain, syncope, TIA, etc. in adults, there is a greater need for cardiac monitoring and ECGs in adults, whereas pediatric patients may have a higher utilization of respiratory treatments, intravenous fluids, steroids, and antibiotics when compared to adults. This may have implications for the pharmacy when stocking medications.

It has also been suggested that the pediatric OU may exhibit a more marked seasonal and monthly or daily variation in OU admissions than adults.[12,19–22] This has been attributed to the pediatric patient population showing greater peaks and valleys in ED visits, inpatient and OU admissions depending on whatever acute infectious illness is in the community. Thus, during rotavirus season, there may be a sudden marked increase in the number of infants and children presenting with dehydration. Similarly, during the winter (in the Northern Hemisphere) when respiratory illnesses are prevalent, there are many cases of pneumonia, croup, and bronchiolitis; during the summer these illnesses are at their nadir and trauma is more prevalent in the ED and OU pediatric patient population.[22] Spikes in the number of asthmatics seen in the ED and, correspondingly, admitted to the OU, may coincide with the occurrence of pollens, air pollutants, and/or the prevalence of respiratory illnesses. With adults, the main diagnoses – chest pain, heart failure, syncope, and TIA – are much less likely to have seasonal variations.

Patient- and family-centered care should be the norm. Accommodations should include the family, for example, parent or guardian, as well as the patient. Dietary requirements need to be age appropriate with formula for infants, appropriate tube feedings for those with feeding tubes and palatable for the child and adolescent as well as considering those with specialized diets: diabetic, cardiac, lactose intolerant, etc. Toys, games, and videos help make the OU "patient friendly" for the child or adolescent. The pediatric OU will need cribs and appropriate size beds depending on the ages admitted. This may allow for more rooms in a fixed space in a pediatric OU than an adult OU, provided there are provisions for the parent(s) in the room. (See Chapter 5 on Design.)

Patient Population: Adult versus Pediatric Patients

As with adults, there are three main categories of patients: those with a known diagnosis who need treatment (e.g., heart failure, asthma), those with a condition or complaint (e.g., chest pain or abdominal pain) who need a diagnostic evaluation, and those with a known diagnosis who need monitoring or observation (including atrial fibrillation, syncope, seizure and overdose).[12] As mentioned, the primary diagnoses differ between the adult and pediatric patients (Table 53.1).

According to the results over 20 years at our large, urban, academic, non-trauma, tertiary care referral center in the United States with a "hybrid" OU, where hybrid is defined as an OU that accepts both adult and pediatric patients, the most common diagnoses for the pediatric patients were (in order of frequency) asthma, dehydration, gastroenteritis, pneumonia, abdominal pain, seizures, fever, bronchiolitis, and croup. Results from other exclusively pediatric OUs in the United States and internationally have similar results.[22–26] For the adults, the leading diagnoses (in order of frequency) were chest pain, heart failure, abdominal pain, syncope, asthma, COPD, dehydration, gastrointestinal bleed, and pneumonia.[12,19–21] Thus, there is less need for cardiac (rhythm strip) monitoring in the pediatric OU.

Patient Population: Pediatric Patients in a Pediatric OU

In the United States, the overwhelming majority of pediatric patients in an OU are "medical," which is consistent with our findings,[19–21] with only 6.0–7.5% of patients in several studies being a surgical or traumatic condition.[9,27] There is one exception, a study from a Pediatric Children's Hospital in Australia with a mixed patient population that included procedural patients in their OU. They still found the majority of patients were medical, although there was a much higher percentage of surgical patients: medical 56%, surgical 30%, and the remainder procedural or psychological.[28]

The percentage of pediatric patients placed in observation status from the ED also varies and has been reported as 2.9%, 4.0%, and 4.8%, respectively, in the United States.[22,25,26] The mean age (years) for pediatric OU patients ranged from 4.36, 4.7, and 6.0 (United States) to 6.23 (Scotland), with one French study having a much lower median age of 26 months.[22,23,25,27,29]

Reported mean LOS (hours) for the pediatric OU patients ranged from 8.4 to 20.5: Australia 17.5 (community hospital) and 20.5 (tertiary care hospital); France 14; United States 8.4, 13, 14.7, 15, and 15.6 hours.[9,22–26,30] The LOS (median) may vary depending on the diagnosis with respiratory patients tending to have longer LOS (median): 21.3 (croup) and 16.5 (asthma) versus poisoning 14.35 or head trauma 13.[9,31–33]

The percentage of patients admitted to the hospital from the pediatric OU is quite variable and ranged from a low of 4% (community hospital, Australia) to a high of 22% (United States)[28,30] with rates in between these two extremes: 10.4%, 12%, and 20.3%.[24–26] The percentage of OU patients admitted to the hospital is likely influenced by multiple variables, of which the diagnosis is one factor. An early study of pediatric OU patients with gastrointestinal illnesses found 81.5% were discharged home, while discharge rates for neurologic illnesses (e.g., seizures, head trauma) were in the 90% range.[34] A more recent study found the highest admission rate to inpatient from the OU was for seizure patients (19%) followed by asthma (16%) and croup (9%), while the lowest inpatient admission rates were for enteritis/dehydration at 5% and poisonings at 4%.[25] Another study had similar findings with respiratory illnesses having the highest inpatient admission rates from the OU at 50% for pneumonia, 46% for bronchiolitis, 33% for infections, 23% for asthma, and 17% for croup. Differing from the other studies, they found a fairly high admission rate for gastroenteritis at 21%, but only 5% for seizures and 2% for trauma.[30]

A study of pediatric closed head injuries found only a 5% admission rate to an inpatient unit from the OU and a study of pediatric poison exposures found a 5.4% hospitalization rate from the OU.[32,33] In general, for pediatric OU patients, it seems that poison exposures (nonintentional) and stable blunt trauma have low hospital admission rates (≤ 5%), while respiratory conditions (asthma, bronchiolitis, croup, pneumonia) and infections have the highest admission rates based on diagnosis.[25,26,30]

Reasons for the differences in LOS and admission rates, etc. may include specific diagnosis or condition, varied setting (academic, tertiary, teaching vs. nonacademic or community hospital), country, and the inclusion of procedural patients and/or "holding" admitted patients.

International Perspective

There may be some differences in the types of pediatric patients placed in a pediatric OU depending on the international location. A questionnaire sent to facilities in the United Kingdom noted that 50% of the accident and emergency departments surveyed had a short-stay ward. Of these, one-fourth admitted small numbers of children, who are "mainly children who have sustained trauma-related problems."[35] This is quite different from other countries (France, Australia, and United States), in which medical patients far outnumbered the surgical patients.[19-21,23,25,26,28,30] In some regions/countries, trauma patients are admitted to the hospital and are not considered for placement in an OU. The United Kingdom study was also a survey and did not report actual patient data from a given OU(s) and may be associated with the usual problems of any survey instrument.

Advantages of Pediatric Observation Medicine

Cost-Effective

Like adult OM, pediatric OM can have many benefits. Pediatric OM has been shown to be cost-effective. Two studies of pediatric asthmatics and one in croup patients documented this fact. One report by O'Brien et al. in asthmatics found the average charge for an inpatient was over five times greater than for the holding unit.[36] The cost for asthmatic patients hospitalized as inpatients for ≤ 1 day was one-and-a-half times greater than the charges for patients in the holding unit in the Willett et al. study.[37] For patients with croup, there was an overall reduction in resource utilization with the median charge significantly decreased (p = 0.03) for OU patients: pre-OU group was $1,685 versus $1,387 for the post-OU group.[31] After institution of a short stay unit, an Australian study estimated a cost savings for 1 year of $1/2 million for one hospital and $2.3 million for another hospital.[28]

Quality of Patient Care

A study evaluating the 16-year experience with croup at an Australian teaching hospital found that the implementation of the mandatory use of corticosteroids in 1991 lead to a decrease in the LOS (from 2.3 days between 1985 and 1990 to 1 day in 1991), number of intubations, and the number of ICU admissions. Next, in 1993, they mandated the use of corticosteroids in their OU and found a marked improvement in their OU discharge rate from 80% in 1991–1992 to 97% in 1993–1995 or conversely a drop in their admission rate from the OU to the inpatient ward from 20% admitted to only 3% admitted.[38] Comparable patient care or improved patient care has been attributed to the pediatric OM. Use of a pediatric OU for pediatric patients with poison exposures and for pediatric blunt head trauma patients, respectively, found no adverse events as a result of OU placement.[3] Multiple studies of pediatric asthma patients have documented that treatment in the OU is medically effective, safe, and cost-effective.[3] In the Gururaj et al. study of pediatric asthmatics treated in a holding unit, only 1.5% returned to the ED and none needed admission. [39]

Decreased Hospital Admissions

Studies have documented that the institution of a pediatric OU does decrease hospital admissions. There was a significant (p < 0.0001) reduction in ward admission rates from 9.5% to 4.2% for children/infants with croup after the introduction of a pediatric OU.[31] A review of pediatric emergency medicine by Knapp also found that OUs were valuable in avoiding a hospital admission for patients with ingestions.[40] A Canadian study in pediatric asthmatic patients found a significant (p ≤ 0.01) decrease in inpatient admissions from 17% (pre-OU) to 10% (post-OU), but with a significantly (p = 0.01) increased rate of repeat visits to the ED after discharge (3% pre-OU vs. 5% post-OU).[41] This increased rate of return appears to be an exception to the rule with all other studies showing no increase or a decrease in return visits to the ED.

Rate of Returns to the Emergency Department and Readmissions

Readmissions for hospitalized asthmatic patients were higher than for holding unit patients. At 1-month follow-up, returns to the ED and readmissions were: those admitted < 1 day had

31.1% returns to ED with 12.5% readmissions, those admitted > 1 day had 13.5% returns to ED with 7.7% readmissions, compared with holding unit patients who had 11.4% returns to the ED with no (0%) readmissions.[37] The study by Guoin et al. looked at the rate of return visits within 72 hours for pediatric asthmatics before and after the initiation of an OU. Their results were pre-observation 12.5% (44/352) returns to the ED with 39% (17/44) readmitted versus post observation 24.3% (85/350) returned to the ED but fewer needed readmission, only 28% (24/85).[41] Another study in asthmatics found no increase in hospital admission rate after opening an OU.[42] Only 1.5% of asthmatics treated in a holding unit returned to the ED and none needed readmission in the report by Gururaj et al.[39] According to the O'Brien et al. study, 7% (5/71) of asthmatics returned to the ED within 1 week of treatment in the holding unit with 5.6% (4/71) readmitted.[36]

Length of Stay

The pediatric OU has a decrease in LOS when compared to inpatient hospitalization. The median LOS for pediatric asthmatic patients treated in an OU is 16.5 hours with a discharge rate of 67–75%.[9,36,37,41] In one study for pediatric blunt head trauma patients, the median LOS was 13 hours with a discharge rate of 95%.[33] A study from the United States found a significant decrease (p = 0.03) from 27.2 to 21.3 hours in median LOS for patients with croup after the introduction of a pediatric OU.[31] A study comparing low-risk hyperbilirubinemia patients treated in an OU with inpatient hospitalization demonstrated 82% of patients were successfully discharged from the OU and OU patients had a shorter LOS of 18 hours compared to 42 hours as an inpatient.[44] Patients with intussusception (successfully reduced by contrast enema) when managed in the ED OU had a significantly shorter LOS than those admitted to the hospital (mean LOS 7.2 vs. 22.7 hours) with no difference in outcome.[45]

Patient, Parental and Physician Satisfaction

Another benefit attributed to OM is increased satisfaction of patients and physicians. The study by Rydman et al. showed adult patients were more satisfied and had fewer problems with the OU than they did with routine hospitalization.[43] Rentz et al. found that the model of a pediatric ED-controlled OU received high satisfaction ratings in all areas by community and subspecialty physicians.[46]

Characteristics of Pediatric OU Patients that Predict Admission

Factors associated with an "inappropriate" OU admission, defined as a prolonged LOS (> 24 hours) or a short stay < 4 hours were evaluated in one study. They found that 3% of patients were discharged home in < 4 hours and 7% of patients were discharged home in > 24 hours. Variables identified as significantly associated with an increased risk of inappropriate admissions were age < 1 year, CT or MRI done, IV fluids or medications, and cardio-respiratory monitoring. One drawback to this study was the inclusion of non-OU patients: some patients were in a holding unit, some in a medical assessment and planning unit, and others (the majority) were in an OU.[23] In another study, age was not seen as a risk factor for inpatient admission.[26] In a study of asthmatics, need for supplemental oxygen at the end of ED management, fever (temperature ≥ 38.5°), and female gender were associated with need for inpatient admission from the OU.[46]

Hybrid Unit

The term "hybrid" unit has several usages.[11,12] If an OU accepts both adult and pediatric patients in the same unit, this is a hybrid unit. If the unit accepts both ED patients for further diagnostic evaluation and/or treatment and other types of patients, specifically, patients undergoing procedures, particularly at a time when the OU may not be "full" with ED patients, this has also been termed a "hybrid" unit. This hybrid unit attempts to make use of the varied admit/discharge cycle of the typical OU which tends to be busiest during the evening shift with ED patients being placed into observation status, and full at night. Most of the patient discharges are in the morning, so there may be some temporary bed availability in the afternoon for non-typical OU patients (post recovery, awaiting procedures, etc.). There is a possible danger with this hybrid plan in that on any given day, if the ED is busy, ED patients may be backed up waiting for an OU bed, although this has not been reported.

The Future

There is tremendous potential for exponential growth in pediatric OM throughout the world. One study from the United States recommends that 70% of all asthmatics be treated in an OU.[47] An editorial from the United States suggests that two-thirds to three-fourths of all asthmatics are potential candidates for an OU instead being treated as an inpatient.[48] A Canadian health policy report estimates that 39% of pediatric and 25% of adult patients could be treated in an OU instead of receiving care as an inpatient.[49]

Summary

Like adult OM, pediatric OM needs the same organizational structure and format. Similarly, no matter what the patient's age, OM has many advantages: cost effectiveness, better patient/family satisfaction, decreased liability, enhanced risk management, psychosocial benefits, decreased LOS, and most importantly, better patient care and improved patient outcomes. There are some differences, however, between OM for infants and children compared to adults: different diagnoses, and different types of needed resources. Unique features of pediatric OM include less need for cardiac monitoring, increased use of respiratory therapy, greater need for IV fluids, and different types of pharmacology usage with antibiotics and antiemetics being the most common medications. It is very likely that pediatric OM, like adult OM, will be expanding in the future.

Some units exclude psychiatric patients from a general OU (as we do) since these patients often need one on one supervision, more intensive nursing observation and it may be disruptive to have a acutely ill psychiatric patient in the bed next to a low risk chest pain patient. An accidental overdose in a nonpsychiatric patient may be acceptable as an appropriate candidate for the OU. There is also the emergence of separate psychiatric OUs specifically for psychiatric patients, who are often intoxicated and need to be observed and reevaluated when they are "sober" and not under the influence of drugs and/or alcohol. (See editor's note on Psychiatric Chapter 60.)

References

1. *Emergency Care for Children: Growing Pains.* Committee on the Future of Emergency Care in the United States Health System. (ISBN: 0–309–65964–7). ch. 1 Introduction, p.18. National Academies Press. www.nap.edu/catalog/11655.html (Accessed February 2016)

2. www.cdc.gov/nchs/fastats/emergency-department.htm (Accessed February 2016)

3. Lamb S, Washington DL, Fink A, et al. Trends in the Use and Capacity of California'a emergency departments 1990-1999. *Ann Emerg Med* 2002; 39:389–396.

4. Zhou JC, Pan KH, Zhou DY, et al. High hospital occupancy is associated with increased risk for patients boarding in the emergency department. *Amer J Emerg Med* 2012; 125(4):416, e1–7.

5. Pines JM, Hilton JA, Weber EJ, et al. International perspectives on emergency department crowding. *Acad Emerg Med* 2011; 18(12); 1358–1370.

6. www.cdc.gov/nchs/data/hus/2011/093.pdf (Table 93) (Accessed February 2016)

7. Nawar EW, Niska RW, Xu J; Division of Health Care Statistics. Advance Data from Vital and Health Statistics. National Hospital Ambulatory Medical Care Survey: 2005 Emergency Department Summary, number 386 + June 29, 2007.

8. Hostetler M, Mace SE, Brown K, et al. Emergency department overcrowding and children. *Pediatr Emerg Care* 2007; 23 (7):507–515.

9. ACEP Observation Medicine Section. State of the Art: Observation Units in the Emergency Department. Policy Resource and Education Paper. American College of Emergency Physicians. Dallas, TX, 2011. www.acep.org/search.aspx?searchtext=observation%20medicine (Accessed February 2016)

10. Mace SE. Pediatric Observation Medicine. In: Graff LG, ed. *Observation Medicine: The Healthcare System's Tincture of Time.* American College of Emergency Physicians, Dallas, TX, 2011, ch. 12. www.acep.org/Search.aspx?searchtext=observation%20medicine%20Observation%20Medicine%20The%20Healthcare%20System%e2%80%99s%20Tincture%20of%20Time.&pgsize=10&filter=acep,news,ecfy,media (Accessed February 2016)

11. Conners GP, Melzer SM, Committee on Hospital Care and Committee on Pediatric Emergency Medicine. *Pediatric Observation Units. Pediatrics* 2012:130:172–179.

12. Mace SE. Pediatric Observation Medicine. *Emerg Med Clin*

North Amer 2001; 19(1): 239–254.

13. Mace SE. Issues in pediatric emergency medicine. *Foresight* 1999; 47:1.

14. Centers for Disease Control: Nationwide Estimates of Specific Health Care Needs Children Qualifiying by Specific Types of Special Health Care Needs Criteria. Atlanta, GA, Centers for Disease Control, 2006.

15. Goske M, Bulas D, Callahan MJ, et al. Image gently: progress and challenges in CT education and advocacy. *Pediatr Radiol* 2011; 41(Suppl 2):S461–S466.

16. Klein BL, Patterson M. Observation unit management of pediatric emergencies. *Emerg Med Clin North Am* 1991; 9:699–676.

17. Graff LG. *Observation Medicine*. Boston: Andover Medical Publishers, Inc; 1993.

18. American College of Emergency Physicians: Report on the Preparedness of the Emergency Department in the Care of Children. American College of Emergency Physicians, Dallas, TX, 1993, p. 1–.

19. Mace SE. A comparison of pediatric versus adult observation medicine patients. Abstract presented at the Ninth Annual Midwest Regional Society for Academic Emergency Medicine Research Forum. Ann Arbor, MI, September 25, 1999.

20. Mace SE. Observing children: can it be done in a general hospital? Presented at Emergency Observation Conference. Harvard School of Medicine. ACEP Short Term Observation Medicine Conference. Boston, MA, October 2, 1999.

21. Mace SE. A comparison of pediatric vs. adult observation medicine patients. Abstract presented at the International Conference of Emergency Medicine. Boston, MA., May 5, 2000. *Ann Emerg Med* 35 (suppl): S61, 2000.

22. LeDuc K. An observation unit in a pediatric emergency department: one children's hospital's experience. *J Emerg Nursing* 2002; 28(5):407–413.

23. Najaf-Zadeh A, Hue V, Bonnel-Mortuaire C, et al. Effectiveness of multifunction paediatric short-stay units: a French multicentre study. *Acta Paediatrica*; e227–e233. DOI:10.1111/j1651-2227.2011.02356a.

24. Wiley JF II, Friday JH, Nowakowski T, et al. Observation units: the role of an outpatient extended treatment site in pediatric care. *Pediatr Emerg Care* 2000; 16: 223–229.

25. Scribano PV, Wiley JF 2nd, Platt K. Use of an observation unit by a pediatric emergency department for common pediatric illnesses. *Pediatr Emerg Care* 2001; 17:321–323.

26. Alpern ER, Calello DP, Windreich R, et al. Utilization and unexpected hospitalization rates of a pediatric emergency department 23- hour observation unit. *Pediatr Emerg Care* 2008; 24(9):589–594.

27. Lamireau T, LLanas B, Dommange S, et al. A short-stay observation unit improves care in the paediatric emergency care setting. *European J Emerg Med* 2000; 7: 261–28.

28. Browne GJ. A short stay or 23-hour ward in a general and academic children's hospital: are they effective? *Pediatric Emerg Care* 2000; 16(4):223–229.

29. Beattie TF, Moir PA. Paediatric accident and emergency short-stay ward: a 1-year audit. *Archives Emerg Med* 1993; 10 (3):181–186.

30. Crocetti MT, Barone MA, Dritt Amin D, et al. Pediatric observation status beds on an inpatient unit: an integrated model. *Pediatr Emerg Care* 2004; 20(1):17–21.

31. Greenberg RA, Dudley NC, Rittichier KK. A reduction in hospitalization, length of stay, and hospital charges for croup with the institution of a pediatric observation unit. *Amer J Emerg Med* 2006; 24 (7):818–821.

32. Calello DP, Alpern ER, McDaniel-Yakscoe M, et al. Observation unit experience for pediatric poison exposures. *J Medical Toxicology* 2009; 5 (1):15–19.

33. Holsti M, Kadish HA, Sill BL, et al. Pediatric closed head injuries treated in an observation unit. *Pediatr Emerg Care* 2005; 21(10):639–644.

34. Ellerstein NS, Sullivan TD. Observation unit in a children's hospital. *NY State J Med* 1980; 80:1684 –

35. Beattie TF, Ferguson J, Moir PA. Short-stay facilitiess in accident and emergency departments for children. *Archives Emerg Med* 1993; 10:177–180.

36. O'Brien SR, Hein EN, Sly RM. Treatment of acute asthmatics attacks in a holding unit in a pediatric emergency room. *Ann Allergy* 1980; 45: 159–162.

37. Willert C, David AT, Herman JJ, et al. Short-term holding room treatment of asthmatics. *J Pediatr* 1985; 106:707–711.

38. Geelhoed GC. Sixteen years of croup in a western Australian teaching hospital. Effects of routine steroid treatment. *Ann Emerg Med* 1996; 28:621–626.

39. Gururaj VJ, Allen JL, Russo RM. Short stay in an outpatient department. *Am J Dis Child* 1972:123:128–132.

40. Knapp JF. What's new in pediatric emergency medicine. *Pediatr Rev* 1997; 18:424–

41. Gouin S, Macarthur C, Parkin PC, et al. Effect of a pediatric observation unit on the rate of hospitalization for asthma. *Ann Emerg Med* 1997; 29(2): 218–222.

42. Marks MK, Lovejoy FH Jr., Rutherford PA, et al. Impact of a short stay unit on asthma patients admitted to a tertiary pediatric hospital. *Quality Management in Health Care* 1997; 6(1):14–22.

43. Rydman RJ, Roberts RR, Albrecht GL, et al. Patient satisfaction with an emergency department asthma observation unit. *Acad Emerg Med* 1999; 6:178–183.

44. Aderonke-Ojo AO, Smitherman HF, Parker R, et al. Managing well-appearing neonates with hyperbilirubinemia in the emergency department observation unit. *Pediatr Emerg Care* 201: 26(5):343–348.

45. Bajaj L, Roback MG. Postreduction management of intussception in a children's hospital emergency department. *Pediatrics* 2003; 112:1302–1307.

46. Miescier MJ, Nelson DS, Firth SD, et al. Children with asthma admitted to a pediatric observation unit. *Pediatr Emerg Care* 2005; 21(10): 645–649.

47. McConnochie AKM, Russo MJ, McBride JT, et al. How commonly are children hospitalized for asthma eligible for care in alternative settings? *Arch Pediatr Adolesc Med* 1999; 153:49–

48. DeAngelis CD. Editor's Note: How commonly are children hospitalized for asthma eligible for care in alternate settings? *Arch Pediatr Adolesc Med* 1999; 153: 49–

49. DeCoster C, Peterson S, Karian P. *Manitoba Centre for Health Policy and Evaluation: Report summary alternatives to acute care.* Winnipeg, Manitoba, Canada. University of Manitoba-Manitoba Centre for Health Policy and Evaluation, 1996.

Chapter

54
Pediatric Observation Medicine at a Children's Hospital

Aderonke Ojo, MBBS

Background

The concepts of observation medicine (OM) and observation units (OUs) are not new; they continue to play a key role in patient flow in the emergency departments (EDs) to which they are attached. In contrast to their longstanding role in adult and community hospitals, pediatric OM and pediatric OUs are relatively new. About 20% of tertiary children's hospitals have pediatric emergency department observation units (ED OUs) (unpublished data from American College of Emergency Physicians survey in 2007).[1] Adult OUs provide optimal and safe care for patients requiring a limited period of hospital care in an outpatient setting; the same is true for the pediatric OU.

As the name implies, pediatric OUs serve only children (newborn to 18 or 21 years or younger, depending on the policy of the unit). These units may be designated as ED OUs (Emergency Department Observation Units), RTUs (Rapid Treatment Units), OUs or CDUs (Clinical Decision Units). These units are typically used to manage or observe patients who require further care for a definite and limited time period (usually less than 24 hours), and also to determine who may require inpatient admission during that time.[2] Most pediatric OUs are located adjacent or close to the ED. Some hospitals have specific units on inpatient floors. A recent survey by Macy et al. confirms that designated OUs are not common in freestanding children's hospitals, with only 12 of 31 responding hospitals reporting their presence. Even in the hospitals with established OUs, not all observation-status patients are managed in these units; all 12 responding hospitals reported providing some form of virtual observation care (in the ED or in an inpatient unit).[3]

Most pediatric OUs are run by ED staff members. However, they function as a separate unit from the ED, serving the needs of other services as well, in response to the limited and decreasing number of inpatient beds.

What makes this an asset in a children's hospital is the more complex and diversified conditions with which patients present. Following care in the ED, most patients are discharged home; 15% or so are admitted; another 3–4% are not ready to be discharged, but are not sick enough to be admitted.[4] Most of these patients (80–90%) are eventually discharged home, but with both ED and inpatient beds becoming increasingly scarce, observing these children in either setting can create problems. The end result is a vicious cycle: limited inpatient beds, increased inpatient holding in the ED, prolonged ED wait times, increased numbers of patients who leave without being seen, and the list goes on. Pediatric ED OUs benefit the hospitals they serve by reducing ED overcrowding, limiting 1-day inpatient admissions, and improving patient satisfaction.[5]

Types and Functions of a Pediatric OU

Pediatric medicine is inherently seasonal, with influenza and other viruses peaking in the winter; this may result in an OU that is full at certain times of the year, while near empty at others. In order to offset this problem, many pediatric OUs have become hybridized. A hybrid unit is one that serves other functions in addition to the primary role of caring for the typical observation patients. These functions may include administration of scheduled blood transfusions, sleep studies, and recovery from procedural sedation.[2] Some pediatric OUs also hold admitted patients awaiting inpatient beds, particularly during the busier winter season; however, this typically is not the

Table 54.1 Texas Children's Hospital – ED OU protocol for patients with abdominal pain

Guidelines for the Management of Children with Abdominal Pain in the ED OU

Time Frame:

Limit of 24 hours for observation and treatment

Appropriate Observation:

Stable vitals
Significant abdominal pain/right lower
  quadrant pain
Ancillary signs and symptoms – anorexia,
  nausea, vomiting, fever, leukocytosis
Normal or equivocal x-rays/ultrasounds or CT scans

Exclusion Criteria:

Unstable vitals (unexplained tachycardia, persistent
  tachycardia despite resuscitation, tachycardia
  > 95th percentile for age)
Surgical abdomen/presence of rebound
Immunocompromised patient
Confirmed appendicitis by diagnostic imaging
  (patients with uncomplicated appendicitis
  can be held in observation unit pending surgery)
Abnormal radiographic studies – except ileus

Observation Unit Intervention:

Keep NPO (nil per os) (nothing by mouth)_
Intravenous (IV) hydration
Serial exams and vital signs Q 4 hours
Repeat laboratory studies/radiographic study
Consultation

Disposition Criteria:

Home: symptomatic improvement of pain
Ability to take fluids/meds per os (PO)
  (by mouth)

Admit:

Deterioration
No improvement
Specific diagnosis identified requiring
  hospitalization
Transfer to the pediatric intensive care
  unit/pediatric clinical unit: Unstable vitals
  (unexplained tachycardia, persistent tachycardia
  despite resuscitation, tachycardia > 95th
  percentile for age)

Table 54.2 Texas Children's Hospital – ED OU protocol for diabetic patients with hyperglycemia

Guidelines for the Management of Children with Diabetes with Hyperglycemia in the ED OU

Timeframe:

Limit of 24 hours for observation and treatment

Appropriate Observation:

Acceptable/ stable vitals for age
No DKA (pH < 7.30, Plasma β-hydroxybutyrate
  < 2.5 mMol/L, HCO3 < 15)
  Initial evaluation completed in ED and formal
  consultation of the endocrine service if
  requested regardless of time of day
Joint agreement of the ED and Endocrine
  Services for placement in the ED OU
  ED OU and Endocrine Services can freely
  communicate as the need arises

Exclusion Criteria:

DKA defined as glucose > 200 mg%, pH < 7.30,
  HCO3 < 15, and plasma β-hydroxybutyrate
  > 2.5 mMol/L
Unstable vital signs for age
Requiring subcutaneous insulin every 2 hours or
  more frequently
Altered mental status/drowsiness
Requirement of an insulin drip
Plasma β-hydroxybutyrate > 2.5 mMol/L
New diagnosis of diabetes mellitus

Observation Unit Interventions:

Subcutaneous insulin
Serial exams
Finger stick blood glucose and β-hydroxybutyrate
  every 2 hours or less frequently
IV hydration
IV glucose

Disposition
Home:

Acceptable/stable vitals for age
Tolerating PO fluids
β-hydroxybutyrate < 0.6 mM/L or trending near
  0.6 mM/L
Reliable family
Clearance by Endocrine Services only required
  for discharge if ED OU has questions or concerns.

Admit to the Hospital:

Persistent emesis
Unstable vitals for age
Persistent hypoglycemia
Persistent β-hydroxybutyrate > 2.5 mMol/L

primary function of a pediatric OU. Carefully set guidelines are needed to determine when holding patients in the OU will be appropriate because it can easily overtake the primary role of the OU.

Clinical Criteria

Pediatric OUs may have more diversified admission diagnoses when compared to adult units. Common diagnoses include gastroenteritis, asthma, croup, cellulitis, abdominal pain, hyperbilirubinemia, ingestions, seizures, urinary tract infections, renal colic, headaches, and aseptic meningitis.[2,4,7–18] Patients are selected based on the guiding principles for all OUs: focused care goals and limited duration and intensity of services, usually 24 hours or less.

Management

Set standards (including admission criteria, documentation, discharge criteria, length of stay, chain of command and proper staffing) and compliance with these standards is necessary to the function of a pediatric OU. Prior to opening such a unit, the goals and objectives of the unit should be set based on the varying needs of the institution. Most OUs in children's hospitals primarily serve the ED, with other functions as described earlier in the hybrid units. Admission criteria are predetermined and are based on the goals and objectives of the unit; discharge criteria and procedures are also predetermined (see following protocol examples for abdominal pain Table 54.1 and diabetes Table 54.2). The various types of documentation and frequency of documentation should be clarified prior to setting up a unit. The unit is a separate unit from the ED and must therefore have appropriate staffing, usually by acute care pediatric nurses. Physician coverage is usually provided by either ED physicians (ideally separate from the physicians actively working in the ED at any given time) or hospitalists; some pediatric OUs have introduced advanced practice clinicians (midlevel providers), for example, nurse practitioners or physician assistants who work under the guidance of the supervising unit physician. Most children's ED OUs are closed units; only ED physicians can place patients in the unit.

Recurring utilization review is required to determine how well the unit is functioning, to prevent inappropriate drain of ED health care resources, and to limit health care costs. Data that should be collected for this purpose include total census, admission rates, and length of stay. An ongoing review of patient care for adherence to standards and quality of patient care follows admission rates, complaints, unscheduled return visits within 48 hours of discharge from the OU, and adverse events including codes and deaths in the unit.[4,12,19–23]

OM in children's hospitals typically operates under the auspices of Emergency Medicine, rather than as an independent section. It is currently not included in the core pediatric curriculum for residents rotating in the ED, and so most of these units have no pediatric residents/learners. However, this is not the case in non-ED settings, especially on the inpatient floors.

Research in the field of OM is increasing, and focuses primarily on resource utilization and the various roles and functions of the OU. This research continues to provide evidence that OUs benefit the hospitals they serve, especially in the areas of patient care, patient and physician satisfaction, ED flow, and cost-effectiveness. Future areas of research include education of health care providers about the various functions and benefits of OUs, standardization of outcome measures, and quality improvement.

References

1. American College of Emergency Physicians Survey. Section of Observation Medicine. Unpublished data from 2007.

2. Zebrack M, Kadish H, Nelson D. The pediatric hybrid observation unit: Aanalysis of 6477 patients. *Pediatrics* 2005; 115: e535–e542.

3. Macy ML, Hall M, Shah SS, et al. Differences in designation of Observation care in US free standing hospitals: are they virtual or real. *J Hospital Med* 2011:1–7.

4. Graff LG. *Observation Medicine*, 1st ed. Andover Medical Publishers, 1993;6–40.

5. Rentz AC, Kadish HA, Nelson DS. Physician satisfaction with a pediatric observation unit administered by Pediatric Emergency physicians. *Ped Emerg Care* 2004; 20: 430–432.

6. Greenberg RA, Dudley NC, Rittichier KK. A reduction in hospitalization, length of stay, and hospital charges for croup with the institution of a pediatric observation unit. *Am J Emerg Med* 2006; 24: 818–821.

7. Mace SE. Pediatric observation medicine. *Emerg Med Clin North Am* 2001; 19: 234–254.

8. Macy ML, Kim CS, Sasson C. Pediatric observation units in the United States: A systematic

review. *J Hospital Med* 2010; 5: 172–182.

9. Mace SE, Graff L, Mikhail M, et al. National survey of observation units in the United States. *American Journal of Emergency Medicine* 2003; 21: 529–533.

10. AmWiley JF. Pediatric clinical decision units: observation, past present and future. *Clin Ped Emerg Med* 2001; 2: 247–252.

11. Holsti M, Kadish HA, Sill BL, et al. Pediatric closed head injuries treated in an observation unit. *P Emerg Care* 2005; 21: 639–644.

12. Mallory MD, Kadish H, Zebrack M, et al. Use of pediatric observation unit for treatment of children with Dehydration caused by gastroenteritis. *P Emerg Care* 2006; 22: 1–6.

13. Alpern ER, Callello DP, Windreich R, et al. Utilization and unexpected hospitalization rates of a pediatric emergency department. *P Emerg Care* 2008: 24: 589–594.

14. Mierscier MJ, Nelson DS, Firth SD, et al. Children with asthma admitted to a pediatric observation unit. *P Emerg Care* 2005; 21: 645–649.

15. Adekunle-Ojo AO, Smithermann HF, Parker R, et al. Managing well-appearing neonates with hyperbilirubinemia in the emergency department observation unit. *P Emerg Care* 2010; 26: 343–346.

16. Adekunle- Ojo AO, Craig AM, Ma L, et al. Intussusception: postreduction fasting is not necessary to prevent complications and recurrences in the emergency department observation unit. *Pediatr Emerg Care* 2011; 27: 897–899.

17. Gouin S, Macarthur C, Parkkin PC, et al. Effect of a Pediatric observation unit on the rate of hospitalization for asthma. *Ann Emerg Med* 1997; 29(2): 218–222.

18. Scribano PV, Wiley JF 2nd, Platt K. Use of an observation unit by a pediatric emergency department for common pediatric illnesses. *P Emerg Care* 2001; 17: 321–323.

19. Cooke MW, Higgins J, Kidd P. Use of emergency observation and assessment wards: a systematic review. *Emerg Med J* 2003; 20: 138–142.

20. Burkhardt J, Peacock WF, Emerman CL, et al. Predictors of ED OU outcomes. *Acad Emerg Med* 2005; 12: 869–874.

21. Mace SE. An analysis of patient complaints in an observation unit. *Journal of Quality in Clinical Practice* 1998; 18(2): 151–158.

22. Mace SE. Resuscitations in an observation unit. *Journal of Quality in Clinical Practice* 1999; 19: 155–164.

23. Mace SE. Continuous quality improvement for the clinical decision unit. *Journal for Healthcare Quality* 2004; 26(1): 29–36.

Chapter 55

Geriatric Observation Medicine

Fredric M. Hustey, MD, FACEP

Background

The proportion of emergency department (ED) visits made by older patients continues to increase at a rate greater than any other demographic group.[1] In the next 20 years, the proportion of ED visits by patients age 65 years and older is expected to rise from approximately 15% to 25%.[1] This is likely to contribute to an increased proportion of older patients being cared for in observation units (OUs). While older ED patients tend to be more complex, require more ED resources, and have longer ED stays,[2] in many cases these patients may be appropriate for ED-based OU care.

Many of the conditions typically managed in OUs are much more common in the older population.[3] Examples of these include chest pain where myocardial infarction is being ruled out,[4] syncope, congestive heart failure, transient ischemic attack evaluation (TIA),[5] atrial fibrillation,[6] and COPD.[3] As the principles of evaluation and management of these conditions are covered elsewhere in this text, this chapter will focus on conditions that are likely to have special issues more unique to the geriatric population. These include falls and injury, altered mental status, and acute abdominal pain.

Discussion

Falls and Injury

ED visits for falls with related injuries are not uncommon in older patients. While many of these patients can be discharged home after a thorough evaluation, some may warrant observation care.

Inclusions

Patients sustaining falls with subsequent injury may have difficulty with mobility. Mobility may be impaired by pain resulting from injury or by the underlying etiology that precipitated the fall (such as lightheadedness). (See Chapter 37 on Dizziness). All older patients for whom ED discharge is being considered should be observed arising and ambulating unless there is a contraindication to do so (such as known or suspected hip fracture). In those patients for whom it is unclear as to whether they will be able to ambulate safely, observation admission may be warranted.

In addition, there is a small subset of patients for whom high-risk fractures cannot be ruled out in the ED. The classic example of this is the older patient with significant hip pain after a fall who undergoes plain radiographs that do not show hip or pelvic fracture. Patients who are discharged with missed femoral neck fractures are at risk for subsequent fracture displacement and avascular necrosis of the femoral head. It is important to exclude hip fracture via obtaining advanced imaging, ideally using MRI.[7] Given the difficulty in obtaining an MRI in the time frame of an ED visit, these patients may also be candidates for OU admission.

Management and Outcome

For patients whose mobility is significantly impaired due to pain, the goal is analgesia. While intravenous opioids may be necessary initially, ideally these should be weaned to oral medications that the patient can use at home. If pain is well-controlled and the patient is able to ambulate safely they may be subsequently discharged. In some cases, however, additional resources may be required that are not immediately available in the ED. In these patients physical therapy assessment and training with ambulatory assistive devices (such as a walker) in the OU may be beneficial. Home health care resources may also be arranged with the assistance of social services when necessary to prevent unnecessary hospitalization.

For patients whose mobility is significantly impaired due to a simple underlying medical condition, the goal is to achieve gait stability through condition management. Patients with orthostatic instability may require an observation stay for continued intravenous hydration and or medication adjustment. In some cases instability may be due to dizziness caused by new medications or medication interactions (especially those with anticholinergic side effects). In patients who have limited home support and are at risk for subsequent falls, medication adjustments can be made followed by observation admission with reassessment of gait prior to discharge. Assessment by a geriatric consult team, if available, may also be beneficial for some patients in this group.

In cases where hip fracture is suspected but not evident on initial radiographs, the goal is to rule out fracture with advanced imaging while attempts are made at pain control. Ideally this should be done with MRI unless there is a contraindication.[7] Once hip fracture has been ruled out, a trial of ambulation should be done with the use of assistive devices as necessary. Patients who can safely ambulate and have adequate pain control may then be discharged to home.

Exclusions

Falls are often a symptom of another underlying process or processes in older patients. Prior to referring these patients to the OU a reasonably thorough ED evaluation should be completed to look for underlying precipitants. While some simple abnormalities may be managed in the ED or OU, more significant problems may require hospital admission. In addition, patients with significant preexisting mobility impairment (such as those already walker dependent), limited home assistance (live alone and no home health care), and persistent severe uncontrolled pain after reasonable attempts in the ED at pain management may be unlikely to progress to an ambulatory state in the appropriate time frame. These patients may require hospital admission directly from the ED. This is confirmed by a recent study that found that frailty was a significant predictor of inpatient admission from the observation unit.[8]

Altered Mental Status

Altered mental status is common in older ED patients.[9] Delirium is a medical emergency requiring emergent evaluation.[10] Previous research has shown that unrecognized delirium is an independent predictor of mortality in older patients seen in EDs and discharged home without admission. In one study by Kakuma et al., there was a statistically significant association between unrecognized delirium and mortality after adjustment for age, sex, functional level, cognitive status, comorbidity, and number of medications for the first 6 months of follow-up (hazard ratio = 7.24, 95% CI = 1.62–32.35). This suggests that in older patients with delirium who are being considered for discharge from the ED, placement in observation status in an ED OU, may be a viable alternative.[11]

Inclusions

Most EDs admit patients with a new alteration in mental status to the inpatient service, instead of placing the patient in the OU. However, in view of the onset of the "extended" or "complex" OU, increasing numbers of geriatric patients, and ED crowding, specific criteria for placing patients with delirium into an OU may be considered. (See Chapters 16 and 17 on extended or complex observation.)

Patients with mild delirium who are being considered for ED discharge may alternatively benefit from evaluation in the ED OU in order to clearly identify or confirm the cause of their delirium and to institute treatment if possible. In addition, patients with mild delirium with a single simple etiology or etiologies identified that is/are potentially correctable during a brief observation stay may be ideal candidates for care in the ED OU. Examples include new medication(s) causing side effects or medication interactions, dehydration with or without mild electrolyte abnormality, drug or alcohol intoxication, or otherwise uncomplicated infection (such as urinary tract).[10]

It is important to remember that delirium is often multifactorial in etiology,[10] and several factors may need to be addressed during observation care. In addition, it is not uncommon for patients with dementia to develop delirium due to a single precipitant.

Management

Management is targeted towards treating precipitating factors. In patients with preexisting dementia it is often only a single additional precipitant requiring management. In others there may be multiple issues requiring intervention. Correcting dehydration and electrolyte deficiencies, treating infection, and managing medications may all play a role depending on the circumstances. Neuroi maging is often not helpful unless other factors point towards a primary central nervous system (CNS) precipitant (such as new focal neurologic deficits, recent head trauma, or concern for CNS infection).

It is important to establish the patient's baseline mental status and to assess for resolution of delirium prior to discharge to home. Family, friends, or caregivers in frequent contact with the patient should be interviewed to establish the baseline. Current mental status is best assessed using a structured tool for delirium such as the Confusion Assessment Method (CAM)[12] or the Confusion Assessment Method for the ICU (CAM-ICU)[13] in addition to a standard short mental status assessment such as the Short Orientation Memory Concentration Test.[14] Both of these tests can be completed in a matter of minutes in the ED and in the OU.[15] Patients should be assessed at a minimum while in the ED, upon admission to the OU, and prior to considering OU discharge. Those individuals who have returned to baseline mental status may be considered for discharge to home. Assessment in the OU by a geriatric consult team, if available, may also be beneficial for some patients in this group.

Exclusions

Patients for whom safety cannot be maintained due to behavioral issues (such as those who are severely agitated or combative) should not be referred for observation care. Severe CNS depression (obtundation due to hypoactive delirium) is unlikely to resolve during an OU stay and should be admitted elsewhere. Patients with severe metabolic abnormalities, potentially life-threatening withdrawal syndromes (alcohol, benzodiazepines, barbiturates), new focal neurologic deficits, and those for whom CNS infection is suspected but has not been ruled out are also not appropriate for OU care.

Acute Abdominal Pain

Acute abdominal pain is a common presenting complaint for older ED patients.[16–17] Those patients with potentially life-threatening etiologies pose a particular challenge in that the diagnosis is often unclear in the ED. Older patients in general tend to have more delayed presentations, vague histories and physical examination findings, and "unimpressive" laboratory results (such as a lack of leukocytosis).[15] In nearly 1 in 5 older patients, the initial ED diagnosis may be inaccurate.[15] Up to 14% of older patients discharged from the ED after presenting with acute abdominal pain may return to the ED within 2 weeks.[15] Given these challenges, a subgroup of older patients with acute abdominal pain may be suitable for care in the ED OU.

Inclusions

Patients who do not have a clear diagnosis at the end of the ED evaluation, those who have moderately poor pain control, or those who are unable to adequately tolerate per os (po) (by mouth) may be candidates for observation-based care. In addition, patients who possess a lack of significant history or physical examination findings but have concerning, nonspecific laboratory findings (such as a marked leukocytosis) may also warrant observation admission for serial abdominal examinations. As cholecystitis is often missed in this population,[15] stable patients for whom the diagnosis is suspected but who have had an unremarkable ED workup (nondiagnostic ultrasonography and unremarkable laboratory findings) may also be candidates for observation. However, this decision should be made in consultation with a surgeon when there is a very high suspicion for the diagnosis. Finally, patients for whom there is a concern for acute coronary syndrome should undergo observation to exclude this possibility if this diagnosis is still in question at the end of the ED visit.

Management

Management is tailored towards providing supportive and symptomatic treatment, careful observation, and serial examinations and further testing as indicated based on the suspected differential diagnosis. For example, patients admitted with a diagnosis of gastroenteritis may receive intravenous fluids, antiemetics, and antidiarrheals, while also undergoing serial abdominal examinations and further diagnostic testing given the relatively higher rate of misdiagnosis in this subgroup. Patients with suspected cholecystitis should receive symptomatic and supportive treatment as well as undergo a hepatobiliary iminodiacetic acid (HIDA) scan if the initial ultrasound was not diagnostic. Patients for whom there is concern for acute coronary syndrome should undergo rule out of myocardial infarction with serial cardiac enzymes and electrocardiograms (ECGs). For those patients in which myocardial infarction has been ruled out, cardiac stress testing may also be indicated prior to discharge based on history, physical examination, and ECG findings.

Exclusions

Patients who are hemodynamically unstable, have serious acute metabolic derangements, or severe uncontrolled pain after ED treatment are not candidates for OU admission. In addition, patients for whom there is a very high suspicion for an acute surgical process in spite of nondiagnostic test results (e.g., those with guarding and rigidity on abdominal examination or patients for whom there is a very high suspicion for mesenteric ischemia in spite of nondiagnostic abdominal CT) should undergo surgical consultation in the ED prior to any consideration of OU admission.

Summary

Older ED patients are typically more complex than younger counterparts. While they generally require more time and resources in the ED, in many cases these patients can be appropriately managed in the OU. While OUs have been caring for older patients for years, there is a lack of evidence regarding OU outcomes for these conditions that are more unique to the geriatric population. Nonetheless appropriate use of the OU in these circumstances may help to avoid unnecessary hospital admissions and ED recidivism for many of these patients.

References

1. Wilber ST, Gerson LW, Terrell KM, et al. Geriatric emergency medicine and the 2006 Institute of Medicine reports from the Committee on the Future of Emergency Care in the U.S. health system. *Acad Emerg Med.* [Review]. 2006 Dec;13(12): 1345–1351.

2. Strange GR, Chen EH. Use of emergency departments by elder patients: a five-year follow-up study. *Acad Emerg Med.* [Research Support, Non-U.S. Gov't]. 1998 Dec;5(12): 1157–1162.

3. Ross MA, Compton S, Richardson D, et al. The use and effectiveness of an emergency department observation unit for elderly patients. *Ann Emerg Med.* [Comparative Study]. 2003 May;41(5):668–677.

4. Madsen TE, Bledsoe J, Bossart P. Appropriately screened geriatric chest pain patients in an observation unit are not admitted at a higher rate than nongeriatric patients. *Crit Pathw Cardiol.* [Comparative Study]. 2008 Dec;7(4): 245–247.

5. Stead LG, Bellolio MF, Suravaram S, et al. Evaluation of transient ischemic attack in an emergency department observation unit. *Neurocrit Care.* [Clinical Trial Research Support, Non-U.S. Gov't]. 2009;10(2):204–208.

6. Decker WW, Smars PA, Vaidyanathan L, et al. A prospective, randomized trial of an emergency department observation unit for acute onset atrial fibrillation. *Ann Emerg Med.* [Randomized Controlled Trial Research Support, Non-U.S. Gov't]. 2008 Oct;52(4):322–328.

7. Chana R, Noorani A, Ashwood N, et al. The role of MRI in the diagnosis of proximal femoral fractures in the elderly. *Injury.* 2006 Feb;37(2): 185–189.

8. Zradzinski MJ, Phelan MP, Mace SE. Impact of frailty and sociodemographic factors on hospital admission froman emeregency department observation unit. *AJMQ* (accepted for publication 2016).

9. Hustey FM, Meldon SW, Smith MD, et al. The effect of mental status screening on the care of elderly emergency department patients. *Ann Emerg Med.* 2003;41(5):678–684.

10. Inouye SK. Delirium in older persons.[see comment] [erratum appears in *N Engl J Med.* 2006 Apr 13;354 (15):1655]. *N Engl J Med.* 2006;354(11): 1157–1165.

11. Katuma R, Galbaud du Fort G, Arsenault L, et al. Delirium in older emergency department patients discharged home: effect on survival. *J Am Geriatr Soc.* 2003;51:443–450.

12. Inouye SK, van Dyck CH, Alessi CA, et al. Clarifying confusion: the confusion assessment method. A new method for detection of delirium. [see comment]. *Annals of Internal Medicine.* 1990;113(12):941–948.

13. Ely EW, Inouye SK, Bernard GR, et al. Delirium in mechanically ventilated patients: validity and reliability of the confusion assessment method for the intensive care unit (CAM-ICU). *JAMA.* 2001;286(21): 2703–2710.

14. Hustey FM, Meldon SW. The prevalence and documentation of impaired mental status in elderly emergency department patients. [see comment]. *Ann Emerg Med.* 2002;39(3):248–253.

15. Lewis LM, Banet GA, Blanda M, et al. Etiology and clinical course of abdominal pain in senior patients: a prospective, multicenter study. *J Gerontol A Biol Sci Med Sci.* [Multicenter Study Research Support, Non-U.S. Gov't]. 2005 Aug;60(8): 1071–1076.

16. Marco CA, Schoenfeld CN, Keyl PM, et al. Abdominal pain in geriatric emergency patients: variables associated with adverse outcomes. *Acad Emerg Med.* [Research Support, Non-U.S. Gov't]. 1998 Dec;5(12): 1163–1168.

Chapter

Abdominal Pain

56

Mark G. Moseley, MD, MHA, FACEP
Miles P. Hawley, MD, MBA

Introduction

Abdominal pain is a frequent cause of emergency department (ED) visits. In many cases the etiology for the pain is unclear. This often requires an extensive evaluation in the ED. In other cases, the cause of the abdominal pain is clear and the focus of the visit is controlling the symptoms. In some cases, patients with differentiated abdominal pain may be placed in the observation unit (OU) for management of their symptoms.

Patients with differentiated abdominal pain can be successfully treated in an OU. The primary goal in this patient population is symptom control. The cause of their symptoms should already be established and therefore observation is used to determine if symptoms can be controlled enough for the patients to be discharged. In some cases, these patients may require some diagnostic workup to determine the severity of their illness. For example, a patient with a Crohn's disease flare may require an abdominal CT scan to determine the extent of the inflammation. A postendoscopy patient with abdominal pain may require an abdominal plain film to rule out perforation. However, in general the primary focus should be on symptom control.

Discussion

Patients frequently present to the ED with an established source of abdominal pain. These patients may include patients with chronic abdominal pain, Crohn's disease, ulcerative colitis, postoperative patients with known ileus and postprocedural patients with abdominal pain. Many of these patients have had frequent evaluations for their pain in the past. Postoperative and postprocedural patients may have had recent inpatient evaluations or outpatient testing. It is unclear exactly how and where to treat this patient population. There is very little evidence to guide

their management and no guidelines exist. There is a subset of these patients who are appropriate for observation care and respond well to treatment in the observation unit. Patient selection is critical in establishing which patients with differentiated abdominal pain are appropriate for treatment in the OU. It is very important to define clear goals and discharge criteria in this population. Chronic abdominal pain without new findings is probably not appropriate for the OU. However, acute on chronic abdominal pain (e.g., acute exacerbation of chronic abdominal pain) may be appropriate. It is very important that this patient population has good outpatient follow-up. Patients with no previously established primary care physician or specialist may benefit from inpatient treatment rather than observation. Symptoms often reoccur and without good follow-up this population will end up back in the ED.

Patient Criteria

Patient selection is critical in this population. Patients must have a good chance of discharge in 24 hours. In addition, there must be clear goals and treatment objectives.

Inclusion Criteria

Patients who have a known cause of abdominal pain and present with worsening of symptoms may be appropriate for observation treatment. These patients need to have a high likelihood that the pain can be controlled in 24 hours.

Exclusion Criteria

Patients with a need for advanced testing such as endoscopic retrograde cholangiopancreatography (ERCP) to evaluate their abdominal pain usually require inpatient admission. Patients with evidence of a surgical abdomen require inpatient admission.

Management

Patients with differentiated abdominal pain require treatment that is often individualized and directed at the underlying disease. This makes treatment of these patients in the OU somewhat more complicated. As mentioned earlier, it is important to define clear goals of care prior to placing these patients in the OU. Often it is necessary to consult subspecialty services prior to placing the patient in the OU. For example, a patient with a flare of Cohn's disease with no clear need for admission may be treated with antibiotics, steroids, and pain control. Alternatively, a patient with gastroparesis who presents with abdominal pain may be treated with IV fluids, pain control, and bowel rest. Postprocedural patients often present to the ED with abdominal pain and fall into this category. Post-endoscopy patients with abdominal pain and bloating can be treated with IV fluids, pain control, and bowel rest. In general, treatment of differentiated abdominal pain focuses on the following principles: treatment of underlying disease process, pain control, and managing diet.

Disease-specific care

Inflammatory Bowel Disease

Patients with inflammatory bowel disease often present with abdominal pain flares. This is frequently accompanied by diarrhea and nausea. Many of these patients will have severe symptoms that require inpatient treatment. Patients with known or suspected abscess, concern for obstruction or perforation, surgical abdomen or signs of severe infection require treatment as an inpatient. Patients with moderate disease with good outpatient follow-up are good candidates for observation treatment. It may be necessary to obtain a CT scan or MRI of the abdomen and pelvis in the ED to determine the extent of disease prior to disposition.[1,2] Treatment of these patients may include the following: steroids, pain control, antibiotics, and antiemetics.[1,2] The primary endpoint in this patient population is pain control and ability to tolerate PO. It is often helpful to discuss the case with the patient's outpatient physician at some point prior to discharge, as these patients often require close follow-up.

Postprocedural Abdominal Pain

Postprocedural patients will often develop abdominal pain. This can occur after upper and lower endoscopy and minor surgery.[3] There are multiple sources of pain in these patients including bloating from endoscopy, anesthesia, constipation related to opioid medications, and the underlying process. Treatment for this patient population often includes bowel rest, IV fluids, and pain control. It is often necessary to obtain an abdominal plain film to rule out free air. Diet should be slowly advanced. Care should be coordinated with the procedural provider. The patient can be discharged when they are tolerating PO and their pain is controlled.

Gastroparesis

Patients with gastroparesis frequently have exacerbations or flares of their symptoms. These flares have many triggers including hyperglycemia, infection, diet, and medication noncompliance. These patients often complain of severe abdominal pain, nausea, and vomiting.[4] They often present with signs of dehydration. Some of these patients can be safely managed in an OU. Treatment of this group of patients usually involves pain control, antiemetics, and IV fluids. Prokinetic medications such as metoclopramide may improve symptoms.[5] Their diet should be slowly advanced. This group can be discharged when their pain is controlled and they are tolerating PO intake. Patients with cyclic vomiting syndrome and chronic abdominal pain can often be treated in a similar manner.

Outcome

The primary goal in this patient population is improvement in symptoms. It is unlikely that the abdominal pain will completely resolve, but rather the goal is that the pain is manageable. In addition, patients should be able to tolerate PO intake and should have an outpatient follow-up plan. Patient's whose pain is not controlled, are unable to tolerate PO, or who require further testing despite treatment in the OU should be made inpatient status.

Conclusion

Patients with differentiated abdominal pain can often be appropriately treated in an OU. This population is diverse and often requires an individualized care plan. It is often necessary to consult or discuss with subspecialty services to ensure that an appropriate plan is established. The primary goals and outcomes in this population include the following: pain management, nausea control, diet management, and establishing outpatient follow-up.

References

1. Carter M, Lobo A, Travis S. Guidelines for the management of inflammatory bowel disease in adults. *Gut.* 2004. 53: v1–v16.

2. Lichtenstein G, Hanauer S, Sandborn W. Management of Crohn's disease in adults. ACG practice guidelines. *American Journal of Gastroenterology.* 2004.

3. Ko C, Riffle S. Incidence of minor complications and time lost of time from minor complications after screening colonoscopy. *Gastrointestinal Endoscopy.* 2007. Apr(4): 648–656.

4. Cherian D, Sachcheva P, Fisher RS, et al. Abdominal pain is a frequent symptom of gastroparesis. *Clinical Gastroenterology and Hepatology.* 2010. Aug(8): 678–681.

5. Parkham H, Hasler W, Fisher R. Diagnosis and treatment of gastroparesis. AGA medical position statement. *Gastroenterology.* 2004. Nov(127), issue 5: 1589–1591.

Chapter

57

Pain Management, Including Musculoskeletal and Low Back Pain

Nathaniel L. Scott, MD, FACEP
James R. Miner, MD, FACEP

Introduction

Pain management is often an important part of treatment in an observation unit (OU). This chapter will discuss general principles of the treatment of pain in the OU, as well as the management of specific painful conditions. Criteria for referral to observation services relevant to acute musculoskeletal pain will be reviewed. Other pain-related complaints that require specific evaluation and treatment, such as chest pain, abdominal pain, and sickle-cell pain, are discussed elsewhere in this text.

Epidemiology

Painful complaints are frequently treated in the observation setting.[1] In one study, back pain was the sixth most common condition treated in an OU, accounting for 4.7% of patients.[2] Nephrolithiasis, abdominal pain, pyelonephritis, cellulitis, traumatic injuries, and headache are also painful conditions routinely treated in OUs.

Principles of Pain Management

The treatment of pain is frequently the reason that patients seek medical care, and satisfaction with care has been correlated with effective analgesia.[3] In addition to the relief of suffering, evidence supports the importance of adequate pain management in the treatment of disease. Unrelieved acute pain has been associated with increased sympathetic nervous system activation, decreased immune function, the development of chronic pain, greater need for subsequent pain treatment, and psychosocial dysfunction.[4–6] From a regulatory standpoint, the Joint Commission mandates documentation of the evaluation and treatment of pain. Clearly, a priority must be placed on effective treatment of pain in the OU.

Assessment

Accurate assessment of pain is critical to effective management. Inadequate treatment is often due to inaccurate assessment.[7] A patient's experience of pain is dependent on the interaction between the patient's physical stimulus, physiology, prior experience and expectation of pain, and their current emotional and cognitive states. It is known that patients presenting with the same injury will often report widely varying levels of pain.[8] Currently, there are no reliable tests or physiologic measurements to objectively assess a patient's level of pain.[9–11] The assessment of pain therefore remains subjective and unique to each individual's experience. To accurately assess pain, it is necessary to consider both verbal and nonverbal communication from the patient, in addition to objective observations. Accordingly, patients who are unable to communicate effectively are at risk for undertreatment. These groups include children, patients with a cultural background different from their provider, patients with mental illness, or patients with emotional or cognitive impairment.[8,12–15]

OUs should have a well-defined method for assessing pain. The Joint Commission has mandated that pain must be assessed using a pain scale as part of routine vital signs. For various developmental reasons, numeric pain scales are difficult to use with children <7 years old. Nonnumeric scales can be utilized, such as the FACES pain scale or color-based pain scales, but it is unclear if children <7 years old, and particularly children <5 years old, can rate pain on a scale. For preverbal children, provider-based scales such as Modified Pre-Verbal, Early Verbal Pediatric Pain Scale (M-PEPPS) and the Children's Hospital of Eastern Ontario Pain Scale (CHEOPS) can be used, but they largely represent a provider's judgment of how much pain the child is observed to have.

Table 57.1 Commonly Used Opioid Medications and Their Pharmacokinetic Properties[17]

Name	Initial Parenteral Dose	Initial Oral Dose	Duration of Action	Equipotent IV Dose	Equipotent Oral Dose
Morphine	0.1 mg/kg	0.5 mg/kg	3–4 hrs	10 mg	50 mg
Hydromorphone	0.015 mg/kg	0.075 mg/kg	2–4 hrs	1.5 mg	7.5 mg
Fentanyl	1.5 µg/kg	3 µg/kg	30–90 min	100 µg	n/a
Oxycodone	0.1 mg/kg	0.15 mg/kg	3–4 hrs	10 mg	15 mg
Hydrocodone	n/a	5–15 mg	3–4 hrs	n/a	30 mg
Codeine	1.3 mg/kg	2.5 mg/kg	2–4 hrs	130 mg	200 mg

Medications

Opioid analgesics are the first-line agents for the management of acute severe pain. Opioids activate endorphin system receptors throughout the peripheral and central nervous system to provide analgesia. Potential side effects can include respiratory depression, constipation, nausea and vomiting, urinary retention, and histamine-mediated urticaria and pruritus. However, most patients tolerate opioids well.

A variety of opioid medications are available. Morphine remains commonly used in clinical practice. Hydromorphone is a semisynthetic derivative of morphine that has been associated with less pruritus and nausea than morphine. Elderly patients and those with liver disease often tolerate hydromorphone better than morphine because its metabolites are less active and accumulate slower than the metabolites of morphine. Fentanyl has a short onset and short duration of action and does not produce active metabolites, but requires frequent monitoring because its associated incidence of respiratory depression is higher than other opioids, limiting its use in the observation setting. Oxycodone is an efficiently absorbed oral agent with a bioavailability approaching 80%, and its effectiveness is comparable to parenteral therapy.[16] Hydrocodone is a weaker opioid than oxycodone, and is commonly used in combination preparations with acetaminophen or nonsteroidal anti-inflammatory drugs (NSAIDs). Codeine is a weak opioid that is associated with a high rate of side effects and has little role in the treatment of pain. Tramadol is a weak mu agonist and has some opioid-like properties, but frequently causes nausea and vomiting with increasing doses, limiting its use as a single agent. Table 57.1 lists opioids that are commonly used and provides an equianalgesic factor using morphine 10 mg as a reference value.

Patients who have been referred to an OU for a painful complaint often have pain that has been refractory to initial treatment, or has required frequent dosing that is not amenable to outpatient treatment, therefore, IV administration is often indicated. Once pain has been effectively treated and a patient's symptoms have stabilized, efforts should be made to transition to oral medications so that an effective regimen can be continued as an outpatient.

Multiple non-opioid medications exist and are appropriate for either first-line or adjunctive treatment of pain in combination with opioids. Acetaminophen is a safe and well-tolerated medication in both children and adults. It can cause hepatic toxicity in the setting of underlying liver disease or concomitant alcohol abuse. Patients with pain who do not have a contraindication should receive acetaminophen as part of any pain treatment strategy.

NSAIDs such as ibuprofen inhibit cyclooxygenase, and therefore decrease prostaglandin, resulting in analgesic effects in patients with inflammation. They have a synergistic effect when administered with opioids and acetaminophen and can reduce the amount of opioid needed to treat a painful complaint. Notably, NSAIDs are the cause of more serious drug-related side effects than any other class of analgesic.[18] Side effects include renal failure, gastrointestinal bleeding, platelet dysfunction, and anaphylaxis. NSAIDS should be used cautiously, or not at all, in patients with preexisting renal disease, cardiovascular disease, gastrointestinal disease, or in pregnant or elderly patients.

Pain Specialists and Pain Clinics

A growing number of physicians are specializing in the practice of pain management, which has been accompanied by a growth in pain clinics that specialize in the treatment of pain. Pain specialists often have advanced training in the medical management of acute and chronic pain. Some are trained to perform procedures such as nerve blocks, steroid injections, or radiofrequency procedures. Depending on local resources, the potential exists for patients being cared for in an OU to engage with these providers. Pain specialists may be available to consult on patients in the OU, or patients can be referred to a pain clinic after discharge. Patients thought to potentially benefit from the services of a pain specialist include those with refractory chronic pain, those who have required a large quantity or the prolonged use of opioids, those with an acute exacerbation of chronic pain, patients with chronic pain of malignancy, and people with a chronic or recurrent painful condition who may benefit from a specific procedure or treatment regimen from a pain specialist.[19]

Special Populations

In general, the principles of pain management for adults are also appropriate to use in a pediatric patient. One of the key differences in the management of pain in children is that assessment is more difficult, increasing the risk of under appreciation and inadequate treatment. It is important for the medical provider to notice both verbal and nonverbal cues in children. Pharmacokinetics of analgesic medications are similar in children, except in neonates and infants, for whom opioid clearance is delayed and plasma levels can be high for a given dose of medication.

The treatment of painful complaints in elderly patients is complicated by more difficult assessment due to underlying medical conditions, the increased accumulation of breakdown products of medications, and increased sensitivity to side effects. Doses of opioids should be reduced to avoid side effects such as confusion, which occurs much more readily in the elderly. Lastly, NSAID medications are best avoided or used in decreased doses due to their potential to cause renal dysfunction or adverse cardiac events in this age group.

Specific Conditions

While much of the discussion in this chapter can be applied to a variety of painful conditions that are treated in the OU, there are several conditions and scenarios that deserve special mention.

Acute Low Back Pain

Back pain is a common symptom that represents a considerable source of lost productivity for workers and a large amount of health care expenditures.[20] Though the vast majority of patients presenting for an evaluation of acute back pain will be ultimately diagnosed with mechanical or nonspecific back pain, several emergent diagnoses must be excluded during the evaluation of this complaint.

While the majority of patients with acute low back pain can be managed as an outpatient, observation may be considered in certain circumstances. For example, if physicians are not able to achieve adequate pain control for a patient with back pain in the emergency department, administration of analgesics can be continued in the observation setting until the pain is controlled sufficiently to permit discharge home. If a neurologic deficit is present and raises concern for serious underlying pathology, a patient could be observed for serial neurologic assessments to assess the progression of the disease and determine the need for additional diagnostic evaluation.

For most patients referred to the OU with low back pain, a careful history and physical examination is sufficient to evaluate their disease state. Plain radiographs have not been found to be useful in the evaluation of uncomplicated back pain of 1–2 months duration.[21] Special attention should be paid to the neurologic and musculoskeletal examination.

Emergent diagnoses that should be considered include abdominal aortic aneurysm, aortic dissection, cauda equina syndrome, epidural abscess or hematoma, spine fracture with cord or nerve root compression, meningitis, osteomyelitis, and tumor. If any of these diagnoses are considered, they should be evaluated for appropriately. Patients who have been determined to have a serious and progressive cause of their back pain should typically be treated in an inpatient setting rather than observation. For patients with a significant or progressive neurologic deficit, advanced imaging is often indicated, while noting that advanced imaging for patients with radicular pain and only sensory deficits does not typically change outcome and an initial course of conservative treatment is recommended.[21,22]

Medical treatment of acute low back pain should include analgesic medications. Either acetaminophen or NSAIDs should be prescribed for all patients, unless a contraindication exists. For moderate to severe pain, opioids can be considered in addition. Muscle relaxants such as benzodiazepines and cyclobenzaprine may benefit some patients demonstrating muscle spasm on examination, but also can cause serious side effects and should be used with caution.[23] Patients should be encouraged to be as active as their level of pain permits, and should be discouraged from sitting or lying down for prolonged periods of time.

Chronic Pain

The evaluation and treatment of patients with chronic pain is challenging. Patients with chronic pain are considered to be those with a pain complaint that has persisted beyond the normal healing of the underlying condition or is not expected to improve with further treatment of the underlying condition. Patients with chronic pain can present with an acute exacerbation of chronic pain, or with untreated/refractory chronic pain. In general, an acute exacerbation of chronic pain can be managed in an OU. There, the patient's pain can be stabilized and their previous treatment plan can be resumed. However, inadequately treated chronic pain should be referred to a primary care provider to develop an outpatient care plan. Because patients with chronic pain can exhibit complex maladaptive behaviors associated with their pain, it can be difficult to develop an effective approach to their pain. For OUs with protocol-based treatment plans, this level of decision making is often too complex for what can be effectively accomplished. Making changes in patients' chronic pain treatment strategies during an acute exacerbation of pain and over the relatively short period of observation is unlikely to provide an effective long-term solution.

Chronic Pain of Malignancy

Chronic pain of malignancy differs from other causes of chronic pain in that it is managed with an approach similar to that used for acute pain. Opioid pain medications are often indicated and associated with improved outcomes and quality of life, in contrast to their use in nonmalignant chronic pain. Patients are commonly prescribed a long-acting opioid medication in addition to a short-acting medication for breakthrough pain.[24] In the OU, opioid medications may be titrated to the desired effect prior to discharge. For a patient with chronic pain of malignancy who is experiencing an acute exacerbation of pain, care must be taken to evaluate appropriately for a new medical condition causing the pain, and to not assume that the pain is secondary to the underlying oncologic process.

Criteria for Observation

Careful consideration must be given to which patients with painful complaints are appropriate for observation. Generally, patients with musculoskeletal pain that may be appropriate for observation are those with 1) an underlying cause of the pain for which inpatient care is not appropriate, and 2) who require multiple doses of IV analgesics without adequate pain relief. Conditions that may require surgery such as a fracture and patients with pain secondary to significant medical illness such as cancer are likely to be most appropriate in an inpatient setting rather than an OU. On the other hand, patients with acute musculoskeletal pain responding to oral analgesics are not likely to be considered appropriate for observation services and could be treated as outpatients. Patients with painful complaints who are unable to ambulate or adequately care for themselves secondary to pain may also be good candidates for observation, as they cannot be safely discharged home.

InterQual® criteria are a commonly used set of criteria to determine the appropriateness of a specific level of care. Though InterQual® or another resource can provide a common foundation for institutions to determine which patients should be referred to observation services, local capabilities, expertise, and resources ultimately require individual OUs to formulate their own criteria.

One of the first steps in determining the appropriate level of care for a patient is to consider whether a specific subset of criteria should be applied. For patients with chest pain of a suspected cardiac etiology, for example, the cardiac criteria should be reviewed. If no other set of criteria seems appropriate, then the following criteria under the "Pain, severe" section may be useful.

To meet InterQual® Severity of Illness criteria for referral to observation services for severe pain, at least one of the following Severity of Illness (SI) criteria should be met.[25]

- Intractable and unresponsive to ≥ 2 doses of parenteral analgesics within the last 6 hours
- Renal calculus or pyelonephritis, suspected
- Migraine, intractable and failed outpatient treatment

- Abdominal pain, unknown etiology
- Sickle cell crisis

For discussion of abdominal pain, headache, renal disease, and sickle cell crisis, please see the appropriate sections elsewhere in this text. (See Chapters 35, 42, 48, 56.) Patients must also meet at least one criteria from the Intensity of Service (IS) section to satisfy InterQual® criteria for observation services. Listed next are common criteria by which patients admitted with painful complaints meet criteria for observation services.

- IV fluids ≥100 ml/hr **or** IV fluids ≥75 ml/hr and age ≥65 or history of chronic heart failure or renal failure
- At least two doses of IV analgesics **or** IV antiemetics **or** IV anxiolytics
- Monitoring of neurologic examination at least six times over 24 hours
- Monitoring of vital signs every 4 hours

Consideration should also be given as to whether patients are most appropriate for an inpatient level of care, as opposed to observation. The CMS Two-Midnight Rule was implemented in 2014 and has provided some guidance in this area. In brief, if it is expected at the time of admission that the patient's length of stay will be at least two midnights or they have another qualifying condition, they should be admitted as an inpatient in most circumstances. In summary, most patients with acute musculoskeletal pain will be deemed appropriate for observation services based on the frequency and route of analgesic medication administration. It is important to note that hospitals are not strictly bound to these criteria, and that by physician review, a patient can be deemed appropriate for observation services even if these criteria are not precisely met. An example of this could be a patient with severe back pain, who is not able to ambulate due to pain, but is not requiring multiple doses of IV analgesic pain medication.

Recommendations for Observation Unit Protocols

While protocols used in OUs must take in to consideration local resources and practice patterns, we have several recommendations regarding the evaluation and treatment of pain in OUs.

- All OU protocols or standing orders should include a mechanism to assess pain at regular intervals. The assessment of pain should be performed at least every 4 hours, and often more frequent assessment is indicated.
- Assessment of pain should be performed using age and developmentally appropriate tools. This can be addressed by having different protocols for the treatment of pain for different age groups.
- The determination of severity of pain should not rely solely on a numeric rating, and should instead take in to account verbal communication with the patient, nonverbal cues, and objective signs as deemed appropriate.
- Orders for appropriate pain medications to be given as needed (prn) should be placed. Only one type of opioid per route of administration should be ordered as a prn medication.
- Patients receiving opioid medications should also receive acetaminophen and NSAIDS if they are not contraindicated.
- The choice of pain medications should be individualized for each patient, therefore, protocols should require medical providers to actively choose which analgesic medications to use in the OU. Contraindications to certain medications, dosing adjustments, the underlying disease process, and multiple other factors must be considered.
- Pulse oximetry monitoring should be considered in patients receiving IV opioids.
- A complete history and physical examination should be performed for all patients referred for observation services, focusing on evaluating for emergent and life-threatening causes of pain.
- Plain radiography and advanced imaging should not be routinely ordered for patients in OUs with uncomplicated back pain, as this information rarely changes care.

Conclusions

The treatment of pain and painful complaints in the OU is dependent on appropriate assessment, frequent reassessment, recognition of any underlying medical conditions, and individualized treatment. Care should be taken that patients referred for observation meet criteria, which are often dependent on the frequency at which intravenous analgesic medications are administered. OU protocols should include provisions for the regular assessment of pain.

References

1. Mace SE, Graff L, Mikhail M, et al. A national survey of observation units in the United States. *The American Journal of Emergency Medicine.* 2003 Nov.;21(7):529–533.

2. Ross M. The use and effectiveness of an emergency department observation unit for elderly patients. *Annals of Emergency Medicine.* 2003 May;41(5):668–677.

3. Fosnocht DE, Swanson ER, Bossart P. Patient expectations for pain medication delivery. *American Journal of Emergency Medicine.* 2001 Sep.;19(5): 399–402.

4. Bayer BM, Brehio RM, Ding XZ, et al. Enhanced susceptibility of the immune system to stress in morphine-tolerant rats. *Brain Behav. Immun.* 1994 Sep.;8(3): 173–184.

5. Beilin B, Shavit Y, Trabekin E, et al. The effects of postoperative pain management on immune response to surgery. *Anesth Analg.* 2003 Sep.;97(3): 822–827.

6. Charmandari E, Kino T, Souvatzoglou E, et al. Pediatric stress: hormonal mediators and human development. *Horm. Res.* 2003;59(4):161–179.

7. Bijur PE, Bérard A, Esses D, et al. Lack of influence of patient self-report of pain intensity on administration of opioids for suspected long-bone fractures. *J Pain.* 2006 Jun.;7(6):438–444.

8. Miner J, Biros MH, Trainor A, et al. Patient and physician perceptions as risk factors for oligoanalgesia: a prospective observational study of the relief of pain in the emergency department. *Acad Emerg Med.* 2006 Feb.;13(2):140–146.

9. Marco CA, Plewa MC, Buderer N, et al. Self-reported pain scores in the emergency department: lack of association with vital signs. *Acad Emerg Med.* 2006 Sep.;13(9):974–979.

10. Bossart P, Fosnocht D. Changes in heart rate do not correlate with changes in pain intensity in emergency department patients. *J Emerg Med.* 2007.

11. Hobbs G. *Assessment, Measurement, History and Examination. Clinical Pain Management: Acute Pain.* London: Arnold; 2003.

12. Todd K, Ducharme J, Choiniere M. Pain in the emergency department: results of the pain and emergency medicine initiative (PEMI) multicenter study. *The Journal of Pain.* 2007.

13. Neighbor ML, Honner S, Kohn MA. Factors affecting emergency department opioid administration to severely injured patients. *Acad Emerg Med.* 2004 Dec.;11(12): 1290–1296.

14. Tamayo-Sarver JH, Hinze SW, Cydulka RK, et al. Racial and ethnic disparities in emergency department analgesic prescription. *Am J Public Health.* 2003 Dec.;93(12): 2067–2073.

15. Todd KH, Samaroo N, Hoffman JR. Ethnicity as a risk factor for inadequate emergency department analgesia. *JAMA.* 1993 Feb.;269 (12):1537–1539.

16. Miner JR, Moore J, Gray RO, et al. Oral versus intravenous opioid dosing for the initial treatment of acute musculoskeletal pain in the emergency department. *Acad Emerg Med.* 2008 Dec.;15 (12):1234–1240.

17. Miner JR, Paris PM, Yealy DM. Chapter 186: Pain Management. In: Marx J, Hockberger R, Walls RM, eds. *Rosen's Emergency Medicine-Concepts and Clinical Practice, 7th Ed.* Philadelphia, PA: Mosby. 2010; 2410–2428.

18. Hersh EV, Pinto A, Moore PA. Adverse drug interactions involving common prescription and over-the-counter analgesic agents. *Clin Ther.* 2007;29 Suppl:2477–2497.

19. Ksionski S. Personal Communication. 2012.

20. Stewart WF, Ricci JA, Chee E, et al. Lost productive time and cost due to common pain conditions in the US workforce. *JAMA.* 2003 Nov. 12;290(18):2443–2454.

21. Chou R, Qaseem A, Snow V, et al. Diagnosis and treatment of low back pain: a joint clinical practice guideline from the American College of Physicians and the American Pain Society. *Ann Intern Med.* 2007. 478–491.

22. Modic MT, Obuchowski NA, Ross JS, et al. Acute low back pain and radiculopathy: MR imaging findings and their prognostic role and effect on outcome. *Radiology.* 2005 Nov.;237(2):597–604.

23. Van Tulder M, Touray T, Furlan A. Muscle relaxants for non-specific low back pain. . . . *Database Syst Rev.* 2003.

24. Fosnocht DE, Swanson ER, Barton ED. Changing attitudes about pain and pain control in emergency medicine. *Emerg Med Clin North Am.* 2005 May;23(2):297–306.

25. InterQual®. *Level of Care Criteria, Acute Care, Adult.* 2011th ed. Newton, MA: McKesson Health Solutions, LLC.

Chapter 58

Trauma

Mark G. Moseley, MD, MHA, FACEP
Miles P. Hawley, MD, MBA

Background

Given the high volume of patients with traumatic complaints that present to most emergency departments (EDs), this patient population is an excellent potential source of observation unit (OU) patient volume. ED-based OUs have been found to be useful and cost efficient in the management of trauma patients.[1] One of the primary reasons for this fact is that it can be difficult to diagnose all injuries on initial presentation to the ED, and as such, many trauma patients require additional diagnostic tests, repeat examinations, and clinical monitoring. Historically, this has often lead to trauma patients being hospitalized to accomplish these patient management goals and to ensure safe dispositions.[2] With this noted, recent studies have demonstrated the feasibility of managing trauma patients including trauma team activation patients at Level 1 trauma centers (clearly a sicker cohort of trauma patients) in the OU setting with favorable outcomes.[3,4]

Trauma patients in the OU can be considered for both diagnostic and therapeutic end points on an observation protocol. Diagnostically, many blunt trauma patients require extensive imaging evaluation and a period of serial examinations. For penetrating or blunt trauma patients, the observation period can afford an environment closely linked to intensive resources available to reevaluate the patient and quickly intervene if clinical deterioration is observed. Therapeutically, some patients arrive in the OU with a clear diagnosis (such as rib fractures) and the goal of the observation period is merely to determine whether the patients are able to manage their symptoms in the outpatient setting sufficient to facilitate discharge.

To this end, it is important to define the goals of the observation period. Is it to diagnose a potential occult injury? Is it to monitor for a complication like vascular compromise or compartment syndrome? These goals will help define the resources necessary to successfully evaluate and disposition a given patient. This is extremely important in the trauma patient population, as local resources and the trauma status of the hospital the clinician works at may lead to distinctly different patient populations managed. At a high-volume, high-acuity trauma center, the majority of trauma patients in the OU will have already been "cleared" by the trauma team of life-threatening injury. Further, extensive resources would be available to reevaluate and resuscitate the patients should they deteriorate. At a nontrauma hospital without trauma team backup, the goals, management resources, and the ability to disposition specific patient populations may differ greatly and should be considered in trauma protocol design.

Patient Selection – Inclusions

Inclusion criteria will vary based on local resources and the capabilities of the OU and its provider team. As noted earlier, there will be variation in the capabilities based on the facility where the clinician works (trauma center or not). While a general observation protocol for trauma can be a catchall for multiple conditions, specific protocols for specific conditions may be considered separately and have distinct criteria. For higher-volume protocols of this subset such as closed head injury, this is prudent since the needs of these patients will differ from patients with more extensive blunt or penetrating trauma. Whether to include pediatric patients, and the age that defines a pediatric patient, will also be an important consideration based on institution and provider preferences. One other important consideration for patient placement is the comfort level of the providers with managing trauma patients. Physicians that are routinely managing trauma patients should be board certified in emergency medicine, trauma surgery, or other appropriate surgical specialty with trauma experience or well versed in Advanced Trauma Life Support (ATLS) or its equivalent. Nurses routinely caring for trauma patients should be certified emergency nurses or well versed in a nursing equivalent of ATLS. This should ensure appropriate knowledge, aptitude, and skill sets in managing trauma patients.

Patient Selection – Exclusions

In the trauma patient population, intoxication and altered mental status are clearly a challenge for appropriate patient selection.[5] Some units and protocols have specific blood alcohol cutoffs, while others prefer to select based upon the perception of clinical sobriety or patients who are directable and compliant with therapy rather than a specific number on the patient's blood alcohol level (BAL). Care should be taken to ensure that violent, belligerent, and nonparticipatory patients with intoxicants on board are not placed in the OU. Setting a Glasgow Coma Scale (GCS) of <14 as an exclusion criteria can assist to this end and also appropriately risk stratify for mild head injury patients. Other exclusion criteria would include hemodynamically unstable patients, patients receiving blood products or aggressive fluid resuscitation, major burn patients, or patients who inevitably need surgical management. Any patient that meets criteria for a transfer to a higher-level trauma center based on ATLS should be excluded at a nontrauma facility.

Pathophysiology

Numerous traumatic conditions are amenable to observation protocols in the OU. As noted earlier, local resources will dictate which protocol populations can be targeted and created based on the demographics and capabilities of the facility where the OU is located. What follows is a listing of some commonly managed traumatic conditions.

Motor Vehicle Collisions

Blunt trauma can be challenging both diagnostically and therapeutically. Occult injuries can be difficult to uncover after initial ED evaluation. As such, patients with blunt trauma from motor vehicle collisions (MVC) are an excellent population to target

for an OU protocol. Benefits of the observation period include the ability to do serial examinations, obtain final readings on imaging studies (which can be significant in this population), monitor the patient's ability to control his or her symptoms, and discharge the patient with a lower risk for significant injury misses.[6,7]

Issues in management for this patient population can include dealing with cervical spine clearance, such as a protocol for who clears the patient's c-spine, when it is important or necessary to establish c-spine clearance, and the criteria for c-spine clearance in significantly injured MVC patients. The occurrence of closed head injury (or concerns sufficient to warrant observation for same) in the MVC population provides adequate justification in most instances to observe a patient and obtain frequent neurologic checks (particularly if imaging is withheld in favor of clinical monitoring).

Patients experiencing more significant blunt trauma from MVC often benefit from serial examinations even if imaging is negative. Repeat Focused Assessment by Sonography for Trauma (FAST) examinations are also recommended.[6,7] Pain and symptom control, intravenous (IV) fluids, and the ability to ambulate and tolerate oral intake are important for disposition considerations in this patient population.

Rib Fractures

Patients with isolated or in some cases even multiple rib fractures are candidates for a trauma protocol with therapeutic end points. Safety, efficacy, and cost-effectiveness of managing these patients has been previously studied.[6,7,8] The goals of the observation period are primarily to determine if the patient can tolerate his or her pain and symptoms assuming life-threatening traumatic injury has been excluded. The focus of the observation period can be therapeutic in terms of providing analgesia and relief from pain as well as a focus on pulmonary toilet. A subset of patients with thoracic trauma has a concern for cardiac or myocardial contusion. In this patient population, cardiac monitoring, serial cardiac enzymes, and even echocardiography are sometimes considered in patient management and disposition decisions and can clearly be accomplished in the OU setting (although the precise workup diagnostically for these patients is still controversial).

Patients with multiple rib fractures and concern for sternal fractures often will need contrast enhanced CT scan to make certain underlying pulmonary or vascular injuries are not present.[6,7] Patients with nondisplaced sternal fractures can be considered for trauma protocol placement, but in most instances, retrosternal hematoma and more significant sternal fractures are not amenable to discharge within 24 hours. Age, medical comorbidities, functional status prior to injury, ability to ambulate, ability to tolerate oral pain medications, and location and number of fractures are all important considerations for disposition decisions in this patient population.

Head Injury

Clinical observation of the head injured patients is one of the most frequently managed patients on a trauma protocol in the OU. This approach has been found to be safe and effective and can reduce inappropriate inpatient admission in this patient population.[9,10] Many such patients have concomitant intoxicants on board that render the observation period invaluable in clinically observing patients to determine if their mental status is appropriate for discharge (determination often not feasible directly from the ED).

The challenge with this patient population is defining (prior to OU placement) the patient's true GCS and making certain more significantly head injured patients are not placed in this care setting. Patients with mild head injuries can also be observed with the benefit of not having to perform a head CT (important for radiation stewardship particularly in younger patients).[9] More advanced OUs with neurosurgical backup have experience managing patients with isolated, mild head trauma on coumadin and other blood thinners. Such patients represent a high-risk cohort of patients to discharge directly from the ED. As long as these patients do not have evidence of significant intra-cranial pathology on initial imaging, monitoring the clinical status in the OU is often appropriate.

Penetrating Trauma

Select patients with penetrating trauma can be successfully managed in the OU. Patient selection is very important with this patient population as certain conditions are inappropriate for the level of care offered in the ED OU and would be more appropriately offered (due to the critical nature and rapid deterioration) in the ICU setting. Patients can have neurovascular checks and be watched for compartment syndrome. Patients with superficial wounds to the thorax and abdomen are appropriate for OU placement and have a low incidence of poor outcome even after brief observation.[11,12] At nontrauma hospitals, most penetrating injuries to the thorax and abdomen will require transfer for initial evaluation by a trauma team prior to OU placement. In general, patients with penetrating neck trauma should not be placed in the OU setting unless cleared by a trauma team at a trauma facility with expertise in managing this patient population in the OU setting.

Isolated extremity penetrating wounds are well managed in most cases in the OU as a high proportion of these patients can be safely monitored and then discharged. Extremity trauma with signs of vascular compromise, compartment syndrome, or delayed presentations of injury with infection should be excluded and require more extensive resources in the inpatient setting.

Mechanical Falls

Patients with significant blunt trauma from mechanical falls can be managed successfully in the OU. Patients with extremity fractures can be included in this patient cohort, but operative fractures like hip fractures and femur fractures should not be placed in the OU. A mechanical fall protocol or accepting fall patients on a general observation protocol for trauma can be particularly beneficial with elderly patients. If such patients have gait instability and risk for further falls, then resources such as physical therapy need to be available for the clinician managing the patient in the OU. Often such patients require additional resources such as case management, social work, and even pharmacists to aid in management and safe disposition. Occult fractures and underlying medical comorbidities can prevent discharge in some cases as can the patient's social situation, living environment, and support system (or lack thereof). (See also geriatric Chapter 55.)

Management/Intervention

Frequent vital signs are the mainstay of observation for the injured trauma patient. Frequent neurologic checks should take place for intoxicated or head injured patients. Specific therapeutic interventions like pain and antiemetic medications, IV fluids, and other needs will be patient and protocol specific. Frequency of vital signs should be consistent with nursing resources and patient acuity. Vascular checks in higher risk patients looking for vascular compromise and compartment syndrome should be delineated. Patients should be transitioned from IV therapies to oral therapies as one data point to determine suitability for discharge and to see if continued outpatient management is appropriate. At trauma facilities it is important to delineate who will be doing repeat examinations, whether the OU providers or members of the trauma team. Cervical spine clearance, if not done initially prior to OU placement, should also be protocolized and consistent with national guidelines. Many trauma patients will need social services support to facilitate follow-up, medication assistance, and even drug and alcohol counseling. As such, social worker coverage for the OU is essential when managing trauma patients. Resources such as physical therapy will depend on the type of patient managed, but can be invaluable in providing information about ongoing fall risk for elderly patients.

Disposition after Observation

A significant majority of trauma patients can be discharged from the OU after an appropriate period of observation.[3,4] All such patients should have stable vital signs, have normal GCS, be clinically sober, be able to ambulate, and be able to tolerate oral intake. The ability to ambulate and tolerate symptoms with oral medications is critical to ensure that such patients do not bounce back to the ED in short order. Imaging studies (which can be significant for this population) should be finalized by radiology and available to the clinician prior to disposition so radiographic abnormalities can be addressed. The patient should have a documented disposition examination; such an examination should be comprehensive from head to toe and include observation of the patient ambulating. Follow-up should be time and action specific related to reevaluation needs and specific for the condition affecting the patient.

For more significantly injured patients, prompt reevaluation is important. This can be a challenge for patients without a primary care physician. Unfortunately in this trauma patient population (younger, more socioeconomically troubled), many will not have access to health care, will be uninsured or underinsured, and will be poorly resourced. As such, bringing the patient back to the ED for wound checks or injury checks in 48–72 hours is a consideration if outpatient follow-up can not be obtained in a timely fashion. Patients are generally discharged with symptom control medications for several days, particularly for blunt trauma patients for whom musculoskeletal soft tissue injury can lead to prolonged pain and symptoms.

Summary

Trauma patients are clearly a very viable patient population to consider for the OU. As with all clinical conditions managed in the OU, careful patient selection is paramount to ensure successful discharge in the majority of managed patients. Clear exclusion criteria should be set to ensure that critically injured patients are not placed in the OU setting. More so than most clinical patient populations managed in the OU, local resources need to be carefully considered to ensure adequate backup is available, particularly at nontrauma hospitals.

References

1. Conrad L, Markovchick V, Mitchiner J, et al. The role of an emergency department observation unit in the management of trauma patients. *J Emerg Med* 1985; 2(5): 325–333.

2. Cowell VL, Ciraula D, Gabram S, et al. Trauma 24-hour observation critical path. *J Trauma* 1998; 45(1): 147–150.

3. Madsen TE, Bledsoe JR, Bossart PJ. Observation unit admission as an alternative to inpatient admission for trauma activation patients. *Emerg Med J* 2009; 26(6): 421–423.

4. Holly J, Bledsoe J, Black K, et al. Prospective evaluation of an ED observation unit protocol for trauma activation patients. *Am J Emerg Med* 2012; 30(8): 1402–1406.

5. Rivara FP, Jurkovich GJ, Gurney JG, et al. The magnitude of acute and chronic alcohol abuse in trauma patients. *Arch Surg* 1993. Aug; 128(8): 907–912.

6. Kendall JL, Kestler AM, Whitaker KT, et al. Blunt abdominal trauma patients are at very low risk for intra-abdominal injury after emergency department

observation. *West J Emerg Med* 2011. Nov; 12 (4): 496–504.

7. Menditto VG, Gabrielli B, Marcosignori M, et al. A management of blunt thoracic trauma in an emergency department observation unit: pre-post observation study. *J Trauma* 2012. Jan; 72(1): 222–228.

8. Ammons MA, Moore EE, Rosen P. Role of the observation unit in the management of thoracic trauma. *J Emerg Med* 1986; 4 (4): 279–282.

9. Holsti M, Kadish HA, Sill BL, et al. Pediatric closed head injuries treated in an observation unit. *Pediatr Emerg Care* 2005. Oct;21(10): 649–644.

10. MacLaren RE, Ghoorahoo HI, Kirby NG. Use of an accident and emergency department observation ward in management of head injury. *Br J Surg* 1993. Feb; 80(2): 215–217.

11. Leppaniemi AK, Voutilainen PE, Haapiainen RK. Indications for early mandatory laparotomy in abdominal stab wounds. *Br J Surg* 1999. Jan; 86(1): 76–80.

12. Ordog GJ, Wasserberger J, Balasubramanium S, et al. Asymptomatic stab wounds of the chest. *J Trauma* 1994. 36 (5): 680–684.

Chapter

59

Toxicology

Steven J. Walsh, MD
Marsha Ford, MD, FACEP

Toxicologic disorders account for over 4 million U.S. emergency department (ED) visits annually.[1] Many patients are discharged to home or to a psychiatric facility after ED evaluation. However, a significant number of poisoned individuals require admission for further observation and management. A large number of these patients do not require an extended hospital stay, making admission to the observation unit (OU) a reasonable disposition option.

The OU should be well-equipped to provide care for the poisoned patient. Continuous cardiopulmonary monitoring, expeditious diagnostic testing (electrocardiography, radiography, laboratory analysis, etc.), a variety of commonly used medications/antidotes (including but not limited to dextrose, antiemetics, analgesics, benzodiazepines, naloxone), a low nurse-to-patient ratio (most OUs have a 1:5 or 1:4 nurse patient ratio), and one-to-one sitters for patient safety/psychiatric observation (if needed) should be available at all times. Any items that could be used for self-harm by suicidal individuals should be placed in a secure location, and all patients should be searched for such prior to admission to the OU. Providers caring for these patients should be familiar with common toxicities and toxidromes (such as opiate/opioid, benzodiazepine, sympathomimetic, and anticholinergic), as well as the dosing, administration, and adverse effects of the aforementioned commonly used medications. All staff should be aware of the Poison Help Hotline (800-222-1222 in the United States), which provides around-the-clock, free, confidential, and expert advice regarding poisoned patients.

A variety of poisonings are appropriate for OU care. In general, toxicologic admissions to the OU should include those patients whose anticipated stay is less than 24 hours and who have normal or near-normal vital signs. Somnolent but arousable patients are appropriate for observation care, as are those with mild central nervous system (CNS) hyperexcitation (hyperreflexia/clonus, mild altered mental status/agitation controlled with benzodiazepines).

Not all poisoned patients are appropriate for observation-type admissions, however. Individuals who will likely require more than 23 hours of observation/management should be admitted to an inpatient service. Those with significant tachycardia (heart rate [HR] > 110/minute) after appropriate toxicologic treatment, severe delirium, agitation and/or psychosis that cannot be controlled with benzodiazepines, significant laboratory and/or EKG derangements (e.g., QRS duration > 120 milliseconds [ms], QTc interval > 500 ms), a high likelihood of clinical deterioration, and patients requiring ICU care should not be admitted to the OU.

While impossible to discuss each and every poisoning that is/is not appropriate for observation admission, some specific toxicities that lend themselves to observation-type care are listed as follows.

Substance: Acetaminophen (APAP)

Observation Admission Criteria:

- Single, acute APAP ingestion (defined as ingestion of the entire amount of APAP within 8 hours[2]) presenting within 24 hours requiring treatment based upon Rumack-Matthew nomogram[3]
- Patients receiving the oral (PO)/intravenous (IV) bolus dose of N-acetylcysteine (NAC) within 8 hours of acute ingestion[3,4]
- Nausea/vomiting/abdominal pain controlled with PO/IV antiemetics/non-APAP analgesics
- Lack of concomitant toxic ingestion that would likely preclude disposition within 24 hours (i.e., salicylate toxicity requiring

bicarbonate infusion, long-acting opiate/opioid toxicity requiring naloxone infusion)

Contraindications to Observation Admission:

- Ingestions other than single acute ingestions[3,5]
- Individuals receiving the bolus dose of NAC greater than 8 hours after acute ingestion[3]
- Patients with baseline hepatic dysfunction (elevated aspartate aminotransferase [AST]/alanine amino transferase [ALT]/international normalized ratio [INR] secondary to alcoholic liver disease, infectious hepatitis, or other underlying pathology)
- Elevated transaminases (AST and/or ALT greater than the upper limit of laboratory reference ranges)
- Coagulopathy (INR greater than the upper limit of laboratory reference range)
- Renal insufficiency (creatinine greater than the upper limit of laboratory reference range, oliguria/anuria)
- Altered mental status
- Gravid patient
- Presence of concomitant toxicity that would likely prevent disposition within 24 hours (i.e., long-acting opiate/opioid toxicity requiring naloxone infusion, salicylate toxicity requiring bicarbonate infusion)
- Provider judgment

Observation Management:

- IV or PO (NAC) per individual facility's protocol[3,4]
- Antiemetics as needed (PRN)
- Psychiatric consultation PRN

Discharge Criteria:

- Patient is clinically well after NAC course (resolution of abdominal pain, no nausea/emesis, normal mentation)[3,4]
- Undetectable [APAP] after NAC course[3,4]
- Normal AST/ALT after NAC course[3,4]

Comments:

- NAC protocols vary between facilities/regions; consult your regional poison center

(800-222-1222 in the United States) for treatment recommendations
- Patients may require extension of NAC course if evidence of liver injury develops (elevated AST/ALT, INR greater than 1.4, etc.; consult your regional poison center for treatment recommendations)[3]

Substance: Benzodiazepines
Observation Admission Criteria:

- Confirmed/suspected symptomatic ingestion (adult or child) after a 6-hour-or-less ED observation period
  - Somnolence/stupor
  - Slurred speech
  - Ataxia

Contraindications to Observation Admission:

- Hypoxia refractory to supplemental oxygen delivered via nasal cannula
- Significant rhabdomyolysis (pressure ulcers/blisters/bullae, creatine phosphokinase [CPK] greater than eight times upper limit of laboratory reference range, myoglobinuria) or compartment syndrome (elevated compartment pressures)
- Clinically significant aspiration pneumonitis (fever, tachypnea, hypoxia, cough productive of sputum, infiltrate on chest radiograph)
- Presence of concomitant toxic ingestion that would likely prevent disposition within 24 hours
- Provider judgment

Observation Management:

- Continuous cardiopulmonary monitoring
- Prevention of respiratory compromise/aspiration (head-of-bed elevation, supplemental oxygen administration)
- Psychiatric consultation PRN

Discharge Criteria:

- Normal mentation
- Fluent (nonslurred) speech
- Ambulatory with a steady gait
- Normal pulse oximetry/respiratory rate

Comments:

- Use caution when considering pharmacologic reversal with flumazenil (may precipitate acute withdrawal, including seizures, in patients with chronic use/abuse of gamma-aminobutyric acid [GABA] agonists [e.g., benzodiazepines])[6]
- Many benzodiazepines are not detected by rapid bedside drugs of abuse screens (high false negative rate)[7]
- Consider aspiration pneumonitis and rhabdomyolysis/compartment syndrome in patients found unresponsive or with altered mental status

Substance: Bupropion

Observation Admission Criteria:

- Any confirmed/suspected symptomatic ingestion responsive to benzodiazepines
  - Mild CNS hyperexcitation (altered mental status, mild agitation, hyperreflexia, clonus)
  - Tachycardia/hypertension
- Confirmed/suspected asymptomatic ingestion of:
  - $\geq$ 10 mg/kg in children
  - $\geq$ 900 mg in adults

Contraindications to Observation Admission:

- Mild CNS hyperexcitation unresponsive to benzodiazepines
- Seizure activity
- QRS interval > 120 ms
- Presence of concomitant toxic ingestion that would likely prevent disposition within 24 hours
- Provider judgment

Observation Management:

- 18- to 24-hour period of observation
- Continuous cardiopulmonary monitoring
- Prevention of respiratory compromise/aspiration
- Benzodiazepines PRN agitation
- Psychiatric consultation PRN

Discharge Criteria:

- Normal mentation/vital signs
- Absence of seizure activity during observation period
- QRS < 120 ms

Comments:

- Many ingestions seize late (hours 15–18)[8,9,10]; 18-hour period of observation is adequate if patient has remained asymptomatic to that point
- All patients who seize should be admitted to the hospital (rather than the OU)
- Consider aspiration pneumonitis in patients found with altered mental status and those who seize

Substance: Sulfonylureas

Observation Admission Criteria:

- Confirmed/suspected symptomatic ingestion (adult or child)[11,12,13]
  - Signs/symptoms of hypoglycemia
    - Altered mental status/confusion/somnolence, generalized weakness, tremor, diaphoresis, piloerection, nausea, etc.
    - Documented hypoglycemia (blood glucose less than lower limit of laboratory reference range)
- Confirmed/suspected asymptomatic ingestion (adult or child)[11,12,13]

Contraindications to Observation Admission:

- Multiple hypoglycemic episodes prehospital and/or in ED
- Signs/symptoms of severe hypoglycemia
  - Hypothermia, focal neurologic deficit, seizure, coma
- Hypoglycemia refractory to dextrose 5% in water (D5W) administration
- Presence of concomitant toxic ingestion that would likely prevent disposition within 24 hours
- Provider judgment

Observation Management:

- Correct hypoglycemia with IV dextrose PRN
  - Empiric dextrose is not indicated in the absence of suspected/documented hypoglycemia (wait until patient becomes symptomatic/hypoglycemic)
- Check blood glucose every 2 hours while awake and every hour while asleep
- Meals/activity as tolerated
- Psychiatric consultation PRN

Discharge Criteria:

- Normal vital signs/blood glucose
- No clinical evidence of hypoglycemia
  - Normal mentation, steady gait, lack of piloerection/diaphoresis, etc.
- No hypoglycemic episodes during a 24-hour observation period
  - Each time the patient requires dextrose, the "clock is reset" and an additional 24-hour observation period is required from time of dextrose administration

Comments:

- After second episode of hypoglycemia requiring dextrose administration, admit for further evaluation/treatment with dextrose/octreotide[11–15]

Substance: Carbon Monoxide (CO)

Observation Admission Criteria:

- Non-gravid patients exposed to CO who may benefit from hyperbaric oxygen (HBO) therapy
  - Syncope/loss of consciousness
  - Altered mental status/confusion
  - Abnormal neurologic (particularly cerebellar) examination
  - Initial carboxyhemoglobin > 25%
  - No evidence of significant end-organ damage
    - Normal EKG
    - Normal troponin
    - No renal insufficiency

Contraindications to Observation Admission:

- Evidence of end-organ damage
  - Persistently abnormal neurologic (particularly cerebellar) examination
    - CT evidence of cerebral ischemia/hemorrhage
    - Abnormal EKG
    - Elevated troponin
    - Renal insufficiency
- Significant rhabdomyolysis and/or compartment syndrome
- Clinically significant aspiration pneumonitis
- Gravid patient
- Presence of concomitant toxic ingestion that would likely prevent disposition within 24 hours
- Provider judgment

Observation Management:

- Continuous cardiopulmonary monitoring
- 100% oxygen administration
- Hyperbaric oxygen (HBO) as indicated
- Symptomatic care (nasal decongestants, etc.) between HBO treatments
- Psychiatric consultation PRN

Discharge Criteria:

- Completion of facility's HBO regimen
- Normal neurologic/cerebellar examination

Comments:

- Consider aspiration pneumonitis and/or rhabdomyolysis/compartment syndrome in patients found unresponsive or with altered mental status
- Indications for HBO are somewhat controversial[16–18]; consult your regional poison center (800-222-1222 in the United States) for recommendations
- Hyperoxygenation therapy is not without risk (fire in the HBO chamber, seizure, hollow organ rupture, pulmonary/middle ear barotrauma, etc.)

Substance: Opiates/opioids

Observation Admission Criteria:

- Confirmed/suspected symptomatic ingestion (adult or child) after 6-hour-or-less ED observation period
  - Somnolence/stupor
  - Slurred speech
  - Ataxia

Contraindications to Observation Admission:

- Hypoxia refractory to supplemental oxygen delivered via nasal cannula
- Significant rhabdomyolysis and/or compartment syndrome
- Clinically significant aspiration pneumonitis
- Signs/symptoms requiring continuous naloxone infusion
- Patients with QTc interval > 500 ms[19]
- Presence of concomitant toxic ingestion that would likely prevent disposition within 24 hours
- Provider judgment

Observation Management:

- Continuous cardiopulmonary monitoring
- Prevention of respiratory compromise/aspiration
- Psychiatric consultation PRN

Discharge Criteria:

- Normal mentation
- Fluent speech
- Ambulatory with a steady gait
- Normal pulse oximetry/respiratory rate

Comments:

- Consider aspiration pneumonitis and rhabdomyolysis/compartment syndrome in patients found unresponsive or with altered mental status
- Use naloxone for bradypnea/hypopnea/hypoxia, not for somnolence
  - Use naloxone with caution in patients with suspected or confirmed tramadol and/or propoxyphene toxicity (may precipitate seizure)
- If patient requires more than two doses of naloxone, begin continuous infusion/admit for further evaluation/management

Substance: Neuroleptics

Observation Admission Criteria:

- Confirmed/suspected symptomatic ingestion (adult or child) after 6-hour-or-less ED observation period

- Altered mental status (somnolence/stupor, agitation/confusion)
- Slurred speech
- Ataxia
- Hyperreflexia/clonus

Contraindications to Observation Admission:

- Tachycardia (HR > 110/min) and/or agitation unresponsive to benzodiazepine administration
- Hypoxia refractory to supplemental oxygen delivered via nasal cannula
- Seizure activity
- Significant rhabdomyolysis and/or compartment syndrome
- Clinically significant aspiration pneumonitis
- Evidence of serotonin syndrome (SS)[20]
  - Fever (core temperature $> 38°$ C)
  - Autonomic instability (tachycardia/bradycardia, hypertension/hypotension)
  - Altered mental status (typically confusion or somnolence/stupor)
  - Tremor/hyperreflexia/clonus and/or hypertonicity (often greater in the lower extremities)
- Evidence of neuroleptic malignant syndrome (NMS)[21,22]
  - Fever
  - Autonomic instability
  - Altered mental status (typically somnolence, confusion, or agitation/hyperactivity)
  - "Lead-pipe" hypertonicity/rigidity
- QRS duration > 120 ms
- QTc interval > 500 ms
- Presence of concomitant toxic ingestion that would likely prevent disposition within 24 hours
- Provider judgment

Observation Management:

- Continuous cardiopulmonary monitoring
- Prevention of respiratory compromise/aspiration
- IV crystalloid hydration
- Benzodiazepines PRN agitation
- Psychiatric consultation PRN

Discharge Criteria:

- Normal mental status
- Fluent speech
- Ambulatory with a steady gait
- QRS duration < 120 ms
- QTc interval < 500 ms
- No signs/symptoms consistent with SS/NMS

Comments:

- Consider aspiration pneumonitis and rhabdomyolysis/compartment syndrome in patients found unresponsive or with altered mental status
- Neuroleptics are a heterogenous group of medications, each with specific toxicities. Contact your regional poison center (800-222-1222 in the United States) for specific recommendations.

Substance: *Latrodectus Mactans* (Black Widow Spider) Envenomation

Observation Admission Criteria:

- Confirmed/suspected symptomatic grade I/II envenomation (defined below) after 6-hour-or-less ED observation/treatment period controlled with PO/IV analgesics and/or benzodiazepines[23]
  - Normal VS
  - Pain at the bite site that may be migratory to the trunk

Contraindications to Observation Admission:

- Grade I/II envenomation requiring continuous infusion of opiates/opioids and/or benzodiazepines
- Grade III envenomation[23,24,25]
  - Autonomic instability, respiratory distress, cardiac ischemia, severe muscle spasm/rigidity, generalized myalgias/diaphoresis, nausea/emesis, headache
- Evidence of superinfection
- Gravid patient

Observation Management:

- PO/IV analgesics/benzodiazepines PRN tachycardia/pain/muscle spasm
- Tetanus prophylaxis

Discharge Criteria:

- Pain/muscle spasm well-controlled with PO analgesics
- No evidence of superinfection

Comments:

- Avoid administration of calcium, dantrolene, and centrally acting "muscle relaxants" (methocarbamol, cyclobenzaprine, metaxalone, etc.)[24,25]
- Consult your regional poison center before administering *Latrodectus* antivenom, which may cause anaphylaxis/anaphylactoid reaction and serum sickness

Substance: Crotalid (Pit Viper) Envenomation

Observation Admission Criteria:

- Progression of swelling halted with elevation in conjunction with antivenom administration (see "Comments" regarding antivenom) and elevation of affected extremity
- Intact neurovascular status
- No evidence of coagulopathy (normal platelet count/PT/INR/fibrinogen)
- Pain controlled with IV/PO analgesics

Observation Admission Contraindications:

- Anaphylaxis to venom/antivenom
- Compartment syndrome (very rare)
- Clinically significant hemorrhage (very rare)
- Pain requiring continuous opiate/opioid infusion

Observation Management:

- Local wound care
- Splinting/elevation/serial circumferential measurements of affected extremity
- Debridement of hemorrhagic blebs PRN
- Tetanus prophylaxis
- IV/PO analgesics PRN
- Antivenom PRN

Discharge Criteria:

- Stable laboratory studies (no worsening thrombocytopenia/hypofibrinogenemia/INR elevation)

- Intact neurovascular status
- Pain controlled with PO analgesics

Comments:

- Consult with your regional poison center prior to antivenom administration; some envenomations may not require antivenom administration; additionally, antivenom can cause anaphylactoid/anaphylactic reactions as well as serum sickness
- Incision and suction of venom and/or ice application to the bite site/affected extremity is not recommended[26–28]

(See also Snakebites Chapters 84 and 85 under Specialized Clinical Protocols)

References

1. Substance Abuse and Mental Health Services Administration, Center for Behavioral Health Statistics and Quality. (July 2, 2012). *The DAWN Report: Highlights of the 2010 Drug Abuse Warning Network (DAWN) Findings on Drug-Related Emergency Department Visits.* Rockville, MD.

2. Dart RC, Erdman AR, Olson KR, et al. Acetaminophen poisoning: an evidence-based consensus guideline for out-of-hospital management. *Clin Toxicol.* 2006;44:1–18.

3. Rumack BH. Acetaminophen hepatotoxicity: the first 35 years. *J Toxicol Clin Toxicol.* 2002;40:3–20.

4. Buckley NA, Whyte IM, O'Connell DL, et al. Oral or intravenous N-acetylcysteine: which is the treatment of choice for acetaminophen (paracetamol) poisoning. *J Toxicol Clin Toxicol.* 1999;37:759–767.

5. Daly FF, O'Malley GF, Heard K, et al. Prospective evaluation of repeated supratherapeutic acetaminophen (paracetamol) ingestion. *Ann Emerg Med.* 2004 Oct;44(4):393–398.

6. Amrein R, Leishman B, Bentzinger C, et al. Flumazenil in benzodiazepine antagonism: actions and clinical use in intoxications and anaesthesiology. *Med Toxicol.* 1987;2:411–429.

7. Dunn W. Various laboratory methods screen and confirm benzodiazepines. *Emerg Med News.* 2000;21–24.

8. Beuhler MC, Spiller HA, Sasser HC. The outcome of unintentional pediatric bupropion ingestions: a NPDS database review. *J Med Toxicol.* 2010 Mar;6(1):4–8.

9. Spiller HA, Bosse GM, Beuhler M, et al. Unintentional ingestion of bupropion in children. *J Emerg Med* 2010; 38:332–336.

10. Harmon T, Jurta D, Krenzelok E. Delayed seizures from sustained-release bupropion overdose. *J Toxicol Clin Toxicol*, 1998;36:522.

11. Quadrani DA, Spiller HA, Widder P. Five-year retrospective evaluation of sulfonylurea ingestion in children. *J Toxicol Clin Toxicol.* 1996;34:267–270.

12. Spiller HA, Villalobos D, Krenzelok EP, et al. Prospective multicenter study of sulfonylurea ingestion in children. *J Pediatr.* 1997;131:141–146.

13. Burkhart KK. When does hypoglycemia develop after sulfonylurea ingestion? *Ann Emerg Med.* 1998;31:771–772.

14. Boyle PJ, Justice K, Krentz AJ, et al. Octreotide reverses hyperinsulinemia and prevents hypoglycemia induced by sulfonylurea overdoses. *J Clin Endocrinol Metab.* 1993;76:752–756.

15. Fasano CJ, O'Malley G, Dominici P, et al. Comparison of octreotide and standard therapy versus standard therapy alone for the treatment of sulfonylurea-induced hypoglycemia. *Ann Emerg Med* 2008 Apr;51(4):400–406.

16. Weaver LK, Gesell LB. Carbon Monoxide Poisoning. In: Gesell LB, ed. *Hyperbaric Oxygen 2009: Indications and Results The Hyperbaric Oxygen Therapy Committee Report.* Durham: Underwater and Hyperbaric Medical Society; 2008:19–28.

17. Myers RAM, Snyder SK, Emhoff TA. Subacute sequelae of carbon monoxide poisoning. *Ann Emerg Med.* 1985;14:1167.

18. Gorman DF, Clayton D, Gilligan JE, et al. A longitudinal study of 100 consecutive admissions for carbon monoxide poisoning to The Royal Adelaide Hospital. *Undersea Hyperb Med.* 1992;20:311–316.

19. Martell BA, Arnsten JH, Krantz MJ, et al. Impact of methadone treatment on cardiac repolarization and conduction in opioid users. *Am J Cardiol.* 2005;95:915–918.

20. Mills KC: Serotonin syndrome. A clinical update. *Crit Care Clin.* 1997;13:763–783.

21. Addonizio G, Susman VL, Roth SD. Neuroleptic malignant syndrome: review and analysis of 115 cases. *Biol Psychiatry.* 1987;22:1004–1020.

22. Caroff SN, Mann SC. Neuroleptic malignant syndrome and malignant hyperthermia. *Anaesth Intensive Care.* 1993;21:477–478.

23. Clark RF, Wethern-Kestner S, Vance MV, et al. Clinical presentation and treatment of black widow spider envenomation: a review of 163 cases. *Ann Emerg Med.* 1992;21:782–787.

24. Key GF. A comparison of calcium gluconate and methocarbamol (Robaxin) in the treatment of latrodectism (black widow spider envenomation). *Am J Trop Med Hyg.* 1981;30:273–277.

25. Clark RF. The safety and efficacy of antivenin Latrodectus mactans. *J Toxicol Clin Toxicol.* 2001;39:125–127.

26. Alberts BM, Shalit M, LoGalbo F. Suction for venomous snakebite: a study of "mock venom" extraction in a human model. *Ann Emerg Med.* 2004;43:181–186.

27. Bush SP, Hegewald KG, Green SM, et al. Effects of a negative pressure venom extraction device (Extractor) on local tissue injury after artificial rattlesnake envenomation in a porcine model. *Wild Environ Med.* 2000;11:180–188.

28. McCollough N, Gennaro J. Evaluation of venomous snakebite in the southern United States. *J Fla Med Assoc.* 1963;49:959–967.

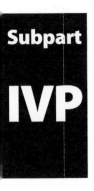

Clinical – Psychosocial

Editor's Comments on Medical Clearance

In the "typical" observation unit (OU), which includes chest pain and other types of stable, "low-maintenance" patients, psychiatric patients or patients undergoing medical clearance are generally excluded from the OU. Psychiatric patients or patients being medically cleared are "high-maintenance" patients who require additional personnel and resources. Moreover, placing an unruly, out-of-control, disruptive individual who is intoxicated from drugs and/or alcohol or high on PCP or a schizophrenic, perhaps, screaming or crying, next to a chest pain patient in the OU for a rule out presents a myriad of challenges. Therefore, the majority of OUs exclude psychiatric patients and/or out-of-control intoxicated patients.[1,2]

However, in view of the extended emergency department (ED) length of stay (LOS) for most psychiatric patients and the increasing numbers of psychiatric patients in the ED, the concept of a ED psychiatric OU has emerged and the presence of ED Psychiatric OUs is likely to increase in the future. Thus, this chapter is intended to address the concept of psychiatric OUs and the medical clearance of ED patients, and is not intended to advocate for the inclusion of these patients into a general or chest pain OU.

References

1. Mace SE, Graff L, Mikhail M, et al. A national survey of observation units in the United States. *Am J Emerg Med* 2003; 21:529–533.

2. Mace SE. Clinical Protocols. (Chapter 82)

Chapter

60

Psychiatric Patients

Jonathan Glauser, MD, FACEP

Introduction

Although patients with primarily psychiatric complaints have not traditionally filled observation units (OUs) in the United States, it is reasonable to think that this tradition will change. It is not uncommon for psychiatric patients to remain in the emergency department (ED) for protracted periods of time awaiting consultation, with disposition dependent upon "medical clearance." Even in settings of over 90% rates of insurance coverage, over 8% of adult psychiatric patients may stay in the ED for over 24 hours.[1] Homelessness, transfer to another hospital, public insurance, and use of restraints or sitters all are associated with prolonged ED stays, and it is unlikely that any of these factors will abate in the foreseeable future. This makes it highly probable that OUs for medical clearance and psychiatric evaluation will play an enhanced role in the health care system. This discussion assumes the capability for monitoring patients with sitters and security as needed.

Aside from protecting a psychiatric patient from him or herself and others, making the decision as to whether or not the patient is "medically clear" is often the principal task in the accurate triage of patients in the ED and subsequently in the OU. A patient may present with severe depression, suicidal or homicidal ideations, psychotic disturbances, or altered mental state that may ultimately lead to admission. It is essential that potentially life-threatening illnesses be detected before a patient is admitted to a setting where resources for diagnosis and treatment are suboptimal. Suicide screening tends to be performed largely on patients with chief complaints of a psychiatric nature, and approximately one-third of these patients in one report had documentation of alcohol abuse, with another third noted to have prescription drug misuse or intentional illegal drug use.[2] Therefore, a large percentage of patients with suicidal ideation or primary psychiatric complaints have confounding substance use that precludes an accurate assessment of risk until a certain amount of time elapses. For example, if a patient metabolizes ethanol at 15–20 mg/dL per hour, many hours may elapse before an accurate risk assessment can be achieved in an inebriated patient.

Many psychiatrists view the patient's initial presentation to the ED as the only opportunity to diagnose an underlying organic process that would otherwise go undetected and potentially lead to morbidity or even mortality if missed. Complaints that appear psychiatric in origin may be manifestations of underlying medical conditions.[3]

The psychiatric patient population represents 2% to 12% of ED visits and behavioral problems have been listed as the presenting complaint in 4% of ED visits.[4,5,6] From 1992 to 2001, there were reported 53 million psychiatric-related ED visits, which is an increase from 17.1 to 23.6 per 1000 visits.[6] Distinguishing whether the patient's signs and symptoms result from a purely psychiatric illness, if a medical disease coexists, or if that disease is the underlying etiology for the patient's presentation will be a continuing concern in any ED and for any ensuing observation stay.

Psychiatric Emergencies: Defined

According to the American Psychiatric Association, a psychiatric emergency is defined as "an acute disturbance in thought, behavior, mood, or social relationship, which requires immediate intervention as defined by the patient, family, or social unit."[7] This umbrella classification covers both functional and organic disease processes, and it is important to recognize certain disorders to think of how medical disease may play a role.

Schizophrenia and other psychoses: These are marked by the presence of delusions (fixed false beliefs that are not amenable to arguments) and by hallucinations. There is loss of reality testing; consciousness is clear. Schizophrenia is characterized by deterioration in functioning, classically with continuous signs of the disturbance for more than 6 months. Onset is usually prior to age 40. The disturbance is not attributable to substance abuse or to a medical disorder. Negative symptoms include social withdrawal, difficulty in functioning in school or at work, lack of volition, blunting of emotion, flattened affect, poor abstract thinking, or apathy.[8]

Anxiety: This disorder is characterized by apprehension, fear, and excessive worry. Feelings of panic or stress might be accompanied by autonomic hyperactivity out of proportion to any real danger to the integrity of the patient's health. It is unlikely that patients would be admitted to an OU or to a psychiatric service for anxiety alone. Symptoms can be induced by a wide variety of legal and illegal substances. Caffeine and nicotine are prominent, as are phencyclidine and cocaine. Over-the-counter medications for cough and colds, including ephedrine and antihistamines, can induce anxiety, as can withdrawal from alcohol, benzodiazepines, barbiturates, and beta-blockers. Palpitations and frank arrhythmias can induce anxiety. Apprehension can be associated with other significant medical illnesses such as hyperthyroidism, hypoglycemia, and hypoxemia.[9]

Panic disorder: This is an anxiety disorder characterized by a sudden surge of anxiety and dread, with changes in autonomic vital signs. Palpitations, tachycardia, chest tightness, shortness of breath, sweating, tremulousness, and subjective dizziness can be present. Organic etiologies, especially entities that may cause cardiac or respiratory compromise, must be ruled out.

Major depression: This diagnosis is characterized by persistent dysphoric mood, or sadness, present most of the day, lasting longer than 2 weeks. The lifetime risk of suicide in depressed patients is approximately 15%.[10] Symptoms should not be attributable to bereavement or to direct physiologic effects of a substance. Patients with major depression without suicidal ideation typically do not meet admission criteria unless the depression is severely limiting the patient's functioning and activities of daily living.

Bipolar disorder: This disorder is characterized by the occurrence of mania (elation or irritability) and grandiosity. An elevated, expansive, or irritable mood should be present for at least 1 week to make the diagnosis. Patients can exhibit a decreased need for sleep, increased activity, rapid or pressured speech, and racing thoughts. They tend to be talkative, with flight of ideas and distractibility. The onset is usually in the third and fourth decades of life.

To make these diagnoses, the symptoms must not be caused by a general medical condition or substance. These medical conditions should be investigated in the OU prior to disposition.

Patients with Altered Mentation

It is necessary to identify which patients have a correctable cause(s) for their disturbed mental status. Determining delirium from dementia is a critical consideration. (Table 60.1)

Delirium: This has also been synonymous with organic brain syndrome, metabolic encephalopathy, toxic encephalopathy, and acute confusional state. It is characterized by global impairment in cognitive function with clouded consciousness and impaired attention. Deterioration is acute,

Table 60.1 Characteristics of Delirium, Dementia, and Psychiatric Illness

Characteristic	Delirium	Dementia	Psychiatric Illness
Onset	Acute – hours/days	Gradual: months/years	Acute
Attention	Impaired	Normal	Disorganized
Consciousness	Decreased	Baseline	Alert
Hallucinations	Typically visual	Absent	Typically auditory
Speech	Rapid, incoherent, hesitant, slow	Inability to find words	Typically coherent
Orientation	Usually impaired	Usually impaired	Rarely impaired
Vital signs	May be abnormal	Usually normal	Usually normal

Table 60.2 *"Can't Miss"* Medical Illnesses Simulating Psychiatric Disease

Meningitis/ encephalitis
Other infections: sepsis, UTI, pneumonia
Diabetic emergencies: hypoglycemia, DKA
Hypoxia or hypercapnia
Encephalopathies (hypertensive, Wernicke, hepatic, uremic)
Head injury
Intracranial hemorrhages
Poisoning
Drug withdrawal (benzodiazepines, barbiturates, ethanol)
Seizures
Neuroleptic malignant syndrome
Serotonin syndrome
Thyroid disturbances
Gross electrolyte abnormalities

measured in hours or days – not months. Hallucinations tend to be visual. By definition, delirium has a medical cause. Changes in cognition and thinking can fluctuate during the day and tend to be more pronounced at night.

Dementia: This diagnosis describes a pervasive disturbance in cognitive functioning in memory, judgment, abstract thinking, personality, and higher cortical functions such as language. Polypharmacy, renal failure, pulmonary disease, endocrine disorders, normal pressure hydrocephalus, slowly growing intracranial mass, hepatic failure, nutritional disease, infectious disease, inflammatory disease, and depression are possible reversible causes. Consciousness is not clouded. Ability to carry out motor functions can be impaired.[11] There is gradual loss of cognitive abilities such as memory or computational skills.[8]

Physicians must always think in terms of the most lethal diagnoses – those entities they can least afford to miss when admitting a patient to a psychiatric ward. The medical entities listed in Table 60.2 can cause serious morbidity or mortality, can masquerade as psychiatric disease, and must be ruled out before physicians can "clear" patients for admission to a psychiatric service. Many can be ruled out clinically.

A partial list of substances potentially causing psychosis includes digitalis, corticosteroids, non-steroidal anti-inflammatory drugs, isoniazid, disulfiram, cyclic antidepressants, anticonvulsants, benzodiazepines, amphetamines, cocaine, narcotics, barbiturates, methyldopa, levodopa, anticholinergic medications, jimson weed, and diphenhydramine. Systemic illnesses that can cause psychosis include systemic lupus erythematosus and tertiary syphilis. Depression can be caused by narcotics, alcohol, and other sedatives; by antihypertensive agents and corticosteroids; and by entities such as thyroid disorders and Cushing syndrome. In 24-hour stay units, physicians cannot formally test for all of these – the workup would be too extensive (lumbar puncture, metabolic evaluation, drug/alcohol screening, neuroimaging, neurologic consultations, endocrine testing). Once the diagnosis of delirium or alteration in mental status is made, the patient is not suitable for observation care and warrants full hospitalization.

A useful mnemonic for discriminating organic from functional psychoses is the MADFOCS scale seen in Table 60.3.[12]

Medical and Psychiatric Illness Coexist

Historically, medical findings have been described in significant numbers of psychiatric patients, including those who were deemed "medically clear." Reasons for errors included inadequate physical examination, failure to obtain indicated laboratory studies, failure to obtain available history, and failure to address abnormal vital signs.[13]

Changes in mental status resulting in psychosis, anxiety or panic, depression, mania, delirium, and dementia have been associated with a broad base of underlying medical etiologies. Historically, these have been categorized into five main groupings: metabolic/endocrine, medications, substances, infectious, and central nervous system (see Table 60.4).[5,14]

History of Present Illness

If the patient is unable to provide a thorough history, it may be obtained from family, police, witnesses, or other health care providers. Focused questioning should determine if the patient has a history of psychiatric or medical disease, if there

Table 60.3 MADFOCS: Mnemonic for Discriminating Organic from Functional Psychosis

	Organic	Functional
M – Memory deficit	Recent impairment	Remote impairment
A – Activity	Hyperactive, hypoactive, tremor, ataxia	Repetitive activity, rocking
D – Distortions	Visual hallucinations	Auditory hallucinations
F – Feelings	Emotional lability	Flat affect
O – Orientation	Disoriented	Oriented
C – Cognition	Lucid thoughts, perceives/attends/ focuses occasionally	No lucid thoughts, unfiltered perceptions, unable to attend/focus
S – Some other findings	Age > 40 Sudden onset Physical exam abnormal Vital signs abnormal Social immodesty Aphasia Consciousness impaired	Age < 40 Gradual onset Physical exam normal Vitals normal Social modesty Intelligible speech Awake/alert

Table 60.4 Medical Conditions with Behavioral Symptoms

Metabolic/ Endocrine	High or low thyroid, blood sugar, parathyroid, cortisol levels
Medications	SSRIs, benzodiazepines, opiates, corticosteroids, anticholinergics, digitalis, others
Substances	Alcohol, amphetamines, benzodiazepines, phencyclidine, LSD, other hallucinogens
Infectious	Meningitis, encephalitis, urinary tract infections, pneumonia, sepsis
Central Nervous System	Seizures, cerebral tumors, CVAs, post-ictal, hydrocephalus, migraines

Table 60.5 Clues Suggesting Organic Medical Illness

- No previous history of psychiatric disorder
- Sudden onset
- Age < 12 or > 40 years at onset
- Disorientation
- Depressed level of consciousness
- Abnormal vital signs
- Focal neurologic deficits
- Visual or tactile hallucinations (not auditory)
- Evidence of exposure to toxins or suspected ingestion

are any new medications, an estimate of the patient's baseline level of alertness and ability to perform activities of daily living, the acuity of onset, and if any substances are involved. Clues suggesting medical illness rather than a primarily psychiatric are listed in Table 60.5.

Physical Examination

The physical examination must note the vital signs. Abnormal vital signs should automatically raise the suspicion that a medical component is playing a role in the patient's presentation. A complete neurological examination should also be performed including cranial nerves, muscle strength, sensation, reflexes, cerebellar function, and orientation assessment prior to observation admission.

Impaired mental status can be the manifestation of a wide range of medical conditions that warrant hospitalization on a medical ward. The Quick Confusion Scale (QCS) has been touted as preferable to the Mini-Mental State Examination for emergency use, because it does not require pencil and paper and is quicker to administer.[15] The QCS may also be useful in determining alteration of cognition:[16,17]

Quick Confusion Scale			
Question	Response	Weight	Score (product)
What year is it?	0 or 1 (0 if incorrect, 1 if correct)	x 2	
What month is it?	0 or 1 (0 if incorrect, 1 if correct)	x 2	
Give memory phrase	John Brown, 42 Market Street, New York (no score given for repetition of phrase)		
What time is it?	0 or 1 (1 if within 1 hour, 0 if not)	x 2	
Count backward from 20 to 1	0, 1, or 2 (2 if no errors, 1 if one error, 0 if two or more)	x 1	
Say the months in reverse	0, 1, or 2 (2 if no errors, 1 if one error, 0 if two or more)	x 1	
Repeat the phrase	0, 1, 2, 3, 4, 5 (score each portion remembered as 1 point)	x 1	

For each response count the number of errors and multiply by the weight to determine the total. The possible score ranges from 0 to 15. A score of less than 12 suggests a need for further evaluation and a score of 7 indicates almost certain cognitive impairment.

If substance abuse or withdrawal is implicated, it should be temporally related to the disturbance. The physical examination should be a head-to-toe assessment looking for evidence of trauma, funduscopic exam looking for papilledema, evidence of prior craniotomy or shunts, enlarged thyroid, meningismus, pneumonia, asterixis, track marks, or other findings.

Routine Testing

Psychiatric consultants may request a myriad of specific tests, although a period of observation may prove more valuable, since toxins in general metabolize and require 4–6 hours of supportive care in an ED or observation setting. The American College of Emergency Physicians (ACEP) suggests that "Focused Medical Assessment" better suits the process of determining if a medical disease is the cause of the patient's symptoms or needs to be acutely treated.[18]

Medical clearance generally entails three components:

1. No physical illness is found in the patient
2. Coexisting medical problems are determined not to be the primary cause of the acute psychiatric symptoms
3. An acute medical condition was stabilized

Laboratory testing may vary depending on each facility, department, and personal practices of the physician and should have input from the

psychiatric service. The history and physical examination is clearly important in medical clearance, while unfocused routine laboratory testing is unnecessary. Pregnancy testing in female patients over the age of 16 should be performed.[19] The presence of an established psychiatric diagnosis coupled with a lack of a specific medical complaint, negative physical findings, and stable vital signs appears to identify a subgroup of patients for whom laboratory testing is not necessary.[20,21]

That said, a recent survey found that such testing was required of 35% of a sample of emergency physicians randomly selected through ACEP membership rolls. Of those required to perform routine testing, 84% were required by the psychiatric service or referral institute. The most commonly required tests were serum alcohol and urine toxicology.[4] If the patient is taking lithium, specific levels may be warranted due to neurologic sequelae, including seizures.

Other commonly requested tests include: complete blood count (CBC); bedside glucose; electrolytes; BUN/creatinine; blood alcohol; pregnancy testing; serum and urine for cocaine, phencyclidine, and amphetamine; urine analysis and culture; arterial blood gases; calcium; creatine phosphokinase (CPK); thyroid function testing; liver function tests; ECG for evaluation of QT interval; and cranial computed tomography. Testing should be directed by the clinical presentation rather than by protocol. Patients with altered mentation may not be appropriate for observation care.

Recent evidence indicates that patient self-reporting is quite accurate regarding drug and ethanol use.[20,21] Testing does increase both cost and time, and patients with straightforward psychiatric complaints have been medically cleared without a urine toxicology screen.[22]

A patient cannot be medically cleared if impaired by alcohol. However, there remains no evidence-based literature supporting the notion that there is a specific blood alcohol concentration where patients regain decision-making capacity or when psychiatric symptoms become more apparent without the confounding influence of alcohol. Cognitive function should be assessed on a case-by-case basis if alcohol is involved. Protocols aside, urine drug screening has seldom proven helpful either in treatment or in influencing disposition.

Imaging and Medical Clearance

One study of healthy military recruits with new onset psychosis revealed no clinically significant findings on head computed tomography (CT) scan.[23] A more recent study of 397 patients with psychiatric complaints and no focal neurological findings indicated that 95% of the head CT scans showed no abnormality. Abnormalities seen in the other 5% were all deemed to be unrelated to the patient's condition. In all, the probability of any relevant abnormality was not greater than finding one in the general population.[24] Head CTs should generally be reserved for patients with HIV, a history of trauma or cancer, focal neurologic findings, or altered behavior or mental status changes. If a head CT is truly indicated, the patient should probably not be primarily managed on a psychiatric service.

It has been suggested that there are groups of patients who are at high risk of medical illness: (1) the elderly, (2) patients with a history of substance abuse, (3) patients without a psychiatric history, (4) patients with preexisting medical disorders, and (5) patients from a lower socioeconomic level.[25] The threshold for testing might be lowered in these individuals.

Summary

Patients with alterations in mental status must receive an appropriate medical diagnostic workup. Any abnormal vital signs must be addressed and should normalize within a 24-hour stay if due to anxiety. History and physical examination is critical, including medication history. Testing should be guided by the history and physical examination findings. No single battery of tests will pick up every metabolic or structural abnormality that might affect patient behavior. Universal laboratory and toxicologic screening of all patients with psychiatric complaints has a low yield and generally does not affect care. It is desirable to coordinate protocols for screening with the desires and needs of one's psychiatric service. Finally, it is notable that the term "medical clearance," cannot ensure that a patient is indeed clear of all medical conditions.

References

1. Chang G, Weiss A, Kosowky JM, et al. Characteristics of adult psychiatric patients with stays of 24 hours or more in the emergency department. *Psychiatr Serv* 2012 Mar 1; 63 (3): 283–286.

2. Ting SA, Sullivan AF, Miller JA, et al. Multicenter study of predictors of suicide screening in emergency departments. *Acad Emerg Med* 2012 Feb; 19 (2): 239–243.

3. Riba M, Hale M. Medical clearance: fact or fiction in the hospital emergency room. *Psychosomatics* 1990;31 (4):400–404.

4. Broderick KB, Lerner EB, McCourt JD, et al. Emergency physician practices and requirements regarding the medical screening examination of psychiatric patients. *Acad Emerg Med* 2002;9(1):88–92.

5. Williams ER, Shepherd SM. Medical clearance of psychiatric patients. *Emerg Med Clin North Am* 2000;18(2):185–198.

6. Larkin GL, Claassen CA, Emond JA, et al. Trends in U.S. emergency department visits for mental health conditions, 1992 to 2001. *Psychiatr Serv* 2005;56:671–677.

7. Allen MH, Forster P, Zealberg J, et al. *APA Task Force on Psychiatric Emergency Services: Report and Recommendations regarding Psychiatric Emergency and Crisis Services.* American Psychiatric Association, 2002.

8. Broder JS, Olshaker JS. Medical clearance of psychiatric patients. *Crit Decis Emerg Med* 2001;16(4):7–11.

9. Dorsey ST. Medical conditions that mimic psychiatric disease: a systematic approach for evaluation of patients who present with psychiatric symptomatology. *Emerg Med Rep* 2002;23(20):233–245.

10. Blumenthal SJ, Kupfer DJ. eds. *Suicide over the Life Cycle: Risk Factors, Assessment, and Treatment of Suicidal Patients.* Washington, DC: American Psychiatric Association, 1990.

11. American Psychiatric Association. *Diagnostic and Statistical Manual of Mental Disorders.* 4th ed. Washington, DC: American Psychiatric Association, 1994.

12. Frame DS, Kercher EE. Acute psychosis. Functional versus organic. *Emerg Med Clin North Am* 1991;9(1):123–136.

13. Reeves RR, Pendarvis EJ, Kimble R. Unrecognized medical emergencies admitted to psychiatric units. *Am J Emerg Med* 2000;18(4):390–393.

14. O'Brien RF, Kifuji K, Summergrad P. Medical conditions with psychiatric manifestations. *Adolesc Med Clin* 2006;17:49–77.

15. Folstein MF, Folstein SE, McHugh PR. "Mini-mental state." A practical method for grading the cognitive state of patients for the clinician. *J Psychiatr Res* 1975;12(3): 189–198.

16. Stair TO, Morrissey J, Jaradeh I, et al. Validation of the quick confusion scale for mental status screening in the emergency department. *Intern Emerg Med* 2007;2:130–132.

17. Irons MJ, Farace E, Brady WJ, et al. Mental status screening of emergency department patients: Normative study of the quick confusion scale. *Acad Emerg Med* 2002;9: 989–994.

18. Lukens TW, Wolf SJ, Edlow JA, et al. Clinical policy: critical issues in the diagnosis and management of the adult psychiatric patient in the emergency department. *Ann Emerg Med* 2006;47:79–99.

19. Korn CS, Currier GW, Herdersen SO. "Medical clearance" of psychiatric patients without medical complaints in the emergency department. *J Emerg Med* 2000;18(2):173–176.

20. Olshaker JS, Browne B, Jerrard DA, et al. Medical clearance and screening of psychiatric patients in the emergency department. *Acad Emerg Med* 1997;4(2):124–128.

21. Shihabuddin B, Hack C, Sivitz A. Role of urine drug screening in medical clearance of psychiatric pediatric patients: is there one? *Ann of Emerg Med* 2010;56(3):144.

22. Fortu JM. Psychiatric patients in the pediatric emergency department undergoing routine urine toxicology screens for medical clearance: results and use. *Pediatr Emerg Care* 2009;25 (6):387–392.

23. Bain BK. CT scans of first-break psychotic patients in good general health. *Psychiatr Serv* 1998;49:234–235.

24. Agzarian MJ. Use of routine computed tomography brain scanning of psychiatry patients. *Australas Radiol* 2006; 50(1):27–28.

25. Gregory, RJ, Nihalani ND, Rodriguez E. Medical screening in the emergency department for psychiatric admission: a procedural analysis. *Gen Hosp Psychiatry* 2004;26: 405–410.

Chapter

61

Disasters

Constance J. Doyle, MD

Introduction

A disaster is defined as occurring when needs outstrip resources, and is dependent on circumstances, as well as on community and mutual aid resources. Preservation of the medical infrastructure and doing the greatest good for the greatest number are the goals of medical surge. Altered standards of care or "crisis standards of care" allows equitable sharing of scarce resources to provide the best possible care for the maximum number of patients. When the local medical infrastructure is overwhelmed during a disaster and hospital capacity is overextended, there must be a plan for allowing hospitals alternate ways of caring for increased numbers of patients and for alternative ways of staffing for these increased needs. The use of observation beds both in the hospital and outside the hospital can provide some of the needed additional bed capacity.

In-Hospital and Inter-Hospital Surge

When hospital beds are full, patients may be accommodated in units within the hospital that would be underutilized in a disaster including elective diagnostic testing units with recovery beds, such as gastroenterology procedural suites for endoscopy and colonoscopy, and outpatient elective ambulatory surgery units. If the disaster is taxing hospital resources, elective surgeries may be cancelled and post anesthesia care unit (PACU) beds would have some capability as well. Community and regional planning among hospitals may allow some movement between hospitals to transfer sicker or more injured patients to hospitals with greater tertiary type capability and to allow the movement of general care floor patients to be "downloaded" to general hospitals.

The Joint Commission requires that hospitals participate in community planning with community partners: emergency management, public health, emergency medical systems (EMS), their medical staffs, and other hospitals.[1,2,3] When hospitals have exceeded capacity, sometimes defined by surge plans as an amount over normal capacity,[4,5,6] then the transfer of patient care to outside resources beyond the local/regional hospital infrastructure may be needed. Regional and state disaster plans will help to define how this patient surge is to occur, as well as identifying transportation resources. A secure, well-integrated patient tracking system is essential to locate and relocate patients, for integrated record keeping, and to allow family access, if needed.

Alternate Care Facilities

Under the grants from the Health Resources Service Administration (HRSA), which is now the Assistant Secretary for Preparedness and Response (ASPR),[7] states have been tasked with the planning and coordination of multiple levels of medical care and the surge of medical care and resources in disasters.[8] This would include expansion of services that can be considered observation, and ward care facilities as well as facilities for triage, prophylaxis, education, and expansion of home care services.

Regional Medical Coordination Centers (MCCs) may be activated for the organization and coordination of hospital and regional resources. Medical coordination and hospital coordination allow sharing of resources and responses and are coordinated by a regional MCC, a regional Emergency Operations Center (EOC) health division or by county medical or public health jurisdictions. Public health is the coordination point in some plans. Regional MCCs then coordinate with the state's medical branch of operations under a state's EOC. State coordination of intra- and interstate resources is part of the National Response Framework.[8] Interstate coordination with federal and state partners occurs at the federal level.

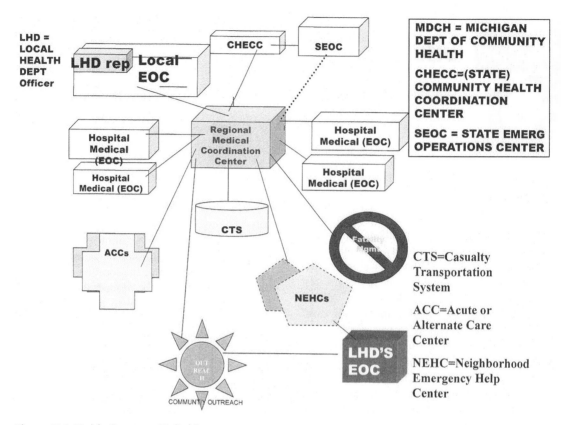

Figure 61.1 Modular Emergency Medical Systems
(Michigan Department of Community Health, Courtesy of Linda Scott BSN, MPH, MEMS and Pandemic Planning [Various Conference Materials] Office of Public Health Preparedness, Lansing Michigan. Diagram used with permission.)

Alternate facilities in disasters have many forms. Some have been set up during domestic disasters such as hurricanes and floods when the health care infrastructure has been compromised or outpatient/home care has not been available or as a place to which special needs and/or medically fragile individuals have been evacuated. Many regular disaster shelters are not capable of providing medical monitoring or observation except by family members *provided* they have been evacuated to the same shelter. Often persons in these shelters have not been evacuated with caregivers, medical records, prescriptions or supplies. These facilities may be only for medical monitoring or observation. Other shelters may be places where some level of active medical observation and treatment occurs. Those who have acute illness or problems may need to be transferred to definitive medical care, for example, the emergency department (ED) or hospital, depending upon the capabilities of the particular shelter for providing medical care.

The Modular Emergency Medical System (MEMS)[9,10] (Figure 61.1 MEMS Diagram) is a system for expanding, in a modular way, community resources to allow community and regional cooperative expansion to meet specific medical and public health needs as they occur. Only needed modules are activated in any particular disaster or all components may be activated in a larger disaster. When first envisioned, MEMS was in response to mass casualty terrorism incidents. The original design was to address the gap in casualty care resources that would exist in most medical care jurisdictions if large numbers of biological warfare casualties were to be present to area hospitals. The concept is based on rapid organization of two types of expandable patient care modules, the Neighborhood Emergency Help Center (NEHC) for screening, triage, education, and possible immunization and prophylaxis elements and the Alternate or Acute Care Center (ACC) for basic medical observation and off-hospital medical care. It also includes a medical command and control element, the Medical Coordination Center (MCC), casualty transportation systems (CTS), expanded outreach/homecare networks, and fatality management systems.[9]

The MEMS concept is integrated into the Incident Command System/National Incident Management System (ICS/NIMS) under the Unified Medical Branch. The United States National Response Plan uses the National Incident Management System (NIMS) for incident command.[12] As federal, state, regional, and local planning has ensued from 2002 to the present, planning has evolved into all hazards planning. The specter of Avian flu and pandemic Influenza brought expanded planning for off-hospital site patient screening and treatment if the medical infrastructure was overwhelmed. Multiple articles on expanded ward care facilities, and possible cohorting of infectious patients, were published after research and community planning.[5,12,14,15] Planning for expanding supplies and equipment and personnel including housekeeping and food service to support these facilities is also needed. In the process of pandemic planning, it was learned that multiple agencies were dependent on the same medical supply chains, which in an emergency would not be able to expand supplies to all hospitals and facilities.[5]

An integrated supply system for all types of hospital materials from linens to pharmaceuticals and intravenous (IV) fluids for these expansion facilities is essential planning for regional and state efforts before the supplies in the Strategic National Stockpile (SNS) would be shipped in to alleviate the shortage and available for backup (usually estimated as 72 hours).[16] Then local distribution points and personnel to handle and process supplies, as well as a plan for unloading and moving supplies, would need to be planned.

Setup of Facilities

The ACC serves as an extension of an already existing facility(s). Planning involves regional hospital groups, state and regional plans, and medical coordination to plan for population-based ACCs. Sponsoring hospitals are identified to coordinate the ACC including identification, setup, and planning for initial staffing prior to mutual aid from other medical staffs. Pre-identification of facilities for off-site treatment will need research to secure appropriate facilities for patient care. Written

interagency and mutual aid agreements and memorandums of understanding/agreement (MOU/MOA) to operate an off-site facility need to be in place before an incident. Considerations for ACCs include parking and access, security, nearness to public transportation, and vehicle and ambulance ingress and egress.

The building would need to have total space for expanding modules of 50 patient "pods" up to a 250 patient capacity (Figure 61.2 ACC). Security, ingress and egress, heating and air conditioning, electricity, sizes of doorways and corridors, lighting, floor coverings, ventilation, sanitation capabilities including hand washing stations, food service capabilities, refrigeration, communications, and patient tracking systems need to be evaluated for each facility. Electronic communication systems sharing with a sponsoring hospital may allow an electronic medical record (EMR) to be used and those records housed by the sponsoring hospital(s).[13]

Determination of Capability and Mission

ACCs may be used for ward type care for infected patients who would be cohorted or noninfected patients who do not need advanced respiratory support; they are designed to create an environment where patients can respond to specific treatments. Patients needing advanced airway support and ventilator support, cardiac monitoring, and intermediate or stepdown care would be referred to the hospital. General ward care, low level oxygen in some ACCs and respiratory treatments would be planned for some facilities. Patients may be cohorted with one particular disease entity, thereby, requiring similar treatment and limiting exposure to noninfected persons, or for general ward type care with limited templated evaluation and treatment options. ACCs may also be used for hospice patients with protocol-driven palliative or comfort care. Planning for ACC patients includes templates for care, especially for personnel who are unfamiliar with an austere environment, and agreed upon pharmaceutical supplies such as IV solutions, limited stocks of antibiotics, antiemetics, and analgesics. Supply exchange with the sponsoring hospital(s) or regional or state caches and plans for supply and resupply, as well as protective supplies for personnel, will need to be planned in advance.

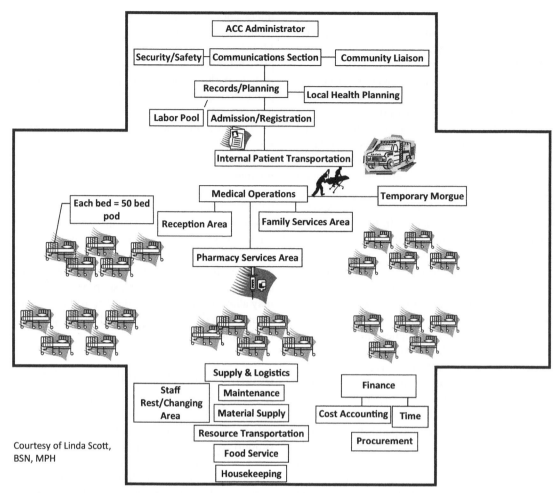

Figure 61.2 Alternate of Acute Care Center (ACC)
(Michigan Department of Community Health, Courtesy of Linda Scott BSN, MPH, MEMS and Pandemic Planning [Various Conference Materials] Office of Public Health Preparedness, Lansing Michigan. Diagram used with permission.)

Staffing Levels

Planned levels of staffing would be part of the plan for the ACC including expanded rolls for nursing, midlevel providers, and students and residents with plans for supervision. Using nontraditional providers such as dentists and veterinarians may be required if personnel resources are scarce.[13] Expanding staffing such as changing 8-hour shifts to 12-hour shifts can increase staffing by almost one-third. Just-in-time training, job action sheets, and templates for treatment can streamline and standardize care. Lean staffing and consideration of/utilization of supportive family members, the caregivers of children and special needs patients, and volunteers are part of the plan. Expansion of personnel and roles of others under direction (students, residents, volunteers) should be written into

the plan. Physician and nurse management for overall operations and designated physician support per shift for each pod and medical staff buy-in will be essential for the smooth operation of this type of facility.

Assurances that a declaration of disaster will alter the standards of care, thereby, creating alternative or "crisis standards of care" would be the expected care model. Acceptance of altered standards of care would help to encourage the staffing of alternate care sites. Declaring a disaster would provide legal relief with the suspension of some laws such as Emergency Medical Treatment and Labor Act (EMTALA). Such a declaration would facilitate staffing by volunteers or assigned staff.

These facilities would only be in operation if a prolonged disaster occurred, such as a pandemic

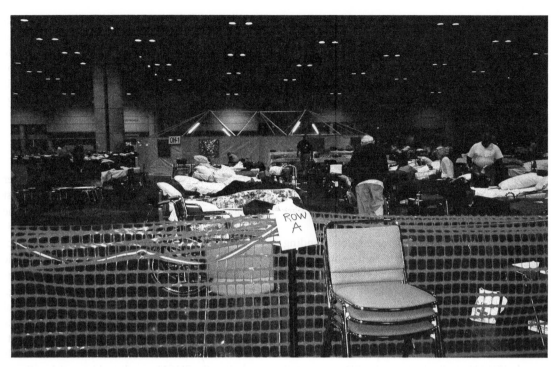

Figure 61.3 Shelter in Florida during a Hurricane Disaster
(Courtesy of CJ Doyle, MD, FACEP, used with permission.)

lasting weeks to months, rather than a traumatic disaster where care could be expanded for a matter of hours to care for casualties.

Since patients are in a large ward type venue, certain patients who may be disruptive to others, security risks, or require extensive supervision may not be appropriate for this type of facility.

The Medical Care or Special Needs Shelter

Special needs facilities have been authorized by local jurisdictions and public health during hurricanes and other disasters. Such facilities have been staffed by medical volunteers, local medical staffs, National Disaster Medical System (NDMS) teams, or Medical Reserve Corps (MRC). Medical care and special needs shelters function under local emergency management and public health. They provide shelter for multiple types of nonambulatory or special needs patients, who cannot be cared for in a shelter where individuals would be expected to care for their own needs including their own medical needs.

Medical shelters can provide electricity for some powered medical equipment and some level of medical care including medication dispensing, dressing changes, and triage to a hospital(s) if a new *medical* problem or need presents. Dialysis patients may need special diets and plans for less frequent intermittent dialysis on an altered schedule. Patients with behavioral needs may need special sheltering and caregivers. If general shelters could be expanded to include care for special needs individuals, then special needs shelters may not need to be established. Mental health needs will need to be included in these shelters as well.

Tracking of patients/clients and reunification also needs to be addressed. Special needs individuals or the vulnerable or at-risk individuals need to be included as part of the overall plan, whether in a special needs shelter or a medical shelter with capabilities for addressing their basic requirements or necessities for functioning or if they are "sheltered in place" with coordination of their acute medical care, along with their routine daily medical needs. (Figure 61.3)

Group homes and long-term care facilities may have limited surge capacity. Disaster plans may provide plans for shelter in place (including disasters when there is no power). In some facilities, common areas could surge to take care of more patients. Adjusting referral criteria to hospitals during a disaster should be included in planning along with the education of staff.[13] If facilities such as group homes or long-term care facilities need to evacuate and plan on moving patients, the relatives, regular caregivers, and/or family may not be available. Transportation may also not be as available. For homebound special needs patients with caregiver support, alternate plans for evacuation may be necessary. Some overall observation and oversight for these facilities, especially regarding special needs patients and sheltering and/or alternate care must be part of community planning.

Some plans in the past have included sending all residents of facilities such as group homes and long term-care facilities to local hospitals even if there is not a new medical need. The problem may be as simple as a lack of a generator for electricity for oxygen concentrators or a ventilator. The solution to avoiding the transportation of such homebound and/or special health care needs (SHCN) individuals to the ED may entail the provision of electricity through an alternate means, for example, a generator, when electrical power is cut off.

Community planning for long-term care facilities, the homebound, and special needs patients will help to allocate sheltering and medical resources for these patients. Integrating long-term care facilities, group homes, and oversight agencies for special needs patients into community disaster plans will aid in sheltering and help distribute medical care to the most appropriate facility or even allow SHCN individuals to remain in their current domicile, whether it is a group home, long-term care facility, or their own home/apartment.

Conclusion

Community, regional, state, and national disaster plans must do the greatest good for the greatest number, preserve the medical infrastructure for the sickest and most injured patients and evenly balance medical care across the entire medical spectrum of observation and acute care. Multiple venues for observation, along with limited evaluation and treatment at off-site facilities (e.g., outside the hospital) with attention to an ethical and equitable distribution system for all patients will allow for appropriate, compassionate, patient- and family-centered treatment of individuals including the SHCN or vulnerable, at-risk patients, and provide quality medical care. Plans made in advance, agreements across medical and community and state entities tailored to the unique disaster and in a tiered modular surge system can facilitate the most appropriate distribution and best care possible for the most patients under the difficult situation and constraints of a disaster.

References

1. JCAHO. Joint Commission on Accreditation of Health Care Organizations. Standards Requiring Hospitals to be Part of Community Planning for Emergencies: Elements of Performance. Communication with Deborah Phillips, March 2012. www.disasterpreparation.net/resources.html.

2. JCAHO. Joint Commission on Accreditation of Health Care Organizations. Hospital Accreditation Standards 2012. Published by Joint Commission Resources. Oakbrook, Ill. 2012. www.ynhhs.com/emergency/commu/JCAHOProposed AdditionstoEMIs

3. JCAHO. Joint Commission on Accreditation of Health Care Organizations. Health Care at the Crossroads: Strategies for Creating and Sustaining Community-wide Emergency Preparedness Systems. Oakbrook Terrace, IL: JCAHO 2003. Recommendations, p. 18.

4. MEMS ACC Plan. www.edgewood.army.mil/downloads/bwirp/ECBC_acc_blue_book.pdf

5. Cinti, S; Wilkerson, W; Holmes, JG. Pandemic influenza and acute care centers: Taking care of sick patients in a non-hospital setting. *Biosecurity and Bioterrorism* 6(4). 2008. DOI: 10.1089/bsp.2008.0030

6. Waldhorn, Richard. What role can alternative care facilities play in an influenza pandemic? *Biosecurity and Bioterrrorism* 6 (4) 2008.

7. Assistant Secretary for Preparedness and Response (ASPR). Health preparedness program. www.phe.gov/preparedness/planning/hpp/Pages/default.aspx

8. ESF #8 Public Health and Medical Services. National Response Framework. National Response Framework Resource Center. www.fema.gov/NRF. Washington DC. Jan 2008.

9. Church, J. Modular Emergency Medical System: Expanding Local Health Care Structure in a Mass Casualty Terrorism Incident. Prepared in Response to the Nunn-Lugar-Domenici Domestic Preparedness Program by the Department of Defense June 1, 2002. Department of Defense www.dqeready.com/UserFiles/MEMS.pdf

10. Nunn-Lugar-Domenici. Domestic Preparedness Acts 1977–2001. (as found in the federal regist. www.investiga tiveproject.org/documents/ testimony/190.pdf and www .gao.gov/archive/1999/ns99016t. pdf

11. Joint Commission Resources. Surge Hospitals-Providing Safe Care in Emergencies. www.jointcommission.org/ assets/1/18/surge_hospitals .pdf

12. National Incident Management System (NIMS). Department of Homeland Security. www.dhs.gov Washington, DC, December 2008.

13. Hanfling, D; Altevogt, BM; Viswanathan, K; Gostin, LO, eds. *Crisis Standards of Care, Volume 4: Hospitals and Alternate Care Systems.* Institute of Medicine, National Academies Press. Downloaded August 28, 2012 from www.nap.edu/catalog.php? record_id=13351

14. Skidmore, S; Wall, WT; Church, JK. *Concept of Operations for the ACC. Modular Emergency Medical System Blue Book 2003.* Homeland Defense Business Unit, Aberdeen Proving Ground, 2003.

15. Goulet, R. *Modular Emergency Medical System, A Regional Response for All- Hazards Catastrophic Emergencies. Planning Guide July 2010.* New England Center for Emergency Preparedness, Lebanon, NH, 2010.

16. Strategic National Stockpile (SNS). www.cdc.gov/phpr/ stockpile/stockpile.htm Accessed March 25, 2012.

17. EMTALA. Emergency Medical Treatment and Labor Act of 1986 American College of Emergency Physicians. Best Practices for Hospital Preparedness. www.ACEP .org Accessed March 20, 2012.

Part V

Financial

Chapter

62

Physician Coding and Reimbursement

Michael A. Granovsky, MD, CPC, FACEP
David A. McKenzie, BS, CAE

Observation Physician Documentation and Coding

Prior chapters have identified clinically appropriate patients for Observation. The general trend has been to extend the universe of patients receiving Observation Services. The concept of Observation has expanded from solely those patients with diagnostic uncertainty to include clinical conditions that classically involved the need for "admission" or short-term treatment in the hospital over several days. As such, the time frame for observation has gradually broadened to include same-day services, up to 24 hours, and now may include multiday stays, with the code sets and reimbursement methodologies evolving to report these services.

With regard to the length of Observation Services that may be compliantly reported, Medicare states in Transmittal 2282, "In only rare and exceptional cases do reasonable and necessary outpatient observation services span more than 48 hours. In the majority of cases, the decision whether to discharge a patient from the hospital following resolution of the reason for the observation care or to admit the patient as an inpatient can be made in less than 48 hours, usually in less than 24 hours."[1]

Of note, Medicare's statement relates to *hours* and does not take into account that the observation period of 24 to 48 hours may take place over three or more calendar days. Consider a patient admitted to observation late on Friday night, observed all day Saturday and discharged Sunday morning. That stay, although less than 36 hours, would span three calendar days. As such the code sets provided by Current Procedural Terminology (CPT) have evolved to accommodate reporting multiday stays.

Justifying the Medical Necessity for Observation in Your Documentation

The Centers for Medicare and Medicaid Services (CMS) defines Observation Care as a well-defined set of specific, clinically appropriate services, which include ongoing short-term treatment, assessment, and reassessment that are furnished while a decision is being made regarding whether patients will require further treatment as hospital inpatients or if they are able to be discharged from the hospital.[2] Those services furnished on a hospital's premises, including use of a bed and periodic monitoring by nursing or other staff, must be reasonable and necessary to evaluate an outpatient's condition or determine the need for a possible admission as an inpatient.[3] Such services are covered only when provided by order of a physician or another individual authorized by State licensure law and hospital bylaws to admit patients to the hospital or to order outpatient tests.

General Documentation Requirements

"The (Observation) codes are used to report encounters by the supervising physician with the patient when designated as Observation status. In this context, this refers to supervision of the care plan for Observation and performance of periodic reassessments."[4]

Based on the aforementioned CMS and CPT directives, some general conclusions can be reached regarding the documentation requirements:

- Chart documentation must contain a risk stratification statement and brief plan that demonstrates the medical necessity for the Observation stay.

Example:

42-year-old male with limited risk factors presenting with vague chest pain. Will place in Observation, obtain serial cardiac enzymes, and plan stress test this evening.

- A clearly dated and timed order to place the patient in Observation.
- Progress notes demonstrating periodic assessments. Of note, there is currently not a proscribed number of progress notes, but rather the frequency of notes should reflect the potential variability in the patient's condition.

Example:

17-year-old female asthmatic:

10:00 Moderate residual wheeze RR 28 O2 saturation 93%

13:00 Improving on Q 1 hour nebs RR 26

17:00 Mild residual wheeze peak flow improved

Coding Scenarios

One of the more confusing aspects related to Observation services is the seemingly myriad of coding scenarios relating to the timing of a patient's Observation care. (See Table 62.1 and Table 62.2.) This discussion will attempt to simplify the scenarios using the following broad constructs:

1. All the care takes place on 1 calendar day
2. The care spans 2 calendar days
3. The care spans more than 2 calendar days

Scenario 1: All the care takes place on a single calendar day. For example: the patient is placed in

Table 62.1 Summary of Coding 1 and 2 Calendar Day Stays in Observation

Observation Complexity	Care All on the Same Day	Care Covers 2 Days
Low	99234	99218 + 99217
Moderate	99235	99219 + 99217
High	99236	99220 + 99217

Table 62.2 Summary of Coding a Multiple Day Observation Stay

Observation Complexity	Initial Day	Subsequent Day(s)	Discharge Day
Low	99218	99224	99217
Moderate	99219	99225	99217
High	99220	99226	99217

Observation at 10 a.m. and discharged home at 9 p.m. the same day. The following codes are used to report the observation services based on the amount of History (Hx), Physical Examination (PE), and Medical Decision Making (MDM). Additionally, whereas CPT typically provides clinical vignettes for Evaluation and Management Services, they have not done so for Observation Services. However, the Relative Value Update Committee (RUC) has developed formal vignettes that were submitted to CMS as part of the RVU valuation process for these services. The specific codes, their requirements, and the corresponding RUC vignette are listed here.

The CPT codes for same-day observation admit and discharge include:

99234 – Observation or inpatient hospital care for presenting problems of low severity. Documentation requires a detailed or comprehensive history, a detailed or comprehensive exam, and straightforward or low-complexity MDM.

> RUC Vignette: 99234 – A 19-year-old pregnant patient (9 weeks gestation) presents to the emergency department (ED) complaining of persistent vomiting for 1 day.

99235 – Observation or inpatient hospital care for presenting problems of moderate severity. Documentation requires a comprehensive history, a comprehensive exam, and moderate-complexity MDM.

> RUC Vignette: 99235 – A 48-year-old patient presents to the ED with a history of asthma in moderate respiratory distress. The patient is admitted for observation and discharged later on the same day.

99236 – Observation or inpatient hospital care for presenting problems of high severity. Documentation requires a comprehensive history, a comprehensive exam, and high-complexity MDM.

> RUC Vignette: 99236 – A 52-year-old patient comes to the ED because of chest pain. The patient is admitted for observation and discharged later on the same day.

Importantly, Medicare requires 8 hours of care to report the same-day Observation code set 99234–99236. As stated in transmittal 2822, "When a patient receives observation care for less than 8 hours on the same calendar date, the Initial Observation Care, from CPT code range 99218–99220, shall be reported by the physician. The Observation Care Discharge Service, CPT code 99217, shall not be reported for this scenario."[1]

Scenario 2: The care spans 2 calendar days. For example, the patient is placed in Observation status at 10 a.m. and discharged home the following day at 9 a.m. Observation provided on calendar date #1 is reported with the code set 99218–99220 based on the documented History, Physician Exam, and Medical Decision Making.

These CPT codes apply to all evaluation and management services that are provided on the same date of initiating "observation status."

99218 – Initial observation care, per day, for presenting problems of low severity. Documentation requires a detailed or comprehensive history, a detailed or comprehensive exam, and straight-forward or low-complexity MDM. Physicians typically spend 30 minutes at the bedside and on the patient's hospital floor or unit.

> RUC Vignette: 99218 – An intoxicated 52-year-old male presents after a fall. He has a blood alcohol concentration of 0.325% and has vomited several times. The patient is admitted for observation.

99219 – Initial observation care, per day, for presenting problems of moderate severity. Documentation requires a comprehensive history, a comprehensive exam, and moderate-complexity MDM. Physicians typically spend 50 minutes at the bedside and on the patient's hospital floor or unit.

> RUC Vignette: 99219 – A 57-year-old woman presents with an allergic reaction after a bee sting complaining that "her throat is constricting" and she is having "difficulty breathing." The patient is admitted for observation.

99220 – Initial observation care, per day, for presenting problems of high severity. Documentation requires a comprehensive history, a comprehensive exam, and high-complexity MDM. Physicians typically spend 70 minutes at the bedside and on the patient's hospital floor or unit.

> RUC Vignette: 99220 – A 78-year-old male with a history of CHF presents complaining of shortness of breath and lower extremity edema. He admits to not taking his "heart pills" and admits to drinking beer and eating hotdogs recently at a baseball game. He is dyspneic, able to complete sentences of three to five words, has rales to mid lung field, and +3 pitting edema in the bilateral lower extremities. His ECG is unchanged from prior. The patient is admitted for observation.

The final day of a 2-day stay is reported with the discharge code 99217.

99217 – Observation care discharge management includes services on the date of observation discharge (can only be used on a calendar day other than the initial day of observation). The documentation for 99217 should include the following: a final exam, discussion of the observation stay, follow-up instructions, and documentation. Do not report in conjunction with a hospital admission.

Scenario 3: The care spans more than 2 calendar days. For example, the patient is placed in Observation status at 10 a.m. on Monday and discharged home on Wednesday at 9 a.m. This scenario incorporates the logic of the 2-day stay but a new set of codes is utilized to report the middle day(s), which are identified as subsequent observation services. The CPT code set 99224–99226 is used to report subsequent observation care based on the History, Physical Exam, and Medical Decision Making.

Subsequent Observation Care As per CPT, utilize these codes for observation care services provided on dates other than the initial or discharge date. These codes include reviewing the medical record and reviewing the results of diagnostic studies and changes in the patient's status since the last assessment by the physician. Of note, because they are subsequent visit codes, only two of the three key components of the History, Physical Exam or Medical Decision Making are required to be satisfied.

99224 – Subsequent observation care, per day, for stable, recovering, or improving patients. Documentation requires a problem-focused interval history, problem-focused examination, and low-complexity MDM. Physicians typically spend 15 minutes at the bedside and on the patient's hospital floor or unit.

> RUC Vignette: 99224 – Subsequent observation care of a 42-year-old male following an uncomplicated mandible fracture who is responding to pain medication; however, he is not controlled on oral medications and requires continued observation.

99225 – Subsequent observation care, per day, for the patient responding inadequately to therapy or has developed a minor complication. Documentation requires expanded problem-focused interval history, expanded problem-focused examination, and moderate-complexity MDM. Physicians typically spend 25 minutes at the bedside and on the patient's hospital floor or unit.

RUC Vignette: 99225 – Subsequent observation care of a 23-year-old female with nausea, vomiting, and crampy abdominal pain, who is responding to therapy. Although the patient's condition has improved, there are concerns regarding the abdominal condition requiring continued observation.

99226 – Subsequent observation care, per day, in which the patient is unstable or has developed a significant complication or a significant new problem. Documentation requires detailed interval history, detailed examination, and high-complexity MDM. Physicians typically spend 35 minutes at the bedside and on the patient's hospital floor or unit.

RUC Vignette: 99226 – Subsequent observation care for a 78-year-old male who fell and suffered contusions to the head and shoulder, but no fractures. He has a history of stroke and is currently on warfarin requiring continued assessment for stability and possible intervention for internal bleeding.

Documentation Requirements

With the implementation of the 1995 CMS documentation guidelines as amended in 1997, physicians providing observation services must be aware of the documentation requirements related to reporting these services. Observation cases are scored primarily based on the key elements of the History, Physical Exam, and Medical Decision Making. With the exception of the lowest level of service, Observation services require a Complex History and Physical Exam.

Summary of Documentation Requirements: 1-Day and 2-Day Observation

Detailed History and Physical Exam for 99218 and 99234

History of Present Illness: 4 elements
Past, Family, or Social History: 1 area
Review of Systems: 2 systems
Physical Exam: 5–7 organ systems/areas

Comprehensive History and Physical Exam for 99219/99220 and 99235/99236

History of Present Illness: 4 elements
Past, Family, or Social History: All 3 areas (Of note, the ED Evaluation and Management (E/M) codes only require 2 of 3 PFSH elements to qualify as comprehensive)
Review of Systems: 10 systems
Physical Exam: 8 organ systems

The subsequent observation codes used to report the "middle days" also have specified documentation requirements.

Table 62.3 summarizes the History, Physical Exam, and Medical Decision Making requirements for each of the individual Observation codes.

Table 62.3 Summary of Observation E/M Code Documentation Requirements

Service	CPT Code	Required Documentation		
		History	Physical	MDM
Same-day observation	99234	D or C	D or C	Straightforward or low
Same-day observation	99235	C	C	Moderate
Same-day observation	99236	C	C	High
Initial observation	99218	D or C	D or C	Straightforward or low
Initial observation	99219	C	C	Moderate
Initial observation	99220	C	C	High
Subsequent observation	99224*	PF	PF	Straightforward or low
Subsequent observation	99225*	EPF	EPF	Moderate
Subsequent observation	99226*	D	D	High

D = Detailed, C = Comprehensive, PF = Problem focused, EPF = Expanded problem focused
*Requires only two of the three key components to meet or exceed stated requirements rather than meeting all three requirements.

Prolonged Services with Observation

Starting in 2012, CPT listed typical times associated with observation code ranges 99218–99220 and 99224–99226 (Table 62.4). With typical times now assigned, those codes sets are eligible for consideration of additionally reporting prolonged services when the time the physician spends performing the service exceeds the typical published time.

CPT offers specific guidance regarding the Prolonged Service codes. Prolonged service refers to direct patient contact, is face-to-face and includes additional non-face-to-face services on the patient's floor or unit in the hospital or nursing facility during the same session, even if the time spent is not continuous. It is reported in addition to the designated evaluation and management services at any level and any other services provided at the same session as evaluation and management services.

The inpatient or observation prolonged code descriptors read as follows:

+99356 – Prolonged service in the inpatient or observation setting requiring unit/floor time beyond the usual service; first hour

(Use 99356 in conjunction with 90837, 99218–99220,

99221–99223, 99224–99226, 99231–99233, 99234–99236,

99251–99255, 99304–99310)

+ 99357 – Each additional 30 minutes (List separately in addition to 99356.)

Prolonged services codes are time-based add-on codes. CPT includes a chart for threshold time requirements (Table 62.5).

The Resource Based Relative Value Scale (RBRVS) Process

When a new code is approved through the CPT process, it is sent to the American Medical Association (AMA) Relative Value Scale Update Committee (RUC) for valuation. Data is provided to the RUC to help members assign an appropriate relative value to the service. The RUC then forwards their recommendations to CMS, which historically has adopted those recommendations over 90% of the time.

An RVU is an abbreviation for Relative Value Unit. Physician services are reported using the Current Procedural Terminology (CPT) coding system. For each CPT code, RVU valuations are calculated for Physician Work, Practice Expense, and Professional Liability Expense. Each of these three components is assigned an RVU value and the sum represents the total RVUs for that CPT code.

RBRVS Formula:

Work RVU
Practice expense RVU
<u>+ Liability insurance RVU</u>
= Total RVUs

> Example for Code 99236
> Work RVU + Practice Expense RVU + Liability Insurance RVU = Total RVU
> 4.20 + 1.64 + 0.29 = 6.13

Table 62.4 Summary of CPT Typical Times Associated with Observation Services

CPT Code	Typical CPT Times
99218	30 minutes
99219	50 minutes
99220	70 minutes
99224	15 minutes
99225	25 minutes
99226	35 minutes

Table 62.5 CPT Time Thresholds for Observation Prolonged Care Services

Total Duration of Prolonged Services	Code(s)
Less than 30 minutes	not reported separately
30–74 minutes (30 minutes – 1 hour 14 minutes)	99356 × 1
75–104 (1 hour 15 minutes – 1 hour 44 minutes)	99356 × 1 and 99357 × 1
105 or more (1 hour 45 minutes or more)	99356 × 1 and 99357 × 2 or more for each additional 30 minutes
Adopted for use with Observation Services	

Table 62.6 RVU Comparison of E/M Codes of Similar Complexity

Emergency Department Codes		Same-Day Observation		2-Day Observation	
CPT code	RVUs	CPT code	RVUs	CPT code	RVUs
99283	1.75	99234	3.76	99218	2.81
99284	3.32	99235	4.76	99219	3.81
99285	4.90	99236	6.13	99220	5.22
				99217	2.05

Table 62.7 Combined RVUs for Patients Admitted on One Day and Discharged on the Next Day

Code Pair: Initial Observation Code + Discharge Code (for following day)	RVUs	Combined RVUs
99218 + 99217	2.81 + 2.05	4.86
99219 + 99217	3.81 + 2.05	5.86
99220 + 99217	5.22 + 2.05	7.27

Table 62.8 RVUs for Subsequent Observation

Subsequent Observation Codes	
CPT code	RVUs
99224	1.12
99225	2.05
99226	2.95

Like other typical Evaluation and Management Services, the Observation Codes have been evaluated by the RUC and CMS has published the Total RVU Values for these services. Typical Observation Code RVUs appear in Table 62.6 with the inclusion of the ED codes of similar complexity to serve as a reference point.

In the scenario where a patient was admitted to observation on one day and discharged on the following day, the 99218–99220 codes would usually be assigned with the discharge code, 99217. The combined RVUs for these code pairs would be as follows: 4.86 for 99218 and 99217; 5.86 for 99219 and 99217; and 7.27 for 99220 and 99217 (see Table 62.7).

As discussed earlier, in the event patient care spans more than 2 calendar days the middle day(s) are reported with the subsequent observation care codes (99224–99226). These codes have also been assigned RVUs (see Table 62.8), which would be additive.[5]

Medicare Payments

To determine the Medicare reimbursement the Total RVUs for a given code are multiplied by a conversion factor (typically published on an annual basis by Medicare) to obtain the resulting Medicare reimbursement for that CPT code (see Table 62.9 and Table 62.10).

Total RVUs × Medicare Conversion Factor = Medicare Payment

Example for 99236 using the updated 2016 Medicare conversion factor:

6.13 Total RVUs × $35.8043 = $219.48

It is important to remember that CPT instructs that when observation status is initiated in the course of an encounter in another site of service such as the emergency department, all E/M services provided by the same physician (usually also defined as a physician of the same specialty from the same group) in conjunction with initiating observation status are considered to be part of the initial observation care when performed on the same date and are not separately reportable. Some groups have considered complex corporate structures to allow reporting both an ED E/M and observation services on the same date. Groups contemplating such complex corporate structures should seek advice from legal counsel before considering such plans.

Modifiers

Many of the same modifiers apply to Observation that would apply to ED E/M service. The most common application would be the 25 modifier (Significant, Separately Identifiable Evaluation and Management Service by the Same Physician

Table 62.9 Sample Medicare Reimbursement for Observation Services

Code	RVUs × Medicare Conversion Factor	Payment	Code	RVUs × Medicare Conversion Factor	Payment	Code	RVUs × Medicare Conversion Factor	Payment
99234	3.76 × 35.8043	$134.62	99218	2.81 × 35.8043	$ 100.61	99224	1.12 × 35.8043	$ 40.10
99235	4.76 × 35.8043	$170.43	99219	3.81 × 35.8043	$136.41	99225	2.05 × 35.8043	$ 73.40
99236	6.13 × 35.8043	$219.48	99220	5.22 × 35.8043	$186.90	99226	2.95 × 35.8043	$105.62
			99217	2.05 × 35.8043	$ 73.40			

Table 62.10 Sample Medicare Reimbursement for ED Services

ED Code	Payment
99281	$21.48
99282	$41.89
99283	$62.66
99284	$118.87
99285	$175.44

on the Same Day of the Procedure or Other Service), to distinguish the observation service from any procedures that were performed during the same encounter.

Consider this scenario: "Presenting patient is a 78-year-old male who fell and suffered contusions to the head and shoulder, but no fractures. He has a history of stroke and is currently on warfarin requiring continued assessment for stability and possible intervention for internal bleeding."

The patient then goes on to develop significant epistaxis requiring complex anterior nasal packing described by CPT code 30903 (Control nasal hemorrhage, anterior, complex [extensive cautery and/or packing] any method). His admission and discharge from observation all occurs on the same calendar day. You would apply the 25 modifier to the 99236 and also report the epistaxis treatment code. Final coding would be:

99236 – 25 and 30903

Keep in mind that the Observation codes may not be used for simple recovery (such as following moderate sedation) particularly if the procedure is part of a global surgical package.

Critical Care Reported with Observation

In the event a patient in observation status suddenly crashed and becomes critically ill, it may be possible to also report the time spent providing critical care, 99291 (Critical care, evaluation and management of the critically ill or injured patient; first 30–74 minutes) if the minimum time thresholds are met. CPT explicitly states that critical care and other E/M services may be provided to the same patient on the same day by the same physician. Additionally, Medicare has stated "When a hospital inpatient or office/outpatient evaluation and management service (E/M) are furnished on a calendar date at which time the patient does not require critical care and the patient subsequently requires critical care both the critical Care Services (CPT codes 99291 and 99292) and the previous E/M service may be paid on the same date of service."[6]

References

1. CMS Manual System Pub 100-04 Medicare Claims Processing Manual, Chapter 12, Section 30.6.8.

2. CMS Manual System Pub 100-04 Medicare Claims Processing Manual, Chapter 4, Section 290.1.

3. CMS Manual System Pub 100-04 Medicare Claims Processing Manual, Chapter 4, Section 290.

4. Current Procedural Terminology CPT®, 2016. Chicago, IL: American Medical Association, 2015.

5. Medicare RBRVS: The Physicians' Guide 2012. Chicago, IL: American Medical Association, 2012.

6. CMS Claims Processing Manual Pub 100-04, Chapter 12, Section 30.6.9.

Hospital Coding and Reimbursement

63

Candace E. Shaeffer, RN, MBA, RHIA
Michael A. Granovsky, MD, CPC, FACEP

OBSERVATION UNIT REIMBURSEMENT: HOSPITAL

Introduction

In addition to understanding the clinical aspects of providing hospital observation services it is important for emergency department (ED) clinical and financial leaders to understand charging, coding, and other aspects of the revenue cycle as they relate to observation reimbursement.

The Healthcare Financial Management Association and others define revenue cycle management as the coordination of "all administrative and clinical functions that contribute to the capture, management, and collection of patient service revenue."[1] While coders manage the coding, and the back-end billing functions remain a patient financial services responsibility, knowledge of these processes – including patient registration, documentation, charging, coding, and some billing related tasks – will be essential to the observation manager as he or she strives to optimize revenue and steer clear of compliance issues.

When examining revenue cycle issues related to observation, managers will discover that the Centers for Medicare and Medicaid Services (CMS) has published an abundance of information, rules and regulations to guide the effort. Commercial payers are often not as transparent so many hospitals have adopted Medicare rules as the standard and apply variations as needed to satisfy specific payer requirements.

The CMS rules for reporting hospital or facility observation are very different from the professional/physician rules discussed in Chapter 62. Being mindful of the fact that different rules come into play on the facility side is a good first step to understanding hospital observation reimbursement.

General Medicare Observation Rules

CMS requires adherence to published guidelines as a condition for payment. As a hospital outpatient service, observation requirements can be found in the Medicare Hospital Manual, various transmittals, and in the Outpatient Prospective Payment (OPPS) rules that are updated annually. As with all billable services, an observation service must be medically necessary and supported with thorough and specific documentation. Because only services that meet CMS requirements are reportable/payable, it is important for providers to be aware of the rules and guidelines to help ensure appropriate reimbursement.

CMS has designated hospital observation, for the purpose of reimbursement, as a "Comprehensive APC" (Ambulatory Payment Classification). This means that generally, all other services provided during the observation stay will be packaged and not paid separately. Under the comprehensive APC payment structure CMS packages payment for items and services that it considers integral, ancillary, supportive, dependent, or adjunctive to the primary service.[2] Observation services require a defined level of supervision based on the stability of the patient. Upon initiation of Observation the services must be provided under *direct supervision* (meaning that the physician or appropriate nonphysician practitioner is immediately available to furnish assistance and direction throughout the performance of the service though he or she does not have to be present in the room where the service or procedure is being performed. *General supervision* (meaning that the service is furnished under the overall direction and control of the physician or appropriate nonphysician practitioner, but his or her physical presence is not required during the performance of the service nor is he/she required to be immediately available) is allowed once the patient is deemed stable. Importantly, the point of transition to general supervision should be documented in the medical record. For example, a 48-year-old asthmatic with labored breathing and moderate wheezing is placed in observation. During this initial stage the patient requires direct supervision. However, with ongoing treatment the patient begins to improve, no longer requires supplemental oxygen and has transitioned to a more stable state requiring only general supervision. Of note, the observation provider can be a physician or nonphysician practitioner as long as the service is within the clinician's scope of licensure, credentialing, and the hospital bylaws.[3]

CMS does not require a specific location for the provision of observation thus allowing a high degree of flexibility to hospitals. Observation areas or beds may be located in the ED, a formal observation unit, an outpatient short-stay area, or even on an inpatient floor.

An observation stay usually follows an ED or clinic visit, but the patient may be directly referred to observation by a physician in the community. Observation services typically last less than 24 hours, and rarely more than 48 hours.[4]

Observation Reimbursement from a Revenue Cycle Perspective

Because the CMS requirements related to registration, documentation, charging, coding, and billing are often found to be confusing, a systematic walk through each of these revenue cycle components as they relate to observation will help provide clarity.

Registration

The physician order determines if a patient is registered as an inpatient or outpatient. Each status has different reporting requirements and implications for reimbursement: registration sets up the downstream charging, coding, and billing processes as either inpatient or outpatient. If caught immediately, a registration error can be changed, but if the patient's care is initiated the back-end process to convert from inpatient to outpatient can be onerous.

An incorrect registration can result from a registration mistake or an incorrect admission order. Registration mistakes are easy to make if the order does not clearly state "place in observation." It is easy to see how a physician's order, "Admit to Observation," could result in an inpatient admission in the registration system.

An incorrect admission order occurs when the patient's intensity of service needs and severity of illness are consistent with outpatient care but the patient is admitted as a formal inpatient. The process for converting an inpatient to an outpatient will be discussed in the Billing section later in this chapter.

Documentation Requirements and Best Practices

Fortunately, the same documentation requirements discussed in the physician section also apply to hospital observation. Interestingly, CMS has published very few observation nursing documentation requirements.

The physician should document a separate observation record that includes:

- A dated and timed order to "place in observation" or "provide observation care"
- Notation of medical necessity, the benefits of observation and/or the risk of discharging the patient home; if observation is for a complication following an outpatient surgery the complication and need for observation should be clearly documented
- A treatment plan
- Progress notes for ongoing care
- A discharge note

In the OPPS rules and Medicare manuals, CMS has further stated that the patient's medical record should include:

- Written orders for observation care and discharge, documentation of a risk assessment by the MD; all notes should be written and signed
- Start and stop times for observation should be documented in the nursing notes

Best practice nursing documentation includes dated and timed initial, progress, and discharge notes that are consistent with the physician's orders; results of "periodic monitoring" by the nurse; responses to any interventions and treatment; notation of communications with the physician or other provider; and nursing signatures.

Charging

Observation charges may be determined by a coder, or a nurse or clerk in the unit where the service was provided. Typical observation "visit" charges include a Current Procedural Technology (CPT) or Healthcare Common Procedure Coding System (HCPCS) code as noted in Table 63.1, units of service in hours, a dollar charge set by the hospital, and observation revenue code 762. Of note, this is a different revenue code than 450, which is typically used for the ED. In addition to the observation visit charge, CPT codes for separately billable procedures and any diagnostic testing would also be reported (Table 63.2). Once determined, each charge will be entered into the billing system and reported on the UB04 hospital claim (an electronic data file) once "coding" has been completed.

Medicare and commercial payers are inconsistent in their observation reporting requirements; Medicare requires the observation

Table 63.1 Medicare Observation HCPCS Codes

Medicare Observation HCPCS Codes	Descriptor
G0378	Hospital observation service, per hour
G0379	Direct referral to observation care

Source: 2016 OPPS Final Rule, Appendix B

HCPCS code, G0378. Some commercial payers will also accept this HCPCS code, but others require an observation CPT code or no code at all and instead expect only the observation revenue code, the duration of the observation stay in

Table 63.2 CPT Private Payer Observation Codes

Observation CPT Code	CPT Descriptor, as Applicable to Hospital Observation
99218	Initial observation care, per day; low-severity presenting problem
99219	Initial observation care, per day; moderate-severity presenting problem
99220	Initial observation care, per day; high-severity presenting problem
99217	Observation care discharge, day management
99224	Subsequent observation care, per day; patient is usually stable, recovering or improving
99225	Subsequent observation care, per day; patient is usually responding inadequately to therapy or has developed a minor complication
99226	Subsequent observation care, per day; patient is usually unstable or has developed a significant complication or a significant new problem
99234	Observation or inpatient hospital care; same day admit and discharge; low-severity presenting problem
99235	Observation or inpatient hospital care; same day admit and discharge; moderate-severity presenting problem
99236	Observation or inpatient hospital care; same day admit and discharge; high-severity presenting problem

Source: 2016 AMA CPT [American Medical Association, CPT Professional Edition, AMA 2016]

OUTPATIENT

1 Any Hospital	2 Any Hospital	3a PAT. CNTL.# 1234		
123 Any Street	456 Any Street	b. MED. REC. # 98765		0131
Bellevue WA 98007	Bellevue WA 98007	5 FED. TAX NO. 221234567	6 STATEMENT COVERS PERIOD FROM 03 10 12 THROUGH 04 11 12	7 RESERVED

8 PATIENT NAME a Patient ID if different from Sub	9 PATIENT ADDRESS a 1234 Main Street				
b Doe, John	b Bellevue			c WA d 98007	Country code if other than USA

10 BIRTH DATE	11 SEX	12 DATE	ADMISSION 13 HR. 14 TYPE 15 SRC	16 DHR	17 STAT	18 19 20 21 CONDITION CODES 22 23 24 25 26 27 28	29 ACDT STATE	30
03 20 1931	M	03 10 12	08 3	3	12 01	Condition Codes Required Identifying Events	WA	RESERVED

31 OCCURRENCE CODE DATE	33 OCCURRENCE CODE DATE	35 OCCURRENCE CODE SPAN FROM THROUGH	36 OCCURRENCE CODE SPAN FROM THROUGH	37
a	Occurrence and Occurrence Span Codes may be used to define a significant event that may affect payer processing			FUTURE USE
b				

38		39 CODE VALUE CODES AMOUNT	41 CODE VALUE CODES AMOUNT
John Doe 1234 Main Street Bellevue, WA 98007		a A1 952:00	
		b Value Codes and amounts required when necessary to process claim	
		c	
		d	

42 REV. CD.	43 DESCRIPTION	44 HCPCS / RATE / HIPPS CODE	45 SERV DATE	46 SERV. UNITS	47 TOTAL CHARGES	48 NON-COVERED CHARGES	49
1 0310	Laboratory N400093723106	88173	03 10 12	1	100:00	0:00	Future 1
2 0402	Ultrasoud	76942	03 10 12	1	100:00	0:00	Use 2
3 0450	ED Services	99284	03 10 12	1	450:00	0:00	3
4 0762	Observation	G0378	03 10 12	14	850:00	0:00	4
5 0260	Infusion	96365	03 10 12	1	180:00	0:00	5
6 0260	Infusion	96366	03 10 12	1	300:00	0:00	6
7							7
8							8
9							9
10							10
11							11
12							12
13							13
14							14
15							15
16							16
17							17
18							18
19							19
20							20
21							21
22							22
23	PAGE 1 OF 1	CREATION DATE	1980:00			0:00	23

50 PAYER NAME	51 HEALTH PLAN ID	52 REL INFO	53 ASG BEN	54 PRIOR PAYMENTS	55 EST. AMOUNT DUE	56 NPI 2222222222	
A Washington State	Report HIPAA National	Y	Y	Required when	Amount	57 1234567890	A
B Secondary Payer	Health Plan Identifier			indicated payer has paid amount to	estimated	OTHER Secondary	B
C Tertiary Payer	when mandatory			Provider	to be due	PRV ID Tertiary	C

58 INSURED'S NAME	59 P.REL	60 INSURED'S UNIQUE ID	61 GROUP NAME	62 INSURANCE GROUP NO.	
A Doe, John	18	ABC1234567800	Employee, Inc.	1234	A
B Secondary					B
C Tertiary					C

63 TREATMENT AUTHORIZATION CODES	64 DOCUMENT CONTROL NUMBER	65 EMPLOYER NAME	
A 02468	491234	Watch Repair, Inc.	A
B Secondary			B
C Tertiary			C

66 DX 3910	Use A through Q to report "Other Diagnosis" if applicable			68 Reserved
9				

69 ADMIT DX 4280	70 PATIENT REASON DX May be used to report reason for visit	71 PPS CODE DRG	72 ECI May be used to report external cause of injury	73 Reserved

74 PRINCIPAL PROCEDURE CODE DATE	b. OTHER PROCEDURE CODE DATE	75	76 ATTENDING NPI 2222222222	QUAL 1G 1234569822
		Reserved	LAST Doctor FIRST MD	
d. OTHER PROCEDURE CODE DATE			77 OPERATING NPI QUAL	
			LAST FIRST	

80 REMARKS	81CC a B3 282N00000X	78 OTHER NPI QUAL
May be used to report additional information.	b Secondary	LAST FIRST
	c Tertiary	79 OTHER NPI QUAL
	d	LAST FIRST

UB-04 CMS-1450   APPROVED OMB NO.   NUBC® National Uniform Billing LIC9213257   THE CERTIFICATIONS ON THE REVERSE APPLY TO THIS BILL AND ARE MADE A PART HEREOF.

Red = Required
Black = Situational/Required, if applicable/Reserved

hours, and a dollar charge. Some hospitals code the observation CPT codes for internal tracking even when they are not required by a payer.

Medicare also requires that CPT/HCPCS codes for the service that led to the observation stay be reported. This would include a CPT code for a qualifying clinic (G0463) or ED visit (99281-992855) or critical care (99291), or the HCPCS code, G0379, if the patient was a direct referral to observation. For example, our asthma patient would have a facility ED code of 99285 and then an additional charge for observation based on the length of the observation services, which will be discussed next.

Correctly calculating the number of reportable observation hours can be challenging. CMS states that facility observation time starts at the clock time documented in the patient's medical record, which "coincides with the time that observation services are initiated in accordance with a physician's order for observation." Observation time ends at the time when all medically necessary services related to observation care are completed – including follow-up after the physician's discharge order is written. For counting partial hours, observation hours are rounded to the nearest hour. For example, our asthmatic patient receives a 99285 ED facility service and is then placed in observation at 7 a.m. The patient receives ongoing treatment for 12 hours with all services completed with discharge at 7 p.m. The facility coding would be 99285 and 12 units of G0378.[5]

The observation start and stop times determine the total duration of observation, but to calculate reportable observation hours, any time that the patient is out of the observation area without an RN and any time spent in a separately billed diagnostic or therapeutic service that requires active monitoring must be subtracted from the total duration of observation. For example, if the same asthmatic patient above received observation services from 7 a.m. to 7 p.m. but departed the observation unit for a bronchoscopy and was gone for 2 hours, only 10 units of G0378 would be coded.[6]

Active monitoring is not defined by CMS; it is left to the hospital to determine, usually by the presence of a physician order requiring such monitoring. CMS does give providers two examples of procedures requiring active monitoring: a colonoscopy and chemotherapy. Other examples might include: certain injections and

infusions, moderate conscious sedation, cardiac catheterization procedures, blood transfusions, and insertion of a central venous access device.

Because the duration of these procedures is not usually documented in the patient's medical record, CMS states that hospitals may subtract an "average" procedure time from the total observation time.[7] Hospitals will need to determine average times for providing these services.

Coding

As with other medical services, the correct coding of ICD-10 diagnostic codes helps to support the medical necessity for an observation service and ensure appropriate reimbursement. Coding is usually performed by professional coders in the Health Information Management (HIM) department and will often include validation of the CPT and HCPCS codes in addition to the coding of ICD-10 codes, modifiers, provider information, and quality reporting if required.

The coding group will also support the billing process by helping to correct claims that did not meet billing requirements or were edited out of the billing system. Coding will research issues causing billing delays and work with the observation manager or other departments to obtain the necessary information or corrections so the claim may be submitted for payment. Coding may also be asked to assist with the appeal process if an observation code on the claim is denied. These codes were detailed earlier in Tables 63.1 and 63.2.

Billing

Most hospital billing is highly automated and includes the consolidation of all observation charges and coding, performing editing or "scrubbing" to create a clean claim, generating the UB04 claim file and other billing forms, and submitting the claim to the payer.

One special observation billing issue deserves mention: condition code 44. Condition code 44 is a CMS utilization review and billing process used to convert an inpatient to outpatient observation if the patient is admitted but is later determined to not meet inpatient criteria. CMS expects this conversion to occur infrequently and only if strict criteria are met:

- The decision to convert from inpatient to outpatient is supported by the Utilization Review committee.

- A physician must concur with the decision and document this with an observation order in the medical record.
- The change is made before the patient is discharged and no claim has been submitted.
- The patient should be informed.

For example, if our asthmatic patient had been admitted to the hospital as an inpatient, and several hours later on utilization review (UR) had been found to not meet inpatient criteria, the case manager would have brought the issue to the UR committee for their review and input. If UR agreed that outpatient services would be more appropriate, the admitting physician would be queried and if she or he concurred an order would be written for placing the patient in observation. Other criteria noted earlier would need to be met and condition code 44 would be added to the outpatient claim form prior to billing.

If all of the above conditions are satisfied, an outpatient, rather than an inpatient, claim is submitted with condition code 44 reported in one of the form locators in fields 24–30 on the UB-04 claim form.[8]

If this condition code 44 situation does occur it is important to remember that the counting of observation hours starts only after the observation order is written. The charges incurred before this conversion may be reported under revenue code 760 or 761.

Other implications of utilizing observation rather than inpatient status include a higher out-of-pocket cost for the patient as they will incur co-pays for outpatient services and the potential loss of a three-day qualifying inpatient stay for skilled-nursing facility coverage. For example, as an inpatient our asthmatic might have had nearly full coverage. However when classified as observation the patient is now responsible for their outpatient deductible and any co-insurance.

Back-end billing processes related to observation reimbursement include the posting of payments, monitoring, and follow-up on denied claims. Not all payers document their policies and sometimes denials occur for unanticipated reasons. It is important that someone monitors payer notification statements to ensure billed charges are reimbursed appropriately.

Facility Observation Reimbursement

After a payer receives the hospital's electronically submitted claim for observation payment, it will be processed or adjudicated and, if all requirements are met, a payment will be issued.

Medicare uses a software claims editor, called the Integrated Outpatient Code Editor (I/OCE), which will determine if observation payment criteria are met and the claim should be paid. In this way, coders do not have to determine if an observation case meets specific criteria in order to code it, the software does this for them. The I/OCE reviews the submitted claim and determines the appropriate reimbursement based on the OPPS rules and the specific Ambulatory Payment Classification (APC) that the submitted CPT and HCPCS codes map to (APCs are the outpatient counterpart to inpatient diagnosis-related groups [DRGs], and each has a designated payment rate).

CMS has designated observation services as a Comprehensive APC or C-APC. They are called comprehensive APCs because observation and the ED or clinic visit or direct referral that preceded it, as well as the vast majority of ancillary studies and treatments, are not reimbursed separately but rather in a single payment for the combination of these multiple services. For example, our asthmatic patient received a 99285 ED service, followed by 8 hours of observation. (Table 63.3) On the UB 04 the facility would report 99285 and 8 units of G0378. The Medicare I/OCE converts those two codes to C-APC 8011, resulting in a single payment for both services to the hospital. Additionally, as a Comprehensive APC the nebulizer treatments as well as typical X-rays and other medications are packaged into the single payment (Table 63.4).

Payment methods for observation vary greatly by payer; the payment may be prospective, such as under Medicare's OPPS rules, hourly, tiered based on blocks of hours, or a case rate. The approximate payment for Medicare observation is $2174 for C-APC 8011.

So, for our asthmatic patient who was initially charged as a 99285 ED visit with reimbursement of $486, with the addition of the 10 units/hours of G0378 the patient now is categorized as Observation, which moves the visit to C-APC 8011 and reimbursement of $2174, representing a roughly $1800 increase.

If observation criteria are not met, the hospital's payment will be based on the service that preceded it – an ED or clinic visit or a direct referral (reported with HCPCS code, G0379).

Most, but not all, commercial payers now recognize and reimburse hospitals for medically necessary observation care. If observation payment policy information is not addressed in the hospital's contract with the payer, the information may be located on the payer's website or in a policy manual. If not found, it will be important for someone at the hospital to query the payer to determine if the observation service is reimbursed and if so, exactly how the payer expects it to be reported. As with all services, it is wise to review payment statements to watch for denials: if all observation payment rules and criteria were met the denial should be appealed.

Compliance Oversight for Observation Services

Recovery Audit Contractors (RACs) and other Medicare contractors, and even private payers, are intensely scrutinizing one-day inpatient stays and use of observation services. Observation has also been identified as an issue of concern in the Office of Inspector General's (OIG's) annual work-plan. For these reasons, and because it is a best practice, hospitals should have written policies and procedures addressing the clinical and revenue cycle aspects of observation services.

These policies should address observation eligibility criteria, medical necessity, and known observation risk areas – physician orders, documentation requirements, physician presence, observation timing issues, standing orders for observation, and excessive lengths of observation over 48 hours. Policies should be based on, and consistent with, internal hospital policies, joint commission standards, state licensure requirements, as well as the Medicare and Medicaid guidelines applicable to the hospital's geographic area.

Observation should be one of the areas monitored under the hospitals compliance plan. Periodic reviews of policies and audits of observation encounters will help identify concerns and opportunities for improvement, and also demonstrate the hospital's commitment to compliance. It is important that someone at the hospital monitors regulatory changes and updates as applicable to observation. This would include CMS's OPPS rules; Medicare Transmittals related to observation; commercial payer, Medicare, and Medicaid website; and commercial payer bulletins. If relevant information is identified it should be communicated internally, added to policies and procedures, and applied to observation revenue cycle practices.

Table 63.3 Typical Medicare Facility Reimbursement Rates

Code	APC	Reimbursement
99284	5024	$326.99
99285	5025	$486.04
99291	5041	$666.27
G0463	5012	$102.12
		$

Source: 2016 OPPS Final Rule

Table 63.4 Medicare Observation Comprehensive APC and Reimbursement

Observation APC and Descriptor	Criteria for Medicare Observation Reimbursement	Reimbursement
C-APC 8011 – Comprehensive Observation Services	Requires at least 8 units of HCPCS code G0378 in addition to 99281–99285, 99291, G0380–G0384, or G0463 on the same day or the day prior.	$2174.14

Source: Medicare Claims Processing Manual; Observation Services

References

1. How Nurses Can Impact the Revenue Cycle. *HFMA–The Business of Caring*, pp.12–13, August, 2007.

2. www.cms.gov/Medicare/ Medicare-Fee-for-Service-Payment/ HospitalOutpatientPPS/ Downloads/Hospital-Outpatient-Therapeutic-Services.pdf (Accessed February 19, 2016)

3. Federal Register, 42 CFR, CMS-1633-FC; CMS Vol. 80, No. 219 November 13, 2015, OPPS Final Rule CY 2016, pp.

4. Medicare Claims Processing Manual 100-04, Chapter 4, Section 290.1 – Observation Services Overview, December 18, 2015 .

5. Medicare Claims Processing Manual 100-04, Chapter 4, Section 290.4.3 – Separate and Packaged Payment for Observation Services, December 18, 2015.

6. Medicare Claims Processing Manual 100-04, Transmittal 1760, Section 290.2.2, July 6, 2009.

7. Medicare Claims Processing Manual 100-04, Chapter 4, Section 290.2.2 – Reporting Hours of Observation, December 18, 2015.

8. Medicare Claims Processing Manual 100-04, Chapter 1, Section 50.3.2 – Policy and Billing Instructions for Condition Code 44, May 8, 2015.

Chapter

64

Determining the Correct Status

BK Kizziar, RN-BC, CCM

Consider the various portals through which patients may enter an acute care hospital. The most common and best known is the Emergency Department. There are also direct admissions from community physician offices. Patients may also be transferred from a lower-level facility to the hospital. Or a hospital-to-hospital transfer may occur. Each of these portals are critical areas for identifying if the patient actually requires an inpatient hospitalization level of care. Often, the admitting physician does not have sufficient clinical information to make the final judgment. However, it may be obvious that the patient does require some level of medical care and further information is required in order to make the determination as to what level of care that might be. In acute care hospitals there are two categories for patients entering through these portals: *Inpatient* and *Observation*.

Inpatient status is given to a patient who requires constant clinical monitoring by licensed professional staff including physicians, nursing, and other care providers. Most hospitals utilize a standardized set of criteria that was developed to assist in the determination of a level of care. The criteria, available from several commercial companies, consists of objective clinical findings and treatments appropriate with the condition and diagnosis. The admission criteria are commonly known as *Severity of Illness (SI)* and includes all of the appropriate levels of care for the condition. During the physician's evaluation of a patient to determine level of care several initial criteria are considered. The criteria are set forth by the *Centers for Medicare and Medicaid Services (CMS)* and include:[1–3]

1. The severity of the signs and symptoms exhibited by the patient,
2. The medical predictability of something adverse happening to the patient,

3. The need for diagnostic studies, acute care level monitoring, medical management, etc.,
4. All available treatment settings and options.

Should a patient not meet the initial screening criteria for an inpatient status but continues to require a significant level of clinical monitoring, the patient may be placed in an Observation status.

Observation is an outpatient designation in which services are provided including the use of a bed, at least periodic monitoring by nursing and other staff, and necessary treatments that are reasonable and necessary to evaluate and treat the patient's condition or determine the need for an inpatient designation and stay. Observation care is rendered in the hospital although classified as outpatient services. It is intended for short-term monitoring, generally less than 48 hours for Medicare patients and 23 hours for managed care patients.

This chapter will speak specifically to Medicare reimbursement criteria as managed companies negotiate various reimbursement systems with their contracting providers. Documentation by the physician is critical in establishing this level of classification. A physician's order must specify "Observation Status" and must be signed and dated by the admitting physician. When the patient has been in Observation Status for 23 hours, physician documentation in the progress notes must include the need to continue observation with a plan for discharge within the next 12–24 hours or the need to convert the patient to an Inpatient Status, documenting the medical necessity for admission or the medical stability of the patient allowing for discharge and a plan for follow-up services a indicated.

"Observation" is a payment category and not an indication of the level of services a patient requires. Should the hospital determine after

Table 64.1 Beneficiary Notices

Type of Notice	Attending or QIO* Concurrence	Patient Liability Begins
Preadmission or Admission HINN	No	Point at which patient enters hospital after receipt of notice is received. However, to hold a patient liable for charges on the day of admission, the notice must be issued no later than 3 p.m. on the day of admission. If the notice is issued after 3 p.m. the patient is liable beginning the following day.
Hospital requested review	Yes	Notification that patient does not qualify for continued stay but the *physician disagrees* and wishes the patient to remain in the hospital. The HRR notifies the patient that the hospital is asking the QIO to review the case and make a determination whether the patient meets clinical criteria to remain in the hospital.
HINN-11	Yes	Noncovered service during covered stay.
HINN-12	Yes	Noncovered continued stay. Includes statement from Business Office estimating the cost to the patient of a continued stay.

* QIO quality improvement organization

admission that the patient did not require an acute level of care there are two options for correcting the status of Medicare beneficiaries. One is known as a "Condition Code 44."[4] The other is "Provider Liable."

Transmittal 299 Change Request 3444 (Condition Code 44) allows the hospital to change a patient status from Inpatient to Observation provided that four criteria are met:

1. The change in patient status from Inpatient to Outpatient/Observation is made prior to discharge or release while the individual is still a patient of the hospital;
2. The hospital has not submitted a claim to CMS for any of the time the patient has spent receiving hospital services;
3. A physician concurs with the utilization review committee's decision; *and*
4. The physician's concurrence with the utilization review committee's decision is documented in the patient's medical records.

The entire episode of care should be treated as though an inpatient admission never took place and should be billed as an outpatient episode of care.

Provider Liable is submitted on a UB-04 claim form indicating the provider is liable for the inpatient admission if the determination that the patient did not meet acute level of care criteria is made after the discharge of the patient.

When a hospital determines that a Medicare beneficiary does not need to be admitted or no longer requires inpatient care, the hospital must notify the beneficiary of this determination. The notification is called a *Hospital Issue Notice of Non-Coverage (HINN)* or a *Medicare Advantage Notice of Discharge and Medicare Appeal Rights (NODMAR)*. If the beneficiary chooses to be admitted or remain in the hospital following this notification, the hospital may charge the beneficiary, rather than Medicare, for the stay. Only the continued stay HINN must be reviewed by the Medicare fiduciary prior to delivery to the patient.

An *Advance Beneficiary Notice (ABN)* is given to a Medicare beneficiary when it is anticipated that the outpatient/observation treatment, care, or services will not be covered by Medicare. The patient must make the decision to forego the intervention or to assume financial responsibility for the cost. This situation is seen typically in the Emergency Department. A patient presents with a condition that does not meet either Inpatient or Observation criteria. However, the patient desires to be admitted and the physician is willing to admit the patient. The patient must be made aware that Medicare will not fund the admission and should the patient be admitted will be expected to pay for all hospital services. If the patient is in Observation status and the physician wishes to change the status to Inpatient although the patient does not meet inpatient criteria, a Pre-Admission Advanced Beneficiary Notice (PAABN) must be issued to the patient indicating that the patient will be financially responsible for all hospital services. In all instances of ABN/PAABN issuances, the patient signature on the form is not required. There must, however, be evidence that the patient was informed as verified by witness signatures on the ABN forms. Claims are submitted with an indication that an ABN was given. (See Table 64.1.)

Medicare has contracted with private auditing firms to review discharged files to determine if patients are classified incorrectly. These auditors, known as *Recovery Audit Contractors (RAC),* review randomly selected discharged charts. Admissions determined to have been inappropriately classified as Inpatient are charged the amount that was paid by Medicare for the inpatient claim. Hospitals may also be fined for continued misclassification. The RACs are reimbursed for their services through a contingency agreement in which they receive a portion of the monies recouped.

Medicare Administrative Contractors (MACs) were put into place to consolidate Medicare Part A and Part B claims processing. The MACs will also compare hospital and physician claims to ensure continuity in billing practices.

The quality of care and treatment of the patient should be the same whether the admission is classified as Inpatient or Observation. The difference is strictly a cost issue. This is an important consideration for patients, hospitals and payers. When admitted under Observation the patient becomes financially responsible for the co-pays associated with their payer requirements. The exact amount varies with the service provided and the payer benefits. Patients may be responsible for more than one co-payment. If the patient's needs are best met in the acute care setting as an Inpatient, the co-pay requirement may be significantly different and deductibles will play a role. However, if after discharge from an acute care inpatient stay the admission was deemed inappropriate, the hospital could be responsible for the entire cost of the stay.

References

1. Centers for Medicaid and Medicare Services (CMS) https://www.cms.gov/Regulations-and-Guidance/Guidance/Transmittals/downloads/R1374CP.pdf (Accessed April 2016)

2. Hospital Inpatient Admission Order and Certification https://www.cms.gov/Medicare/Medicare-Fee-for-Service-Payment/AcuteInpatientPPS/Downloads/IP-Certification-and-Order-09-05-13.pdf (Accessed April 2016)

3. Final Comments for Acute Inpatient Services versus Observation (Outpatient) Services (Hosp-001) DL322. https://downloads.cms.gov/medicare-coverage-database/lcd_attachments/32222_1/DL32222_HOSP001_Final Comments.pdfA (Accessed April 2016)

4. Clarification of Medicare Payment Policy When Inpatient Admission is Determined Not to be Medically Necessary, Including the Use of Condition Code 44: "Inpatient Admission Changed to Outpatient"Transmittal #: R299CP https://www.cms.gov/Outreach-and-Education/Medicare-Learning-Network-MLN/MLNMattersArticles/downloads/SE0622.pdf (Accessed April 2016)

Chapter

65

Case Management: Care Coordination

Nancy E. Skinner, RN-BC, CCM

Observational Status: Care Coordination Through Each Transition of Care

When establishment of the medical necessity and appropriateness of care based on intensity of services and severity of illness fails to meet criteria for admission to an acute care facility, medical management and the consistent monitoring of the patient's health status may be provided as an outpatient service. Deemed observational status, these services are generally utilized to gain additional information regarding the acuity, significance, and/or potential impact of presenting symptoms or to provide continued care or interventions during a prolonged recovery following an outpatient procedure.[1]

Any decision regarding appropriate patient status is based on established criteria, supported by specific and documented clinical rationale, and follows a signed and dated physician order. Determinations regarding the appropriateness of inpatient admission or observational status must be consistent with that physician order, the medical interventions or management to be provided, and the established medical necessity and appropriateness of those services.

Although the hospital utilization review committee and utilization management plan is defined in the hospital Condition of Participation (CoP), the process of adhering to that Plan and following the criteria that supports that Plan is a vital function of the hospital case manager or utilization manager. These health care professionals (HCP) are charged with coordination of each step within the process in order to facilitate effective utilization review and advance appropriate reimbursement for provided services. This is a role that should not be considered to be intermittent or cursory. To be successful, utilization managers should be available within most facilities at least 16 hours each day, every day of the year.

Although observational status is billed as an outpatient service, the quality of provided care is mandated to be the same whether the patient is admitted to the acute care facility or determined to be appropriate for outpatient observation. In March 2011, the U.S. Department of Health and Human Services released its National Strategy for Quality Improvement in Health Care (National Quality Strategy). The strategy presents three aims for the health care system:

- Better Care: Improve the overall quality, by making health care more patient-centered, reliable, accessible, and safe.
- Healthy People and Communities: Improve the health of the U.S. population by supporting proven interventions to address behavioral, social, and environmental determinants of health in addition to delivering higher-quality care.
- Affordable Care: Reduce the cost of quality health care for individuals, families, employers, and government.[2]

The six priorities identified to support these aims include:

- Making care safer by reducing harm caused in the delivery of care.
- Ensuring that each person and family are engaged as partners in their care.
- Promoting effective communication and coordination of care.
- Supporting better health in communities.
- Prevention and treatment of the leading causes of mortality.
- Making quality care more affordable for individuals, families, employers, and governments by developing and spreading new health care delivery models.[3]

As today's health care facilities and providers look to following these strategies and to provide care that is "safe, timely, effective, efficient, equitable and patient-centered," the focus on quality of care, cost of provided services and patient satisfaction has never been higher.[4] To achieve this delicate balance, many hospitals have established specific protocols that are designed to address the efficient movement of patients to an appropriate level of care. These steps include a focus on gaining physician direction regarding the appropriate level of patient care based on a comprehensive assessment of the patient's history and physical exam, any risk factors that are present or probable due to the patient's condition, and the care required to address patient-specific continuing needs. Additionally, the physician must document the order to provide observational care and confirmation that similar criteria is utilized for all patients regardless of payer.

While each step in the utilization review process is generally well scripted and supported by established criteria, the process that encourages patient/family engagement in their care and facilitates an efficient and timely transition to the next level of care is often fragmented and haphazard. Patients sometimes move from one environment or provider to another with little advocacy, no established transitional care plan, and absolutely no idea that it should not be that way. We "treat 'em and street 'em." We "diagnosis and adios" and rarely consider affecting an appropriate transition of care. In many instances, this lack of care continuity may negatively impact the goals we desire for our patients and the goals our patients have established for themselves.

To be more successful in facilitating enhanced patient engagement and promoting effective communication across all levels of care, it is vital that the role of the case manager is not limited to utilization review. Case management is defined by the Case Management Society of America (CMSA) as:

> Case management is a collaborative process of assessment, planning, facilitation, and advocacy for options and services to meet an individual's health needs through communication and available resources to promote quality cost-effective outcomes.[5]

To fulfill this role and adhere to the intent if not the content of this definition, the case manager is charged with coordination of transitional services as the patient moves to the next level of care and the next provider of services. This function is not limited to traditional discharges that occur at the end of inpatient admissions but also includes the coordination of care as the patient moves from the portal of entry to observational status and from observation to following level or site of care.

The multidisciplinary treatment team is charged with both the provision of care and patient empowerment, engagement, and education during any hospital stay or intervention. This includes every patient who receives observational monitoring and care. Some outpatient environments employ case managers to provide effective care coordination. Other hospitals utilize members of the care delivery team to achieve this role. But, in every health care setting, care coordination must be an essential element of the stay and never be an afterthought or intended intervention that is not consistently delivered.

Care coordination as defined by the National Quality Forum (NQF) is a "function that helps ensure that the patient's needs and preferences for health services and information sharing across people, functions, and sites are met over time. It maximizes the value of services delivered to patients by facilitating beneficial, efficient, safe, and high-quality patient experiences and improved health care outcomes."[6] Care coordination typically encompasses the assessment of the patient's needs, the development and implementation of a plan of care, and an evaluation of the care plan.

Transitional care, a more targeted form of care coordination, is a set of actions designed to advance the coordination and the continuity of health care services as patients transfer between different locations or different levels of care within the same location.[7] In order to deliver efficient and effective care coordination services, an appropriate "handover" of the patient to subsequent care providers and care givers is absolutely necessary. The initial step in this process begins when the patient enters the acute care facility seeking health care services and includes the following:

- What is the patient's primary concern regarding their health status?
- Did a member of the team perform a comprehensive evaluation of past history and current physical condition?

- What is the name or names of HCP who provide or provided care to the patient in the past?
- Has a member of the health care team attempted to reach out to that HCP to gain further information regarding the patient's health status?
- Has the patient made any decision regarding advance directives?
- Which medications are currently being prescribed for the patient? Which medications have been prescribed in the past?
- What medication regimen does the patient currently follow including over-the-counter medications?
- Does a local pharmacy or pharmacy benefit manager fill current prescriptions?
- What is the patient's understanding of their current diagnosis or diagnoses?
- Does the patient possess and maintain a personal health record?

After a determination is made regarding placement to observational status, who is primarily responsibility for assuring an appropriate handover of the patient to the HCP that will be managing that patient's care during an observational stay? Additionally, the process of patient engagement, empowerment, and education must begin if it had not already been initiated in the emergency department or other portal to care. Education minimally includes information regarding the diagnosis and what that diagnosis means. It is vital that all education be provided based on the patient's health literacy and cultural beliefs. Subsequent education is generally focused on moving the patient to self-management of their disease state and active participation in their plan of care.

As the patient prepares to transition out of observation to the next level of care, it is vital that each patient receives the following:

- Verbal and written information regarding their diagnosis and what that diagnosis means.
- A copy of the prescribed treatment plan including a medication list that has been reconciled.
- A list of the potential signs of disease exacerbation and the steps to take if that increase in symptoms occurs.
- A referral to community-based care management if those services are available in

Table 65.2 Key Measures for National Quality Strategy Priority – Promoting Effective Communication and Coordination of Care[8]

Measure Focus	Key Measure Name/ Description
3-item care transition measure	- During this hospital stay, staff took my preferences and those of my family or caregiver into account in deciding what my health care needs would be when I left - When I left the hospital, I had a good understanding of the things I was responsible for in managing my health - When I left the hospital, I clearly understood the purpose for taking each of my medications

the geographic region in which the patient resides.

- An appointment for physician care in the community.

Although the following measures have not been implemented for outpatient environments as yet, the consistently changing and expanding regulations and reimbursement associated with a satisfactory patient experience are expected to touch outpatient services in the future.[8] To prepare for that probability, it is recommended that HCPs and acute care facilities that serve patients in outpatient settings begin to consider the Key Measures for the National Quality Strategy Priority.[9] One set of those measures is detailed in Table 65.2.

Consider who within your current health care delivery environment advances the patient's ability to positively respond to those three key descriptors. If no one member of the team shoulders that responsibility, it is time to reengineer the transition of care in order to facilitate the timely movement of the patient through the health care continuum. It is my belief that the one member of the team who is this facilitator is the care coordinator or case manager. Their role must minimally include a role that reflects the established definition of case management while achieving that delicate balance of fiscal responsibility and patient advocacy.

References

1. Medicare Benefit Policy Manual, CMS Pub. 100-02, Chapter 6, §20.6.

2. DHHS. National Strategy for Quality Improvement in Health Care. www.healthcare .gov/center/reports/national qualitystrategy032011.pdf March 2011.

3. Ibid.

4. O'Reilly, K. Health Reform Law Will Boost Care Quality. Amednews.com. www .ama-assn.org/amednews /2010/12/20/prse1221.htm. June 2012.

5. Case Management Society of America Standards of Practice for Case Management, Revised 2010. www.cmsa.org/SOP. June 2012.

6. National Quality Forum (NQF) - Endorsed definition and framework for measuring care coordination. Available at www.qualityforum.org/ projects/care_coordination .aspx. June 2012.

7. Coleman EA, Berenson RA. Lost in transition: challenges and opportunities for improving the quality of transitional care. *Ann Intern Med.* 2004;141:533–536.

8. 2012 Annual Progress Report to Congress – National Strategy for Quality Improvement in Health Care. Corrected August 2012 and May 2014. www .ahrq.gov/workingforquality/ nqs/nqs2012annlrpt.pdf. June 2012. (Accessed April 2016)

9. Ibid.

Chapter

66

Medical Necessity

Robert H. Leviton, MD, MPH, FACEP, Diplomate, ABPM, Clinical Informatics

In 1965, President Eisenhower suffered an uncomplicated anterior wall myocardial infarction and spent 7 weeks convalescing in a hospital where he was not permitted any physical activity, allowed only to be carried to and from his bed by two corpsmen; the same treatment was equally provided to less notable individuals.[1] Hospital length of stay was highly individualized and prolonged; no two physicians or hospitals followed any particular regimen, often adhering to their own judgment about tests that were needed or the amount of time a patient would remain hospitalized. Patients would stay in hospitals for weeks or months for treatments that today would require only a few days.

In that same year, President Johnson signed into law the Social Security Act of 1965 where Title XVII and XIX enacted the formation of Medicare and Medicaid to provide health insurance coverage to more than 19 million people. Within the many provisions of the law, regulation 42 CFR 482.30, section 1861 (k) required "each hospital to develop a utilization review plan to review hospital admissions, the duration of hospital stays, the professional services provided (including drugs and biological) furnished, (A) with respect to the medical necessity of the service and (B) for the purpose of promoting the most efficient use of available health facilities and services."

In the early years of utilization review, guidance for making admission and length of stay decisions was provided by the Professional Activity Study, a principal service of the Commission on Professional and Hospital Activities. While an early important source for the research, evaluation, planning, and management of patient care and monitoring regional trends in diseases and in medical procedures, some studies suggested that there were operational problems with the methods in performing reviews.[2] Regional differences in the approach to care[3] led to a government request for assistance developing a quality assurance program based upon severity of illness and intensity of service criteria, later including appropriateness of admissions, levels of service, and discharge screens. Responding to this request, the InterQual criteria was first published in 1978 and by the 1990s, the Centers for Medicare and Medicaid Services (CMS) licensed InterQual criteria for use in reviewing Medicare hospital inpatient services.[4]

Since its inception in 1965, the Medicare program has only paid for those health care items and services that are considered to be medically necessary and relevant to improving or maintaining the health of a beneficiary. In particular, Section 1862(a)(1) of the Social Security Act prohibits payment for services or procedures that are not "reasonable and necessary for the diagnosis or treatment of an illness or injury or to improve the functioning of a malformed body member." Accordingly, Medicare carriers have generally used the following criteria to determine the medical necessity of specific items and services:

- Consistent with the symptoms or diagnoses of the illness or injury under treatment.
- Necessary and consistent with generally accepted professional medical standards (i.e., not experimental or investigational).
- Not furnished primarily for the convenience of the patient, the attending physician, or another physician or supplier.
- Furnished at the most appropriate level that can be provided safely and effectively to the patient.

With the rise of third-party payers and managed care health care coverage programs, there was increasing concern in contract reviews that revealed language imposing "lower cost" criteria being included in the definition of medical necessity. This raised the question whether some health plans were basing their medical necessity determination on a standard that provided patients a lower quality of care than most physicians would provide without the cost-of-services concerns. Lawsuits abounded and alleged that since 1990, Aetna, CIGNA, Health Net, Prudential, Anthem/WellPoint, and Humana engaged in a conspiracy to improperly deny, delay, or reduce payment to physicians by engaging in several types of improper conduct, including failing to pay for "medically necessary" services in accordance with member plan documents.[5] Under the terms of the settlement agreements between 2003 and 2006, each company agreed to accept a definition of medical necessity.

The American Medical Association (AMA) has numerous policies regarding medical necessity and strongly recommends that physicians should review their health insurance plan's medical services agreements for their specific definition of medical necessity. The AMA policy defines medical necessity as:

> Health care services or products that a prudent physician would provide to a patient for the purpose of preventing, diagnosing or treating an illness, injury, or disease or its symptoms in a manner that is: (a) in accordance with generally accepted standards of medical practice; (b) clinically appropriate in terms of type, frequency, extent, site, and duration; and (c) not primarily for the economic benefit of the health insurers and purchasers or for the convenience of the patient, treating physician, or other health care provider.[6]

In its original intent, Congress sought to define medical necessity as a means to assure physicians and hospitals were paid for services they provided their patients. As health care costs continued to rise, both the public and private sector began to seek new methods for controlling costs while managing increasingly complex, new and expensive technologies and treatments. Emergency physicians must be aware of the complex and widening array of programs that seek to define how their care decisions may be scrutinized and questioned. The following list of programs, reports, and activities serve as a reference point to begin more detailed study and preparations to best manage your department's policy and procedures relating to medically necessary care,

appropriate test ordering, coding, and patient disposition status.

National and Local Coverage Determinants

National Coverage Determinants (NCDs) are developed by CMS to describe circumstances for Medicare Coverage for a specific medical service, procedure, or device. NCDs generally outline the conditions for which a service is considered to be covered or not covered under Medicare coverage and is limited to items and services that are reasonable and necessary for the diagnosis or treatment of an illness or injury. The primary authority for all coverage provisions and subsequent policies is the Social Security Act, section 1862(a)(1). NCDs are made through evidence-based processes[7] that allow for public comment periods. It is important for emergency physicians to be aware of those tests or medications that may not be covered for a patient's visit.

For example, a finger stick glucose determination often necessary for the management of patients with diabetes mellitus may be denied payment because repeat testing may not be indicated unless abnormal results are found and documented or there is a documented change in a patient's condition. If repeat testing is performed, a specific diagnosis code should be reported to support medical necessity.

Computed tomography requires that sufficient medical record documentation be provided with claims to insure that the requested CT scan is reasonable and necessary for the individual patient; that is, the use of CT scanning must be found to be medically appropriate considering the patient's symptoms and preliminary diagnosis. A case reviewer may determine that the use of a CT scan as the initial diagnostic test was not reasonable and necessary because it was not supported by the patient's symptoms or complaints as stated in the medical record or claims form.

In the absence of a national policy, Medicare contractors may use their discretion to establish medical policy, earlier described as Local Medical Review Policies (LMRPs) but now referred to as Local Coverage Determinants (LCDs). Each Medicare contractor may develop LCDs pertinent to its area of jurisdiction when a validated, widespread problem demonstrates a significant risk to the Medicare Trust Fund, identified as potentially high-dollar and/or high-volume services.

Emergency physicians are expected to be aware of both current NCDs and LCDs coverage policies. The Medicare Coverage Database (MCD)[8] contains all NCDs and LCDs, local articles, and proposed NCD decisions. The database also includes several other types of National Coverage policy-related documents, including National Coverage Analyses (NCAs), Coding Analyses for Labs (CALs), Medicare Evidence Development & Coverage Advisory Committee (MEDCAC) proceedings, and Medicare coverage guidance documents.

Remember, when a patient's medical care may not be covered because it is not medically necessary and reasonable in a particular case, you are obliged to provide the patient with an Advanced Beneficiary Notice (ABN).[9] The ABN indicates the patient's choice to receive the item or service and accept the financial liability for the care.

National Correct Coding Initiative (NCCI)

CMS developed the NCCI to promote national correct coding methodologies and to control improper coding leading to inappropriate payment in Part B claims. These coding polices are based upon coding conventions defined by the American Medical Association's Current Procedural Terminology (CPT) manual, national and local policies and edits, coding guidelines developed by national societies, analysis of standard medical and surgical practices, and a review of current coding practices. CMS annually updates the National Correct Coding Initiative Coding Policy Manual for Medicare Service and is used by carriers and Fiscal Intermediaries as a general reference that explains the rationale for NCCI edits.

For example, a patient who has chronic pain to the foot after sustaining a contusion was noted to have a normal plain film radiography study on a previous admission. The emergency physician elected to order an MRI to evaluate the potential for stress fracture of the foot. The claim form was submitted and ICD-10 code S90.30 (contusion of unspecified foot) and the procedure code 73721, (Magnetic Resonance Imaging, any joint of the lower extremity, without contrast material). The claim was rejected because "coverage of this procedure with the given diagnosis is not covered, based upon the official Medical Review Policy."

The purpose of the NCCI edits is to prevent improper payment when incorrect code combinations are reported.

Office of Inspector General Annual Work Plan[10–12]

The Office of the Inspector General (OIG) was created to protect the integrity of the Health and Human Services (HHS) programs and operations as well as the well-being of beneficiaries by detecting fraud, waste, and abuse; identifying opportunities to improve program economy, efficiency, and effectiveness; and holding accountable those who do not meet program requirements or who violate Federal laws.

The OIG collaborates with HHS and its operating staff divisions, the Department of Justice (DOJ) and other executive branch agencies, Congress, and States to bring about systemic changes, successful prosecutions, negotiated settlements, and recovery of funds. Each year, the OIG considers mandatory requirements for reviews as described by laws, regulations, or other directives; requests made by Congress, HHS Management, and the Office of Management and Budget; and work to be performed in collaboration with partner organizations.

The OIG Work Plan outlines the current focus areas and states the primary objectives for each review. The plan is published annually usually during the first week of October. Reviews slated to begin in 2015 could result in 2015 or 2016 reports.[11,12]

It is important for emergency physicians to know the study and review areas within the OIG Work Plan to ascertain whether a study topic will impact on the policies and procedures of their practices and departments. For example, in the 2012 Work Plan the following reviews impact on the Emergency Department (ED):

- Hospital admissions with conditions coded Present on Admission (POA) – review claims to determine which facilities most frequently transfer patients with certain diagnoses, for example, pressure ulcers that were coded as being present when patients were admitted. For certain diagnoses specified by CMS, hospitals will receive a lower payment if the specified diagnoses were acquired in the hospital.

- Accuracy of POA Indicators Submitted on Medicare Claims – hospitals do not receive additional payments for certain conditions that were not present when the patient was admitted. Recent law provides that hospitals with high rates of hospital acquired conditions (HACs) will receive reduced payments. Accurate POA indicators are needed for CMS to implement the requirements of the Act when reviewing medical records and Medicare claims.

- Observation services during outpatient visits – OIG will review Medicare payments for observation services provided by hospital outpatient departments, including EDs, to assess the appropriateness of the services and their effect on Medicare beneficiaries' out-of-pocket expenses for health care services. Part B covers hospital outpatient services and reimbursement for such services under the hospital outpatient prospective payment system.

Hospital Payment Monitoring Program[13]

(Hospital Payment Monitoring Program HPMP) was created by CMS to measure, monitor and reduce the incidence of improper fee-for-service inpatient Medicare payments. This includes the provision of medically unnecessary services, the provision of services in inappropriate settings, errors in Diagnosis-Related Group (DRG) assignment and or coding, errors in billing, and errors in prepayment denials.

During 2002, the Peer Review Organizations were renamed Quality Improvement Organizations (QIOs). As specified in 42CFR 476.71(a)(6), QIO reviews of hospital medical records must indicate that inpatient hospital care was medically necessary, reasonable, and appropriate for the diagnosis and condition of the patient at any time during the stay. The patient must demonstrate signs and or symptoms severe enough to warrant the need for medical care and must receive services of such intensity that they can be furnished safely and effectively only on an inpatient basis. Similarly, these reviews seek to determine whether a patient has been prematurely discharged from the hospital, that is, the patient was not medically stable and/or discharge was not consistent with the patient's need for continued acute inpatient hospital care.[14]

The HPMP Compliance Workbook provides numerous suggestions and tools for hospitals to develop programs to control activities that can lead to citation by their QIO or other regulatory agency.

Program for Evaluating Payment Patterns Electronic Report[15]

Under contract with the CMS, the TMF Health Quality Institute (web site: www.tmf.org) provides hospitals with an electronic data report that contains a single hospital's claims data statistics for Medicare severity DRGs and discharges at high risk for improper payment due to billing, coding, and or admission necessity issues. Data in (Program for Evaluating Payment Patterns Electronic Report PEPPER) such as 30-Day Readmission to same hospital, 2-day stays for heart failure and shock (DRG 291,292,293), cardiac arrhythmia (DRG 308, 309), and esophagitis or gastroenteritis (DRG 391, 392) are some of the data elements presented in tabular form as well as in graphs that depict the hospital's target areas percentages over time. The PEPPER report is designed to assist hospitals to identify potential overpayments as well as potential underpayments.

Comprehensive Error Rate Testing

CMS developed the Comprehensive Error Rate Testing (CERT) program[16] to determine national, contractor specific, provider compliance error rates, paid claim error rates, and claims processing error rates. The CERT measures error rate claims submitted to Medicare Administrative Contractors (MACs). The CERT Methodology includes randomly selecting a sample of approximately 120,000 submitted claims, requesting medical records of providers who submitted claims, and reviewing the claims and medical records for compliance with Medicare coverage, coding, and billing rules.

Medicare Administrative Contractors

Under the recent Medicare contracting reform initiative, Fiscal Intermediaries and carriers are being replaced by Medicare Administrative Contractors (MACs).[17] Through the initial series of

Part A/B MAC procurements, Medicare's claim processing operations have realized significant operational savings from the consolidation of state workloads. Emergency physicians should be knowledgeable of their MAC work plans[18] and efforts to manage the administration of all Medicare services. MAC jurisdictions are awarded regionally and currently comprise 15 regions but will be consolidated to 10 in the next several years. New York, Connecticut, Illinois, Indiana, Michigan, and Wisconsin are managed by National Government Services whose website, www.ngsmedicare.com/wps/portal/ngsmedicare, provides valuable content for Medicare providers.

Recovery Audit Program

Section 302 of the Tax Relief and Health Care Act of 2006 made the Recovery Audit Program (RACs)[19] a permanent and required expansion of the program in all 50 states no later than 2010. Each RAC is responsible for identifying overpayments and underpayments in our country. RAC jurisdictions match the Durable Medical Equipment MAC jurisdictions.

RACs review claims on a post payment basis and may be automated where no medical record is needed or manually reviewed where the medical record is required. A demand letter is issued by the RAC requesting the hospital to supply medical records for review; if there is an improper payment determination, the RAC will offer an opportunity for the provider to discuss the improper payment determination. Issues identified by the RAC will be approved by CMS prior to widespread review posting on the RAC's website. If you agree with the RAC's determination, you may pay by check, allow recoupment from future payments, request for an extended payment plan, or appeal the determination.

It is important for the emergency physician to review their jurisdiction's RAC website for new issues, vulnerabilities, and detailed result reviews. Previous improper payment determinations are also listed in the OIG and CERT reports. If you are familiar with these findings, you can protect your practice by assuring proper policies and procedures are in place for documenting the medical necessity and appropriateness of care. Keep track of denied claims, look for patterns of errors, then determine what corrective actions you need to take to avoid improper payments.

Observation Care and Medical Necessity

In a 2010 communication, the U.S. Attorney's Officer for the Western District of New York, in conjunction with the U.S. Department of Health and Human Services, Office of Inspector General, the DOJ reviewed certain zero and 1-day chest pain admissions. The review involved assessments of the medical necessity of chest pain admissions and the claim submission related to the procedures treating the patient's chest pain. After reviewing the records from the hospital, the US DOJ determined that there were concerns with the billing for 1-day stays applying Medicare rules for inpatient services.

The DOJ wrote, "Medicare generally describes that an inpatient site of service is appropriate for a patient who is admitted to a hospital for the purposes of receiving inpatient hospital services." When assessing whether a patient requires inpatient level of services, the provider must consider whether the "patient demonstrate[s] signs and/or symptoms severe enough to warrant the need for medical care and must receive services of such intensity that they can be furnished safely and effectively in an inpatient basis."

The letter continued by citing the Medical Benefit Policy Manual (ch.1, section 10) and the Medicare Quality Improvement Organization Manual (section 4110), describing that "inpatient care rather than outpatient (or observation status) care is required only if the patient's medical condition, safety, or health would be significantly and directly threatened if care was provide in a less intensive setting." The author of the letter concluded by describing, "the critical assessment as to whether patient safety or health would have been significantly and directly threatened by care in a less intensive setting requires more than a monotonous physician provider's decision to admit all patients with chest pain. The medically necessary and documented treatment will be a significant factor in assessing the credibility of any safety or health claim offered by the institutional or individual practitioner."

One can readily appreciate why there is a growing consensus to use observation services to meet the needs and requirements of our patient's care while remaining within the guidelines and definitions of medical necessity and the appropriateness of services.

When providing Observation care[20] – which includes certain short-term services such as treatment, assessment, and reassessment that are furnished while a decision is being made regarding whether patients will require further treatment as hospital inpatients or if they are able to be discharged from the hospital – it is important to accurately document the reasons for placement in the Observation Service. Have you adequately documented within the patient's medical record:

- Current medical needs
- Patients medical history
- Stability/instability of vital signs
- Presence or absence of severe pain
- Current diagnosis, including chronic and acute conditions
- Laboratory and other test results relating to the need for an observation stay
- Severity of other signs/symptoms
- Physician concerns from a clinical perspective
- Medical likelihood of an adverse outcome if the patient is not placed in an observation setting
- Risks if the patient is discharged home
- Patients' reaction to treatment
- Discussions with the patient and family
- Communication with patient/family concerning the rationale behind the treatment decisions.

Observation services must be reasonable and necessary to be covered by Medicare. In only rare and exceptional cases do reasonable and necessary outpatient observation services span more than 48 hours. In the majority of cases, the decision whether to discharge a patient from the hospital following resolution of the reason for the observation care or to admit the patient as an inpatient can be made in less than 48 hours, usually in less than 24 hours.

Improper use of observation services may subject beneficiaries to high cost sharing. It is extremely important to remember the need to advise the patient that they are being placed in an observation service and not admitted to the hospital. Many patients remaining in the hospital overnight may believe they are admitted to the hospital rather than being kept for observation services. This will make a difference on their hospital bill as patients may be obligated for an unexpected co-payment while medications may also not be covered. A handy guide to provide patients is the pamphlet, "Are You a Hospital Inpatient or Outpatient?"[21]

In other instances, a patient may insist upon being admitted to the hospital when, in fact, there is not a medically necessary reason to substantiate the admission. In these instances it is best to provide the patient with a Hospital Issued Notice of Noncoverage (HINN) model letter[22] that describes the financial liability protections provided under the patient's policy coverage.[23]

Observation services should not be billed concurrently with other diagnostic or therapeutic services for which active monitoring is a part of the procedure (e.g., colonoscopy for acute gastrointestinal bleeding, Cardiac Stress Testing). In situations where such a procedure interrupts observation services, hospitals may determine the most appropriate way to account for this time. For example, a hospital may record the beginning and ending time during the outpatient observation encounter for each period of diagnostic or therapeutic service, then add the total length of time for each period of observation services together to obtain the total number of units reported on the claim for the hourly observation services using the Healthcare Common Procedure Coding System (HCPCS) code G0378 (Hospital observation service, per hour). A hospital would then deduct the average length of time of the interrupting procedure from the total duration of time that the patient receives observation services.

Observation time ends when all medically necessary services related to observation care are completed. For example, this could be before discharge when the need for observation has ended, but other medically necessary services not meeting the definition of observation care are provided (in which case, the additional medically necessary services would be billed separately or included as part of the ED or clinic visit).

Alternatively, the end time of observation services may coincide with the time the patient is actually discharged from the hospital or admitted as an inpatient. Observation time may include medically necessary services and follow-up care provided after the time that the physician writes the discharge order, but before the patient is discharged. However, reported observation time would not include the time patients remain in the hospital after treatment is finished for reasons such as waiting for transportation home.

There are instances where a physician may order a patient to be admitted to the hospital to an inpatient bed, and not an observation bed. However, upon subsequent review by a utilization review committee, it is determined that an inpatient level does not meet the hospital's admission criteria. The National Uniform Billing Committee (NUBC) provided CMS a new condition code that all emergency physicians should be aware of, the Condition Code 44, applied when an inpatient admission is changed to outpatient or observation service.[24]

When a Condition Code 44 has been applied, there are several conditions that must be met to successfully submit an outpatient claim for Medicare Part B services:

a) The change in patient status from inpatient to outpatient is made prior to discharge or release, while the patient is still in the hospital;

b) The hospital has not submitted a claim to Medicare for the inpatient admission;

c) A physician concurs with the utilization review committee's decision; and

d) The physician's concurrence with the utilization review committee's decision is documented in the patient's medical record.

When the hospital has determined that conditions above have been met, it may submit an outpatient claim and the entire episode of care should be treated as though the inpatient admission never occurred.

Creating a check list or electronic guidance using an electronic health record (EHR) clinical decision support will often assist you in determining whether a patient is a candidate for observation services or inpatient admission and avoid many of the reviews, citations, and denials described here. Some suggestions for your medical record:

- Does the patient's placement in observation services comply with the hospital's bylaws and admission policies?
- Is the patient acutely ill?
- Does the patient require an observation level of care?
- Does the patient require observation care monitoring?
- Dose the patient require observation care services?
- Does the patient require hospital services that can be provided only in an observation setting?

- Are observation services medically required based upon the patient's medical condition?
- Based upon the patient's medical condition, can care be provided safely and effectively within the observation setting?
- Do diagnostic studies used to assess the medical necessity of inpatient admission require a hospital stay of less than 24 hours?
- Are the facilities needed by the physician to perform the procedure/test available in an outpatient setting in the local community?
- Is the procedure to be performed medically necessary with regard to relevant community standards of practice?
- Does the patient's history prior to observation support the need for observation services?
- Could the patient's treatment have been performed safely in an outpatient setting?
- Does this patient's initial clinical presentation indicate the need for observation service?
- Does the patient care record contain medically justified explanations of why the patient's condition requires at least a 24-hour stay?
- Do later tests results support a finding that admission was medically necessary, that is, following the evaluation is it likely that the patient will need inpatient services for more than 24 hours?
- Does the patient condition or care receiving in the observation setting substantiate the need for inpatient admission?

Once these conditions have been met, you are certain to have met the criteria of medical necessity.

Summary

As our health care system continuously transforms, seeking new methods to provide our patients with the highest quality of care, with complex medical conditions, requiring new services and technology, it will always be incumbent on the emergency physician to deftly describe the medical necessity for the patient's admission to avoid the consequences of denied care or payment. Use of Observation Services as described in the following chapters will certainly provide a successful pathway to assure optimal outcomes for our patients.

References

1. Curfman, G. Shorter hospital stay for myocardial infarction. *N Eng J Med.* 1988 Apr 28; 318:1123–1125.

2. Buford, R, Averill, RF. The relationship between diagnostic information available at admission and discharge for patients in one PSRO setting: implications for concurrent review. *Med Care.* 1979 Apr;17 (4):369–381.

3. Lanska, DJ. Length of hospital stay for cerebrovascular disease in the United States: Professional Activity Study, 1963–1991. *J Neurol Sci.* 1994 Dec 20;127(2):214–220.

4. Mitus, AJ. The birth of InterQual, evidence based decision support criteria that helped change healthcare. *Professional Case Management* 2008;13(4):228–233.

5. OLR Research Report, Defining Medical Necessity; www.cga.ct.gov/2007/rpt/2007-r-0055.htm (last accessed February 20, 2016)

6. Statement of the American Medical Association to the Institute of Medicine's Committee on Determination of Essential Health Benefits. January 14, 2011. http://iom.nationalacademies.org/~/media/8D03963CAEB24450947C1AEC0CAECD85.ashx (Accessed February 20, 2016)

7. Medicare Coverage Determination Process; www.cms.gov/Medicare/Coverage/DeterminationProcess/index.html (last accessed February 20, 2016)

8. Medicare Coverage Database; www.cms.gov/medicare-coverage-database/overview-and-quick-search.aspx (last accessed February 20, 2016)

9. Advance Beneficiary Notice of Noncoverage; www.cms.gov/Outreach-and-Education/Medicare-Learning-Network-MLN/MLNProducts/downloads/ABN_Booklet_ICN006266.pdf (last accessed February 20, 2016)

10. Office of the Inspector General Work Plan, Fiscal Year 2012; http://oig.hhs.gov/reports-and-publications/archives/workplan/2012/Work-Plan-2012.pdf (last accessed February 20, 2016)

11. Office of the Inspector General Work Plan, Fiscal Year 2015; http://oig.hhs.gov/reports-and-publications/archives/workplan/2015/FY15-Work-Plan.pdf (last accessed February 20, 2016)

12. Office of the Inspector General Work Plan, Fiscal Year 2016; http://oig.hhs.gov/reports-and-publications/archives/workplan/2016/oig-work-plan-2016 (last accessed February 20, 2016)

13. Hospital Payment Monitoring Program; www.metastar.com/Web/Portals/0/Documents/HPMP/HPMP-ComplianceWorkbook.pdf (last accessed February 20, 2016)

14. Quality Improvement Organization Manual, Chapter 4, Case Reviews; www.cms.gov/Regulations-and-Guidance/Guidance/Manuals/downloads/qio110c04.pdf (last accessed February 20, 2016)

15. PEPPER, Short-term Acute Care Program for Evaluating Payment Patterns Electronic Report; www.pepperresources.org/LinkClick.aspx?fileticket=HaExUlAgiVo%3d&tabid=92 (last accessed February 20, 2016)

16. Comprehensive Error Rate Testing; www.cms.gov/Research-Statistics-Data-and-Systems/Monitoring-Programs/CERT/index.html?redirect=/CERT/ (last accessed February 20, 2016)

17. Medicare Contracting Reform; www.cms.gov/Medicare/Medicare-Contracting/Medicare/ContractingReform/index.html (last accessed February 20, 2016)

18. MAC Jurisdictions Map and Contacts; www.cms.gov/Medicare/Medicare-Contracting/MedicareContracting Reform/PartAandPartBMAC Jurisdictions.html (last accessed February 20, 2016)

19. Recovery Audit Contractor; www.cms.gov/Research-Statistics-Data-and-Systems/Monitoring-Programs/recovery-audit-program/index.html?redirect=/Recovery-Audit-Program/ (last accessed February 20, 2016)

20. Outpatient Observation Services, Medicare Claims Processing Manual Chapter 4 Part B Hospital; www.cms.gov/Regulations-and-Guidance/Guidance/Manuals/downloads/clm104c04.pdf (last accessed February 20, 2016)

21. CMS; Are You a Hospital Inpatient or Outpatient?; www.medicare.gov/publications/pubs/pdf/11435.pdf (last accessed February 20, 2016)

22. Hospital Issued Notice of NonCoverage/HINN; www.cms.gov/Medicare/Medicare-General-Information/BNI/downloads/HINNs1to10.pdf (last accessed February 20, 2016)

23. https://www.cms.gov/Regulations-and-Guidance/Guidance/Manuals/downloads/clm104c30.pdf (last accessed February 20, 2016)

24. CMS Manual System, Pub.100-04 Medicare Claims Processing, Transmittal 299, "Use of Condition Code 44, Inpatient Admission Changed to Outpatient," September 10, 2004.

Denials and Appeals

Robert H. Leviton, MD, MPH, FACEP

There will soon come a day when you arrive on your shift to find a letter from a health care plan or perhaps your hospital's Utilization Management Department describing that the care you provided to your patient has been denied; the health care plan wants to take back several thousands of dollars of paid reimbursement because your care was determined to be "medically unnecessary." What are you to do?

If your original medical record documentation has been clear and consistent with current standards of care and practice, you may be okay; if not, it's time to brush up on how to meet the standards of medical necessity and be relieved that all initial claims determinations have the right to be appealed. Processes have been defined by the patient's health care insurance plan or by the Medical Administrative Contractors (MAC), the Fiscal Intermediaries (FIs) who contract with Medicare or Medicaid to provide services, and assure all health care services claims are processed, corrected, adjusted, or cancelled. These same FIs may make inquiries for the status of claims, make requests for additional information, determine patient eligibility, and review the various codes applied to the bill for services.

There are many reasons that the care you provided a patient may be denied:

- Mutually exclusive, incidental, down coding, or bundling of procedure codes
- Health Care Insurance Plan contract or fee schedule or reimbursement terms
- Modifier used for reimbursement; Current Procedural Terminology (CPT) modifier 25 (e.g., a significant, separately billable service is provided on the same day by the same physician) or 59 (e.g., procedures or services that are commonly bundled together but are appropriate to report separately under some circumstances) from the medical code set maintained by the American Medical Association

- Inpatient facility denial due to level of care, length of stay, delayed treatment day
- Experimental or Investigational procedure
- Medical necessity of service
- Timely claim filing
- Precertification/Authorization not obtained
- Request for in-network benefits
- Benefit plan exclusion or limitation
- Benefit plan administration (i.e., co-pay, deductible, etc.)
- Maximum reimbursable amount attained

Generally, there are denials for billing or coding issues and for care that was determined to be medically unnecessary. Each carrier will have a defined number of days to appeal the denied services and several levels of process that a physician may follow to successfully overturn the denial for services.[1] Blue Cross Blue Shield allows providers 90 calendar days from the claim adjudication date to submit Level 1 billing, coding, or Medical Necessity Provider Appeals. Cigna[2] allows 180 calendar days from the date of the initial payment or denial decision.[3] These time periods are critical to know so you do not lose the opportunity to appeal a denial. Other contractual language may describe that a third party, such as your billing agency, cannot act on your behalf in the appeals process; you have to write the letter yourself. Be sure to have someone in your practice create a health insurance plan denials management log that lists each carrier's appeals process.[4]

Once receiving your appeal information, the insurer has a contractually defined period, in some instances 30 calendar days to complete the Level 1 Provider Appeal review and respond to your letter. Each carrier may have a nurse reviewer determine whether the appeal may be reversed or not; if not reversed, the appeal will be turned over to their physician reviewer or plan Medical Director.

If you are not satisfied with the First Level review decision, always request a Second Level Payment Review. In general, the Second Level review must be initiated within 60 calendar days of the date of the First Level review decision letter. These Second Level reviews must be handled by a reviewer who was not involved in the initial decision or First Level review. In the case of medical necessity denials, the reviewer must be in same specialty (but not necessarily in the same subspecialty) as the ordering or treating provider. In some instances, Second Level review may be associated with a filing fee determined by the amount of reimbursement in dispute; a medical necessity dispute valued at less than $1,000 may require a $50 filing fee while a dispute in excess of $1,000 may require a filing fee of $250 or more. Again, it's important to review every detail of your contracts with health care insurers to understand how they have structured their denial and appeals process.

The appeals process does not end with a Second Level review as all health care insurance plans must offer an External Review process as well. The External Review will be provided by an independent medical review organization described by the health care insurance plan. These independent review organizations (IROs) have no affiliation with the insurance company other than a vendor-contract relationship. Again, the IRO must use a practitioner of the same specialty as the ordering or treating provider. Most health care insurance plans will describe that providers must exhaust the internal appeals processes, then the request for the External Review must take place within a specified period of time, in some instances, within 180 days of the of the Second Level denial letter. The decision by the IRO's external appeal is usually binding for both parties in the process where the insurer must comply with the decision of the external reviewer.[5,6]

The Medicare Appeals process is more detailed, offering five levels to the Part A and B processes.[7,8]

- First Level of Appeal: Redetermination – an examination of a claim by the FI, carrier, or MAC personnel different from the individual who made the initial determination. You have 120 days from the date of receipt of the denial to file the appeal. A decision must be provided within 60 days of the redetermination appeal request.
- If not using CMS Form 20027; be prepared to include the beneficiary's name, Medicare Health Insurance Claim (HIC) Number, specific service and or items for which the appeal is being requested, specific date(s) of service, name and signature of the provider or their representative. Be sure to include any supporting documentation to add strength to your appeal letter.
- Second Level Appeal: Reconsideration – if you are dissatisfied with the First Level redetermination, a Qualified Independent Contractor (QIC) will conduct the reconsideration by a panel of physicians or other health care professionals. If you are taking this route, it is very important to be sure to include any and all evidence to support your appeal as evidence not submitted may be excluded from consideration at subsequent levels of appeal unless you show good cause for submitting the evidence late. You will hear a decision from the QIC within 60 days of receipt of the request for reconsideration.
- Third Level Appeal: Administrative Law Judge (ALJ)Hearing – if at least $130 remains in controversy following the QIC's decision, you may request an ALJ hearing within 60 days of receipt of the reconsideration appeal letter. If you go this route, be prepared to send your ALJ request to all previous level contacts; also the ALJ reviews are generally by video-teleconference or telephone, although you may ask for an in-person hearing. The ALJ will usually issue a decision within 90 days of receipt of the hearing request, but may be extended due to a variety of reasons.
- Fourth Level Appeal: Appeals Council Review – if you are still dissatisfied with the decisions rendered by the ALJ, you may request a review by the Appeals Council by submitting a request in writing within 60 days of receipt of the ALJ's decision and specify the issues and findings that are being contested. You should hear the decision of the Appeals Council within 90 days of receipt of a request for review.
- Fifth Level Appeal: Judicial Review in U.S. District Court – if at least $1,260 or more is still in controversy following the Appeals Council's decision, you may request judicial review before a U.S. District Court judge by filing a request for review within 60 days of receipt of the Appeals Council's decision.

Medical Necessity Denials

Most denials that Emergency Physicians will encounter concern medically unnecessary admissions to a hospital. The American Medical Association (AMA) defines medical necessity as:

> Health care services or products that a prudent physician would provide to a patient for the purpose of preventing, diagnosing or treating an illness, injury, disease or its symptoms in a manner that is: (a) in accordance with generally accepted standards of medical practice; (b) clinically appropriate in terms of type, frequency, extent, site and duration; and (c) not primarily for the economic benefit of the health plans and purchasers or for the convenience of the patient, treating physician or other health care provider.[9]

When confronted with a denial for medical necessity, the Emergency Physician must be prepared to write a strong letter of appeal by providing clear, concise medical facts to support the services and care provided while avoiding comments of criticism of the health care plan or health care system.[10,11,12]

Begin by describing your role in the patient's care, for example, "I am a Board Certified Emergency Physician licensed to practice medicine in [your] State, with XX years of experience treating patients presenting with [the diagnosis]."

State the reason the patient required hospitalization using succinct statements that give support to your medical decision making and evidence from your chart such as ancillary services results (laboratory, cardiology, radiology), consultation notes, conversation with family members, EMS, or significant others.

Describe in detail how the hospitalization was imperative to prevent progression of the patient's illness, injury, or disability. What treatments did you attempt that did/or did not provide the patient relief from his or her presenting problem or chief complaint; did the patient fail to respond to intravenous antiemetics for his or her nausea and vomiting; did the patient's pain fail to respond to analgesia despite repeated and escalating doses of medications? Was the patient compliant with home medication regimens; did he or she have the necessary social network of support to manage his or her illness safely in his or her home environment; did the patient have the necessary coping skills to manage the complexity of his or her illness, disease or injury that would assure no further deterioration, placing him or her at increased risk to succumb to his or her disease or condition?

Explain how the hospitalization will improve the patient's physical, mental, or developmental effects of his or her underlying illness, disease, or injury. Explain how previous hospitalizations impacted on the patient's ability to manage his or her disease, overcome obstacles of care, or improve as a result of hospital-provided services. Identify failed treatment regimens and what changed in the patient's condition during this visit. . . this visit that led to your decision to admit. It is always beneficial to cite articles from the literature that support your medical decision making. Provide descriptions of psychological and social factors that impacted your decision to admit: was there sufficient support structures in the home environment to provide surveillance of the patient, did the patient lack cognitive ability to provide his or her own care and supervision, etc.

Ultimately, it is incumbent upon the Emergency Physician to be able to substantiate that the hospitalization would reasonably benefit or prevent the deterioration of the patient's illness, injury, or disability, and that the outcome of hospitalization would assist the patient in achieving his or her functional capacities that are appropriate for individuals of the same age to regularly participate in activities of daily living.

Clearly, having a well-documented emergency medical record during the patient's initial encounter will go a long way to avoiding a denial letter. Having a departmental practice manager review the details of your health care insurance plan contracts listing the number of calendar days for each level of appeal and external appeal is imperative. Using an electronic program that can track and trend reasons for denials by physician, diagnosis, and health care insurance plan goes a long way to developing department policies and procedures in conjunction with your hospital's Utilization Review and Case Management Department that will promote enhanced patient care efforts, improve quality, reduce denials, and preserve revenue.

References

1. Fidelis Care New York Provider Manual, Section Thirteen, Provider Appeals, V12.1-1/20/12.

2. Cigna HealthCare Reference Guide, TriState Region, 801759g; 7/2011.

3. Request for Payment Review and Appeal Form, Cigna Corporation, 2011.

4. Appeal that Claim, Take an Active Approach to the Claims Revenue Cycle, AMA Practice Management Center, Kristie L. Martinez, CMM, CCS-P, American Medical Association, 2011.

5. New York State, Department of Financial Services, External Appeals, 2012.

6. New York State Insurance Law, Article 49.

7. Olaniyan O; Brown I; Williams K. Managing Medical Necessity and Notification Denials, *Healthcare Financial Management*, **63**.8 (2009), Aug;63(8);62–67.

8. The Medicare Appeals Process, Five Levels to Protect Providers, Physicians, and Other Suppliers, Department of Health and Human Services, Centers for Medicare and Medicaid Services, January 2011.

9. Statement of the American Medical Association to the Institute of Medicine's Committee on Determination of Essential Health Benefits.

January 14, 2011. http://iom.nationalacademies.org/~/media/8D03963CAEB24450947C1AEC0CAECD85.ashx (Accessed February 20, 2016)

10. How to Prepare a Winning RAC Appeal, Craneware InSight Consulting, 2011.

11. Brown, R, Lagorio, N et al. *Mistaken Admission: Establishing Medical Necessity for Inpatient Procedures*, CAN Health Pro, Chicago, IL, March 2009.

12. Moore, K. Navigating the Patient Appeals Process, *Fam Pract Manag.* 2000, Oct; 7(9);43–46.

Chapter

Ensuring Financial Viability

The Business Case for Observation Units

Christopher W. Baugh, MD, MBA FACEP
J. Stephen Bohan, MD, MS FACEP, FACP

Observation Use is Increasing

The use of observation services and presence of observation units (OUs) have been rapidly accelerating over the past decade. A 2003 survey found that about 19% of Emergency Departments (EDs) had an OU, with another 12% planning to open one.[1] Subsequent data from the 2007 National Hospital Ambulatory Medical Care Survey (NHAMCS) revealed that about 36% of EDs had a dedicated OU.[2] An analysis of Medicare claims data shows that observation hours increased from 23 million in 2006 to 36 million in 2009.[3] Finally, another analysis of the NHAMCS data shows that between 2001 and 2008, ED visits resulting in a disposition to observation increased from 642,000 (0.60%) to 2,318,000 (1.87%).[4] The number of observation stays per 1,000 Part B beneficiaries almost doubled with an increase from 28 to 53 between 2006 and 2012.[5]

Reasons behind Trend

Several forces have united to drive these increases in observation use. In addition to the publication of additional evidence supporting greater efficiency and lower costs with equivalent or better clinical outcomes using pathway-driven observation care in dedicated units versus standard inpatient admission,[6-8] other actions by the government and payers have encouraged wider use of observation in recent years. Investigations of short-stay inpatient admissions by the Office of the Inspector General (OIG) threaten fines and bad publicity, audits by Recovery Audit Contractors (RAC) put past revenue at risk, and new Medicare penalties for inpatient readmissions encourage alternative management strategies.[9,10] In addition, the health care reform legislation of 2011 encourages the formation of Accountable Care Organizations (ACOs), a model of care

driven by efficiency, not volume of health care services.[11] In this model, the efficiency of pathway-driven observation care is getting the attention of hospital administrators looking for opportunities to better manage patients eligible for this care. (See Chapter 20 on ACOs.)

The Business Model of Observation Care

SWOT Analysis

Many forces impact the strategic value of observation services, as illustrated in Figure 68.1. In this figure, an analysis of Strengths, Weaknesses, Opportunities and Threats (SWOT) illustrate the internal and external forces that contribute to the value of observation services. A SWOT analysis is a strategic analytical tool used to better understand the benefits and challenges of a particular business.[12]

Stakeholder Analysis

Many stakeholders play a key role in the delivery of observation care. These include the patients and their advocates, physicians, nurses, hospital administrators, and payers. Communicating the value proposition of observation care to each of these unique audiences is critical to gaining and sustaining a supportive environment for the delivery of observation services.

For **patients and their advocates**, a robust evidence base demonstrates that observation care offers less time in the hospital with an equivalent or better medical outcome for many conditions (e.g., chest pain, transient ischemic attack, asthma, congestive heart failure and many others).[6,8, 13-17] In addition, several studies have also shown that patient satisfaction is higher with the observation experience than with the standard inpatient

	Helpful	Harmful

Internal	• <u>Strengths:</u>
	  ➢ Established model of care
	  ➢ Large body of literature supporting use
	  ➢ Hospitals incentivized to support in current climate
	  ➢ A "triple win" across the CMS three-part aim of better care, better health and lower costs
	  ➢ Relies on Advanced Practice Providers, with less input from physicians (looming physician shortage)
		• <u>Weaknesses:</u>
		  ➢ Vulnerable to misuse, underuse and overuse (i.e., inappropriate patient selection – use of observation units for patients who should be directly sent home from ED; care of patients too sick/complicated for OU care, etc.)
		  ➢ Lack of stakeholder buy-in can mitigate efficiency advantages (i.e., nurse blocking admissions)

External	• <u>Opportunities:</u>
	  ➢ Increasing volume of observation patients managed outside of an observation unit that would be better managed in a dedicated unit
	  ➢ Creating new pathways of care, expanding scope of illnesses managed in an observation unit
	  ➢ Rise of ACOs puts emphasis on more efficient patient management strategies
		• <u>Threats:</u>
		  ➢ Unstable payment policies threaten model sustainability (i.e., if CMS decides not to pay for observation tomorrow, the entire model of care is jeopardized)
		  ➢ Medicaid generally does not pay or pays very low for observation services
		  ➢ Perception of patient cost shifting and patient advocacy group litigation against CMS

Figure 68.1 SWOT analysis

admission for equivalent illnesses.[18,19] Finally, an observation stay often accomplishes the equivalent evaluation that would usually take many outpatient visits to accomplish. For example, a patient undergoing a transient ischemic attack evaluation could have an MRI of the brain, an echocardiogram, laboratory studies, Neurology consultation and physical therapy evaluation, all within 24 hours before discharge to home. An equivalent outpatient evaluation could potentially take weeks of coordination, placing a much higher burden on the patient and risking noncompliance with the recommended follow-up plan.

Although most observation patients are covered by private insurance, Medicare's policy on the subject is very influential and closely monitored. Recently, Medicare patient advocates have drawn attention to the potential for a high amount of patient cost sharing for observation care (a result of Centers for Medicare and Medicaid Services [CMS] categorizing observation as outpatient care), especially for long stays. For example, the rate of long observation admissions (over 48 hours) has increased from 3% in 2006 to 6% in 2008.[20] Such long stays can potentially generate higher out of pocket costs than an inpatient admission since Medicare Part B is used for observation services, which typically requires patients to pay a 20% coinsurance payment of the negotiated Medicare rates in a fee-for-service billing model.[21] In contrast, the 2012 Medicare Part A deductible for 2016 is $1,288, which effectively caps the patient out-of-pocket costs for a short-stay inpatient admission.[22] This is not an annual deductible, so patients are at risk of paying this for multiple hospitalizations if sufficient time (60 days) passes in between illnesses.[23] However, the 2016 CMS outpatient prospective payment system final rule introduced a composite facility payment that is anticipated to mitigate the potential for outlier patient costs. (See Chapter 63 on comprehensive APCs of C-APCs.) In addition, as opposed to an inpatient admission, time spent in observation does not count toward the three-day minimum for Medicare patients to qualify for coverage of subsequent skilled-nursing facility care. As a result of perceived unfair cost shifting, in November of 2011 a patient advocacy group filed a lawsuit against CMS.[24]

Physicians are the providers choosing to use observation services as an alternative to discharge to home or inpatient admission. Emergency physicians are being challenged with an aging and more complex patient population, and observation management provides a third disposition option for patients that do not fit neatly into the false dichotomy of home versus admission after an initial ED evaluation. **Advanced Practice Providers**, such as Physician Assistants and Nurse Practitioners, often serve as a continuous presence in the OU and play a key role as part of the care team. Observation creates another setting for these providers to work, increasing demand for their services and ensuring a favorable job market persists despite increasing numbers of new graduates.

Nurses caring for patients in an OU are usually the only providers with continuous patient contact during that stay. As a result, it is key to have nursing support for observation care, as they are the caregivers that most patients will associate with their observation experience. Since nurses are continuously staffed in the OU, the costs of nursing care are typically the most expensive component of unit staffing.

Hospital administrators need to value OUs in order to support the resources needed to establish and sustain a unit. OU care that is pathway driven has been shown to much more efficiently manage patients.[7] As previously discussed, the OIG and RAC have been a constant threat to audit, recover, and fine hospitals for the inappropriate classification and billing of patients as inpatients when observation care was warranted.[8]

Payers benefit for the efficiency created by observation care, as outpatient payments are less costly than inpatient payments. If payers did not support observation services, physicians would be forced back into a home versus discharge decision, and many patients that would have otherwise been managed at much lower cost in an OU would then be forced into an inpatient admission. Additionally, appropriate use of observation care can also avoid costly readmissions. This is an area of heightened scrutiny, as upcoming quality measures connecting readmissions to payments as well as new ACO global payment models strongly penalize readmissions.[25] CMS and other payers will be watching to make sure providers are not using observation to circumvent penalties in cases where an inpatient level of care is needed. However, when observation is most appropriate, the observation setting can offer additional time and resources for patients recently discharged with needs outside of the scope of an ED visit. Finally, as the use of observation services increases, payers will surely begin to focus more attention on the patient eligibility for observation services versus the alternative of discharge home with a more traditional outpatient follow-up plan.

Appropriate use of observation in a dedicated space with well-designed protocols of care benefits all stakeholders because it is an efficient alternative to inpatient care. Efficiency translates into lower costs, which is an important component of any model of care in today's health care environment. In addition, by avoiding inpatient admissions, the use of observation is building additional inpatient capacity for patients needing that level of care. This virtual capacity increases the value of an observation admission, possibly by as much as 40% for capacity-constrained hospitals that regularly use ambulance diversion and turn down transfer patients due to crowding.[26] The ED plays a crucial role in keeping observation-eligible patients out of inpatient beds and deserves fiscal recognition by hospital leadership for their management of these patients.

References

1. Mace SE, Graff L, Mikhail M, Ross M. A national survey of observation units in the United States. *Am J Emerg Med* 2003 Nov;21(7):529–533.

2. Wiler JL, Ross MA, Ginde AA. National study of emergency department observation services. *Acad Emerg Med* 2011 Sep;18(9):959–965.

3. Medicare Payment Advisory Committee. *A Data Book: Healthcare Spending and the Medicare Program.* June 2011:112.

4. Venkatesh AK, Geisler BP, Gibson Chambers JJ, Baugh CW, Bohan JS, Schuur JD. Use of Observation Care in US Emergency Departments, 2001 to 2008. *PLoS ONE* 2011 09/14;6(9):e24326.

5. MedPac (Medicare Payment Advisory Commission). Report to the Congress Medicare and the Health Delivery System. http://medpac.gov/documents/reports/june-2015-report-to-the-congress-medicare-and-the-health-care-delivery-system.pdf?sfvrsn=0 (Accessed February 20, 2016)

6. Ross MA, Compton S, Medado P, Fitzgerald M, Kilanowski P, O'Neil BJ. An emergency department diagnostic protocol for patients with transient ischemic attack: a randomized controlled trial. *Ann Emerg Med* 2007 Aug;50(2):109–119.

7. Baugh CW, Venkatesh AK, Bohan JS. Emergency department observation units: A clinical and financial benefit for hospitals. *Health Care Manage Rev* 2011 Jan–Mar; 36(1):28–37.

8. Greenberg RA, Dudley NC, Rittichier KK. A reduction in hospitalization, length of stay, and hospital charges for croup with the institution of a pediatric observation unit. *Am J Emerg Med* 2006 Nov; 24(7):818–821.

9. Bissey B. *Observation, admission, and RAC - The next perfect storm?* IMA Consulting 2008;12.

10. OIG reports reveal Medicare overpayments at several hospitals. Healthcare Finance News. Available at: www.healthcarefinancenews.com/news/recent-oig-reports-reveal-medicare-overpayments-several-hospitals. Accessed February 4, 2016

11. H.R.3590. Patient Protection and Affordable Care Act. 2010: Section 1302.

12. Bradford RD, Duncan J, Tarcy B. *Simplified Strategic Planning: A No-Nonsense Guide for Busy People Who Want Results Fast!* Chandler House Press.

13. Peacock WF, 4th, Young J, Collins S, Diercks D, Emerman C. Heart failure observation units: optimizing care. *Ann Emerg Med* 2006 Jan;47(1):22–33.

14. Jagminas L, Partridge R. A comparison of emergency department versus inhospital chest pain observation units. *Am J Emerg Med* 2005 Mar; 23(2):111–113.

15. Storrow AB, Collins SP, Lyons MS, Wagoner LE, Gibler WB, Lindsell CJ. Emergency department observation of heart failure: preliminary analysis of safety and cost. *Congest Heart Fail* 2005 Mar–Apr;11(2):68–72.

16. Shen WK, Decker WW, Smars PA, Goyal DG, Walker AE, Hodge DO, et al. Syncope Evaluation in the Emergency Department Study (SEEDS): a multidisciplinary approach to syncope management. *Circulation* 2004 Dec 14; 110(24):3636–3645.

17. Ross MA, Compton S, Richardson D, Jones R, Nittis T, Wilson A. The use and effectiveness of an emergency department observation unit for elderly patients. *Ann Emerg Med* 2003 May;41(5):668–677.

18. Rydman RJ, Zalenski RJ, Roberts RR, Albrecht GA, Misiewicz VM, Kampe LM, et al. Patient satisfaction with an emergency department chest pain observation unit. *Ann Emerg Med* 1997 Jan; 29(1):109–115.

19. Rydman RJ, Roberts RR, Albrecht GL, Zalenski RJ, McDermott M. Patient satisfaction with an emergency department asthma observation unit. *Acad Emerg Med* 1999 Mar;6(3):178–183.

20. Tavenner M. Centers for Medicare & Medicaid Services' letter to American Hospital Association on extended observation services 2010 July 7th; Letter from CMS Acting Administrator and Chief Operating Office Marilyn Tavenner to AHA President Richard Umbdenstock.

21. Medicare.gov – Your Medicare Coverage. Available at: www.medicare.gov/coverage/html Accessed February 4, 2016.

22. Medicare: FAQs. Available at: https://questions.medicare.gov/. Accessed February 4, 2016.

23. Centers for Medicare & Medicaid Services (CMS). Medicare Benefit Policy Manual: Chapter 3 – Duration of Covered Inpatient Services. 2003.

24. The Advisory Board Company. Patients sue HHS over hospital 'observation status' – The Advisory Board Daily Briefing. 2011. Available at: www.advisory.com/Daily-Briefing/2011/11/04/Patients-sue-HHS-over-observation-status-rules. Accessed February 4, 2016.

25. Berenson RA, Paulus RA, Kalman NS. Medicare's Readmissions-Reduction Program — A positive alternative. *N Engl J Med* 2012, March 28; 2012/04.

26. Baugh CW, Bohan JS. Estimating observation unit profitability with options modeling. *Acad Emerg Med* 2008;15(5):445–452.

Chapter

69

Observation Services in the Eyes of the Payers

Sandra Sieck, RN, MBA

Reimbursement for observation unit (OU) services has been evolving over the last several years. Hospital facilities must stay abreast of the ever changing criteria for this level of care and the factors that drive optimal reimbursement. Facilities and providers will deal with multiple payers on the commercial side as well as Medicare and Medicaid. Rather than play a passive or reactive role, facilities must take an active stance toward OU reimbursements and adhere to the rules under which such reimbursement is defined.

Medical Necessity Guidelines

Scientifically sound medical necessity criteria form the foundation for determining appropriate level of care. Many payers will use nationally known criteria for considering OU as an appropriate level of care for payment. InterQual or Milliman & Robertson are nationally known sets of criteria that can assist case managers and payers to more specifically define acceptable standards for considering when a patient meets criteria for an acute level of care, ICU status, telemetry, or observation.[1] The Centers for Medicare and Medicaid Services (CMS) Guidance does not require RAC (Recovery Audit Contractor) and MAC (Medicare Administrative Contractor) auditors to use only these guidelines for determining medical necessity. Auditors can use their clinical judgment, CMS coverage guidelines, coding guidelines, interventional guidelines, or nationally accepted community standards.

The disease states or medical conditions that are appropriate for observation status are no longer limited as they once were in the Medicare world several years ago. The only current requirement is that the condition meets criteria for a short stay as an outpatient with a reasonable expectation that the condition can be sufficiently improved with focused treatment as an outpatient

or an expeditious determination made for inpatient care within 24–48 hours.

Payment and Coding

CMS has led the way in observation medicine reimbursement.[2] CMS has pushed for more outpatient services where medically appropriate and has instituted review of inappropriate one-day hospital admissions. Medicare patients make up a large segment of the OU patient population. In the CMS model, the rules are very specific for what criteria define an appropriate OU stay and billing procedure. CMS is quite strict in requiring facilities to adhere to its guidelines, so it is crucial that providers and coders understand and follow the guidelines in order to secure reimbursement.[3]

CMS uses the Outpatient Prospective Payment System (OPPS) for coverage of OU care. The OU is considered an outpatient service by CMS. Revenue Code 0762 is appropriate and place of service code is 21 for outpatient. CMS reimburses for OU care under the composite Ambulatory Payment Classification (APC) codes, 8002 and 8003, for extended assessment and management (see Table 69.1).[4] The appropriate APC code depends on the concomitant utilization of a clinic visit, emergency department (ED) visit, or critical care visit occurred on the day of or day before the OU status, or if the OU stay resulted as a direct referral from a physician. APC 8003 is a composite payment that covers both the ED visit and OU stay.

The degree of supervision for diagnostic and therapeutic services in the outpatient setting is important for OU reimbursement. CMS requires direct supervision by a physician or nonphysician provider at the initiation of OU care. Direct supervision requires that the provider is immediately available if needed. However, this does not require continuous physical presence in the room. Once the physician has determined that the

Table 69.1 Medicare Coding Issues for Observation Status[5]

APC	Definition and Requirements	Payment (2012)
8002 – Level I	• Coding for a clinic visit (99205 or 99215) the same day or day prior to OU admit is required. The associated evaluation and management (E&M) code must be billed with modifier 25 and on the same claim form as G0378. • A minimum of 8 units of observation services (G0378) must be coded. • No procedures with a T code status indicator can be billed.	$393.15[6]
8003 – Level II	• A Type A ED visit (99284 or 99285), G0384 level 5 Type B ED visit, or critical care (99291) code on the day of or day before admit to OU is required. The associated E&M code must be billed with modifier 25 and on the same claim form as G0378. • A minimum of 8 units of observation services (G0378) must be coded. • No procedures with a T code status indicator can be billed.	$720.64[7]

patient is stable, general supervision is sufficient. General supervision means the services are rendered under the provider's direction, again without the need for continual physical presence.

CMS APC 8002–8003 requires at least 8 hours to be provided in observation, up to 24 unit hours. While a stay may last up to 48 hours, no further reimbursement is made for any hours spent after 24 hours. Procedures and tests performed during the OU stay can be billed in addition to the APC codes but no T status procedure (surgical procedure) can be performed.

Additionally, the OU records must show pristine documentation of the physician orders, risk stratification used (nationally accepted standards or individual hospital guidelines), and hourly care provided (see Table 69.2). Since OU status can be provided anywhere in the facility physically, orders must state, "Place in Observation" rather than "Admit to Observation." This will avoid confusion regarding whether the patient has been admitted to acute level of care or truly observation status. The Medicare Outpatient Code Editor (OCE) is the final determinant of what services will be covered under the APC composite.

What if a patient's clinical condition changes? Condition 44 occurs when a patient's status changes. A patient may start in observation status and later be admitted to inpatient status if medically necessary. In this case, the OU time is incorporated into the hospital stay. For Medicare, the appropriate diagnosis-related group (DRG) will be reimbursed and no separate OU billing is allowed. Conversely, at times a patient may change from inpatient to outpatient observation status. CMS does not allow a retrospective admit to OU; OU can only be billed from the exact time of transfer to OU status. Condition 44 requires billing either as an inpatient or outpatient; it does not recognize OU as a third option. OU is considered an outpatient encounter. The hospital cannot change the claim from inpatient to outpatient without involving the UR Committee with physician concurrence. A facility cannot retrospectively bill for G0378 (OU) for the time the patient was an inpatient. G0378 can only be billed upon the time of arrival to observation status. However, facilities may bill for charges for all hospital resources used during the entire patient encounter.[9]

Payers Focus on Double Dipping

Payers are well aware of the practice of double dipping in billing. The Medicare Claims Processing Manual (Pub 100–4) does not allow OU time billing for those services provided in OU that would otherwise require active monitoring. Such services include colonoscopy, chemotherapy, administration of certain drugs, etc. The hospital must determine if a procedure or intervention would normally require monitoring. If so, G0378 cannot be billed during the times these services are administered.

Table 69.2 Medicare Criteria for Medical Necessity of Observation Status[8]

Criteria	Specific Documentation
Physician order	Order to place patient in observation status
Specific codes	Ops code G0378 for the observation level Visit code: G0384 ED (Level 5 Type B ED) or 99284 or 99285 (Type A ED) or 99205 or 99215 (Clinic visit) or 99291 (Critical Care visit) or G0379 for direct referral to OU E&M code with modifier 25 if same Date of Service (DOS) as G0378
Time units	• Minimum of 8 hours up to 24 hour maximum for billing (can stay up to 48 hours but no additional reimbursement beyond 24 hours) • Time must be clocked • Does not include time out of OU for obtaining any tests
Documentation of care provided	Must be included in OU records by MD or nonphysician practitioner: • Admission note • Progress notes for each hour • All notes must be timed and signed • Discharge instructions
Risk stratification	Physician must document in records that a risk stratification assessment was made that showed OU status as appropriate
Additional services provided	Any additional tests or treatments can be coded and must be documented

Table 69.3 Physician Coding for OU Services[10]

Service	Code	Description
OU same-day admit/ discharge	99234 99235 99236	E&M for OU care with same date of admit and discharge with Low severity Moderate severity High severity
Initial OU care	99218 99219 99220	Initial E&M for OU care per day, with duration of visit: ~30 minutes ~50 minutes ~70 minutes
Subsequent OU care	99224 99225 99226	Subsequent E&M for OU care per day, with duration of service ~15 minutes ~25 minutes ~35 minutes
Discharge	99217	OU discharge management when discharge is not same day as admit

Physician Considerations

Physicians caring for patients in the OU have a set of appropriate billing codes based on the patient's length of stay in the OU, severity/ complexity of the E&M services, and discharge management (see Table 69.3). Physicians (i.e., specialty consultants) who provide services other than observation are to bill the appropriate outpatient code for the service.

The commercial payers often follow Medicare guidelines for reimbursable OU coding, however, certain payers will define their own criteria for OU level of care and payment. Facilities and providers should engage payers in defining the details of such criteria in contracts, if possible, or at least become aware of the guidelines that affiliated payers use. Physicians' documentation on admission notes, progress notes, orders, and treatments are most important when reviewing care for medical necessity.

Payment Denial Issues

In an attempt to eliminate waste, Medicare has targeted several situations that have represented payment error and under/overcoding in the past. These areas include one-day hospital stays, 7-day readmits, 3-day nursing home admits, coding of complications and comorbidities, and problematic diagnoses (heart failure, shock, sepsis, stroke with infarct, gastroenteritis, complex pneumonia, etc.). Medicare uses its own hospital data and provides results quarterly in the Program for Evaluating Payment Patterns Electronic Report (PEPPER). Hospitals can use this information to assess the efficiencies of their programs and find areas for improvement.

Areas with a high presence of managed care may present additional challenges for providers and facilities. Many managed care payers have prior authorization requirements for admissions or require authorization for level of care at the time of admission. Care managers within the facility and physicians in the OU should have access to such criteria and work with payers on the authorization process, preferably concurrent to the admission.

A payer may retrospectively review an OU stay for coverage. Facilities should submit detailed records for such post-service authorization reviews to cover observation status. A letter of support that explains the criteria a patient meets is important, but additional record documentation is especially important. All clinical information, orders, progress notes, admit note, clock time in and out, supporting diagnostic and ancillary tests, discharge note, nurses' notes, and delineation of the criteria used to verify that the patient met guidelines for an OU stay should be submitted. Denials by payers for observation status can be costly to the organization if full payment is denied. Additionally, the cost and time-consuming efforts of the appeal process also add to the hospital's cost. If the regulatory statutes or payers' rules allow for an appeal of a denied OU stay, it is worthwhile to provide key clinical information regarding the patient's condition, status, criteria met for OU, and proper admission criteria for such coverage to the respective payer. An appeal request should detail specifically why the facility believes OU stay was medically necessary and then include the medical record documentation that supports this justification as well as for all services provided.

Reimbursement rates for OU services are an important consideration for facility viability.

Contracted rates for OU services may be agreed upon in advance between payers and facilities or providers in certain geographies. These contracts are common in areas of high-managed care penetration. The contractual language should detail the specific criteria for admission to and reimbursement for observation status. As contractual arrangements between hospitals and payers become more specific, it behooves the facility to negotiate acceptable definitions for what constitutes observation level care, which specific criteria or guidelines will become the arbitrator for OU, and how these services will be reimbursed. The facility should consider actuarial analysis of prior observation practice patterns, ancillary utilization rates, and status costs prior to negotiating fair rates with contracting payers.

Future Directions

As the cost of health care continues to increase and outpace the general inflation, payers are challenging the current payment model to provide built-in guarantees of quality and value. The era of automatic reimbursement in a fee-for-service mode is quickly becoming a historic past. Unbridled reimbursement of submitted charges has fostered, at least in part, the runaway health care costs of the past decades. The evolution of managed care has tempered runaway costs to some extent, however, providers complain that the capitated, discounted, and DRG models are unfair in the other direction.

Future health care reimbursement will pay for evidence-based, medically necessary, and efficient services that will afford the patient optimal health for the underlying medical condition. Medicare has been the frontrunner in the search for a payment model that rewards quality and value rather than quantity of service.[11] Beginning in 2013, Medicare will enact a new Value Based Performance (VBP) program for hospital payments. If this program is perceived as successful in reimbursement that rewards quality care, it is likely to extend to other treatment venues as well, including OU.

References

1. InterQual Level of Care Criteria 2011, McKesson Health Solutions, LLC.

2. Medicare Benefit Policy Manual. Chapter 6 – Hospital Services Covered Under Part B. 20.6- Outpatient Observation Services. (Rev. 152, 12–29-1) www.cms.gov/manuals/Downloads/bp102c06.pdf (Accessed February 4, 2016).

3. Pub 100-04 Medicare Claims Processing Manual. Chapter 4. Section 290. Outpatient Observation Services. www.cms.gov/manuals/downloads/clm104c04.pdf (Accessed February 4, 2016).

4. American College of Emergency Physicians. Clinical and Practice Management. FAQ. www.acep.org/content.aspx?id=30486 (Accessed February 4, 2016).

5. American College of Emergency Physicians. Clinical and Practice Management. FAQ. www.acep.org/content.aspx?id=30486 (Accessed February 4, 2016).

6. Highlights of the 2012 OPPS Final Rule. www.acep.org/content.aspx?id=35402 (Accessed February 4, 2016).

7. Highlights of the 2012 OPPS Final Rule. www.acep.org/content.aspx?id=35402 (Accessed February 4, 2016).

8. American College of Emergency Physicians. Clinical and Practice Management. FAQ. www.acep.org/content.aspx?id=30486 (Accessed February 4, 2016).

9. Centers for Medicare and Medicaid Services. Answers. https://questions.cms.hhs.gov/app/answers/detail/a_id/9973/kw/9973 (Accessed February 4, 2016).

10. American College of Emergency Physicians. Clinical and Practice Management. FAQ. www.acep.org/content.aspx?id=30486 (Accessed February 4, 2016).

11. Department of Health and Human Services, Centers for Medicare and Medicaid Services, 42 CFR Parts 422 and 480, Medicare Program: Hospital Inpatient Value-Based Purchasing Program. Federal Register/Vol.76, No. 88/Friday, May 6, 2001/ Rules and Regulations.

Chapter 70

The Business of Observation Medicine

Sandra Sieck, RN, MBA

Introduction

In an era in which health care costs appear to be unmanageable and quality of care has not been consistently attained, the delivery of health care services is in need of a total redesign.[1] The practice models of the last century are no longer adequate to ensure quality care at an affordable price. On a smaller scale, the observation unit (OU) represents a piece of the transformation of the delivery model to more efficiently and cost-effectively bridge the outpatient and inpatient care for serious medical conditions. But as with many advances in medicine, the OU has taken on different forms in its evolution and now finds itself requiring refinement in how best to design its structure and operation into an optimal business model to meet quality and financial performance measures.

The Need for a Business Model

Traditionally, patients who required more than a short course of treatment in the emergency department (ED) were admitted to the acute hospital setting. In an era when reimbursements favored quantity of service, this posed no adverse financial impact to the hospital. In fact, the opposite was true. In a cost constrained, diagnosis-related group (DRG)-based or capitated environment, utilization of high-cost inpatient services for every patient no longer is associated with favorable financial payments. This result is a mismatch between services required for optimal outcomes and intensity of effort provided – in other words wasteful overutilization. The mantra of medicine in the current environment is to have the "right patient" in the "right place" at the "right time."

While medicine has often been averse to thinking in terms of operating under a business model, it is imperative to do so these days. A business model for health care services must combine financial viability with delivery of a quality product. Early studies showed that use of an OU can result in fewer unnecessary hospital admissions with roughly only 20–25% of patients needing to be admitted following OU status care.[2] The OU has been associated with reduced hospital readmission rates, increased ED discharges, shorter length of stay (LOS), better clinical outcomes, and increased patient satisfaction.[3,4,5,6,7]

Cost savings have also been demonstrated for certain medical conditions, particularly chest pain.[8] An OU can contribute to profit margins by increasing revenues for select patient conditions while reducing costs through more efficient use of resources.[9] Revenues may be increased by avoiding an inpatient admission, particularly in conditions for which reimbursement may not fully cover costs of care, such as in certain DRG-based or capitated situations. For instance, Medicare will reimburse for the OU stay and separately cover most performed tests in addition. An OU stay can thus turn what would otherwise be a loss for the hospital into a profitable stay.

First Steps

A successful OU is defined as one that provides efficient, quality, and cost-effective care for those conditions requiring short-term but focused treatment. The facility must strategically determine what steps are required to create such a unit. The design of the unit operationally requires collaboration between the medical staff and administrative departments in order to be successful. It requires fully committed leadership, both administrative and medical.

A facility must provide a sound argument justifying creation of an OU. While studies show clinical and financial benefits of an OU in selected settings and conditions, each facility must analyze its own data to determine how best to operationalize an OU to ensure maximal benefit.

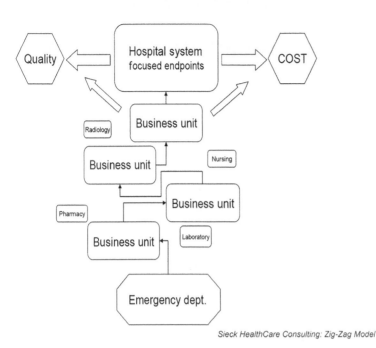

FIGURE 70.1 The Zig-Zag Model of Care2008 Update: Sieck S. Cost effectiveness of chest pain units. *Cardiol Clin* 2005; 23(4):598.

Sieck HealthCare Consulting: Zig-Zag Model

The first critical step to creating a successful OU is to determine if an OU is a viable and feasible option based on the current patient mix and volume. Forecasting involves performing an analysis of the facility's current ED and acute care utilization and estimating the volume and diagnostic types of cases that would be routed to the OU. Anticipation of future trends in usage and patient mix is part of the strategic development process. An OU in a high-volume facility may evolve quickly to a fully operational OU, whereas a small low-volume facility may not find that an OU is an economically sound approach.

The majority of costs associated with patients admitted to acute care are related to admission time.[10] If roughly half of patients admitted with chest pain do not have acute coronary syndrome (ACS) and could have been safely evaluated in an OU, substantial savings would result. However, such savings might not be realized for all facilities. For instance, in some countries where hospital costs are not as high as in the United States, savings from preventing an unnecessary admission could be substantially less.[11] This is why each facility contemplating establishing or expanding an OU must analyze its own data.

Financial projections of revenue and cost can be made based on current estimates of patient mix, reimbursements specific to the OU, and costs of running the unit. Fixed unit cost estimates are related to space, dedicated equipment, and staffing needs. Nursing needs are generally less for the OU than the acute level as a nurse can care for more patients in the OU. (See Chapters 1 – Clinical, 6 – Staffing and 7 – Nursing.) Variable cost estimates for supplies related to care, medications, and testing also impact overall cost projections.

Merging Quality and Finances

Most acute care admissions follow a zigzag approach of delivering care/services from the point of entry to discharge. (See Figure 70.1.) A patient's 'flow' through the hospital care system is not linear but often quite disconnected through various diagnostic or therapeutic care units, each of which functions more as an independent unit than as an integrated part of a cohesive strategy. Although the zigzag model can eventually result in appropriate care, it is generally an inefficient and resource wasteful process.

Y-Model: Y3 – CHF Details

Development elements

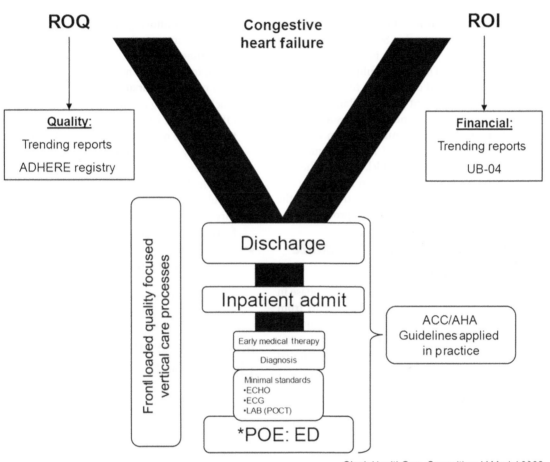

Sieck HealthCare Consulting: Y-Model 2008

*POE = Point of entry
ROI = return on investment
ROQ = return on quality
ACC = American college of cordiology
AHA = American heart association
Congestive heart failure

FIGURE 70.2 Quality and Cost Focus of the Y-Model2008 Update: Sieck S. Cost effectivenss of chest pain units. *Cardiol Clin* 2005;23(4):597.
*POE = Point of Entry

Facilities must design a methodology to merge quality of care and finance to ensure long-term viability. The Y-Model approach affords a blueprint for this merger.[12] The Y-Model sets up the overall design of OU operations by focusing on the desired end points of quality and costs. (See Figure 70.2.) In the business environment, the optimal route to attaining a quality end product at the maximal contribution margin is to streamline the overall process and reduce variances in the route of production. Similarly in medicine, focusing on the methods to ensure a quality end result for a patient requires adherence to evidence-based evaluations and treatments performed expeditiously and efficiently through a streamlined process.

The Y-Model involves placing proper sequencing of services 'up front' at the point of entry into the medical care track. Seamless integration between operating care units is the essential core of the Y-Model. The successfully designed OU focuses on front-end compliance toward a subsequent tailored treatment pathway. Randomness of care, and therefore, unnecessary resource consumption, is essentially eliminated from the path. The basic concept of an OU meets the methodology espoused in the Y-Model. Indeed, the OU may represent the initial redesign in acute health care delivery that will ultimately transform the entire system into a more efficient process.

Operational Elements to Maximize Efficiencies in the OU

Once a strategic plan is in place, the next phase in setting up an OU is to obtain solid support from the hospital to provide the infrastructure, resources, and strong leadership. Each implementation step requires a strategy focused on tailored treatment and efficient resource utilization.

- Regardless of where in the facility the OU is housed, the facility must be fully committed to the operation of the unit on par with other units within the organization. The OU cannot be deemed perfunctory or expendable. Additionally, a clear-cut path to and through the OU must be developed and adhered to.
- While an OU can be located anywhere within the facility and even be virtual in nature, the OU is best located in a known and defined physical place to experience optimal financial efficiencies. The physical layout, design, flow, and equipment (or proximity to ancillary services) should also foster expedient flow. (See Chapter 5 Observation Unit Design.) Time/flow studies may be an integral part of the planning process.
- The ideal OU requires a dedicated staff that has been trained in OU requirements and policy. Physicians could be emergency physicians, internists, hospitalists, or critical care specialists. Mid-level practitioners such as nurse practitioner (NP) or physician assistant (PA) are often included on staff. Their use may help financial integrity of the unit while supporting the mandates of the CMS new outpatient (OP) quality and structural measures. Nursing ratios should allow for frequent monitoring of patient status and treatment interventions. The OU lends an opportune time to integrate patient education into a teachable moment. (See Chapters 6 Staffing and 7 Nursing.)

- Ancillary testing can be either dedicated to the OU or shared with other departments, such as the ED. The most efficient is a dedicated set of laboratory and imaging departments. However, this may not always be financially feasible. If such services are shared, the OU should at least have dedicated time slots throughout a 24-hour period based on the forecasted data analysis.
- Patients can be referred to OU from the ED or directly from a physician's office. Efficient ED assessment to route to the OU requires education in the ED for such transfer to higher level of service.

Medical Necessity Review and Disease Specific Issues

- Acceptable OU criteria should be created and implemented. (See Chapter 82 Clinical Protocols.)
- Assessment should be made by the OU physician to verify criteria are met. Either internal criteria can be developed or external criteria such as InterQual or Milliman & Robertson guidelines can be used.
- Case managers placed in the ED 24/7 can lend assistance to the physician to ensure appropriate patient status. In the initial stages of establishing a new OU, the unit can focus on standard medical conditions that have been deemed appropriate for OU such as chest pain, heart failure, asthma, GI bleed, syncope, dehydration, some infections, etc.
- As the unit establishes itself and maintains efficiencies and improved clinical outcomes, more complex conditions should be considered.
- Clear placement (inclusion/exclusion) criteria, protocols, and clinical pathways are an

important piece of an efficient OU. Criteria can be based on national guidelines or developed locally per diagnostic condition. Pre-printed orders assist with facilitating timely assessments and interventions. (See Chapters 89–96.) Because the OU focuses on patients needing 24–48 hours of care, all actions in the OU must be considered time-sensitive.

- Maximal reimbursement, especially for Medicare patients, requires pristine documentation of care, often on an hourly basis. A physician order necessitates documentation of the continuation of care. The OU should have a relatively straightforward, but sufficiently detailed documentation protocol. An electronic health record (EHR) is ideal but not required. Documentation provisions for outpatient (OP) measures, coding and billing, and unit validation requires staff education to ensure that optimal outcomes will be attained.

- Upfront Case Management (CM) and Discharge Planning techniques should be instituted upon first patient contact rather than midstream or at the back end. Significant time is lost if waiting until the patient's care course is hours into the process to only discover the patient status is incorrect according to criteria. This back-end CM process can be costly for the patient, physician, and the hospital. A well-defined coordinated care model will reduce risk.

Operational Oversight

Once a functional and efficient structural design has been developed and implemented, continued operational oversight of the processes is necessary to align strategic goals with outcomes. Ongoing data analysis of outcomes and costs of operation, near real time measures if possible, is important to identify trends and make any adjustments to the OU operation.

- Monitor clinical outcomes related to the diagnostic mix of the OU. Include measures involved in any pay for performance activities or accreditation parameters.

- Patient satisfaction is one component of outcomes that is being measured by Medicare and health plans. Although not directly related to quality of care, it is a key measure in many pay-for-performance programs and also impacts public relations for the facility.

- Financial outcomes and fixed and variable costs of operation, patient volume, and trends in utilization should be assessed periodically.

- Coding oversight is essential for maximal reimbursements. Adherence to payer requirements and correction of any missteps must be implemented expeditiously.

- Quality Improvement initiatives should be aligned within the OU. (See Chapter 9 Metrics and Performance.)

- The financial analysis should be used to optimize contractual reimbursements for capitated and noncapitated clients based on actuarial forecasting when possible.

Future Trends

Two major emerging trends occurring in the United States will alter reimbursements for providers. The first is value-based purchasing (VBP). Medicare reimbursement has previously rewarded the quantity of health care services provided but is quickly moving toward a patient-centric value proposition that will reward providers for delivering high quality efficient care.[13] As of October 2012 (FY2013), the VBP payment methodology focuses on hospitals through the Medicare Inpatient Prospective Payment System. Facilities can "earn back" the payment reductions through meeting targets for selected conditions and predetermined performance measures. If this program shows promise, it is likely that other payers will begin to pay for value. A well-designed OU should be integrated into the process improvement objectives to assist in meeting these goals.

The second shift is the development of Accountable Care Organizations (ACO).[14] An ACO integrates physicians, facilities, and other health care providers with the intent of providing high quality collaboratively efficient care. ACO participants will share in any resultant cost savings. The positive impact of an OU in an ACO is the reduction in unnecessary admissions, reduced LOS, decreased readmission rate, and reduced subsequent ED visits.[15] Thus, an OU is poised to play an important role within the evolving ACO concept. A dedicated outpatient OU by design is meeting the needs of placing patients in a low-rent district. (See Chapter 20 Accountability Care Organizations.)

Conclusion

While the future of the health care reimbursement system may be difficult to predict, the OU appears to be here to stay. The OU aligns with the ever-increasing need to develop more efficient strategies to deliver the best individualized care in the right care setting to attain optimal outcomes. As the shift to outpatient care and services marches on, the use of the OU will continue to increase. A facility that fails to adjust its treatment design to meet these needs will be competitively disadvantaged in the health care marketplace.

References

1. Committee on Quality of Health Care in America, Institute of Medicine, Crossing the Quality Chasm: A New Health System for the 21st Century. Consensus Report, March 1, 2001.

2. Graff LG, Dallara J, Ross MA, et al. Impact on the care of the emergency department chest pain patient from the chest pain evaluation registry (CHEPER) study. *Am J Cardiol* 1997;80: 563–568.

3. Graff L, Zun LS, Leikin J, et al. Emergency department observation beds improve patient care: Society for Academic Emergency Medicine debate. *Ann Emerg Med* 1992;21:967–975.

4. Graff L, Prete M, Werdmann M, et al. Improved outcomes with implementation of emergency department observation units within a multihospital network. *J Qual Improv* 2000;26:421–427.

5. Mace SE. Asthma therapy in the observation unit. *Emerg Med Clin North Am* 2001;19:169–185.

6. Ng CW, Lim GH, McMaster F, et al. Patient satisfaction in an observation unit: the Consumer Assessment of Health Providers and Systems Hospital Survey *Emerg Med J* 2009 Aug;26(8):586–589.

7. Peacock WF. Management of acute decompensated heart failure in the emergency department. *J Am Coll Cardiol* 2003;3:336A.

8. Baugh CW, Venkatesh AK, Bohan JS. Emergency department observation units: A clinical and financial benefit for hospitals. *Health Care Management Review* 2011; Jan–Mar;36:26–37.

9. Venkatesh A. ED Observation units lower health care costs. Emergency Medicine Residents' Association. www.emra.org/emra_articles.aspx?id=42328 (Accessed March 7, 2010).

10. Forberg JL, Henriksen LS, Edenbrandt L, et al. Direct hospital costs of chest pain patients attending the emergency department: a retrospective study. *BMC Emerg Med* 2006;6:6.

11. Goodacre S, Morris F, Arnold J, et al. Is a chest pain observation unit likely to be cost saving in a British hospital? *Emerg Med J* 2001 Jan; 18(1):11–4.

12. Sieck S. Cost-effectiveness of chest pain units. *Cardiol Clin* 2005; 23(4): 589–599, ix.

13. Department of Health and Human Services, Centers for Medicare and Medicaid Services, 42 CFR Parts 422 and 480, Medicare Program: Hospital Inpatient Value-Based Purchasing Program. Federal Register/Vol.76, No. 88/Friday, May 6, 2001/ Rules and Regulations.

14. www.cms.gov/ACO/ (Accessed February 4, 2016).

15. Suri P. The role of observation units in Accountable Care Organizations. *Emergency Physicians Monthly* July 27, 2011.

Part VI

International

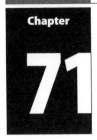

Chapter

71

South Africa

Heather Tuffin, MD, MBChB (UCT), DipPEC (CMSA)
LA Wallis, MBChB (Edin), MD (Edin), FRCS (A&E) (Edin),
DIMCRCS (Edin), Dip Sport Med (Glasgow), FCEM (London),
FCEM (SA), FIFEM

Emergency Medicine in South Africa

Emergency medicine is still in its infancy in South Africa. The specialty having been first recognized in 2003, there are now 108 registered specialists: just more than 1 for each million of the approximately 55 million people living in South Africa. There are four emergency medicine training programs in the country, the oldest a mere 13 years old at the time of this writing (2016). At the National Department of Health, hospital emergency medicine has yet to find a champion and accordingly is underprioritized.

There are about 150 private hospitals in South Africa that have emergency centers (ECs), very few of which have dedicated observation wards. In the public sector, there are approximately 300 hospitals, only about 100 of which justify having a dedicated observation ward. The remainder are small, district-level hospitals in which the ECs are manned by family practitioners who also run the inpatient areas, and where EC load would not justify the ring-fencing of space and resources for a separate stream of patients.

At the time of this writing it is for the most part only the ECs in regional and central hospitals (larger hospitals attracting more complex patients from larger regions) that have their own observation wards under the jurisdiction of emergency medicine specialists. This is a small pool of hospitals. However, there is room for expansion. As emergency medicine becomes better accepted as a specialty in its own right, more specialists are registered, and emergency patient loads continue to rise, there will be both need and opportunity for each EC to be manned by emergency medicine specialists who will also run their own observation units.

While it is understood that observation medicine is not the exclusive realm of emergency medicine, with the exception of some isolated cases, emergency medicine is the only group in South Africa who are currently making forays into this aspect of medicine.

Emergency Center Observation Wards

Following what seems to be a worldwide trend, South African hospitals have been experiencing ever-increasing EC presentation and hospital admission rates over the past few years. With no concomitant rise in inpatient bed numbers, emergency center observation wards (ECOWs) have come under the spotlight, both as a potential answer to the increasing admission rates and because those in existence have quickly lost their core functionality secondary to housing patients waiting for admission to inpatient beds. As part of a strategy to decrease EC and hospital overcrowding, ECOWs, properly utilized, house subgroups of patients fitting specific clinical criteria who need treatment for longer periods than normal for the EC, but who are deemed likely to stay for less than 24 hours. This frees up an EC space for receiving an incoming emergency or an inpatient ward bed for accepting a patient with more complex pathology, and thus an anticipated longer length of stay. At the same time the patient remains under the care of the people best equipped to give that care, who routinely review patients on a far more frequent basis than the traditional daily inpatient ward review, thus allowing for the high turnover that is necessary to maintain this stream.

In 2010 the Provincial Department of Health in the Western Cape published a standard operating procedure (SOP) covering the functions of ECOWs in Western Cape public hospitals (Appendix 1).[1] The Emergency Medicine Society of South Africa (EMSSA) has endorsed this document as a best practice for all EC observation wards.[2]

As delineated by the SOP, appropriate admissions to the ECOW include patients requiring evaluation of high-risk chief complaints or short-term therapy of an emergency condition with:

- limited need for intense medical services
- pathology involving only one system
- clinical conditions appropriate for observation
- limited severity of illness, anticipation of discharge home within time limits (24 hours or less)

Categories of appropriate patients for admission include:

- Patients requiring diagnostic evaluation, for example, patients with chest pain, but a low probability of myocardial infarction
- Patients requiring short-term therapy, for example, asthmatic patients, patients with dehydration
- Patients requiring psychosocial needs to be met, for example, patients with acute alcohol withdrawal. These needs are met in conjunction with appropriate support services.

All patients admitted to the ECOW remain the responsibility of the EC staff. Clear, focused, patient care goals must be set upon admission and reviewed at least q 12 hours. A time limit should be monitored and strictly enforced in order to ensure that patients are either discharged or admitted to the appropriate inpatient team within a maximum of 48 hours.

As well as delineating who should be admitted to the ECOW, the SOP equally importantly delineates who should *not* be accommodated:

- Patients referred to, or admitted to, an in-patient speciality
- Psychiatric patients at any point of their admission
- Patients for planned surgery
- Postoperative patients
- Patients admitted from out-patient clinics, awaiting an in-patient bed

Unfortunately, the reality is that ECOWs rarely reflect the stipulated delineations, with anecdotal evidence highlighting up to 70% of staffed spaces taken up by psychiatric patients or patients waiting for admission, and ECOWs running at well over 100% capacity. We have no information about the use of ECOWs in other provinces, but it is reasonable to infer that a similar picture is likely elsewhere in the country.

The Way Ahead

While the situation is presently less than ideal, with an increased focus on improving the flow of patients, as well as the rise of emergency medicine as a specialty, the future of ECOWs looks reasonably optimistic. With good guiding documents available and a growing cadre of specialists to implement positive changes and maintain control of the governing parameters, observational medicine promises to move into its own in South Africa in the foreseeable future.

References

1. Emergency Centre Observation Wards. Cape Town: Western Cape Department of Health; 2010.

2. Emergency Centre Observation Wards. Pretoria: EMSSA; 2010.

Appendix 1: Emergency Center Observation Wards

Introduction

Every Western Cape Department of Health hospital with an EC is to have a dedicated observation ward adjacent to the EC. The aim of the observation ward is to improve the quality of care for patients through extended evaluation and treatment, while reducing inappropriate admissions. The ward should have:

- dedicated observation beds (number to be determined by annual patient census in EC, at a rate of 2.5–5 beds per 10,000 attendees)
- dedicated nursing staffing (on rotation through the ward from the EC)
- dedicated ablution facilities
- dedicated support staff

This SOP DOES NOT apply to rural District level hospitals: the guidance in here may be something for these facilities to work towards, but is not currently achievable. A similar service, however, should be provided within existing bed configurations.

The aim of the SOP is to define the process for the observation ward.

Management Procedures

The EC Clinical Lead is to institute clearly defined written policies and procedures for the management of the observation ward and patients admitted therein. The absolute criteria for admission to the Observation Ward will vary according to local need, but the contents of this SOP should guide these decisions. All decisions are to be in line with the Western Cape Package of Care for Emergency Medicine. The following are key management principles:

- patients are the responsibility of the EC medical staff
- only EC doctors are allowed to admit to Observation Ward beds
- clearly identified patient care goals must be in place

- patients may require:
  - evaluation of high-risk chief complaints
  - short-term therapy of an emergency condition
  - psychosocial needs meeting (in conjunction with appropriate support services)
- patients should have:
  - limited need for intense medical services
  - clinical conditions appropriate for observation
  - limited severity of illness, anticipation of discharge home within time limits
- the period of observation should be for a maximum of 48 hours (unless in exceptional circumstances): at that time, discharge or admission to the appropriate in-patient team is required
- the period of observation should have a focused goal

In deciding on admission criteria, consider that:

- Some patients require evaluation of specific chief complaints that may be indicative of conditions with high mortality or morbidity (e.g., the patient with chest pain and a low probability of myocardial infarction; the patient with right lower quadrant abdominal pain and low probability of appendicitis). It may not be necessary to admit such a patient to a formal ward bed, but discharge after initial examination places the patient at risk of an adverse event. Such patients are best served by an overnight Observation Ward bed admission.
- Many patients with emergency conditions such as asthma or dehydration have not improved enough after the first few hours to be discharged, but are very likely to improve enough for discharge after a few hours of therapy.

- Some patients have pressing psychosocial problems but cannot be admitted to the hospital because of restricted admission criteria.

The intensity of service needs should be limited and consistent with the staffing pattern of the ward. This must be matched to the patient's illness severity (which should be limited to one organ system).

The severity of illness must not preclude the expectation that the patient will be discharged within established time limits. A time limit is very important and should be carefully monitored and strictly enforced.

Observation Ward Admission Paperwork

An admission note must be generated, detailing:

- time admitted in EC
- time admitted into Observation Ward
- the reason for observation
- the working diagnosis (and other possible conditions needing exclusion)
- treatment plan and aims
- outstanding special investigations results
- a clearly defined end point for patient disposition

Documentation (both medical and nursing) should be simple and goal driven.

- All medical and nursing notes, drug cardex, fluid charts and observation sheets should transfer with the patient from the EC to the Observation Ward; they should continue until discharge.
- There should be standardized designed cover sheets, which only get completed upon admission to the EC obs ward. Segments should be kept simple and aim driven.
  1) Time admitted in EC
  2) Time admitted in Observation Ward
  3) Working Diagnosis (and other possible conditions needed exclusion)
  4) Outstanding special investigations results
  5) Treatment plan and aims

Suggested Admission Criteria

The following are ideal for Observation Ward admission:

Diagnostic evaluation of haemodynamically stable patients with:

- Abdominal pain
- Chest pain with low probability of myocardial infarction (following a diagnostic pathway)
- Flank pain (evaluation and pain management of suspected kidney stones)
- Gastrointestinal bleeding (with no evidence of ongoing bleeding)
- Chest trauma (normal initial evaluation and CXR)
- Drug overdose (clinically stable)
- Syncope (negative initial evaluation following diagnostic pathway)
- Nonpregnancy related vaginal bleeding awaiting Ultrasound/Gynaecological evaluation
- Trauma patients with minor injuries but significant mechanism of injury
- Mixed alcohol intoxication and minor head injury

Short-term therapy of patients with:

- Allergic reactions
- Asthma/COPD
- Acute exacerbation of chronic congestive cardiac failure
- Dehydration
- Hyperglycemia
- Hypertensive urgencies
- Selected infections (e.g., pyelonephritis, cellulitis, pneumonia with low CURB score, etc.)
- Blood transfusion
- Seizure disorders requiring anticonvulsant loading or observation

Meeting psychosocial needs of patients with:

- Acute alcohol withdrawal
- Depression with ongoing suicide ideation (with documented risk assessment; after discussion with Psychiatry)

All patients remain the responsibility of the EC.

Patients who should not be admitted:

The following patients SHOULD NOT be accommodated in Observation Ward bed:

- Patients referred to, or admitted to, an inpatient speciality
- Psychiatric patients at any point of their admission

- Patients for planned surgery
- Postoperative patients
- Patients admitted from outpatient clinics, awaiting an inpatient bed

Chapter 72

Singapore

Malcolm Mahadevan, MD FRCS (A&E), MRCP (Int Med), FAMS
Chew Yian Chai, MD, MCEM, FAMS

Introduction

Origins

It was in 1998 and early 1999 after reading the first edition of *Observation Medicine* by Louis Graff that the author was first introduced to the concept of observation medicine. This concept was presented and the possibility explored with the hospital administration of setting up such a unit at the National University Hospital Singapore. With their blessing an application for a scholarship under the human manpower development award was made and obtained. The author (MM) successfully completed a fellowship program in Observation Medicine with Louis G. Graff, MD, FACEP at the University of Connecticut Medical School in Hartford, Connecticut. Subsequently the first formal observation medicine unit in Singapore was approved and set up in 2004 at the National University Hospital, and was named Extended Diagnostic Treatment Unit (EDTU) as a pilot project.

Challenges

The hurdles initially encountered in setting up and running the unit included reimbursement for observable conditions, acceptance by the local hospital as a recognized site for continued care, as well as establishing its role and utility in a hospital system. For reimbursement there needed to be approval from the government that patients could utilize their medical savings (called medisave).

When the first protocols were being written there was consultation with relevant specialties related to the observed conditions. Examples included cardiology for chest pain patients to rule out myocardial injury. Utilizing repeat enzyme testing was done by our unit, but the investigation for possible coronary artery or ischemia by treadmill stress test, dobutamine echo or technetium sestamibi scan was done by the cardiology service. There had to be a meeting of minds as well as agreement for continuity of care.

Following the National University Hospital, most of the major restructured government hospitals in Singapore started developing their own observation units (OUs). Also fostering the growth of observation medicine in Singapore, two additional physicians from Singapore completed fellowships in observation medicine in Cleveland, Ohio in 2006–2007 with the editor of this textbook, Dr. Mace. To date, six major hospitals offer formal observation services. As all OUs are in various stages of their development, hospital-to-hospital variation occurs in terms of size, number of protocols available, staffing ratio, and extended services available; however, they all work on the same fundamentals of observation medicine and are largely protocol driven.

The National University Hospital's EDTU started with 8 beds and 8 protocols. Over the years, we have expanded to 16 beds, and we now have 32 protocols in place. We are still continuously seeking improvement and refining our workflows and processes. Table 72.1 lists the protocols we have in place.

Guidelines on Concept, Staffing

OUs are generally housed adjacent to the emergency department (ED) and are staffed and run by ED physicians. Rounds are made twice daily. The staffing ratio of nurses to patients is kept at 1:5, thus allowing close monitoring of patients. In our current model of care, no provision for additional physician staff has been factored in for running the OU. This has limited the size of the units and placed some strain on manpower. Moving forward there should be better rationalization of needed resources to enable more efficient safe care delivery.

Table 72.1 EDTU Protocols, National University Hospital

Diagnostic Conditions	Therapeutic Conditions	Diagnostic & Therapeutic Conditions
Appendicitis	Atrial fibrillation	Dehydration
Chest pain	Anaphylaxis	Dyspepsia
	Pneumothorax – Apical and rim	Headache
	Asthma	Seizure
	Back pain	Stable head injury
	Blunt chest trauma	Syncope
	Cellulitis	Vertigo/Dizziness
	Colorectal conditions	
	Congestive heart failure	
	Chronic obstructive pulmonary disease (COPD)	
	Dengue	
	Deep vein thrombosis	
	Gastroenteritis	
	Gastrointestinal bleeding	
	Hyperglycemia	
	Hypoglycemia	
	Pneumonia	
	Renal or ureteric colic	
	Toxic smoke inhalation	
	Transient Ischemic attack	
	Urinary tract infection/pyelonephritis	
	Vertebral compression fracture	

Unique Features of Observation Medicine in Singapore

Our protocols are evidence based as far as possible. On occasion we have discovered that there is a dearth of evidence available and this has led us to push the boundaries through research and publication of observable conditions. One example would be the management of primary spontaneous pneumothorax. We initially placed a normal bore chest drain utilizing open dissection with the drain being connected to an underwater seal. This was a painful procedure and patients experienced discomfort with the drain. We then tried aspirating and observing but soon realized that many

reaccumulated their pneumothorax. We then went on to utilize a small bore drain inserted with a seldinger technique and aspirated the pneumothorax after we which we connected to an underwater seal and observed the patients over 24 hours. This has proven to be much more favorable, with a 39% reduction in insertion of chest tubes; 65% of our patients were managed with mini chest tubes and 56% of those admitted to our OU were successfully discharged within 24 hours.

The utility of our abdominal pain protocol allows us to observe those with moderate probability of appendicitis (Alvarado score) hence minimizing unnecessary CT scans of the abdomen.

Our asthma and COPD pathways involved the input and assistance of inpatient nurses specially trained to assess and follow up with these patients at home. This helps us discharge our patients safely with timely follow-up. The management of our COPD patients presenting to the ED in the EDTU is part of a continuum of care, which includes early recognition in ED for noninvasive ventilation (NIV) (which we initiate) and has shown a mortality reduction from 11.8% to 1.7%. This decision is based on posttherapy arterial blood gas. If the initial pH is below 7.25 then NIV is initiated. If the patient has a pH of greater than 7.25 posttherapy and is deemed suitable for EDTU care, then he or she is admitted to the EDTU for further treatment and assessment.

The advent of observation medicine in Singapore has also greatly helped limit our inpatient admissions. As many of our facilities like those in other countries have access block issues with bed limitations, it has helped us as part of the hospital system to cope better.

What is the Role of Observation Medicine in the Health System?

The introduction of observation medicine has seen increased merits in the health care system. A review of the statistics over the past 2 years shows that on the average, 444 patients in a month are placed in our OU, which amounts to 4% of our ED volume. Discharge rates are as high as 82%. This has greatly helped to reduce overall length of stay in the hospital, thus freeing up more inpatient beds for the needy and sicker patients. In addition, patients admitted to the OU get earlier access to short-term specialized services such as cardiac stress tests, gastroduodenoscopies, abdominal ultrasound, electroencephalograms, and doppler ultrasounds (to exclude deep vein thrombosis). Early follow-up can be arranged in our early access clinics called "Hot Clinics." All these improve the continuity of care and translate to overall high-quality patient care in a cost-effective environment.

References

1. Wilder JL, Ross MA, Ginde AA. National Study of Emergency Department Observation Services. *Acad Emerg Med* 2011 Sep; 18(9): 959–965.

2. Venkatesh AK, Geisler BP, Gibson Chambers JJ, et al. Use of Observation Care in US Emergency Departments, 2001 to 2008. *PloS One* 2011; 6(9):e24326.

3. Baugh CW, Venkatesh AK, Bohan JS. Emergency Department Observation Units. A clinical and financial benefit for hospitals. *Health Care Manage Rev.* 2011 Jan–Mar; 36(1):28–37.

4. Graff L, Mucci D, Radford MJ. Decision to hospitalize: Objective diagnosis-related group criteria versus clinical judgement. *Ann Emerg Med* 1988; 17:943–952.

5. Ng CW, Lim GH, McMaster F, et al. Patient satisfaction in an Observation Unit: the Consumer Assessment of Health Providers and Systems Hospital Survey. *Emerg Med J.* 2009 Aug; 26(8):586–589.

6. American College of Emergency Physicians. Management of Observation Units. *Ann Emerg Med* 1988; 17:1348–1352.

7. Realdi G, Giannini S, Floretto P, et al. Diagnostic pathways of the complex patients: rapid intensive observation in an acute medical unit. *Intern Emerg Med* 2011 Oct; 6 Suppl 1:85–92.

8. Graff LG, Radford MJ. Formula for emergency physician staffing. *Ann Emerg Med* 1990; 8:194–199.

9. Observation Medicine Guidelines 2009. Victorian Government Department of Human Services, Melbourne, Australia.

10. Graff LG. The observation patient in the DRG era. *Am J Emerg Med* 1988; 6:93–103.

11. Neville L, Rowland RS. Short stay unit solves emergency overcrowding. *Dimens Health Serv* 1983; 60:26–27.

12. Kellerman A, Andrulis A, Hackman B. Hospital and emergency medicine department overcrowding. Results of a National Survey. *Ann Emerg Med* 1990; 19:447.

Chapter 73

Australia

John Burke, FACEM

Introduction

Observation Medicine has become an essential adjunct to emergency medicine practice in Australasia, and dedicated Observation Wards (OW) are now featured in the design of most modern metropolitan hospitals. While their function may vary according to local flow models and resource constraints, their common focus is the rapid turnover of selected patient groups for the purposes of admission avoidance and early discharge. Successful implementation requires not only well-defined operational parameters but also a clear understanding of how the unit contributes to overall patient flow.

Australasian Model of Care

While many international authors endorse an expanded role for observation facilities, the Australasian OW is typically based in the emergency department (ED) and does not provide care for inpatients under normal circumstances. It may, however, coexist with short-stay units governed by internal medicine departments (Emergency Medical Units, Medical Assessment and Planning Units, etc.) that focus upon more complex inpatient services. The different responsibilities (and governance) of each of these units need to be explicitly stated to avoid confusion.

Australasian OWs target specific patient groups whose care may be augmented by early intensive workup and/or treatment that falls within the resources and skill set of Emergency Physicians (EPs). These include:

- Undifferentiated presentations that may benefit from serial examination and/or further diagnostic studies;
- Stable patients who require a brief period of specific therapy prior to outpatient management;

- Vulnerable or socially disadvantaged patients who require additional supports in place prior to discharge.

Boarding inpatients are not a preferred category of OW patients and the use of the OW as a holding unit compromises the efficiency of the main department. For similar reasons, patients who clearly require admission for > 24 hours are unlikely to benefit from interim care in the OW and their presence reduces the functional capacity of the unit.

Minimum Requirements

A sustained improvement in patient flow outcomes is dependent upon several key features:

- *Geographical proximity to the Emergency Department*, which provides all medical/ nursing/allied health personnel. This maintains the emphasis on regular review and early decision making with respect to disposition. Provision for optimal staffing is normally made in the main departmental roster, which ensures that personnel are competent to perform duties in all areas.
- *Admitting rights for specialist emergency physicians* who retain clinical responsibility and provide regular review. If the patient stays beyond the end of a staff specialist's shift, case knowledge is handed over to ED-based house staff who maintain care on behalf of the admitting doctor.
- *Strict inclusion/exclusion criteria to identify suitable patients.* Some departments are more prescriptive than others in their approach to patient selection. As mentioned earlier, patients whose trajectory may be changed or improved by OW admission should be considered, while those with a high chance of eventual admission should be referred directly

to inpatient services, particularly those requiring specialized beds.

- *Well-defined assessment/management plans with clear end-points.* Further workup should address a specific differential diagnosis and revolve around simple binary decision points. Management should be limited to a single clinical problem with clearly documented therapies and discharge criteria.
- *Priority access to diagnostic services such as pathology and medical imaging.* Larger departments typically have co-located radiology services and early reporting.
- *Priority referral to allied health services.* Poor mobility and a need for social supports are significant predictors of failed discharge planning.
- *A nominal time limit (usually 24 hours) enforced by an unambiguous transfer policy.* Inpatient review on the wards traditionally occurs during once-daily rounds, meaning that the inpatient length of stay (IPLOS) tends to be measured in whole days once the patient leaves the ED. Not only does the OW offer an alternative pathway measured in hours, but it identifies and discharges diagnostic groups that are not funded for longer stays under activity-based business models.
- *Consistent management guidelines for the most common diagnostic groups,* such as:
  - Chest pain for investigation
  - Asthma
  - Renal colic
  - Overdose
  - Cellulitis
  - Pyelonephritis
  - Minor head injuries
  - Migraine, etc.

Impact of Observation Wards

In 2000 Williams et al.[1] reported on the ability of Australasian OWs to reduce total length of stay for certain diagnostic-related groups (DRGs) by reducing ward admissions (at the expense of a greater number of short-stay admissions). Since that time there have been few prospective interventional trials examining the utility of Australian OWs. The implementation of OWs is frequently part of a greater structural and operational redesign that makes it difficult to control for confounders.

Local experience supports the commonly held international view that OWs may safely reduce LOS and inappropriate admissions, while increasing staff and patient satisfaction. Areas of uncertainty in the literature include the ideal size/capacity of an OW and the overall financial benefit of observation medicine across a range of economic conditions.

Observation Medicine Culture

In order for any short-stay unit to improve the performance of a hospital, its beds must function as more than simply additional capacity – they must add something of value that is not available further along the patient journey. In this case, the advantage is discharge facilitation via front-loaded senior expertise. This opportunity is lost by passively allowing boarding inpatients to be "held" in the OW, a practice that demonstrates a lack of understanding of hospital bed dynamics.

In addition to clinical support, the OW model of care requires the advocacy of emergency physicians, who can demonstrate the value of observation medicine by way of example. A proactive approach to patient selection and early discharge will prevent the OW from becoming an easy target during times of economic hardship or bed shortage.

Case Study – Royal Brisbane and Women's Hospital

Royal Brisbane & Women's Hospital
Brisbane, Queensland.

Hospital	
Bed capacity (no Pediatrics)	Total beds ~ 850 Acute overnight beds ~ 600
Emergency admissions	~24,000
Average inpatient LOS	5.5 days

Emergency Department	
Annual ED presentations (adult)	74,000
Admission rate	32%
ED capacity	Resuscitation + Trauma bays: 7 Acute cubicles: 27 Fast-track bays: 5 + Physiotherapy
Observation Ward	
Bed capacity	18 (unmonitored)
Staffing (0800–1800 hours)	5 nurses, 1 Registrar, 1 Staff Specialist
Admissions	ED ~ 8000 per annum (LOS 10 hours) Inpatient (boarding) ~ 500 per annum (LOS 23 hours)
Discharge rate (ED patients)	86%
Top 10 DRGs	Chest pain (15%) Headache Abdominal pain Syncope Cellulitis Pharmaceutical overdose Pyelonephritis Asthma Acute back pain Renal colic
Chest pain pathway (protocol)	~ 1,000 intermediate risk patients (negative biomarkers and ECG) 0.2% admitted with positive markers at 6 hours 5% admitted with positive exercise stress test (EST)
Novel patient groups	Post-aspiration of spontaneous pneumothorax Snake bite* Decompression illness (hyperbaric unit)** Hospital in the Nursing Home*** (HINH)

LOS = length of stay

* Snakebites that do not produce clinical or biochemical envenomation are observed in the OW during a 12-hour serial assessment and treatment program. (See snakebite protocols in Chapters 84 and 85)

** The hyperbaric patients are managed by a visiting hyperbaric specialist who admits to the OW under a special arrangement with the hospital.

*** HINH = Hospital in the Nursing Home is a locally developed hospital avoidance program that features a team of ED specialists and registered nurses who liaise with local aged care facilities. Many presentations to the hospital ED can be avoided by way of nursing home visits, phone consultation, or brief ED assessment and OW management.

References

1. Williams A, Jelinek G, Rogers I, et al. The effect of establishment of an observation ward on hospital admission profiles. *Med Journal Aust* 2000; 173:411–414.

2. Ross M, Graff L.. Principles of observation medicine. *Emerg Med Clin Nth Am* 2001; 19(1) 1–17.

3. Williams, A. Emergency department observation wards. In: Cameron et al. (ed). *Textbook of Adult Emergency Medicine.* 2nd ed. Churchill Livingstone; 2004. pp. 710–712.

4. Cooke MW, Higgins J, Kidd P. Use of emergency observation and assessment wards: a systematic literature review. *Emerg Med J* 2003;20: 138–142.

5. Chan T, Arendts G, Stevens M. Variables that predict admission to hospital from an emergency department observation unit. *Emerg Med Aust* 2008; 20: 216–220.

6. Lucas BP, Kumapley R. A hospitalist-run short-stay unit: features that predict length-of-stay and eventual admission to traditional inpatient services. *J Hosp Med* 2009; 4(5): 276–283.

7. Clinical Epidemiology & Health Service Evaluation Unit. Models of care to optimise acute length of stay – Short Stay/Observation Unit (SOU), Medical Assessment and Planning Unit (MAPU), Emergency Medical Unit (EMU). Available from www.royalmelbourne hospital.org/project-reports/ w1/i1017258/ (Accessed March 2016).

Chapter

74

New Zealand

Michael Ardagh, ONZM, PhD, MbChB, DCH, FACEM

National Overview

In 2009 overcrowding of New Zealand (NZ) emergency departments (EDs) prompted the adoption of an ED length of stay (LOS) target. The 'Shorter Stays in Emergency Departments' health target is one of six government health priorities and is defined as follows: 95% of patients will be admitted, discharged or transferred from an ED within 6 hours of arrival. Admission, in this regard, includes admission to an ED observation unit (OU). Consequently the target has encouraged, among many other things, the development of observation units.

ED LOS targets have the potential for both good and bad consequences and an explicit part of pursuing the target in NZ has been to discourage mere compliance and instead to encourage changes which result in genuine improvements in the quality of patient care.[1] To this end a government sponsored advisory group, composed mostly of Emergency Physicians and Emergency Nurses, published a document[2] intended to encourage the development of these units for the right reasons. Specifically it states:

> ED Observation Units are valuable for reasons of efficiency, patient comfort and patient safety. They allow prolonged ED care in a more conducive environment (on a bed rather than a stretcher, with less light and noise than the main ED), and provide an alternative to either the admission of patients to inpatient wards or the discharge of patients when it may be unsafe or inappropriate to do so (e.g., elderly patients at night).

The document suggests ED OUs should

- allow a short period of observation, further treatment, or further investigation by ED staff;
- be for patients who are perceived to be safe for discharge at the end of that period;
- be for patients for whom there is usually no need, or an unlikely need, for input from inpatient staff/teams;
- have a duration of stay of usually 6 to 8 hours, but up to a maximum of 24 hours.

It recommends that governance of an ED OU, including resourcing, clinical management, standards, policies, and procedures, should be with the ED. It goes on to define the circumstances under which admission to an ED OU should allow "stopping the clock" for the purposes of the Shorter Stays in the ED Health Target, emphasizing that units should have dedicated staffing, patients in beds rather than trolleys, and be located in a dedicated space. Consequently, observation medicine in NZ is not intended to be practiced in corridors or waiting rooms.

In early 2010 just over half of NZ EDs, including most of the busiest EDs, had an OU and others are planning them.[3] In 2011, there was a major earthquake in Christchurch, NZ so populations changed and services were affected. We are now back to a reasonably stable state with services resurrected.

An Example

Christchurch Hospital serves a population of approximately 500,000 for secondary care and provides tertiary services for much of the population of the South Island of NZ. In 2010, the ED saw 72,000 presentations per annum. Currently, the ED sees in excess of 90,000 presentations per annum. It has approximately 40 treatment cubicles and 10 beds in a co-located OU. It is unable to "divert" to other local EDs, and historically has been prone to considerable peaks of demand and episodes of overcrowding.

Observation beds have been operational since 1995, and in their current form since 2008. Patients will be admitted to the unit under the following conditions, according to the guidelines for admission to the unit:

- The patient has an 80 to 90% perceived chance of discharge home from the observation unit.

- The patient will likely be ready for discharge within 8 hours of admission to the OU (although with the expectation that they will stay overnight if the 8 hours finishes late at night).
- The patient will be under the care of ED doctors and is unlikely to need input from inpatient specialist teams.
- The patient should have one of the following conditions (or some other condition consistent with the above criteria, at the discretion of the senior doctor on duty):
  - Clinically stable drug overdose
  - Clinically stable allergic reaction
  - Minor head injury (GCS 14 or 15) without skull fracture or significant other injuries
  - Acute alcohol intoxication with no other significant illness
  - Social disposition problem
  - Mild asthmatic promptly responsive to treatment
  - Single seizures with full recovery
  - Hypoglycemia with full recovery

An increasing trend has been the overnight admission of elderly after falls or other presentations not mandating hospital admission. An emergency physician does a round each morning and a multidisciplinary team, consisting of social workers, physiotherapists and occupational therapists, helps facilitate discharge. A Psychiatric Emergency Service assesses relevant patients routinely in the mornings or on call. A community-based "acute demand" team, funded by the District Health Board to provide a number of admission avoidance/discharge facilitation services, often will assist with discharge arrangements.

Like most NZ OUs there is not a specific pathway for rule out acute coronary syndrome (ACS) in low-risk chest pain. This function tends to be undertaken in the ED itself, or after referral to Cardiology or Internal Medicine inpatient services. However, an accelerated pathway for rule out of ACS in low–risk patients is the subject of research[4] and the practice is likely to change in the future.

In the calendar year of 2010 the Christchurch Hospital ED OU admitted 5,154 patients, with an average LOS of 7.3 hours (median of 6 hours) and a subsequent admission rate to hospital of 15%. Common diagnostic groups included deliberate self-poisoning, alcohol intoxication (often associated with assault or falls with head and/or facial injuries), elderly with falls or syncope (often associated with soft tissue injury or minor fractures limiting mobility), minor head injuries, gastroenteritis requiring intravenous rehydration, renal colic, back pain, and constipation.

Summary

Observation medicine in NZ is active, but variable and evolving. Our challenge is to ensure that the growth of this service is guided by good reason.

References

1. Ardagh M. How to achieve New Zealand's shorter stays in emergency departments health targets. *New Zealand Medical Journal*. 11 June 2010, Vol. 123 No. 1316; ISSN 1175 8716 www.nzma.org.nz/journal/123–1316/4152/ (Accessed March 2016).

2. Streaming and the use of Emergency Department Observation Units and Inpatient Assessment Units. www.hiirc.org.nz/page/18737/guidance-statement-ed-obervation-and-inpatient/?tab=4179&contentType=451&section=9088

3. Ardagh M, Tonkin G, Possenniskie C. Improving acute patient flow and resolving emergency department overcrowding in New Zealand hospitals—the major challenges and the promising initiatives. *New Zealand Medical Journal*. 14 October 2011, Vol. 124 No. 1344; ISSN 1175 8716 http://journal.nzma.org.nz/journal/124–1344/4904/

4. Than M, Cullen L, Reid CM, et al. A 2-h diagnostic protocol to assess patients with chest pain symptoms in the Asia-Pacific region (ASPECT): a prospective observational validation study *The Lancet*. 26 March 2011, Vol. 377, No. 9771, Pages 1077–1084. DOI: 10.1016/S0140-6736(11) 60310-3.

France

Said Laribi, MD, PhD
Patrick Plaisance, MD, PhD

Context

Over the past 30 years there has been on average a 30% decrease in the number of hospital beds in France from 11.1 to 7.7 per 1,000 inhabitants.[1] On the other hand, the number of Emergency Department (ED) visits has doubled over the past decade.[2] As an example, we used to receive in our ED 52,000 visits in 2005, in 2011 we received 72,000 patients. Around 15% of our ED patients are hospitalized. In this context, it was decided 20 years ago to create ED observation units (OUs).[3] The initial aim of these units was to admit patients in need of 24-hour hospitalization either to do additional examinations or for surveillance/monitoring. In our ED, ~12,000 patients (17% of the total visits) had to be hospitalized in 2011; half of these patients were directly admitted to the hospital, the other half being admitted to our ED OU. Around 8% of our ED patients are more than 75 years old with a lot of comorbidities. Another specificity of our ED is that it is located in a poor neighborhood of Paris. As a consequence, we receive many patients with social difficulties: the homeless, elderly patients without relatives, etc. Of note, most of the hospitals change their conventional hospital beds into beds that can be used only during weekdays, (e.g. Monday morning to Friday evening) which decreases the beds available to the EDs on weekends. In this context, we are going to describe the daily organization of our ED OU.

Emergency Department Observation Unit organization

Our ED OU is composed of 13 beds with a possible extension to 21 beds. It is located nearby the ED. Patients admitted to this unit are in need of 24-hour surveillance/monitoring before discharge, for example: psychiatric patients, patients who wait for some specialized tests (MRI, scan, etc.), and patients who need an inpatient bed when no bed is available in the hospital. Two nurses are dedicated to this unit 24/7. From 9 a.m. to 6 p.m. a senior emergency physician and a resident in emergency medicine are dedicated to this area. Their work consists of an evaluation of all patients admitted to this unit the previous night, doing further examinations if needed and deciding the best destination for each patient: going back home, admission to an in hospital unit, or direct transfer to a rehabilitation center, etc.

To help physicians and nurses achieve this task, we have during the weekdays two dedicated social workers. They help in the social evaluation of the patients, especially the elderly and homeless people. With their help, it is sometimes possible to send back home some elderly patients. Our social workers organize a nurse visit to these patients in their home following discharge. They also are in contact with rehabilitation centers. If a patient is too weak to go back home but doesn't need to be hospitalized, our social workers prepare a request to the rehabilitation centers. This system allows us to keep the beds in the hospital for the patients who need further exploration.

We also have the possibility of calling during weekdays a geriatric mobile unit composed of a physician and a nurse specialized in geriatrics.[4] They help the emergency physician in the evaluation of some elderly patients with a lot of comorbidities. Rarely, it is possible to send back home some of these patients with a geriatrics consultation organized at follow-up.

Another issue that emergency physicians have to face is the care of patients with a chronic disease in need of palliative care. Over the last years we have had to keep these patients in our OU until their death because no palliative bed is available.

Ideally the ED OU should be empty at the beginning of the night shift: from 6 p.m. to 9 a.m. Due to the shortage in inpatient beds and the overcrowding of our ED, elderly patients with comorbidities are admitted to the ED OU.[5] We have on a regular basis four to five patients that spend more than 24 hours in our OU.

During the night shift, from 6 p.m. to 9 a.m, if needed, the nurses call the emergency physician on shift to see a patient or review a test result.

Perspectives

Our main objective is to maintain the length of stay in the OU below 48 hours. To achieve this goal, we work closely with the other departments of our hospital so everybody in the institution knows that our ED needs around 35 beds every 24 hours. We also work with the other departments on the kind of patients that they would like to take charge of. The principle difficulty that persists concerns the elderly patients in need of a bed in the geriatric department. Due to the lack of beds in the geriatric department and the resistance of some of the other departments to take charge of these patients, these patients may spend more than 48 hours in our OU, increasing the mean length of stay.

To conclude, the ED OU has become, over the last few years, a mandatory tool to manage patients in need of hospitalization. The presence of a senior emergency physician seven days a week allows hospitalizing only the patients that really need it. The presence of social workers appears to be very helpful in our ED OU.

References

1. World Health Organization: www.who.int/en/ (Accessed March 2016).

2. French Society for Emergency Medicine (SFMU). [Situation of emergency departments in France] (French) www.sfmu.org/documents/ressources/referentiels/Aval_SU_SFMU_mai_2005.pdf (Accessed March 2016).

3. French Society for Medicine Emergency on establishment, management, use and evaluation of ED observation units (French): www.sfmu.org/documents/ressources/referentiels/ref_uhcd.pdf (Accessed March 2016).

4. Ross MA, Compton S, Richardson D, et al. The use and effectiveness of an emergency department observation unit for elderly patients. *Annals of Emergency Medicine* May 2003; 41(5):668–677.

5. Pines JM, Weber JA, Alkemade AJ, et al. International Perspectives on Emergency Department Crowding. *Acad Emerg Med* 2011; 18:1358–1370.

Chapter 76

Germany

Martin Mockel, MD, PhD, FESC, FAHA
Julia Searle, MD, Phd

Background and Clinical Need

In Germany, of the adults with medical emergencies seen in the emergency department (ED), around 10% of patients present with a chief complaint of chest pain. Of these, around 50% suffer from an acute coronary syndrome (ACS), and an acute myocardial infarction (AMI) is diagnosed in roughly 20% of the chest pain patients.[1] It is one of the most difficult challenges in Emergency Medicine (EM) to identify chest pain patients with or in acute danger of an AMI and those with non-ischemic or non-cardiac underlying problems. Both the incorrect classification into the high-risk group and the erroneous classification into a low-risk group can have negative consequences for the patient as well as for the health care system. The rate of patients who were mistakenly discharged from the ED with myocardial infarction has been described to lie between 2 and 8% and the risk-adjusted mortality ratio for those who were not hospitalized, as compared with those who were, was significantly increased.[2] On the other hand, the admission of chest pain patients without ACS puts patients at risk of inappropriate or unnecessary diagnostic testing and treatment with the potential for side effects from the treatment, and poses a burden to costs for the health care system and resource availability in the ED. In summary, chest pain is a frequent symptom in adults seen with a medical emergency in the ED and can be caused by life-threatening diseases, which need to be diagnosed or excluded in a standardized patient workup.

The Establishment of Chest Pain Units in Germany

Aware of the diagnostic challenges, specialized observation units (OUs) or chest pain centers (CPCs) have been set up in the United States and the United Kingdom since the beginning of the 1990s and clinical trials have shown their great success in improving patient outcome as well as economic resource utilization.[3,4]

In Germany, the first Chest Pain Units (CPUs) were established at the beginning of this century. In 2008, the Task Force CPU of the German Society of Cardiology (Deutsche Gesellschaft für Kardiologie [DGK]) defined minimal standard criteria for a CPU and started a certification campaign to avoid misuse of the term Chest Pain Unit and to guarantee a systematic approach.[5] The DGK standards follow the Guidelines of the DGK for patients with ACS[6,7] and include requirements regarding the premises of the CPU, technical equipment, diagnostic measures, therapeutic strategies, cooperating partners, and institutions as well as training and professional experience of staff.[5] Since the first certification in October 2008, 141 German CPUs have been certified by the DGK (as of April 17, 2012) and numbers are rising. The DGK estimates that 250 CPUs are necessary to cover the whole German territory.[8]

The Concept of a CPU

The overall aim of a CPU is to optimize the diagnostic and therapeutic management process for patients with acute chest pain whilst meeting the requirements of current evidence-based guidelines to improve patient outcome and reduce costs. Figure 76.1 illustrates the standardized flowchart of patient management in a CPU. It is important to stress that the starting point for standardized patient care involves all patients with all kinds of chest pain and not only patients with ACS. Optimized care is delivered not only to patients with ACS but also to those with non-ischemic and extra-cardiac chest pain.

Important prerequisites to fulfill certification requirements are the availability of a cardiac catheterization laboratory 24 hours a day, 365 days a year, a minimum of four monitored beds, and

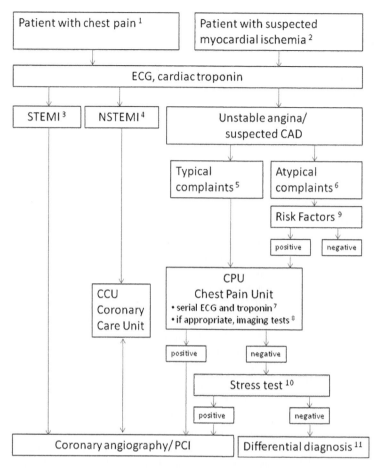

Figure 76.1 Chest Pain Unit:[1] Chest pain of all kinds,[2] Angina pectoris equivalents. This could be dyspnea, atypical chest pain, or other symptoms and needs to be judged individually. Suspicion of myocardial ischemia can also result from a series of events, e.g., arrhythmogenic syncope in a patient with a high-risk cardiac profile,[3]
There are three categories of patients: STEMI, NSTEMI and chest pain patients without elevated cardiac markers or acute ST elevation MI. STEMI and NSTEMI patients are monitored in a Coronary Care Unit. Stable chest pain patients without elevated cardiac markers or acute ST elevation MI can be monitored in a chest pain unit.
ST-elevation myocardial infarction (STEMI). Patients with STEMI are treated according to current guidelines. Standard operating procedures (SOPs) need to be available at a Chest Pain Unit (CPU) and regular training needs to be available,[4]
Non-ST-elevation myocardial infarction (NSTEMI). Patients with NSTEMI are treated according to the current guidelines. Standard operating procedures (SOPs) need to be available at a CPU and regular training needs to be available.Patients with NSTEMI are monitored on a Coronary Care Unit (Intensive or Intermediate Care Unit).[5]
Patients with typical complaints but without elevated cardiac markers (troponin) and without ST-elevation are immediately transferred to the CPU.[6] Patients with atypical complaints are in most cases transferred to the CPU, unless myocardial ischemia is extremely unlikely.[7] Cardiac markers.
Patients on a CPU should be tested for cardiac markers, preferably troponin, at admission and again after 6–8 hours; earlier time points (e.g., 3h) are discussed with high-sensitive troponin assays,[8] Imaging. In addition to serial ECG and marker testing, imaging techniques can be indicated (e.g., echocardiography, cardiac MRI, cardiac CT, SPECT).[9]
Risk factors. Risk factors in this sense are refractory angina, diabetes mellitus, TIMI risk score > 3 points or GRACE-score > 140.[10] Stress test. After exclusion of acute myocardial infarction, a stress test should be performed as soon as possible (bicycle stress test, stress echocardiography, stress myocardial scintigraphy, stress-MRI).[11]
Differential diagnosis. In case of a negative evaluation the differential diagnoses of the acute chest pain should be sought. The most important diagnoses are pulmonary embolism, peri/myocarditis, and aortic dissection. Orthopedic correlates and gastrointestinal diseases can mostly be evaluated in the primary care system.

24-hour availability of a laboratory as well as availability of echocardiography, but also the availability of computerized tomography (CT), magnetic resonance imaging (MRI) and abdominal ultrasound for the evaluation of differential diagnoses.

An important aspect of the CPU concept is to create an environment that assures the implementation of evidence-based guidelines. Minimal standard criteria of the DGK include the introduction of algorithms for STEMI (divided in pre-announced and unannounced STEMI), NSTEMI, stable and unstable angina pectoris, hypertensive crisis, acute pulmonary embolism, acute aortic syndrome, cardiogenic shock and resuscitation; and recommendations for implementation of additional standard operating procedures (SOPs) and algorithms. Additionally door-to-balloon times for patients with STEMI and NSTEMI have to meet the guideline requirements.[5]

The Effect of CPUs in Germany

A number of secondary data analyses and clinical trials have shown the beneficial effect on patient outcome and on resource utilization of patient management in a CPU as opposed to management in a conventional inpatient setting in the United States and the United Kingdom.[3,4] The same is true for results of the evaluation of CPUs in Germany. The University of Mainz was the first institution with a certified CPU in Germany. They retrospectively evaluated patient outcome

(combined endpoint of AMI, stroke, or death of all causes within 1 year after the initial event), length of stay (LOS) as a criterion for economic benefit, and patient satisfaction in their institution, using patient data from before and after the implementation of their CPU.[9–11] In the population of all patients with chest pain, no outcome benefit could be shown. In the group of patients with ACS though, treatment in a conventional ED showed a significantly increased hazard ratio for the combined endpoint and a reduced 1-year survival rate as compared to CPU treatment.[9] Likewise, the LOS of patients with ACS was significantly shorter after CPU implementation[10] and patient satisfaction was markedly increased.[11]

Conclusion

The concept of specialized Chest Pain Units in Germany is relatively new and nation-wide coverage still has to be achieved. Due to the dedicated work of a Task Force of the German Society of Cardiology and the certification process, the term CPU is standardized and institutions have to meet at least defined "minimal" requirements. Evidence for the prognostic and economic benefit of German CPUs has only been evaluated by retrospective data analysis in one center. Large prospective controlled clinical trials as well as the evaluation of guideline adherence, management processes, and the economic benefit considering all patients with of all kinds of chest pain are still lacking.

References

1. Mockel M, Searle J, Muller R, et al. Chief complaints in medical emergencies: do they relate to underlying disease and outcome? The Charite Emergency Medicine Study (CHARITEM). *Eur J Emerg Med* 2012 Mar 1.

2. Pope JH, Aufderheide TP, Ruthazer R, et al. Missed diagnoses of acute cardiac ischemia in the emergency department. *N Engl J Med* 2000 Apr 20;342(16):1163–1170.

3. Farkouh ME, Smars PA, Reeder GS, et al. A clinical trial of a chest-pain observation unit for patients with unstable angina. Chest Pain Evaluation in the Emergency Room (CHEER) Investigators. *N Engl J Med* 1998 Dec 24;339 (26):1882–1888.

4. Goodacre S, Nicholl J, Dixon S, et al. Randomised controlled trial and economic evaluation of a chest pain observation unit compared with routine care. *BMJ* 2004 Jan 31;328 (7434):254.

5. Breuckmann F, Post F, Giannitsis E, et al. Kriterien der Deutschen Gesellschaft für Kardiologie - Herz- und Kreislaufforschung für "Chest-Pain-Units." *Kardiologe* 2008 Sep 15;5(2):389–394.

6. Hamm CW. Guidelines: Acute coronary syndrome (ACS). II: Acute coronary syndrome with ST-elevation. *Z Kardiol* 2004 Apr;93 (4):324–341.

7. Hamm CW. [Guidelines: acute coronary syndrome (ACS). 1: ACS without persistent ST segment elevations]. *Z Kardiol* 2004 Jan;93(1):72–90.

8. Post F, Gori T, Senges J, et al. Establishment and progress of the chest pain unit certification process in Germany and the local experiences of Mainz. *Eur Heart J* 2012 Mar;33 (6):682–686.

9. Keller T, Post F, Tzikas S, et al. Improved outcome in acute coronary syndrome by establishing a chest pain unit. *Clin Res Cardiol* 2010 Mar;99 (3):149–155.

10. Keller T, Tzikas S, Scheiba O, et al. The length of hospital stay in patients with acute coronary syndrome is reduced by establishing a chest pain unit. *Herz* 2011 Nov 5.

11. Tzikas S, Keller T, Post F, et al. Patient satisfaction in acute coronary syndrome. Improvement through the establishment of a chest pain unit. *Herz* 2010 Sep;35(6):403–409.

Chapter

Italy

77

Salvatore Di Somma, MD, PhD
Angelo Ianni, MD
Cristina Bongiovanni, MD

Emergency Medicine is deputed to manage clinical emergencies. At the end of this process the Emergency Department (ED) physician must decide for final disposition: discharge or admission of the patient. Today, ED overcrowding represents an international crisis that may negatively affect the quality and the access to health care and is associated with an increased risk of in-hospital mortality.[1,2] As a consequence of the lack of available beds for acute patient's hospitalization and the request of more appropriate disposition, the ED mission gradually changed from "Admit to work" to

"Work to admit," indicating the need to create a new filter system for hospital admission.[3]

The Observation Unit (OU) is the third opportunity for ED physicians to manage clinical emergencies, in an attempt to avoid the risk of inappropriate discharge and/or hospitalization. In Italy, observation practice in the ED is very common and widespread, trying to face off the problem of the acute patient's long length of stay (LOS) in the ED, waiting for bed allocation, with consequent ED overcrowding.[4] According to Italian data, about 5 to 7% of patients referring to the

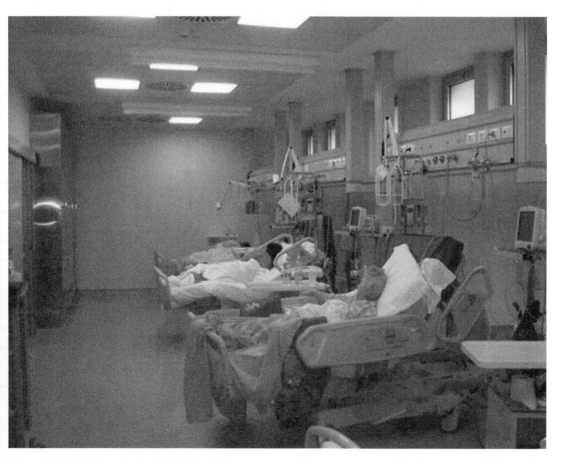

Figure 77.1 The OU ward in Sant'Andrea Hospital, Rome.

ED need to be observed for a time, requiring care for 24–36 hours. Of these patients, 10 to 30% are admitted, while 70–90% are discharged.[3]

In the 1990s, the National Health System (NHS) decided to introduce in Italy observation medicine (OM) with the aim to impact the in-hospital admission decision. The Italian Presidential Decree of March 27, 1992, enhanced the power of the local regional government in terms of public health activities planning, funding, organization, and control.[5,6] In this document the activation of OU wards was introduced with the objective to ameliorate the decision for hospital admission from the ED, through an intensive and accurate stabilization of critical patients who often do not need subsequent hospitalization. This project was also coupled with a common teaching process for ED doctors and nurses to better use the emergency "evidence based medicine." The proper use of the OU was aimed to:[7]

– decrease the risk of medical mistakes through accelerated management protocols;
– reduce inappropriate admissions by improving the function of the filter;
– decrease the LOS;
– reduce the costs;
– improve the quality of health care perceived by users.

Systematic guidelines were created and approved in the attempt to unify the different approach of every Italian region to OU management.[8] These guidelines introduced the all-comprehensive daily reimbursement, of the value of 220€/patient not hospitalized after observation in ED. Exceptions are Region Lazio (275€),[9] Region Veneto (200€),[10] and Region Alto Adige (250 €).[11]

In the OU, accelerated management protocols allow facilitation of patient care for selected ED patients and improve the observation quality of patients at "low risk" for complications.[8] The

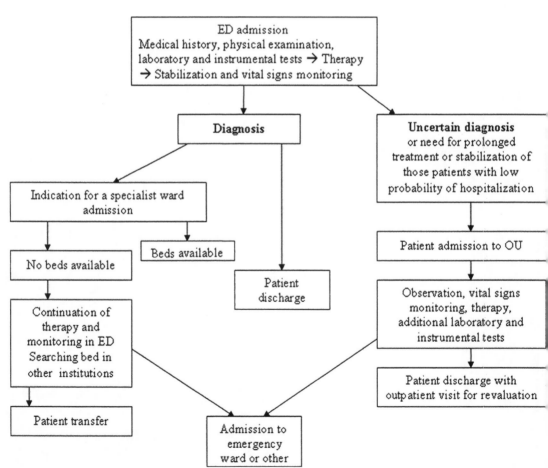

Figure 77.2 Proposed protocol for the management of patient care in emergency department.

LOS in the OU is usually not less than 6 hours and not more than 24 hours, with exceptions arising from the requirements of individual regions or specifically of the single hospital (maximum of 36 hours).[9,12,13,14]

From a structural point of view, the OU is a dedicated area nearby the ED, providing the same services as the ED. In particular, there must be available a fair and appropriate (relative to inpatient beds), highly skilled, dedicated, 24-hour nursing staff, support staff, and medical staff; a laboratory providing for quick laboratory tests with an ability to respond 24 hours a day; and a conventional radiology and CT scan for the total body 24 hours a day with real time x-ray responses. All medical and nursing activity must be computerized and available: there should be a clinical diary for each patient and, at discharge time, a brief report for the general practitioner must be delivered.

Depending on the existing buildings, there are two different possible settings: 1) an open space with center console and 2) individual rooms or compartments with central monitoring. The number of beds in each OU is identified using two equivalent criteria: 2% of the hospital's total number of beds or one bed for every 4,000–8,000 access to the ED. A portion of beds, on average 50%, must be provided with hemodynamic and respiratory monitoring with pulse oximeter. Each bed should be provided with oxygen and vacuum and at least one monitor defibrillator/pacer, one noninvasive mechanical ventilator able to work in PSV/PEEP mode, one multidisciplinary ultrasound, one electrocardiograph, an appropriate number of glucometers, of sphygmomanometers, of infusion pumps, and intubation/CPR staff.[4] (See Chapter 5 on Observation Unit Design)

In particular, in Sant'Andrea Hospital, Rome, the OU is provided with eight multiparametric monitored beds divided into two rooms with a central core working station. (Figure 77.1) Point-of-care laboratory system test for blood gas

Table 77.1 Conditions for Admission to OU

Asthma, COPD	Paroxysmal atrial
Abdominal pain	fibrillation
Renal colic	Intoxication
Chest pain	Congestive heart failure
Infections	Syncope
Allergic reactions	Transient ischemic
Dehydration	attack
Headache	Vertigo
Deep vein	Minor head trauma
thrombosis	Minor chest trauma
Hypertensive crisis	Hypo/Hyperglycemia

analysis, troponin, brain natriuretic peptide (BNP), neutrophil gelatinase-associated lipocain (NGAL), and urine drug abuse test are included. Furthermore, point-of-care ultrasound equipment are available for abdominal, thoracic, and cardiac disease dedicated protocols. Moreover, a continuous data recording system for EKG (24 hours) is provided for detecting complex cardiac arrhythmias and an online system allows the prompt visualization of x-ray imaging and reports. Ventilator systems for invasive and noninvasive ventilation are also provided.

In Italy differences exist between each regional state on the lists of diseases eligible for OU admission (but these lists should be interpreted with some flexibility). In every hospital and in particular in every ED dedicated structure, appropriate diagnostic and therapeutic paths are drawn for more common diseases, shared after the appropriate contextualization as the Guidelines National Plan also provides.[8] (Figure 77.2)

Table 77.1 shows the most suitable conditions for short observation admission in Italy.[8,15] Each region has its own protocols for the management of the listed acute conditions.

Monitoring the quality of care and service delivery differs in each region, and it is important for the development and implementation of "best practice" models for OM.

References

1. Bernstein SL. The effect of emergency department crowding on clinically oriented outcomes. *Acad Emerg Med.* 2009 January; 16(1):1–10.

2. Kellermann AL. Crisis in the emergency department. *N Engl J Med.* 2006 September 28; 355 (13):130.

3. Ministero della salute: documento commissione urgenza-emergenza 2008. Available at: www.salute.gov.it/imgs/C_17_pubblicazioni_856_ulterioriallegati_ulterio reallegato_0_alleg.pdf (Accessed March 2016).

4. Hoot NR. Systematic review of emergency department crowding: causes, effects, and solutions. *Ann Emerg Med.* 2008 August; 52(2):126–36. 0–3.

5. Il futuro della osservazione breve intensiva e della medicina d'urgenza. 2010. Available at: www.simeu.it/ basilicata/convegnoOBi Matera/2_Guerra.pdf (Accessed March 2016).

6. DPR 27 marzo 1992. Atto di indirizzo e coordinamento alle Regioni per la determinazione dei livelli di assistenza sanitaria di emergenza pubblicato sulla G.U. n. 76 del 31/3/92 - Serie Generale. 1992. Available at: www.118italia.net/lex/dpr 920327.asp (Accessed March 2016).

7. Section of Short Term Observation Services (ACEP): "Missed diagnosis and observation", vol. 12, no. 1, April 2003; "Observation unit lecture", vol. 13, no. 1, August 2004.

8. Ministero della Sanità. Gazzetta Ufficiale N. 114 Serie Generale del 17 maggio1996. Atto di intesa tra Stato e regioni di approvazione delle linee guida sul sistema di emergenza sanitaria in applicazione del decreto del Presidente della Repubblica 27 marzo 1992. 1996. Available at: www.ars.marche.it/nuovo/ html/download/emergenza/ documenti%20nazionali/ int1705_96.pdf (Accessed March 2016).

9. DGR 946/07. Introduzione dell'osservazione breve intensiva nel Lazio dal 1 gennaio 2008: adempimento rif.1.3.3 del piano di rientro DGR 65/2007 e DGR 149/07. 2007. Available at: www.asplazio.it/asp_online/ att_ospedaliera/files/file_ emergenza/obi/elenco_quadri_ clinici%20.pdf (Accessed March 2016).

10. Borella L. L'osservazione breve intensiva nel Veneto. Available at: www.simeu.it/download/ convegni/2010/Relazioni_ Congresso_SIMEU_2010/ Osservazione%20Breve% 20Intensiva/L.Borella_ Osservazione%20Breve% 20Intensiva%20nel%20veneto .Pps (Accessed March 2016).

11. Linee guida per la rilevazione delle prestazioni di specialistica ambulatoriale, di diagnostica strumentale e di laboratorio (SPA) e linee guida per la procedura informativa "scheda di pronto soccorso" (SPS) Available at: www.provincia .bz.it/oep/download/unione_ SPS_PS.pdf (Accessed March 2016).

12. Proposta di linea guida istituzionale per l'Osservazione Breve in Abruzzo. 2004. Available at: www.simeu.it/ abruzzo/PropostaLineaGuida .pdf (Accessed March 2016).

13. Piemonte e Valle d'Aosta. Osservazione Breve. 2006. Available at: www.simeu.it/ piemonte/OBI_finale.pdf (Accessed March 2016).

14. DGR 24/05 Regione Emilia Romagna. Approvazione linee guida regionali per la funzione di osservazione breve intensiva (obi). Determinazione della tariffa di remunerazione dell'attivita' e definizione degli adempimenti correlati ai flussi informativi. 2005. Available at: http://utenti.unife.it/giampaolo .garani/OssBreveIntensiva/ OssBreveIntensiva-24-2005ER- evidenziato.doc (Accessed March 2016).

15. ACEP (American College Emergency Physicians) Policy Statement: Management of observation units, July 1994; Emergency Department Observation Unit, Oct 1998; Management of observation Units. *Ann Em Med* 1998, 17; 1348–1352; Emergency Care Guidelines, September 1996.

78

United Kingdom

Louella Vaughan, MBBS, MPhil, DPhil, FRACP

Dylan Jenkins, MBBS

Emergency Medicine (EM) services in the United Kingdom (UK) have supported high-quality Observation Medicine (OM) for many years. However, the context of OM is internationally unique, with UK Emergency Departments (EDs) being subject to complex national performance targets and the recent development of Acute Medicine as a subspecialty branch of General Medicine that deals solely with the first 12–72 hours of care of the medically unwell patient (see Chapter 21 Acute Medicine in the United Kingdom, Chapter 16 Extended and Complex Observation and Chapter 17 Extended Observation Services). This chapter will provide a brief overview of EM in the UK and describe the development of a new model of care.

Overview

The structure and functioning of EDs in the UK has been heavily influenced over the past decade by the need to meet governmental performance targets.[1] The 'four hour rule' was introduced in 2003/2004 and this mandated that 98% of patients presenting to an ED must be seen, treated, and then admitted or discharged in under 4 hours. As a result, many EDs have ED-led Observation Units (OUs) or Clinical Decision Units (CDUs). However, the development of Acute Medicine (AM) as a new specialty in the UK (see Chapter 21) has meant the task of Observational Medicine varies from hospital to hospital and is dictated by local circumstances.[2] Decisions about which area is most appropriate for any given patient tends to be determined by considerations regarding patient safety, rather than by given condition. Given that many EDs in the UK remain relatively understaffed,[3] OUs and CDUs have tended to be small and to take very well-defined groups of low-risk patients.

St Thomas' Hospital has one of the busiest EDs in the UK, seeing about 170,000 patients each year. The ED incorporates a 24-bed space, immediately adjacent to the main department. In the past, this space was used as a CDU, which utilized protocols to manage a range of diseases for periods of up to 72 hours. Although the CDU offered a high standard of care, its smooth functioning was often challenged by the demands of the 4-hour target, with the CDU seen as an option to avoid patients "breaching" their ED length of stay target. This problem was compounded by the relatively strict criteria for entry to the unit mandated by the protocols, resulting in the CDU being relatively underutilized or inappropriately utilized at times when bed demand was otherwise high.

In July 2012, the model of care was changed, with a focus on Goal Directed Outcomes (GDO), for both admission and discharge. Eight beds within the new Emergency Medical Unit (EMU) are now dedicated to Goal Directed Therapy, with the remainder for rapid Goal Directed Discharge. The approach within the EMU is multidisciplinary, with the EMU coordinating whatever aspects of care are required to facilitate discharge. Patients with conditions/ presentations that can be assigned to a clear investigative or management pathway are identified as early as possible within the main ED and are ideally referred to the EMU within 2 hours. Although there are no longer any rigid criteria for admission, patients with low/intermediate risk chest pain, possible pulmonary embolism, renal colic, pyelonephritis, and biliary colic represent conditions where expected outcomes and parameters for safe and effective care are clear to both Emergency and Speciality staff. The Goal Directed Therapy area of the unit has monitored beds and will accept more complex patients for stabilization before inter-hospital transfer (certain specialities are located on a second hospital site), admission to a hospital ward, or discharge home. (See Chapter 16

Extended and Complex Observation and Chapter 17 Extended Observation.) In all cases, the aim is for the patient to have a stay of less than 12 hours.

The care of patients with sickle cell disease is particularly well developed and suited to the ethos of the new unit. Care is aimed at normalizing physiology, reducing pain, and investigating to exclude treatable precipitants of the crisis and/or sinister complications (such as embolism). All patients with sickle cell who regularly attend the main ED have individualized care plans and are managed in conjunction with the Hematology Team and the dedicated Sickle Cell Nurse. This substantially reduces the time that these patients spend in the main department, improves their pain management, and facilitates their early discharge. The care plans and cooperative approach to management is being used as a model to develop services for other patient groups with relapsing disease, such as inflammatory bowel disease, who would usually be managed on a hospital ward.

Although there are no strict admission criteria, the EMU does not accept children (under 16 years) or violent/aggressive patients. For patients between the ages of 16 and 18, suitability depends on the individual patient and presenting condition. Psychiatric patients are occasionally accepted, although there must be a clear plan for the patient's management. (See Chapter 60 Psychiatric Patients.) The EMU will accept pregnant patients under 20 weeks; patients over 20 weeks go directly to obstetrics. (See Chapter 52 Hyperemesis Gravidarum.) The unit no longer accepts patients from the main ED who are awaiting beds in the hospital in order to avoid breaching performance targets.

The shift from the CDU to the EMU model of care was accompanied by an increase in both medical and nursing staff. There are two 12.5 hour long nursing shifts, with seven registered nurses (RNs) during the day and six RNs and one health care assistant (HCA) at night. There are four junior (PGY2-3) and middle grade (PGY4-8) doctors covering staggered shifts from 08:00 to 24:00 hours. Overnight, the unit has a single junior doctor covering, supported by the middle grade doctors in the main ED. There is a consultant on the floor from 08:00 to 18:00 hours, who conducts three ward rounds per day and is responsible for the gatekeeping of the EMU during the day. There is an emphasis on the maintenance of an appropriately high level of skills-mix on the EMU at all times, with an intensive program of education focused on patient safety and advanced skills. To facilitate the cross-disciplinary approach and support education, it is intended that nursing staff will rotate with staff from the main ED, as well as the Acute Medical Admission Wards. The EMU has its own clerical staff 12 hours per day.

The EMU is supported by excellent access to diagnostics and support services. The main ED hosts its own dedicated CT scanner and all EMU requests are considered urgent. Further, scans for certain conditions, such as possible head injury or renal colic, can be approved by the senior radiographers, who are present permanently within the department. The EMU is able to access the ED pathology laboratory for rapid blood results and also has its own point of care biomarker analyser for troponins and brain natriuretic peptide (BNPs). The EMU is visited twice daily by support outreach teams, including those from the Respiratory and Elderly Care departments, and these teams can be accessed quickly at other times. The co-location of the Acute Physician service and a surgical registrar (PGY4-8) within the main ED means that advice from specialist services can be quickly obtained. Medically unwell patients can be referred from the EMU into a series of "Hot Clinics" (e.g., General Medicine, Returning Traveler, Falls/Syncope, Acute Chest Pain, etc.) for review within 2–10 days of discharge, ensuring robust patient follow-up.

Outcomes

The design and the increased staffing levels resulted in rapid improvement in departmental performance. The flow through the department has increased from 15–20 patients per day to 30–35 patients per day, managing 40–45 patients on days of high demand. The performance of the main department has improved, with the department now consistently able to meet complex governmental targets and a substantial decrease on the level of "access block" and overcrowding within the department. The EMU also has positively impacted on the rest of the hospital, with reductions in admissions by 15–20 patients per day (i.e., 15–20%). Safety on the EMU has been improved, with a reduction in clinical incidents, despite more and sicker patients being admitted.

Conclusion

The CDU at St Thomas' functioned for many years as a place to deliver effective and safe protocolized care. The shift from the CDU to EMU model of care, with a focus on patient physiology and multidisciplinary input, has resulted in better care being delivered to a wider spectrum of patients and considerable improvement in departmental and hospital performance.

References

1. Mason S. United Kingdom experiences of evaluating performance and quality in Emergency Medicine. *Acad Emerg Med* 2011; 18:1234–1238.

2. Goodacre SW. Role of short stay observation ward in accident and emergency departments in the United Kingdom. *J Accid Emerg Med* 1998; 15:26–30.

3. Paw RC. Emergency department staffing in England and Wales, April 2007, *Emerg Med J* 2008; 25:420–423.

Colombia

Carlos-Hernan Camargo-Mila, MD, EAES, ACEP

Observation Medicine at Fundacion Cardio Infantil Emergency Department

Fundacion Cardio Infantil Institute of Cardiology is one of the main high-complexity teaching hospitals in Bogotá D.C. (Colombia, South America) and a national and regional research and referral center for Cardiology and Cardiovascular Surgery, Transplant Medicine, and Neurosciences. It is a nonprofit private foundation.

Our Emergency Department (ED) provides care to 110,000 patients a year, with an adult/pediatric ratio of 1.9 to 1. Initially, each patient comes in contact with the Emergency Advisor (Nursing Technician) who makes a quick visual assessment and collects initial demographic data if the patient's condition allows it. The critically ill patients (Triage 1 and 2)[1] are treated immediately either in the resuscitation room or in the Observation Unit (OU). Stable patients arriving by ambulance (Triage 3) are also treated directly in the OU. The Emergency Advisor completes the initial assessment of walking patients (Triage 3, 4, and 5)[1] with a rapid interrogation and directs them to the waiting room. From there, patients are called to Triage consultation where they are assessed by a General Physician. After this, with an initial diagnostic impression, part of the patients classified Triage 4 or 5 are redirected to Priority Care Centers (lower-complexity centers outside our hospital managed by health insurance companies). The rest (Triage 3 and some of 4 and 5) return to the waiting room after completing administrative admission. Then they are called to consultation rooms in decreasing order of complexity (with the most complex patients seen first). At this instance our General Physician decides if the patient is discharged or continues to the OU where – after medical treatment, laboratory results, images and/or specialist assessment – the patient is discharged, admitted for hospitalization, or sent to another institution for further definitive treatment. (Figure 79.1)

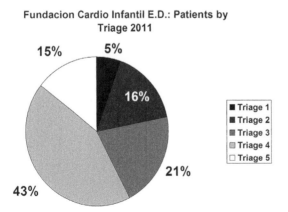

Fundacion Cardio Infantil E.D.: Patients by Triage 2011

15% 5% 16% 21% 43%

- Triage 1
- Triage 2
- Triage 3
- Triage 4
- Triage 5

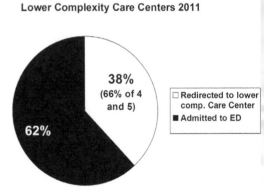

Fundacion Cardio Infantil E.D.: Redirection to Lower Complexity Care Centers 2011

38% (66% of 4 and 5) 62%

- Redirected to lower comp. Care Center
- Admitted to ED

Like in the rest of the world, Colombian emergency services have to face daily the consequences of the lack of sufficient health networks in primary care and the lack of opportunity in outpatient care, which result in congestion at the entrance.[2] This input overcrowding generally does not affect the OU and is faced with diverse strategies that are not the subject of this chapter.[3]

Fifteen percent of our patients (24% of those patients who are not redirected to a Priority Care Center) are treated in the OU. Of the 16,500 patients observed each year, 86% are discharged home and 14% are either hospitalized or referred for hospitalization in another institution at the same level of complexity.

As in all high-complexity EDs all over Colombia, the OU is directly attached to the ED[4,5] and its operation is organized in three main shifts: morning, afternoon, and night, with some additional coverage of peak situations. In our OU each shift is managed by an Emergency Specialist, two Internal Medicine Specialists, two Pediatricians, and an Orthopedist, leading the rest of the OU team composed by five General Physicians, an Internal Medicine resident, an Orthopedics resident, two Pediatrics residents, five Nurses, and eight Nursing Technicians.[6] Our observation area has a capacity of 38 patients.

The biggest challenge in our OU, common to all of Colombia, is the exit door (Output):[7] with a shortage of hospital beds throughout the country. Patients awaiting inpatient care stay in the OUs, pending a hospital bed in the health network. This situation means that every day we have between 45 and 60 patients (7 to 22 overcapacity) of which 40% to 50% have waited more than 12 hours for a hospital bed. In the end, on average 20% of patients with a hospitalization order are discharged home directly from the OU. (Figure 79.2). This situation shifted the average stay in the OU from 4.8 hours to 8.1 hours in 2011.

In order to deal with it, we developed strategies that increased our internal efficiency (throughput) and opened the exit door (output):

Fundacion Cardio Infantil ED OU: Success Rate of Hospitalization and Referral 2011

	Total 2010	Jan	Feb	Mar	Apr	May	Jun	Jul	Aug	Sep	Oct	Nov	Dec	Total 2011
■ Not affected	2,237	142	136	276	159	217	232	151	245	200	147	163	73	2,141
▨ Referred	1,900	172	173	178	136	201	173	191	192	199	260	244	199	2,318
▢ Hospitalized	6,447	528	550	595	521	543	552	565	515	462	473	473	491	6,268

In addition to normal rounds, we perform a clinical-administrative round each shift by a team composed of the ED Medical Coordinator, Physician and Nurse in charge of the patient, ED Patient's Service Coordinator, ED Quality Officer, and ED Administrative Supervisor. This multidisciplinary team verifies clinical evolution and pending laboratory studies and procedures, contributes in defining medical conduct earlier, detects and manages any administrative problem, brings accurate and understandable information to the patients and family about ED processes, and resolves any doubt about the ED care of each patient.

We empower our team to manage ED patients as much as possible without the consult of other specialties, supported on clinical guidelines and clinical pathways.

We manage special units inside the OU based on a virtual model depending on the demand: Chest Pain Unit (Average Door to Needle time 37 minutes, average Door to Balloon time 69 minutes),[8] Cerebrovascular Stroke Unit (Average Door to Needle time 117 minutes) and Hydration Unit.[9]

We establish and constantly update service agreements with the Laboratory and Imaging Departments and Consulting Specialists, in order to improve their response time.

We are improving mobile technology to support clinical records in real time.

We are working on monitoring technology with direct connection and recording to the electronic medical record (EMR).

We recently completed the construction of a Pneumatic Tube Transport System for laboratory samples and blood products. This system has a preferential pathway for ED and Intensive Care Units (ICUs) controlled by radiofrequency (RF) sensors. It was fully operational in April 2012. It has reduced laboratory management time by 25 minutes per sample.

Our administrative team is permanently aware of the management of the authorization of the services and procedures involved in the OU care process.

Once the decision of inpatient care is taken, our strong Admission and Referral Department simultaneously begins the referral process, in order to take the first open available hospital bed for our patient either inside or outside Fundacion Cardio Infantil.[10]

As soon as possible we coordinate home care with health insurance companies.

Fundacion Cardio Infantil is also working on institutional strategies that could improve OU performance. We just built a new tower that will increase our current number of inpatient beds from 340 to 400 and we are strengthening an "early discharge task force" to improve the turnover of these beds.

References

1. Gilboy N, Tanabe P, Travers D et al. Emergency Severity Index (ESI): A Triage Tool for Emergency Department Care. AHRQ Publication No. 12-0014, 2012.

2. Trzeciak S, Rivers EP. Emergency Department overcrowding in the United States: an emerging threat to patient safety and public health. *Emergency Medicine Journal* 2003; 20: 402–405.

3. Asaro PV, Lewis LM, Boxerman SB. The impact of input and output factors on emergency department throughput. *Academic Emergency Medicine* 2007; 14(3): 235–242.

4. Daly S, Campbell DA, Cameron PA. Short-stay units and observation medicine: a systematic review. *Medical Journal of Australia* 2003; 178: 559–563.

5. Graff L., 2. Principles of Observation Medicine. *Observation Medicine: The Healthcare System's Tincture of Time.* 2011. www.iep.org/Our%20Physicians/Journal%20Club/Observation%20Medicine%2002.03.11/Observation%20Medicine.pdf (Accessed January 2012).

6. Baugh CW, Graff L. 8. Management – Staffing. *Observation Medicine: The Healthcare System's Tincture of Time.* 2011. www.iep.org/Our%20Physicians/Journal%20Club/Observation%20Medicine%2002.03.11/Observation%20Medicine.pdf (Accessed January 2012).

7. Oldshaker JS. Managing emergency department overcrowding. *Emergency Medicine Clinics of North America* 2009; 27(4): 593–603.

8. Gabrielli L, Castro P, Corbalán R, et al. Long term follow up of patients consulting in a Chest Pain Unit. *Revista Médica*

Chilena 2010; 138(9): 1117–1123. Spanish.

9. Appendix 2: Types of conditions most often managed in observation medicine units. Observation Medicine Guidelines 2009. Victorian Government Department of Human Services, Melbourne, Victoria, Australia. www.health.vic.gov.au/emergency/obs09.pdf (Accessed January 2012).

10. Olshaker JS, Rathlev NK. Emergency Department overcrowding and ambulance diversion: the impact and potential solutions of extended boarding of admitted patients in the Emergency Department. *Journal of Emergency Medicine* 2006; 30(3): 351–356.

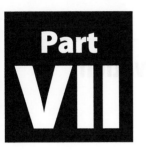

Part VII

Evidence Basis for Observation Medicine

80

The Evidence Basis for Observation Medicine in Adults Based on Diagnosis/Clinical Condition

Christopher W. Baugh, MD, MBA, FACEP
Sharon E. Mace, MD, FACEP, FAAP
Margarita E. Pena, MD, FACEP
J. Stephen Bohan, MD, MS, FACEP, FACP

Abstract

This chapter deals with critical issues in observation medicine for adult patients based on a given diagnosis or clinical condition, such as chest pain or asthma. A separate chapter deals with critical issues in observation medicine based on age, for example, observation medicine for pediatric and geriatric patients. The critical questions addressed in this chapter are:

1: In adult patients, when compared with inpatient treatment does the provision of observation services, specifically in a dedicated, protocol-driven observation unit (OU), improve patient outcomes, decrease length of stay (LOS), reduce costs, increase patient satisfaction, and have other benefits, including (but not limited to) decreased readmissions?

2: In adult patients, does the use of OU clinical and administrative methodology (by aggressive early diagnostic and therapeutic management using tools such as protocol-driven therapy) produce equivalent or better results (e.g., patient outcomes, LOS, costs, and adverse events) compared with routine inpatient care?

3: In the adult emergency department (ED), does use of an OU improve key measures of department efficiency, such as decreases in ED LOS, door-to-doctor time, ambulance diversion, and the left-without-being-seen rate?

Introduction

Recently, health care reform efforts have renewed the international dialog surrounding improving patient outcomes, cutting health care costs, improving patient safety, and increasing patient satisfaction. One of the largest drivers of these factors is reducing hospital length of stay (LOS), which results in decreased costs and fewer patient errors due to decreased exposure to the hazards of hospitalization and thus fewer opportunities for patient errors or risks such as falls and nosocomial infections. By decreasing LOS and preventing "avoidable admissions" through dedicated and efficient observation units (OUs) that use evidence-based protocols of care, OUs can achieve all of these goals. This chapter summarizes the extensive literature supporting wider use of OUs as a key strategy in our health care system.

An important concept to understand about observation care is that although observation services may occur anywhere in a hospital, under the care of any physician, the best practice is to provide observation services in a dedicated, protocol-driven unit. These well-managed units are very different from observation services occurring in a bed elsewhere in the hospital, which most often do not employ the same evidence-driven patient management strategies. Rather, these dedicated units specialize in the care of observation patients, using clinical and administrative resources and methods to use diagnosis and/or complaint-specific protocols, typically achieving a LOS that is a fraction of the time needed elsewhere for the same patient populations.

The purpose of an observation stay is to provide additional time, typically up to 24 hours but sometimes longer, for additional monitoring, diagnostics, and treatments to evaluate if a patient will require inpatient admission. In the absence of an available OU, emergency department (ED) patients who need this additional time are typically managed in inpatient beds even though most will not end up qualifying for an inpatient billing status; otherwise, providers in the ED would quickly lose the capacity to care for new patients. However, when an OU is available, it can serve as the setting of care for these patients who would have otherwise been sent to an inpatient bed. Observation services are considered outpatient services, yet are recognized as distinct and separate from either the ED visit or an inpatient admission – as recognized by both Current Procedural Terminology (CPT) and the Centers for Medicare and Medicaid Services (CMS).

The research confirming the value and success of such OUs is extensive. Over the past several decades, an increasingly robust evidence basis demonstrating the advantages of delivering care in an OU setting has developed across a wide variety of specific conditions. This chapter, using an evidence-based approach to the literature, delineates the specific research dealing with observation medicine in adults. The following chapter addresses the same critical questions for patients based on age, for example, the use of such protocol-driven, dedicated units for children and infants and the elderly.

Methodology

We created this summary of the currently available peer-reviewed literature on observation care after careful review and critical analysis of the medical literature. Additional studies were found by searching the reference lists of included papers. All articles listed in this chapter were graded by two authors for quality and strength of evidence. If there was a difference between two authors, a third author provided a tie-breaking grade to settle on a final grade. We classified the articles into three classes of evidence on the basis of the design of the study. Design 1 represents the strongest evidence for therapeutic, diagnostic, and prognostic studies, respectively and Design 3 represents the weakest evidence (Appendix A). Authors of this chapter did not grade papers they authored themselves. Articles were then graded on dimensions related

to the study's methodological features: blinded versus nonblinded outcome assessment, blinded or randomized allocation, direct or indirect outcome measures (reliability and validity), biases (e.g., selection, detection, transfer), external validity (e.g., generalizability), and sufficient sample size. Articles received a final grade (Class I, II, III) on the basis of a predetermined formula, taking into account the design and study quality; articles irrelevant to the question or with a fatal flaw were given an "X" and were not utilized in creating the final recommendation (Appendix B). Finally, patient management recommendations were made according to the criteria in Appendix C (Level A, B, or C).

The literature reviewed included articles worldwide and not just in the United States. Therefore, the scope of application could be international, in addition to the myriad of articles from the United States. The inclusion criteria are adult patients presenting to the ED. We excluded pediatric patients, who are addressed in another chapter.

We adjusted reported cost data to 2013 U.S. dollars using the medical portion of the Consumer Price Index and prevailing international currency exchange rates as of February 2013.

Articles are organized by condition and listed by level of evidence first and chronologically second; for papers published in the same year, they are further listed by strength of evidence and then grouped by use of a dedicated OU (Table 80.1) and use of OU tools/methodology, such as protocol-driven care (Table 80.2).

Results

Of the 102 articles reviewed, there were 83 articles that dealt directly with adult patients managed in an OU. The number of evidence-based articles was greatest for cardiac diagnoses with 43 articles (chest pain 29, congestive heart failure 7, atrial fibrillation 6, deep vein thrombosis 1). The remaining 40 articles included trauma 7 (general/abdominal trauma 4, head injury 3), asthma 6, ED efficiency 6, toxicology 3, pyelonephritis 3, abdominal pain 3, transient ischemic attack 3, syncope 2, and the following with 1 article each: pneumonia, COPD exacerbation, cellulitis, and decompression illness, plus 3 systematic reviews (Table 80.1A).

Table 80.1 Evidentiary Table for Critical Questions #1 and #2

Author/Year	Design	Outcomes			Other Metrics	Limitations/Comments	Class
		Length of Stay (LOS)	Cost	Patient Satisfaction			
Chest pain							
de Leon et al.[2] 1989	Prospective cohort study of CP patients placed in a CPOU utilizing a cardiac profile enzyme screen (N=495) compared to a historical inpatient group	LOS 11.1h CPOU, 3 days for historical inpatient group	Average cost for discharged non-MI patients $589 CPOU vs. $3,103 historical inpatient group 2013 USD $1,635 CPOU vs. $8,614 inpatient		Rate of discharge from CPOU after serial cardiac profile enzyme screen and non-diagnostic ECG 66%; rate of hospitalization 48h after discharge from CPOU 0%; serial cardiac profile enzyme screen false negative rate 0.6% and false positive rate 2%	Limited 48h f/u on 31% of patients	I
Gibler et al.[3] 1992	Prospective multicenter cohort study utilizing a Heart ER protocol in low-intermediate risk CP patients (N=1010)				Discharge to home rate 82.1%, AMA 2.8%, admission rate 15.1% with ACS confirmed in 33.9% of these; rate of AMI patients with initial nondiagnostic ECG 63.9%; sensitivity 79.7% and NPV 96.2% of serial CK-MB in AMI patients with nondiagnostic ECG; sensitivity of combined ECG and serial CK-MB at 3h 98.4%	Patient population not consecutive; possible false positive results of elevated CK-MB due to other noncardiac causes	I

Study	Description	LOS	Cost	Outcomes		Limitations
Gaspoz et al.[4] 1994	Prospective study of clinical outcomes and cost of patients placed in a CPOU (N=592) vs. comparison group of inpatients and discharged ED patients (N=924)	Mean, median LOS 2.3 days, 1 day CPOU vs. 6.3 days, 4 days inpatient	Median total cost/patient index visit $1,318 CPOU vs. $3,589 inpatient Median total cost at 6-month f/u $1,927 CPOU vs. $4,712 inpatient 2013 USD Index visit $3,941 CPOU vs. $10,731 inpatient 6-month f/u $5,762 CPOU vs. $14,089 inpatient	72h post-CPOU discharge AMI rate 0.8%; 6-month post-CPOU discharge AMI rate 1.7%, mortality rate 2.2%, cardiac mortality rate 1.7%, and overall survival rate 97.8%	—	Non-randomized, variation in unit setting and staffing
Gomez et al.[5] 1996	Prospective cohort of 100 low-risk CP patients assigned to rapid rule-out protocol in CPOU compared to low-risk CP historical inpatient care control group	LOS 12.1h ED OU vs. 22.3h inpatient	Index visit hospital charges $893 ED OU vs. $1,349 inpatient; hospital charges through 30-day f/u $898 ED OU vs. $1,522 inpatient 2013 USD Index visit $1,623 ED OU vs. $2,452 inpatient; 30-day f/u $1,632 ED OU vs. $2,766 inpatient	No diff in ACS between groups during index visit; no death or missed ACS diagnosis after discharge through 30-days f/u in either group	—	Low rate of ACS in either group; charges vs. cost data used; possible bias due to non-blinded study
Roberts et al.[6] 1997	Prospective, randomized controlled trial to compare ED CP patients treated using an accelerated diagnosis protocol (ADP) in an ED OU (N=82) vs. inpatient controls (N=83)	LOS 33.1h ADP vs. 44.8h inpatient; 15.7h in ADP subgroup sent home	Mean total cost per patient $1,528 ADP vs. $2,098 inpatient; $803 for ADP subgroup sent home 2013 USD $3,148 ADP vs. $4,322 inpatient; $1,654 for ADP subgroup sent home	Discharge to home rate 55% in ADP group vs. 0% in control group. No diff in readmission rates (6.1% vs. 4.8%)	—	Unable to measure differences in mortality or morbidity due to small sample size of patients with poor outcomes

Table 80.1 (cont.)

Author/ Year	Design	Outcomes				Limitations/ Comments	Class
		Length of Stay (LOS)	Cost	Patient Satisfaction	Other Metrics		
Chest pain							
Rydman et al.[7] 1997	Prospective study of low-risk CP patients randomized to a CPOU (N=52) or an inpatient unit (N=52)			Mean score for overall satisfaction 3.57 CPOU vs. 3.06 inpatient on 4-point Likert scale (1 is lowest, 4 is highest)	Mean scores for quality of service 3.67 CPOU vs. 2.98 inpatient, recommendation of service 3.38 CPOU vs. 3.08 inpatient, effective handling of problem 3.63 CPOU vs. 3.20 inpatient unit	Non-blinded study	I
Zalenski et al.[8] 1997	Prospective, cohort of low-risk CP patients undergoing a 12-h rule out AMI protocol and immediate exercise stress testing in a CPOU (N=317)				CP diagnostic protocol patients with ACS 9.5% and AMI 3%; protocol sensitivity 90%, specificity 50.5%, PPV 16%, NPV 98%; CK-MB, serial ECGs, and stress testing improved protocol sensitivity and accuracy	No standard criteria for diagnosis of ACS	I
Farkouh et al.[9] 1998	Prospective, controlled trial of intermediate-risk CP patients with unstable angina randomized to either CPOU or to inpatient care (N=424)	LOS 9.2h in CPOU group (no data for inpatient group)	Inpatient group ~61%; more costs related to cardiac care during index visit and 6-month follow-up period		No diff in MACE (8.5% vs. 7.1%)	Majority of patients white (~95%) and middle class	I

434

Goodacre et al.[10] 2004	Prospective randomized controlled trial comparing protocol-directed CPU care (N=479) vs. non-protocol-directed routine care (N=493)	Mean cost per patient for CP-related care over 6-month f/u £478 CPU vs. £556 routine care 2013 USD $1,050 CPU vs. $1,221 routine care	Discharge to home rate 63% for CPU care vs. 46% for routine care 0.0137 QALYs gained for CPU care group compared to routine care; no diff in MACE (3.8% vs. 3.4%)	Possible selection bias
Goodacre et al.[11] 2004	Prospective randomized controlled trial comparing effect of assessment with protocol-directed CPU care (N=479) vs. non-protocol-directed routine care (N=493) upon psychological symptoms and health-related quality of life		HADS depression scores at 2 days and 1 month follow-up 4.3, 4.42 CPU care vs. 5.23, 5.43 routine care, CPU care was associated with significant improvements (p<0.05) in all dimensions of health related QOL measures at 1 month except the emotional role dimension, incidence and severity (visual analog scale) of subsequent chest pain at 1 month 45%, 36.5mm CPU care vs. 53.5%, 43mm routine care; no diff in time taken off work at 1 month 15.6% CPU care vs. 18.4% routine care	Patients not blinded to intervention; possible selection bias

Table 80.1 (cont.)

Author/ Year	Design	Length of Stay (LOS)	Cost	Outcomes Patient Satisfaction	Other Metrics	Limitations/ Comments	Class
Chest pain							
Miller et al.[12] 2010	Prospective study of intermediate- and high-risk CP patients randomized to OU/ stress cardiac MRI (N=53) vs. inpatient (N=57)	Median LOS 25.7h OU with cardiac MRI vs. 29.9h inpatient	Median direct cost $2,062 OU with cardiac MRI vs. $2,680 inpatient; Median total revenue $1,854 OU with cardiac MRI vs. $897 inpatient 2013 USD $2,350 OU with cardiac MRI vs. $3,055 inpatient; Median total revenue $2,113 OU with cardiac MRI vs. $1,022 inpatient		No diff in rate of ACS after 30-day f/u (0%)	Selection bias – select times of MRI availability; limited external validity – single institution	I
Sayre et al.[14] 1994	Retrospective cost analysis of CP patients evaluated in an ED OU (N=751) vs. inpatient (N=132)		Mean cost all patients $1,299 ED OU vs. $2,748 inpatient; mean cost discharged patients $995 ED OU vs. $2,026 inpatient 2013 USD All patients $2,554 ED OU vs. $5,402 inpatient; discharged patients $1,956 ED OU vs. $3,983 inpatient		Discharge to home rate 82.4% ED OU		II

Study	Study description	CPOU LOS	Cost outcomes	Satisfaction	Clinical outcomes	Limitations	Level of evidence
Graff et al.[15] 1997	Multiple site registry study of 8 CPOUs to assess for effectiveness and cost (N=23,407)		Saved cost from avoided hospital admissions $4,093,466 and estimated overall true cost savings $2,873,966 for the 8 OU study hospitals 2013 USD $7,237,202 saved from avoided admissions, $5,081,140 in true cost savings		Discharge to home rate after initial ED evaluation 59% OU study population vs. 43% comparable population; proportion of CP patients with rule-out MI evaluation after initial ED evaluation 67% OU study population vs. 57% comparable population; proportion of missed AMI 0.4% OU study population vs. 4.5% comparable population	Very large N; variable OU criteria among CPOU sites; missed AMI and cost data estimated	II
Mikhail et al.[16] 1997	Prospective observational study of low- to moderate-risk CP patients with immediate stress testing after AMI ruled out in a CPOU (N=502)	CPOU LOS 12.75h	Average total cost-per-case $894 CPOU vs. $2,364 inpatient. Cost of mandatory stress testing to identify one patient with IHD after AMI ruled out $3,125 2013 USD $1,757 CPOU vs. $4,647 inpatient. cost to identify IHD patient: $6,143	99.5% moderate or very satisfied with CPOU care	CPOU discharge home rate 86%; discharged patients with negative CPOU work-up 0% mortality/AMI at 5-month f/u	No prospective control group; possible inability to extrapolate cost analysis to other institutions	II
Zalenski et al.[17] 1997	Observational study of a low-risk CPOU protocol with stress test (N=63)				ED patients admitted for chest pain with low probability for AMI	Use of historical reports for diagnosis of AMI	II

Table 80.1 (cont.)

Author/Year	Design	Outcomes				Limitations/Comments	Class
		Length of Stay (LOS)	Cost	Patient Satisfaction	Other Metrics		
Chest pain							
					53.3% (Goldman's algorithm); proportion appropriate for CPOU 14%; eligible patients excluded due to CAD history (46%) and inability to perform a valid exercise stress test (42%)	or angina; population bias	
Stomel et al.[18] 1999	Retrospective study to assess effects of implementing a CPOU and a patient management algorithm for evaluation of CP patients (N=140 low-risk CP; N=333 intermediate-risk CP)	LOS 12.7h low-risk CP vs. 18.2h intermediate-risk CP; mean LOS 16.6h	Total charges (cost) for intermediate-risk patients $3,113 ($1,071) CPOU vs. $5,840 ($2,568) inpatient 2013 USD $5,153 ($1,773) CPOU vs. $9,667 ($4,251) inpatient		Admission rate 27% before vs. 21% after management algorithm implemented; CP risk discharged from CPOU 70.4% intermediate-risk CP vs. 29.6% low-risk CP; MACE at 1-year f/u 2.4%	Inability to conclude intervention wholly responsible for changes	II
Lai et al.[19] 2003	Retrospective chart review of managed care CP patients discharged from OU without stress testing (N=344)				Rate of 60-day f/u MACE 6%, mortality 2%; rate of ED return for CP after discharge within 60days 7%; rate of primary care f/u 55.2%; rate of stress	Retrospective small study size; selection bias – study population limited to patients with	II

438

Study	Design	LOS	Cost	Results	Limitations	
				test performed within 60 days after OU discharge 43.3%	PCP and a high likelihood of f/u	
Jagminas et al.[20] 2005	Retrospective, observational study of CP patients placed in an ED OU (N=440) vs. an inpatient OU (N=973) during separate time periods		Mean charge $890 ED OU vs. $1,040 inpatient OU 2013 USD $1,524 ED OU vs. $1,781 inpatient OU	Discharge to home rate 92.1% for ED OU, 80.8% for inpatient OU	Patient selection uncontrolled in both groups	=
Diercks et al.[21] 2007	Retrospective study of CPOU patients (N=4568) presenting with associated cocaine and amphetamine use (N=224)			5% CPOU patients Utox positive for cocaine or amphetamines (N=224); CAD diagnosis 9% Utox negative vs. 12% Utox positive	Possible selection bias of Utox patients place in CPOU; not all CPOU patients had Utox and/or diagnostic testing; No f/u period	=
Chang et al.[22] 2008	Retrospective convenience study comparing evaluation of ED CP patients with immediate CTA without serial biomarkers (N=98); OU with serial biomarkers and CTA (N=102); OU with serial biomarkers and stress testing (N=154); usual care (admission with serial biomarkers and hospitalist-directed evaluation) (N=289)	LOS 8.1h immediate CTA vs. 20.9h OU with serial biomarker and CTA vs. 26.2h OU with serial biomarker and stress test vs. 30.2h usual care	Median facility cost $1,240 immediate CTA vs. $2,318 OU with serial biomarkers and CTA vs. $4,024 OU with serial biomarkers and stress test vs. $2,913 usual care 2013 USD $1,413 immediate CTA vs. $2,642 OU with serial biomarkers and CTA vs. $4,586 OU with serial	No diff in CAD diagnosis, death or MI rates; 30-day readmission rate 0% immediate CTA vs. 3.2% OU with serial biomarkers and CTA vs. 2.3% OU with serial biomarkers and stress test vs. 12.2% usual care	Selection bias – decision of which group patient is placed by physician	=

Table 80.1 (cont.)

Author/ Year	Design	Length of Stay (LOS)	Cost	Outcomes Patient Satisfaction	Other Metrics	Limitations/ Comments	Class
Chest pain			biomarkers and stress test vs. $3,320 usual care				
Limkakeng et al.[23] 2010	Retrospective study to assess prevalence of renal dysfunction in CP OU patients and effect on cardiac evaluation outcomes (N=529)				Rate of patients with GFR ≥90 43.3%, GFR <90 and ≥60 43.7%, GFR <60 13%; rate of patients with abnormal evaluation for ACS 12.1%; majority of patients 43/64 (67%) with abnormal evaluation for ACS had at least mild renal impairment (GFR <90); rate of positive or indeterminate ST 9.1% GFR ≥90, 13.4% GFR<90 and ≥60, 17.4% <60	Small sample size, selection bias	II
Maag et al.[24] 1997	Observational descriptive study of a process improvement initiative to implement	LOS 12h in best-practice CPOU			Use of a five phase process and best practice modeling allowed 5 of 9		III

440

Study	Description	Results	Limitations	Level
	a CPOU in 9 area hospitals	hospitals to successfully implement a CPOU; range of admission rates for CP 16–54% pre-implementation; lack of financial hospital support in participating hospitals contributed to inability to implement a CPOU		
Kirk et al.[25] 1998	Prospective case series of low-risk CP patients to assess safety and utility of immediate stress testing in a chest pain unit (N=212)	Low-risk CP patients undergoing immediate stress testing after ED evaluation without biomarkers 50%; Immediate stress test results 64% negative 25% indeterminate 11% positive; PPV of immediate stress test 57%; MACE of discharged patients with negative immediate stress test at 30-day f/u 0%	Convenience study – stress test available only 14h/day; incomplete patient f/u	III
Goodacre et al.[26] 2001	Prospective case series of CPOU patients measuring psychological	Rate of CPOU patients with moderate anxiety at baseline and at	Brief f/u period, no control group, individual	III

Table 80.1 (cont.)

Author/Year	Design	Outcomes				Limitations/Comments	Class
		Length of Stay (LOS)	Cost	Patient Satisfaction	Other Metrics		
Chest pain							
	morbidity and health-related QOL using 3 questionnaires (N=192)				1 month 19%, 19% vs. moderate depression 13%, 12%; health utility and all dimensions of quality of life scores substantially below age-adjusted normal values at baseline, improvement of pain score and deterioration of physical role and mental health dimensions score at 1-month f/u; rate of CPOU patients reassured after evaluation 86%	patient baselines unknown	
Weber et al.[27] 2003	Prospective case series of CPOU patients with CP and reported or test positive cocaine use (N=302)				Rate of MACE at 30-day f/u after CPOU d/c for cocaine-associated CP cohort 1.6% (all non-fatal MI in patients that continued to use cocaine)	F/u not available for all cohort patients (2 patients not in National Death Index and detailed f/u available for 256 patients)	III
Goodacre et al.[28] 2005	Extrapolation study of data from a prospective		Mean ED costs £116 CPU care vs. £73 routine care,		QALYs 0.3936 CPU vs. 0.3799 routine care (=2.7%	ESCAPE trial limitations, use	III

Study	Description	Results	Limitations	Level
	randomized controlled trial (ESCAPE) to create a model that compares cost-effectiveness of protocol-directed CPU care (N=479) with nonprotocol-directed routine care (N=493)	mean cost of inpatient hospital stay £312; mean cost per patient for CP-related care over 6 months £478 CPU vs. £556 routine care 2013 USD $225 CPU vs. $142 routine care, mean inpatient stay $605, CP-related care over 6 months $927 CPU vs. $1,080 routine care	improvement in quality of life over 6 months). Discharge to home rate 63% for CPU vs. 46% for routine care	of model assumptions
Madsen et al.[29] 2009	Retrospective case series of chest pain patients managed in an ED OU to determine baseline rate of positive stress test and CTA findings (N=353)	11% of stress tests were positive; assuming only 70% of patients referred to outpatient testing actually f/u, one could extrapolate that about 3.3% of positive stress tests are missed because patients are sent home without one	Single-center, rate of missed positive stress test extrapolated from mix of case series data and assumption	III
Madsen et al.[30] 2010	Retrospective chart review of OU CP patients comparing outcomes of those with a CAD history	Discharge to home rate 74% of OU patients with CAD history vs. 91.4% OU patients without CAD history;	Study type; not all patients underwent stress test or CTA; possible selection bias	III

Table 80.1 (cont.)

Author/ Year	Design	Outcomes				Other Metrics	Limitations/ Comments	Class
		Length of Stay (LOS)	Cost	Patient Satisfaction				
Chest pain								
	(N=125) vs. no CAD history (N=406)					positive stress test or CTA 32.3% if CAD history vs. 6.9% no CAD history; rate of cardiac cath, revascularization 12%, 7.2% CAD history vs. 5.9%, 2.2% no CAD history		
Pines et al.[31] 2010	Prospective study surveying ED physician (N=31) risk tolerance in patients presenting with CP syndrome and effect of opening an ED OU (N=2872)					Association between risk tolerance and decision to admit ED CP patients to inpatient or OU/use CTA and order biomarkers 78%, 83% most risk-averse quartile of the risk–taking scale vs. 68%, 78% least risk-averse quartile; no diff in CP admission rate before and after OU implementation for entire cohort 73% vs. 73% and with TIMI 0–1 62% vs. 62%	Study limited to one physician group at one institution; CP admission rate higher than benchmarks	III

Study	Description	LOS/Disposition	Cost	Satisfaction	Outcome	Comments	Level
Mcdermott et al.[32] 1997	Randomized study of adult ED patients with asthma sent to EDTU or inpatient (N=222)	Inpatient control subgroup LOS 39h vs. d/c from EDTU 8.8h	Mean EDTU $1,202 (± $1,343) Inpatient $2,247 (± $1,110) P<0.001 2013 USD EDTU $2,125 (± $2,374) Inpatient $3,973 (± $2,374)	EDTU was higher on 4 of 7 global satisfaction criteria p<0.05	8 week relapse rate EDTU 40%, Inpatient 42% P=0.74 NS QOL EDTU higher in 5 of 8 domains (p≤0.02)	F/u appts 1, 8 weeks; Telephone interviews 3, 5, 7 weeks; Equivalent baseline clinical and historical measures 2 groups similar acuity	I
Rydman et al.[33] 1998	Randomized study of adult ED patients with asthma sent to EDTU vs. inpatient (N=113)		EDTU $1,202 Inpatient $2,247 (p<0.001) 2013 USD EDTU $2,059 Inpatient $3,849		Significantly higher QOL in 5 of 8 domains (p≤0.02). No diff in relapse, peak flows, 1 week health comparisons	Used standardized Medical Outcomes Study SF 36, equivalent baseline measures	I
Rydman et al.[34] 1999	Randomized study of adult ED patients with asthma sent to AOU vs. inpatient (N=163)			Global satisfaction better for AOU than inpatient in 6 of 7 categories (p<0.05) 1 category (p=.09, NS)	For problems with care processes: AOU better in 4 categories (p≤ 0.03); no diff in 4 (NS), 1 category (financial info) worse (p=.02)	Patients "more satisfied, fewer problems with OU than (inpatient admission)"	I
Zwicke et al.[35] 1982	Cohort study of adult ED patients with asthma (N=46) d/c home =12, admit from ED =7 HOSTT =27 (18 discharged + 9 admitted to hospital)	LOS 20h on HOSTT Inpatient 3.3 days	HOSTT $459 Inpatient $1,347 HOSTT =34% of inpatient cost 2013 USD HOSTT $2,057 Inpatient $6,037		Clinical variables have little predictive value. Historical data (symptoms >24h, prior HOSTT or hospital admission) predicted disposition (need hospital admission)	Equivalent baseline criteria Downgrade for small N (only 27 HOSTT patients) and HOSTT patients included holding patients not just observation patients	III

Table 80.1 (cont.)

Author/ Year	Design	Outcomes			Limitations/ Comments	Class
		Length of Stay (LOS)	Cost	Patient Satisfaction	Other Metrics	

Asthma exacerbation

Author/ Year	Design	Length of Stay (LOS)	Cost	Patient Satisfaction	Other Metrics	Limitations/ Comments	Class
Brillman et al.[36] 1994	Case series of ED patients with asthma (mainly adults) before and after opening OU (N=1224). Used historical controls pre-observation 834 post-observation 390		Median admission charge $2,968. Savings $57,705/year for 2.7% ↓ in hospital admission rate. OU charge $210 for 12h x 48.3 patients/year = $10,143; net savings of $47,542/year 2013 USD Median admission charge $8,240. Savings $160,199/year for 2.7% ↓ in hospital admission rate. OU charge $583 for 12h x 48.3 pts/year =$28,159; net savings of $132,040/year		Hospital admission rate pre-observation 16.1%, post-observation 13.4% (p=0.25, NS). Discharged from ED pre-observation 83.9%, post-observation 77.2% (p=0.01)	Did not include charges for OU patients discharged home so downgraded since difficult to compare pre-observation and post-observation	III
Mace et al.[37] 2001	7 studies (3 pediatric, 4 adult) of OU treatment of asthma reviewed	LOS in OU < inpatient when compared (2 peds, 2 adult studies). Short LOS for OU in 2 other peds studies but not compared with inpatient	Inpatient costs > than OU in all studies that evaluated cost (2 peds, 4 adult studies)	Patient satisfaction for OU > inpatient when compared (2 adult studies)	Better QOL/ decreased problems with care (2 adult studies). Readmission rate no diff in 1 adult and 1 peds study (OU vs. inpatients)	Includes OU protocol on asthma	III

Syncope

Study	Description	LOS	Cost	Results	Limitations	Level
Shen et al.[38] 2004	Patients with intermediate risk for serious disease as cause of syncope randomized to special "syncope unit" care or standard care (N=103)			Diagnostic yield 67% in ED OU patients and 10% in standard care patients. Hospital admission rate 43% for ED OU patients, 98% for standard care patients	Small numbers and sophisticated evaluation protocol limit use in other hospitals	I
Stockley et al.[39] 2009	Survey of 177 EDs in UK and Ireland on approach to syncope			18% of EDs had syncope guidelines, 55% had an ED OU		III

Transient ischemic attack

Study	Description	LOS	Cost	Results	Limitations	Level
Ross et al.[40] 2007	Randomized trial of ADP in ED OU or admitted to standard care (N=149)	ADP 25.6h; Admit 61.2h	ADP $844; Admit $1,529 2013 USD ADP $998; Admit $1,807	Stroke within 90 days=3.3% in both groups. Compliance with protocol, e.g., carotid imaging ADP=97% Admit=91%	Small numbers limit power	I
Brown et al.[41] 2007	Prospective cohort study of patients to assess the impact of a TIA protocol in ED (N=75)			46.7% of patients discharged home after TIA protocol. Compliance with recommendation for antithrombotic and carotid imaging was 85.3%	Convenience sample; Hawthorne effect	II
Stead et al.[45] 2009	Case series of patients who underwent a TIA protocol in an ED OU (N=418)			30.4% of patients discharged home from ED OU; risk of stroke after ED OU stay at 2 days was 0.96%, at 7 days 1.2%, at 30 days		III

Table 80.1 (cont.)

Author/Year	Design	Outcomes				Limitations/Comments	Class
		Length of Stay (LOS)	Cost	Patient Satisfaction	Other Metrics		
Transient ischemic attack							
					1.9%, and 2.4% at 90 days		
Deep vein thrombosis							
Koopman et al.[46] 1996	Randomized trial of LMWH vs. UF heparin (N=400)	LOS for UF heparin 8.1 days; LMWH 50% not admitted and 25% of rest sent home in <48h			No decrement in QOL with LMWH	No mention of ED OU, though concept is apparent	I
Atrial fibrillation							
Decker et al.[52] 2008	Prospective randomized trial of patients for an ED OU pathway for cardioversion vs. traditional admission (N=153)	Median LOS ED OU 10.1h Inpatient 25.2h			ED OU ↑12% patients in NSR at discharge	No diff in tests/procedures/adverse events, or rehosp at 6-month f/u	1
Cristoni et al.[53] 2011	Prospective comparison of two cohorts at two different hospitals, comparing a chemical protocol vs. an electrical protocol for cardioversion, using a "short observation unit" (N=322)	LOS same in patients who converted within 6h but many more chemical pathway patients admitted (44% vs. 6%)			93% of electrical protocol sent home in NSR within 24h vs. 51% for chemical protocol	Patients not randomized; electrical cardioversion protocol mixed chemical and electrical Rx	I

Study	Description	ED OU LOS	Results	Limitations	Level
Conti et al.[55] 2012	Observational study of patients before and after the implementation of an observation protocol and outpatient clinic (N=3,475)		Before OU 50% admitted, decreasing to 38% and eventually to 24%, with the addition of a specific f/u clinic.	Patients not randomized, single institution	II
Koenig et al.[56] 2002	Case series of patients in an ED OU protocol for atrial fibrillation (N=67)	LOS in ED 4.7h; LOS in ED OU 11.8h for those who convert and 17h for those admitted	While in ED OU 83% converted to NSR. Complications – none; positive diagnostic outcomes –2 AMI, 2 fever, and 1 VT	No comparison group	III
Ross et al.[57] 2004	Case series of patients with an ED OU protocol for atrial fibrillation (N=74)	Mean ED OU LOS was 14.9h	81% of patients sent home after ED OU stay; 73% converted with chemical treatment; 6% needed electrical cardioversion		III
Stiell et al.[58] 2008	Case series patients managed with an ED-based atrial fibrillation protocol involving chemical cardioversion and if unsuccessful, followed by electrical cardioversion (N=660)	ED LOS 4.9h (3.9h for successful chemical and 6.5h if electrical cardioversion required)	95% discharged home; 90% in NSR. 7.6% adverse events mostly transient hypotension; 3% admission rate, no death or stroke in 7 days	Retrospective and observational; All in ED	III

Abdominal pain

Study	Description	ED OU LOS	Results	Limitations	Level
Graff et al.[62] 1991	Retrospective cohort study of patients who underwent a period of	Mean ED OU LOS 10.4h	True and false positives and negatives	Retrospective; antedates	II

Table 80.1 (cont.)

Author/Year	Design	Outcomes				Limitations/Comments	Class
		Length of Stay (LOS)	Cost	Patient Satisfaction	Other Metrics		
Abdominal pain							
	observation in an ED OU increased diagnostic accuracy; used Alvarado appendicitis score (N=252)				(regarding the presence of appendicitis at surgery)	widespread use of CT	
Graff et al.[63] 2000	Retrospective two-arm cohort study at 12 acute care hospitals examining consecutive appendectomy patients and consecutive ED patients with abdominal pain (N=1,026)				Subset of patients who were observed had 18% false negative rate with marked inter institution variability; presence of OU improved processes of care but did not affect other outcomes	Retrospective; antedates widespread use of CT	II
Saunders et al.[65] 1988	Retrospective cohort study of patients with recurrent alcoholic pancreatitis managed under an ED OU protocol (N=27)	Mean LOS of ED OU patients sent home was 14.4h; mean LOS of directly admitted patients was 5.8 days			52% of ED OU patients sent home within 24h	Downgraded for small number of patients	III
Head injury							
Fabbri et al.[66] 2004	Prospective cohort study of patients with "high-risk" mild head	Median obs LOS 96h			No diff in intracranial injuries between groups, no	Uncontrolled patient selection;	I

	injury and negative CT scan, managed in an OU vs. discharged home with monitoring (N=1,408)	diff in deaths at 6 months	patients kept in the hospital were more severely injured. Observation period was much longer than typical ED OU evaluation	
Menditto et al.[69] 2012	Prospective case series of patients testing an ED OU protocol including a repeat CT at 24h if initial head CT normal in patients on warfarin with minor head injury (N=97)	% of patients w/ intracranial lesions after 24h of observation following normal CT (N=87) was 6% (N=5), with an additional 2 patients who had normal 2nd CT developed bleed (both had INR >3)	Small number	II
MacLaren et al.[70] 1993	Case series of patients with minor head injury and variable access to an OU, depending on the day of the week (N=405)	23.5% of patients who met high-risk criteria for further observation were sent home when the unit was unavailable compared with only 9.9% when it was an option	Study antedates the most widely used current decision rules for minor head trauma (e.g., Canadian, New Orleans criteria)	III

Congestive heart failure

Peacock et al.[72] 2005	Multicenter, randomized controlled study in ED OU patients with CHF,	Nesiritide patients had fewer 30-day	Additional cost of Nesiritide was balanced by the	Nesiritide not currently recommended	I

Table 80.1 (cont.)

Author/Year	Design	Outcomes				Limitations/Comments	Class
		Length of Stay (LOS)	Cost	Patient Satisfaction	Other Metrics		
Congestive heart failure							
	looking at the impact of Nesiritide on index hospitalization, repeat hospitalization at 30 days and other outcomes (N=237)	readmits, with shorter LOS	shorter LOS and fewer readmits			for routine use in CHF patients	
Graff et al.[73] 1999	Retrospective cohort study of patients with CHF in 12 hospitals to identify patient characteristics associated with low-risk for poor outcomes (N=1,674)				Patients with 0 or 1 admission criteria combined with physician judgment of safe outpatient plan were low risk	Study helps identify potential ED OU candidates, but did not test ED OU care	II
Storrow et al.[74] 2005	Prospective cohort study of patients with CHF managed sequentially in an ED OU and versus a matched group on an inpatient service (N=64)	Mean ED OU LOS 25.7h vs. 58.5h for inpatient	Use of ED OU estimated to save $3,600 per visit 2013 USD Savings of $4,620 per visit		79% of ED OU patients discharged home. No significant diff in outcomes at 30 days between ED OU and inpatient groups	Not enough power in study to detect outcome differences between groups	II
Peacock et al.[75] 2002	Case series of patients before and after an ED OU CHF protocol was implemented in a single hospital (N=154)				↓ 90-day ED revisit rate for CHF by 56% after ED OU; ↓90-day readmit rate for CHF by 64% after ED OU	Inclusion and exclusion criteria of ED OU protocol detailed in paper	III

Study	Description			Level
Burkhardt et al.[76] 2005	Case series of patients with CHF exacerbation in an ED OU protocol (N=385)		74% of ED OU patients discharged home; BUN >30 mg/dl significantly predicted ED OU management failure	III
Diercks et al.[77] 2006	Case series of patients to determine which factors are associated with appropriate patient selection for a 24h ED OU CHF pathway (N=499)		Factors associated with prolonged LOS and 30-day adverse outcomes were SBP >160 m Hg at ED presentation and positive TnI	Actual study patient dispositions varied; only 50 patients managed in ED OU, many more identified as "OU appropriate"	III
Collins et al.[78] 2009	Decision model of alternative disposition options for a low-risk CHF patient presenting to the ED: home, ED OU, and inpatient admission	ED OU costs were $44,248 per QALY and inpatient costs were $684,101 per QALY 2013 USD ED OU costs were $48,869 per QALY and inpatient costs were $755,539 per QALY	Risk of readmission if sent home directly from ED 26% at 5 days and 74% at 30 days	ED OU shown to be optimal balance of cost and risk versus alternatives	III
Pyelonephritis				
Schrock et al.[79] 2010	Retrospective cohort study of patients, before and after the opening of an ED OU (N=633)	Median ED OU LOS was 22h, median inpatient LOS was 3 days	72% of ED OU patients discharged home. Percentage of patients admitted to the hospital dropped from 35% to 26% (p<.05) after the ED OU opened	Uncontrolled design	II

Table 80.1 *(cont.)*

| Author/ Year | Design | Outcomes | | | | Limitations/ Comments | Class |
		Length of Stay (LOS)	Cost	Patient Satisfaction	Other Metrics		
Pyelonephritis							
Israel et al.[80] 1991	Case series of patients with pyelonephritis who underwent a 12h ED OU protocol (N=87)				72% of patients with confirmed pyelonephritis discharged home	Only about 80% of patients sent to the ED OU for pyelonephritis actually had the disease	III
Ward et al.[81] 1991	Case series of patients with pyelonephritis who underwent a 24h ED OU protocol (N=44)				43 of 44 (98%) patients discharged home after two doses of IV antibiotics	Authors excluded patients retrospectively if urine culture from index visit was negative	III
Cellulitis/soft tissue infections							
Schrock et al.[82] 2008	Case series of patients with skin and soft tissue infections who were managed in an ED OU (N=179)				62% of patients discharged home after observation stay; female gender OR 2.33 and WBC >15,000; OR 4.06 significantly associated with failure to discharge		III
Abdominal and general trauma							
Conrad et al.[83] 1985	Case series of mixed trauma patients who underwent an ED OU protocol (N=485)	Mean LOS was 6h	Nearly 50% ↓ in cost vs. inpatient stay		80% of patients discharged home after observation stay		III

Study	Study design (N)			Outcome	Comment	LOE
Henneman et al. [84] 1989	Case series of mixed blunt and penetrating abdominal trauma patients who underwent 12h of ED OU monitoring after a negative initial DPL (N=230)		Mean cost savings of $224 2013 USD Mean cost savings of $869	81% of patients discharged home after observation stay	DPL not routinely used today	III
Cowell et al. [85] 1998	Case series of mixed trauma patients who underwent a 24h ED OU protocol (N=122)			80% of patients discharged home after observation stay		III
Madsen et al. [86] 2009	Case series of mixed trauma patients who underwent an ED OU protocol (N=364)	Mean LOS was 12h 46 minutes		88.5% of patients discharged home after observation stay; at 30-day f/u, there were no significant missed injuries	There were no deaths, intubations, loss of vital signs or other adverse events	III
Toxicology/drug overdose						
Hollander et al. [88] 1999	Case series of stable, minimally symptomatic or asymptomatic patients in ED observation with potentially toxic ingestions at two hospitals (N=215)			167 (77%) patients were deemed medically clear after only 2–4h of observation	Findings suggest asymptomatic patients with selected acute intentional ingestions can be released from observation in <6h	III
Sivilotti et al. [89] 2005	Case series of acetaminophen overdose registry patients modeled with a 20h intravenous N-acetylcysteine protocol (N=1,270)	20h protocol versus 72h protocol	Authors estimate switching from 72h to 20h protocol would save 40,000 patient-days annually in the U.S., with an		Low-risk patients may be identified at the beginning of therapy using the published nomogram, given a 20h course of	III

Table 80.1 (cont.)

Author/Year	Design	Outcomes				Limitations/Comments	Class
		Length of Stay (LOS)	Cost	Patient Satisfaction	Other Metrics		
Toxicology/drug overdose							
			annual cost savings of >$100 million			treatment, and released without further testing	
Sztajnkrycer et al.[90] 2007	Case series of patients with various toxic exposures managed under a new ED OU protocol (N=6)				2 of 6 patients required subsequent inpatient medical admission	Very low number of patients; higher number identified as potential ED OU candidates	III
Pneumonia							
Chan et al.[91] 2001	Case series of patients with community acquired pneumonia in an ED OU (N=14)	Median ED OU LOS 15h			71% of patients discharged home after observation stay		II
COPD							
Salazar et al.[92] 2007	Case series of patients with COPD in an ED short-stay unit (N=545)	Mean LOS 3.4d for short-stay unit vs. 12d for inpatient			Short-stay unit group had lower mortality (1.7%) vs. inpatient (8.1%) but also higher hospital readmission rate (9.9% vs. 7%)	Study performed in Spain, where concept of ED OU is different (LOS was over 3d); short-stay patients were significantly less sick than inpatients	III

ED efficiency

Baugh et al.[1] 2012	Model of cost savings of a single ED OU visit, entire ED OU, and potential national savings from increased ED OU use	Cost savings from a single ED OU visit was $1,572; annual hospital savings $4.6M, and national savings of $3.1B from increased ED OU use	I
Hadden et al.[93] 1996	Retrospective cohort analysis of 107 patients managed in an observation ward, which was later closed for administrative reasons compared with 107 similar observation patients subsequently managed in inpatient areas	99% of OU patients discharged within 2 days, vs. only 77% of patients managed in inpatient areas	Number of "investigations" of OU patients was 1.3, much lower than for patients in inpatient areas (3.3); 97% of OU patients seen by senior doctor within 24h versus 71% for the other group	II
Baugh et al.[94] 2008	Model of financial value of an observation visit using an optional analysis framework and considering indirect benefits of observation, such as freeing inpatient beds, and thus transfer capacity	Revenue created by an average ED OU visit was $2,908; 40% of which was indirect value 2013 USD Revenue of $3,314	II
Bazarian et al.[95] 1996	Before and after study of an inpatient short-stay unit, which treated 4 types of patients: asthma, chest pain, sickle-cell crisis and seizure	After short-stay unit opened, LOS for ED boarders >8h ↓ from 9.6h to 2.3h, LOS for treat and release ↑13.4% in ED pro billing after short-stay unit opened	# of ED patients left without being seen ↓42% Mean LOS for short-stay unit was 2.4 days, significantly longer than the target of a typical ED OU	III

Table 80.1 (cont.)

Author/Year	Design	Outcomes				Limitations/Comments	Class
		Length of Stay (LOS)	Cost	Patient Satisfaction	Other Metrics		
ED efficiency							
Kelen et al.[96] 2001	Before and after study of adding a remote ED OU at a single academic medical center	ED chest pain patients ↓24%, and ↓15% for asthma patients			LWBS ↓ from 10.1% just prior to opening of the ED OU to 5.0%. Ambulance diversion ↓ from 6.7h per 100 patients to 2.8h per 100 patients		III
Chandra et al.[97] 2011	Before and after study of patient satisfaction scores after adding an ED OU at a single academic medical center			Mean overall PG scores pre-ED OU was 75.2 and post-ED OU was 802 (p<.05)		Other key factors (i.e., physician and nursing staffing, wait times, etc.) all remained the same during this period	III
Other							
Cook et al.[99] 2003	Systematic literature review and critical assessment of the observation medicine literature	14 studies identified showing shorter LOS and more rapid disposition though OU use	5 studies across various conditions show lower costs through OU use	3 studies showed higher satisfaction in asthma and chest pain patients		Included pediatric studies	III

Study	Description	LOS	Cost	Satisfaction	Outcomes / Comments		Level
Daly et al.[100] 2003	Systematic literature review of how short-stay observation units (SOUs) affect the efficiency of health care delivery and the quality of services provided	1 study showed no change, another 1 showed shorter LOS with OU use	1 study in asthma patients was found to show lower costs of care through OU use	2 studies showed higher satisfaction in asthma and chest pain patients	2 studies showed no change, 2 others showed a decrease in medical admissions, 2 studies showed equivalent clinical outcomes with OU use vs. routine care		III
Tempel et al.[101] 2006	Retrospective case series of consecutive patients with decompression illness presenting to a major hyperbaric facility (N=102)				42 patients (41.2%) had neurological sequelae requiring further hyperbaric oxygen treatments; 38 of these had their treatments completed within 24h, which is an ideal OU time frame	Single center; retrospective analysis to see if OU protocol would have been appropriate	III
Ross et al.[102] 2012	Historical overview of the development of OUs and literature synthesis summarizing the benefits of OU care across many clinical conditions	Cite numerous studies showing shorter LOS with OU use	Cite numerous studies showing less cost with OU use	Cite numerous studies showing higher patient satisfaction with OU use	Recent, thorough, and concise review with helpful supporting information, such as OU management strategies		III

Table 80.2 Evidentiary Table for Critical Question #2

Author/ Year	Design	Outcomes				Limitations/ Comments	Class
		Length of Stay (LOS)	Cost	Patient Satisfaction	Other Metrics		
Other							
Kerns et al.[13] 1993	Prospective cohort study of ED low-risk CP patients undergoing immediate stress test (N=32) vs. comparison inpatient group (N=26)	LOS 5.5h immediate stress test group vs. 2 days for inpatient group	Average patient charge $467 ED protocol vs. $2,340 inpatient 2013 USD $962 for ED protocol vs. $4,821 inpatient		No diff in MACE at 6-month f/u: 0% ED protocol and inpatient	Selection bias of low-risk patients with atypical CP, low pretest probability of CAD and normal ECG; inpatient group retrospectively selected. Downgrade for small number of patients	II
Transient ischemic attack							
Rothwell et al.[42] 2007	Population based before and after establishment of walk-in clinic for evaluation and treatment of TIA or minor stroke (N=1,278)				Rate of stroke within 90 days after TIA or prior minor stroke pre- vs. post-intervention: Before intervention rate=10.3%, After intervention 2.1%	Same-day diagnostics and Rx, but clinic mimics OBS; No exclusions is a strength as is large numbers	II
Luengo-Fernandez et al.[43] 2009	Before and after study of patients referred to an outpatient TIA clinic in the UK; no appointment needed in the second phase (N=1,278)				Delay to assessment fell from 3 days to less than 1; 90-day risk of recurrent stroke fell by 80%	Implication that timing of assessment important implies role for ED OU	II
Lavallee et al.[44] 2007	Case series of patients to assess the impact of an intervention (24/7 TIA clinic; N=1,085)				Rate of stroke within 90 days of attendance at clinic (1.24%) compared to expected rate based on ABCD2 score (5.96%)	Not randomized and no comparative group, i.e., measured against a score; mimics rapid assessment 24/7; large numbers an asset	III

Deep vein thrombosis

Levine et al.[47] 1996	Prospective, randomized study of patients with proximal DVT either to UF heparin in the hospital vs. LMWH at home (N=500)	LOS 1.1 days for LMWH group, 6.5 days for UF heparin group		No significant diff in recurrent DVT or major bleeding at 90 days	I
O'Brien et al.[48] 1999	Randomized trial comparing cost of standard hospital-based treatment for DVT with LMWH (N=300)		Saving of $2,617 Canadian per patient for outpatient Rx 2013 USD Savings of $4,524 per patient for outpatient Rx	disposition choices were home vs. admit	I
Vinson et al.[49] 2001	Observational study of patients before and after the implementation of a DVT protocol using LMWH at two EDs (N=274)	Total hospital days for group before pathway was 383d, total for after pathway was 6 days		No significant diff in outcomes between groups	No mention of ED OU, though concept is apparent	II
Rodger et al.[50] 1998	Observational, retrospective evaluation of effectiveness and safety of protocol for management of DVT with output LMWH (N=105)		Total case costs for hospitalization for UF heparin was $3,048 vs. output cost of $1,641 for LMWH 2013 USD UF heparin $5,734 vs. $3,087 for LMWH	No diff in bleeding risk, lower risk of recurrence and death in LMWH group	Patients who had difficulty with initial injections received a 12h visit	III
Gould et al.[51] 1999	Modeling cost-effectiveness of LMWH vs. UF heparin		If half of patients were eligible for full or partial outpatient Rx: $790 savings per patient 2013 USD $1,486 savings per patient		Small mention of "outpatient" Rx, and "partial" outpatient Rx	III

Atrial fibrillation

Kim et al.[54] 2002	Prospective randomized trial of patients for a	Mean costs were $879 and $1,706 for pathway			Small numbers, but some statistically	II

Table 80.2 (cont.)

Author/ Year	Design	Outcomes				Limitations/ Comments	Class
		Length of Stay (LOS)	Cost	Patient Satisfaction	Other Metrics		
Atrial fibrillation							
	rapid pathway for cardioversion of atrial fibrillation vs. traditional admission (N=18)	LOS in pathway 4.8h and 29.8h in admitted group	and admission; savings of $827 per visit and 40% of costs of pathway were for LMWH 2013 USD Costs of $1,276 and $2,477 for pathway and admission; savings of $1,201 per visit			significant findings Downgrade for small number of patients	
Vinson et al.[59] 2012	Case series of patients in 3 community EDs in same system to test ED-based cardioversion protocol (N=206)				89% of patients discharged home after protocol; 2 patients with embolic event at 30-day follow-up	Patients selected as convenience sample	III
Abdominal pain							
Lopez et al.[60] 2007	Prospective randomized trial of female patients to either observation or CT scan if appendicitis was suspected; used Alvarado appendicitis score (N=90)	No significant diff in LOS	No significant diff in hospital charges		The two groups were similar in diagnostic accuracy, sensitivity, and specificity	Observation was performed in an inpatient setting	I
White et al.[61] 1975	Retrospective cohort study of pediatric patients with intermediate suspicion of acute appendicitis before and after the routine use of an observation period prior to surgery (N=136)				Negative laparotomy rate fell from 15% to 1.9% Rate of death and ruptured appendicitis unchanged	Historical controls; antedates widespread use of CT	II

Reference	Methods		Outcome	Comments	Level
Thomson et al.[64] 1986	Prospective observational study. One clinician did serial examinations over 12h on all patients (adult and children) at two hospitals; (N=252)		Negative laparotomy rate was 5% vs. historical 20%	Single examiner; historical controls; antedates wide spread use of CT	III
Head injury					
Geijerstam et al.[67] 2006	Randomized patients between CT during ED visit and home if negative vs. no CT and observation according to local custom (N=2,602)	Satisfaction equal in both groups	No significant diff in outcomes at 3 months		I
Norlund et al.[68] 2006	Randomized patients between CT during ED visit and home if negative vs. no CT and observation according to local custom (N=2,602)	Cost per patient for CT group was €461; for observation group €677, 32% less 2013 USD Cost per patient for CT group was $756; for observation group $1,110	No diff in death or disability at 90 days	Does not account for indirect costs associated with CT scan, such as exposure to ionizing radiation	I
Geijerstam et al.[71] 2004	Modeling cost difference between observation of patients with minor head injury vs. immediate CT	Cost saving of immediate CT and home could be £170 per case, 36% lower than observation, 2013 USD Savings of $343 per case		Superseded by Norland et al.[68] 2006	III
Toxicology/drug overdose					
Foulke et al.[87] 1995	Case series of patients with antidepressant overdose, classified as high or low risk (N=67)		28 (42%) of patients were low risk; no subsequent complications identified in this group	Potential to apply screening criteria and divert low-risk antidepressant overdose patients away from inpatient care	III

Table 80.2 (cont.)

Author/Year	Design	Outcomes				Limitations/Comments	Class
		Length of Stay (LOS)	Cost	Patient Satisfaction	Other Metrics		
Sickle cell crisis							
Benjamin et al.[98] 2000	Case series of visits at a specialty outpatient clinic delivering a care protocol for uncomplicated sickle cell pain crisis as an alternative to standard ED care (N=2,554)	Mean clinic visit LOS was 4.5h, vs. 13h for ED visits	Total single-hospital savings estimated at $1.7M over 5 years 2013 USD Savings of $2.7M over 5 years		81% of patients discharged home after clinic visit Inpatient admissions ↓ by 40% after clinic opened	Setting was specialty clinic, not ED OU, but suggests a standard protocol can be successfully used in these patients	III

Tables 80.1 and 80.2

ACS: Acute coronary syndrome
ADP: Accelerated diagnostic protocol
AMA: Against medical advice
AMI: Acute myocardial infarction
AOU: Asthma observation unit
Appts: Appointments
CAD: Coronary artery disease
CK-MB: Creatine kinase MB isoenzyme
COPD: Chronic obstructive pulmonary disease
CP: Chest pain
CPU: Chest pain unit
CPOU: Chest pain observation unit
CT: Computed tomography
CTA: Computed tomography angiogram
d/c: Discharged
Diff: Difference
DPL: Diagnostic peritoneal lavage
DVT: Deep venous thrombosis
ED OU: Emergency department observation unit
EDTU: Emergency department treatment unit
F/u: Follow-up

GFR: Glomerular filtration rate
GI: Gastrointestinal
h: Hours
HADS: Hospital anxiety depression scale
Hosp: Hospital
HOSTT: Holding, observation, short-term therapy
IHD: Ischemic heart disease
Info: Information
LMWH: Low molecular weight heparin
LOS: Length of stay
LWBS: Left without being seen
MACE: Major adverse cardiac events
NPV: Negative predictive value
NSR: Normal sinus rhythm
Obs: Observation
OR: Odds ratio
OU: Observation unit
PED: Pediatric emergency department
Peds: Pediatric
PG: Press Ganey
PPV: Positive predictive value
pro: Professional
QALY: Quality-adjusted life year
QOL: Quality of life
Rehosp: Rehospitalization
Rx: Treatment
SBP: Systolic blood pressure
TIMI: Thrombolysis in myocardial infarction
TnI: Troponin I
UF: Unfractionated
USD: United States Dollar
Utox: Urine toxicology
VT: Ventricular tachycardia
WBC: White blood cell count

Table 80.3 Summary of Evidence-Based Articles for Critical Question #1 and #3

	# Articles	# Articles	# Articles	# Articles
Level of evidence	Class I	Class II	Class III	Total
Cardiovascular: Chest pain	11	10	8	29
Cardiovascular: CHF	1	2	4	7
Cardiovascular: Atrial fibrillation	2	1	3	6
Cardiovascular: DVT	1	-	-	1
Respiratory: Asthma	3	-	3	7
Respiratory: COPD exacerbation	-	-	1	1
Respiratory/infection: Pneumonia	-	1	-	1
Infections: Pyelonephritis	-	1	2	3
Infections: Cellulitis	-	-	1	1
Neurologic: TIA	1	1	1	3
Neurologic: Syncope	1	-	1	2
Abdominal Pain	-	2	1	3
Trauma – Head injury	1	1	1	3
Trauma – General/abdominal	-	-	4	4
Toxicology	-	-	3	3
Decompression illness	-	-	1*	1
ED efficiency	1	2	3	6
Systematic review articles	-	-	3*	3
Total number of articles	22	21	40	83

Decompression Illness is also a systematic review so there
were 4 systematic reviews but is counted under
decompression illness

Summary of Evidence-Based Articles for Critical Question #2

	# Articles	# Articles	# Articles	# Articles
Level of Evidence	Class I	Class II	Class III	Total
Cardiovascular: Chest Pain	-	1	-	1
Cardiovascular: DVT	2	1	2	5
Cardiovascular: Atrial Fibrillation	-	1	1	2
Neurologic: TIA	-	2	1	3
Abdominal Pain	1	1	1	3
Trauma – Head Injury	2	-	1	3
Sickle Cell	-	-	1	1
Toxicology	-	-	1	1
Total Number of Articles	5	6	8	19

Summary of Evidence-Based Articles for Critical Questions #1, #2, #3

	# Articles	# Articles	# Articles	# Articles
Level of evidence	Class I	Class II	Class III	Total
Cardiovascular: Chest pain	11	10	8	29
Cardiovascular: CHF	1	2	4	7
Cardiovascular: Atrial fibrillation	2	1	3	6
Cardiovascular: DVT	1	-	-	1
Respiratory: Asthma	3	-	3	6
Respiratory: COPD exacerbation	-	-	1	1
Respiratory/Infection: Pneumonia	-	1	-	1
Infections: Pyelonephritis	-	1	2	3
Infections: Cellulitis	-	-	1	1
Neurologic: TIA	1	1	1	3
Neurologic: Syncope	1	-	1	2
Abdominal Pain	-	2	1	3
Trauma – Head injury	1	1	1	3
Trauma – General/abdominal	-	-	4	4
Toxicology	-	-	3	3
Decompression illness	-	-	1*	1
ED efficiency	1	2	3	6
Systematic review articles	-	-	3*	3
Total number of articles	22	21	40	83

*Decompression illness is also a systematic review so there were 4 systematic reviews but is counted under decompression illness

In addition, there were 19 articles that demonstrated the utility of standardized diagnostic protocols and/or an accelerated "upfront" loading of patient diagnostic and/or therapeutic interventions that are an integral part of current OU management of patients. These clinical conditions/disorders (and the number of articles) that were dealt with were as follows: deep vein thrombosis (5), transient ischemic attack (3), abdominal pain (3), head injury (3), atrial fibrillation (2), chest pain (1), sickle cell disease (1), and toxicology[1]. These are all conditions/disorders that have been successfully managed in OUs (Table 80.2).

Moreover, if we add the 37 articles in the following chapter on the evidence-based literature for pediatrics (33 articles) and geriatrics (4 articles), there are 139 articles encompassing many different diseases and conditions and all ages of patients. A summary of the literature by diagnosis and condition is listed in Table 80.3 (excludes the articles from the next chapter).

Overall Summary

Of all the 102 adult articles (and 37 pediatric/geriatric studies for 139 studies, see Chapter 81), which include the 19 articles employing OU-type protocols and/or methodology, the advantages of OU management were noted in every one of these studies. Even when separating out the studies based on a specific disorder (i.e., cardiac disease or respiratory disorders, trauma, infections, etc. or by diagnostic category, such as cardiac vs. noncardiac) there is overwhelming Level A evidence supporting the use of OUs. The many advantages include, but are not limited to, better patient outcomes, decreased LOS, lower costs, fewer readmissions, and increased patient satisfaction. A summary of level of recommendation for selected clinical conditions is listed in Appendix D.

Critical Questions

1. *In adult patients, when compared with inpatient treatment does the provision of observation services, specifically in a dedicated, protocol-driven OU, improve patient outcomes, decrease LOS, reduce costs, increase patient satisfaction and have other benefits, including (but not limited to) decreased readmissions?*

Recommendations

Level A recommendations. In adult ED patients, when compared with standard inpatient therapy, the use of a dedicated, protocol-driven OU decreases LOS, reduces costs, and increases patient satisfaction.

Level B recommendations. In adult ED patients, when compared with standard inpatient therapy, the use of a dedicated, protocol-driven OU improves patient outcomes.

Level C recommendations. In adult ED patients, when compared with standard inpatient therapy the use of a dedicated, protocol driven OU decreases hospital readmissions.

2. *In adult patients, does the use of OU clinical and administrative methodology (by aggressive early diagnostic and therapeutic management using tools such as protocol-driven therapy) produce equivalent or better results (e.g., in patient outcomes, LOS, costs, and adverse events) compared with routine inpatient care?*

Recommendations

Level A recommendations. In adult ED patients, when compared with standard inpatient therapy, the use of OU methodology with aggressive early diagnostic and therapeutic management, such as using protocol-driven patient management, decreases LOS and reduces costs when compared with standard inpatient therapy.

Level B recommendations. In adult ED patients, when compared with standard inpatient therapy, the use of OU methodology with aggressive early diagnostic and therapeutic management, such as using protocol-driven patient management, improves outcomes when compared with standard inpatient therapy.

Level C recommendations. None specified.

3. **In the adult ED, does use of an OU improve key measures of department efficiency, such as decreases in the ED LOS, door-to-doctor time, ambulance diversion, and the left-without-being-seen rate?**

Recommendations

Level A recommendations. None specified.

Level B recommendations. In the adult ED, use of an OU improves key measures of department efficiency, such as door-to-doctor time and a decrease in the left-without-being-seen rate.

Level C recommendations. In the adult ED, use of an OU improves key measures of department efficiency, including professional billing rates, ED LOS for both inpatient boarders and treat and release patients, and ambulance diversion time.

Future Research

The use of dedicated OU and employing aggressive, early management and protocol-driven care is still a relatively new but promising care delivery model. It has the potential to have a major positive impact, not only on patient outcomes and cost savings, but also on the entire health care system. However, only about one-third of the hospitals in the United States have an OU. For a given hospital, the implementation of such an OU could result in about $4.6 million dollars in annual savings, and for the U.S. health care system, $3.1 billion dollars in overall savings in one year alone if eligible hospitals opened these units.[1]

Appendix A: Literature Classification Schema

Design/ Class	Therapy	Diagnosis	Prognosis
1	Randomized, controlled trial or meta-analysis of randomized trials	Prospective cohort using a criterion standard or meta-analysis of prospective studies	Population prospective cohort or meta-analysis of prospective studies
2	Nonrandomized trial	Retrospective observational	Retrospective cohort; Case control
3	Case series; Case report; Other (e.g., consensus, review)	Case series; Case report; Other (e.g., consensus, review)	Case series; Case report; Other (e.g., consensus, review)

Appendix B: Approach to Downgrading Strength of Evidence

	Design/Class		
Downgrading	1	2	3
None	I	II	III
1 Level	II	III	X
2 Levels	III	X	X
Fatal flaw	X	X	X

Appendix C: Criteria Used for Clinical Findings and Strength of Recommendations

Level A recommendation Generally accepted principles for patient management that indicate a high degree of clinical certainty (i.e., based on strength of evidence Class I or overwhelming evidence from strength of evidence Class II studies that directly address all of the issues).

Level B recommendation Generally accepted principles for patient management that indicate a moderate degree of clinical certainty (i.e., based on strength of evidence Class II studies that directly address all of the issues, decision analysis that directly addresses the issue, or strong consensus of strength of evidence Class III studies).

Level C recommendation Patient management strategies that are based on strength of evidence Class III studies.

Appendix D: Critical Questions Based on Specific Diagnosis or Condition

Critical Questions

1. In adult patients, when compared with inpatient treatment does the provision of observation services, specifically in a dedicated, protocol-driven OU, improve patient outcomes, decrease LOS, reduce costs, increase patient satisfaction, and have other benefits, including (but not limited to) decreased readmissions?

Recommendations Based on Specific Diagnosis or Condition

Level A Recommendations

In adult ED patients with chest pain, asthma, transient ischemic attack, syncope, or congestive heart failure, when compared with standard inpatient therapy, the use of a dedicated, protocol-driven OU decreases LOS and reduces costs.

In adult ED patients with chest pain and asthma, when compared with standard inpatient therapy, the use of a dedicated, protocol-driven OU increases patient satisfaction.

In adult ED patients with atrial fibrillation, when compared with standard inpatient therapy, the use of a dedicated, protocol-driven observation decreases LOS.

In adult ED patients with traumatic head injury, when compared with standard inpatient therapy, the use of a dedicated, protocol-driven OU decreases LOS.

Level B Recommendations

In adult ED patients with chest pain, when compared with standard inpatient therapy, the use of a dedicated, protocol-driven OU improves patient outcomes.

In adult ED patients with abdominal pain, when compared with standard inpatient therapy the use of a dedicated, protocol-driven OU decreases LOS.

In adult ED patients with pyelonephritis, when compared with standard inpatient therapy the use of a dedicated, protocol-driven OU decreases LOS.

Level C Recommendations

In adult ED patients with abdominal trauma, when compared with standard inpatient therapy the use of a dedicated, protocol-driven OU decreases LOS and reduces cost.

In adult ED patients with toxic exposures, when compared with standard inpatient therapy the use of a dedicated, protocol-driven OU decreases LOS and reduces cost.

In adult ED patients with COPD and pneumonia, when compared with standard inpatient therapy the use of a dedicated, protocol-driven OU decreases LOS.

In adult ED patients with congestive heart failure, when compared with standard inpatient therapy the use of a dedicated, protocol-driven OU decreases hospital readmissions.

Critical Question 2:

In patients, does the use of OU clinical and administrative methodology (by aggressive early diagnostic and therapeutic management using tools such as protocol-driven therapy) produce equivalent or better results (e.g., patient outcomes, LOS, costs, and adverse events) compared with routine inpatient care?

Recommendations

Level A Recommendations

In adult ED patients with deep venous thrombosis, when compared with standard inpatient therapy the use of OU methodology with aggressive early diagnostic and therapeutic management, such as using protocol-driven patient management, decreases LOS and reduces costs when compared with standard inpatient therapy.

Level B Recommendations

In adult ED patients with chest pain, when compared with standard inpatient therapy the use of OU methodology with aggressive early diagnostic and therapeutic management, such as using protocol-driven patient management, decreases LOS and reduces costs when compared with standard inpatient therapy.

In adult ED patients with transient ischemic attack, when compared with standard inpatient therapy the use of OU methodology with aggressive early diagnostic and therapeutic management, such as using protocol-driven patient management, improves outcomes when compared with standard inpatient therapy.

In adult ED patients with atrial fibrillation, when compared with standard inpatient therapy, the use of OU methodology with aggressive early diagnostic and therapeutic management, such as using protocol-driven patient management, decreases LOS and reduces costs when compared with standard inpatient therapy.

In adult ED patients with sickle cell disease, when compared with standard inpatient therapy, the use of OU methodology with aggressive early diagnostic and therapeutic management, such as using protocol- driven patient management, decreases LOS and reduces costs when compared with standard inpatient therapy.

Level C Recommendations
None specified.

Critical Question 3: In the adult ED, does use of an OU improve key measures of department efficiency, such as decreases in ED LOS, door-to-doctor time, ambulance diversion, and the left-without-being-seen rate?

Level A Recommendations
None specified.

Level B Recommendations
In the adult ED, use of an OU improves key measures of department efficiency, such as door-to-doctor time and a decrease in the left-without-being-seen rate.

Level C Recommendations
In the adult ED, use of an OU improves key measures of department efficiency, such professional billing rates, ED LOS for both inpatient boarders and treat and release patients, and ambulance diversion time.

References

1. Baugh CW, Venkatesh AK, Hilton JA, et al. Making greater use Of dedicated hospital observation units for many short-stay patients could save $3.1 billion a year. *Health Aff* 2012;31(10):2314–2323.

2. de Leon AC, Jr, Farmer CA, King G, et al. Chest pain evaluation unit: a cost-effective approach for ruling out acute myocardial infarction. *South Med J* 1989 Sep;82 (9):1083–1089.

3. Gibler WB, Young GP, Hedges JR, et al. Acute myocardial infarction in chest pain patients with nondiagnostic ECGs: serial CK-MB sampling in the emergency department. The Emergency Medicine Cardiac Research Group. *Ann Emerg Med* 1992 May;21(5):504–512.

4. Gaspoz JM, Lee TH, Weinstein MC, et al. Cost-effectiveness of a new short-stay unit to "rule out" acute myocardial infarction in low risk patients. *J Am Coll Cardiol* 1994 Nov 1;24(5):1249–1259.

5. Gomez MA, Anderson JL, Karagounis LA, et al. An emergency department-based protocol for rapidly ruling out myocardial ischemia reduces hospital time and expense: results of a randomized study (ROMIO). *J Am Coll Cardiol* 1996 Jul;28 (1):25–33.

6. Roberts RR, Zalenski RJ, Mensah EK, et al. Costs of an emergency department-based accelerated diagnostic protocol vs hospitalization in patients with chest pain: a randomized controlled trial. *JAMA* 1997 Nov 26;278(20):1670–1676.

7. Rydman RJ, Zalenski RJ, Roberts RR, et al. Patient satisfaction with an emergency department chest pain observation unit. *Ann Emerg Med* 1997 Jan;29(1):109–115.

8. Zalenski RJ, Rydman RJ, McCarren M, et al. Feasibility of a rapid diagnostic protocol for an emergency department chest pain unit. *Ann Emerg Med* 1997 Jan;29 (1):99–108.

9. Farkouh ME, Smars PA, Reeder GS, et al. A clinical trial of a chest-pain observation unit for patients with unstable angina. Chest Pain Evaluation in the Emergency Room (CHEER) Investigators. *N Engl J Med* 1998 Dec 24;339(26):1882–1888.

10. Goodacre S, Nicholl J, Dixon S, et al. Randomised controlled trial and economic evaluation of a chest pain observation unit compared with routine care. *BMJ* 2004 Jan 31;328(7434):254.

11. Goodacre S, Nicholl J. A randomised controlled trial to measure the effect of chest pain unit care upon anxiety,

depression, and health-related quality of life [ISRCTN85078221. *Health Qual Life Outcomes* 2004 Jul 29;2:39.

12. Miller CD, Hwang W, Hoekstra JW, et al. Stress cardiac magnetic resonance imaging with observation unit care reduces cost for patients with emergent chest pain: a randomized trial. *Ann Emerg Med* 2010 Sep;56(3):209–219.e2.

13. Kerns JR, Shaub TF, Fontanarosa PB. Emergency cardiac stress testing in the evaluation of emergency department patients with atypical chest pain. *Ann Emerg Med* 1993 May;22(5):794–798.

14. Sayre MR, Bender AL, Dey CC, et al. Evaluating chest pain patients in an emergency department rapid diagnostic and treatment center is cost-effective. *Academic Emergency Medicine* 1994;1:A45.

15. Graff LG, Dallara J, Ross MA, et al. Impact on the care of the emergency department chest pain patient from the chest pain evaluation registry (CHEPER) study. *Am J Cardiol* 1997 Sep 1;80(5):563–568.

16. Mikhail MG, Smith FA, Gray M, et al. Cost-effectiveness of mandatory stress testing in chest pain center patients. *Ann Emerg Med* 1997 Jan;29(1):88–98.

17. Zalenski RJ, McCarren M, Roberts R, et al. An evaluation of a chest pain diagnostic protocol to exclude acute cardiac ischemia in the emergency department. *Archives of Internal Medicine* 1997;157(10):1085–1091.

18. Stomel R, Grant R, Eagle KA. Lessons learned from a community hospital chest pain center. *Am J Cardiol* 1999 Apr 1;83(7):1033–1037.

19. Lai C, Noeller TP, Schmidt K, et al. Short-term risk after initial observation for chest pain. *J Emerg Med* 2003 Nov;25(4):357–362.

20. Jagminas L, Partridge R. A comparison of emergency department versus inhospital chest pain observation units. *Am J Emerg Med* 2005 Mar;23(2):111–113.

21. Diercks DB, Kirk JD, Turnipseed SD, et al. Evaluation of patients with methamphetamine- and cocaine-related chest pain in a chest pain observation unit. *Crit pathw cardiol* 2007 Dec;6(4):161–164.

22. Chang AM, Shofer FS, Weiner MG, et al. Actual financial comparison of four strategies to evaluate patients with potential acute coronary syndromes. *Acad Emerg Med* 2008 Jul;15(7):649–655.

23. Limkakeng AT, Jr, Chandra A. Impact of renal dysfunction on acute coronary syndrome evaluation in observation unit patients. *Am J Emerg Med* 2010 Jul;28(6):658–662.

24. Maag R, Krivenko C, Graff L, et al. Improving chest pain evaluation within a multihospital network by the use of emergency department observation units. *Jt Comm J Qual Improv* 1997 Jun;23(6):312–320.

25. Kirk JD, Turnipseed S, Lewis WR, et al. Evaluation of chest pain in low-risk patients presenting to the emergency department: the role of immediate exercise testing. *Ann Emerg Med* 1998 Jul;32(1):1–7.

26. Goodacre S, Mason S, Arnold J, et al. Psychologic morbidity and health-related quality of life of patients assessed in a chest pain observation unit. *Ann Emerg Med* 2001 Oct;38(4):369–376.

27. Weber JE, Shofer FS, Larkin GL, et al. Validation of a brief observation period for patients with cocaine-associated chest pain. *N Engl J Med* 2003 Feb 6;348(6):510–517.

28. Goodacre S, Dixon S. Is a chest pain observation unit likely to be cost effective at my hospital? Extrapolation of data from a randomised controlled trial. *Emerg Med J* 2005 Jun;22(6):418–422.

29. Madsen T, Mallin M, Bledsoe J et al. Utility of the emergency department observation unit in ensuring stress testing in low-risk chest pain patients. *Crit Pathw Cardiol* 2009 Sep;8(3):122–124.

30. Madsen T, Bossart P, Bledsoe J, et al. Patients with coronary disease fail observation status at higher rates than patients without coronary disease. *Am J Emerg Med* 2010 Jan;28(1):19–22.

31. Pines JM, Isserman JA, Szyld D, et al. The effect of physician risk tolerance and the presence of an observation unit on decision making for ED patients with chest pain. *Am J Emerg Med* 2010 Sep;28(7):771–779.

32. McDermott, M F, Murphy, D G, Zalenski, R J, et al. A comparison between emergency diagnostic and treatment unit and inpatient care in the management of acute asthma. *Archives of Internal Medicine* 1997;157(18):2055–2062.

33. Rydman RJ, Isola ML, Roberts RR, et al. Emergency department observation unit versus hospital inpatient care for a chronic asthmatic population: a randomized trial of health status outcome and cost. *Med Care* 1998 Apr;36(4):599–609.

34. Rydman RJ, Roberts RR, Albrecht GL, et al. Patient satisfaction with an emergency department asthma observation unit. *Acad Emerg Med* 1999 Mar;6(3):178–183.

35. Zwicke DL, Donohue JF, Wagner EH. Use of the emergency department observation unit in the treatment of acute asthma. *Ann Emerg Med* 1982 Feb;11(2):77–83.

36. Brillman JC, Tandberg D. Observation unit impact on ED admission for asthma. *The American Journal of Emergency Medicine* 1994;12(1).

37. Mace SE. Asthma therapy in the observation unit. *Emerg Med Clin North Am* 2001 Feb;19(1):169–185.

38. Shen WK, Decker WW, Smars PA, et al. Syncope Evaluation in the Emergency Department Study (SEEDS): a multidisciplinary approach to syncope management. *Circulation* 2004 Dec 14;110(24):3636–3645.

39. Stockley CJ, Bonney ME, Gray AJ, et al. Syncope management in the UK and Republic of Ireland. *Emerg Med J* 2009 May;26(5):331–333.

40. Ross MA, Compton S, Medado P, et al. An emergency department diagnostic protocol for patients with transient ischemic attack: a randomized controlled trial. *Ann Emerg Med* 2007 Aug;50(2):109–119.

41. Brown MD, Reeves MJ, Glynn T, et al. Implementation of an emergency department based transient ischemic attack clinical pathway: a pilot study in knowledge translation. *Acad Emerg Med* 2007 Nov;14 (11):1114–1119.

42. Rothwell PM, Giles MF, Chandratheva A, et al. Effect of urgent treatment of transient ischaemic attack and minor stroke on early recurrent stroke (EXPRESS study): a prospective population-based sequential comparison. *Lancet* 2007 Oct 20;370(9596):1432–1442.

43. Luengo-Fernandez R, Gray AM, Rothwell PM. Effect of urgent treatment for transient ischaemic attack and minor stroke on disability and hospital costs (EXPRESS study): a prospective population-based sequential comparison. *Lancet Neurol* 2009 Mar;8(3):235–243.

44. Lavallee PC, Meseguer E, Abboud H, et al. A transient ischaemic attack clinic with round-the-clock access (SOS-TIA): feasibility and effects. *Lancet Neurol* 2007 Nov;6(11):953–960.

45. Stead LG, Bellolio MF, Suravaram S, et al. Evaluation of transient ischemic attack in an emergency department observation unit. *Neurocrit Care* 2009;10(2):204–208.

46. Koopman MMW, Prandoni P, Piovella F, et al. Treatment of venous thrombosis with intravenous unfractionated heparin administered in the hospital as compared with subcutaneous low-molecular-weight heparin administered at home. *N Engl J Med* 1996 03/14; 2013/02;334(11):682–687.

47. Levine M, Gent M, Hirsh J, et al. A comparison of low-molecular-weight heparin administered primarily at home with unfractionated heparin administered in the hospital for proximal deep-vein thrombosis. *N Engl J Med* 1996 Mar 14;334(11):677–681.

48. O'Brien B, Levine M, Willan A, et al. Economic evaluation of outpatient treatment with low-molecular-weight heparin for proximal vein thrombosis. *Arch Intern Med* 1999 Oct 25;159(19):2298–2304.

49. Vinson DR, Berman DA. Outpatient treatment of deep venous thrombosis: a clinical care pathway managed by the emergency department. *Ann Emerg Med* 2001 Mar;37(3):251–258.

50. Rodger M, Bredeson C, Wells PS, et al. Cost-effectiveness of low-molecular-weight heparin and unfractionated heparin in treatment of deep vein thrombosis. *CMAJ* 1998 Oct 20;159(8):931–938.

51. Gould MK, Dembitzer AD, Sanders GD, et al. Low-molecular-weight heparins compared with unfractionated heparin for treatment of acute deep venous thrombosis. A cost-effectiveness analysis. *Ann Intern Med* 1999 May 18;130(10):789–799.

52. Decker WW, Smars PA, Vaidyanathan L, et al. A prospective, randomized trial of an emergency department observation unit for acute onset atrial fibrillation. *Annals of Emergency Medicine* 2008;52 (4):322–328.

53. Cristoni L, Tampieri A, Mucci F, et al. Cardioversion of acute atrial fibrillation in the short observation unit: comparison of a protocol focused on electrical cardioversion with simple antiarrhythmic treatment. *Emerg Med J* 2011 Nov;28(11):932–937.

54. Kim MH, Morady F, Conlon B, et al. A prospective, randomized, controlled trial of an emergency department-based atrial fibrillation treatment strategy with low-molecular-weight heparin. *Ann Emerg Med* 2002 Aug;40(2):187–192.

55. Conti A, Canuti E, Mariannini Y, et al. Clinical management of atrial fibrillation: early interventions, observation, and structured follow-up reduce hospitalizations. *Am J Emerg Med* 2012 Nov;30 (9):1962–1969.

56. Koenig BO, Ross MA, Jackson RE. An emergency department observation unit protocol for acute-onset atrial fibrillation is

feasible. *Ann Emerg Med* 2002 Apr;39(4):374–381.

57. Ross MA, Davis B, Dresselhouse A. The role of an emergency department observation unit in a clinical pathway for atrial fibrillation. *Crit Pathw Cardiol* 2004 Mar;3(1):8–12.

58. Stiell IG, Clement CM, Perry JJ, et al. Association of the Ottawa Aggressive Protocol with rapid discharge of emergency department patients with recent-onset atrial fibrillation or flutter. *CJEM* 2010 May;12(3):181–191.

59. Vinson DR, Hoehn T, Graber DJ, et al. Managing emergency department patients with recent-onset atrial fibrillation. *J Emerg Med* 2012 Feb;42(2):139–148.

60. Lopez PP, Cohn SM, Popkin CA, et al. Appendicitis Diagnostic G. The use of a computed tomography scan to rule out appendicitis in women of childbearing age is as accurate as clinical examination: a prospective randomized trial. *Am Surg* 2007 Dec;73(12):1232–1236.

61. White JJ, Santillana M, Haller JA, Jr. Intensive in-hospital observation: a safe way to decrease unnecessary appendectomy. *Am Surg* 1975 Dec;41(12):793–798.

62. Graff L, Radford MJ, Werne C. Probability of appendicitis before and after observation. *Ann Emerg Med* 1991 May;20 (5):503–507.

63. Graff L, Russell J, Seashore J, et al. False-negative and false-positive errors in abdominal pain evaluation: failure to diagnose acute appendicitis and unnecessary surgery. *Acad Emerg Med* 2000 Nov;7(11):1244–1255.

64. Thomson HJ, Jones PF. Active observation in acute abdominal pain. *Am J Surg* 1986 Nov;152(5):522–525.

65. Saunders CE, Gentile DA. Treatment of mild exacerbations of recurrent alcoholic pancreatitis in an emergency department observation unit. *South Med J* 1988 Mar;81(3):317–320.

66. Fabbri A, Servadei F, Marchesini G, et al. Which type of observation for patients with high-risk mild head injury and negative computed tomography?. *Eur J Emerg Med* 2004 Apr;11(2):65–69.

67. af Geijerstam JL, Oredsson S, Britton M, OCTOPUS Study I. Medical outcome after immediate computed tomography or admission for observation in patients with mild head injury: randomised controlled trial. *BMJ* 2006 Sep 2;333(7566):465.

68. Norlund A, Marke LA, af Geijerstam JL, et al. Immediate computed tomography or admission for observation after mild head injury: cost comparison in randomised controlled trial. *BMJ* 2006 Sep 2;333(7566):469.

69. Menditto VG, Lucci M, Polonara S, et al. Management of minor head injury in patients receiving oral anticoagulant therapy: a prospective study of a 24-hour observation protocol. *Ann Emerg Med* 2012 Jun;59(6):451–455.

70. MacLaren RE, Ghoorahoo HI, Kirby NG. Use of an accident and emergency department observation ward in the management of head injury. *Br J Surg* 1993 Feb;80(2):215–217.

71. Af Geijerstam JL, Britton M, Marke LA. Mild head injury: observation or computed tomography? Economic aspects by literature review and decision analysis. *Emerg Med J* 2004 Jan;21(1):54–58.

72. Peacock WF, 4th, Holland R, Gyarmathy R, et al.

Observation unit treatment of heart failure with nesiritide: results from the proaction trial. *J Emerg Med* 2005 Oct;29(3):243–252.

73. Graff L, Orledge J, Radford MJ, et al. Correlation of the Agency for Health Care Policy and Research congestive heart failure admission guideline with mortality: peer review organization voluntary hospital association initiative to decrease events (PROVIDE) for congestive heart failure. *Ann Emerg Med* 1999 Oct;34(4 Pt 1):429–437.

74. Storrow AB, Collins SP, Lyons MS, et al. Emergency department observation of heart failure: preliminary analysis of safety and cost. *Congest Heart Fail* 2005 Mar–Apr;11(2):68–72.

75. Peacock WF, 4th, Remer EE, Aponte J, et al. Effective observation unit treatment of decompensated heart failure. *Congest Heart Fail* 2002 Mar–Apr;8(2):68–73.

76. Burkhardt J, Peacock WF, Emerman CL. Predictors of emergency department observation unit outcomes. *Acad Emerg Med* 2005 Sep;12(9):869–874.

77. Diercks DB, Peacock WF, Kirk JD, et al. ED patients with heart failure: identification of an observational unit-appropriate cohort. *Am J Emerg Med* 2006 May;24(3):319–324.

78. Collins SP, Schauer DP, Gupta A, et al. Cost-effectiveness analysis of ED decision making in patients with non-high-risk heart failure. *Am J Emerg Med* 2009 Mar;27(3):293–302.

79. Schrock JW, Reznikova S, Weller S. The effect of an observation unit on the rate of ED admission and discharge for pyelonephritis. *Am J Emerg Med* 2010 Jul;28(6):682–688.

80. Israel RS, Lowenstein SR, Marx JA, et al. Management of acute

pyelonephritis in an emergency department observation unit. *Ann Emerg Med* 1991 Mar;20(3):253–257.

81. Ward G, Jorden RC, Severance HW. Treatment of pyelonephritis in an observation unit. *Ann Emerg Med* 1991 Mar;20(3):258–261.

82. Schrock JW, Laskey S, Cydulka RK. Predicting observation unit treatment failures in patients with skin and soft tissue infections. *Int J Emerg Med* 2008 Jun;1(2):85–90.

83. Conrad L, Markovchick V, Mitchiner J, et al. The role of an emergency department observation unit in the management of trauma patients. *J Emerg Med* 1985;2(5):325–333.

84. Henneman PL, Marx JA, Cantrill SC, et al. The use of an emergency department observation unit in the management of abdominal trauma. *Ann Emerg Med* 1989 Jun;18(6):647–650.

85. Cowell VL, Ciraulo D, Gabram S, et al. Trauma 24-hour observation critical path. *J Trauma* 1998 Jul;45(1):147–150.

86. Madsen TE, Bledsoe JR, Bossart PJ. Observation unit admission as an alternative to inpatient admission for trauma activation patients. *Emerg Med J* 2009 Jun;26(6):421–423.

87. Foulke GE. Identifying toxicity risk early after antidepressant overdose. *Am J Emerg Med* 1995 Mar;13(2):123–126.

88. Hollander JE, McCracken G, Johnson S, et al. Emergency department observation of poisoned patients: how long is necessary? [see comment].

Acad Emerg Med 1999 Sep;6(9):887–894.

89. Sivilotti ML, Yarema MC, Juurlink DN, et al. A risk quantification instrument for acute acetaminophen overdose patients treated with N-acetylcysteine. *Ann Emerg Med* 2005 Sep;46(3):263–271.

90. Sztajnkrycer MD, Mell HK, Melin GJ. Development and implementation of an emergency department observation unit protocol for deliberate drug ingestion in adults - preliminary results. *Clin Toxicol (Phila)* 2007 Jun–Aug;45(5):499–504.

91. Chan SS, Yuen EH, Kew J, et al. Community-acquired pneumonia–implementation of a prediction rule to guide selection of patients for outpatient treatment. *Eur J Emerg Med* 2001 Dec;8(4):279–286.

92. Salazar A, Juan A, Ballbe R, et al. Emergency short-stay unit as an effective alternative to in-hospital admission for acute chronic obstructive pulmonary disease exacerbation. *Am J Emerg Med* 2007 May;25(4):486–487.

93. Hadden DS, Dearden CH, Rocke LG. Short stay observation patients: general wards are inappropriate. *J Accid Emerg Med* 1996 May;13(3):163–165.

94. Baugh CW, Bohan JS. Estimating observation unit profitability with options modeling. *Acad Emerg Med* 2008;15(5):445–452.

95. Bazarian JJ, Schneider SM, Newman VJ, et al. Do admitted patients held in the emergency department impact the

throughput of treat-and-release patients? *Acad Emerg Med* 1996 Dec;3(12):1113–1118.

96. Kelen GD, Scheulen JJ, Hill PM. Effect of an emergency department (ED) managed acute care unit on ED overcrowding and emergency medical services diversion. *Acad Emerg Med* 2001 Nov;8(11):1095–1100.

97. Chandra A, Sieck S, Hocker M, et al. An observation unit may help improve an institution's Press Ganey satisfaction score. *Crit Pathw Cardiol* 2011 Jun;10(2):104–106.

98. Benjamin LJ, Swinson GI, Nagel RL. Sickle cell anemia day hospital: an approach for the management of uncomplicated painful crises. *Blood* 2000 Feb 15;95(4):1130–1136.

99. Cooke MW, Higgins J, Kidd P. Use of emergency observation and assessment wards: a systematic literature review. *Emerg Med J* 2003 Mar;20(2):138–142.

100. Daly S, Campbell DA, Cameron PA. Short-stay units and observation medicine: a systematic review. *Med J Aust* 2003 Jun 2;178(11):559–563.

101. Tempel R, Severance HW. Proposing short-term observation units for the management of decompression illness. *Undersea Hyperb Med* 2006 Mar–Apr;33(2):89–94.

102. Ross MA, Aurora T, Graff L, et al. State of the art: emergency department observation units. *Crit Pathw Cardiol* 2012 Sep;11(3):128–138.

Chapter

The Evidence Basis for Age-Related Observation Care

Sharon E. Mace, MD, FACEP, FAAP
Christopher W. Baugh, MD, MBA, FACEP
Madeline Joseph, MD, FACEP, FAAP

Abstract

In this chapter, we examine and summarize the evidence for observation care based on age, for example, the pediatric and geriatric population, as the previous chapter did for adults with a given condition or diagnosis, such as chest pain or asthma. The critical questions addressed in this chapter are:

1. Can infants and children (e.g., pediatric patients) be successfully and safely treated in an observation unit setting?
2. Can geriatric patients be successfully and safely treated in an observation unit setting?

Introduction

The key components in any discussion of health care and health care reform include patient outcomes, patient safety, quality, and cost.[1] When a safe and efficient alternative exists, avoiding inpatient hospital admissions can have benefits for the individual patient, as well as more efficient use of the health care system. Avoiding hospital admissions and/or decreasing length of stay (LOS) improves patient safety and outcomes by decreasing the opportunities for patient error and other risks to the patient, including medication errors, nosocomial infections, adverse drug events, use of restraints, delirium, pressure sores, falls, and a deterioration in functional status.[2–5] Nearly one-third of the health care cost in the United States is attributable to inpatient hospital care[6] and over 50% (55% excluding maternal/neonatal admissions according to the Healthcare Cost and Utilization Project) of hospitalizations in the United States begin in the emergency department (ED).[7] Obviously, avoiding hospital admissions, improving patient flow through hospitals, and decreasing hospital readmissions should decrease the cost of health care.[8] Thus, there is a critical need for any process or system of care that prevents "avoidable admissions" and/or decreases LOS, while maintaining high-quality, cost-effective patient care, increased patient satisfaction and providing a critical link to accountable care organizations (ACOs)[6,7] (See ACO Chapter 20). Observation units (OUs) can meet this need.[5, 9–11]

Observation medicine is designed to improve the patient throughput process, increase patient safety and quality, and improve outcomes by the efficient use of systems of care and key clinical and administrative methods or techniques. Such techniques include clinical protocols and pathways, order sets, observation unit guidelines, monitoring of performance metrics, appropriate staffing, and the coordination or streamlining of hospital systems (see Clinical Protocols Chapters 82–87, Administrative Policies Chapter 88, Order Sets Chapter 89–96). The Institute of Medicine in its 2006 report endorsed the use of emergency department observation units (ED OUs) as a method for decreasing ambulance diversion, ED boarding, and avoidable hospital admissions.[9] A recent policy by the American College of Emergency Physicians on ED OUs identifies the provision of care "in a dedicated ED observation area, instead of a general inpatient bed or acute care ED bed" as a "best practice."[10]

Properly designed and managed OUs have been proposed as a solution to the health care crisis including escalating costs and concerns for patient safety and quality, since they can provide high-quality patient care at a lower cost with increased patient satisfaction.[5, 8–11] It is estimated that hospital systems in the United States alone could save an additional $3.1 billion per year through the avoidance of 3.6 million annual inpatient hospital admissions just by opening more observation units.[11]

Protocol-driven, dedicated OUs for specific diagnoses and/or complaints in adults have been studied. There is robust evidence that such units, by efficiently utilizing clinical and administrative resources and methodology, attain a LOS that is a small fraction of the time required elsewhere for the same patient population (see The Evidence Basis for Observation Medicine Chapter 80). This leads us to examine the question of whether there are the same advantages, such as decreased LOS, for patients in the extremes of age: children and elderly patients.

Methodology

We systematically evaluated the literature to develop evidence-based recommendations to answer the following critical questions: 1. "Can infants and children (e.g., pediatric patients) be successfully and safely treated in an observation unit setting?" A related secondary question is "In pediatric patients, does the provision of observation services, using observation unit methodology characterized by aggressive early diagnostic and therapeutic management, usually in the setting of a dedicated, protocol-driven observation unit, decrease LOS, decrease costs, decrease inpatient admissions, and have other benefits when compared with inpatient hospital care?" 2. "Can geriatric patients be successfully and safely treated in an observation unit setting?" A related secondary question is "In the elderly does the provision of observation services, using observation unit methodology characterized by early aggressive diagnostic and therapeutic management, usually in the setting of a dedicated, protocol- driven observation unit, decrease LOS, decrease costs, decrease inpatient admissions and have other benefits when compared with inpatient hospital care?"

We performed a literature search, graded the evidence, and provided recommendations based on the strength of the available data in the medical literature.

We created this document regarding the currently available peer-reviewed literature on observation care after careful review and critical analysis of the medical literature. Additional studies were found by searching the reference lists of included papers. All articles listed in this chapter were graded by two authors for quality and strength of evidence. If there was a difference between two authors, a third author provided a tie-breaking grade to settle on a final grade. We classified the articles into three classes of evidence on the basis of the design of the study. Design 1 represents the strongest evidence. Design 3 represents the weakest evidence for therapeutic, diagnostic, and prognostic studies, respectively (Appendix A). Authors of this chapter did not grade papers they authored themselves. Articles were then graded on dimensions related to the study's methodological features: blinded versus non-blinded, outcome assessment, blinded or randomized allocation, direct or indirect outcome measures (reliability and validity), biases (e.g., selection, detection, transfer), external validity (i.e., generalizability), and sufficient sample size. Articles received a final grade (Class I, II, III) on the basis of a predetermined formula, taking into account the design and study quality (Appendix A). Articles irrelevant to the question or with a fatal flaw were given an "X" and were not utilized in creating the final recommendation (Appendix B). Clinical results and strength of the recommendation were made according to the criteria in Appendix C.

The literature we reviewed included articles worldwide and not just from the United States. Therefore, the scope of application is international, not just within the United States. The inclusion criteria are for pediatric patients (age ≤ 21 years old) and geriatric patients (age ≥ 65 years old) presenting to the ED. The exclusion criteria are for adult non-geriatric patients, who are addressed in the previous chapter.

We adjusted reported cost data to United States dollars using the medical portion of the Consumer Price Index and prevailing international currency exchange rates as of February 2013.

We divided the articles into pediatric and geriatric sections and listed them by level of evidence first and then chronologically by year of publication.

Results: Pediatric

There were six class I studies, 20 Class II studies and 7 Class III studies.[12–44]

In the various clinical studies, pediatric patients in all age groups from infants to adolescents, even neonates, were successfully managed in an OU setting.[12–40] Direct comparison of similar patient populations in an OU versus inpatient setting revealed significantly shorter LOS in OUs in all five studies (one Class I, four Class II) for various common pediatric illnesses. In the Class I study of infants 3–24 months old with dehydration from gastroenteritis who were treated with IV fluids, the LOS was 9.9 hours for the ED holding unit versus 103.2 hours for inpatients (p < 0.00001).[12] In the Class II study of infants with hyperbilirubinemia, the observation unit median LOS of 17.8 hours was significantly different (p < 0.0001) from the inpatient comparison of 41.8 hours.[13] For pediatric patients status post an uncomplicated barium enema for the reduction of intussusception (Class II study), the mean observation unit LOS was 7.1 hours vs. 22.7 hours inpatient (p < 0.001).[14] A Class II study of pediatric patients with croup comparing the pre- versus post-observation LOS reported a 27.2 hour pre-observation LOS and 21.3 hour post-observation LOS (p < 0.03).[15] Another Class II study reported a mean LOS for pediatric asthmatic patients in a short-stay unit (SSU) of 35.3 hours, which was significantly different at p < 0.0001 from the 47.2 hours LOS for non-short-stay unit patients.[16] This was not an ED OU but an inpatient SSU adjacent to the pediatric ward, which may explain the relatively longer LOS than in other reports. Some SSU allow up to 48 hours for patient management, whereas most OUs have a 24-hour set criteria for maximum LOS.

In all seven studies (three Class I, four Class II) that evaluated cost, the observation unit charges and/or costs were significantly less than the inpatient costs[12, 15–20] For the Class I study of infants with dehydration from acute gastroenteritis who were treated with intravenous fluids, the costs for observation was $1,481, while the costs for the an inpatient stay was $8,920 (p < 0.00001).[12] The Class I study of pediatric asthmatics found significantly (p < 0.001) higher costs for inpatients: $9,939 compared to $5,667 for the ED holding room.[17] In the Class I report from Australia, the cost was $302 per bed day and the hospital cost savings was $509,690 for one year for the general hospital, and $408 per bed day and hospital cost savings of $4,213,363 for two years for the Children's hospital.[18] Four Class II studies

also found significantly lower costs for children and infants treated in an OU setting versus inpatient hospitalization. One Class II study of asthmatics at a children's hospital using the median per diem hospital costs of $2,496 and direct costs of $1,012 for the non-ICU asthmatic patients estimated the annual decrease in hospital charges to be $628,739 and in direct costs of $254,914 if the short-stay unit managed half of the 1,016 asthma patients admitted in one year.[16] In another Class II study of asthmatic infants and children, the costs per patient were $885 for ED holding unit vs. $5,716 for admitted patients.[19] The results for pediatric patients with croup were $2,110 if an observation unit patient and $2,679 if an admitted patient (p = 0.03).[15] This study appears not to have differentiated the OU patients from the inpatients in their post-OU data when comparing with the pre-OU charges. Thus, it is possible, even likely, that the actual savings may be even greater than reported if they separated out the OU patients from the inpatients in their post-OU charges. In another study of pediatric patients with all types of conditions/illnesses in a SSU, the cost per patient was no greater than $390 (and may have been < $390 for some patients) for the SSU and $1,378 if an inpatient.[20] This yielded decreased charges of $3,320,720 for one year.[20] All costs were adjusted to 2013 USD.

In all of the studies (two Class I, four Class II) that reported admission rates to the inpatient hospital following the introduction of an OU or SSU, the admission rates all showed decreases. There was a reduction in hospital admissions for the Class I Australian study by 10.3% (from 5,315 in 1993 to 4,766 in 1994) at the teaching hospital and 14.7% (from 8,065 in 1997 to 6,873 in 1998) at the children's hospital after the introduction of a SSU.[18] A Class I multi-center French study found that the introduction of a SSU "reduced inpatient hospitalizations."[21] In the Class II study of patients with croup, the admission rate after the introduction of a pediatric OU dropped by more than half from 9.5% to 4.2% (p < 0.0001).[15] In another Class II study from Canada, after the introduction of a pediatric OU, the admission rate for asthmatics declined significantly from 31% to 24% (p ≤ 0.01) and 1-day admissions decreased from 17% to 10% (p ≤ 0.01).[22] According to a Class II French study, referrals to the pediatric ED had been increasing by 8.25% per year and hospitalizations on pediatric wards were increasing by

5% annually.[23] But after the opening of a SSU, although the number of referrals to the pediatric ED continued to increase, the "increase in hospitalizations was stopped and even decreased slightly."[23] In another Class II study of pediatric asthmatics, inpatient admissions fell from 9.5% to 7.7% (SSU opened in August of that year) and 7.0% the following year SSU was open for the entire year).[16]

For other metrics, there were thirteen studies: three Class I and ten Class II.[12–14, 16–18, 20,22, 24–26, 38,44] Time to initiate treatment (and LOS) was markedly reduced with admission to an OU compared to inpatient admission. In the Class II study of hyperbilirubinemia in neonates, the median time to beginning treatment (e.g., phototherapy) was more than four times greater for the inpatients (N=105) at 6.7 hours compared to 1.6 hours for the OU (N=62) patients (p < 0.001).[13]

In another class I study, there was no increase in morbidity and a decreased percentage of returns to the hospital within 28 days was noted with the treatment of asthmatics of comparable severity (by 39 pretreatment and treatment variables including asthma scores) in an ED holding unit versus those admitted to the hospital.[17] Returns within 28 days occurred in 11.4% (4/35) of holding unit patients and in 17.6% (12/68) of inpatients.[17] For dehydrated infants with acute gastroenteritis treated with IV fluids (N=14) in the ED holding unit or as a hospital inpatient, both groups were successfully rehydrated clinically, and by laboratory and clinical parameters there were no significant differences either at baseline or at 24 hours between the ED holding unit patients versus the inpatients except for the significantly decreased costs and LOS for the ED holding unit patients (Class I study).[12] In the Class I study from Australia with two hospitals (one "teaching" hospital and one "children's" hospital), there were "no adverse events or critical incidents" for 6,248 patients and observation was "considered safe."[18] Unscheduled visits within 72 hours of discharge at the teaching hospital were 0.4% (4/1300) and at the children's hospital 0.9% (44/4948).[18] The authors noted that all the return visits within 72 hours of discharge were "all with minor problems, which were mostly due to parental anxiety".[18]

Readmission rates within 72 hours of discharge for pediatric asthmatics admitted to a SSU on a pediatric ward was 0.6% (2/298) versus 2.0% (2/102) for those not admitted to the SSU (Class II study).[16] In a Class II study of SSU patients in the United States, there were no fatalities and only 1% of 437 patients needed readmission to the hospital.[20] A similar rate of returns to the ED within 72 hours that were admitted was found in a Class II study of pediatric gastroenteritis patients (1.6%, 7 out of 430 OU admissions).[34] In general, studies in pediatric patients from neonates to adolescents all reported a decrease or no difference in returns to the ED or hospital when observation/short-stay patients were compared with inpatients. One outlier was a Class II Canadian study in asthmatics that found repeat ED visits after treatment for asthma was 3% before the OU and 5 % (p- 0.01) after opening of the OU.[22] This study had an extremely short OU LOS of 5.3 hours if discharged home and 6.5 hours if admitted, which may help explain this exception to the findings in other studies of a decreased or equivalent rate of return to the ED or hospital for OU patients when compared to inpatients.

In the Class II study of pediatric patients who had a barium enema for intussusception, there were no adverse events in either group (observation N=51 or inpatient N=27) and the reoccurrence rates were less for the observation patients (7.8%, 4/51) than for the inpatients (14.8%, 4/27).[14] A second Class II study of infants status post barium enema reduction of intussusception confirmed these findings with no complications (such as perforation, sepsis or shock) in any of their 149 OU patients.[28] A Class II study that included pediatric patients (N=363) as well as adults in an OU reported no mortalities, 0.8% of pediatric patients went to the operating room, and no pediatric patients signed out against medical advice.[24]

An Australian Class II study of infants and children with croup compared OU and mandatory steroid use with pre-observation and non-mandatory steroid use (i.e., optional steroid use per individual physician discretion): average number of ICU transfers 2.6% versus 11.6%, average number of intubated patients 4 versus 8, and average ICU days 24 versus 129.[25] The drawback to this study is that it is difficult to separate out the effect of mandatory steroids from the initiation of OU. It does point out that the institution of "best practices" may be easier in a dedicated, protocol-driven observation unit than for inpatients comingled with other patients throughout the inpatient wards.

One Class III study evaluated "satisfaction." On a 1 (lowest) to 4 (highest) Likert scale, parental satisfaction was 3.49 ± 0.79 and referring physician satisfaction was 3.63 ± (0.79). Others also reported "high parental satisfaction."[18]

In all of the studies in infants and children treated in observation units or observation unit settings, no deaths and "no critical incidents or major adverse events" were reported.[12–44]

Discussion: Pediatric

In the United States, there were 136.1 million ED visits in 2009.[45] This number has been steadily increasing over the past few decades. In 1991 there were 85 million ED visits, representing an increase of 60.1% from 1991 to 2009.[45, 46] The increase in ED visits is almost double what would be expected from population growth.[47]

In recent years, ED visits for pediatric patients have also been increasing.[48] Infants and children are responsible for more than one-fourth (27%) of all ED visits.[49] Infants (i.e., those less than 12 months of age) are the segment of the population with the highest annual per capita ED visit rate.[50]

Pediatric patients from neonates to adolescents and young adults with various common conditions or diseases have been monitored, diagnosed, and treated in an OU with admission rates similar to the benchmark inpatient admission rate of about 22.3% noted in adults.[51] Similar to the adult literature, the inpatient admission rate varies depending on the clinical condition, with a trend for higher admission rates for respiratory illnesses (e.g., pneumonia, bronchiolitis, and asthma) and the lowest incidence of admissions for accidental ingestions/overdoses, with other diagnostic categories (e.g., gastrointestinal, neurologic, trauma, and infections) having intermediate admission rates.[29–31, 37,38] The LOS for pediatric patients (when considering all categories of diseases and conditions), seems to be about the same[27,37,38] or somewhat less[17,20,21,24,30,33,36,39] than the benchmark noted in adult studies of 15.3 hours.[51] There is only one study (from Australia) that found a longer LOS (17.5 and 20.5 hours, respectively at two different hospitals), although the LOS was still < 24 hours.[18] Psychiatric patients were allowed to be admitted to this short-stay unit with

14% of admissions being "psychosocial" and "an alarmingly high number of behavioral, overdose, psychiatric, suicidal and violent cases."[18] This is very different from most OUs, which exclude psychiatric diagnoses[39,40,51] or have a small percentage of psychosocial care,[20,27,30,31] which are generally known to have a prolonged LOS in the ED and a high rate of inpatient admission. This finding may explain why the LOS was an outlier in this one study. The majority of pediatric studies occurred in the setting of a pediatric children's hospital, although there is evidence that children and infants can be successfully managed in a location other than a children's hospital and in even a combined ("hybrid") unit where both adults and children are cared for in the same observation unit.[24,40] (See Chapter 10 on Community Hospitals and Pediatric Chapter 53.)

These findings in infants and children do not seem to change over the last several decades. Studies performed in the 1970s and 1980s demonstrate similar findings to the studies conducted in the 1990s and from 2000 to the present. This suggests that although diagnostic and therapeutic management may differ over decades, the benefits of observation unit methodology and observation units remain irrespective of the time frame. This trend suggests that the positive results of OUs may be due to the systems of care or processes that are unique to OUs and not merely to drugs or other therapies that tend to change significantly over time.

The use of OUs to manage infants and children is not exclusive to the United States, but is an international occurrence with reports from Canada,[22] Australia[18,25] and Europe.[21,23,36,41]

Since a considerable number of inpatient admissions in children and infants are for a relatively short time frame or duration, placing children and infants in OUs could potentially have a major impact on inpatient admisssions.[52–56] Various research studies[52–54] seem to confirm a recent editorial[55] and a Canadian health policy report[56] that recommended placing children and infants in an alternative setting (e.g., observation unit) instead of being admitted to the hospital. One of these studies found that "nearly one-third of children hospitalized in the United States experience a high-turnover stay" and "may be eligible for care in an alternative setting."[52] A study of hospitalized asthmatics concluded that "more than 70% of asthma hospitalizations in this community could be cared for in alternate settings."[53] Another report of dehydrated children and infants had similar conclusions, indicated that "nearly all children hospitalized for simple acute gastroenteritis might be eligible for care in alternative settings designed to provide hospital-level care for short periods."[54] According to a Canadian health policy report, 25% of adult patients and 39% of pediatric patients could be managed in an OU instead of being admitted to the hospital as an inpatient.[56]

Results: Geriatric

Geriatric patients were successfully managed in an observation unit/short-stay unit in all four studies that focused on this population, with no major adverse events noted and "overall good results."[57–60] The overwhelming majority of elderly patients who received care in an OU were discharged home (71%, 72%, 83%, 84%); conversely only 16.1% to 29% were subsequently admitted as hospital inpatients. The two studies with somewhat higher admission rates (28% and 29%) and lower discharge rates of 71% and 72% were earlier studies (published in 1985 and 1997) in SSUs in Wales and the United Kingdom;[57,58] the later studies (published in 2003 and 2008) were from OUs in the United States.[59,60] These differences may be due to time (differences over the years), location (United Kingdom vs. United States), the type of unit (short-stay vs. observation unit), and the age used to define geriatric, a combination of these factors or some other unknown variable(s). One of the SSUs used age > 70 years as their definition of geriatric patient,[57] whereas the other three studies used > 65 or ≥ 65 years as their age cutoff.[58–60] These geriatric admission rates compare favorably with national cited rates of about 77.7% of OU patients being discharged home and 22.3% being admitted to an inpatient bed from an OU.[51]

The LOS for elderly patients managed in an OU of 15.8 hours in the Ross et al. study[59] is consistent with the quoted average LOS of 15.3 hours for OUs in general.[51]

It may be that the critical factor is comorbidity and not age as a determinant of LOS. A study comparing elderly (≥ 65 years old) versus non-geriatric (< 65 years of age) adults with chest pain in an ED OU found no significant difference in inpatient hospital admission rate from the ED OU

for geriatric patients with no history of coronary artery disease (CAD) (12%) versus non-geriatric patients (7.7%) (p = 0.2), where CAD was defined as previous myocardial infarction, coronary artery stent or coronary artery bypass graft.[60] A recent study found that frailty and sociodemographic factors but not age to be a predictor of hospital admission from an OU.[61]

There were no reported deaths in the OU or SSU in these four studies.[57–60] One of the four studies evaluated returns to the ED within 30 days for the younger vs. older patients.[59] No deaths were reported in the younger ED OU patients (< 65 years of age) who returned (0%), while two of the elderly ED OU patients, aged 75 and 77 years old, who returned to the ED within 30 days expired (0.6%). Both deaths were related to existing comorbid conditions and unrelated to the index visit or management received on that visit.

Discussion: Geriatric

Currently, those over 65 years old comprise 12% of the population and by 2030, that figure is anticipated to nearly double to 21%.[62,63] Although they are only 12% of the population at present, those over 65 years old account for at least one-third of hospital stays and one-fourth of doctors' office visits.[64] The fastest growing age group is the population aged ≥ 80 years old.[65,66] Moreover, this is the very portion of the population that uses the most health care resources, requiring the most expensive and intensive medical care.[62,66]

This "impending crisis" in senior care[62–64, 66] is attributed to the aging of the population as baby boomers head toward old age and to a growth in age-specific consumption of health care. The segment of the population over 65 years old has become 8 times more numerous and those over 85 years old have become 21 times more numerous in society since the start of the twenty-first century.[67] In addition to the exponential growth in the number of the elderly, the older individual consumes a much larger percentage of health care consumption. In recent decades, spending in the United States on geriatric health care has outpaced the gross domestic product (GDP) by 4.0% per year. In dollar amounts, geriatric health care consumption in 1995 was $9,200 in 1995 and based on previous trends is projected to be $25,000 per person in 2020, a 171% increase in 25 years.[68]

In the near future, more than half of all medical care in the United States will go to the elderly if current trends continue. These trends for the geriatric population are true not just for the United States, but are a worldwide phenomenom.[66]

Older patients are increasing exponentially as a segment of the population, are consuming a greater and disproportionate share of health care expenditures, "require more time and resources while in the ED," and are admitted to the hospital and to high technology, labor intensive, resource demanding, expensive critical care units more often than their younger counterparts.[66] The looming crisis in the provision of geriatric health has caused some to consider health care rationing for the elderly.[67,68]

Currently, health care spending in the United States accounts for 17% of GDP and is growing. If current trends persist, 38% of GDP will be spent on health care by the year 2075.[69]

Moreover, geriatric patients are particularly vulnerable to inpatient complications and are known to have higher rates of nosocomial infections, adverse drug events, falls, delirium, restraint usage, pressure sores, and a decline in functional status.[59, 70–73]

Although there is no panacea for the crisis in geriatric health care, any system or program such as OUs that can prevent hospital admissions and decrease LOS in elderly patients, while maintaining patient quality of care and patient satisfaction, must be considered and endorsed. Although there needs to be more research in this area, it seems intuitive that the provision of observation medicine (i.e., in a dedicated, protocol-driven unit employing early aggressive monitoring, diagnostics, and therapy) will prove to be as successful in the elderly as it has been in other age groups (see The Evidence Basis for Observation Medicine Chapter 80 and this chapter's section on pediatrics).

Summary and the Future

EDs are portals for health care, not just as a source of outpatient care, comprising about one-quarter of all acute care outpatient visits in the United States,[74] but also as an increasing source of hospital admissions, now accounting for about one-half of all inpatient hospital admissions.[7] In the United States, from 1993 to 2006, the number of hospital admissions increased by 15% and the number of admissions from the ED increased by 50.4%.[74] For the conditions most frequently admitted to the hospital, 12 of the 13 conditions had an increased proportion of admitted patients who came through the ED, with the exception of "coronary atherosclerosis for which rapid 'rule out' protocols and ED based chest-pain observation units have reduced the need for inpatient admission."[74] If similar protocols and observation medicine methodology with the processes and systems of care practiced in observation units could be applied to all ages of patients including the sizable pediatric and the growing geriatric patient populations and for non-chest pain conditions and diseases as well as chest pain, the potential benefits, not just in cost savings to the health care system but also in improved patient quality of care and patient safety with better patient outcomes, would be enormous. This chapter on age-related observation, similar to the previous chapter regarding observation for adults based on a disease or clinical condition, provides documentation for the evidence-based medicine rationale for observation units and their integrated, efficient systems of care.

Critical Questions

1. Can infants and children (e.g., pediatric patients) be successfully and safely treated in an observation unit setting?

Recommendations

Level A Recommendations:

(1) Pediatric patients can be successfully and safely managed in an observation unit.

(2) Infants and children in an observation unit setting have a shorter LOS when compared with admitted patients for the same diseases.

(3) If infants and children are treated in an observation unit setting, costs are lower than with an inpatient admission.

(4) After the implementation of an observation unit, inpatient hospital admission rates for infants and children decreased.

Clinicians should consider placing appropriately selected infants and children in an observation unit instead of an inpatient admission due to a shorter LOS and decreased costs with equivalent or better outcomes.

Level B Recommendations:

When other metrics are considered, there are additional benefits of treating infants and children in an observation unit setting compared to an inpatient admission. These include shorter time to treatment, decreased returns to ED or hospital, decreased re-admissions to the hospital, improved patient outcome; decrease in morbidity, and improved parent satisfaction.

Level C Recommendations:
None specified.

2. Can geriatric patients be successfully and safely treated in an observation unit setting?

Recommendations

Level A Recommendations:
None specified.

Level B Recommendations:

Geriatric patients can be successfully and safely managed in an observation unit.

Level C Recommendations:

Admission rates to the hospital from an observation unit for geriatric patients are consistent with generally accepted benchmarks for non-geriatric patients.

Table 81.1 Evidentiary Table for Pediatric and Geriatric Patients

Author/ Year Published/ Country/ Setting/ Time Frame*	Design	Patient Population	Outcomes		Effect of Observation Unit on Inpatient Admissions	Other Metrics	Limitations/ Comments	Class
			Length of Stay (LOS)	Cost				
Willert C[17] 1985 United States Children's Hospital Holding Room (HR) in ED Oct 5 – Dec 11, 1981	RCT compared HR to hospital admission for asthmatics	N = 103 Age >1 year, asthma score ≤ 5, no comorbidity HR N = 52, inpatients N = 51	LOS (hours ± SD) discharged from HR = 11.8 (± 4.61) inpatients 45.6 (± 12)	Cost (± SD): HR $1,133 (± $980) Inpatient $1,987 (± $799) p <0.001 For ≤ 1 day admits HR $526 Inpatient $1,439 (excludes those with recurrent episodes) In 2013 USD Cost (± SD) HR $5,667 (± $4,902) Inpatient $9,939 (± $3,996) For ≤ 1 day admits HR $2,630.96, inpatients $7,197.62	——	For HR, 67% (35/52) discharged, 33% admitted (17/52) Reoccurrence rates within first week and 1 month were not statistically different Reoccurrence rates within 28 days after discharge: HR 11.4% vs. 17.6% inpatients	Equivalent baseline and severity for two groups. "Two treatment groups were comparable with regard to all 39 pretreatment, treatment and calculated medical variables including asthma scores." Reoccurrence rate for all patients = 15.5%, HR is five bed ward in PED, asthma score >5 is severe asthma with respiratory failure, patients received "standardized" protocolized therapy to treat asthma	I
Listernick R[12] 1986 United States Children's Hospital	RCT of dehydrated infants from	N = 14 treated with IV, randomized to HR N =	Mean LOS HR 9.9 hours Inpatient 103.2 hours p <0.00001	Mean cost HR $379. Inpatient $2,300. p <0.00001 In USD 2013	——	Age 3 to 24 months with no chronic diseases with acute gastroenteritis "compared efficacy, safety	IV was subgroup of larger study of 29 patients (15 oral rehydration, 14 IV) Small N, groups had	I

486

Study	Design	N / Diagnoses	Mean LOS	Cost	Results	Admissions	Comments
ED holding room (HR) Jan 1983–May 1984	acute gastro enteritis	7 or inpatient N = 7		HR $1,481. Inpatient $8,920.	and costs" to assess use of ED holding room		equivalent baseline and severity. Similar labs at baseline and at 24 hours for both groups —
Browne GJ[18] 2000 Australia SSW in ED General teaching hospital April 1994–April 1995, Children's Hospital Nov 1996–Nov 1997	— Prospective cohort of all children with all diagnoses admitted to SSW in ED at two hospitals	N = 1,300 general teaching hospital (GH) N = 4,948 Children's Hospital (CH) All diagnoses Total N = 6,248	Mean LOS 17.5 hours (GH) 20.4 hours (CH)	Daily bed cost $231 per bed day, savings of $2,383,138.80 for 2 years CH $171 per bed day, savings of $288,288 for 1 year for GH In 2013 USD $408. per bed day, savings of $4,213,363 for 2 year CH, $302.32 per bed day, savings of $509,690 for 1 year GH	Decreased inpatient admits by 14.7 % (8,065 in 1997 to 6,873 in 1998) (CH), by 10.3 % (5,315 in 1993 to 4,766 in 1994) (GH)	Both hospitals 56% medical, 30% surgical, 10% procedural psychiatric 4% Admissions from SSW to inpatient 4% (GH), 6% (CH) Returns to ED within 72 hours 0.4% GH, 0.9% CH	"No critical incidents or adverse events" "high parental satisfaction" at both GH and CH Age < 2 years 52.1% GH, 49.9% CH;, age 2–3 years 22.3% GH, 19.9% CH;, age 4–8 years 14.9% GH, 20.0% CH; age > 8 years 10.7% GH, 10.2% CH
Martineau O[21] 2003 France Children's Hospital Short-Stay SOU (SSOU) in PED Sept 4–Oct 31, 2001	— Prospective cohort, MD indicated decision he/she would make in absence of SSOU	N = 509 All diagnoses	Mean LOS 14 ± 8 hours			66% of SSOU admitted were discharged Questionnaire: Decision if no SSOU available was inpatient hospitalization 77%, if no inpatient beds transfer to another hospital 7%, discharge home 10%, prolonged stay in ED 4%, unknown 2%	Median age 4 years Trauma 34%, chronic disease 26% —
Alpern ER[27] 2008 United States Children's	— Prospective cohort,	N = 4,453 All diagnoses	Mean LOS 15 hours			Hospital admission rate = 20.3% (903/4,453), OU patients = 2.9% of PED patients	Age, gender, ethnicity, insurance status not associated with

Table 81.1 (cont.)

PEDIATRIC

Author/ Year Published/ Country/ Setting/ Time Frame*	Design	Patient Population	Outcomes				Limitations/ Comments	Class
			Length of Stay (LOS)	Cost	Effect of Observation Unit on Inpatient Admissions	Other Metrics		
Hospital ED POU Jan 1999 - June 2001	data form on all OU patients					Mean age = 4.7 (SD ± 4.7) years	hosp adm. Resource use: IV fluids, IV meds, CR monitoring, RT, supplemental oxygen, subspecialty consults, esophageal FB were assoc with hosp adm	
Najaf-Zadeh A[36] 2011 France Multicenter 9 Children's Hospitals Ped SSU Mar 2001– Apr 2001	I Prospective cohort data form completed on all SSU patients during their SSU stay	N = 718 for OU, N = 225 for MAPU N = 141 for HU	OU Mean LOS (hours) all dx 14, pneumonia 19, dehydration 19, asthma or bronchiolitis 11, head trauma 8		—	% OU appropriate admit* by diagnosis: head trauma 82%, seizure 82%, accidental OD 79%, upper airway infection 76%, dehydration 70%, others 70%, nonsurgical GI 69%, asthma or bronchiolitis 69%, fever/viral illness 68%, bone injury 64%, pneumonia 56% *appropriate OU admit defined as LOS > 4 and < 24 hours and discharged home	Age <1 year, need for IV fluids or meds, CT scan or MRI, CR monitoring were associated with increased risk of inappropriate admission, SSU are multifunctional, include OU, MAPU (accepts patients for 24–48 hours) and HU (HU defined as admitted patients waiting for a bed)	I

Study	Level/Design	Population	LOS	Cost analysis	Results	Deaths/Hospitalization	Most common diagnoses	Level
Gururaj VJ[20] 1972 United States SSU in Pediatric emergency area of outpatient dept, 1 year Dec 1, 1969 –Nov 30, 1970	II Retrospective cohort of all patients, all diagnoses seen in SSU	447 pts in SSU 252 (58%) discharged 185 (42%) admitted	80% LOS ≤ 16 hours ~ 50% LOS < 8 hours	Daily average inpatient charge $113 SSU charge = routine outpatient visit = income based but no >$32 (may be less) Decreased charges of $272,304 for 1 year = (248 × 10 × 113 − 248 × 32) In 2013 USD Daily average inpatient charge = $1,378 SSU charge = routine outpatient visit = income based but no > $390 (may be less) Decreased charges of $3,320,720 for 1 year = (248 × 10 × 1,378 − 248 × 390)	Prevented 248 admits (average 20.6 admits per month), saving 2,480 hospital days	No deaths, of those discharged from SSU about 1% required subsequent hospitalization	Most common diagnoses: asthma 35%, gastroenteritis 20%, ingestion 10%	II
Ellerstein NS[31] 1980 United States Children's Hospital ED POU Jan 1, 1973– Dec 31, 1978 (5 years)	II Retrospective cohort, all OU patients, all diagnoses	N = 5,858 OU Short-stay elective surgery 1,403 Total 7,261 includes elective surgery ages 0–21 years	LOS by criteria all were discharged or admitted by 24 hours (No mean LOS given)		Mean age 74 months Median age 58 months 82.9% discharged home 17.1% admitted to inpatient hospital No difference in hospital admission rate for age groups (very young infants did not have higher admission rates), highest admission rates for respiratory diseases		% of total patients: Resp 17.6%, GI 12.5%, Neuro 18.3%, Ingestion 4.9%, Social- Psych 4.8%, Trauma 9.9%, Infection 4.0%, Miscellaneous 1.1% % admitted to hospital: Resp 31.5%, GI 18.5%, Neuro 10.2%, Ingestion 3.9%, Social-Psych 21.4%,	II

Table 81.1 (cont.)

				PEDIATRIC				
Author/Year Published/Country/Setting/Time Frame*	Design	Patient Population	Outcomes Length of Stay (LOS)	Cost	Effect of Observation Unit on Inpatient Admissions	Other Metrics	Limitations/Comments	Class
							Trauma 13%, Infection 18.7%, Miscellaneous 16.9%	
O'Brien SR[19] 1980 United States Children's Hospital PED Holding Unit (HU) May 1979	II Retrospective cohort asthma	N = 106 in HU 434 seen in PED, 24% (106/434) to HU asthma	—	Average cost HU $144 Inpatient = $930 In 2013 USD HU $885 Inpatient $5,716		67% (71/106) discharged 33% (35/106) admitted Returns within 7 days 7% (5/71): 1 home, 4 hospitalized	Average cost of hospitalization for admitted patients was more than 5 times the average cost of OU care Age range (ED patients) 8 months to 19 years	II
Gouin S[22] 1997 Canada Children's hospital POU Pre July 1, 1991–June 30, 1992 Post July 1993–June 30, 1994	II Retrospective cohort asthma age 1–18 years	N = 702 randomly selected ~17% of PED asthma visits in each group, pre-OU 352, post-OU 350 age 1–18 years	OU LOS if discharged home 5.3 hours If admitted 6.5 hours	—	Hospital admission rate: pre-OU 31%, post-OU 24% (p <0.01), 1 day (<24 hours) admissions: pre-OU 17%, post-OU 10% (p ≤0.01)	PreOU vs. postOU: ED asthma visits 1,979 vs. 2,248, Repeat ED visits in < 72 hours pre-OU 3% vs. post-OU 5% (p = 0.01)	None of the returns to ED within 72 hours were admitted to OU or to hospital, all were treated in the ED Equivalent baseline measures and acuity for OU and inpatient groups	II
Marks MK[16] 1997 United States Retrospective cohort asthma	II	N = 400 SSU 298 Non-SSU 102	Mean LOS SSU 35.3 hours	Median per diem hospital charges $1,327	Hospital admissions from ED (Sept 1 to Jan 31) for asthma	Readmission to hospital within 72 hours of discharge SSU 0.6% (2/	30.8% (298/968) of SSU admits had asthma	II

Children's Hospital SSU adjacent to pediatric ward Aug 30, 1994–Jan 1995	Non-SSU 47.2 hours p = 0.0001 Note: SSU was adjacent to ped ward not an ED OU	Direct costs $538 Yearly savings for 1993 of $334,239 in hospital charges and $135,513 for direct costs if SSU managed half of hosp admissions In 2013 USD, Median per diem hospital charges $2,496.22 Direct costs $1,012 Yearly savings for 1993 of $628,739 in hospital charges and $254,914 for direct costs	pre-SSU (1993–1994) 9.5% (667/7,055), post-SSU (1994–1995) * 7.7% (555/7,212), (1995–1996) 7.0% (475/6,806) *SSU opened August 30, 1994	298), non-SSU 2.0% (2/102) At presentation to ED, initial RR was similar for both SSU and non-SSU, but initial oxygen saturation was lower in SSU patients	Mean age months (± SD) SSU 47.2 (± 61.2) Non-SSU 65.3 ± (51.8) Compared SSU with non-SSU and historical controls for asthma
Wiley JF[39] 1998 United States Children's Hospital POU Apr 2, 1996 –Apr 1, 1997	II Retrospective cohort, all pediatric OU patients. All diagnoses	N = 805 All pediatric OU patients	Average LOS 14.7 hours (range (6–23)	"Price of service is less than hospital per diem charge. Rates typically range from $50 to $70 per hour. A minimum charge of 2 to 3 units of time may also be applied."(actual charges not given)	Common diagnoses: asthma, gastroenteritis/ dehydration, seizures, head trauma/concussion, ingestions, abdominal pain, psychiatric disorder, fracture (not skull), croup 88% discharged, 12% of OU patients admitted	Psychiatric patients needing 1:1 observation were not admitted to OU. 3.5% (805/22,977) of PED census were admitted to OU, 6.3% (1,645/ 22,297) of PED census direct inpatient admissions

II

Table 81.1 (cont.)

			Outcomes					
Author/Year Published/Country/Setting/Time Frame*	**Design**	**Patient Population**	**Length of Stay (LOS)**	**Cost**	**Effect of Observation Unit on Inpatient Admissions**	**Other Metrics**	**Limitations/Comments**	**Class**
					PEDIATRIC			
Lamireau T[23] 2000 France Children's Hospital Short-Stay OU 1992 (sampled 13 weeks during year)	II Retrospective cohort, all diagnoses Sample: every 4th week in 1996 for total 13 weeks	N = 442 (excludes patients awaiting inpatient bed)			From 1987 to 1991, # hospitalized children increased 5% per year on average, after opening of SSOU, "this increase stopped and even decreased slightly" although # referrals to PED was still going up	79% (349/442) discharged home, admitted to hospital 21% (93/442).	Included patients awaiting an inpatient bed in their OU, also did not give details for non-admitted patients in OU except for % admit or discharge	II
Scribano PV[37] 2001 United States Children's Hospital POU Oct 1, 1996 –Sept 30, 1998	II Retrospective cohort All children in OU over 2 years	N = 1,798 All diagnoses	Mean OU LOS 15.6 (SD ± 6.1) hours				Admits to OU from ED 4% (1,798/ 44,459), inpatient admits 7.4% (3241/ 44,459) of all ED visits, OU mean age 6 (SD ± 5.3) years, 31% age <2 years	II
Hostetler B[24] 2002 United States Academic Hospital General OU	II Retrospective cohort All ages of patients in OU compared:	Pediatric (age < 17 years) N =363 Adult (age 17–65)	Average LOS (hours) Peds 11.2 Adult 15.1 Geriatric 15.4			No mortalities # to operating room: Peds 0.8% (3/363) Adults 0.1% (3/4,084) Geriatric 0% (0/941) # signed out against	ED OU termed Acute Diagnostic and Treatment Unit (ADTU), admitted all ages of patients (whether there was	II

Study / Setting / Dates	Design	Population	LOS	Results	Comments	LOE
Oct 1996–July 12, 2000; pediatric, adult, geriatric		N = 4,084; Geriatric (> 65 years); N = 941		medical advice; Peds 0% (0/363); Adults 0.4% (17/4,084); Geriatric 0.1% (1/941)	a lower age limit was unknown)	
LeDuc K[33] 2002 United States Children's Hospital POU Oct 1998–Mar 1999	Retrospective cohort; All OU patients over 6 months	N = 686 OU patients, all diagnoses (Note: they may include admitted patients waiting for a bed in OU)	Average LOS 8.4 (range 1 to 62) hours (In 80% of the cases, stays beyond the average were due to no inpatient beds)	Most common diagnoses: respiratory illnesses 41.4% (284/686), gastrointestinal illness 38% (261/686), trauma 6.6% (45/686), neurological diagnosis 4.5% (31/686), ingestions 2.6%, fever 2.3%, infection 1.9%, hematologic 1.0%, other 1.5% Respiratory and hematologic disorders had the longest LOS	4.8% (33/686) of all ED patients were put in OU. Average age 4.36 years, Census increased during winter months (Jan, Feb, Mar) Did not separate out admitted patients waiting a bed from OU patients	II
Bajaj L[14] 2003 United States Children's Hospital ED POU Jan 1997–July 31, 2001	Retrospective cohort s/p umcomplicated BE for intussusception	N = 78 age ≤ 18 years 27 inpatient 51 OU	Mean LOS (range) hours OU = 7.12 (0–21) inpatient = 22.7 (10–50) p <0.001	No adverse events in either group 11 reoccurrences (10%) in 8 of 78 patients, 7.8% = 4/51 in OU, 14.8%, = 4/27 inpatients All first reoccurrences occurred after discharge from inpatient or OU	OU and inpatient groups had equivalent baseline Mean age 19 months, range 14 months – 12.6 year	II
Crocetti MT[30] 2004 United States Community hospital Obs Status (OS) on inpatient	Retrospective cohort All OS patients admitted to pediatric ward	N = 800 age 0–18 years, OS patients on pediatric ward had different	Mean LOS 13 (± 6) hours, median 12 hours	75% discharged, 23% admitted or transferred Admission rates by diagnosis: pneumonia 50%, bronchiolitis 46%, infection 33%, asthma	Most common diagnoses: asthma 27%, gastroenteritis-dehydration 16%, infectious diseases (ID) 12%	II

Table 81.1 (cont.)

Author/Year Published/Country/Setting/Time Frame*	Design	Patient Population	Outcomes			Effect of Observation Unit on Inpatient Admissions	Other Metrics	Limitations/Comments	Class
			Length of Stay (LOS)	Cost					
					PEDIATRIC				
floor Apr 1, 1997–Apr 30, 1999		chart from inpatients					23%, gastroenteritis-dehydration 21%	bronchiolitis 9%; Cellulitis was most common ID. Community hospital with inpatient pediatric ward, no PICU, no ped subspecialist	
Holsti[32] 2005 United States Children's Hosp POU Aug 1999–2001	II Retrospective cohort Closed head injury (CHI) patients in OU	N = 285 CHI patients patients in OU	Median LOS 13 hours	—		—	5% (13/285) admitted from OU OU to inpatient 827 CHI patients with CHI: 34% (285/827) to OU, 33% (273/827) admitted, 33% discharged (269/827)	Age 2 weeks to 17 years median age 5.2 year 60.9% male, basilar skull fractures (OR 11.91), lacerations (scalp or facial) (OR 7.52), need for IV fluids (OR 4.26) were associated with need for hospital admission	II
Mierscier MJ[35] 2005 United States Children's Hospital POU	II Retrospective cohort asthma	N = 161 Age ≥2 years	Median LOS 16.5 hours	—		—	75% (121/161) of OU patients discharged home, 25% (40/161) admitted to hospital 9.9% (301/3,029) of PED asthma patients admitted to OU, 140 failed inclusion criteria	Factors associated with hospital admission: female gender (P = 0.03), fever (T > 38.5°) (p < 0.01), need for oxygen treatment at	II

Study / Setting	Design	N / Population	LOS	Charges	Results	Additional results	Quality / Notes
Aug 1999 – July 2001					mainly due to age < 2 years	end of ED treatment (p < 0.01) Mean age 5.7 years Median age 4.0 years	=
Zebrack[38] 2005 United States Children's Hospital Aug 1999– July 2001 ED POU	= Retrospective cohort All diagnoses, all patients	N = 4,189 OU N = 2,288 elective procedures "Hybrid" unit includes elective procedures and OU patients	Median LOS 15.5 hours	——	Excluding elective patients: 85% discharged Common OU diagnoses: Enteritis/dehydration 17.2% (722/4,189), orthopedic injuries 8.6% (362/4,189), asthma 7.8% (327/4,189), closed head injury 6.9% (289/4,189), urgent transfusion 5.3% (221/4,189), bronchiolitis 5.1% (212/4,189), croup 4.9% (207/4,189) abdominal pain 4.8% (199/4189) cellulitis 4.2% (177/4,189) s seizures 2.3% (98/4,189) Median OU age 2.5 years	Rate of inpatient admission from OU: hematochezia 60%, viral pneumonia 46%, bronchiolitis 43%, VP shunt issues 40%, bacterial pneumonia 30%, abd pain 27%, fever 26%, cyclic vomiting 25%, r/o sepsis 22%, asthma 22% "Hybrid unit" included scheduled elective procedures and "acutely ill and injured" OU patients, >85% discharge rate for aseptic meningitis, DKA, neonatal hyperbilirubinemia	=
Greenberg[15] RA 2006 United States Children's Hospital POU	= Retrospective cohort ED pts with croup(non-ICU patients)	Year 1 preOU = historical control N = 66 inpatients	Median LOS 27.2 hour, post-OU (includes OU + inpatients)	Median charges pre-OU $1,685, post- OU $1,327 p = 0.03 In 2013 USD pre-OU $ $2,679, post-OU $	Inpatient admits of all ED croup patients PreOU 9.5% (66 adm/694 ED patients)	7.9% (5/76) of OU croup patients were admitted to inpatient service PreOU = 66/694 = 9.5% ward adm, PostOU = OU adm + ward adm = (76 OU + 28 ward)/	= Median age 1.5 years for pre- and PostOU Age range PreOU 0.16 to 11.9 years. PostOU 0.2 to 11.0

Table 81.1 (cont.)

PEDIATRIC

Author/Year Published/Country/Setting/Time Frame*	Design	Patient Population	Outcomes Length of Stay (LOS)	Cost	Effect of Observation Unit on Inpatient Admissions	Other Metrics	Limitations/Comments	Class
over 2 years Pre-OU = Aug 1998 – Jul 1999 PostOU Aug 1999– Aug 2000		Year 2 post-OU N = 76 in OU + 33 inpatients	21.3 hour p = 0.03	$2,110 Note: Actual savings may be even greater if be greater if just considered OU patients and not both OU and inpatients for post-OU year	PostOU 4.2% (33 adm /789 ED patients) = (28 directly from ED + 5 from OU/789 p <0.0001, Post-OU 76/789 = 9.6% of ED croup patients are admitted to OU	789 ED croup patients = 104/789 = 13.2% total adm	years Treatment (pre- and post- OU) was the same (all got dexamethasone) Post-OU charges do not seem to differentiate charges between OU adm and inpatients	
Mallory MD[34] 2006 United States Children's Hospital POU Aug 2000 – July 2001	II Retrospective cohort Dehydrated gastroenteritis patients with vomiting ± diarrhea	N = 430 OU admissions, 417 patients met inclusion criteria patients Age <11 years No comorbidity	—	—		81% discharged from OU, 19% admitted from OU, 5 patients readmitted to OU with same diagnosis within 5 days of initial discharge home, one was admitted to hospital from OU, 7 patients readmitted as inpatients to hospital within 72 hours of discharge from OU	Mean age 1.8 years Median age 1.2 years Range 2 weeks–10 years No relationship between historical, PE, lab variables, and need for inpatient admission	II
Calello DP[29] 2009 United States Children's Hospital, ED	II Retrospective cohort Children with poison exposure	N = 86 patients with poison exposures	Mean LOS (hours) Overall (15.0 (± 5.9),		98 exposures in 86 pts; Only 2 pts (4% = 2/53 with normal mental status and VS) developed abnormal VS in OU and needed adm		Most common exposures: psychoactive drugs (25.3%), cardiovascular	II

POU Jan 1999–June 2001 30 months		98 toxicants implicated	If discharged 14.4 (± 6.6)		(2.2% = 2/91) unexpected admission rate (for hydrocarbon/charcoal aspiration), 3 pts planned adm for endoscopy or psychiatry, total admitted from OU to inpatient 5.5% (5/91)	drugs (19.2%). 6.1% unknown exposure For all ED visits (all diagnoses), 2.9% (4,453/153,351) were admitted to OU over 30 months of study	
Adekunle-Ojo[13] 2010 United States Children's Hospital ED POU over 2 years 2004 and 2006	II Retrospective cohort Infants hyper-bilirubinemia historical control = year 2004, OU year = 2006	N = 167 neonatal hyper bili rubin emia pre-OU N = 105, OU N = 62	LOS pre-OU 41.8 hours, post-OU 17.8 hours p <0.0001		Median time to phototherapy pre-OU 6.7 hours, OU 1.6 hours p <0.0001	Even adjusting for baseline bilirubin, still a significant difference in LOS between pre-OU and OU Baseline bilirubin is the only significant cofounder p= 0.046 Two groups had equivalent baseline Median age 5 days	II
Adekunle-Ojo[28] 2011 United States Children's Hospital ED POU Apr 1, 2003–Aug 31, 2009	II Retrospective cohort Fed early <2 hours vs. fed late ≥2 hours	N =149 s/p radiologic reduction of intussception Fed early N = 61, fed late N = 88	LOS fed early 15.6 hours fed late 16.1 hours p = 0.58		Fed early vs. late: symptoms 13% vs. 16%, repeat imaging 20% vs. 22%, hospital admission 3% vs. 8%, reoccurrence 8% vs. 15% No complications No difference in symptoms: fever, emesis, abdominal pain, Repeat imaging, hospitalization, reoccurrence	Two groups equivalent baseline Median age 16 months Range 3–95 months No complications (no perforation, shock, sepsis)	II
Geelhoed GC[25] 1996	II Retrospective compared	Impossible to give exact N for croup	Average LOS: Post-OW and mandatory		Post-OW and mandatory steroids vs. pre-OW: discharged home 97%	Mandatory use of steroids in 1993 makes it	III

Table 81.1 (cont.)

				PEDIATRIC				
Author/Year Published/Country/Setting/Time Frame*	Design	Patient Population	Outcomes Length of Stay (LOS)	Cost	Effect of Observation Unit on Inpatient Admissions	Other Metrics	Limitations/Comments	Class
Australia Children's Hospital Short-stay Obs Ward (OW) in ED Pre used 1980–1989, Post 1990–1995 or 1994–1995	outcomes for croup by years pre- and post-mandatory steroid use	pts Years compared differed: # intubated and ICU days: pre-OW 1980–1989, post-OW 1990–1995, For LOS and ICU transfers: pre-OW 1980–1989, post-OW 1994–1995	steroids 1.1 days vs. pre-OW 2.03 days from 1992–1995, mandatory steroids in OW in 1993			vs. 80%, average # transfers to ICU 2.6% vs.11.6%, average # intubated 4 vs. 8, average total ICU days 129 vs. 24	difficult to separate out effects of steroids with effects of OW and difficult to give exact N for years of study. Strong case for steroid use in croup, used OW extensively for croup and had good outcomes in 1994–1995, shows benefits of "standardized" protocol type care	
Beattie TF[41] 1993 United Kingdom Accident & Emergency departments (A&E)	III Survey in 1992 Sent to 100 randomly selected A&E consultants	90% (90/100) return rate	—	—	—	12.2% (11/90) admitted children: 9 exclusively under A&E care, 2 joint care with pediatricians 1 institution admitted 450 children per year, 4 admitted between 50 and 450 children per year, 2 admitted < 50 children per year, 4 not known	50% of A&E have short-stay wards, of these only 25% accept children For children, mainly trauma-related problems, bulk of diagnoses were fractures, soft tissue injuries, head injuries	III

Study	Design	Methods/Scale	LOS	Cost	Results	Conclusions	Level
Rentz AC[26] 2004 Children's Hosp POU pts were treated from Aug 1999 to Jan 2002 survey mailed Jan 2002	III Survey N = 198 Pediatricians, family practitioners, ped subspecialists who had patients in OU	Likert scale 1 (lowest) to 4 (highest) 198/248 = 80% return rate	—	—	Median (mean ± SD) all MDs overall satisfaction 4 (3.63 ± 0.79) parental satisfaction 4 (3.49 ± 0.79) notification 4 (3.33 ± 0.88) quality of care 4 (3.70 ± 0.78)	In > 50% of respondents: diagnoses for which that OU was perceived to be most helpful in managing were dehydration, gastroenteritis, reactive airways disease, bronchiolitis	III
Klein B[43] 1991	III Review	—	—	—	OU "is an extension of the ED, preferably adjacent to it, where children can be observed and treated for a limited period of time. Its principal function is to enable the emergency physician to better decide whether admission or discharge is warranted."	The OU "should not be used as a holding area for patients requiring hospital admission when beds are not available."	III
Mace SE[40] 2001 United States General Hospital (combined adult and pediatric OU) 1995–1999	III Review included experience in general ED OU where adult and pediatric patients are cohorted	—	LOS in OU < inpatient (two peds, two adult studies), in two other peds studies there was a short LOS for OU but didn't compare with inpatient	Costs for OU << inpatient in all studies that looked at cost (two peds, four adult studies)	Better QOL and decreased problems with care (two adult studies) for OU compared with inpatient No difference in readmission rate (one adult, one ped study)	In general OU with adults and children/ infants, the most common pediatric diagnoses for 1994–1999 were asthma, dehydration, gastroenteritis, pneumonia, abdominal pain, seizures, fever, bronchiolitis, croup Experience with	III

Table 81.1 (cont.)

Author/Year Published/Country/Setting/Time Frame*	Design	Patient Population	Outcomes Length of Stay (LOS)	Cost	Effect of Observation Unit on Inpatient Admissions	Other Metrics	Limitations/Comments	Class
PEDIATRIC								
							"hybrid" or "general" OU where both adult and pediatric patients can be cohorted	
Connor GP[44] 2012	III Review of pediatric observation medicine				"A benefit of OUs may reduce the rates of admissions to inpatient units"	"OUs may have an especially important effect on pediatric inpatient admissions, in part because a significant number of inpatient admissions among children are of relatively short duration."	AAP Policy Statement	III
Macy ML[42] 2012 United States 42 Children's Hospitals	III Survey 2 web-based surveys of PHIS database	PHIS = Pediatric Hospital Information System of 42 Children's Hospitals				39% (12/31) had designated OUs, Observation status varies in duration and criteria, observation time <48 hours in 77%, Observation is delivered in a variety of settings	Respondents report no difference in clinical care delivered to virtual observation status patients when compared to other patients. Response rate: survey 1 was 88%, survey 2 was 45.2%	III

GERIATRIC						
Author/ Year Published Country/ Setting/ Time Frame*	Design	Patient Population	Outcomes		Limitations/ Comments	Class
			LOS	Other Metrics		
Ross MA[59] 2003 United States ED OU over 5 years 1996–2000	II Compared adults in ED OU >65 years (Ger) vs. <65 years (NG)	N = 22,530 in ED OU 37.2% Ger N = 8,381 NG N = 14,149 All diagnoses	Ger 15.8 hour (95% CI 15.7 to 16) vs. NG 14.5 hour (95% CI 14.3 to 14.5)	Admit rate <30% for both: Ger 26.1% vs. NG 18.5% 30-day return visit: Ger 9.4% vs. NG 7.6% Comparable mean LOS <18 hour for Ger and NG adults	#1 diagnosis was CP for both Ger or NG Other top diagnoses differed Very large N Elderly use OU for different reasons, different outcomes, overall good results.	II
Madsen[60] 2008 United States ED OU Apr 2006–June 2007	II Compared adults with chest pain in ED OU > 65 years (Ger) vs. < 65 years (NG)	N = 528 394 were < 65 years 134 were >65 years Chest pain patients only	____	inpatient admission (no CAD + CAD) Ger 17%, NG 10.7% p=0.048 CAD Ger 31.3%, NG 20.8% p = 0.013 Subgroup of no CAD: Ger N = 92, NG N = 312, total = 404 Inpatient admission for no CAD: Ger 12%, NG 7.7%, p = 0.2	"Geriatric patients without a history of CAD are admitted at a rate consistent with generally accepted obs failure rate of 10%" CAD = previous MI, stent, or CABG	II
Harrop SN[57] 1985 Wales Short-stay unit*** of A&E Sept–Nov 1983	II Evaluated 100 geriatric patients	N = 100 Age > 70 years All diagnoses	Not specifically listed, < half in hospital for > 24 hours	72% discharged home	100 patients admitted to short-stay unit when no geriatric inpatient beds available so some patients met inpatient criteria, these patients were not separated out from other patients	III
Khan SA[58]1997 United Kingdom over 9 months Apr–Dec 1993 Short-stay unit of A&E	II Evaluated geriatric patients ≥ 65 years in SSU of A&E	N = 502 Age ≥65 years	Usually discharged within 24 hours (no exact # given)	71% (355/502) discharged home, 29% (147/502) admitted Admission rates by diagnosis: falls/injury 35%, infections 15%, collapse 6%, constipation 5%, stroke/TIA 3%, social 2%, other 34%	Most common diagnoses: fall/ injury 45%, infections 11%, constipation 5%, collapse 4%, stroke/TIA 3%, social 2%, others 30% No exact data on LOS	III

Since there were numerous international studies and the various studies and data collection were over many different years and sometimes in different settings (e.g., ED OU vs. short-stay unit), the country, time frame and setting are included in the evidentiary table.

* Time frame = time period in which patient data was collected.

** The early short-stay units may have had some different characteristics from later observation units.

*** In the Harrop study et al, the short-stay ward was in the ED but did not have a rigid time limit such as 24 hours. Indeed, over half the patients had a LOS >24 hours. This is quite different from most ED OUs, which strictly adhere to a <24-hour time frame.

Abbreviations

Abd: Abdominal
Adm: Admission
AAP: American Academy of Pediatrics
A&E: Accident and Emergency Department
Assoc: Associated
BE: Barium enema
CABG: Coronary artery bypass graft
CAD: Coronary artery disease
CH: Children's hospital
CI: Confidence interval
CP: Chest pain
CR: Cardiorespiratory
Dept: Department
DKA: Diabetic ketoacidosis
Dx: Diagnosis
ED: Emergency department
Feb: February
FB: Foreign body
Ger: Geriatric
GI: Gastrointestinal
GH: General hospital
Hosp: Hospital
HR: Holding room
HU: Holding unit
ICU: intensive care unit
IV: Intravenous
Lab: Laboratory
MAPU: Medical assessment and planning unit, usually accepts patients for 24- 48 hours while OU accepts patients for <24 hours
Mar: March
MI: Myocardial infarction
Misc: Miscellaneous
Neuro: Neurologic
NG: Nongeriatric
NIS : Nationwide Inpatient Sample
OU: Observation unit
OW: Observation ward
PE: Physical examination
Ped: Pediatric
PED: Pediatric emergency department
POU : Pediatric observation unit
Psych: Psychiatric
Pts: Patients
QOL: Quality of life
RCT: Randomized controlled trial
Resp: Respiratory
RT : Respiratory therapist involved in their care
SD: Standard deviation
s/p: Status post
SSOU: Short-stay observation unit
SSU: Short-stay unit
SSW: Short-stay ward
TIA: Transient ischemic attack
USD: United States dollars
VS: Vital signs

Appendix A: Literature Classification Schema

Design/ Class	Therapy	Diagnosis	Prognosis
1	Randomized, controlled trial or meta-analysis of randomized trials	Prospective cohort using a criterion standard or meta-analysis of prospective studies	Population prospective cohort or meta-analysis of prospective studies
2	Nonrandomized trial	Retrospective observational	Retrospective cohort Case control
3	Case series Case report Other (e.g., consensus, review)	Case series Case report Other (e.g., consensus, review)	Case series Case report Other (e.g., consensus, review)

Appendix B: Approach to Downgrading Strength of Evidence

	Design/Class		
Downgrading	1	2	3
None	I	II	III
1 Level	II	III	X
2 Levels	III	X	X
Fatal flaw	X	X	X

Appendix C: Criteria Used for Clinical Findings and Strength of Recommendations

Level A recommendation

Generally accepted principles for patient management that indicate a high degree of clinical certainty (i.e., based on strength of evidence Class I or overwhelming evidence from strength of evidence Class II studies that directly address all of the issues).

Level B recommendation

Generally accepted principles for patient management that indicate a moderate degree of clinical certainty (i.e. based on strength of evidence Class II studies that directly address all of the issues, decision analysis that directly addresses the issues, or strong consensus of strength of evidence Class III studies).

Level C recommendation

Patient management strategies that are based on Class III studies.

References

1. Rosenbaum L. The whole ball game – overcoming the blind spots in health care reform. *N Eng J Med* 2013; 368 (10):959–962.

2. Creditor MC. Hazards of hospitalization of the elderly. *Ann Intern Med* 1993; 118: 219–223.

3. Rothschild JM, Bates DW, Leape LL. Preventable medical injuries in older patients. *Arch Intern Med* 2000; 160:2717–2728.

4. Gill TM, Allore HG, Gahbauer EA, et al. Change in disability after hospitalization or restricted activity in older persons. *JAMA* 2010; 304:1919–1928.

5. Ross MA, Aurora T, Graff L, et al. State of the art: emergency department observation units. *Crit Pathways in Cardiol* 2012; 11:128–138.

6. www.kaiseredu.org/issue-modules/us-health-care-costs/background-brief.aspx (Accessed March 2016)

7. www.hcup-us.ahrq.gov/reports/statbriefs/sb1.jsp (Accessed March 2016)

8. Woodhams V, de Lusignan S Mughal S, et al. Triumph of hope over experience: learning from interventions to reduce avoidable hospital admissions identified through an academic health and social care network. *BMC Health Services Research* 2012; 12:253–262.

9. Institute of Medicine. IOM report: the future of emergency care in the United States health system. *Acad Emerg Med* 2006; 13:1081–1085.

10. American College of Emergency Physicians Policy Statement.Emergency department observation services. *Ann Emerg Med* 2008; 51: 686.

11. Baugh CW, Venkatesh AK, Hilton JA, et al. Making greater use Of dedicated hospital observation units for many short-stay patients could save $3.1 billion a year. *Health Aff* 2012;31(10):2314–2323.

12. Listernick R, Zieseri E, Davis AT. Outpatient oral rehydration in the United States. *AJDC* 1986; 140:211–215.

13. Adekunle-Ojo AO, Smitherman HF, Parker R, et al. Managing well-appearing neonates with hyperbilirubinemia in the emergency observation unit. *Pediatr Emerg Care* 2010; 26: 343–348.

14. Bajaj L, Roback MG. Postreduction management of intussception in a children's hospital emergency department 2003: *Pediatrics* 112(6): 1302–1307.

15. Greenberg RA, Dudley NC, Rittichier KK. A reduction in hospitalization, length of stay, and hospital charges for croup with the institution of a pediatric observation unit. *Amer J Emerg Med* 2006; 24:818–821.

16. Marks MK, Lovejoy FH, Rutherford PA, et al. Impact of a short stay unit on asthma patients admitted to a tertiary pediatric hospital. *Quality Management in Health Care* 1997; 6(1): 14–22.

17. Willert C, David AT, Herman JJ, et al. Short-term holding room treatment of asthmatics. *J Pediatr* 1985; 106: 707–711.

18. Browne GJ. A short-stay or 23 hour ward in a general and academic childrens hospital: are they effective? *Pediatric Emergency Care* 2000; 16 (4):223–229.

19. O'Brien SR, Hein EW, Sly RM. Treatment of acute asthmatic attacks in a holding unit of a pediatric emergency room *Annals of Allergy* 1980; 45 (3):159–1162.

20. Gururaj VJ, Allen JE, Russo RM. Short stay in an outpatient department: an alternative to hospitalization. *Amer J Dis Childn*1972; 123:128–133.

21. Martineau O, Martinot A, Chatier A, et al. Effectiveness of a short-stay observation unit in a pediatric emergency department. *Archives de Pediatrie* 2003; 10:410–416.

22. Gouin S, Macarthur C, Parkki PC, et al. Effect of pediatric observation unit on the rate of hospitalization for asthma. *Ann Emerg Med* 1997; 29(2): 218–222.

23. Lamireau T, Lanas B, Dommange S, et al. A short-stay observation unit improves care in the paediatric emergency care setting. *European J Emerg Med* 2000; 7: 261–265.

24. Hostetler B, Leikin JB, Timmons JA, et al. Patterns of use of an emergency department-based observation unit. *Amer J Therapeutics* 2002; 9:499–502.

25. Geelhoed GC. Sixteen years of croup in a Western Australian teaching hospital: effects of routine steroid treatment. *Ann Emerg Med* 1996; 28 (6):621–626.

26. Rentz AC, Kadish HA, Nelson DS. Physician satisfaction with a pediatric observation unit administered by pediatric emergency medicine physicians. *Pediatr Emerg Care* 2004; 20(7):430–432.

27. Alpern ER, Callello DP, Windreich R, et a Utilization and unexpected hospitalization rates of a pediatric emergency department 23 hour observation unit. *Pediatr Emerg Care* 2008; 24(9): 589–594.

28. Adekunle-Ojo, Craig AM, Long Ma, et al. Intussusception: postreduction fasting is not necessary to prevent complications and recurrences in the emergency department observation unit. *Pediatr Emerg Care* 2011; 27 (10):897–899.

29. Calello DP, Alpern ER, McDaniel Yakscoe M, et al. Observation unit experience for pediatric poison exposures. *J Medical Toxicology* 2009: 5 (1):15–19.

30. Crocetti MT, Barone MA, Dritt Amin D, et al. Pediatric observation status beds on an inpatient unit : an integrated care model. *Pediatr Emerg care* 2004; 20(1):17–21.

31. Ellerstein NS, Sullivan TD. Observation unit in a children's hospital: adjunct to delivery and teaching of ambulatory pediatric care. *New York State Journal of Medicine* 1980; 80 (11):1684–1686.

32. Holsti M, Kadish HA, Sill BL, et al. Pediatric closed head injuries treated in an observation unit. *Pediatr Emerg Care* 2005; 21(10):639–644.

33. LeDuc K, Haley-Andrews S, Rannie M. An observation unit in a pediatric emergency department: one children's hospital's experience. *JEN* 2002:407–413.

34. Mallory MD, Kadish H, Zebrack M, et al. Use of a pediatric observation unit for treatment of children with dehydration caused by gastroenteritis. *Pediatr Emerg Care* 2006; 22(1):1–6.

35. Miescier MJ, Nelson DS, Firth SD, et al. Children with asthma admitted to a pedictric observation unit. *Pediatr Emerg Care* 2005: 112: 1302–1307.

36. Najaf-Zadeh A, Hue V, Bonnel-Motuaire C, et al. Effectiveness of multifunction paediatric short-saty units: a French multicentre study. *Acta Paediatrica* 2001; 100: e227–e225.2011.

37. Scribano PV, Wiley JF 2nd, Platt K. Use of an observation unit by a pediatric emergency department for common pediatric illnesses. *Pediatric Emergency Care* 2001; 17: 321–323.

38. Zebrack M, Kadfish H, Nelson D. The pediatric hybrid observation unit: analysis of 6477 consecutive patient encounters. *Pediatrics* 2005; 115(5): e535–e542.

39. Wiley JF. Pediatric clinical decision units: observation, past, present and future. *Clin Ped Emerg Med* 2001: 2:247–252.

40. Mace SE. Pediatric Observation Medicine.*Emerg Med Clin North Amer* 2001; 19(1): 239–254.

41. Beattie TF, Ferguson J, Moir PA. Short-stay facilities in accident and emergency departments for children. *Archive of Emergency Medicine* 1993; 10: 177–180.

42. Macy ML, Hall M, Dshah SS, et al. Differences in designations of observation care in US freestanding children's hospitals: are they virtual or are they real? *Journal of Hospital Medicine* 2012; 7:287–293.

43. Klein BL, Patterson M. Observation unit management of pediatric emergencies. *Emerg Med Clin North Amer* 1991; 9(3): 669–676.

44. Connor GP, Melzer SM. Pediatric Observation Units. *Pediatrics* 2012; 130(1): 172–179.

45. Emergency Department Visits. Centers for Disease Control and Prevention. www.cdc.gov/nchs/fastats/ervisits.htm (Accessed March 2016)

46. http://hcupnet.ahrq.gov/HCUPnet.jsp?Id=64ADDB30DDA5FA72&Form=DispTab&JS=Y&Action=%3E%3ENext%3E%3E&__InDispTab=Yes&_Rhttp://hcupnet.ahrq.gov/HCUPnet.jsp?Id=64ADDB30DDA5FA72&Form=DispTab&JS=Y&Action=%3E%3ENext%3E%3E&__InDispTab=Yes&_Results=Print&SortOpt= (Accessed March 2016)

47. Tang N, Stein J, Hsia RY, et al. Trends and characteristics of US emergency department visits, 1997–2007. *JAMA* 2010; 304(6):664–670.

48. www.cdc.gov/nchs/data/hus/2011/093.pdf (Table 93) (Accessed March 2016)

49. Committee on the Future of Emergency Care in the United States Health System. *Emergency Care for Children: Growing Pains* (ISBN: 0-309-65964-7). ch.1 Introduction, pp.18. National Academies Press. www.nap.edu/catalog/11655.html (Accessed March 2016)

50. Nawar EW, Niska RW, Xu J; Division of Health Care Statistics. Advance Data from Vital and Health Statistics. National Hospital Ambulatory Medical Care Survey: 2005 Emergency Department Summary, number 386. June 29, 2007.

51. Mace SE, Graff L, Mikhail M, et al. A national survey of observation units in the United States. *Am J Emerg Med* 2003; 21:529–533.

52. Macy ML, Stanley RM, Lozon MM. Trends in high turnover stays among children hospitalized in the United States, 1993–2003. *Pediatrics* 2009; 123(3):996–1002.

53. McConnochie KM, Russo MJ, McBride JT, et al. How commonly are children hospitalized for asthma eligible for care in alternative settings? *Arch Pediatr Adolesc Med* 1999; 153:49–55.

54. McConnochie KM, Connors GP, Lu E. How commonly are children hospitalized for dehydration eligible for care in alternative settings? *Arch Pediatr Adolesc med* 1999; 153:1233–1241.

55. DeAngelis CD. Editor's Note: How commonly are children hospitalized for asthma eligible for care in alternate settings?

Arch Pediatr Adolesc Med 1999; 153: 49.

56. DeCoster C, Peterson S, Karian P. Manitoba Centre for Health Policy and Evaluation: Report summary alternatives to acute care. Winnipeg, Manitoba, Canada. University of Manitoba – Manitoba Centre for Health Policy and Evaluation, 1996.

57. Harrop SN, Morgan WJ. Emergency care of the elderly in the short-stay ward of the accident and emergency department. *Arch Emerg Med* 1985; 2:141–147.

58. Khan SA. Benefits of an accident and emergency short stay ward in the staged hospital care of elderly patients. *J Accid Emerg Med* 1997; 14: 151–152.

59. Ross MA, Compton S, Richardson D, et al. The use and effectiveness of an emergency department observation unit for elderly patients. *Ann Emerg Med (compartative study)* 2003 May: 41(5):668–677.

60. Madsen TE, Bledsoe J, Bossart P. Appropriately screened geriatric chest pain patients in an observation unit are not admitted at a higher rate than nongeriatric patients. *Crit Pathways in Cardiol* 2008: 7:245–247.

61. Zdradzinski MJ, Phelan MP, Mace SE. Impact of frailty and sociodemographic factors on hospital admission from an emergency department observation unit. *Amer J Medical Quality* (accepted for publication 2016).

62. Andre C, Velasquez M. Age based health care rationing. Santa Clara University. www.scu.edu/ethics/publications/iie/v3n3/age.html (Last accessed March 21, 2013)

63. Cipriano PF. Senior care: are we prepared for the impending health care crisis? *Amer Nurse Today* 3(8):8.

64. Francis T, Fuhrmans V. Geriatric care is facing crisis. *The Wall Street Journal* April 15, 2008.

65. Fischer JE, Zeiss AM, Carstensen LL. Psychopathology of the aging. In: Sutker PB, Adams HE (eds.). *Comprehensive Handbook of Psychopathology*, 2002, ch. 32, pp 921–951.

66. Wilber ST, Gerson LW, Terrell KM, et al. Geriatric emergency medicine and the 2006 Institute of Medicine Reports from the Committee on the Future of Emergency Care in the U.S. Health System. *Acad Emerg Med* 2006; 13:1345–1351.

67. Smith GP. The elderly and health care rationing. *Pierce Law Review* 2009; 171–182.

68. Fuchs VR. Health care for the elderly. How Much? Who will pay for it? *Health Affairs. SMR* 1(1):12–16.

69. Gruber J. The cost implications of health care reform. *N Engl J Med* 2010: 2050–2051.

70. Creditor MC. Hazards of hospitalization of the elderly. *Ann Intern Med* 1993; 118: 219–223.

71. Rothschild JM, Bates, DW, Leape LL. Preventable injuries in older patients. *Arch Intern Med* 2000; 160:2717–2728.

72. Gill TM, Allore HG, Gahbauer EA, et al. Change in disability after hospitalization or restricted activity in older persons. *JAMA* 2010; 304:1919–1926.

73. Boltz M, Resnick B, Capezuti E, et al. Functional decline in hospitalized older adults: can nursing make a difference? *Geriatric Nursing* 2012: 33(4): 272–279.

74. Schur JD, Venkatesh AK. The growing role of emergency departments in hospital admissions. *N Engl J Med* 2012;367(5):391–393.

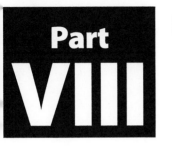

Part VIII

Clinical Protocols

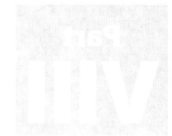

Author's and Editor's Comments: Protocols and Order Sets

This next section deals with protocols and order sets. These are not meant to be mandatory policies, but guidelines that are suggested best practices to follow in a particular set of circumstances to reach optimal outcomes. Although they are written as separate chapters, they can and should be integrated. Historically, the protocols come first. The clinical protocols set the inclusion and exclusion criteria, the interventions (what can be done in the observation unit), and the decision criteria for disposition, specifying the conditions when patients need to be admitted as an inpatient to the hospital or can be discharged from the observation unit (OU). The administrative protocols are essential to establishing the organizational framework and efficient functioning of the OU. Next are the order sets.

Clinical Protocols

Although the protocols are specific for a given condition or diagnosis, such as chest pain or asthma, there are a set of general or generic principles and interventions for any illness or injury that apply to observation patients. By definition, patients appropriate for observation should have stable vital signs, be "non-critical", stable and "low-maintenance." They should *not* need "intensive" nursing care or "intensive" physician care. They should have a disposition suitable to admit as an inpatient to the hospital or discharge home in a "reasonably short" time frame, specifically, less than 24 hours.

Based on these principles, a list of acceptable diagnoses for observation patients would include (but not be limited to) cardiac: chest pain, syncope, atrial fibrillation; respiratory: asthma, pneumonia, COPD exacerbation, acute bronchitis, bronchiolitis; gastrointestinal (GI): gastroenteritis, vomiting, diarrhea, dehydration, stable GI bleeding; genitourinary: kidney stones, pyelonephritis; infections: cellulitis, lymphangitis; hematologic: anemia, sickle cell crisis, hemophilia; toxicology: ingestions, accidental overdoses; and stable trauma patients.

Conversely, patients excluded from observation would include critically ill patients, intensive care unit patients, those with unstable vital signs, anyone needing "intensive "nursing or "intensive" physician care, and anyone whose anticipated length of stay would be greater than 24 hours. Thus, patients who are *not* candidates for observation would be patients with shock or respiratory failure, who are comatose, who have neutropenic fever or bacterial meningitis, or any intensive care unit patient, to name a few examples. (See specific Observation Exclusions.) If the generic exclusion protocol is applied to any given illness or injury, a specific clinical protocol can be derived for any condition or disease. Clinical protocols can include scoring systems, such as TIMI scores for chest pain, PORT or CURB or PSI scores for pneumonia, or the ABCD2 scores for transient ischemic attacks (see TIA protocol). We have tried them (such as TIMI scores) in the past. Currently clinical criteria that risk stratify seem to be preferred, although risk stratification by specific scoring systems as part of the OU protocol may become more widespread as scoring systems become validated and easy to use.

Since a given disease is a spectrum, some patients with the same diagnosis will be critical and some stable although both groups may need additional diagnostic or therapeutic measures. For example, chest pain can be an acute myocardial infarction (MI), unstable angina or cardiogenic shock, all of which are *not* appropriate for observation. Or it may be a stable patient with a negative initial set of enzymes and a negative or unchanged ECG who needs telemetry and a stress test. Thus, someone on a heparin drip (indicating treatment for an MI) or on a nitroglycerin drip (signifying unstable angina) may be exclusions from the OU and the statement could be made that "no one on an IV drip is a candidate for observation." Similarly, patients with an acute exacerbation of asthma can be placed in an OU, while asthmatic patients with respiratory failure, significant hypoxia (e.g., saturation < 90%), or in status asthmaticus should *not* be put in observation status. However, there may be a trend toward higher acuity patients in the OU which reflects the trend in the emergency department (ED) with more severely ill and injured patients over the past decades, and there is the development of "complex" or "extended" observation. (See Chapters 16 and 17.)

Although we use the term "observation" patient or "observation" unit, by no means is the observation patient a patient who is "just being observed." For every patient placed in observation, he or she is undergoing a rapid aggressive diagnostic testing and/or treatment regimen. Thus, other names, such as "Clinical Decision Unit" (CDU), a term coined at and first used at our institution that denotes the importance of quickly evaluating patients in order to make a decision or disposition in an expeditious time frame, or "Rapid Diagnostic and Treatment Unit" (RDTU) or "Accelerated Diagnostic and Treatment Center" (ADTC) may be better terms. The goal is to be actively doing something for the patient in the OU. The core principle of the CDU or RDTU or "Obs" Unit is to provide an efficient, cost-effective and expedited approach to patient evaluation and management.

OUs can provide benefits in any locale or type of hospital, and is not unique to the United States but is an international occurrence. As the former director of ED(s) in several community hospitals for nearly a decade, I understand the value of observation medicine, not just in large academic urban institutions, but also in community hospitals in suburban, rural, and urban locations.

Virtually, every OU has a protocol for chest pain. If you are starting an OU, I recommend starting with what is known, established and relatively easy to do, which is chest pain. Once your unit is established and functioning well, then you can add other diagnoses and protocols, but it usually takes months to get established and for the OU to be accepted and then the census will grow exponentially. As a guide, about 10% of all adult ED patients could be managed in an OU.

The OU can be tailored to accommodate your patients and the physicians and/or services that your hospital offers. For example, we have set up with our gastroenterologists a protocol whereby stable patients with GI bleeding are made NPO (nil per os) after midnight, are given IV fluids, have serial hemoglobin/hematocrits done, and undergo an esophagastroduodeno-scopy (EGD) and/or colonoscopy (with a bowel prep completed prior to procedure) the next a. m. and return after the procedure for appropriate disposition based on their test results. Other protocols such as on snakebites or on Dengue are included to also emphasize the fact that the CDU can be adapted to fit the needs of your local patient population and the services provided by your physicians and hospital.

Protocols and order sets are not static but can and should be added, deleted or modified and reviewed on a regular basis. They should be revised to accommodate the changes in clinical practice and health care.

The protocols and order sets originally were designed for the "uncomplicated" OU patient, focusing on one or a limited number of complaints or problems. However, for the "complex" or "extended" OU patient, combining several protocols or order sets could be done to accommodate these patients as well. These are a different patient population from the "uncomplicated" OU patient and it may be that there are two OUs in the hospital of the future: one for the "simple or uncomplicated" OU patient with a LOS < 24 hours and one for the complicated OU patient in an "extended or complex" OU with a LOS < 48 hours. (See Chapters 16 and 17 on Extended and Complex Observation.)

Administrative Policies

There are two administrative policies that are essential for observation medicine: one is the overview or mission statement, which establishes the *raison d'etre* for observation, and the second is the chain of command, which sets up the administrative structure for observation. I have included other policies that could be valuable in setting up and maintaining a successful OU.

Order Sets

The order sets for a given condition or illness evolved from the specific protocols and enumerate the common diagnostic procedures/tests and the usual monitoring and therapy including drug regimens. The order sets have been designed in modular fashion based on grouped orders: activity, diet, nursing interventions including vital signs and when to notify the physician, respiratory interventions, laboratory, radiology studies, cardiac studies, intravenous fluids, medications, and patient/family education.

The order sets are intended to include a large number of possibilities that can be narrowed down to fit the given diagnosis. For example, cardiac studies, stress tests, and serial ECGs or enzymes are not indicated in a patient with a kidney stone but are essential for a chest pain patient. The reader is encouraged to modify the order sets (and protocols) as appropriate according to the patient's diagnosis and their own physician(s) and hospital practice.

In view of the recent unpredictable shortages of medications, we intentionally listed multiple drugs in the various pharmacologic categories since lack of availability has forced us to substitute other drugs when one(s) we usually use are unavailable. This does not mean we stock everything on the list. Indeed, generally, we only stock one or two drugs in any given category, such as antiemetics or antibiotics, for various reasons including cost and space.

The brand names for commercially available drugs in the United States are given because health care providers often recognize and order medications by the brand name instead of the pharmacologic name. This is not meant to endorse or recommend any given drug. Some medications were not included for various reasons. Observation patients should not be "critically" ill so certain drugs usually restricted to the critically ill would not be stocked in the CDU. Medications that are difficult to switch within 24 hours from an IV to oral form that the patient could be discharged home with would also not be standard CDU medications and are not in the order sets.

The drugs, dosages, etc. in the order sets have been derived from many sources and recommendations; including but not limited to standard textbooks and references, such as the *Red Book of Pediatrics* and the *Drug Information Handbook* published by Lexi-Comp, as well as the package labeling from pharmaceutical manufacturers. Where guidelines exist, such as with the Infectious Disease Society of America (IDSA) or the American College of Obstetricians and Gynecologists (ACOG), we tried to incorporate them. The protocols, policies, procedures, and order sets are meant to be guidelines and are not mandatory.

There are many advantages to using order sets. Presenting preferred choices or options to a clinician via an order set assists in therapeutic decisions for patient care. While clinicians have multiple options within a given order set and can generate additional orders outside of order set recommendations, the order set provides specific guidance related to selected orders and the management of specific disease states. The benefits of order sets include ease of use, increased provider efficiency, increased medication safety, increased patient safety, and promotion of best practices.

Chapter

Clinical Protocols

Sharon E. Mace, MD, FACEP, FAAP

Protocol: Abdominal Pain

Criteria for Observation

1. Abdominal pain with or without associated symptoms, such as nausea, vomiting, diarrhea, and/or anorexia. Dehydration may or may not be present.
2. Stable vital signs
3. Probability of discharge in < 24 hours is ≥ 80%

Exclusion from Observation

1. Patients with indications for emergent surgery
2. Peritonitis on physical examination
3. Free air on x-ray except for patients recently post-surgery or peritoneal dialysis
4. Bowel obstruction
5. Ileus
6. Chronic abdominal pain
7. Unstable vital signs

Observation Unit Interventions (may include)

1. NPO as necessary
2. Intravenous (IV) hydration
3. Parenteral antiemetics
4. Parenteral analgesics
5. Serial exams and vital signs as ordered
6. Repeat labs including CBC and differential as ordered
7. Consults as indicated
8. Radiology studies including CT scan or ultrasound of abdomen as indicated
9. Patient/family education

Disposition Criteria (Disposition from the Observation Unit)

Admission to Hospital as Inpatient

1. Worsening of symptoms or no significant improvement in symptoms
2. Clarification of diagnosis requiring admission
3. Unstable vital signs

Discharge from Observation Unit

1. Significant symptomatic improvement of pain and other symptoms, if present
2. Ability to tolerate oral intake and oral medications
3. Someone to take patient home (if sedating drugs are given such as opioids)
4. Stable vital signs

Time Frame

< 24 hours for diagnostic evaluation and/or treatment, which may include IV fluids and medications and/or diagnostic testing and to show resolution or significant improvement (decrease in abdominal pain

Originated by: ___ Date: ___
Approved by: Observation Unit Director
Date: ___
Endorsed by: Observation Unit Committee
Date: ___
Reviewed and Reaffirmed by: Date: ___

Protocol: Allergic Reaction/ Angioedema

Criteria for Observation

1. Allergic reaction and/or angioedema
2. No actual or impending airway compromise or stridor
3. No respiratory failure or respiratory distress
4. Stable vital signs
5. Probability of discharge in < 24 hours is ≥ 80%

Exclusion from Observation

1. Stridor
2. Evidence of actual or impending airway obstruction/airway compromise

3. Oxygen saturation < 90% and/or arterial blood gas (ABG) with pO2 < 90 mmHg
4. Respiratory distress or respiratory failure
5. Progression (worsening) of allergic reaction or angioedema while undergoing treatment in the emergency department
6. Unstable vital signs

Observation Unit Interventions (may include)

1. Cardiac/respiratory monitoring including pulse oxygen saturation and cardiac monitoring
2. Monitor vital signs including respiratory status
3. Respiratory treatments/aerosols
4. IV fluids
5. IV antihistamines
6. IV corticosteroids
7. IV H2 blockers
8. Serial examinations including respiratory/pulmonary systems
9. Consults, such as ENT or pulmonary for laryngoscopy
10. If known, stop the offending medication (such as ace inhibitor)
11. Patient/family education

Disposition Criteria (Disposition from the Observation Unit)

Admission to Hospital as Inpatient

1. Hypoxia: oxygen saturation < 90%
2. Airway compromise or development of stridor
3. Respiratory failure or respiratory distress
4. Failure of symptoms (such as respiratory symptoms or skin irritation: swelling/hives/rash) to resolve or improve significantly
5. Unstable vital signs: such as systolic BP < 90 mmHg or RR > 24/min

Discharge from Observation Unit

1. Significant improvement in clinical condition
2. Significant improvement in or resolution of respiratory symptoms and/or skin irritation: swelling, hives, rash
3. Stable vital signs

Time Frame

< 24 hours for IV fluids, IV medications, and other treatment and for resolution of or significant improvement in clinical symptoms (e.g., decrease in swelling, rash)

Originated by: ___ Date: ___
Approved by: Observation Unit Director
Date: ___
Endorsed by: Observation Unit Committee
Date: ___
Reviewed and Reaffirmed by: Date: ___

Protocol: Altered Level of Consciousness Secondary to Acute Intoxication and/or Substance Abuse

Criteria for Observation

1. Acute intoxication
2. Lethargy/somnolence but not comatose
3. Toxicology screen positive for substance abuse, if obtained
4. May have dehydration: mild to moderate
5. May have mild electrolyte and/or metabolic abnormalities
6. Stable vital signs including afebrile
7. Probability of discharge in < 24 hours is ≥ 80%

Exclusion from Observation

1. New focal neurologic deficit
2. Abnormal CT head scan positive for acute injury or illness
3. Comatose or severe alteration in mental status
4. Severe dehydration
5. Markedly abnormal laboratory values
6. Acute psychiatric illness or problems
7. Disruptive behavior
8. Other acute coexisting illnesses, such as pneumonia, pancreatitis
9. Fever
10. Multiple or significant trauma
11. Significant comorbidity
12. Clinically unstable

Observation Unit Interventions (may include)

1. Monitor vital signs
2. Neurologic checks

3. IV fluids
4. IV antiemetics
5. When awake, advance diet as tolerated
6. When awake, ambulate as tolerated
7. Social work consult for substance abuse, if indicated
8. Patient/family education

Disposition Criteria (Disposition from the Observation Unit)

Admission to Hospital as Inpatient

1. No improvement in or deterioration of mental status
2. Any new significant abnormalities detected on CT scan, if done
3. No improvement in dehydration and electrolyte abnormalities, if present
4. Significant laboratory values uncorrected or worsening
5. Inability to tolerate oral fluids and/or oral medications
6. Inability to ambulate unassisted or at baseline
7. Clarification of diagnosis requiring admission
8. Unstable vital signs

Discharge from Observation Unit

1. Alert and oriented, normal mental status or at baseline mental status
2. Ability to take po fluids
3. Ability to ambulate without assistance or at baseline
4. Significant improvement in or resolution of vomiting/nausea, if present
5. Significant improvement in or resolution of dehydration, if present
6. Significant improvement in or resolution of laboratory abnormalities, if present
7. Stable vital signs

Time Frame

< 24 hours for monitoring, IV fluids and medications, improvement in mental status, and ability to ambulate without assistance or return to baseline

Originated by: ___ Date: ___
Approved by: Observation Unit Director
Date: ___
Endorsed by: Observation Unit Committee
Date: ___
Reviewed and Reaffirmed by: Date: ___

Protocol: Asthma
Criteria for Observation

1. Acute asthmatic attack
2. Pulse oximetry $\geq 90\%$ on room air
3. Baseline mentation
4. Mild or moderate asthma by symptom severity classification
5. Stable vital signs
6. Probability of discharge in < 24 hours is $\geq 80\%$

Exclusion from Observation

1. Actual or impending respiratory failure
2. Significant respiratory distress (such as: RR > 40, use of accessory respiratory muscles in the neck, marked or severe intercostal retractions)
3. New change in mental status
4. Pulse oximetry < 90%
5. Severe asthma by symptom severity classification
6. Significant new ECG changes and/or acute ischemic changes
7. Pneumothorax or multi-focal infiltrates on chest radiograph
8. ABG parameters: marked acidosis pH ≤ 7.20, or hypercarbia with $pCO_2 > 50$, or hypoxia with $pO_2 < 80$, if done
9. Peak flow (PF) or peak expiratory flow rate (PEFR) < 20% of expected or < 20% improvement in initial PF/PEFR with ED bronchodilator, if patient is able to cooperate for PF/PEFR
10. Unstable vital signs

Observation Unit Interventions (may include)

1. Vital signs
2. Respiratory assessment
3. Mental status assessment
4. Respiratory monitoring and pulse oximetry (continuous monitoring/pulse oximetry if continuous beta$_2$-agonists are administered)
5. Serial examinations
6. Inhaled beta2-agonists
7. Inhaled anticholinergics
8. Corticosteroids
9. Supplemental oxygen
10. Hydration, as indicated

11. Other medications as ordered
12. Diagnostic interventions, such as chest radiograph, if indicated
13. Evaluation, such as peak flows or spirometry, as ordered
14. Patient/family education

Disposition Criteria (Disposition from the Observation Unit)

Admission to Hospital as Inpatient

1. Deterioration of condition: worsening vital signs, mental status, respiratory distress/failure
2. Minimal or no clinical improvement and/or in PEFR after 24 hours of therapy
3. Inability to maintain saturation > 90% on room air or return to baseline
4. Asthma symptom classification of severe
5. Significant new ECG changes
6. Worsening ABG values despite therapy, if ABG obtained
7. Unstable vital signs

Discharge from Observation Unit

1. Resolution of signs and symptoms and/or return to baseline
2. PEFR > 75% predicted or return to baseline
3. Saturation > 92% on room air or return to baseline
4. Contact Respiratory Therapist or Nursing for asthma education
5. Stable vital signs

Time Frame

< 24 hours for monitoring and treatment of acute asthmatic attack and to show resolution of or significant improvement in asthmatic symptoms

Originated by: ___ Date: ___
Approved by: Observation Unit Director
Date: ___
Endorsed by: Observation Unit Committee
Date: ___
Reviewed and Reaffirmed by: Date: ___

Protocol: Atrial Fibrillation

Criteria for Observation

1. Atrial Fibrillation
2. Stable vital signs

3. Probability of discharge in < 24 hours is ≥ 80%

Exclusion from Observation

1. Myocardial infarction (MI) (ST elevation MI [STEMI] or nonST elevation MI [NSTEMI]), unstable angina, crescendo angina
2. Cardiac tamponade
3. New embolic disease (pulmonary emboli, arterial emboli, or stroke)
4. Progression or worsening of excessively rapid or slow ventricular response and/or symptoms (such as chest pain or dyspnea) while undergoing treatment in the emergency department
5. Significantly abnormal blood value, such as severe hypokalemia (K < 2.0)
6. Hemodynamic instability
7. Unstable vital signs

Observation Unit Interventions (may include)

1. Vital signs including pulse oximetry
2. Serial examinations
3. EKG monitoring
4. Supplemental oxygen (maintain SPO_2 > 90%)
5. Elective cardioversion: pharmacologic or electrical cardioversion
6. Medications administered for control of heart rate/ventricular response
7. Prophylactic anticoagulant medications
8. Other medications as ordered
9. Serial ECG and enzymes, as indicated
10. Cardiology consult
11. Patient/family education

Disposition Criteria (Disposition from the Observation Unit)

Admission to Hospital as Inpatient

1. Uncontrolled heart rate
2. Rule in of exclusionary causes (such as MI, new embolic disease, tamponade)
3. Unstable vital signs

Discharge from Observation Unit

1. Control of heart rate or conversion to normal sinus rhythm
2. Stable vital signs

Time Frame

< 24 hours for monitoring and control/conversion of heart rate

Originated by: ___ Date: ___
Approved by: Observation Unit Director
Date: ___
Endorsed by: Observation Unit Committee
Date: ___
Reviewed and Reaffirmed by: Date: ___

Protocol: Acute Back Pain/Spine Pain

Criteria for Observation

1. Acute severe back pain without a history of significant acute trauma
2. Inability to ambulate because of pain
3. Inability to control pain by oral medications
4. Stable vital signs
5. Probability of discharge in < 24 hours is ≥ 80%

Exclusion from Observation Criteria

1. Back pain with unstable fractures
2. Multiple trauma
3. Acute dissecting aneurysm
4. Known metastatic disease to the spine and/or in palliative care
5. Significant new neurological symptoms except patients may be placed in observation while evaluation is in progress if clinically stable
6. Chronic back pain without new neurologic symptoms and/or signs
7. Unstable vital signs

Observation Unit Interventions (may include)

1. Monitoring of vital signs
2. Serial examinations
3. Parenteral analgesics
4. Other medications, such as steroids, as ordered
5. Diagnostic studies including MRI, if indicated
6. Consultation as ordered, e.g., spine service, pain management
7. Physical therapy (assessment), if indicated
8. Patient/family education

Disposition Criteria (Disposition from the Observation Unit)

Admission to Hospital as Inpatient

1. No significant improvement in symptoms
2. Inability to ambulate or unable to return to baseline
3. Inability to tolerate pain on oral medications
4. Deterioration in clinical status or neurological examination
5. Clarification of diagnosis requiring admission (such as epidural abscess, acute dissecting aneurysm)
6. Unstable vital signs

Discharge from Observation Unit

1. Ability to tolerate pain on oral medication(s)
2. Ability to ambulate or at baseline
3. No worsening of or deterioration in neurological examination or clinical status
4. Someone to take patient home (if sedating drugs are given such as opioids)
5. Stable vital signs

Time Frame

< 24 hours of evaluation and therapy with ability to show improvement in ambulation, significant decrease in pain and ability to tolerate oral pain therapy

Originated by: ___ Date: ___
Approved by: Observation Unit Director
Date: ___
Endorsed by: Observation Unit Committee
Date: ___
Reviewed and Reaffirmed by: Date: ___

Protocol: Cellulitis

Criteria for Observation

1. Skin/soft tissue infection
2. Stable vital signs
3. Probability of discharge in < 24 hours is ≥ 80%

Exclusion from Observation

1. Sepsis or shock
2. Toxic appearance
3. No evidence for necrotizing fasciitis, Fournier's gangrene, or other serious, life-threatening skin, or limb-threatening skin infection

4. Significant comorbidity, including HIV, malignancy, immunosuppression
5. Unstable vital signs

Observation Unit Interventions (may include)

1. Monitor vital signs
2. Neurovascular checks
3. Serial examinations
4. Laboratory studies such as complete blood count (CBC), sedimentation rate, C-reactive protein, electrolytes, renal function tests
5. Diagnostic studies such as x-rays, ultrasound
6. IV antibiotics
7. Pain medications
8. Consults, as indicated (such as plastic surgery, general surgery, infectious disease)
9. Patient/family education

Disposition Criteria (Disposition from the Observation Unit)

Admission to Hospital as Inpatient

1. Failure of infection to improve significantly
2. Diagnosis of infection requiring admission (necrotizing fasciitis, Fournier's gangrene, etc.)
3. Unstable vital signs

Discharge from Observation Unit

1. Significant improvement in clinical condition and symptoms
2. Significant improvement in infection
3. Stable vital signs

Time Frame

< 24 hours for IV antibiotics and to show significant improvement in infection

Originated by: ___ Date: ___
Approved by: Observation Unit Director
Date: ___
Endorsed by: Observation Unit Committee
Date: ___
Reviewed and Reaffirmed by: Date: ___

Protocol: Chest Pain

Criteria for Observation

1. Chest pain or chest pain/anginal equivalent (such as shortness of breath)

2. ECG: normal (e.g., without significant abnormalities) or unchanged from previous ECG
3. Initial cardiac enzymes (CK-MB and troponin) within normal range*
4. Stable vital signs
5. Probability of discharge in < 24 hours is ≥ 80%

Exclusion from Observation

1. ECG evidence of acute MI
2. Significant new ECG changes when compared to previous ECG (such as new ischemic changes)
3. Enzyme evidence of acute MI (e.g., elevated cardiac enzymes, the exception may be a renal failure patient with elevated troponin but normal CK-MB)*
4. Unstable angina, crescendo angina
5. Significant dysrhythmia
6. High- or moderate-risk cardiac patients; including history of angioplasty with stents, recent bypass surgery, recent MI
7. No one with any IV drip; such as IV nitroglycerin or IV heparin
8. Unstable vital signs

Observation Unit Interventions (may include)

1. Cardiac monitoring including rhythm strip monitoring
2. Serial cardiac enzymes
3. Serial ECGs
4. CXR
5. Other laboratory studies, as indicated
6. Aspirin 325 mg po daily (if no allergy or contraindication)
7. Supplemental oxygen
8. Stress test
9. Echocardiogram
10. Other diagnostic studies, such as CT chest, as indicated
11. Cardiology consult
12. Nursing to contact ED MD with any elevated enzymes
13. Nursing to contact ED MD with any new significant ECG abnormalities
14. Patient/family education

Disposition Criteria (Disposition from the Observation Unit)

Admission to Hospital as Inpatient

1. Uncontrolled heart rate
2. Rule in of exclusionary causes
3. Unstable vital signs

Discharge from Observation Unit

1. Negative cardiac enzymes
2. Negative or unremarkable stress test, if obtained
3. Negative or unremarkable CT chest, if obtained
4. No significant changes on ECG
5. No significant dysrhythmias
6. No ongoing cardiac chest pain (no unstable angina, no crescendo angina)
7. Stable vital signs

Time Frame

< 24 hours for cardiac monitoring, diagnostic evaluation and treatment

Originated by: ___ Date: ___
Approved by: Observation Unit Director
Date: ___
Endorsed by: Observation Unit Committee
Date: ___
Reviewed and Reaffirmed by: Date: ___

---

* Renal failure patients may have an elevated troponin secondary to their renal disease and not from cardiac disease. Renal failure patients, however, may be at risk for cardiac disease and in need of an evaluation for chest pain. Clinically stable renal failure patients who meet the above criteria, with an elevated creatinine and normal CK-MB and whose elevated troponin is stable (e.g., not increasing and not higher than previous levels) may be admitted to the observation for a rule out protocol with serial enzymes and ECGs and a stress test, if indicated. (See Chapter 89 for chest pain order set.)

Note: The decision for which patients with chest pain get referred to observation is usually defined by high- and moderate- risk patients being admitted to the hospital, while low-risk patients are referred to or placed in observation. Some institutions use specific criteria such as the TIMI score or the Goldman criteria, while others use clinical criteria. For example, any patient needing a drip to treat their chest pain or anginal equivalent symptoms, such as any patient on a nitroglycerin (NTG) drip can*not be placed in observation* since patients on a NTG drip have ongoing chest pain, which indicates they have ongoing or unstable angina and need to be *admitted to the hospital.* Patients with a heparin drip have an acute coronary syndrome and need to be *admitted to the hospital.*

As part of the ongoing performance improvement process, patients who rule in for MI (e.g., positive enzymes and/or ECG), go to the cardiac catheterization laboratory, have a positive stress test, or are admitted to cardiology should be looked at as part of the ongoing process improvement (PI) or continuous quality improvement (CQI) program. Similarly, the percentage of chest pain patients admitted to the hospital should also be evaluated as part of the PI or CQI program to determine if appropriate patients are being placed in observation and admitted to the hospital, respectively. (See Chapter 9 on Metrics and Performance Improvement)

Protocol: Chronic Obstructive Pulmonary Disease (COPD)

Criteria for Observation

1. Acute exacerbation of COPD
2. Pulse oximetry $\geq$ 90% on room air
3. Baseline mentation
4. Mild to moderate COPD exacerbation
5. Stable vital signs
6. Probability of discharge in < 24 hours is $\geq$ 80%

Exclusion from Observation

1. Actual or impending respiratory failure
2. Significant respiratory distress (such as: RR > 40, use of accessory respiratory muscles in the neck, marked or severe intercostal retractions)
3. New change in mental status
4. Pulse oximetry < 90%
5. Severe COPD by symptom severity classification
6. Significant new ECG changes and/or acute ischemic changes
7. Pneumothorax or multi-focal infiltrates on chest radiograph, if done
8. ABG parameters: marked acidosis pH $\leq$ 7.20, or hypercarbia with pCO_2 > 50, or hypoxia with pO_2 < 80, if ABG done

9. Acute ischemic changes on ECG or elevated cardiac enzymes, if done
10. On home oxygen
11. Unstable vital signs

Observation Unit Interventions (may include)

1. Vital signs
2. Respiratory assessment
3. Mental status assessment
4. Respiratory monitoring and pulse oximetry
5. Cardiac monitoring
6. Serial examinations
7. Inhaled beta2-agonists
8. Inhaled anticholinergics
9. Corticosteroids
10. Cardiac monitoring
11. Supplemental oxygen to maintain saturation > 90% or at patient's baseline
12. Hydration, as indicated
13. Additional medications as ordered (antibiotics, etc.)
14. Diagnostic interventions, such as chest radiograph, if indicated
15. ABG or repeat ABG if ordered
16. Patent/family education: consult respiratory therapy or nursing

Disposition Criteria (Disposition from the Observation Unit)

Admission to Hospital as Inpatient

1. Deterioration of condition: worsening vital signs and/or mentation
2. Minimal or no clinical improvement even with OU therapy
3. Inability to maintain saturation > 90% on room air
4. COPD symptom classification of severe
5. Significant new ECG changes
6. Worsening ABG values despite intervention, if ABG done
7. Unstable vital signs

Discharge from Observation Unit

1. Resolution of signs and symptoms and/or return to baseline
2. PEFR returns to baseline

3. Symptom Classification mild or return to baseline
4. Stable vital signs

Time Frame

< 24 hours for treatment of acute exacerbation of COPD and to show significant improvement in COPD symptoms and clinical condition and/or with return to baseline

Originated by: ___ Date: ___
Approved by: Observation Unit Director
Date: ___
Endorsed by: Observation Unit Committee
Date: ___
Reviewed and Reaffirmed by: Date: ___

Protocol: Dehydration and/or Vomiting and/or Diarrhea

Criteria for Observation

1. Volume deficit treatable and expected to resolve in 24 hours
2. Mild to moderate dehydration
3. Mild to moderate changes in electrolytes
4. Stable vital signs
5. Probability of discharge in < 24 hours is ≥ 80%

Exclusion from Observation

1. Severe dehydration
2. Severe electrolyte changes (such as; Na < 125 mEq/L, Na > 150 mEq/L)
3. Renal failure, renal insufficiency, or marked changes in renal function
4. Severe hypotension or hypotension refractory to IV fluid administration
5. Associated with causes not usually correctable within a 24-hour treatment time frame such as: adrenal insufficiency, bowel obstruction, heat stroke, burns, diabetes insidious, post obstructive diuresis)
6. Significant cardiac dysrhythmias
7. Unstable vital signs

Observation Unit Interventions (may include)

1. Monitor vital signs
2. Serial examinations

3. IV fluids
4. IV electrolytes
5. IV antiemetics, if vomiting
6. Antidiarrheal medications, if indicated
7. Stool for c. difficile, if indicated
8. Stool for culture and sensitivity, if indicated
9. Stool for ova and parasites, if indicated
10. Patient/family education

Disposition Criteria (Disposition from the Observation Unit)

Admission to Hospital as Inpatient

1. No significant improvement in clinical condition
2. Inability to take po fluids
3. Rule in of exclusionary causes
4. Unstable vital signs

Discharge from Observation Unit

1. Resolution of or significant improvement in symptoms and clinical condition (e.g., marked improvement in or no longer dehydrated, vomiting, or having diarrhea)
2. Normal (or near normal) electrolytes or significantly improved, if obtained
3. Ability to take po fluids
4. Stable vital signs

Time Frame

< 24 hours for IV fluids, IV medications, etc. and to show significant improvement in symptoms and clinical condition and in degree of dehydration

Originated by: ___ Date: ___
Approved by: Observation Unit Director
Date: ___
Endorsed by: Observation Unit Committee
Date: ___
Reviewed and Reaffirmed by: Date: ___

Protocol: Dizziness/Vertigo

Criteria for Observation

1. Symptoms of dizziness or peripheral vertigo
2. Symptoms may impair ability to ambulate without assistance
3. Symptoms suspected to be due to or consistent with peripheral vertigo
4. Stable vital signs
5. Probability of discharge in < 24 hours is $\geq$ 80%

Exclusion from CDU Criteria

1. New focal neurologic deficits
2. New abnormal cerebellar examination
3. Symptoms suspected to be due to or consistent with central vertigo
4. Severe headache or head trauma associated with vertigo
5. Fever
6. Unstable vital signs

Observation Unit Interventions (may include)

1. Monitor vital signs
2. IV hydration
3. IV antiemtics for nausea/vomiting
4. Orthostatic vital signs (if patient can tolerate)
5. Trial of medications to treat symptoms:
    Antihistamines: meclizine, diphenhydramine
    Prokinetic, antiemetic, gastrointestinal agent: metoclopramide
    Benzodiazepines: ativan, low dose valium
6. Other medications, as ordered
7. Diagnostic testing: consider blood work (CBC glucose, renal function tests, electrolytes including calcium and magnesium, urinalysis and consider head CT scan or MRI/MRA, as indicated
8. Consults, as indicated (such as otolaryngology, neurology)
9. Advance diet as tolerated
10. Ambulation as tolerated
11. Patient/family education

Disposition Criteria (Disposition from the Observation Unit)

Admission to Hospital as Inpatient

1. Inability to ambulate at baseline
2. Inability to tolerate oral fluids and oral medications
3. Deterioration in neurological examination
4. Clarification of diagnosis requiring admission (such as CNS mass or infection)
5. Unstable vital signs

Discharge from Observation Unit

1. Ability to ambulate at baseline and care for self safely in home environment

2. Ability to take oral fluids and oral medications
3. Resolution of or significant improvement in symptoms
4. Stable vital signs

Time Frame

< 24 hours of diagnostic evaluation and therapy with ability to show significant improvement in ambulation, ability to tolerate po medications and have adequate po intake

Originated by: ___ Date: ___
Approved by: Observation Unit Director
Date: ___
Endorsed by: Observation Unit Committee
Date: ___
Reviewed and Reaffirmed by: Date:___

Protocol: Electrolyte Abnormality (Hypercalcemia, Hyperkalemia, Hypernatremia)*
Criteria for Observation

1. Mild to moderate electrolyte abnormalities
2. No significant and/or new dysrhythmias
3. No new significant ECG changes
4. New onset of altered mental status
5. May have mild or moderate dehydration, but not severe dehydration
6. Stable vital signs
7. Probability of discharge in < 24 hours is ≥ 80%

Exclusion from Observation

1. Significant cardiac dysrhythmias or new ECG changes
2. New onset of altered mental status
3. Serious precipitating cause(s) not usually correctable within a 24-hour treatment time frame (such as: adrenal insufficiency, acute renal failure, diabetes insipidus, new diagnosis of malignancy)
4. Severe dehydration
5. Serum potassium > 7.0 mEq/dl, calcium > 13.0 mEq/dl, sodium > 150 mEq/dl
6. Unstable vital signs

Observation Unit Interventions (may include)

1. Monitor vital signs
2. Cardiac monitoring
3. ECG
4. Serial measurement of electrolytes
5. Other laboratory studies as indicated, such as renal function tests
6. IV fluids
7. Therapy for specific elevated electrolytes:
   For hyperkalemia: calcium, insulin with glucose, beta 2 adrenergic agents, sodium bicarbonate
   For hypercalcemia: saline infusion, bisphosphonates, calcitonin, glucocorticoids
   For hypernatremia: IV fluids
8. Serial examinations including cardiopulmonary examination and mental status
9. Consults as indicated (such as endocrinology)
10. Patient/family education

Disposition Criteria (Disposition from the Observation Unit)
Admission to Hospital as Inpatient

1. Failure of electrolyte abnormalities to improve significantly
2. Significant side effects/complications of electrolyte abnormalities (such as ECG abnormalities or dysrhythmias)
3. Deterioration of clinical condition
4. Clarification of diagnosis requiring admission (such as adrenal insufficiency)
5. Unstable vital signs

Discharge from Observation Unit

1. Significant improvement in or resolution of electrolyte abnormalities
2. Significant improvement in or resolution of dehydration or fluid deficits/imbalances
3. Stable vital signs

Time Frame

< 24 hours for IV fluids, IV electrolyte solutions to be administered and to show significant improvement in electrolytes and fluid status

Originated by: ___ Date: ___
Approved by: Observation Unit Director
Date: ___
Endorsed by: Observation Unit Committee
Date: ___
Reviewed and Reaffirmed by: Date: ___
*Hypermagnesemia is excluded from observation since the treatment of elevated levels includes

hemodialysis as a first-line therapy in addition to restriction of magnesium-containing medications

Protocol: Electrolyte Abnormality (Hypocalcemia, Hypokalemia, Hyponatremia)

Criteria for Observation

1. Mild to moderate electrolyte abnormalities
2. Is not in diabetic or hyperosmolar ketoacidosis
3. No significant dysrhythmias
4. No new significant ECG changes
5. No altered mental status
6. Stable vital signs
7. Probability of discharge in < 24 hours is 80%

Exclusion from Observation

1. Significant cardiac dysrhythmias or new ECG changes
2. Altered mental status which is new
3. Serious precipitating cause (such as adrenal insufficiency)
4. Diabetic or hyperosmolar ketoacidosis
5. Serum pH < 7.30, or anion gap > 15, or total CO_2 < 15
6. Severe dehydration
7. Serum potassium < 2.0 mEq/dl, serum calcium < 7.0 mEq/dl, serum magnesium < 1.2 mEq/dl, serum sodium < 125 mEq/dl,

Observation Unit Interventions (*may include*)

1. Monitor vital signs
2. Cardiac monitoring
3. ECG
4. Intravenous fluids
5. Intravenous electrolyte solutions
6. Intravenous medications
7. Patient/family education

Disposition Criteria (Disposition from the Observation Unit)

Admission to Hospital as Inpatient

1. Failure of electrolyte abnormalities to improve significantly

2. Significant side effects/complications of electrolyte abnormalities (such as ECG abnormalities or dysrhythmias)
3. Clarification of diagnosis requiring admission (such as adrenal insufficiency)
4. Unstable vital signs

Discharge from Observation Unit

1. Significant improvement in or resolution of electrolyte abnormalities
2. Significant improvement in or resolution of dehydration or fluid deficits/imbalances
3. Stable vital signs

Time Frame

< 24 hours for IV fluids, IV electrolyte solutions to be administered and to show significant improvement in electrolytes and fluid status

Originated by: ___ Date: ___
Approved by: Observation Unit Director
Date: ___
Endorsed by: Observation Unit Committee
Date: ___
Reviewed and Reaffirmed by: Date: ___

Protocol: Extremity Infections (Including Hand Infections, Cellulitis, Abscess)

Criteria for Observation

1. Infection/abscess of extremity
2. Patient is not toxic, in shock or septic
3. No evidence for acute ischemia or acute arterial occlusion
4. Stable vital signs
5. Probability of discharge in < 24 hours is ≥ 80%

Exclusion from Observation Criteria

1. Sepsis or shock
2. Toxic appearance
3. No evidence for necrotizing fasciitis or other serious, life-threatening infection/injury or limb threatening infection/injury
4. Significant comorbidity; including HIV, malignancy, immunosuppression
5. Unstable vital signs

Observation Unit Interventions (may include)

1. Monitor vital signs
2. Neurovascular checks
3. Serial examinations
4. IV antibiotics
5. IV analgesics
6. Other medications, as ordered
7. Diagnostic studies including x-rays, CT scan or MRI, if indicated
8. Consultations as ordered (e.g., hand service, plastic surgery, orthopedics, general surgery, infectious disease)
9. Measurement of tissue pressure (e.g., assessment for compartment syndrome)
10. Drainage of abscess
11. Elevation of extremity
12. Wound care and dressing changes
13. Physical therapy (assessment), if indicated
14. Patient/family education

Disposition Criteria (Disposition from the Observation Unit)

Admission to Hospital as Inpatient

1. Failure of infection to improve significantly
2. Inability to complete required wound care, medication treatment, physical therapy, etc. as an outpatient
3. Clarification of diagnosis requiring admission (such as necrotizing fasciitis)
4. Unstable vital signs

Discharge from Observation Unit

1. Significant improvement of infection
2. Ability to complete required wound care, medication therapy, physical therapy, etc. as an outpatient
3. Someone to take patient home (if sedating drugs are given such as opioids)
4. Stable vital signs

Time Frame

< 24 hours of evaluation and management therapy with ability to show significant improvement in clinical condition (e.g., extremity infection), significant decrease in signs and/or symptoms such as pain, extremity swelling, fever, etc. and ability to complete required outpatient management/therapy

Originated by: ___ Date: ___
Approved by: Observation Unit Director
Date: ___
Endorsed by: Observation Unit Committee
Date: ___
Reviewed and Reaffirmed by: Date: ___

Protocol: Gastrointestinal Bleeding
Criteria for Observation

1. Gastrointestinal (GI) bleeding
2. Hemodynamically stable
3. Stable vital signs
4. Probability of discharge in < 24 hours is ≥ 80%

Exclusion from Observation

1. Coexisting acute severe medical condition (such as sepsis, acute coronary syndrome, renal disease, liver disease, malignancy, transient ischemic attack)
2. New change in mental status
3. New ECG changes
4. History of coagulopathy including coumadin use with increased INR > 5.0
5. Acute ongoing GI bleeding associated with acute significant drop in hematocrit/hemoglobin with symptoms (such as shortness of breath, chest pain)
6. Hematocrit < 20, hemoglobin < 7.0
7. Unstable vital signs

Observation Unit Interventions (may include)

1. Monitor vital signs
2. Serial examinations
3. Serial hematocrit/hemoglobin
4. Coagulation studies
5. Hemoccult stools
6. Type and screen for blood type
7. IV fluids
8. IV H2 blockers
9. Other medications (GI agents, etc.)
10. Endoscopy in a.m.: NPO after midnight (notify: gastroenterology, check INR, hold anticoagulants)
11. Colonoscopy in a.m.: NPO after midnight, bowel preparation with go-lytely or other

(notify: gastroenterology, check INR, hold anticoagulants)

12. Consults, as indicated (such as gastroenterology, hematology)
13. Type and cross for transfusion of __ units of packed bed blood cells
14. Patient/family education

Disposition Criteria (Disposition from the Observation Unit)

Admission to Hospital as Inpatient

1. Failure of significant GI bleeding to resolve or improve significantly
2. Significantly abnormal laboratory values, or uncorrected or worsening laboratory values
3. Identification of causes of GI bleeding that warrant inpatient evaluation and treatment
4. Unstable vital signs

Discharge from Observation Unit

1. Resolution of or significant improvement in GI bleeding
2. Resolution of symptoms after treatment (e.g., transfusion), if present (such as shortness of breath, dyspnea on exertion, chest pain)
3. Negative or nonsignificant findings on endoscopy or colonoscopy, if done
4. Stable hematocrit/hemoglobin
5. Stable vital signs

Time Frame

< 24 hours for diagnostic evaluation, treatment and to document hemodynamic and clinical stability

Originated by: ___ Date: ___
Approved by: Observation Unit Director
Date: ___
Endorsed by: Observation Unit Committee
Date: ___
Reviewed and Reaffirmed by: Date: ___

Protocol: Generic Protocol

Criteria for Observation

1. No evidence of actual or impending airway obstruction
2. No hypoxia (pulse oxygen saturation < 90%)
3. No significant respiratory distress/failure
4. No shock or acute hypotension (systolic BP < 90 mmHg in an adult)

5. No acute change in/altered mental status not due to acute intoxication from alcohol or drugs
6. No acute psychiatric illness and/or disruptive behavior and/or uncooperative patient
7. Not pregnant or pregnancy < 20 weeks
8. No acute significant illness/injury (e.g., patient with active treatment for significant comorbidity including HIV, malignancy, immunosuppression, acute organ transplant)
9. Stable vital signs
10. Probability of discharge in 24 hours is ≥ 80%

Exclusion from Observation

1. Evidence of actual or impending airway obstruction
2. Hypoxia (pulse oxygen saturation < 90%)
3. Significant respiratory distress/failure
4. Shock or acute hypotension (systolic BP < 90 mmHg in an adult)
5. Acute change in/altered mental status not due to acute intoxication from alcohol or drugs
6. Acute psychiatric illness and/or disruptive behavior and/or uncooperative
7. Pregnancy > 20 weeks
8. Acute significant illness/injury in a patient with active treatment for significant comorbidity including HIV, malignancy, immunosuppression, acute organ transplant
9. Unstable vital signs
10. Probability of discharge in 24 hours is < 80%

Observation Unit Interventions (may include)

1. Serial vital signs including pulse oxygen saturation
2. Serial examinations
3. Neurologic checks, neurovascular checks
4. Continuous monitoring: cardiac/telemetry, pulse oximetry
5. Laboratory studies, such as cardiac enzymes
6. Cardiology studies, such as stress test or echocardiogram
7. Radiology studies, such as CT scan, ultrasound, MRI/MRA
8. Consults
9. IV hydration
10. IV analgesics
11. IV antiemetics

12. IV antibiotics
13. Other IV medications
14. Other medications (not IV)
15. Aerosols
16. Wound care and dressing changes
17. Patient/family education

Disposition Criteria (Disposition from the Observation Unit)

Admission to Hospital as Inpatient

1. Diagnostic change requiring hospitalization
2. Rule in of exclusionary causes
3. Minimal or no improvement in clinical condition
4. Inability to control pain
5. Inability to control symptoms such as nausea and vomiting
6. Inability to take po fluids and diet
7. Inability to take po medications
8. New inability to ambulate
9. Need for continued evaluation and/or treatment beyond 24 hours
10. Airway obstruction or stridor
11. Respiratory failure/distress
12. Hypoxia (pulse oxygen saturation < 90% or < baseline)
13. Shock
14. New onset of altered mental status
15. Unstable vital signs

Discharge from Observation Unit

1. Ability to control pain
2. Ability to control symptoms, such as nausea and vomiting
3. Ability to ambulate without assistance (or at baseline)
4. Ability to tolerate po fluids and diet or to resume baseline feedings
5. Ability to comply with outpatient management/therapy
6. Outpatient follow-up arranged
7. Stable vital signs
8. Someone to take patient home (if sedating drugs are given such as opioids)

Time Frame

< 24 hours for diagnostic evaluation and treatment, to show significant improvement in or resolution of symptoms (such as pain, nausea, vomiting), ability to tolerate po fluids/diet, and ability to ambulate

Originated by: ___ Date: ___
Approved by: Observation Unit Director
Date: ___
Endorsed by: Observation Unit Committee
Date: ___
Reviewed and Reaffirmed by: Date: ___

Protocol: Headache

Criteria for Observation

1. Persistent benign headache
2. Stable vital signs
3. Probability of discharge in < 24 hours is ≥ 80%

Exclusion from Observation

1. CT scan demonstrating need for immediate surgery
2. Acute/subacute intracerebral bleed
3. Acute/subacute stroke
4. CT scan showing intracranial lesion or mass
5. Increased intracranial pressure
6. Evidence for bacterial meningitis
7. Unstable vital signs

Observation Unit Interventions (may include)

1. Monitor vital signs
2. Serial neurologic checks
3. Serial examinations including mental status examinations
4. Laboratory studies: CBC, ESR, chemistry, etc. as indicated
5. CT scan of head, if indicated
6. MRI/MRA of head, if indicated
7. Other diagnostic studies, as indicated
8. Lumbar puncture, if indicated
9. Consults as indicated (such as neurology, pain management)
10. IV antiemetics
11. IV hydration
12. Parenteral therapy for migraines/"benign" headaches (Note: opioid analgesics are not part of the "routine" therapy for benign headaches, see Headache Chapter 35 and Headache Order Set Chapter 89)
13. Epidural blood patch if spinal headache
14. Patient/family education

Disposition Criteria *(Disposition from the Observation Unit)*

Admission to Hospital as Inpatient

1. No significant improvement in pain
2. Deterioration in clinical course or worsening of symptoms despite therapy
3. Clarification of diagnosis requiring admission
4. Unstable vital signs

Discharge from Observation Unit

1. Resolution of or significant improvement in clinical condition and symptoms
2. No deterioration in clinical course
3. Someone to take patient home (if sedating drugs are given such as diphenhydramine or valproate)
4. Stable vital signs

Time Frame

< 24 hours for diagnostic evaluation and treatment and to show significant improvement in clinical condition and headache symptoms

Originated by: ___ Date: ___
Approved by: Observation Unit Director
Date: ___
Endorsed by: Observation Unit Committee
Date: ___
Reviewed and Reaffirmed by: Date: ___

Protocol: Heart Failure

Criteria for Observation

1. Evidence of heart failure based on history, physical examination, chest radiograph, and/or laboratory studies
2. Stable vital signs
3. Probability of discharge in < 24 hours is ≥ 80%

Exclusion from Observation

1. Hemodynamic instability or unstable vital signs
2. MI or ischemia by ECG and/or cardiac enzymes
3. Unstable angina, crescendo angina, refractory angina
4. Significant dysrhythmias
5. Chronic renal failure requiring dialysis
6. New or worsening renal failure
7. New change in mental status
8. Severe electrolyte imbalance
9. Need for mechanical support (e.g., intra-aortic balloon pump, left ventricular assist device [LVAD])
10. Need for ventilatory support (e.g., intubation, BiPAP, CPAP)
11. Status post cardiac transplantation
12. Persistent severe vital sign abnormalities: systolic BP > 220 mmHg, diastolic BP > 130 mmHg, systolic BP < 90 mmHg (without vasodilators), HR > 140 bpm, HR < 50 bpm
13. Unstable vital signs

Observation Unit Interventions *(may include)*

1. Monitor vital signs
2. Cardiac monitoring
3. Serial examinations
4. Laboratory studies: (such as BNP, electrolytes, cardiac enzymes, lactate)
5. Treatment of electrolyte abnormalities (especially, potassium and/or magnesium replacement), follow nomograms (see heart failure order set)
6. Supplemental oxygen
7. IV diuretics
8. IV vasodilators
9. Additional cardiac medications
10. Serial ECGs
11. Serial cardiac enzymes
12. Cardiac evaluation/diagnostic studies, e.g. transthoracic echocardiogram (if not done within last 12 months)
13. Consults, as indicated (such as cardiology, heart failure service)
14. Patient/family education

Disposition Criteria *(Disposition from the Observation Unit)*

Admission to Hospital as Inpatient

1. No improvement in or worsening of heart failure symptoms
2. Persistent symptomatic failure without significant improvement (e.g., treatment plan failure)
3. Development of cardiac ischemia, significant hypotension, uncontrolled hypertension, rhythm and/or conduction disturbances, renal failure/insufficiency

4. Symptomatic end-stage heart failure or heart failure complicated by concomitant disease(s) that requires additional evaluation and disposition that cannot be performed on an outpatient basis (due to the patient's physical condition or treatment plan)
5. Unstable vital signs

Discharge from Observation Unit

1. Good response to cardiac medications (diuretics and vasodilators) with good diuresis
2. Improvement in or resolution of symptoms of heart failure (such as dyspnea, peripheral edema)
3. No evidence of new rhythm or conduction disturbances
4. No evidence of significant hypotension
5. No worsening of renal function (e.g., increasing BUN/creatinine)
6. Improvement in or resolution of electrolyte abnormalities
7. Stable vital signs

Time Frame

< 24 hours for treatment of heart failure and to show significant improvement in heart failure symptoms and clinical condition and/or with return to baseline

Originated by: ___ Date: ___
Approved by: Observation Unit Director Date: ___
Endorsed by: Observation Unit Committee Date: ___
Reviewed and Reaffirmed by: Date: ___

Protocol: Hematuria
Criteria for Observation

1. Grossly bloody urine
2. Stable vital signs
3. Probability of discharge in < 24 hours is ≥ 80%

Exclusion from Observation

1. Hemodynamically unstable
2. Acute renal failure or renal insufficiency
3. Urosepsis
4. Evidence of coagulopathy
5. Unstable vital signs

Observation Unit Interventions (may include)

1. Monitor vital signs

2. Serial examinations
3. IV fluids
4. Laboratory studies including urinalysis, urine culture, hematocrit/hemoglobin or CBC, coagulation studies (e.g., PT, INR, PTT)
5. Diagnostic studies including ultrasound, CT scan or MRI, if indicated
6. Insertion of foley catheter
7. Continuous bladder irrigation with three-way irrigation set attached to foley catheter
8. Serial hematocrit/hemoglobin
9. Repeat urinalysis or coagulation studies, if indicated
10. Stop any anticoagulants, if possible
11. Consultation as ordered (e.g., urology)
12. Patient/family education

Disposition Criteria (Disposition from the Observation Unit)
Admission to Hospital as Inpatient

1. Significant blood loss
2. Marked decrease in hematocrit/hemoglobin
3. Continued gross hematuria even with continuous bladder irrigation
4. Persistent coagulopathy
5. Clarification of diagnosis requiring admission
6. Unstable vital signs

Discharge from Observation Unit

1. Resolution of or significant improvement in gross hematuria
2. Improvement in abnormal supratherapeutic coagulation studies if obtained and patient on anticoagulants
3. Stable vital signs

Time Frame

< 24 hours of evaluation and therapy with ability to show improvement in (decrease in) gross hematuria

Originated by: ___ Date: ___
Approved by: Observation Unit Director Date: ___
Endorsed by: Observation Unit Committee Date: ___
Reviewed and Reaffirmed by: Date: ___

Protocol: Hyperemesis Gravidarum
Criteria for Observation

1. Nausea and/or vomiting during pregnancy

2. Inability to take po fluids
3. Pregnancy < 20 weeks
4. Stable vital signs
5. Probability of discharge in < 24 hours is $\geq 80\%$

Exclusion from Observation

1. Pregnancy ≥ 20 weeks
2. Severe dehydration
3. Markedly abnormal laboratory values
4. Unstable vital signs
5. Preeclampsia or eclampsia

Observation Unit Interventions (may include)

1. Monitor vital signs
2. Serial examinations
3. Laboratory studies, if indicated, such as: glucose, BUN, creatinine, electrolytes, quantitative beta HCG, urinalysis
4. Diagnostic studies including ultrasound, if indicated
5. IV fluids
6. IV antiemetics
7. Consultation as indicated (e.g., obstetrics/gynecology)
8. Patient/family education

Disposition Criteria (Disposition from the Observation Unit)

Admission to Hospital as Inpatient

1. Failure of symptoms (nausea, vomiting) to resolve or improve significantly
2. Failure of dehydration to resolve or to improve significantly
3. Laboratory values uncorrected or worsening
4. Inability to tolerate oral fluids and/or oral medications including oral antiemetics
5. Clarification of diagnosis requiring admission
6. Unstable vital signs

Discharge from Observation Unit

1. Ability to take po fluids
2. Ability to po medications (e.g., oral antiemetics)
3. Improvement in or resolution of vomiting/nausea
4. Improvement in or resolution of laboratory abnormalities (including resolution of urinary ketosis), if obtained and present
5. Stable vital signs

Time Frame

< 24 hours of evaluation and therapy with ability to show improvement in symptoms and dehydration and ability to tolerate oral fluids and oral medications therapy

Originated by: ___ Date: ___
Approved by: Observation Unit Director Date: ___
Endorsed by: Observation Unit Committee Date: ___
Reviewed and Reaffirmed by: Date: ___

Protocol: Hyperglycemia
Criteria for Observation

1. Elevated glucose with bicarbonate > 15 and ph > 7.20
2. Readily treatable precipitating cause
3. Normal mental status and normal or baseline neurologic exam
4. Stable vital signs
5. Probability of discharge in < 24 hours is $\geq 80\%$

Exclusion from Observation

1. Bicarbonate < 15 and/or pH < 7.20
2. Hyperosmolar hyperglycemic state (nonketotic hyperglycemia state)
3. Severe diabetic ketoacidosis
4. Precipitating cause not readily treatable
5. New change in mental status or new abnormality on neurologic exam
6. No insulin drips
7. Unstable vital signs

Observation Unit Interventions (may include)

1. Monitoring of vital signs
2. Serial examinations including mental status
3. Capillary blood glucose within 1 hour of arrival in OU and serial capillary blood glucose
4. IV fluids (e.g., Normal Saline [NS]),
5. IV electrolytes
6. Laboratory tests, such as glucose, BUN, creatinine, electrolytes (may include magnesium and phosphate), serum ketones, urinalysis, CBC
7. Treatment of glucose and electrolyte abnormalities
8. Treatment of any precipitating cause, such as an infection (urinary tract infection, etc.)
9. Consultation as ordered (e.g., endocrinology, internal medicine)
10. Patient/family education (e.g., diabetic teaching

Disposition Criteria *(Disposition from the Observation Unit)*

Admission to Hospital as Inpatient

1. Diabetic ketoacidosis
2. Hyperosmolar hyperglycemic state (nonketotic hyperglycemic state)
3. Moderate to severe acidosis (bicarbonate < 15 and/or pH < 7.20)
4. Altered mental status and/or new focal neurologic abnormality
5. No or minimal improvement in elevated blood glucose level
6. Unstable vital signs

Discharge from Observation Unit

1. Significant improvement in or resolution of hyperglycemia
2. Treatment of precipitating factor(s)
3. Significant improvement in or resolution of symptoms, if present
4. Stable vital signs

Time Frame

< 24 hours of therapy with ability to show improvement in (decrease in) blood glucose level, improvement in or resolution of accompanying symptoms, and initiation of treatment of precipitating factors such as infection

Originated by: ___ Date: ___
Approved by: Observation Unit Director
Date: ___
Endorsed by: Observation Unit Committee
Date: ___
Reviewed and Reaffirmed by: Date: ___

Protocol: Hypertensive Urgency

Criteria for Observation

1. Previous or new onset of hypertension
2. BP < 220/140 after initial ED treatment and other vital signs stable
3. Probability of discharge in < 24 hours is ≥ 80%

Exclusion from Observation

1. BP > 220/140 after initial ED treatment and/or other vital signs unstable
2. Eclampsia or preeclampsia
3. ECG with new ischemic changes
4. Cardiac enzymes indicative of infarction or acute coronary syndrome
5. Hypertensive emergency
6. Evidence of acute end-organ injury: intracranial hemorrhage, acute renal failure, focal neurologic abnormalities, aortic dissection, etc.
7. New change in mental status (altered mental status)
8. Unstable vital signs

Observation Unit Interventions *(may include)*

1. Monitor vital signs including BP and neurologic checks
2. Cardiac monitoring
3. Serial examinations including neurologic and cardiovascular examination and mental status
4. Laboratory studies including renal function tests (BUN, creatinine), urinalysis, CBC, cardiac enzymes, BNP
5. Radiology studies including CXR
6. Cardiac studies including ECG, echocardiogram
7. Serial ECGs and cardiac enzymes
8. Anti-hypertensive medications
9. Consultation as ordered, such as nephrology, cardiology, or internal medicine
10. Patient/family education

Disposition Criteria *(Disposition from the Observation Unit)*

Admission to Hospital as Inpatient

1. Symptoms worsen or persist
2. Persistent systolic BP > 200 mmHg and/or diastolic BP > 120 mmHg in spite of therapy
3. Clarification of diagnosis requiring admission
4. Other vital signs unstable

Discharge from Observation Unit

1. Resolution of or significant improvement in acute symptoms referable to hypertension resolve
2. Improvement in BP (e.g., systolic BP < 200 mmHg and/or diastolic BP < 120 mmHg)
3. Other vital signs stable

Time Frame

< 24 hours of evaluation and therapy with ability to show improvement in BP and resolution of symptoms

Originated by: ___ Date: ___

Approved by: Observation Unit Director
Date: ___
Endorsed by: Observation Unit Committee
Date: ___
Reviewed and Reaffirmed by: Date: ___

Protocol: Hypoglycemia
Criteria for Observation

1. Blood glucose < 60 mg % in the emergency department (ED) or per emergency medical services (EMS)
2. Symptoms in ED improved with administration of glucose
3. Insulin, oral hypoglycemic medication or alcohol as etiology
4. Stable vital signs
5. Probability of discharge in < 24 hours is ≥ 80%

Exclusion from Observation

1. Intentional overdose of hypoglycemic medications
2. Intake of long-acting oral hypoglycemic medications (e.g., sulfonylureas)
3. Inadequate decrease in symptoms with administration of glucose
4. New alteration of mental status
5. Unstable vital signs

Observation Unit Interventions (may include)

1. Capillary blood glucose obtained within 1 hour of admission to observation unit
2. Serial capillary blood glucose
3. Monitoring of vital signs
4. Serial examinations including mental status
5. Laboratory tests including glucose, electrolytes
6. IV glucose administration as needed
7. IV electrolytes and/or IV fluids as indicated
8. Repeat laboratory tests such as glucose
9. Diabetic counseling
10. Patient/family education

Disposition Criteria (Disposition from the Observation Unit)

Admission to Hospital as Inpatient

1. No or minimal improvement
2. Continued hypoglycemia (blood sugar < 60 mg %)
3. Deterioration in clinical status
4. Altered mental status that is new
5. Inadequate oral intake or inability to take po
6. Clarification of diagnosis requiring admission
7. Deterioration in neurological examination
8. Unstable vital signs

Discharge from Observation Unit

1. Resolution of or significant improvement in symptoms
2. Blood sugars over 80 mg %
3. Resolution or treatment of precipitating factor
4. Stable vital signs

Time Frame

< 24 hours for treatment of hypoglycemia and any precipitating causes and to show ability to maintain blood sugar and have adequate po intake

Originated by: ___   *Date:* ___
Approved by: Observation Unit Director
Date: ___
Endorsed by: Observation Unit Committee
Date: ___
Reviewed and Reaffirmed by: Date: ___

Protocol: Kidney Stones/ Uretero Nephrolithiasis
Criteria for Observation

1. Flank pain/abdominal pain with clinical impression of kidney stone
2. Hematuria may or may not be present*
3. Radiologic study; such as CT scan, ultrasound, plain x-ray showing a stone**
4. Stable vital signs
5. Probability of discharge in < 24 hours is ≥ 80%

Exclusion from Observation

1. Stone > 6 mm (stone > 6 mm unlikely to pass)
2. New or worsening abnormal renal function tests as indicated by elevated creatinine
3. Significant hydronephrosis
4. Unstable vital signs

Observation Unit Interventions (may include)

1. Monitor vital signs
2. Serial examinations
3. IV antiemetics

4. IV pain medications
5. IV fluids
6. Laboratory studies including urinalysis, urine culture, BUN, creatinine, electrolytes, CBC
7. Diagnostic studies including ultrasound, CT scan or MRI, if indicated
8. Strain all urine (send stone for analysis)
9. Consult urology as indicated
10. Patient/family education

Disposition Criteria (Disposition from the Observation Unit)

Admission to Hospital as Inpatient

1. No improvement or worsening of systemic symptoms
2. Inability to take po medications and po fluids
3. Clarification of diagnosis requiring admission
4. Unstable vital signs

Discharge from Observation Unit

1. Resolution of or significant improvement in symptoms such as pain, nausea, vomiting
2. Ability to take po fluids and medications
3. Stable vital signs

Time Frame

< 24 hours of evaluation and therapy with ability to show improvement in symptoms and ability to transition to oral intake and oral medications

Originated by: ___ Date: ___
Approved by: Observation Unit Director
Date: ___
Endorsed by: Observation Unit Committee
Date: ___
Reviewed and Reaffirmed by: Date: ___

   * It is recognized that not all patients with kidney stones may have hematuria.
   ** Patients do not need a radiologic study prior to placing the patient in the observation unit

Protocol: Overdose

Criteria for Observation

1. Accidental drug overdose or
2. Toxicologic ingestion/exposure
3. Stable vital signs
3. Probability of discharge in < 24 hours is ≥ 80%

Exclusion from Observation

1. Hypoxia (pulse oxygen saturation < 90%)
2. Respiratory failure or respiratory distress
3. Apnea
4. Intentional overdose/exposure
5. Acute psychiatric illness or problems
6. Disruptive behavior and/or uncooperative
7. Other acute co-existing illnesses, such as pneumonia
8. Fever
9. Multiple or significant trauma
10. Significant comorbidity
11. Clinically unstable and/or unstable vital signs

Observation Unit Interventions (may include)

1. Serial vital signs
2. Neurologic checks
3. Cardiac monitoring
4. Respiratory monitoring including pulse oximetry
5. Serial examinations including respiratory, neurologic and mental status
6. Laboratory studies including urine toxicology screen, blood toxicology, drug levels, urinalysis, electrolytes, renal function tests (BUN, creatinine), liver function tests, CBC, coagulation studies (e.g. PT, INR, PTT), ABG, carbon monoxide level, etc., if indicated
7. Diagnostic studies including Ultrasound, CT scan, or MRI, if indicated
8. Contact Poison Center and/or obtain toxicology consult
9. Other consults as indicated
10. IV fluids
11. IV medications
12. Patient/family education

Disposition Criteria (Disposition from the Observation Unit)

Admission to Hospital as Inpatient

1. Abnormal mental status or neurologic function
2. Respiratory distress or failure or instability
3. Hypoxia
4. Significant dysrhythmias

5. Abnormal toxicologic laboratory value requiring further treatment
6. Clarification of diagnosis requiring admission
7. Unstable vital signs

Discharge from Observation Unit

1. Normal or baseline mental status
2. No respiratory distress or respiratory status at baseline
3. Normal neurologic function or at baseline
4. Return to pre-ingestion/pre-exposure clinical state
5. Toxicology laboratory tests in normal range and/or no need for further treatment of toxicologic ingestion/exposure
6. Stable vital signs

Time Frame

< 24 hours of monitoring, diagnostic studies, IV fluids, to administer medications/antidotes and to show hemodynamic, respiratory, cardiac and neurologic stability

Originated by: ___ Date: ___
Approved by: Observation Unit Director Date: ___
Endorsed by: Observation Unit Committee Date: ___
Reviewed and Reaffirmed by: Date: ___

Protocol: Pelvic Inflammatory Disease (PID)
Criteria for Observation

1. Abdominal pain/pelvic pain
2. Inability to take po fluids
3. Inability to take po medications
4. Stable vital signs
5. Probability of discharge in < 24 hours is ≥ 80%

Exclusion from Observation

1. Sepsis
2. Pregnancy
3. Acute peritonitis
4. Unstable vital signs

Observation Unit Interventions (may include)

1. Monitor vital signs
2. Serial examinations
3. Laboratory studies including urinalysis, pregnancy test, urine culture, CBC, cultures

4. Diagnostic studies including ultrasound, CT scan, or MRI, if indicated
5. IV fluids
6. IV antibiotics
7. IV anti-emetics
8. Consultation as ordered, such as gynecology, infectious disease
9. Patient/family education

Disposition Criteria (Disposition from the Observation Unit)
Admission to Hospital as Inpatient

1. Failure of symptoms (such as pain or vomiting/nausea) to resolve or improve significantly
2. Inability to tolerate oral fluids and/or oral medications including oral antibiotics
3. Clarification of diagnosis requiring admission
4. Unstable vital signs

Discharge from Observation Unit

1. Ability to take po fluids
2. Ability to take po medications (e.g., antibiotics)
3. Significant improvement in or resolution of abdominal pain/pelvic pain
4. Stable vital signs

Time Frame

< 24 hours of therapy with IV fluids, IV antibiotics and other medications and to show ability to tolerate oral fluids and po antibiotics and ability to show improvement in (decrease in) clinical symptoms

Originated by: ___ Date: ___
Approved by: Observation Unit Director Date: ___
Endorsed by: Observation Unit Committee Date:___
Reviewed and Reaffirmed by: Date:___

Protocol: Acute Pharyngitis / Peritonsillar Abscess
Criteria for Observation

1. Acute severe pharyngitis and/or peritonsilar abscess
2. Inability to take oral fluids
3. Inability to take oral antibiotics
4. Inability to take oral pain medications
5. Stable vital signs
6. Probability of discharge in < 24 hours is ≥ 80%

Exclusion from Observation

1. Stridor
2. Respiratory distress
3. Hypoxemia: oxygen saturation < 90% and/or ABG with pO2 < 90 mmHg
4. Significant comorbidity, such as HIV, malignancy, immunosuppression, diabetes, steroids or other imunosuppressive drugs
5. Unstable vital signs; such as hypotension/shock, tachypnea/bradypnea, severe tachycardia (HR > 180)

Observation Unit Interventions (may include)

1. Monitor vital signs
2. Respiratory monitoring including pulse oxygen saturation
3. Serial examinations including respiratory/pulmonary systems
3. IV antibiotics
4. IV fluids
5. IV pain medications
6. Respiratory treatments/aerosols
7. Corticosteroids
8. Incision and drainage of abscess
9. Consults, as indicated (such as otolaryngology for incision and drainage of abscess)
10. Patient/family education

Disposition Criteria (Disposition from the Observation Unit)

Admission to Hospital as Inpatient

1. Hypoxia: oxygen saturation < 90%
2. Stridor
3. Respiratory failure/distress
4. Failure of symptoms (such as pain, inability to take oral fluids and medications) to resolve or improve significantly
5. Unstable vital signs

Discharge from Observation Unit

1. Improvement in clinical condition
2. Ability to take oral fluids
3. Ability to take oral medications
4. Stable vital signs

Time Frame

< 24 hours for IV fluids, IV medications and to show improvement in clinical symptoms with abiltiy to take po fluids and medications

Originated by:___ Date:___
Approved by: Observation Unit Director Date:___
Endorsed by: Observation Unit Committee Date:___
Reviewed and Reaffirmed by: Date:___

Protocol: Pneumonia/Acute Bronchitis

Criteria for Observation

1. Pneumonia or acute bronchitis
2. Pulse oximetry ≥ 90% on room air
3. Stable vital signs
4. Baseline mentation
5. Probability of discharge in < 24 hours is ≥ 80%

Exclusion from Observation

1. Actual or impending respiratory failure
2. Significant respiratory distress (such as: RR > 40, use of accessory respiratory muscles in the neck, marked or severe intercostal retractions)
3. New change in mental status
4. Pulse oximetry < 90% on room air
5. Unstable vital signs

Observation Unit Interventions (may include)

1. Vital signs
2. Respiratory assessment
3. Mental status assessment
4. Respiratory monitoring and pulse oximetry
5. Serial exams and vital signs as ordered
6. Antibiotics, as indicated
7. IV fluids, as indicated
8. Supplemental oxygen
9. Respiratory treatments, if indicated
10. Patient/family education

Disposition Criteria (Disposition from the Observation Unit)

Admission to Hospital as Inpatient

1. Deterioration of condition: worsening vital signs, mental status, respiratory distress/failure

2. Worsening of symptoms or no significant improvement in symptoms
3. Inability to maintain saturation > 90% on room air or return to baseline
4. Unstable vital signs

Discharge from Observation Unit

1. Significant symptomatic improvement
2. Ability to tolerate oral intake and oral medications
3. Saturation > 90% on room air or return to baseline
4. Stable vital signs

Time Frame

< 24 hours for monitoring and/or treatment, which may include IV fluids and IV antibiotics, and to show resolution or significant improvement

Originated by:___ Date:___
Approved by: Observation Unit Director Date:___
Endorsed by: Observation Unit Committee Date:___
Reviewed and Reaffirmed by: Date:___

Protocol: Pyelonephritis/Urinary Tract Infection

Criteria for Observation

1. Signs and symptoms consistent with the diagnosis of pyelonephritis or urinary tract infection, such as: frequency, urgency, dysuria, flank pain, fever
2. Urinalysis consistent with urinary tract infection (UTI)/pyelonephritis
3. Stable vital signs
4. Probability of discharge in < 24 hours is ≥ 80%

Exclusion from Observation

1. Septic shock
2. New change in mentation/abnormal mental status
3. Unstable vital signs

Observation Unit Interventions (may include)

1. Monitor vital signs
2. Serial examinations
3. IV antibiotics
4. IV analgesics
5. IV anti-emetics, if needed
6. IV hydration

7. Antipyretics, as needed
8. Other medications, as ordered
9. Laboratory studies including urinalysis, urine culture, CBC, renal function tests (creatinine, BUN), electrolytes, glucose
10. Diagnostic studies including ultrasound of kidneys, if indicated
11. Consults, if indicated
12. Patient/family education

Disposition Criteria (Disposition from the Observation Unit)

Admission to Hospital as Inpatient

1. No significant improvement in or worsening of signs and symptoms
2. Inability to take po medications and/or to maintain adequate po fluid intake
3. Diagnostic change requiring hospitalization
4. Unstable vital signs

Discharge from Observation Unit

1. Resolution or significant improvement of symptoms
2. Ability to take po medications including antibiotics and maintain adequate po fluid intake
3. Someone to take patient home (if sedating drugs are given such as opioids)
4. Stable vital signs

Time Frame

< 24 hours for IV antibiotics, IV fluids and other medications and to show ability to take oral medications and maintain po fluid intake

Originated by: ___ Date: ___
Approved by: Observation Unit Director Date: ___
Endorsed by: Observation Unit Committee Date: ___
Reviewed and Reaffirmed by: Date: ___

Protocol: Renal Colic (Flank Pain)
Criteria for Observation

1. Flank pain consistent with the diagnosis of renal colic
2. Flank pain may be with or without associated symptoms, such as nausea or vomiting. Dehydration may or may not be present.
3. Pain unrelieved by oral medications and/or patient unable to take oral medications
4. Stable vital signs
5. Probability of discharge in < 24 hours is ≥ 80%

Exclusion from Observation

1. Sepsis
2. Evidence of acute renal failure or renal insufficiency (e.g., elevated creatinine)
3. Suspected pyelonephritis with obstructive stone
4. Significant hydronephrosis
5. Kidney stone not likely to pass and that will likely need urologic intervention (such as renal stent)
6. Unstable vital signs

Observation Unit Interventions (may include)

1. Monitoring vital signs
2. Serial examinations
3. Parenteral analgesics
4. Parenteral anti-emetics
5. Other medications, as ordered, such as tamsulosin
6. IV hydration
7. Laboratory studies including renal function test (creatinine, BUN), electrolytes, glucose, CBC
8. Diagnostic radiology studies such as ultrasound of kidneys or CT scan renal stone protocol, if indicated
9. Consults as indicated, such as urology
10. Patient/family education

Disposition Criteria (Disposition from the Observation Unit)

Admission to Hospital as Inpatient

1. Acute renal failure/insufficiency
2. Inability to control symptoms including pain, nausea, and vomiting with oral medications
3. Diagnosis of renal calculi with significant hydronephrosis and/or obstruction with stone not likely to pass and that will likely need urology intervention such as renal stent
4. Diagnostic change requiring hospitalization
5. Unstable vital signs

Discharge from Observation Unit

1. Diagnosis of renal calculi without complications
2. Ability to control symptoms: pain, nausea, and vomiting, etc. with oral medications
3. Someone to take patient home (if sedating drugs are given such as opioids)
4. Stable vital signs

Time Frame

< 24 hours for diagnostic evaluation and treatment, to show significant improvement in or resolution of symptoms (pain, nausea, vomiting), and if a stone is present for the kidney stone to pass

Originated by: ___   Date: ___
Approved by: Observation Unit Director Date: ___
Endorsed by: Observation Unit Committee Date: ___
Reviewed and Reaffirmed by: Date: ___

Protocol: Seizure

Criteria for Observation

1. History of seizures with breakthrough seizure
2. New onset or previous seizure with a negative CT scan, if done and a normal or baseline neurologic examination
3. Seizure after blunt head trauma with normal or baseline neurologic examination
4. Stable vital signs
5. Probability of discharge in < 24 hours is $\geq$ 80%

Exclusion from Observation

1. CT scan or MRI demonstrating need for immediate surgical intervention
2. Status epilepticus
3. Acute/subacute stroke
4. Acute or subacute intracranial bleed, or subdural hematoma, or epidural hematoma, or subarchnoid hemorrhage
5. Evidence of bacterial meningitis or encephalitis
6. Eclampsia
7. Alcohol withdrawal seizures
8. Unstable vital signs

Observation Unit Interventions (may include)

1. Monitoring vital signs
2. Neurologic checks
3. Serial examinations
4. Cardiac/respiratory monitoring
5. Laboratory studies
6. Diagnostic studies if indicated; such as glucose, electrolytes, EEG, CT scan, MRI/MRA, if indicated and not done in the ED
7. Consults, such as neurology, if ordered
8. Administration of medications, including anti-convulsants as indicated
9. Patient/family education

Disposition Criteria *(Disposition from the Observation Unit)*

Admission to Hospital as Inpatient

1. Symptoms unresolved or worsening
2. Positive CT scan or MRI with significant findings
3. Deterioration in mental status
4. Deterioration in neurological examination
5. Clarification of diagnosis requiring admission
6. Unstable vital signs

Discharge from Observation Unit

1. Resolution of symptoms, e.g. adequate control of seizures
2. Negative CT scan and/or MRI
3. No worsening of or deterioration in neurological examination
4. Stable vital signs

Time Frame

< 24 hours for obtaining necessary diagnostic studies and to initiate antiplatelet treatment, if indicated

Originated by: ___ *Date:* ___
Approved by: Observation Unit Director Date: ___
Endorsed by: Observation Unit Committee Date: ___
Reviewed and Reaffirmed by: Date: ___

Protocol: Sickle Cell Disease

Criteria for Observation

1. Symptoms consistent with acute sickle cell crisis
2. Stable vital signs
3. Probability of discharge in < 24 hours is ≥ 80%

Exclusion from Observation

1. Acute chest syndrome
2. Aplastic crisis
3. Hyperhemolytic crisis
4. Acute splenic sequestration crisis
5. Serious infection (such as meningitis, sepsis, pneumonia, osteomyelitis)
6. Fever
7. Heart failure
8. Pregnancy
9. Complications of sickle cell disease other than acute pain crisis such as new CNS signs/symptoms, priapism, acute chest syndrome

10. Acute cholangitis, acute cholecystitis
11. Hepatic crisis
12. Altered mental status that is acute
13. Need for exchange transfusion
14. Hematocrit < 20, hemoglobin < 7.0
15. Unstable vital signs

Observation Unit Interventions *(may include)*

1. Monitoring vital signs
2. Continuous pulse oximetry (especially if on high doses of opioids)
3. Serial examinations
4. Parenteral analgesics
5. Other medications if ordered such as folic acid
6. Intravenous hydration, if indicated
7. Supplemental oxygen, if indicated
8. Laboratory studies such as CBC, reticulocyte count, glucose, renal function tests, liver function tests, urinalysis, pregnancy test (if female in childbearing age)
9. Radiology and other diagnostic studies if indicated
10. Consults, such as hematology
11. Transfusion if indicated (e.g., significant decrease in hematocrit/hemoglobin, symptomatic with anemia)
12. Patient/family education

Disposition Criteria *(Disposition from the Observation Unit)*

Admission to Hospital as Inpatient

1. Minimal or no improvement in pain or inability to tolerate pain on oral medications
2. Inability to take oral therapy
3. Deterioration of clinical course
4. Rule in of exclusionary causes or clarification of diagnosis requiring admission
5. Unstable vital signs

Discharge from Observation Unit

1. Significant improvement in pain
2. Ability to tolerate oral intake and oral medications
3. No worsening of or deterioration in clinical condition
4. Normal or baseline vital signs

5. Someone to take patient home if sedating drugs are given such as opioids
6. Stable vital signs

Time Frame

< 24 hours for diagnostic evaluation and/or treatment and to show resolution or significant improvement (decrease) in sickle cell pain

Originated by: ___ Date: ___
Approved by: Observation Unit Director Date: ___
Endorsed by: Observation Unit Committee Date: ___
Reviewed and Reaffirmed by: Date: ___

Protocol: Syncope / Near Syncope
Criteria for Observation

1. Transient loss of consciousness (syncope) or near syncope
2. No acute neurologic deficits
3. No new ECG changes indicative of acute infarction/ischemia or significant dysrhythmia
4. Stable vital signs
5. Probability of discharge in < 24 hours is $\geq$ 80%

Exclusion from Observation

1. New acute neurologic deficit
2. Abnormal head CT scan or MRI with acute injury, infarct, or illness
3. Abnormal ECG or cardiac enzymes consistent with acute MI
4. New acute significant ECG changes or significant dysrhythmia
5. Syncope associated with known significant etiology; such as: GI bleed, pulmonary emboli, MI, dissecting aortic aneurysm
6. Syncope with associated high-risk factors including cyanosis, apnea, significant cardiac history of family history of sudden death, new significant ECG abnormalities: dysrhythmias or prolonged QT interval, prolonged LOC > 10 minutes, etc.
7. Unstable vital signs

Observation Unit Interventions (may include)

1. Monitoring of vital signs including pulse oximetry and orthostatic vital signs
2. Neurologic checks

3. Serial examinations including neurologic examination
4. Continuous cardiac monitoring with serial EKG, cardiac enzymes
5. Diagnostic testing, as indicated, depending upon the history and physical examination
6. Consults as indicated
7. IV hydration as needed
8. Patient/family education

Disposition Criteria (Disposition from the Observation Unit)
Admission to Hospital as Inpatient

1. Deterioration of clinical course
2. Rule in of an exclusionary cause
3. Significantly abnormal diagnostic test
4. Clarification of diagnosis requiring admission
5. Unstable vital signs

Discharge from Observation Unit

1. Benign course in observation unit
2. Diagnostic testing negative or findings stable with ability to further evaluate as an outpatient
3. Additional outpatient evaluation as indicated (e.g., 30-day King of Hearts monitor, syncope clinic)
4. Stable vital signs

Time Frame

< 24 hours for monitoring, diagnostic evaluation and treatment where appropriate and to show benign observation unit course without significant findings

Originated by: ___ Date: ___
Approved by: Observation Unit Director Date: ___
Endorsed by: Observation Unit Committee Date: ___
Reviewed and Reaffirmed by: Date: ___

Protocol: Transient Ischemic Attack
Criteria for Observation

1. Mild focal or transient neurological deficit(s)
2. Stable vital signs
3. Probability of discharge in < 24 hours is $\geq$ 80%

Exclusion from Observation

1. Acute/subacute stroke
2. Significant dysrhythmias
3. New inability to perform ADLs (activities of daily living)

4. Acute alteration of mental status
5. Acute intoxication
6. Unstable vital signs

Observation Unit Interventions
(may include)

1. Monitoring vital signs
2. Neurologic checks
3. Serial examinations
4. Cardiac monitoring
5. Laboratory studies
6. Diagnostic studies if indicated; such as carotid ultrasound, echocardiogram, CT scan, MRI/MRA
7. Consults, such as neurology if ordered
8. Begin antiplatelet therapy when indicated
9. Patient/family education

Disposition Criteria (Disposition from the Observation Unit)

Admission to Hospital as Inpatient

1. Symptoms unresolved or worsening
2. Positive CT scan or MRI with significant findings
3. Deterioration in mental status
4. Deterioration in neurological examination
5. Clarification of diagnosis requiring admission
6. Unstable vital signs

Discharge from Observation Unit

1. Resolution of symptoms
2. Negative CT scan and/or MRI
3. No worsening of or deterioration in neurological examination
4. Stable vital signs

Time Frame

< 24 hours for obtaining necessary diagnostic studies and to initiate antiplatelet treatment, if indicated

Originated by: ___ Date: ___
Approved by: Observation Unit Director Date: ___
Endorsed by: Observation Unit Committee Date: ___
Reviewed and Reaffirmed by: Date: ___

Protocol: Transfusion
Criteria for Observation

1. Anemia
2. Pulse oximetry $\geq$ 90% on room air

3. Stable vital signs
4. Baseline mentation
5. Probability of discharge in < 24 hours is $\geq$ 80%

Exclusion from Observation

1. Any respiratory distress
2. New change in mental status
3. Pulse oximetry < 90% on room air
4. Unstable vital signs

Observation Unit Interventions
(may include)

1. Vital signs and pulse oximetry
2. Laboratory studies, as indicted
3. Transfusion
4. Patient/family education

Disposition Criteria (Disposition from the Observation Unit)

Admission to Hospital as Inpatient

1. Deterioration of condition: worsening vital signs, mental status, respiratory distress/failure
2. Worsening of symptoms or no significant improvement in symptoms
3. Active significant bleeding
4. Unstable vital signs

Discharge from Observation Unit

1. Improvement in hematocrit/hemoglobin, if obtained
2. Significant symptomatic improvement
3. Stable vital signs

Time Frame

< 24 hours for obtaining laboratory studies, transfusion, and monitoring, which may include transfusion, and repeat hematocrit/hemoglobin, and to show resolution or significant symptomatic improvement

Originated by: ___ Date: ___
Approved by: Observation Unit Director Date: ___
Endorsed by: Observation Unit Committee Date: ___
Reviewed and Reaffirmed by: Date: ___

Protocol: Vaginal Bleeding
Criteria for Observation

1. Vaginal bleeding
2. Negative pregnancy test

3. Stable vital signs
4. Probability of discharge in < 24 hours is ≥ 80%

Exclusion from Observation

1. Patients with indications for emergent surgery
2. Positive pregnancy test
3. Severe anemia (Hematocrit < 20, hemoglobin < 7.0)
4. Unstable vital signs

Observation Unit Interventions (may include)

1. Monitoring vital signs
2. Serial examinations
3. NPO as necessary
4. Laboratory studies: such as hematocrit, hemoglobin, CBC, coagulation studies, pregnancy test
5. Repeat or serial hematocrit/hemoglobin
6. IV hydration, as indicated
7. Transfusion, as indicated
8. Diagnostic radiologic studies: pelvic ultrasound, CT scan of pelvis/abdomen, MRI of pelvis/abdomen, as indicated
9. Gynecology consultation
10. Initiation of therapy, as appropriate with gynecology consult (such as hormonal therapy)
11. Patient/family education

Disposition Criteria (Disposition from the Observation Unit)

Admission to Hospital as Inpatient

1. Worsening of or no significant improvement in vaginal bleeding and/symptoms
2. Clarification of diagnosis requiring admission
3. Unstable vital signs

Discharge from Observation Unit

1. Improvement (decrease) in vaginal bleeding and in symptoms (e.g., dizziness, weakness, syncope, near syncope)
2. Hemodynamically stable
3. Stable vital signs

Time Frame

< 24 hours for diagnostic evaluation and/or treatment and to show resolution or significant improvement (decrease) in vaginal bleeding and other clinical symptoms

Originated by: ___ Date: ___
Approved by: Observation Unit Director Date: ___
Endorsed by: Observation Unit Committee Date: ___
Reviewed and Reaffirmed by: Date: ___

Protocol: Venous Thromboembolic Disease/Deep Vein Thrombosis

Criteria for Observation

1. Acute deep vein thrombosis (DVT) documented or suspected
2. No evidence for pulmonary emboli
3. Stable vital signs
4. Probability of discharge in < 24 hours is ≥ 80%

Exclusion from CDU Criteria

1 Documented pulmonary embolus
2. Hypoxia (pulse oxygen saturation < 90%) or < baseline
3. Contraindication to anticoagulation
4. Unstable vital signs

Observation Unit Interventions (may include)

1. Monitor vital signs
2. Pulse oximetry
3. Serial examinations
4. Obtain definitive diagnostic test
5. Obtain laboratory (e.g., coagulation) studies
6. Initiate anticoagulation
7. Other medications, such as pain medications, as ordered
8. Consultation as ordered, e.g. vascular medicine, internal medicine
9. Patient/family education

Disposition Criteria (Disposition from the Observation Unit)

Admission to Hospital as Inpatient

1. Pulmonary emboli diagnosed
2. Hypoxia and/or respiratory distress
3. Bleeding complications from therapy
4. Patient/family unable to administer anticoagulant medications
5. Unstable vital signs

Discharge from Observation Unit

1. Negative for DVT upon completion of diagnostic tests such as ultrasound
2. DVT diagnosed, patient/family education done, documentation of ability for patient and/or family to appropriately administer anticoagulant medication
3. No worsening of or deterioration in clinical condition
4. Stable vital signs

Time Frame

< 24 hours for evaluation (e.g., to obtain appropriate laboratory and diagnostic studies), to initiate treatment and educate the patient/family
Originated by: ___ Date: ___
Approved by: Observation Unit Director Date: ___
Endorsed by: Observation Unit Committee Date: ___
Reviewed and Reaffirmed by: Date: ___

Protocol: Abdominal Trauma

Criteria for Observation

1. No airway compromise
2. No respiratory failure/distress
3. No alteration of mental status or change from baseline mental status (excluding acute intoxication from drugs or alcohol)
4. Hemodynamically stable/stable vital signs
5. Patient is cooperative, able to take directions, compliant with therapy (e.g., not violent, disruptive or with acute psychiatric issues)
6. Seen by trauma service (or general surgery)* and deemed appropriate for observation
7. Probability of discharge in < 24 hours is ≥ 80%

Exclusion from Observation

1. Diagnostic study, such as CT scan or ultrasound demonstrating need for immediate surgery
2. Hemodynamically unstable/unstable vital signs
3. Patients receiving blood products
4. Patients on vasopressor drugs
5. Patients receiving aggressive fluid resuscitation
6. Significant acute decrease in hematocrit/hemoglobin
7. Evidence of actual or impending airway obstruction or compromise or stridor
8. Respiratory distress or respiratory failure
9. Hypoxia (oxygen saturation < 90%) and/or ABG with pO2 < 90 mmHg
10. Markedly abnormal laboratory studies
11. Glasgow coma scale ≤ 14
12. Trauma score criteria**
13. Major burn patients
14. Suicidal, acute psychiatric illness and/or disruptive behavior and/or uncooperative patient
15. Altered mental status not attributable to drug or alcohol intoxication
16. Trauma service (or general surgery) deems patient should be inpatient admission
17. Unstable vital signs

Observation Unit Interventions (may include)

1. Monitoring vital signs
2. Neurologic checks
3. Vascular checks
4. Cardiac monitoring
5. Pulse oximetry, continuous
6. Serial examinations
7. Laboratory studies including CBC, glucose, renal function tests, liver function test, urinalysis, toxicology screens, blood alcohol, amylase/lipase, etc.
8. Diagnostic studies including plain x-rays, CT scan, ultrasound, MRI, as ordered
9. Other studies as indicated, such as ECG, echocardiogram
10. Consults: trauma surgery, general surgery, orthopedics, neurosurgery, vascular surgery, others*
11. Serial laboratory studies such as hematocrit/hemoglobin
12. IV fluids
13. Parenteral analgesics
14. Parenteral antiemetics
15. Social work consult/assistance
16. Patient/family education

Disposition Criteria (Disposition from the Observation Unit)

Admission to Hospital as Inpatient

1. Indication for immediate surgery
2. Hemodynamically unstable/unstable vital signs
3. Airway compromise or respiratory failure/distress or hypoxia
4. Deterioration in clinical condition

5. Clarification of diagnosis requiring admission
6. Inability to tolerate pain on oral medications
7. No significant improvement in symptoms

Discharge from Observation Unit

1. No worsening of or deterioration in clinical condition
2. Resolution of or significant improvement in symptoms
3. Ability to take po fluids and oral medication(s)
4. Ability to complete physical therapy on outpatient basis if indicated
5. Someone to take patient home (if sedating drugs are given such as opioids)
6. Stable vital signs

Time Frame

< 24 hours of evaluation and therapy with ability to show improvement in symptoms and clinical condition with ability to take po fluids and tolerate oral pain therapy if needed

Originated by: ___ Date: ___
Approved by: Observation Unit Director Date: ___
Endorsed by: Observation Unit Committee
Date: ___
Reviewed and Reaffirmed by: Date: ___

    * There should be a mechanism in place for the trauma service (or general surgery or whatever service is designated at the given hospital facility) to see these patients in the emergency department and verify the appropriateness for observation. The protocols for observation of trauma patients should be developed in conjunction with the trauma service, just as similar criteria for risk stratification are determined jointly with other services such as cardiology for chest pain patients. These and other services can evaluate and follow these patients in the observation unit in conjunction with the observation unit physicians similar to how patients are co-managed in intensive care units.

    **There are various trauma triage scoring systems, such as trauma score, revised trauma score, pediatric trauma score, abbreviated injury scale, trauma injury severity score and others. Similar to using the Glasgow Coma scale with a set cutoff (e.g., patients with a score ≤ 14 are excluded from observation), a given injury severity score can be used to exclude trauma patients from observation (e.g., patients with a score less than a set number will be excluded from observation). This is a method of risk stratification for trauma patients similar to risk stratification for chest pain patients, for example.

Protocol: Chest Trauma
Criteria for Observation

1. No airway compromise
2. No respiratory failure/distress
3. No alteration of mental status or change from baseline mental status (excluding acute intoxication from drugs or alcohol)
4. Hemodynamically stable/stable vital signs
5. Patient is cooperative, is able to take directions, compliant with therapy (e.g., not violent, disruptive or with acute psychiatric issues)
6. Seen by trauma service (or general surgery)* and deemed appropriate for observation
7. Probability of discharge in < 24 hours is ≥ 80%

Exclusion from Observation

1. Diagnostic study, such as CT scan or ultrasound demonstrating need for immediate surgery
2. Hemodynamically unstable/unstable vital signs
3. Patients receiving blood products
4. Patients on vasopressor drugs
5. Patients receiving aggressive fluid resuscitation
6. Significant acute decrease in hematocrit/hemoglobin
7. Evidence of actual or impending airway obstruction or compromise or stridor
8. Respiratory distress or respiratory failure
9. Hypoxia (oxygen saturation < 90%) and/or ABG with pO_2 < 90 mmHg
10. Markedly abnormal laboratory studies
11. Glasgow coma scale ≤ 14
12. Trauma score criteria**
13. Major burn patients
14. Suicidal, acute psychiatric illness and/or disruptive behavior and/or uncooperative patient
15. Altered mental status not attributable to drug or alcohol intoxication
16. Trauma service (or general surgery) deems patient should be inpatient admission
17. Unstable vital signs

Observation Unit Interventions (may include)

1. Monitoring vital signs
2. Cardiac monitoring
3. Continuous pulse oximetry
4. Serial ECGs

5. Serial cardiac enzymes
6. Cardiac diagnostic studies, such as transthoracic echocardiogram
7. Serial examinations
8. Other laboratory studies including CBC, glucose, renal function tests, liver function test, urinalysis, toxicology screens, blood alcohol, amylase/lipase, ABG, etc.
9. Radiology studies including plain X-rays, CT scan, V/Q scan, ultrasound, MRI, as ordered
10. Consult: trauma surgery, general surgery, orthopedics, neurosurgery, vascular surgery, cardiology, others*
11. Other serial laboratory studies such as: hematocrit/hemoglobin
12. IV fluids
13. Parenteral analgesics
14. Parenteral antiemetics
15. Social work consult/assistance

Disposition Criteria (Disposition from the Observation Unit)

Admission to Hospital as Inpatient

1. Indication for immediate surgery
2. Hemodynamically unstable/unstable vital signs
3. Airway compromise or respiratory failure/ distress or hypoxia
4. Deterioration in clinical condition
5. Clarification of diagnosis requiring admission
6. Inability to tolerate pain on oral medications
7. No significant improvement in symptoms

Discharge from Observation Unit

1. No worsening of or deterioration in clinical condition
2. Resolution of or significant improvement in symptoms
3. Ability to take po fluids and oral medication(s)
4. Ability to complete physical therapy on outpatient basis if indicated
5. Someone to take patient home (if sedating drugs are given such as opioids)
6. Stable vital signs

Time Frame

< 24 hours of evaluation and therapy with ability to show improvement in symptoms and clinical condition with ability to take po fluids and tolerate oral pain therapy if needed

Originated by: ___ Date: ___
Approved by: Observation Unit Director Date: ___
Endorsed by: Observation Unit Committee Date: ___
Reviewed and Reaffirmed by: Date: ___

* There should be a mechanism in place for the trauma service (or general surgery or whatever service is designated at the given hospital facility) to see these patients in the emergency department and verify the appropriateness for observation. The protocols for observation of trauma patients should be developed in conjunction with the trauma service, just as similar criteria for risk stratification are determined jointly with other services such as cardiology for chest pain patients. These and other services can evaluate and follow these patients in the observation unit in conjunction with the observation unit physicians similar to how patients are co-managed in intensive care units.

** There are various trauma triage scoring systems, such as trauma score, revised trauma score, pediatric trauma score, abbreviated injury scale, trauma injury severity score and others. Similar to using the Glasgow Coma scale with a set cutoff (e.g., patients with a score ≤ 14 are excluded from observation), a given injury severity score can be used to exclude trauma patients from observation (e.g., patients with a score less than a set number will be excluded from observation). This is a method of risk stratification for trauma patients similar to risk stratification for chest pain patients, for example.

Protocol: Extremity Wounds / Traumatic Injuries (Including Hand Wounds / Injuries)

Criteria for Observation

1. Patient is not a multiple trauma patient
2. Patient is not in shock
3. Isolated extremity injury/wound
4. No evidence for acute ischemia or acute arterial occlusion
5. Stable vital signs
6. Probability of discharge in < 24 hours is ≥ 80%

Exclusion from Observation

1. Multiple trauma
2. Shock
3. No evidence for serious, life-threatening or limb-threatening injury

4. Significant comorbidity, including HIV, malignancy, immunosuppression
5. Unstable vital signs

Observation Unit Interventions (may include)

1. Monitor vital signs
2. Neurovascular checks
3. Serial examinations
4. IV antibiotics
5. IV analgesics
6. Other medications, as ordered
7. Diagnostic studies including X-rays, CT scan or MRI, if indicated
8. Consultations as ordered (e.g., hand service, plastic surgery, orthopedics, general surgery, infectious disease)
9. Measurement of tissue pressure (e.g., assessment for compartment syndrome)
10. Elevation of extremity
11. Wound care and dressing changes
12. Physical therapy (assessment), if indicated
13. Patient/family education

Disposition Criteria (Disposition from the Observation Unit)

Admission to Hospital as Inpatient

1. Failure of injury/wound to improve significantly
2. Inability to complete required wound care, medication therapy, physical therapy, etc. as an outpatient
3. Clarification of diagnosis requiring admission (such as compartment syndrome, acute arterial occlusion)
4. Unstable vital signs

Discharge from Observation Unit

1. Significant improvement of injury/wound
2. Ability to complete required wound care, medication therapy, physical therapy, etc. as an outpatient
3. Someone to take patient home (if sedating drugs are given such as opioids)
4. Stable vital signs

Time Frame

< 24 hours of evaluation and management therapy with ability to show significant improvement in clinical condition (e.g., extremity injury/

wound), significant decrease in symptoms such as pain, extremity swelling, etc. and ability to complete required outpatient management/therapy

Originated by: ___   Date: ___
Approved by: Observation Unit Director Date: ___
Endorsed by: Observation Unit Committee Date: ___
Reviewed and Reaffirmed by: Date: ___

Protocol: Head Trauma

Criteria for Observation

1. No airway compromise
2. No respiratory failure/distress
3. No alteration of mental status or change from baseline mental status (excluding acute intoxication from drugs or alcohol)
4. Glasgow coma scale ≥ 14
5. Hemodynamically stable/stable vital signs
6. Patient is cooperative, able to take directions, compliant with therapy (e.g. not violent, disruptive or with acute psychiatric issues)
7. Seen by neurosurgery and/or trauma service * and deemed appropriate for observation
8. Probability of discharge in < 24 hours is $\geq 80\%$

Exclusion from Observation

1. Diagnostic study, such as CT scan or ultrasound demonstrating a need for immediate surgery
2. Hemodynamically unstable/unstable vital signs
3. Acute or subacute: intracerebral bleed, epidural hematoma, subdural hematoma, subarachnoid hemorrhage or diffuse axonal injury
4. Patients receiving blood products
5. Patients on vasopressor drugs
6. Patients receiving aggressive fluid resuscitation
7. Significant acute decrease in hematocrit/ hemoglobin
8. Evidence of actual or impending airway obstruction or compromise or stridor
9. Respiratory distress or respiratory failure
10. Hypoxia (oxygen saturation < 90%) and/or ABG with pO2 < 90 mmHg
11. Markedly abnormal laboratory studies
12. Glasgow coma scale ≤ 14
13. Trauma score criteria**
14. Major burn patients
15. Suicidal, acute psychiatric illness and/or disruptive behavior and/or uncooperative patient

16. Altered mental status not attributable to drug or alcohol intoxication
17. Neurosurgery/Trauma service deems patient should be inpatient admission
18. Unstable vital signs

Observation Unit Interventions (may include)

1. Monitoring vital signs
2. Neurologic checks
3. Vascular checks
4. Cardiac monitoring
5. Continuous pulse oximetry
6. Serial examinations
7. Laboratory studies including CBC, glucose, renal function tests, liver function test, urinalysis, toxicology screens, blood alcohol, amylase/lipase, etc.
8. Diagnostic studies including plain x-rays, CT scan, ultrasound, MRI, as ordered
9. Other studies as indicated, such as ECG, echocardiogram
10. Consults; neurosurgery, trauma surgery, general surgery, orthopedics, vascular surgery, others*
11. Serial laboratory studies such as; hematocrit/hemoglobin
12. IV fluids
13. Parenteral analgesics
14. Parenteral antiemetics
15. Supplemental oxygen
16. Social work consult/assistance
17. Patient/family education

Disposition Criteria (Disposition from the Observation Unit)

Admission to Hospital as Inpatient

1. Indication for immediate surgery
2. Hemodynamically unstable/unstable vital signs
3. Airway compromise or respiratory failure/distress or hypoxia
4. Deterioration in clinical condition
5. Deterioration in mental status
6. Deterioration in Glasgow coma scale
7. Clarification of diagnosis requiring admission
8. Inability to tolerate pain on oral medications
9. No significant improvement in symptoms

Discharge from Observation Unit

1. No worsening of or deterioration in clinical condition
2. Resolution of or significant improvement in symptoms e.g. nausea/vomiting and headache as with post-concussive syndrome
3. Ability to take po fluids and oral medication(s)
4. Ability to complete physical therapy on outpatient basis if indicated
5. Someone to take patient home (if sedating drugs are given such as opioids)
6. Stable vital signs

Time Frame

< 24 hours of evaluation and therapy with ability to show improvement in symptoms and clinical condition with ability to take po fluids and tolerate oral pain therapy if needed

Originated by: ___ *Date:* ___
Approved by: Observation Unit Director Date: ___
Endorsed by: Observation Unit Committee Date: ___
Reviewed and Reaffirmed by: *Date:* ___

   * There should be a mechanism in place for the neurosurgery and/or trauma service (or general surgery or whatever service is designated at the given hospital facility) to see these patients in the emergency department and verify the appropriateness for observation. The protocols for observation of trauma patients should be developed in conjunction with the trauma service, just as similar criteria for risk stratification are determined jointly with other services such as cardiology for chest pain patients. These and other services can evaluate and follow these patients in the observation unit in conjunction with the observation unit physicians similar to how patients are co-managed in intensive care units.

   ** There are various trauma triage scoring systems, such as trauma score, revised trauma score, pediatric trauma score, abbreviated injury scale, trauma injury severity score and others. Similar to using the Glasgow Coma scale with a set cutoff (e.g. patients with a score ≤ 14 are excluded from observation), a given injury severity score can be used to exclude trauma patients from observation (e.g. patients with a score less than a set number will be excluded from observation). This is a method of risk stratification for trauma patients similar to risk stratification for chest pain patients, for example.

Specialized Clinical Protocols

These following chapters are an excellent example of how observation medicine can be tailored to your specific community and the diseases/illnesses/injuries physicians will encounter and manage in their daily practice. This also demonstrates the value of observation medicine at an international level. Because we see a lot of hemodynamically stable patients with the complaint of epigastric abdominal pain or vomiting blood (small amount) or blood in the stools (small amount), we have arranged with our gastroenterologists to place such patients in our observation unit, make them NPO after midnight, do a colon prep if necessary, give IV fluids overnight since they are NPO, and do the esophagogastroduodenoscopy or colonoscopy the next morning. If a polyp or other abnormality is found, then it is removed, etc. We can then take the findings and note whether the patient has colitis, diverticulitis, an ulcer, gastritis, etc. and treat the specific disorder. Rarely an initially stable patient placed in the observation unit may decompensate in the observation unit and then that patient would be admitted to the appropriate inpatient floor.

Spontaneous Pneumothorax

Chew Yian Chai, MD, MCEM, FAMS

Table 83.1 Inclusion and Exclusion Criteria for Observation Unit Management of Spontaneous Pneumothorax

INCLUSION CRITERIA
Hemodynamically stable
Primary Spontaneous Pneumothorax (PSP)

EXCLUSION CRITERIA
Secondary pneumothorax
Hemopneumothorax
Tension pneumothorax
Bilateral pneumothorax
Pneumothorax with a large pleural effusion
Recurrent pneumothorax (on ipsilateral or contralateral side)
Hemodynamically unstable
History of video-assisted thorascopic surgery
High risk of air leak

National University Hospital Extended Diagnostic Treatment Unit (EDTU)

Pre-Observation Criteria Checklist for: Apical Pneumothorax

Inclusion Criteria

1. Clinically stable Apical Pneumothorax
   - SBP > 90 mm Hg
   - SpO2 > 92%

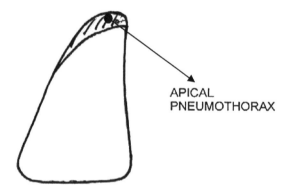

APICAL
PNEUMOTHORAX

Table 83.2 Management of Spontaneous Primary Pneumothorax

Pneumothorax	Management	Repeat CXR	Level of Evidence	Comments
Small, minimal symptoms	OU for high flow oxygen and for pain control or Outpatient treatment	At hour 14	B	Oxygen: 4-fold ↑ in rate of resolution
Symptomatic of any size	Needle aspiration or chest tube	Immediately post procedure and hour 14 for NA, or hour 14 for chest tube (following clamping of tube at hour 12)	A	
Apical < 2 cm	OU for high flow oxygen	At hour 14		
Apical > 2 cm	Needle aspiration	Immediately post NA and hour 14		
Rim	12F seldinger chest drain, OU for high flow oxygen	Immediately post tube insertion. Clamp tube at hour 12, repeat CXR hour 14		

CXR = chest radiograph, COPD = chronic obstructive pulmonary disease, NA = needle aspiration, SBP = systolic blood pressure, SpO2 = pulse oxygen saturation, VATS = video-assisted thorascopic surgery, PMHX = past medical history, VS = vital signs, hrly = hourly, Snr = senior, ISQ = in status quo, FU = follow-up, EMD = emergency department

Exclusion Criteria

1. Clinically stable
2. Hemothorax
3. Multiple comorbidities
4. COPD
5. Trauma
6. High risk of air leak
7. Past medical history of VATS

ED Interventions

- Oxygen supplementation
- Conservative Management versus needle aspiration technique (if apex cupola distance > 2 cm)
- Repeat chest radiograph post aspiration

Table 83.3 Tips on Needle Thoracocentesis

Equipment

- Dressing pack
- Large bore cannula (12 or 14 gauge)
- 50 mL syringe
- 3 way stopcock

- Antiseptic solution
- 1% lignocaine ampoule
- Tegaderm x 2

Analgesia, Anesthesia, Sedation

Analgesia and local anesthesia are advised.

- Use local anesthetic
- Consider oral or parenteral analgesia pre-procedure

Procedure

- Place patient on continuous cardiac monitoring and pulse oximetry
- Patient position: should be placed in 45-degree sitting position
- Palpate landmark – 2nd Intercostal Space midclavicular line (the upper border of the 3rd rib is preferable) and antiseptically prepare the area
- Attach a 5 mL syringe to the catheter device
- Puncture the skin at the level of above landmark
- Carefully insert the needle at a slightly downwards angle into the pleural space while aspirating the syringe, you may feel a change of resistance
- Withdraw the needle while gently advancing the cannula downwards into position
- Secure cannula with Tegaderm
- Attach 3 way stopcock and 50 mL syringe
- Drain until no further drainage

Post-Procedure Care

Reassess Airway, Breathing, Circulation (ABCs)

- Consider need for further analgesia (oral or parenteral)
- Obtain Post-Aspiration CXR
- If vital signs stable – admit to EDTU

PRIMARY SPONTANEOUS APICAL PNEUMOTHORAX WORKFLOW

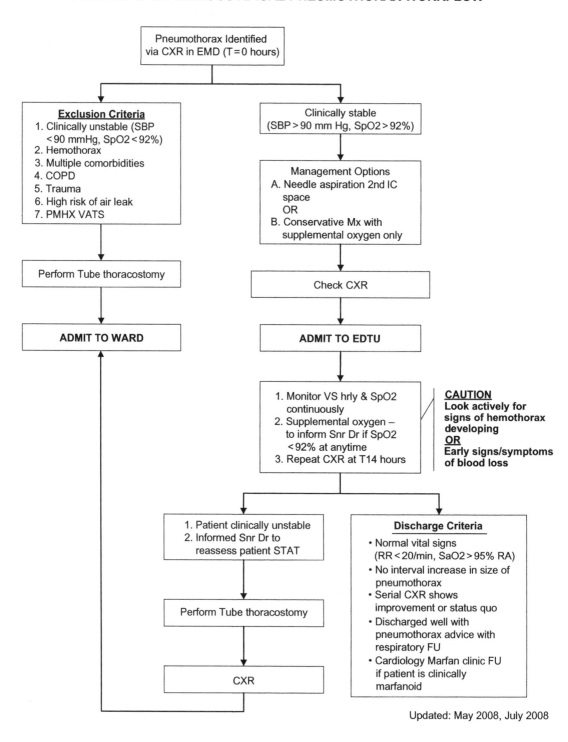

Pneumothorax Identified via CXR in EMD (T = 0 hours)

Exclusion Criteria
1. Clinically unstable (SBP < 90 mmHg, SpO2 < 92%)
2. Hemothorax
3. Multiple comorbidities
4. COPD
5. Trauma
6. High risk of air leak
7. PMHX VATS

Clinically stable (SBP > 90 mm Hg, SpO2 > 92%)

Management Options
A. Needle aspiration 2nd IC space
OR
B. Conservative Mx with supplemental oxygen only

Perform Tube thoracostomy

Check CXR

ADMIT TO WARD

ADMIT TO EDTU

1. Monitor VS hrly & SpO2 continuously
2. Supplemental oxygen – to inform Snr Dr if SpO2 < 92% at anytime
3. Repeat CXR at T14 hours

CAUTION
Look actively for signs of hemothorax developing
OR
Early signs/symptoms of blood loss

1. Patient clinically unstable
2. Informed Snr Dr to reassess patient STAT

Discharge Criteria
• Normal vital signs (RR < 20/min, SaO2 > 95% RA)
• No interval increase in size of pneumothorax
• Serial CXR shows improvement or status quo
• Discharged well with pneumothorax advice with respiratory FU
• Cardiology Marfan clinic FU if patient is clinically marfanoid

Perform Tube thoracostomy

CXR

Updated: May 2008, July 2008

National University Hospital Extended Diagnostic Treatment Unit (EDTU)

Pre-Observation Criteria Checklist for: RIM (Homogeneous) Pneumothorax

Inclusion Criteria

1. Homogeneous RIM – Primary spontaneous pneumothorax requiring aspiration
2. Clinically stable
   - SBP > 90 mm Hg
   - SpO2 > 92%

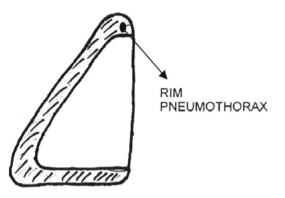

RIM PNEUMOTHORAX

Exclusion Criteria

1. Clinically unstable
2. Hemothorax
3. Multiple comorbidities
4. COPD
5. Trauma
6. High risk of air leak
7. Past medical history of VATS

ED Interventions

- Oxygen supplementation
- Modified aspiration techniques
- Repeat chest radiograph post aspiration

RIM (HOMOGENEOUS) PNEUMOTHORAX WORKFLOW

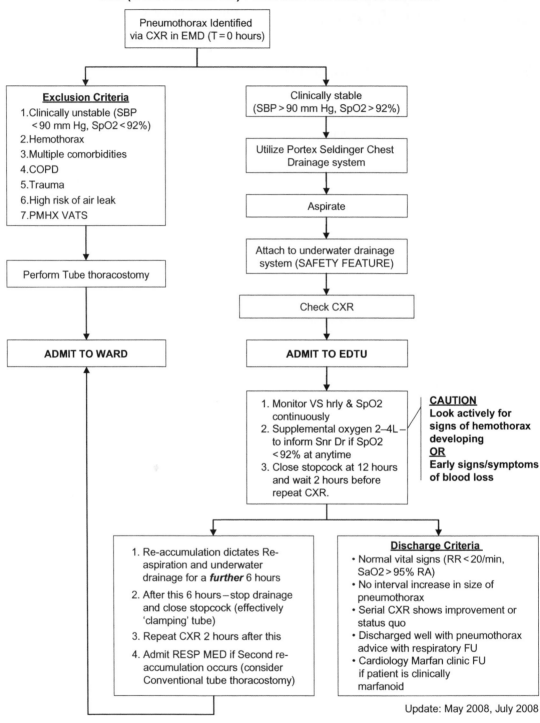

Pneumothorax Identified via CXR in EMD (T = 0 hours)

Exclusion Criteria

1. Clinically unstable (SBP < 90 mm Hg, SpO2 < 92%)
2. Hemothorax
3. Multiple comorbidities
4. COPD
5. Trauma
6. High risk of air leak
7. PMHX VATS

Perform Tube thoracostomy

ADMIT TO WARD

Clinically stable (SBP > 90 mm Hg, SpO2 > 92%)

Utilize Portex Seldinger Chest Drainage system

Aspirate

Attach to underwater drainage system (SAFETY FEATURE)

Check CXR

ADMIT TO EDTU

1. Monitor VS hrly & SpO2 continuously
2. Supplemental oxygen 2–4L to inform Snr Dr if SpO2 < 92% at anytime
3. Close stopcock at 12 hours and wait 2 hours before repeat CXR.

CAUTION
Look actively for signs of hemothorax developing
OR
Early signs/symptoms of blood loss

1. Re-accumulation dictates Re-aspiration and underwater drainage for a *further* 6 hours
2. After this 6 hours – stop drainage and close stopcock (effectively 'clamping' tube)
3. Repeat CXR 2 hours after this
4. Admit RESP MED if Second re-accumulation occurs (consider Conventional tube thoracostomy)

Discharge Criteria

• Normal vital signs (RR < 20/min, SaO2 > 95% RA)
• No interval increase in size of pneumothorax
• Serial CXR shows improvement or status quo
• Discharged well with pneumothorax advice with respiratory FU
• Cardiology Marfan clinic FU if patient is clinically marfanoid

Update: May 2008, July 2008

Portex Seldinger Chest Drainage Kit
(Instructions for use)

Kit Contents (see figure)

1. Scalpel, Size 11
2. 10 mL syringe
3; 16G × 80 mm Introducer needle (blunt tip)
4. J-tip guidewire and Introducer
5. 14F blue dilator
6. 12F pleural catheter
7. 4-way stopcock
8. Luer lock male taper connector

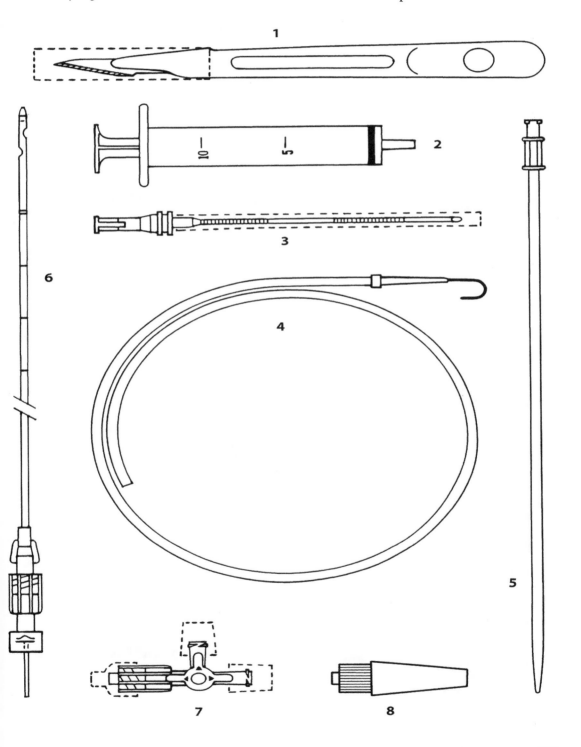

Procedure (Conventional Seldinger Technique)

1. Identify the insertion site (Triangle of safety) and clean the area with antiseptic solution.
2. Infiltrate the skin and subcutaneous tissues down to the parietal pleura with local anesthetic, avoiding the lower margins of the rib (and thus avoiding neurovascular bundle).

3. Make a small (4 mm) incision in the skin with a Size 11 scalpel blade (or equivalent) over the insertion site (**FIG. 2**).
4. Attach the syringe to the 16G Introducer needle. Advance the needle slowly through the skin and subcutaneous tissue over the upper rib margin until puncture of the parietal pleura is sensed either by a 'pop' and

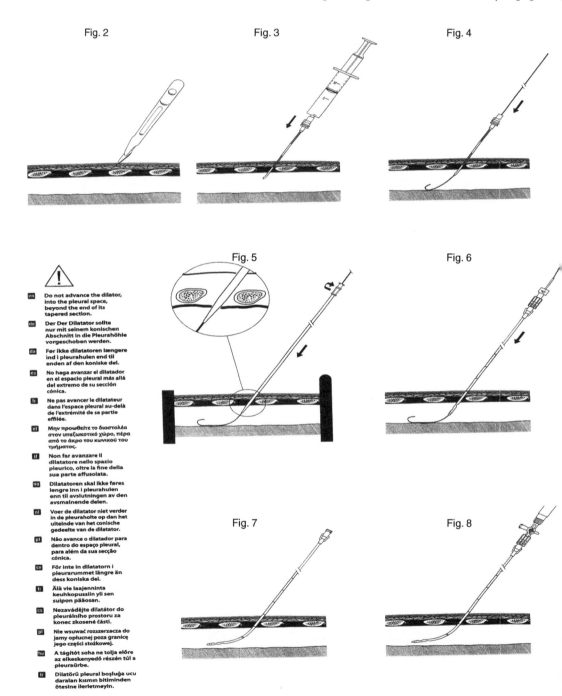

Fig. 2

Fig. 3

Fig. 4

Fig. 5

Fig. 6

Fig. 7

Fig. 8

en Do not advance the dilator, into the pleural space, beyond the end of its tapered section.

de Der Der Dilatator sollte nur mit seinem konischen Abschnitt in die Pleurahöhle vorgeschoben werden.

da Før ikke dilatatoren længere ind i pleurahulen end til enden af den koniske del.

es No haga avanzar el dilatador en el espacio pleural más allá del extremo de su sección cónica.

fr Ne pas avancer le dilatateur dans l'espace pleural au-delà de l'extrémité de sa partie effilée.

el Μην προωθείτε το διαστολέα στον υπεζωκοτικό χώρο, πέρα από το άκρο του κωνικού του τμήματος.

it Non far avanzare il dilatatore nello spazio pleurico, oltre la fine della sua parte affusolata.

no Dilatatoren skal ikke føres lengre inn i pleurahulen enn til avslutningen av den avsmalnende delen.

nl Voer de dilatator niet verder in de pleuraholte op dan het uiteinde van het conische gedeelte van de dilatator.

pt Não avance o dilatador para dentro do espaço pleural, para além da sua secção cónica.

sv För inte in dilatatorn i pleurarummet längre än dess koniska del.

fi Älä vie laajenninta keuhkopussiin yli sen suipon pääosan.

cs Nezavádějte dilatátor do pleurálního prostoru za konec zkosené části.

pl Nie wsuwać rozszerzacza do jamy opłucnej poza granicę jego części stożkowej.

hu A tágítót soha ne tolja előre az elkeskenyedő részén túl a pleuraűrbe.

tr Dilatörü pleural boşluğa ucu daralan kısmın bitiminden ötesine ilerletmeyin.

aspiration of air indicates entry into the pleural space. (FIG. 3) Then remove the syringe and discard while maintaining the insertion depth.* Observe the distance from the skin to the pleural cavity using the 20 mm graduations on the needle as a visual guide.

* Warning – Insert only as far as necessary to enter pleural cavity, guidance is 30 mm insertion, but patient anatomy will dictate changes to this rough guide.

5. Direct the Introducer needle in the appropriate orientation and insert the J-tip guidewire through the Introducer needle into the pleural space. Ensure an adequate length of guidewire (50 mm minimum) is inserted into the pleural cavity and confirm free forward movement of the guidewire before removing the Introducer needle, whilst holding the guidewire to prevent its displacement. (FIG. 4)

6. Whilst maintaining the guidewire position, introduce the dilator over the guidewire, dilate the track opening, as required, into the pleural space to the depth observed from the insertion of the Introducer needle. Do this by advancing and rotating the dilator over the Guidewire in the same plane as the guidewire so as to prevent kinking. (FIG. 5)

The guidewire should be free to move at all times as the dilator is inserted. A loss of resistance may be felt when the dilators full width has successfully entered the pleural cavity. Confirm free movement of the guidewire, and then, whilst maintaining the guidewire insertion depth, remove the dilator.

7. Ensure the pleural catheter internal stiffener is fully located at the catheter tip. Whilst maintaining the guidewire position, advance the pleural catheter assembly over the guidewire into the pleural space in the same plane as the guidewire to prevent it kinking, ensuring the guidewire is free to move at all times.

Do not advance the catheter if resistance to insertion is felt at any stage. (FIG. 6)

If resistance is encountered, stop procedure and investigate cause before proceeding.

8. Remove the guidewire and pleural catheter stiffener by unlocking the assembly (Haemostasis valve) from the catheter, leaving the pleural catheter in the pleural space. (FIG. 7)

9. Where required, attach a 3-way stopcock and Luer lock male connector to the pleural catheter and attach the Luer lock connector firmly to the tubing of a chest drainage system. (FIG. 8) Alternatively, attach the stopcock to a syringe for aspiration.

10. Anchor the catheter securely using elastoplast or any strong sticky tape.

11. Check all connections and obtain a chest radiograph to confirm correct positioning of the catheter.

Aftercare

Reassess Airway, Breathing, Circulation (ABCs)

- Consider need for further analgesia
- Obtain chest radiograph
- If vital signs stable – admit to EDTU
- Consider reaspiration for reaccumulations of air OR Attach to a underwater drainage system.
- If resolution of pneumothorax is deemed satisfactory and before contemplation of discharge, consider closure of 3-way stopcock (rather than physical clamping of tube) for 2–4 hours before final chest radiograph, chest drain removal, and ultimate discharge.

Workflow protocols courtesy of Dr. Amila Clarence A. C. Y. Punyadasa of Yong Loo Lin School of Medicine, NUS, Singapore.

Chapter 84

Snakebites: Rattlesnake Bites

Sean Bush

Guidelines for Treating Patients with Rattlesnake Bites

Airway support and/or ACLS protocol should be provided as needed.

ADMIT to Emergency Department Envenomation Service

DIAGNOSIS: rattlesnake bite

VITALS: Q 1–20 minutes until stabilized, then Q 1–2 hours

Allergies:

- Be sure and ask if the patient has an allergy to sheep serum, papain (papaya), or latex.

Nursing:

- Provide oxygen
- Place monitors (cardiac, blood pressure, and pulse oxygen).
- Start 2 intravenous lines. Minimize sticks.
- Remove jewelry or tight-fitting clothing in anticipation of severe swelling.
- Measure from the most distal fang mark to the leading edge of advancing edema. Mark the leading edge with a permanent marker and write the time alongside. Document your measurement in your notes. Repeat this measurement often enough to gauge progression. Measure every 15 to 20 minutes initially. Once CroFab is started, measurements should be followed every 1 to 2 hours.
- Maintain the extremity in a neutral position of comfort (not elevated or below the level of the heart).
- Record urine output.
- Obtain a comfortable bed.

Diet:

- NPO until it is clear patient will not need endotracheal intubation.

IV Fluids:

- Give a fluid bolus.
- Maintenance fluids should follow boluses. Give more or less fluids as indicated.

Medications:

CroFab (Crotalides Polyvalent Immune Fab [Ovine]) Antivenom

- Determine the need for antivenom. Antivenom should be given promptly for best results (remember: "Time is tissue!"), although it may have benefit for 2 weeks or more after a snakebite.
- Obtain informed consent when possible. Explain risk, benefits, and alternatives.

Mixing CroFab:

- **A starting dose of CroFab is 4 to 6 vials.** No change in dose for pediatrics (although fluid volumes may need to be adjusted for very small infants and children).
- **Reconstitute each vial of CroFab with 20 mL sterile water for injection, USP.**
- Swirl or roll the vials between your hands rather than shake them. It can take anywhere from about 10 to 30 minutes to go into solution.
- Once dissolved, **all vials should be added into a total volume of 250 mL of normal saline.** First remove 40 to 60 mL of saline from a 250-mL bag. Then inject each vial into the bag.

Infusing CroFab:

- Prepare to manage immediate adverse reactions (i.e., have difficult airway equipment and medications to treat anaphylaxis immediately available). While the infusion is started, a physician skilled in resuscitation should be readily available.
- No skin test is required. Instead, **start the infusion slowly – at a rate of 50 mL per hour**

for the first 10 minutes. As the infusion is initiated, watch for signs of any adverse reactions.

- If the infusion is tolerated for the first 10 minutes without evidence of an adverse reaction, **the rate should be increased to a maximum of 250 mL in an hour. IF THERE IS A PROBLEM AT ANY TIME, STOP THE INFUSION, TREAT THE ADVERSE REACTION ACCORDINGLY, AND REASSESS THE NEED TO CONTINUE ANTIVENOM TREATMENT.**

During CroFab:

- Assess 1 hour after infusion for INITIAL CONTROL, defined as arrest of progression of venom-induced effects (i.e., no further advancement of local effects, improvement of systemic effects and a trending of abnormal coagulation parameters toward normal).
- **Repeat doses of 4–6 vials until INITIAL CONTROL is achieved.**
- MAINTENANCE DOSING is no longer considered effective. Instead, observe closely for delayed-onset venom effects and recurrence phenomena (see below), and give additional antivenom PRN.
- **DELAYED-ONSET VENOM EFFECTS AND RECURRENCE PHENOMENA** are emergence or reemergence of any venom effect after initial control. **Treat with additional 2 vials of CroFab.**
  - If there are delayed-onset or recurrent progressive **local effects.**
  - If there are delayed-onset or recurrent **coagulopathy** with abnormal bleeding, fibrinogen less than 50 mcg/mL, platelet count less than 25/cu mm, international normalized ratio (INR) greater than 3.0, multi-component coagulopathy, worsening trend, inpatient with prior severe coagulopathy, high-risk behavior for trauma and/or comorbid conditions that increase bleeding risk.
- Repeat 2-vial doses as necessary.
- Coagulopathy can develop new-onset or recur 2 weeks or more after envenomation and may be responsive to additional antivenom.
- Consider transfusion if CroFab doesn't correct coagulopathy/thrombocytopenia and/or if imminent risk of serious bleeding. Consider a Head CT if patient has a headache or altered level of consciousness (ALOC) with a severe coagulopathy/thrombocytopenia.
- Provide **pain relief** with opioid analgesics. Nonsteroidal anti-inflammatory drugs (NSAIDS) are contraindicated.
- Update **tetanus** prophylaxis.
- Prophylactic antibiotics are generally not necessary. See discharge instructions below. Clean snakebite wounds and irrigate copiously.

Labs:

- **Initial labs: Complete Blood Count,** Prothrombin Time/Partial Thromboplastin Time/International Normalized Ratio, **fibrinogen, and Type & Screen.** Replace labs often enough to gauge response to therapy and anticipate coagulopathy recurrence.
- **Recheck labs: the same as initial labs plus creatinine kinase (CK), electrolytes, BUN, and creatinine.** Patients with snakebites can develop rhabdomyolysis, which usually responds to aggressive fluid hydration, but can require dialysis if myoglobinuric renal failure develops.
- Other diagnostic studies (such as an ECG) may be indicated on the basis of a patient's age or medical history.

Consults:

- Compartment syndrome is diagnosed using clinical exam and compartment pressure. Treat with additional antivenom and monitor pressures. Surgical (i.e., hand or orthopedic) consultation may be needed. Fasciotomy and/ or digit dermatomy should be considered last resort.
- **Contact Dr. _____, envenomation specialist, pager ____, with questions.**
- Alternatively, call Poison Control at 800-411-8080.
- Transfer to MICU or PICU: patients on a ventilator, patients with persistent hypotension, patients who receive fasciotomy, or otherwise at the emergency attending physician's discretion.

- Patients with snakebites should not be transferred to other facilities until fully stabilized.

Disposition:

- **All adult patients with rattlesnake bites should be admitted to the Emergency Department Observation Unit or the MICU. Children should remain in the Pediatric Emergency Department and/or be admitted to the Observation Unit or the PICU.** Very close observation for local recurrence and frequent measurements (every 1 to 2 hours) of swelling **for 24 hours after initial control** is recommended.

Discharge:

- Patients with **dry bites and/or non-envenomations** may be discharged **after at least 8 hours of** observation. A "dry bite" is a snakebite without any signs or symptoms of envenomation. It occurs in less than 10% of patients presenting to Loma Linda University Medical Center.
- Patients with rattlesnake **envenomations** may be discharged **24 hours after initial control** with CroFab.
- Give **Snakebite Discharge Instructions** to patient.
  - The patient should be instructed to return immediately if further swelling or severe pain.
  - Instruct the patient to **watch for any abnormal bleeding, bruising,** melena, several headache, or petechiae. The patient should return immediately for any concerns. No contact sports, elective surgery, or dental work for 2 weeks.
  - Have the patient **watch for signs of infection.** Prophylactic antibodies are generally not necessary, but antibiotics would be indicated if a bite wound became infected. A fang may "break off" in a bite wound but they usually work themselves out (like a splinter). X-rays would possibly be indicated if a wound became infected to rule out the possibility of retained fangs.
  - Warn patients about **serum sickness.** Serum sickness is an allergic reaction that can occur as late as 3 weeks after treatment with antivenom. Serum sickness may manifest with a low-grade fever, itchy rash, swollen lymph nodes, and/or joint pain. It is usually treated on an outpatient basis with diphenhydramine, an H2-blocker (such as cimetidine), and oral steroids.
  - For **pain control** after discharge, prescribe an oral opiate or plain acetaminophen. Aspirin and NSAIDs should be avoided for at least 2 weeks after a rattlesnake bite because they could contribute to venom-induced coagulopathies.
  - Patients should drink plenty of fluids and return for decreased urination, hematuria, or cola-colored urine.
  - Blisters, blebs, and bullae should be left in place, but may need debridement along with necrotic tissue after several days, and so surgical referral as appropriate is suggested. Skin grafting is sometimes necessary.
  - If bitten on the foot or leg, crutches and crutch training should be provided. Elevate and mobilize affected extremity as tolerated.
  - Refer the patient to a physical therapist as needed.

Follow-up:

- Next day wound check at MD discretion on a case-by-case basis.
- Follow-up or recheck in ED every 3 days for 2 weeks with repeat Complete Blood Count, Prothrombin Time, Partial Thromboplastin Time, International Normalized Ratio, and fibrinogen. Retreat with antivenom as above if there is delayed-onset or recurrent coagulopathy thrombocytopenia.

Disclosure: These are guidelines and clinicians should use judgment for individual patient encounters.

Rattlesnake Bite Physician Orders

Instructions: Check (✓) boxes and fill out the blanks as appropriate

✓ **Attending Physician:** **Weight:** **kg:**

Diagnosis: Rattlesnake bite

Condition: Stable

Admit to Outpatient Observation:

Allergies: NKDA Other

Routine Observation Orders:

Cardiac monitoring: Patient may be off monitoring for tests/procedures/bathroom privileges

Continuous pulse oximetry

Vital signs every 2 hours with progress note documentation by nurse or physician

Activity: Bathroom privileges with assistance

Diet: Regular

Measure and mark leading edge of edema every 2 hours, and if swelling progresses, notify physician

Diagnostics:

Repeat CBC: without differential PT/PTT/INR, fibrinogen, CK, electrolytes, 2 hours after dose of CroFab

STAT CBC without differential, PT/PTT/INR, fibrinogen if any abnormal bleeding or bruising or petechiae at any time

Medications:

CroFab 2 vials in 250 mL NaCl IV run over 1 hour PRN recurrence or increase in area of pain/swelling

Pain medication (NO NSAIDS)

Push oral fluids

If unable to take oral fluids, start 0.9% NaCl IV to run as _____mL per hour

Additional Orders:

Provide patient with printed SNAKEBITE DISCHARGE INSTRUCTIONS **Date Time**
(from Snakebite folder in ED)

Consult hand surgery if compartment syndrome and/or a threatened digit suspected

Contact Dr. _____ (pager _____) PRN

Date	Time	Verified By _____		
		Signature/Title	Pager number	Name of attending
Date	Time	Verified By_____RN	Date Time	Protocol by Unit Secretary/RN/

Chapter

85

Snakebites: North American Crotalid Snake (Pit Viper)

Bret A. Nicks, MD, MHA, FACEP

Indication:

Bite from a North American crotalid snake (pit viper) of moderate to severe grade

Examples: Copperheads, Rattlesnakes, or Water Moccasins/Cottonmouths

*CroFab not indicated for coral snake bite, "dry" bites or most mild envenomations

Consider consultation with Toxicologist or Poison Center:

Envenomation Specialist/Toxicologist
Dr. _____
Poison Control Center 1-800-222-1222

Signs and Symptoms	Severity Grading		
	Mild*	**Moderate**	**Severe**
Local	Swelling, pain, and/or ecchymosis limited to the immediate bite site	Swelling, pain, and/or ecchymosis extending beyond bite site	Swelling, pain, and/or ecchymosis involving the entire extremity or threatening the airway
Systemic	Absent	Non-life-threatening signs and symptoms (nausea/vomiting, oral paresthesia, mild hypotension, mild tachycardia, mild tachypnea*	Markedly abnormal or life-threatening signs and symptoms (alteration of mental status, severe hypotension, severe tachycardia, respiratory insufficiency)
Coagulation parameters	Normal	Abnormalities without clinically significant bleeding*	Abnormalities with clinically significant bleeding

* Mild envenomations, transient systemic symptoms, or isolated coagulation abnormalities without clinically significant bleeding DO NOT necessarily need CROFAB

Contraindications:

No absolute contraindications

Relative contraindications: treatment may be warranted if benefits outweigh the risks

Allergy to sheep products; allergy to papaya, papain, pineapple, or latex; or allergy to prior CroFab antivenom

Snakebite Treatment Algorithm

Patient with indication for CroFab antivenin therapy
(Moderate to severe envenomation)

Administer 4 to 6 vials of CroFab
to establish initial control

Has initial envenomation syndrome **control** been achieved?

* Refer to Page 3, instruction 8

Copperhead Envenomation

Administer 2-vial dose as needed for recurrence of symptoms

Rattlesnake or Cottonmouth Envenomation

Consider administration of SCHEDULED CroFab to prevent recurrence of symptoms (discuss with toxicology on call): 2-vial dose at 6, 12, and 18 hours after initial control

Repeat doses of 4-6 vials at a time and

~Consider alternate diagnosis

~Consider if envenomation warrants continued antivenom therapy

Yes, initial control has been achieved

No, initial control not yet achieved

1. **Initial Assessment**

   Remove tight clothing and jewelry in anticipation of extreme swelling
   Baseline ECG
   Elevate and extend the affected extremity
   Monitor extremity measurements (next page)

2. **Laboratory Orders**

   Routine: Complete Blood Count, Prothrombin Time/International Normalized Ratio, Partial Thromboplastin Time, Fibrinogen
   Optional: Creatinine **kinase**, urinalysis, Type and Screen, Comprehensive Metabolic Panel

3. **CroFab Administration**

   2 peripheral IVs (one dedicated for CroFab)
   Telemetry until completion of CroFab therapy
   Do not piggyback CroFab (FabAV) with other medications or fluids
   Normal initial dose is 4–6 vials diluted to a final volume 250 mL in 0.9% Sodium Chloride
   Start initial infusion rate at 25–50 mL/hour for the first 10 minutes; if no hypersensitivity reaction apparent, increase rate to infuse 250 mL/hour.
   Consider maintenance dosing for rattlesnake or cotton mouth (NOT indicated for copperhead bites).

   Discuss with toxicology on call: 2 vials diluted to final volume 250 mL in 0.9% Sodium Chloride.

   Infuse at 250 mL/hour at 6, 12, 18 hours from time of initial control.

4. **Hypersensitivity/Allergic Reactions**

   Stop infusion, but DO NOT discard solution (Antivenom therapy may still be warranted if benefits outweigh risks, as determined by physician after controlling hypersensitivity reaction.) **Discuss with attending.**
   Maintain CroFab IV site with 0.9% Sodium Chloride at KVO.
   Hypersensitivity treatment to include as needed: Oxygen, NS bolus, Benadryl, Solumedrol, Zantac, Epinephrine
   For anaphylactoid reactions, CroFab is usually tolerated at a slower infusion rate. Consider consultation with a toxicologist or the poison center.

5. **Comfort Treatment**

   NO NSAIDs for 2 weeks after envenomation
   For pain: Tylenol, Vicodin, morphine, Dilaudid prn
   For nausea: Zofran or other antiemetic prn

6. **Vaccination**

   Address tetanus status and administer tetanus vaccination. (Tdap 11–64 yo, Td for 7–10 yo or 65+ yo)

7. **Disposition**

   Observe patient for minimum of 8 hours in ED prior to disposition

Dry bites may be safely discharged to home
For adults: mild envenomations maybe
discharge to home with pain management;
≥ moderate envenomations should be
admitted
For pediatrics: ≥ mild envenomations
should be admitted
If patient tolerates CroFab infusion in the
ED and is clinically stable, the patient may be
admitted to a monitored bed

8. **Monitoring**

Measure circumference of affected extremity at:

1) bite site
2) location distal to bite on same extremity
3) two locations proximal to bite on same
   extremity

Record:

Every 30 minutes for 2 hours from arrival

1 hour after CroFab administration and
every hour until control of envenomation i
achieved, then every 2–4 hours

*Control of envenomation syndrome is
achieved when:*

- Swelling at the bite has halted
  (measurements at the bite site are
  fairly stable, while measurements
  proximal to the bite site WILL
  increase if the extremity is
  appropriately elevated)
- The patient has clinically
  improved
- The patient has no clinically
  significantly coagulation
  abnormalities (CroFab *will not*
  completely normalize coagulation
  parameters and is not an endpoint to
  treatment)

Extremity Measurements

Time	Circumference of Extremity Distal to Bite	Circumference of Extremity at Bite Site	Circumference of Extremity Proximal to Bite	Groin or Axillary Tenderness?

Wake Forest Baptist Medical Center Adult Emergency Department Clinical Decision Unit*: Snake Bite

*All patients will be evaluated in the ED prior to consideration for Clinical Decision Unit placement.

ED Evaluation:

1) Complete blood count (CBC), basic metabolic panel (BMP), Coagulation tests including prothrombin and platelet count, **creatinine kinase** (CK) total, UA and type and screen (if indicated)
2) Chest radiograph (if indicated)
3) Pregnancy test (if indicated)
4) Skin marking to follow serial extremity measurements

*Patients with dehydration secondary to decreased oral intake, over-diuresis, unrelenting nausea, vomiting, and diarrhea need careful evaluation prior to OU placement. This is especially true in the elderly, patients with preexisting renal disease, and patients with known heart disease.

ED Clinical Decision Unit Criteria:

Acceptable vital signs
Mild to moderate dehydration
Self-limiting or treatable cause not requiring hospitalization
Mild electrolyte abnormalities (if done)

Exclusion Criteria:

Unstable vital signs
Cardiovascular compromise
Severe dehydration or marked electrolyte abnormalities

ED Clinical Decision Unit Potential Interventions:

IV hydration (as indicated)
Serial exams and vital signs
Antiemetics
Tolerance of orals prior to disposition
Continuation of CroFab infusion

ED Clinical Decision Unit Disposition:

Home:

Acceptable vital signs
Resolution of symptoms, able to tolerate oral fluids
Normal electrolytes (if done)

Hospital:

Unstable vital signs
Inability to control swelling with CroFab or recurrence of swelling after cessation of CroFab
Inability to tolerate oral fluids

Time Frame:

Less than 24 hours

NCBH Physician Order Form

NCBH PHYSICIAN ORDER FORM

PHYSICIANS:

All orders should be written generically and using the metric system; **include the physician's signature, PRINTED name, ID number, beeper number, and the date/time.** A generically and therapeutically alternative drug as approved by the P & T Committee may be dispensed <u>unless the order is specifically</u> designated "Dispense as Written."

Pt. ID Sticker

ED Clinical Decision Unit Patient Care Orders – SNAKE BITE

DATE:	TIME:	ALLERGIES/REACTION:

ED Clinical Decision Unit Status

Initiated: _____ : _____   Date: _____ / _____ / _____

1. DIAGNOSIS: Snake Bite

  Other: _____

2. Attending: _____ Phone: _____

ED Clinical Decision Unit NP: _____
Phone: _____

3. Condition: Stable

4. Observation Orders: General Order Set
☐ Vital Signs with O$_2$ Sat, q4 hr
☑ Telemetry
☐ Oxygen _____ L/min
☐ Activity ☐ Bed rest with BRP ☐ Ad lib ☐ Other_____
☐ Diet ☐ Regular ☐ ADA ☐ NPO
     ☐ Clear liquids ☐ Other _____

☐ IV: Saline Lock ☐ IV Fluids _____

☐ Call MD/NP with: ☐ T > 38.3^{0}c
     ☐ HR < 50 or > 120 ☐ RR < 10 or > 28
     ☐ SBP < 90 or > 180 ☐ DBP < 50 or > 100
     ☐ O$_2$Sat < 93%
☐ Check I&O every shift
☐ Monitor circumferential extremity measurements per protocol

5. Lab Orders: (as indicated)
☐ CBC q12h ☐ Type and Screen
☐ CK total q12h ☐ BMP
☐ PT/PTT q12h
☐ UA

6. Tests/Evaluations:
☐ EKG Reason for test _____
☐ CXR Reason for test _____
☐ Other _____

7. Code status: ☐ Full ☐ Other: _____ * Confirm status on arrival to ED Clinical Decision Unit

8. Medications:
☐ GI Cocktail _____ ml (30ml) PO q4 hr prn indigestion
☐ Morphine Sulfate _____ mg IV q _____ hr prn severe pain
☐ Dilaudid _____ mg IV q _____ hr prn for severe pain
☐ Milk of Magnesia _____ ml (30ml) PO q12 hr prn constipation
☐ Acetaminophen _____ mg (650mg) PO q4 hr prn pain/T>101°F
☐ Ondansetron _____ mg (4mg) IV q6 hr prn N & V
☐ Zolpidem _____ mg (5mg or 10mg) PO qhs prn insomnia

☐ Other: _____
☐ Other: _____

DO NOT GIVE NSAIDS OTHER THAN TYLENOL DUE TO PLATELET DYSFUNCTION! ALERT ATTENDING IMMEDIATELY WITH SIGNS OR SYMPTOMS OF ALLERGIC REACTION.

9. Home Medications: Continue the following medications (including dose, route & frequency):

DATE:	TIME:		
MD/NP Computer ID #	**MD/NP SIGNATURE:**	**PRINT** MD/NP NAME:	Beeper/Phone #:
Unit Secretary SIGNATURE:	**TIME Sent to Pharmacy:**	**RN SIGNATURE:**	

ORDERS

Chapter

Dengue

Chew Yian Chai, MD, MCEM, FAMS

National University Hospital Extended Diagnostic Treatment Unit (EDTU)

Pre-Observation Criteria Checklist for Dengue Fever

Inclusion Criteria

1. Platelet > 50,000 and Hct > 49% (males), 43% (females) or unable to tolerate oral fluids
2. Platelets < 50,000 but serial platelets showing increasing trend.

Exclusion Criteria

1. Sepsis, Malaria
2. Immunocompromised (oncology patients, steroids usage, etc.)
3. Significant comorbidities
4. Altered mental status
5. Bleeding or shock
6. Poor social support

ED Interventions

1. Symptomatic treatment
2. IV hydration 1–2L if no contraindication (e.g., poor ejection fraction [EF], elderly)

EDTU Interventions

1. IV normal saline 500 mL every 4 hours
2. Symptomatic treatment (e.g. paracetamol, IV metoclopramide)
3. Complete rest in bed/rest in bed
4. No intra-muscular injections
5. Repeat full blood count at T20 hours
6. Ensure notification done

7. Please call admitting consultant if there is any query on admission or management of this patient.

Discharge Criteria

1. Normal vital signs and no postural drop in BP
2. Patient symptomatically better and able to tolerate oral feeds
3. Platelets on upward trend or above 50,000
4. Platelets 50–80K: refer Dengue outpatient management next day
5. Platelets > 80K: refer outpatient service next day

Admission Criteria

1. Abnormal vital signs
2. Unwell patients (e.g. significant abdominal pain or postural drop BP)
3. Platelets below 50,000. Please note that patients with falling trend but platelets above 50–80K may be referred to Dengue outpatient management if well.
4. Unable to tolerate oral fluids.

_____ _____
Doctor's stamp and signature   Nurse's name and signature
Arrival in EDTU: _____(date) Time: _____(hours)

Discharge Advice for Dengue

Return Immediately If:

1. Fainting spells
2. Black stools
3. Increasing abdominal pain
4. Active bleeding except minor gum bleed
5. Vomiting
6. Feeling increasingly unwell

You are encouraged to consume more than 3.0 L of water daily unless otherwise indicated by your physician.

I have received and understand these instructions.

Patient name and signature

Date: _____

Staff name and signature

Time:_____(hours)

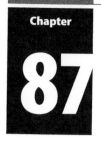

Low-Risk Pulmonary Embolism (PE)

David G. Paje, MD, FACP, SFHM

Observation Unit Checklist for Pulmonary Embolism

Inclusion Criteria

1. Patients diagnosed with Pulmonary Embolism (PE) based on positive findings on computed tomography angiogram (CTA)
2. Patients diagnosed with PE based on a combination of high clinical probability and high probability ventilation-perfusion scintigraphy (V/Q scan)

Exclusion Criteria

1. Shock or hypotension (SBP < 90 mmHg)
2. Evidence of right ventricular dysfunction
3. Evidence of myocardial injury
4. Class III–V Pulmonary Embolism Severity Index (PESI) or high-risk Geneva Risk Score
5. Severe renal dysfunction
6. High-risk of bleeding
7. Questionable compliance
8. Unavailability or inaccessibility of outpatient regimen for immediate anticoagulation

Diagnostic Interventions

1. Complete blood count, including platelet count
2. Basic blood chemistry, including creatinine
3. Coagulation profile, including prothrombin time and international normalized ratio (INR)
4. Brain natriuretic peptide (BNP)
5. Cardiac troponin T or I

Treatment Interventions

1. Immediate anticoagulation with rivaroxaban or apixaban for initial and longterm treatment
2. Or immediate anticoagulation with a parenteral anticoagulant for 5–10 days, then switch to edoxaban or dabigatran
3. Or immediate anticoagulation with a parenteral anticoagulant while initiating oral vitamin K antagonist (VKA)

Indications for Admission

1. Development of shock or hypotension (SBP < 90 mmHg)
2. Evidence of right ventricular dysfunction
3. Evidence of myocardial injury
4. Class III–V PESI or high-risk Geneva Risk Score
5. Bleeding complication

Goals for Discharge

1. Stable vital signs
2. Patient and family education
3. Availability and accessibility of outpatient anticoagulation regimen
4. Close follow-up with outpatient physician or anticoagulation clinic within 2–3 days

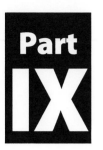

Part IX

Administrative Policies

Chapter

88

Administrative Policies

Sharon E. Mace, MD, FACEP, FAAP

Care Coordinator (Case Manager) of the Observation Unit (Observation Services)

Background

The care coordinator (case manager) assists the physician, nursing, and other personnel in the provision of value-based patient care that meets existing regulations and standards.

Objectives (Purpose)

The care coordinator (case manager) provides timely and accurate information not only to the physicians, nursing and other personnel involved in the delivery of care to patients in the observation unit (OU) and the emergency department (ED); but also to patients, families, payers, regulatory agencies, and government. The care coordinator is responsible for the coordination and integration of utilization management, screening of patients for appropriate designation or placement, facilitation of care, and discharge planning.

Policy

The following is a summary of the role of the Care Coordinator for the OU (observation status patients).

Job Description

* *Overall role:* Is responsible for screening of assigned patients based on clinical appropriateness, utilization review, monitoring length of stay (LOS), and resource usage and discharge planning

* *Specific duties:*

- Screens assigned patients for appropriate disposition including placement in the OU (observation status)

- Performs utilization review and is responsible for utilization management
- Implements discharge planning
- Utilizes clinical appropriateness criteria to screen for appropriateness of admissions and for continued stays
- Documents and communicates his or her findings
- Monitors LOS and ancillary usage of resources
- Recognizes at-risk patients and mobilizes resources to assist in their care and disposition
- Coordinates and facilitates patient care throughout the continuum from arrival in the ED, to placement in the OU (in observation status), to the patient's disposition from observation either being discharged or becoming an inpatient admission, to care following discharge
- Provides accurate and timely information to health care providers involved in the care of patients in the OU (observation status)
- Provides accurate and timely information to patients, their families, payers, regulatory agencies, and government regarding the care of patients in the OU (in observation status)
- Is knowledgeable in relevant guidelines, mandates, requirements, standards, regulations, and laws pertinent to care coordination (case management) and utilization review
- Other duties as assigned

Training/Education

- Bachelor of Science in Nursing (BSN) or Master of Science in Nursing (MSN) and/or certification in Case Management (If no certification in nursing then other appropriate relevant experience and training is acceptable)

Licensure/Certification

- Current license to practice as a nurse or other health care provider
- Certification as a case manager is preferred. If no certification in case management when starting the position, it is encouraged for the individual in this position to attain certification in case management within 2 years.

Discussion

Although not all hospitals and/or OUs are large enough or have enough observation status patients to necessitate a separate, full-time care coordinator (case manager) for the OU or for the observation status patients, this does not imply there is no role or need for the care coordinator to be involved with observation patients. There is every indication that OUs and observation status patients will be increasing in the future, so to ignore observation would be a mistake. There should be some ongoing involvement with case management and utilization review for observation. The exact mechanisms of how this is accomplished may vary based on local needs and resources. This job description is not intended to determine or mandate staffing, but is intended to delineate the multifaceted and significant aspects of this important position and highlight the many roles and responsibilities performed by case management and utilization review. Since there is a shortage of care coordinators (case managers), other relevant, appropriate training or education and work experience other than nursing (such as social work, etc.) is acceptable. Although those with a background in nursing comprise the majority of case managers, others with appropriate background, training, and work experience including social workers have functioned as and are working as case managers.

Policy approved: Date:
Policy reaffirmed: Date:

Charge Nurse for the Observation Unit

Background

The charge nurse serves as a resource for physicians, advanced practice providers, nursing staff, and other health care providers involved in the care of patients in the OU. The charge nurse is essential to maintaining the plan of care for patients in the OU. The charge nurse acts to ensure the principles of observation care: the best possible patient care achieved through patient- and family-centered, efficient processes of care delivered in a timely manner (< 24 hours).

Objectives (Purpose)

To define the position and specify the responsibilities of the charge nurse for the OU.

Policy

The following is a summary of the role of the charge nurse for the OU:

Job Description

* *Overall role:* provides direct nursing patient care, serves as a resource person for nursing and ancillary personnel, and is available to assist the physicians and advanced practice providers (midlevel providers) in the provision of care to the patients in the OU
* *Specific duties:*

- Works with the physician and the advanced practice providers in the provision of care to patients in the OU
- Serves as a resource to coworkers: nurses and ancillary personnel in the OU
- Addresses issues raised by the physicians, advanced practice providers, nurses, and ancillary personnel in the OU
- Is available to deal with patient complaints and concerns
- Assigns incoming patients to primary nurses and patient care technicians working in the OU
- Problems that occur during their clinical shift
- Deals with staffing and coverage issues that may occur
- May assist with the ordering of supplies and equipment needed in the OU
- Assists the nurse manager of the OU with clinical and administrative duties
- Other duties as assigned

Training/Education

- Bachelor of Science in Nursing (BSN) or Master of Science in Nursing (MSN)
- Training/Experience: clinical expertise in observation nursing, emergency nursing, or equivalent

Licensure/Certification

- Current state licensure as a registered nurse (RN)

Reporting Structure

- Reports to nurse manager of the OU

Additional Requirements

RN who

- has successfully completed the hospital, ED, and OU orientation;
- has experience as a primary nurse in the OU;
- knows the OU Policies and Procedures and has the ability to administer the policies and procedures in an equitable manner;
- knows the nursing and physician philosophy, the objectives and the organizational leadership of the OU, the ED and the hospital;
- knows current nursing practice;
- has demonstrated the ability to function as a team member as well as provide nursing leadership;
- promotes good public relations for the OU, the ED, and the hospital;
- maintains good communications with the medical staff, the physician director of the OU, the nurse manager of the ED, other nurse managers, and all personnel working in the OU and ED;
- exhibits the following qualities: has leadership skills, performs his or her duties in a fair and equitable fashion, maintains his or her composure under stress, exhibits good judgment, and has excellent nursing skills.

Policy approved: *Date:*
Policy reaffirmed: *Date:*

Change of Shift
Background

At change of shift, patient care is transferred to an oncoming emergency physician(s) who is then assigned to and assumes responsibility for their patients in the OU, which is then documented in the medical record. In a similar manner, there is a transfer of nursing care to the oncoming primary nurse(s) who will be assigned to and responsible for the nursing care of the OU patients.

Objectives (Purpose)

To ensure a smooth transition of care at all times including at change of shift and to maintain a

clear delineation of responsibility for patient care at all levels.

Policy

At change of shift, an appropriate hand off is done for each patient in the OU.

This should be done by the attending physician staff, the advanced practice providers, the nursing staff, as well as by any residents/fellows involved in the care of patients in the OU.

The oncoming physician, nursing staff, advanced practice providers and residents/fellows responsible for the patient will be documented in the patient's medical record.

Policy approved: *Date:*
Policy reaffirmed: *Date:*

Communication Boards for Patient Rooms
Background

It is important for patients and their families to understand the goals of the OU, which are to provide optimal patient care in a time-limited fashion (e.g. < 24 hours) and for health care providers to communicate with patients and their families.

Objectives (Purpose)

One tool for communication is the use of a communication board (e.g., a "blackboard" or "greaseboard") placed in every patient's room in the OU.

Policy

A "greaseboard" or "blackboard" will be placed in each patient's room in the OU. The board will contain the following information

Room number
Attending physician
Advanced practice provider*
Resident*
Nurse
Clinical Technician*
Phone number for the room*
Date and time patient placed in observation**
Date and time of anticipated disposition (when patient is expected to be discharged or if unable to be discharged, when he/she is to be admitted)***

* Every patient will have an attending physician and primary nurse and clinical technician assigned to him or her. In addition, there may or may not be an advanced practice provider and/or resident involved in a patient's care.

** Placing the date and time the patient is placed in observation on the board in the patient's room emphasizes the time-limited nature of the OU to everyone involved in the patient's care in addition to the patient and his or her family.

*** The date and time the patient is expected to be ready for discharge (or if needed to be admitted) is 24 hours or less after the time the patient is placed in observation.

Additional information, such as the patient's diagnosis (e.g. chest pain or asthma could be added to the communication board).

Any communication board will maintain patient confidentiality and meet the Health Insurance Portability and Accountability Act (HIPPA) and/or any other laws or regulations. For example, the communication board is within the patient's room and does not contain patient information but instead contains the health care provider information (e.g. physician and nurse) for the patient and family.

The communication board may also add another "patient safety" check, as another tool for identifying the patient's treating physician and the nurse (e.g. those caring for him or her in the unit); if there is an emergent need to contact the physician, the name is readily available to any nurse or health care provider seeing or caring for the patient.

The communication board will be updated when any changes occur, such as change of shift when there is a new primary nurse or physician assigned to the patient.

Information on the communication board will be deleted when the OU patient is discharged from the OU or is admitted as an inpatient and transported to the inpatient unit.

When a new patient is placed in a room in the OU, then the appropriate information should be entered on the communication board.

In the future, it is likely that an electronic version of the blackboard or greaseboard will be available.

Policy approved: *Date:*
Policy reaffirmed: *Date:*

Continuing (Ongoing) Care of Patients Placed in Observation Status

Background

Once the patient is placed in the OU (in observation status), after the appropriate forms have been signed, registration completed, and orientation of the patient (and family) has been done, then the initial and continuing care of the patient begins. Some of these nursing tasks may be delegated to other members of the health care team in the OU, as appropriate for their respective job descriptions.

Objectives (Purpose)

To describe the continuing care of the patient in the OU. Tasks encompassing the initial and ongoing care of the OU patient will be outlined.

Policy

The nursing plan of care should include, but is not limited to the following:

- Initial set of vital signs
- Patients will be placed on telemetry if cardiac monitoring is ordered
- Patients will be placed on pulse oximetry if continuous pulse oximetry is ordered
- Initial telemetry strip will be obtained and placed in the nursing flow sheet if the patient is on a cardiac monitor
- Initial orders will be acknowledged and completed (including a date and time)
- Initial nursing assessment and or nursing assessments will be performed, as ordered
- Procedures will be completed as ordered (e.g., placement of IVs, placement of foley catheter, placement of nasogastric tubes, venipuncture for blood samples)
- Diagnostic tests will be done as ordered, for example, ECGs will be done, and laboratory samples (blood, urine) will be obtained as per hospital policy
- Intravenous lines will be flushed to keep the IV line open as per hospital policy
- Intravenous fluids (IVF) will be administered as ordered
- Medications will be administered as ordered
- An initial patient safety and comfort evaluation will be completed

- Participation in physician and/or advanced practice provider rounds, as requested, on OU patients
- Monitoring laboratory, radiology, and other ancillary test reports and consultant notes and reporting to the responsible physician and/or advanced practice provider
- Arranges patient transport to procedures, tests, etc. as needed
- Performs standard nursing care (as outlined in other nursing policies)
- Updates the patient and family on the patient's progress
- Performs monitoring and observation of the patient, such as vital signs, neurologic checks, vascular checks, etc., as ordered
- Notifies the physician or advance practice provider of any significant changes in the patient's vital signs or condition
- Provides education for the patient and family
- Participates in discharge planning, as indicated
- Other responsibilities, as assigned
- Documents the nursing care in the nursing flow sheets, graphics, etc.

Discussion

This is not an all-inclusive list but summarizes the many important functions and responsibilities of nursing in the care of the patient in the OU.

Policy approved: Date:
Policy reaffirmed: Date:

Database for the Observation Unit

Background

A database for the OU is essential for many reasons. For patients it is important for follow-up care and referrals, coordinating care with their primary care providers and specialists and their health care insurance or plan, and providing a smooth transition of care. For the hospital it is essential in order to meet regulatory and governmental regulations and to provide information to insurers/payers. A database is also necessary for performance improvement (PI)/continuous quality improvement (CQI). A database can also be used for education and research. A database is useful as a tool to track the OU census and other trends, which can be valuable in resource utilization including staffing, budgeting, and strategic planning.

Objectives (Purpose)

To devise a useful and user friendly database that can be utilized for many purposes by appropriate individuals in order to gather information for external sources – including information required by insurers/payers, regulatory agencies, and government – and for internal use: resource utilization, budgeting, planning, education, research, and ongoing PI.

Policy

The following are some key elements in a data set for the OU:

- Patient identifiers
- Demographics: age, gender, ethnicity*
- LOS in OU
- Disposition from OU: admission to inpatient, discharge, expired, other (left against medical advice)
- Number (and percentage) of patients placed in the OU from the ED
- Number (and percentage) of patients admitted to the hospital from the OU
- Patient contact information (address, phone, etc.)**
- Insurance/payer information**
- Procedures and time for procedures**

Additional elements that are useful:

- Types of patients placed in the OU***
- Ancillary services used by OU patients: laboratory, radiology, others****
- Resources used by OU patients****
- Clinical information: final diagnosis, chief complaint, procedures, consults, radiology studies (CT scans, ultrasound, MRI, etc.), laboratory tests, significant comorbidity

The OU medical director, nurse manager, and administration will meet with the informatics department in order to set up and maintain a database for the OU that has information that can be used not only for billing/reimbursement, but also for patient care (especially for follow-up and longitudinal care), resource utilization and management, PI (involving patient quality and safety), education, and research.

Discussion

* Demographic data (such as age, gender, ethnicity) may help to define the patient population you serve so hospital programs could be tailored to serve your community.

** Needed for reimbursement/billing. Although this may seem intuitive, it is not a rare occurrence that the OU has been set up and is accepting patients yet the data capture has not been put in place at the beginning. Prospective data is ideal. Patient contact information is also needed for follow-up of various test or procedures, for example, culture results.

*** Data on the types of patients would be useful for determining what ancillary services might be needed. For example, knowing the number of chest pain patients would be useful to decide on the number of patients who need cardiac monitoring (vs. nonmonitored patients) or how many stress tests to plan for on a daily basis. The number of OU patients with "stable" gastrointestinal bleeding could be useful to determine the number of OU patients who need an endoscopy and/or colonoscopy.

**** Keeping track of "special studies" done on OU patients, such MRI or echocardiograms, would allow other departments to plan for accommodating the OU patients and keeping the LOS as short as possible.

Policy approved: *Date:*
Policy reaffirmed: *Date:*

Physician Responsibilities and Delegation of Care

Background

The physician is ultimately responsible for the patient's management in the OU.

Objectives (Purpose)

To outline the physician responsibilities for patients in the OU.

Policy

Responsibility: The management of the patient in the OU is the responsibility of the ED attending on duty. There will be clear delineation of which physician is responsible for each patient at all times. The patient's attending will be documented in the patient's medical record.

Change of Shift: Sign-in /sign-out rounds must be done at change of shift with an appropriate hand-off done for each patient. The oncoming physician responsible for the patient will be documented in the patient's medical record.

Placement in Observation/Refer to Observation: When a patient is placed in observation status or referred to observation, there must be an initial history and physical examination with a preliminary diagnosis and a plan of management for the patient while in observation; initial orders must be written and signed (this may be done electronically). The initial diagnosis, goals of management, and time frame for response (e.g., < 24 hours) should be noted in the initial history and physical examination. The medical decision making and expected clinical course should be noted. Patients will not be placed in observation without an order from the attending physician.

Ongoing Management: Whenever there is a significant change in the patient's condition, or new significant information available as a result of ongoing management, then this should be noted in a progress note and/or in the discharge note. The attending physician should be available at all times to respond promptly when warranted by changes in the patient's clinical condition.

Disposition from Observation: Prior to disposition of the patient, either when discharged or when admitted to the hospital as an inpatient, a disposition note will be done. The note should include an updated history and physical examination; the clinical course while the patient has been in observation; the results of monitoring, diagnostic testing and/or treatment while in observation; and the medical decision making, the diagnosis, and the treatment plan. The treatment plan for patients admitted as inpatients to the hospital should include the service and the attending to which the patient is being admitted. If the patient is being discharged, the medications for discharge, discharge instructions, any follow-up diagnostic testing or treatment, and the follow-up service(s) and/or physician(s) should be documented.

Advanced Practice Providers (Midlevel Practitioners): Physician assistants and/or nurse practitioners may be involved in the management of observation patients, provided an attending physician provides oversight, is readily available for consultation when necessary, and provides clinical care when needed.

575

Physicians in Training: Residents and/or fellows may be involved in the management of observation patients, provided the attending physician is providing oversight, is readily available for consultation, and provides clinical care when needed.

Policy approved: *Date:*
Policy reaffirmed: *Date:*

Disposition of Patients Placed in the Observation Unit: Admission to an Inpatient Floor from the Observation Unit

Background

In order to maintain a continuum of care for the patient, disposition from the OU requires a smooth transition of the patient from the OU to admission on an inpatient floor of the hospital.

Objectives (Purpose)

To ensure continuity of care for OU patients being admitted to an inpatient floor.

Procedure: Admission to an Inpatient Floor from the Observation Unit

- The attending physician will write an order for admission of the patient to an inpatient floor of the hospital, which is dated and timed.
- The OU RN responsible for the patient will validate that an admission order has been signed by the attending.
- The OU secretary will notify patient registration so that the patient can be assigned an inpatient bed.
- Patient registration will notify the OU RN who is caring for the patient that the bed has been assigned.
- When the inpatient bed is available, the OU RN will call report to the inpatient nursing unit.
- Prior to transport to the inpatient floor, a set of vital signs will be done. If the RN has any concerns or questions prior to transfer of the patient to the inpatient floor, he or she should contact the responsible physician in the OU.

- Prior to transfer to the floor, the usual procedures as done in the ED before transferring a patient to the inpatient floor will be done, such as collecting the patient's belongings in a hospital patient bag for transport with the patient to the floor, sending the patient's chart with the patient to the floor, and calling report to the RN on the inpatient floor who will be responsible for the patient's care when he or she is admitted. The OU RN should follow the ED policy on transferring a patient to the inpatient floor.
- If the patient is going to an Intensive Care Unit (ICU) or stepdown unit, then the RN will accompany the patient to the ICU or stepdown unit. If the patient is stable and not going to a monitored stepdown or ICU bed, then, if the physician approves, the patient care technician or hospital transport may transport the patient to the inpatient floor.
- After the patient is transferred to the inpatient floor, the OU secretary will notify housekeeping of the patient's inpatient admission and the need to clean the patient's room, and patient registration so they are aware of the bed availability.*

* If there is no OU secretary, then the ED secretary who is covering the OU will notify housekeeping and patient registration. If there is no OU secretary or other secretarial support staff covering the OU, then the OU RN will notify housekeeping and patient registration.

Policy approved: *Date:*
Policy reaffirmed: *Date:*

Disposition of Patients Placed in the Observation Unit: Discharge from the Observation Unit

Background

In order to maintain a continuum of care for the patient, disposition from the OU requires a smooth transition of the patient from the OU to admission on an inpatient floor of the hospital; or for patients discharged from the OU, a coordinated postdischarge plan of care. A coordinated disposition plan of care generally includes a discharge plan including patient instructions and medications, if needed, as well as follow-up appointment and/or additional outpatient testing and procedures, as indicated.

Objectives (Purpose)

To ensure appropriate discharge and follow-up for OU patients.

Procedure: Discharge from Observation Status

Physician Responsibilities

- The attending physician is responsible for the formulation of a *coordinated discharge plan* that includes: *discharge instructions* for the patient, *medications/prescriptions* if needed, any *additional tests or procedures* to be done as an outpatient, and *follow-up* with physicians and other health care providers or clinics if necessary.*

The attending physician will write a *discharge order*, which is dated and timed.* Nursing Responsibilities

- The primary RN responsible for the patient will validate that a discharge order has been signed by the attending.
- The RN will confirm and review with the patient and/or family, as appropriate, the patient's discharge instructions, home going medications, prescriptions, wound care or other therapy, additional outpatient tests or procedures, and follow-up.

Care Coordination (Case Management)/ Social Work

- Care coordination (case management) or social work, if available, will assist with the discharge planning, which may or may not include placement, transportation, and outpatient services including home health care, if needed.

Other Health Care Providers

- The pharmacist, if available, may review the medications with the patient and his or her family, if indicated, and reconcile any medications prior to the patient's discharge.**
- Respiratory therapy, if available, may review the use of home-going respiratory medications or treatments, including inhalers, spacers, nebulized treatments, etc.**
- The dietician, if available, may review any dietary recommendations including

special diets as recommended by the physician.**

- After the patient is discharged, the OU secretary will notify housekeeping of the patient's discharge and the need to clean the patient's room and patient registration so they are aware of the bed availability.

Discussion

* Depending on the individual resources, some of these responsibilities may be delegated to an advance practice provider and/or a fellow/resident in training, if appropriate. In our institution, orders need to be countersigned and patient management sanctioned by an attending physician. Administrative/secretarial personnel and/or nursing may assist in the set-up and scheduling of the follow-up tests, procedures, and appointments. Input from nursing, social work, care coordination (case management), and others may be invaluable in developing a coordinated discharge plan for patients. With the advent of accountability care organizations (see Chapter 20 on ACOs) this is becoming increasingly important.

** Not all institutions have the resources, such as a pharmacist, respiratory therapist, or dietician who are available to assist in patient /family education. However, there does appear to be a growing trend to include a multidisciplinary team to assist in the longitudinal care of the patient.

Past experience, for example, our experience with our heart failure patients, has demonstrated the value of such teaching with videos, pamphlets, and other educational tools, which, in this example, discussed ways to limit a patient's salt intake, thereby, decreasing the risk of an exacerbation of the heart failure. Similarly, the education of asthmatics or COPD patients in the OU by respiratory therapy in how to take their medications is another example of using the OU as "a teachable moment" in order to improve patient outcomes and decrease readmissions.

Policy approved: Date:

Policy reaffirmed: Date:

Nursing Documentation for Patients Placed in the Observation Unit

Background

Documentation provides a description of the ongoing care and plan of management that is being provided to patients and details what is occurring over time regarding any patient in the OU. Such documentation is essential for communication of the patient's plan of care.

Objectives (Purpose)

To outline the key elements of the documentation for patients in the OU (in observation status).

Policy

The following documentation should be noted in the patient's medical record by nursing or other appropriate personnel.*

1. The date and time the patient was placed in the OU (or observation status) and the attending OU physician as indicated by the dated and timed physician's order.
2. In addition to the responsible attending physician, and if appropriate, the advanced practice provider(s) and/or resident(s) involved in the patient's care.**
3. A brief summary of the patient's initial or provisional diagnosis, and the overall plan for observation.***
4. The date and time that the initial orders and all additional orders are acknowledged by the RN.
5. The initial set of vital signs when the patient is placed in observation status and all subsequent vital signs including a set of vital signs prior to the patient's disposition from the OU.
6. When the patient is seen by the attending physician, resident/fellow, advanced practice clinician, or a consultant, the date and time should be noted as well the name(s) of the individual(s) seeing the patient and their medical specialty or service.
7. When a patient has a diagnostic or therapeutic procedure, the specific procedure or treatment with the date and time.
8. If the patient leaves the OU for any reason including diagnostic studies and/or treatment – such as, stress test, esophagogastroduodenoscopy, EEG, CT scan, MRI, or interventional radiology procedure – the procedure or test, along with the date and time the patient leaves the OU and the date and time the patient returns to the OU, should be noted.****

9. Any relevant, significant phone calls or other communication to or from physicians or other health care providers involved in the patient's care.
10. Whenever there is a significant change in the vital signs or the patient's condition, the physician (and/or advanced practice provider) should be notified and this should be recorded in the chart.
11. Any other significant and/or relevant occurrences that may affect the patient's outcome or plan of care.
12. The date and time of the patient's disposition either discharge from the OU or admission to an inpatient service.*
13. The follow-up service(s) and/or physician(s) or clinic(s) for when patients are discharged from the unit, and any follow-up tests or treatments and discharge medications.*****
14. The service and physician the patient is being admitted to as an inpatient.*****

Discussion

Nursing documentation begins when the patient is placed in observation status. (The date and time that the patient is placed in observation status is indicated by the dated and timed physician's order.)

* Some of the information may be documented by other appropriate personnel. For example, the technicians can obtain and record vital signs. Registration may be responsible for documenting the attending physician for the OU patient, the attending physician for the OU patient who is admitted as an inpatient, and the times the patient is placed in observation, etc.

** As part of the education and training residents/fellows may be involved in the care of a patient(s) in the OU. Advanced practice providers as part of their job description and professional duties also may be involved in the care of OU patients and this should be duly noted.

*** The brief summary or notation of the patient's initial or provisional diagnosis and the overall plan for observation may include the essentials of the report given by the ED nurse prior to transferring the patient to the OU. This is a method of informing everyone of the plan of care and helps ensure that there are specific diagnostics and therapeutic aims for each patient placed in observation. This might be as simple is follows: 45-year-old male with chest pain placed in observation by Dr. Smith at 2100 hours on Monday the 10th for rule out and stress test, or 16-year-old asthmatic placed in observation by Dr. Jones at 1100 hours on Saturday the 12th to receive aerosols and steroids in the OU. The initial history, physical examination, clinical course in the ED, provisional diagnosis and plan as detailed in the physician or advanced practice provider's note could also serve as the summary of the patient's initial or provisional diagnosis and the overall plan of care while the patient is in observation.

The attending physician and other health care providers including nursing who are caring for the patient should also be noted on the "communication board" in the patient's room. This is a good communication tool and is discussed in another administrative policy.

**** For billing and reimbursement, the time patients are not in the OU (as for a stress test, etc.) should be subtracted from what is billed for their care as part of the hospital charges. Generally, the government and other payers will accept an average time for a given procedure instead of the exact time for a given patient. However, charting this information (i.e., the time the patient is away from and returns to the OU) is useful as part of the chart, which is a medical-legal document.

***** This may be noted in the physician documentation and/or by registration; if so, nursing may not need separate duplicate documentation but should have this information so it can be included in patient/family education prior to the patient's disposition from the OU.

Policy approved: *Date:*
Policy reaffirmed: *Date:*

Physician Documentation for Observation Unit Patients

Background

Patient care depends on a careful evaluation and plan of care based upon a history, physical examination, and appropriate testing and/or therapy, as well as communication of that plan to others involved in that patient's care.

Objectives (Purpose)

To establish physician documentation guidelines for patients in the OU.

Policy

Placement in Observation/Refer to Observation

When a patient is placed in observation status or referred to observation, there must be an initial history and physical examination with a preliminary diagnosis and a plan of management for the patient while the patient is in observation, and initial orders must be written and signed (this may be done electronically).

If a resident/ fellow or advanced practice provider is involved in the patient's care, the attending physician must review and countersign the initial note and the orders.

The initial note should include the following components: history of present illness, allergies, medications, review of systems, past medical history, social history, family history, provisional or initial diagnosis, goals of management, specific plan of monitoring/diagnostic evaluation/treatment, and time frame for response (e.g., < 24 hours). The medical decision making and expected clinical course should be noted.

Ongoing Evaluation

Whenever there is a significant change in the patient's condition, or new significant information available as a result of ongoing management, then this should be noted in a progress note and/or in the discharge note.

Progress notes should be done at regular intervals when indicated.

This may be done electronically.

If a resident/ fellow or advanced care practitioner is involved in the patient's care, the attending physician must review and countersign the progress notes.

Disposition from Observation

Prior to disposition of the patient, either when discharged or when admitted to the hospital as an inpatient, a disposition note will be done. The note should include an updated history and physical examination; the clinical course while the patient has been in observation; the results of monitoring, diagnostic testing, and/or treatment given while in the OU; the medical decision making, the final diagnosis, and the treatment plan. The treatment plan for patients admitted as inpatients to the hospital should include the attending and service to which the patient is being admitted. If the patient is being discharged, the medications for discharge, discharge instructions, any follow-up diagnostic testing or treatment, and the follow-up service and/or physician should be documented.

This may be done electronically. If a resident/fellow or advanced practice provider is involved in the patient's care, the attending physician must review and countersign the disposition note and the discharge or admission to inpatient service orders.

Policy approved: Date:
Policy reaffirmed: Date:

Patients with Infectious Diseases: Placement in the Observation Unit

Background

Patients with various infectious diseases may be placed in the OU.[1] Patients with infectious diseases belong to two groups: those with a communicable or contagious disease and those with a noncommunicable or noncontagious disease. Communicable or contagious diseases are transmitted by direct contact, droplet spread, or contaminated fomites. Examples of communicable diseases include HIV, herpes, tuberculosis, hepatitis, pertussis, various infectious diarrhea/gastroenteritis (rotavirus, Norwalk virus, salmonella, etc.), most respiratory infections (e.g., various pneumonia, bronchitis, bronchiolitis), and acute pharyngitis (strep pharyngitis, mononucleosis, viral, etc.). Examples of infections that are not communicable or not contagious would be cellulitis, urinary tract infection, or lymphangitis. Patients with any communicable or contagious disease should have appropriate infection control measures to prevent the spread of communicable diseases.

Purposes (Objectives)

To allow patients with various infectious disease including communicable or contagious diseases to be placed in the OU, provided that they meet other appropriate criteria for the OU (refer to Administrative Policies on "Patient Criteria for Placement in the Observation Unit"), while ensuring appropriate infection control to avoid the spread of contagious disease.

Policy

Patients with infections may be placed in the OU provided they are appropriate for placement in the observation unit based on clinical criteria (see other administrative policies on "Patient Criteria for Placement in the Observation Unit") and applicable infection control policies. Specific infection control policies are modeled after the Center for Disease Control (CDC) guidelines.[2] Patients with infections who are excluded from the OU are (1) those with a communicable disease caused by a newly recognized/emergent and/or epidemiologically important pathogen and/or (2) those needing a negative pressure room.

Discussion

After chest pain/cardiac, the most common conditions placed in an OU are gastrointestinal (GI)/abdominal and asthma/respiratory and dehydration (which is often due to poor oral intake often occurring with respiratory illnesses and/or increased fluid loss generally found with gastrointestinal complaints: nausea/vomiting/diarrhea). These two categories in the top three of common OU conditions generally improve within ≤ 24 hours, but may need appropriate infection control measures to prevent the spread of infectious respiratory or gastrointestinal diseases.

This policy is intended to answer the question "Can the following patient with an infection be placed in the OU?" The answer is almost always yes if other observation patient criteria are met, infection control policy is followed, and the contagious patients are placed in a private room.

The same infection control policies for inpatients apply to the OU patients and entail various methods such as hand hygiene, gloves, gown, mask, and private room; these should follow the CDC standard precautions, contact precautions, droplet precautions, and airborne precautions.

There are only a few exceptions to the placement of patients with infections in the OU. The exceptions include newly recognized/emergent and/or epidemiologically important pathogens, such as SARS. Any patient needing a negative pressure room, such as a patient with tuberculosis, would be excluded since negative pressure rooms are quite expensive and generally not included as part of the design of an OU. (See Chapter 5 on Design) Moreover, such patients would be excluded from observation because they would be more severely ill and unlikely to be discharged from the OU within 24 hours (as the case with an active tuberculosis patient).

Of course, patients who are critically ill or unlikely to improve and be discharged within 24 hours or less are not candidates for the OU, such as patients with sepsis or shock.

Other patients with a communicable or contagious disease, such as those with acute pharyngitis or a peritonsilar abscess or a patient with pneumonia (who is not significantly hypoxic, e.g., pulse oxygen saturation is $\geq 90\%$) may be appropriate for the OU if proper infection control practices are followed. Patients with infections that are not contagious, such as pyelonephritis or cellulitis, may also be appropriate for the OU.

References

1. Mace SE, Graff L, Mikhail M, et al. A national survey of observation units in the United States. *Am J Emerg Med* 2002; 21:529–533.

2. CDC Guideline for Isolation Precautions: www.cdc.gov/hicpac/2007IP/ 2007isolationPrecautions.html. Siegel JD, Rhinehart E, Jackson M, Chiarello L, and the Healthcare Infection Control Practices Advisory Committee, 2007 Guideline for Isolation Precautions: Preventing Transmission of Infectious Agents in Healthcare Settings http://www.cdc.gov/ncidod/dhqp/pdf/isolation2007.pdf and http://quinarie.com/Cdc_Isolation_ Appendix_A_Pdf (Accessed April 2016)

3. See also chapters on Infections (Chapter 44 Skin and Soft Tissue Infections, Chapter 49 Pyelonephritis/Acute Cystitis), Pulmonary (Chapter 29 Community Acquired Pneumonia) and Gastrointestinal (Chapter 47 Dehydration, Gastroenteritis, and Vomiting) in this textbook.

Policy approved: *Date:*
Policy reaffirmed: *Date:*

Medical Director of the Observation Unit

Background

In order for the OU to be successful, there needs to be a physician director in charge of the OU, who serves as the administrative and clinical leader of the unit.

Objectives (Purpose)

The medical director of the OU is a physician who provides leadership for the OU. The physician medical director oversees the provision of care for patients in observation status and works closely with the nurse manager of the OU. He or she has a dual role and provides both clinical oversight of patients in the OU and has administrative responsibility for the OU.

Policy

The following is a summary of the role of the Medical Director of the OU.

Job Description

* Overall role: Provides medical direction for the OU

- Dual function: both clinical and administrative responsibilities

* Specific duties: clinical

- Oversees the provision of patient care in the OU
- Provides physician direction for the OU
- Works clinical shifts in the OU
- Reviews patient care delivered in the OU and may refer to quality management, patient safety, peer review or other appropriate venue for further input and discussion
- If not working clinically in the OU, may "round" with the physician(s), advanced practice provider(s), nursing and ancillary personnel working in/covering the OU in order to maintain a direct presence in the OU
- Identifies issues or problems, addresses any concerns and answers questions

* Specific duties: administrative

- Works with the nurse manager of the OU to ensure the efficient operation of the OU
- Serves as a resource for administration on issues relevant to the OU
- Refers to nursing management, when indicated (e.g., observation nurse manager and/or other nursing personnel, as appropriate), any issues specific to nursing care or nursing personnel
- Chairs the OU meetings including setting the agenda, studying the topics, researching agenda items, and preparing a summary of agenda items
- Writes clinical guidelines, protocols, policies, procedures, and order sets
- Reports on metrics and benchmarks for the OU

- Reports to hospital administration
* Other Responsibilities: as assigned

Training/Education

- Doctor of Medicine degree (MD) or Doctor of Osteopathic Medicine (DO) degree
- Completion of approved residency

Licensure/Certification

- Current license to practice medicine
- Board certification in emergency medicine (Note: If the OU is managed by the hospitalists, then board certification in internal medicine or family practice if an adult OU, or board certification in pediatrics if a pediatric OU)

Additional Qualifications

- Clinical experience in observation medicine preferred
- Administrative experience preferred
- Demonstrated leadership ability
- Knows current medical practice
- Knows and supports the medical philosophy, the objectives/goals of the hospital, the ED and the OU
- Knows the OU Policies, Procedures and Guidelines and has the ability to administer the policies and procedures in an equitable manner
- Maintains good communications with the medical staff, the nurse manager of the ED, and other nursing units, other managers, and personnel working in the OU and the ED
- Promotes good public relations for the OU, the ED, and the hospital
- Exhibits the following qualities: has leadership skills, performs his or her duties in a fair and equitable manner, works well under stress and maintains his or her composure under stress, and exhibits good judgment
- Works with the nurse manager of the OU in order to maintain the mission of the OU and the efficient daily functioning of the OU

Discussion

Reporting structure may vary depending on the specific institution. If under the ED, may report to the Director of the ED; or if under the hospitalists, may report to the Department of Internal Medicine; or may report directly to hospital administration as a separate division or department.

The physician medical director of the OU should have administrative time to oversee the provision of medical care in the OU and to maintain the day-to-day functioning of the OU in conjunction with the nurse manager of the OU.[1] The physician medical director of the OU should be able to treat patients in the OU, but needs protected time to deal with the many clinical and administrative functions. The physician medical director and the nurse manager of the OU the work closely together to maintain the goals of observation medicine – which is focused on cost-effective, quality patient care delivered in a relatively short time frame – and together foster a climate for the best possible patient care in the OU.

Reference

1. Mace SE, Graff L, Mikhail M, et al. A national survey of observation units in the United States. *Am J Emerg Med* 2003; 21: 529–533.

Policy approved: Date:
Policy reaffirmed: Date:

Metrics
Background

A metric is any measurement. Metrics can refer to patient care, operational, or administrative issues. There may be overlap between clinical, operational, and administrative metrics, as well as between quality indicators and metrics since quality indicators can be used as metrics.* Metrics can refer to patient care directly or indirectly. The recent use of core measures, sometimes linked to performance ("pay for performance"), may be associated directly or indirectly to patient care and performance. Core measures may also be considered as metrics.** Metrics can be used in the PI or quality improvement (QI) process and by administration to determine staffing, equipment, supplies, and other needs for the OU and to assist in the budgetary process. Metrics may be clinically focused, operational, administrative, or a combination and may be used to determine any trends in the OU that may be occurring over time.

Objectives (Purpose)

The goal of this policy is to delineate metrics or measures that can be used for many purposes: clinical for PI to evaluate patient care, operational to assess the processes in the delivery of care, and administrative to plan for use of resources including staffing, supplies, and equipment. Clinical indicators emphasize metrics dealing with direct patient care, while other metrics may deal with more of the operational and administrative aspects, although there is overlap. Operational, administrative, and clinical metrics are the focus of this policy.

Policy

The following are three core administrative metrics for the OU:

- Number (and percentage) of ED patients placed in the OU***
- Number (and percentage) of patients admitted to the hospital from the OU****
- LOS in the OU****
- Additional administrative metrics for the OU are

Types of patients placed in the OU*****

Ancillary services used by patients*****

Resources used by OU patients*****

Time (hour) of day of patient placement in and discharge from the OU (OU bed occupancy hourly rate)*****

Discussion

Some prefer to separate the QI indicators from metrics since the metrics as outlined earlier tend to be used more for planning staffing needs and resources utilization, which can be considered more "operational" or "administrative" than the QI indicators, which tend to measure clinical outcomes. However, others may decide to put all the metrics and clinical indicators together.

Quality indicators or clinical metrics are further discussed in Chapter 9 on Metrics and Performance Improvement.

Demographic data (such age, gender, and ethnicity) may help to define the patient population you serve so hospital programs could be tailored to serve your community. Insurance data may be useful in determining who needs referrals and to what physicians or group for follow-up.

Following trends may be useful in planning. For example, an increasing ED volume and a growing ED census might suggest the need for additional observation beds.

* An example of a "clinical" metric could be the rule-in-rate for the OU. The rule in rate for OU patients according to the literature is 6.9%.[1] Knowing this national average and allowing for some institutional variation, a threshold or benchmark rule in rate of 10% might be selected as a quality indicator with high rule in rates suggesting that patients with too many risk factors are placed in observation (and maybe should have been admitted as inpatients directly from the ED instead of to the OU) and conversely, a very low rule in rate of say 2% might indicate that that very low risk patients are being placed in observation. Either a very high or very low comparative rule in rate suggests that the risk stratification of chest pain patients should be evaluated. This could be used as a clinical performance indicator or benchmark in the PI process. Since this 10% quality indicator is a measurement, it is also a "metric."

** The length of time patients are in the ED has been proposed as a core metric. This can be considered an "operational" metric. Although this measure, LOS, is affected by what happens to the patient in the ED and the provision of care, this is a somewhat circuitous or indirect measure of the quality of patient care. LOS in the ED or in the OU is a common operational metric. Having an OU decreases the ED LOS (see Chapter 80 on the Evidence Basis for Observation Care in Adults). The national average of 15.7 hours LOS in the OU is often used as an operational benchmark.[2]

*** The number or percentage of ED patients placed in the OU could be an administrative metric that may be used to determine the number of observation beds needed for a given ED patient volume or census.

In general, the number of patients or percentage of ED patients that could be placed in observation status depends on the patients' age. For adults seen in the ED, about 10% of all adult ED patients would be likely candidates for the OU. Thus, if the daily ED census is 200, then 10% of 200 or 20 patients a day would be eligible for the management in the OU.

The percentage is different for pediatric patients and may vary depending on whether the setting is a free-standing children's hospital ED or a general ED where both adult and pediatric patients are seen. For a children's hospital, about 5% of infants and children seen in the ED can be placed in an OU. (See pediatric Chapter 53.) For the general ED, the percentage may be lower in the range of 2–3%. This may reflect the tendency for referrals of sicker pediatric patients to the children's hospital ED from other institutions as well as a tendency for pre-hospital care providers and Emergency Medical Services by protocol to selectively refer sicker patients to the children's hospital.

Early data from our institution showed a rate of pediatric inpatient admissions from our OU, about 16%, which was less than our admission rate for adult OU patients at about 20%, but higher than reported for pediatric admissions at most other institutions. This likely reflects our tertiary or quaternary referral status with a high acuity of our patients, including pediatric and adult patients, as well as the shortage of pediatric inpatient beds at the time. More recently, our rate of pediatric admissions has decreased since opening additional pediatric inpatient beds.

These percentages are external benchmarks and the pattern is probably more important than a single number and each institution should follow its own numbers and trends.

Pediatric observation units, whether at a children's hospital or in a community or non-children's hospital setting that cares for children, are a valuable resource just like adult OUs. Indeed, there may be some advantages to avoiding a transfer to a tertiary care children's hospital and keeping a hospitalized child in his or her own community for the child, family, community hospital, and tertiary care facility provided there are adequate resources including qualified pediatricians and/or family practitioners who can care for such children. Pediatric census also reflects a much greater seasonal variation than adults, likely due to the greater incidence of acute infectious illnesses (e.g., bronchiolitis, croup, and gastroenteritis) in children and infants.

**** The general rule for admissions to the hospital from the OU is about 18–20% with 80–82% of OU patients being discharged.[2,3]

***** Types of patients would be useful for determining what ancillary services might be needed. For example, the number of chest pain patients would be useful to decide on the number of stress tests to plan for on a daily basis. The number of OU patients with "stable" gastrointestinal bleeding could be useful to determine the number of OU patients who need an endoscopy and/or colonoscopy.

The hourly or daily OU bed occupancy rate might determine if post procedure patients could be placed in the OU in the early afternoon and discharged from the OU before the main influx of ED patients into the OU occurs in the late afternoon or early evening; it might also be used to plan nursing staffing.

References

1. Graff LG, Dallara J, Ross MA, et al. Impact on the care of the emergency department chest pain patient evaluation registry (CHEPER) study. *Amer J Card* 1997; 80(5): 563–568.

2. Mace SE, Graff L, Mikhail M, et al. A national survey of observation units in the United States. *Am J Emerg Med* 2003; 21: 529–533.

3. Wiler JL, Ross MA, Ginde AA. National study of emergency department observation services. *Acad Emerg Med* 2011; 18: 959–965.

Policy approved: Date:
Policy reaffirmed: Date:

Advanced Practice Providers in the Observation Unit

Background

The scope of practice for advanced practice providers (also referred to as advanced practice clinicians or midlevel providers): physician assistants and nurse practitioners) is defined by state regulations and hospital policy.

Objectives (Purpose)

Advanced practice providers: physician assistants and nurse practitioners may be involved in the management of observation patients, provided an attending physician is readily available for consultation and to provide clinical direction and oversight when necessary and in accordance with their scope of practice.

Policy

Advanced practice providers: physician assistants and nurse practitioners can be employed to provide patient care for OU patients.

There is an emergency physician attending on duty at all times (24 hours a day, 7 days a week, 365 days a year) who is available on site to provide consultation and direct assistance to the advanced practice providers who are working in the OU whenever necessary. The medical director of the OU is also available to provide consultation and assistance.

Discussion

According to the literature, a national survey reported that 21.4% of OU in the United States used midlevel providers.[1] In the United States at present, the reimbursement for midlevel providers, either in the ED or in the OU, is 85% of that for the physician.[2] (See Chapter 1 Clinical Issues)

References

1. Mace SE, Graff L, Mikhail M, et al. A national survey of observation units in the United States. *Am J Emerg Med* 2003; 21: 529–533.

2. Granovsky M. Personal communication (7/10/2016) (see also Financial Section: Reimbursement Chapters)

Relevant Policies

See Policy on Physician Delegation.
Policy approved: *Date:*
Policy reaffirmed: *Date:*

Mission Statement
Background

The goal of the OU is to allow the physician the ability to diagnose and treat selected appropriate ED patients over a slightly longer time frame than would otherwise be possible.

There are many advantages of an OU. These include but are not limited to: a decrease in inpatient admissions, a shorter patient LOS for patients admitted to the hospital from the OU (compared to patients admitted directly from the ED), improved ED patient flow with a shorter ED turn around time and shorter ED LOS, greater patient/family satisfaction, better risk management, and the ability to provide a concise efficient diagnostic evaluation and treatment in a caring, pleasant, patient/family-centered environment at a lower cost.

Objectives (Purpose)

The purpose of the OU is to improve patient outcomes by providing high quality, cost-effective patient care.

Policy

The existence of the OU provides for the longitudinal monitoring, assessment, and management of the patient, allowing for a more specific diagnosis, additional treatment, more cost-effective and better patient care with improved patient outcomes.

Discussion

If I had to select only one administrative policy, it would be the mission statement since this gives the purpose or reason for observation medicine or the why of observation medicine.
Policy approved: *Date:*
Policy reaffirmed: *Date:*

Nurse Manager of the Observation Unit
Background

In order for the OU to be successful, there needs to be a nurse manager responsible who manages the practice of nursing and the delivery of nursing care in the OU.

Objectives (Purpose)

The nurse manager of the OU provides nursing management for the OU. The nurse manager works closely with the physician medical director of the unit. He or she provides clinical and administrative oversight for the practice of nursing and nursing care in the OU.

Policy
Job Description

* Overall role: Provides clinical and administrative nursing direction for the OU

- Dual function: both clinical and administrative responsibilities for nursing care in the OU

** Specific duties

- Oversees the provision of nursing care in the OU
- Provides nursing direction for the OU
- Ensures that nursing practice standards are maintained
- Collaborates with other departments to maintain nursing standards of care and to maintain the efficient delivery of quality patient care for OU patients
- Identifies and resolves problems or issues related to the OU

- Refers to the physician medical director of the OU any problems or issues related to the physician care of patients
- Works to meet appropriate regulations relevant to the including (but not limited to) Joint Commission (Joint Commission on the Accreditation of Health Care Organizations [JCAHO]), federal, state, and local regulations
- Deals with operational aspects of the OU that pertain to nursing including staffing, equipment, supplies, and other resources
- Is the supervisor for non-physician/non-midlevel personnel who work in the OU including nurses, nursing assistants, patient care technicians, secretarial personnel, and others
- In his or her capacity as supervisor of non-physician/non-midlevel provider personnel in the OU, evaluates performance, assists human resources in recruitment and hiring of new employees and termination of employees, and maintains the scheduling of employees
- Develops a budget for the OU
- Other responsibilities as assigned by hospital administration

Training/Education

- Bachelor of Science in Nursing (BSN) or Master of Science in Nursing (MSN)
- Training/Experience: clinical expertise in observation nursing, emergency nursing, or equivalent

Licensure/Certification

- Current state licensure as a RN

Reporting Structure

- Reports to hospital nursing administration and to physician medical director of OU

Additional Qualifications

- Minimum of 5 years clinical nursing experience preferred
- Minimum of 2 years nursing management experience preferred
- Clinical and/or administrative experience in OU nursing preferred
- Demonstrated leadership ability
- Knows current nursing practice

- Knows and supports the nursing and physician philosophy, and the objectives/goals of the hospital, the ED, and the OU
- Knows the OU Policies, Procedures and Guidelines and has the ability to administer the policies and procedures in an equitable manner
- Maintains good communications with the medical staff, the nurse manager of the ED and other nursing units, other managers, and personnel working in the OU and the ED
- Promotes good public relations for the OU, the ED, and the hospital
- Exhibits the following qualities: has leadership skills, performs his or her duties in a fair and equitable manner, works well under stress and maintains his or her composure under stress, and exhibits good judgment
- Works with the physician medical director of the OU in order to maintain the mission of the OU and the efficient daily functioning of the OU

Discussion

The nurse manager should have administrative time to maintain the day-to-day functioning of the OU, especially in terms of staffing the unit, equipment, supplies, etc. The nurse manager should be able to function as a charge nurse and primary nurse in the OU, but needs protected time to deal with the many administrative functions. The nurse manager of the OU and the physician medical director work closely together to maintain the goals of observation medicine – which is focused on cost-effective, quality patient care delivered in a relatively short time frame – and together foster a climate for the best possible patient care in the OU.

Policy approved: *Date:*
Policy reaffirmed: *Date:*

Nursing Scope of Patient Care (Nursing Services Provided to Patients in the Observation Unit)

Background

The purpose of the OU is to provide monitoring, diagnostic evaluation and treatment for ED patients with various diseases and conditions. To accomplish these goals, patients are monitored and various diagnostic and therapeutic services are provided based on the clinical situation.

Objectives (Purpose)

In addition to being monitored or "observed," patients in the OU generally undergo a wide variety of diagnostic and therapeutic procedures in order to arrive at a disposition within a short, limited time frame, usually < 24 hours. The provision of nursing care and nursing services as ordered by a physician is integral to achieving this goal.

Policy

The following encompasses some of the many nursing services and nursing care provided to patients in the OU. This is not an all-inclusive list but gives some of the common elements of nursing practice grouped according to observation/monitoring, diagnostics, and therapy as ordered by a physician in addition to "standard" or "routine" nursing care. In some instances, individual tasks may be delegated to other personnel, as appropriate to their scope of practice. When nursing care or nursing services are provided this should be documented in the medical record. Some of the nursing care and services include the following:

Standard Nursing Care

- Availability for "rounds" and other discussion with the physician
- Education of patient/family
- Notify the physician of any changes in the patient's condition including abnormal vital signs
- Notify the physician of the results of various consults, significant tests or evaluations including laboratory tests, radiology studies, and procedures: stress tests, colonoscopy, esophagogastroduodenoscopy, echocardiograms, and other studies
- Provision of meals/nutrition
- Routine hygiene
- Social services
- Transport of patients to other diagnostic and treatment areas (such as radiology, stress testing, endoscopy, etc.)
- Wound care

Monitoring/Observation

- Episodic noninvasive hemodynamic monitoring: blood pressure, heart rate or pulse, respirations, pulse oxygen saturation
- Continuous noninvasive hemodynamic monitoring of vital signs: heart rate, respirations, blood pressure, pulse oxygen saturation
- Continuous monitoring of rhythm: electrocardiogram monitor strips
- Monitoring of vital signs including temperature, heart rate, respiratory rate, blood pressure, and pulse oximetry
- Neurologic checks: alertness, orientation, motor, sensory, pupils, speech, and gait (as indicated)
- Respiratory checks: respiratory rate, auscultation, work of breathing, oxygen saturation
- Vascular checks of extremities: skin color, temperature, pulses, motor, and sensory

Diagnostic

- I and O: input and output
- Obtain urine samples
- Obtain cultures
- Obtain ECGs

Procedures

- Obtain blood: draw blood samples from peripheral (venipuncture) or central lines
- Placement of foley catheter
- Placement of nasogastric (or orogastric tubes)
- Start peripheral intravenous lines

Therapeutic:

- Administer aerosolized medications (respiratory treatments)
- Administer electrolytes: potassium, calcium, magnesium, etc.
- Administer IVF
- Administer intravenous medications
- Administer oral medications
- Administer intramuscular medications
- Administer subcutaneous medications
- Administer topical medications

Discussion

Patients should not be merely placed in observation, but should be undergoing active monitoring, diagnostic evaluation, and treatment in the OU or while in observation status. As this extensive list of services and care provided indicates, patients are not merely placed in observation, but are monitored ("observed"), and undergo diagnostic and/or therapeutic activities. This is why many years ago we created the term "clinical decision unit" or CDU to emphasize the comprehensive patient management activities that are occurring and that the goal is to determine in a short-time frame (< 24 hours) the disposition of the patient, whether to be admitted to an inpatient service or discharged.

I have been quoted "Although I am the Medical Director of the Observation Unit, the nurses actually run the unit" in the sense that the nurses are continually with the patient(s), monitoring them and are making sure that all the tests and treatments are being done and reporting back to physician the results. They truly act as our agents on behalf of the patients and their families.

Policy approved: Date:
Policy reaffirmed: Date:

Nursing Responsibilities
Background
The OU nursing staff is key to implementing each OU patient's plan of care.

Objectives (Purpose)
To outline the nursing responsibilities performed daily

Policy
Patient Care
- Perform nursing assessment(s) to include at a minimum: initial nursing assessment for patients placed in the OU upon their arrival in OU, disposition nursing assessment (for patients just prior to discharge or prior to inpatient admission), and ongoing nursing assessments
- Obtain vital signs (including pulse oximetry) and pain scales, if appropriate of patients upon arrival to the OU, during their stay in the OU, and prior to disposition of patients from the OU
- Monitoring of patients in the OU including vital signs, pain scales, telemetry (if the patient is on a cardiac monitor), procedures, and therapy
- Assess patients for safety risks including falls
- Nursing report: takes report from ED nursing staff on new patients placed in the OU, gives report to inpatient nursing on OU patients who are admitted to the hospital or to other services, such as catheterization lab or operating room, as indicated
- When a primary nurse for a given OU patient, gives report to another nurse who will serve temporarily as primary nurse for that patient and gives report to oncoming primary nurse (s) at change of shift
- Assess patients for comfort and nutrition
- Offer meals and snacks to patients based on the diet ordered, assuming patients are not NPO
- Offer morning care, which includes assistance with bathing, as appropriate
- Restocking of supplies for equipment carts, bedside carts, linen carts, cupboards, etc.
- Acknowledge and complete physician orders:

  - Place patients on telemetry if cardiac monitoring is ordered
  - Place patients on pulse oximetry if continuous pulse oxygen saturation is ordered
  - Complete procedures as ordered: for example, respiratory treatments, placement of foley catheters and nasogastric tubes
  - Complete tests as ordered: for example, draw blood samples for laboratory tests, obtain 12-lead ECGs
  - Administer medications as ordered and documents in the medicine administration record
  - Administer IVF as ordered and documents in the medicine administration record
  - Flush the peripheral IV keep vein open (KVO) line with normal saline as per the hospital policy

- Monitor the patient and notifies the physician or advanced practice provider of any significant changes or concerns
- Monitor laboratory, radiology, and other ancillary test reports and consultant evaluations/notes and report to the physician or advanced practice provider any significant findings*

- Assess the patient and request additional orders, if indicated
- Participate in rounds with the physicians or advanced practice providers on the observation medicine patients and/or update them on the patient's progress as requested by the physician or advanced practice provider

Documentation

- Document patient care: vital signs, telemetry strips (if the patient is on a cardiac monitor), pain scales, intake and output, medications and IV therapy (see nursing documentation policy)**

Discussion

Currently, we do not have physicians or advanced practice providers stationed solely in the OU on all shifts (specifically late evenings and nights) so the primary nurses are responsible for reviewing reports on their patients in the OU and reporting to the covering physician any significant findings. For example, the primary nurses will look at all laboratory tests, radiology reports, cardiology reports (stress tests, echocardiograms) and other ancillary test reports (such as EEG) and notify the physician in the ED to let him or her know that the tests results are back for the patient. If there are positive cardiac enzymes, the primary nurse immediately notifies the OU attending and/or the advanced practice provider (during the day shift) and in the evening or night shifts the emergency physician who is covering, who then has the unit secretary page cardiology for a stat consult. We have a physician or advanced practice provider assigned solely to the OU during the day shift but on other shifts (evenings and nights) the respective emergency physician(s) "covers" the OU. This is probably good nursing practice under any type of physician coverage for the primary nurse to look at any results or consult notes on their patients since primary nurses may notice the abnormal test or that a test result is back before the physician or advanced practice provider sees the result. Thus, the primary nurse may realize that the patient may be able to be discharged or may need inpatient admission before the physician or advanced practice provider is aware of the findings. It is a team effort.

We are currently evaluating and planning to add additional coverage for the additional shifts to improve our ability to further expedite care in the OU.

Relevant Policies

**Administrative policy on Nursing Documentation
Policy approved: Date:
Policy reaffirmed: Date:

Nursing and Ancillary Staffing for the Observation Unit

Background

There needs to be adequate nursing and ancillary staffing for the OU.

The usual nurse to patient ratio for OU patients is 1:4 or 1:5.*

Objectives (Purpose)

To establish nursing staffing guidelines for the OU

Policy

Nursing Staffing

The preferred nursing staffing ratio is one RN for every four patients during the day and evening and one RN for every five patients at night. One of these RNs will also serve as the charge nurse. There will be a designated charge nurse for the OU 24 hours a day, 7 days a week, 365 days a year. The OU nursing staff is augmented by ancillary staff, including clinical technicians and unit coordinators. (See Chapter 6 Staffing Considerations.)

Clinical Technicians

The clinical technicians will assist the RN staff in the nursing care of patients. This may include, but is not limited to, obtaining ECGs, drawing blood, transporting patients to and from testing and procedures, and obtaining vital signs. The preferred staffing is one clinical technician at night and two technicians during the day and evening shifts.

Unit Coordinators

The unit coordinators for the OU provide secretarial support and assist the RNs in the scheduling and coordination of tests and procedures for the observation patients, in the preparation of documents needed for patient disposition, follow-up appointments, transfers, and in the stocking and ordering of certain supplies. The preferred staffing is one unit coordinator on all shifts.

Reference

*Mace SE, Graff L, Mikhail M, et al. A national survey of observation units in the United States. *Am J Emerg Med* 2003; 21:529–533.

Policy approved: Date:
Policy reaffirmed: Date:

Organizational Structure of the Observation Unit

Background

Administrative support is essential for the functioning of the OU. A clearly defined management structure identifies the individuals responsible for the operations of the unit and delineates the "chain of command."

Objectives (Purpose)

To provide administrative support and leadership for the OU

Policy

The organizational structure and leadership of the OU is defined as the following (Figure 88.1):

Discussion

Depending on institutional considerations, the reporting structure may vary. For example, the OU director may report directly to hospital administration (Figure 88.2) and bypass reporting to the ED director and/or the ED administrator (Figure 88.3).

If the OU is managed by hospitalists and not the ED, then the hospitalist in charge of the OU would likely report to the department of internal medicine. If a pediatric OU, then the medical director of the OU would likely report to the ED director or the chair of the department of pediatrics.

There are many advantages of an OU. There are benefits for the providers (both primary care and specialists), the ED, the hospital, and the health care system, but most importantly, for the patient and his or her family. However,

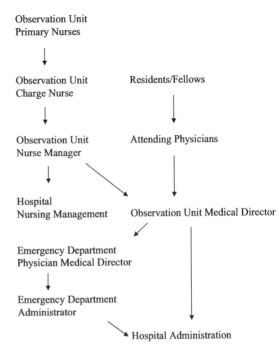

Figure 88.1 Observation Unit Director Reports to Emergency Department Director and to Hospital Administration

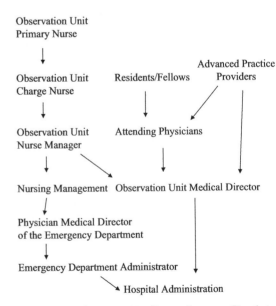

Figure 88.2 Observation Unit Director Reports to Directly to Hospital Administration and Advanced Practice Providers Also Work in the Observation Unit

selection of the appropriate patients for observation is critical and having systems in place for management of these patients is also essential. Patients placed in the OU must be undergoing

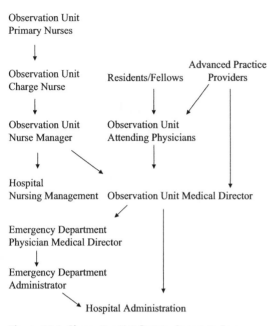

Observation Unit
Primary Nurses

↓

Observation Unit   Advanced Practice
Charge Nurse   Residents/Fellows   Providers

↓

Observation Unit   Observation Unit
Nurse Manager   Attending Physicians

↓

Hospital
Nursing Management   Observation Unit Medical Director

Emergency Department
Physician Medical Director

↓

Emergency Department
Administrator

Hospital Administration

Figure 88.3 Observation Unit Director Reports to Emergency Department Director and to Hospital Administration and Advanced Practice Providers Also Work in the Observation Unit

active management that encompasses any one of or combination of the following: monitoring, diagnostics, and/or treatment.

In some cases, the same individual may serve as the both the director of the OU and the director of the ED. However, having the director of the OU be different from the ED director may be preferable to having one individual serve both functions in that this allows the OU director to have additional time and the ability to focus or concentrate on the OU instead of splitting time between many other responsibilities.

Moreover, the medical director of the OU should have some protected time for his or her administrative responsibility for the OU.[1]

In some institutions, advanced practice providers may play a role in the administrative structure. The administrative structure would be modified to include these advanced practice providers as follows (Figures 88.2 and 88.3):

Reference

1. Mace SE, Graff L, Mikhail M, et al. A national survey of observation units in the United States. *Am J Emerg Med* 2003; 21: 529–533.

Policy approved: *Date:*
Policy reaffirmed: *Date:*

Patient Criteria for Placement in the Observation Unit (in Observation Status): Patients Meeting Specific Clinical Protocol(s)

Background

Although patients placed in the OU (in observation status) may have a variety of diseases and/or conditions, patients placed in the OU are anticipated to have a disposition in 24 hours or less. Moreover, patients placed in the OU (in observation status) are expected to be discharged in ≤ 24 hours. In general, about 80–82% of patients placed in an OU will be discharged and only 18–20% admitted (national average).[1,2] Thus, any patient placed in the OU should have about an 80% chance of being discharged.

Objectives (Purpose)

Patients with the various conditions or diagnoses outlined in a specific clinical protocol/guideline should meet the inclusion criteria for that given condition (e.g., chest pain protocol/guideline) or diagnosis (e.g., asthma protocol/guideline) in order to be placed in the OU. Similarly, patients who have any of the exclusions for a given condition (e.g., chest pain protocol/guideline) or diagnosis (e.g., asthma protocol/guideline) should not be placed in the OU. (Refer to clinical protocols/guidelines.) This is to encourage the appropriate selection of patients for the OU.

Policy

In general, patients placed in the OU will meet the specific inclusion criteria for that given clinical protocol/guideline. In general, patients with any one or more of the exclusion criteria for that given clinical protocol/guideline will not be placed in the OU.

Overall, patients appropriate for an OU are patients who meet the following criteria. The patient placed in observation should be

1. Clinically stable
2. Not critically ill
3. Do not need intensive nursing care
4. Do not need intensive physician care

Discussion

Clinical protocols/guidelines are intended to promote best practices and to maintain the core philosophy of observation medicine, which is the provision of the best possible care and most efficient, cost-effective diagnostic evaluation and/or treatment in a limited time frame (< 24 hours) with predetermined resources. Thus, preserving and adhering to the various clinical protocols/guidelines is essential for the functioning of the OU.

However, clinical protocols are guidelines and are not intended to take the place of clinical judgment by the clinician. Review and discussion of any variations from the protocols or guidelines can be an integral part of the PI or CQI for the OU and is a valid way to modify or reaffirm various protocols/guidelines and/or policies.

Indeed, my recommendation would be to rename "clinical protocols" to "clinical guidelines." Guidelines are not mandatory, but instead are suggested best practices that outline processes to follow in a certain set of circumstances in order to reach defined quality outcomes.

Clinical protocols/guidelines should distinguish between patients with mild to moderate disease or illness severity, who are likely appropriate for the OU, from those with a severe disease or condition, who are not appropriate for the OU. For example, a patient with mild or moderate asthma may be appropriate for the OU but not if he/she has severe asthma and is intubated or has been emergently placed on bilevel positive airway pressure (BiPaP). Specific parameters for a given protocol should distinguish clinically between those with mild to moderate disease versus those with severe disease or who are critically ill. For example, patients excluded from the OU would include anyone intubated or acutely placed on noninvasive ventilation. Those on continuous positive airway pressure (CPAP) at night for sleep apnea and not acutely placed on CPAP or BiPAP may be appropriate for observation. Inclusion/exclusion criteria for pneumonia patients might be delineated by a scoring system (such as PORT score) or by clinical parameters (heart rate, saturation, CXR findings, etc.)

References

1. Mace SE, Graff L, Mikhail M, et al. A national survey of observation units in the United States. *Am J Emerg Med* 2003; 21: 529–533.

2. Wiler JL, Ross MA, Ginde AA. National study of emergency department observation services. *Acad Emerg Med* 2011; 18: 959–965.

Policy approved: Date:
Policy reaffirmed: Date:

Patient Criteria for Placement in the Observation Unit (in Observation Status): Patients Not Meeting Specific Clinical Protocol(s)

Background

Although the clinical protocols include the majority of conditions and diseases that are encountered in clinical practice, it is anticipated that there will be patients who do not fall into one of the categories of clinical protocols. However, these patients may be appropriate for placement in the OU and can be placed in the OU.

Objectives (Purpose)

Patients who do not belong to a given clinical protocol may be suitable for placement in the OU and may be appropriately placed in the OU. The same general considerations apply to these patients. These patients, similar to those included in a specific clinical protocol, are anticipated to have a disposition in 24 hours or less and 80–82% are expected to be discharged in ≤ 24 hours from the OU with only 18–20% needing to be admitted as a hospital inpatient.[1,2]

Policy

In general, patients appropriate for an OU are patients who meet the following criteria. The patient placed in observation should be

1. Clinically stable*
2. Not critically ill
3. Do not need intensive nursing care
4. Do not need intensive physician care

Discussion

Clinically stable does not necessarily imply that the vital signs must be completely normal. For example, an OU patient may have a fever but should not be septic or in shock. An asthmatic appropriate for observation may have mild tachycardia and/or mild tachypnea and/or a pulse oxygen saturation $< 95\%$ but should not have an oxygen saturation ≤ 89%. Mild tachycardia from pain, anxiety, or underlying disease may be acceptable if it is not causing hemodynamic compromise and is expected to significantly improve or resolve with treatment within 24 hours. A patient who has mild bradycardia from over-medication with a normal blood pressure and baseline mental status, who should improve by holding medication and monitoring, may be a suitable patient for observation.

References

1. Mace SE, Graff L, Mikhail M, et al. A national survey of observation units in the United States. *Am J Emerg Med* 2003; 21: 529–533.
2. Wiler JL, Ross MA, Ginde AA. National study of emergency department observation services. *Acad Emerg Med* 2011; 18: 959–965.

Policy approved: Date:
Policy reaffirmed: Date:

Patient Placed in Observation Status

Background

There are multiple steps involving various personnel that occur when a patient is placed in the OU. In order for the transition of the patient from the ED to placement in the OU (or in observation status) to occur, the personnel and steps in the process should be identified.

Objectives (Purpose)

To delineate the roles and responsibilities when a patient is placed in the OU (in observation status).

Policy

Physician Responsibility

The ED attending makes the decision to place a patient in the OU (observation status). The decision may be made after discussion with the primary care physicians and/or specialty physicians. In general, the emergency physician attending should follow the guidelines set forth in the Observation Unit Clinical Guidelines and Administrative Policies. If there are any questions or concerns, the physician director of the OU or other designated physician administrative personnel may be contacted for advice and clarification of the OU Clinical Guidelines and Administrative Policies and for advice regarding the appropriateness of placement of the patient in the OU (in observation status).

The order to place the patient in observation status and the initial orders for management of the patient while in observation status must be signed by the ED attending.

Nursing Responsibility: Observation Unit Charge Nurse

The OU charge RN will be contacted by the ED RN to determine OU bed availability. If an OU bed is available, then the OU charge nurse will notify patient registration that there is an order for a patient to be placed in the OU. He/she will assign an RN to be the primary RN responsible for the nursing care of the patient while the patient is in the OU and assign the patient to a room in the OU.

Nursing Responsibility: Emergency Department Nurse

The ED nurse will call the charge nurse in the OU to determine if an OU bed is available. If a bed is available, then he/she will give report on the patient to the OU primary nurse who is assigned to that patient and then have the patient transported to the OU.

Nursing Responsibility: Observation Unit Primary Nurse

The OU primary nurse responsible for the patient in the OU will orient the patient to the OU and will begin documentation of the patient's care in the nursing flow sheets.

Patient Registration

Patient registration will obtain the necessary contact information, insurance data, and other relevant information; obtain the required signatures; and complete the necessary forms or paperwork and documentation as needed. Patient registration will notify the care coordinator (case manager) that the patient has been placed in observation status.

Care Coordinator (Case Manager)

The care coordinator (case manager) will meet with the patient and family, if appropriate, and distribute an informational booklet on observation status to the patient and/or their family and answer any questions that they may have. If the care coordinator (case manager) is not available, then other appropriate personnel (such as nursing or patient registration) will distribute the informational booklet on observation status to the patient and/or their family and answer any questions that they may have and begin the referral to the care coordinator (case management).

Discussion

Depending on availability and various job descriptions, steps in the process may vary depending on the specifics of the local hospital. For example, if a care coordinator (case manager) is not available, nursing or patient registration may assume some of the initial steps in the process. For multiple reasons including regulations, etc. it is best to use the term "place in observation" or "refer to observation" instead of "admit to observation" because observation is considered an outpatient service and not an inpatient service. Thus, the better term is place in observation so I would recommend using this phrase in an order set instead of admit to observation. When a patient is placed in observation, there needs to be some easily identified method to identify this event since this is when the "clock begins." There are multiple ways to accomplish this, whether using a different nursing flow sheet or demarcating a section of the ED record, etc. The purpose is to easily and readily identify when a patient is placed in observation and that events will be occurring as part of the patient's plan of management when in observation status.

Relevant Policies

See also the Administrative Policies on Orientation to the Unit, Responsibilities of the Physician, Responsibilities of the Charge Nurse, Responsibilities of the Primary Nurse and Case Manager.

Policy approved: *Date:*

Policy reaffirmed: *Date:*

Patients Placed in the Observation Unit (Observation Status) or Appropriate Selection of Patients for the Observation Unit

Background

A patient in need of monitoring might be a patient with syncope who needs monitoring of their vital signs and cardiac rhythm to determine whether their syncope is benign or due to a significant dysrhythmia.

An example of a patient with a specific diagnosis who would be likely to improve with treatment within a short time frame, specifically ≤ 24 hours, would be an asthmatic (with a pulse oxygen saturation $> 90\%$) who might be improved but still be wheezing after treatment in the ED. Such a patient with continued aerosols and steroids has a high probability of being discharged in < 24 hours.

An example of a patient without a specific diagnosis but who needs further diagnostic evaluation would be a patient with chest pain. An ED patient with negative initial cardiac enzymes and a normal ECG or ECG without significant ECG changes or a baseline ECG unchanged from previous ECGs would be an appropriate candidate for the OU. Such a patient with chest pain may be placed in the OU on a cardiac monitor, have serial cardiac enzymes and ECGs done, and have a stress test done if the ECGs and enzymes remain negative. A positive evaluation would yield the more specific diagnosis of cardiac chest pain (with positive enzymes and/or ECGs or stress test) versus noncardiac chest pain (with enzymes, ECGs and stress test all negative).

Patients may need any combination of these modalities: monitoring, diagnostics, and therapy. A patient with an extremity infection or traumatic hand injury may need monitoring (neurovascular checks), diagnostics (radiology studies: plain x-rays, CT scan, MRI), laboratory studies, consults, and treatment (IV antibiotics, IV analgesics).

Objectives (Purpose)

There are many advantages of an OU. There are benefits for the clinicians (both primary care and specialists), the ED, the hospital, and the health care system; but most importantly, for the patient and their family. However, selection of the appropriate patient for observation is critical and having systems in place for management of these patients is also essential. Patients placed in the OU must be *undergoing active management* that encompasses any one of or combination of the following: *monitoring, diagnostics, and/or treatment.*

Policy

Although many different types of patients can be placed in an OU (or observation status), these patients all have the same overriding characteristics. OU patients are acutely ill, but not critical; do not require intensive physician or nursing care; and are expected to have a disposition within < 24 hours. They can be grouped into several categories: (1) those in whom monitoring is needed in order to determine the severity of illness or injury and thus, inpatient admission or discharge, (2) those in whom additional time (< 24 hours) for further evaluation or workup is needed in order to determine the specific diagnosis (and thus, disposition), or (3) those in whom the diagnosis is known but are not quite ready to be discharged from the ED and require additional treatment but are expected to improve within 24 hours and be able to be discharged from the OU. Patients placed in observation should have an 80% or better chance of having being discharged from the OU within 24 hours or less.

Policy approved: *Date:*
Policy reaffirmed: *Date:*

Performance Improvement/ Continuous Quality Improvement

Background

PI, also referred to as CQI is a mechanism for ongoing evaluation of the operations of the OU and of the care provided to patients in the OU.

Objectives (Purpose)

The goal of CQI is continual improvement in the functioning of the OU and in the ability to provide the best care possible to patients placed in the OU.

Policy

CQI for the OU will be done on a regular ongoing basis and used to make improvements in the operations of the OU and in the provision of patient care in the OU. This may include, but is not limited to, the use of performance indicators and metrics as a tool for the assessment of the operations and patient care in the OU.

Discussion

The purpose of CQI is to make improvements in systems of care instead of focusing on individual provider(s). Patient care and processes are monitored and reviewed on a regular basis. This information is then analyzed in order to advance systems of care and is not meant to be punitive toward any given individual or health care provider, but is intended to "close the loop" and be used to "make the system" better. Data should not be isolated but instead used to foster constructive change. Once a process or processes are identified to be modified, then they are monitored both before and after the changes are made in order to assess the expected improvement in patient care or in the delivery of that care. The importance of an ongoing PI or CQI process is delineated in the chapter on PI.

References

1. Mace SE. Continuous quality improvement for the clinical decision unit. *Journal for Healthcare Quality* 2004; 26(1): 29–36.

2. Mace SE. Patient quality (continuous quality improvement), safety, and experience for the observation unit. In: *Observation Medicine*. American College of Emergency Physicians, www.acep.org (last accessed May 2016).

Relevant Policies

See also Policies on Quality Indicators and on Metrics.

Policy approved: *Date:*
Policy reaffirmed: *Date:*

Physician Availability

Background

Responsibility: The overall management including observation/monitoring, diagnostic evaluation and treatment, and disposition of the patient in the OU is the responsibility of the ED attending on duty.

Objectives (Purpose)

There must be a designated physician responsible for patient care in the OU at all times: 24 hours a day, 7 days a week, 365 days a year.

Policy

The responsible physician must be available and able to respond to any nursing concerns and any emergencies in the OU, write orders, as well as make a disposition on OU patients and document the patients' care, as necessary and per the administrative policy on physician documentation.

The attending physician should be available at all times to respond expeditiously when warranted by changes in the patient's clinical condition.

This responsible attending should be documented in the medical record.

Policy approved: *Date:*
Policy reaffirmed: *Date:*

Physician Responsibilities for the Observation Unit: Delegation of Care

Background

Although other health care providers may be actively involved in the care of patients in the OU, the ultimate responsibility lies with the attending ED physician.

Objectives (Purpose)

To establish physician responsibility for patient care in the OU.

Policy

There will be an attending emergency physician (s) assigned to and responsible for the care of every patient in the OU.

Physicians in Training: Residents and or fellows may be involved in the management of observation patients, provided the attending physician is providing oversight and is readily available on site for consultation and to provide clinical care when necessary.

Advanced practice providers (advanced practice clinicians, midlevel providers): Physician assistants and nurse practitioners may be involved in the management of observation patients, in accordance with their scope of practice, and provided an attending physician is readily available on site for consultation and to provide clinical direction, oversight, and consultation when necessary.

Discussion

Responsibility: The overall management including observation/monitoring, diagnostic evaluation, and treatment of the patient in the OU is the responsibility of the ED attending on duty who is assigned to the OU. (If it is a hospitalist run unit, then the attending hospitalist on duty who is assigned to the OU is responsible for the overall management of the patient(s) in the OU.)

Relevant Policies

See also Policy on Physician Responsibility and Physician Documentation.

Policy approved: *Date:*
Policy reaffirmed: *Date:*

Physician Staffing (Coverage) of the Observation Unit

Background

There must be a designated physician responsible for patient care in the OU at all times; 24 hours a day, 7 days a week, 365 days a year.

Objectives (Purpose)

To establish physician staffing or coverage guidelines for the OU. When a patient is placed in observation status or referred to observation, there must be a specific physician who accepts responsibility for the care of that given patient.

Policy

There will be clear delineation of which physician is responsible for each patient in the OU at all times.

Prior to placement in the OU, the patient's attending will be documented in the patient's medical record.

No patient will be allowed to be placed in the OU unless they have an attending physician of record who is ultimately responsible for the care delivered.

The attending physician should be available at all times to respond expeditiously when warranted by changes in the patient's clinical condition. If there are any changes in the attending physician or coverage for the OU, the OU nursing staff must be notified and the change in coverage documented.

Discussion

Physician coverage may be delegated to advanced practice providers, specifically, physician assistants or nurse practitioners. However, even if some coverage is allocated to advanced practice providers, there still must be attending staff physician oversight and on-site availability.

Policy approved: *Date:*
Policy reaffirmed: *Date:*

Quality Indicators
Background

As noted in the PI/CQI policy, quality indicators are a component of the ongoing PI process for the OU. Quality indicators are a tool for the evaluation of patient care and for the assessment of the processes involved in the delivery of care. Quality indicators can be utilized to develop benchmarks. Benchmarks, which can be external or internal, may be used to set goals for the OU.

Objectives (Purpose)

Quality indicators are part of the PI process and are valuable in monitoring patient care and the processes or systems of care for patients placed in observation status. Quality indicators and benchmarks are a method for reviewing patient care and the processes of delivering that care and are used to make recommendations for continuing or modifying current practices.

Policy

The following are some key quality indicators that have been determined to be useful in the PI process for the OU:[1,2]

- LOS > 24 hours
- LOS < 6 hours
- Deaths
- Codes/resuscitations[3]
- Invasive airway interventions/Unplanned need for mechanical ventilation
- Admissions to intensive care unit (ICU)
- Admissions to the operating room (OR)
- Admissions to the cardiac catheterization unit
- Chest pain that rules in
- Complaints[4]
- Left without treatment completed (LWTC), left against medical advice (LAMA)

- Returns to the ED within 72 hours
- Readmissions to the hospital within 30 days
- Incident/SERS reports

Discussion

Quality indicators should be integrated into PI on a regular basis. This is usually done on a monthly and yearly basis so trends can be tracked over time.

References

1. Mace SE. Continuous quality improvement for the clinical decision unit. *Journal for Healthcare Quality* 2004; 26(1): 29–36.

2. Mace SE. Patient quality (continuous quality improvement), safety, and experience for the observation unit. In: *Observation Medicine.* American College of Emergency Physicians, www.acep.org (last accessed 2/2014)

3. Mace SE. Resuscitations in an observation unit. *J Qual Clin Practice* 1999; 19:155–164.

4. Mace SE. An analysis of patient complaints in an observation unit. *J Qual Clin Practice* 1998; 18 (2):151–158.

Relevant Policies

See also Policies on PI/CQI and on Metrics.
Policy approved: *Date:*
Policy reaffirmed: *Date:*

Residents in the Observation Unit
Background

Residents and fellows have an important role within the institution. Education and training is an integral part of the hospital mission. As consistent throughout the institution, physicians in training (e.g., residents and fellows) must have appropriate supervision in the OU. Residents and fellows in the OU may be on rotation in the OU/ED or from other services and serving as consultants or evaluating patients admitted as inpatients to the hospital from the OU.

Objectives (Purpose)

To ensure appropriate supervision and provide the best possible educational experience for physicians in training, while maintaining optimal patient care, all residents and fellows must have their evaluations (such as history/ physical examinations, consult notes, progress notes, etc.), orders, and any other recommendations for patient care confirmed by an attending physician.

Policy

I. For emergency medicine residents/fellows and residents on other specialties on rotation in the ED and/or in the OU

1. All notes must be countersigned by an ED attending.
2. All orders on OU patients must be countersigned by an ED attending.
3. Patients will be placed in the OU only if there is a note (history, physical examination with a plan of care for the patient in the OU) and orders for the patient's OU care. A note and/or orders by the resident or fellow is acceptable provided the note and or orders are countersigned by the emergency medicine attending.

II. For consults from other services, the consult note by a resident or fellow must be countersigned by an attending from the respective service.

III. Orders by residents or fellows who are in the process of evaluating OU patients who are admitted to inpatient services must also have their orders approved and countersigned by attending.

IV. Nursing will not follow or complete any orders by residents or fellows unless the orders are countersigned by an attending, except for emergency situations and/or other extenuating circumstances.

Discussion

Residents and fellows are an integral part of any teaching institution. They are expected to evaluate and care for patients, but appropriate guidance is essential to any educational program. There is an attending available in the ED 24 hours a day, 7 days a week, 365 days a year, who can and is available for oversight of physicians in training who are caring for patients in the OU.

Policy approved: *Date:*
Policy reaffirmed: *Date:*

Time in the Observation Unit: Length of Stay > 24 HOURS

Background

The premise underlying observation units is that an efficient, proactive, well-specified plan of management for a specific group of ED patients can determine their disposition as to whether they can be discharged or need inpatient hospitalization within the targeted goal of 24 hours or less. The timely disposition is contingent on there being monitoring of the patient's clinical condition, and/or diagnostic evaluation, and/or a treatment regimen focused on establishing whether it is safe for the patient to be discharged (or needs an inpatient admission), at arriving at a definitive diagnosis, and/or achieving significant improvement in the patient's clinical condition. A previous study reported an average LOS in the OU of 15.3 hours with 75% having a LOS ≤ 18 hours.[1]

Objectives (Purpose)

To promote the timely disposition within < 24 hours of patients placed in the OU.

Procedure

Patients placed in observation will have an initial history, physical examination, medical decision making/clinical course, and a set of orders prior to the patient being placed in the OU or observation status that includes an active plan of management while the patient is in the OU. At any time during the patient's observation stay, the RN may notify the physician medical director of the OU or physician administrator regarding delays in patient care and if there is any need for assistance in the disposition of the OU patient or any other patient care concerns or issues. When a patient's LOS becomes > 20 hours, this will be flagged as part of the electronic tracking system for the OU and the advanced practice provider, resident, and/ or attending in charge of the patient's care will be notified regarding the patient's LOS and for the need to determine a disposition for the patient. If the patient is still in observation at 24 hours then this will be again flagged as part of the electronic tracking system for the OU and the advanced practice provider, resident, and/or attending in charge of the patient's care will be notified regarding the patient's LOS > 24 hour and for the need to determine a disposition for the patient. Patients with an OU LOS > 24 hours are a metric for the OU and will be referred as part of the OU PI or CQI.

Reference

1. Mace SE, Graff L, Mikhail M, et al. A National Survey of Observation Units in the United States. *Am J Emerg Med* 2002; 21: 529-533.

Policy approved: *Date:*
Policy reaffirmed: *Date:*

Vital Signs
Background

Vital signs are an important part of nursing care for any patient including those placed in the OU. Vital signs may be part of the information used to determine the patient's disposition from the OU, whether to be admitted to an inpatient floor or to be discharged from the OU.

Objectives (Purpose)

To establish baseline vital signs on patients placed in OU.

Policy

- Vital signs will be done when the patient is placed in the OU (in observation status)

- Vital signs will be done prior to the patient's disposition from the OU. A recent set of vital signs will be obtained prior to the patient being transported to an inpatient unit or prior to discharge from the OU. Thus, a minimum of two sets of vital signs will be obtained on patients placed in the OU, unless otherwise indicated (such as patient refusal).
- Vital signs include: temperature, pulse, respirations, blood pressure and pulse oximetry, unless otherwise specified by the physician.
- Pain assessment will be included in the vital signs, if appropriate.
- Vital signs will be done as per physician orders.
- If not specified by the physician, vital signs will be every 4 hours for monitored patients (e.g., patients on telemetry) and every 8 hours if the patient is not on telemetry.
- The RN may do vital signs more frequently, as he/she deems appropriate.
- Abnormal vital signs will be reported to the responsible physician or advanced practice provider as specified in the physician's orders and/or as deemed appropriate by the nursing staff.

Policy approved: *Date:*
Policy reaffirmed: *Date:*

Part X

Order Sets

Chapter

89

Medical Center Department of Emergency Medicine Observation Unit Manual: Adult Order Sets by Diagnosis/Clinical Condition

Sharon E. Mace, MD, FACEP, FAAP
Matthew J. Campbell, PharmD, BCPS, BCCCP

Abdominal Pain Order Set

Place in Emergency Department (ED)
   Observation _____
Diagnosis *ACUTE ABDOMINAL PAIN*,
   _____, _____, _____
ED Attending _____
Resident (if applicable) _____
Advanced Practice Provider (if applicable)
_____

Allergies: Yes _____ No _____

If yes, what _____, _____, _____, _____,
   _____, _____

Vital Signs

Temperature__ Pulse __ Respiration __BP__
   Pulse oximetry ____
__ q 2 hours ___ q 4 hours ___ q 6 hours q ___
   hours ___ q shift ___ qd ____ other
Cardiac monitoring (telemetry) _____
Orthostatic vital signs _____
Continuous pulse oximetry _____
Other _____

Notify Physician if

Temperature (°C) > 38.0° ___ 38.5°___ 39° ___
   40° ____ other _____
Systolic blood pressure (mmHg) ≤ 90 ___ ≥
   160 ___ ≥ 180 ___ ≥ 200 ___ other _____
Diastolic blood pressure (mmHg) ≥ 120 ____
   other _____
Heart rate ≤ 50 ___ ≥ 120 ___ ≥ 150 ___ ≥
   200 ___ other ____
Oxygen saturation < 90% _____
   other _____
Any change in mental status _____
Any respiratory distress _____

Activity

Up ad lib _____
Assisted _____
Out of bed to chair _____
Bedrest with bathroom privileges _____
Bedrest with bedside commode _____
Bedrest _____
Other _____

Diet

NPO _____
Regular _____
Advance diet as tolerated _____
Clear liquids ____
Dental, mechanical soft _____
Diabetic _____
Formula _____
Full liquids _____
Low added fat/No added salt _____
Low cholesterol _____
Pureed _____
Sodium: 1 gram ___ 2 grams ___
   unrestricted____
Per feeding tube _____
Other _____

Nursing Interventions

Weight ____ on admission ____ qd ____ prior
   to discharge ____ other
Height ____
I & Os _____ routine _____ strict _____
Fluid restriction ____ mL/hour ____ mL/shift
   ____ mL/24 hour ____ other
Fall precautions _____
Seizure precautions _____
Capillary blood glucose ___ × 1 q ___ hours
   ___ before meals and at bedtime

Respiratory Interventions

Oxygen __ liters nasal cannula __ venti mask at ___ liters per minute _____ other

Wean oxygen as tolerated without dyspnea, stridor, or oxygen saturation < 90% ____

Peak flow __ on admission ___ prior to discharge ___ pre and post aerosols

Sleep apnea qhs __ CPAP BiPAP settings cm H_2O ___ inspiratory ___ expiratory

Laboratory Tests

CBC _____ with differential

Amylase ___ Lipase ___

Basic metabolic panel _____

Cardiac enzymes ___ × 1 ___ q 4 hours × 3 ___ q 4 hours × 4 ____ other

Complete metabolic panel _____

Lactate _____

Liver function tests _____

Pregnancy test (qualitative urine) _____

Pregnancy test (quantitative blood) _____

Renal function tests (e.g., BUN, creatinine) _____

Type and screen _____

Urinalysis _____

Urine culture _____

Other _____, _____, _____, _____, _____, _____, _____, _____

Repeat _____, _____, _____, _____, _____ in a.m. _____ in _____ hours

Radiology Studies

Acute abdominal series ____

CXR portable_____

CXR (PA and lateral) _____

KUB (kidneys, ureters, bladder) X-ray _____

CT scan abdomen/pelvis ____ with contrast: __ IV __ PO ___ PR ___ CT enterography

Ultrasound Pelvis _____

Ultrasound RUQ _____

Cholescintigraphy (hepatic iminodiacetic acid [HIDA] scan) _____

MRI _____

Other _____, _____, _____

Cardiac Studies

ECG __ × 1 __ q 4 hours × 3 ___ q 4 hours × 4 ___ other ____ with cardiac enzymes

Echocardiogram (transthoracic) __ with agitated (bubble) study __ without agitated (bubble) study

Consultants

Care coordination (Case management) _____ Notified: Name _____ Time _____

Colorectal surgery_____ Notified: Name _____ Time _____

Gastroenterology_____ Notified: Name _____ Time _____

General surgery _____ Notified: Name _____ Time _____

Gynecology _____ Notified: Name _____ Time _____

Social work_____ Notified: Name _____ Time _____

Other _____ Notified: Name _____ Time _____

Abdominal Pain Medications (Adult Dosage)

Analgesics

Acetaminophen (Paracetamol) (Tylenol®) 325 mg tab __ 1 tab __ 1–2 tabs __ 2 tabs PO __ q 4 hours __ q 6 hours ___ prn pain ___ prn fever (maximum 4 g daily)

____ If unable to take tablet formulation, may give suspension

____ If unable to take PO, may give suppository PR __ 325 mg __ 650 mg __ q 4 hours ___ q 6 hours

IV ___ mg __ q 4 hours __ q 6 hours __ prn pain __ prn fever (maximum adult dose: if weight < 50 kg is 15 mg/kg up to 750 mg for a single dose, 75 mg/kg up to 3750 mg for daily dose; if weight > 50 kg is 650 mg q 4 hours or 1000 mg q 6 hours up to 1000 mg for a single dose and 4000 mg for a daily dose)

Acetaminophen-Hydrocodone (Vicodin®) 300 mg/5 mg tabs __ 1 tab __ 1–2 tabs __ 2 tabs PO __ q 4 hours __ q 6 hours ___ prn pain (maximum 4 grams daily based on acetaminophen dose)

Acetaminophen-Oxycodone (Endocet®, Percocet®, Roxicet®) 325 mg / 5 mg tab __ 1 tab __ 1–2 tabs __ 2 tabs PO __ q 4 hours

__ q 6 hours ___ prn pain (maximum
4 grams daily based on acetaminophen dose)
Hydromorphone (Dilaudid®) __ 0.5 mg __
1 mg __ 2 mg __ mg: ___ IV __ q 2 hours __
q 4 hours __ q 6 hours q ___ hours __
prn pain
Ibuprofen (Advil®, Motrin®) __ 400 mg __
600 mg __ 800 mg PO __ q 4 hours __ q
6 hours __ q 8 hours ___ prn pain
Ketorolac (Toradol®) __ 30 mg IV __ q 6 hours
__ prn pain (maximum 120 mg daily)
Morphine __ 0.5 mg __ 1 mg __ 2 mg __ 4 mg
__ mg: ____ IV __ q 2 hours __ q 4 hours __
q 6 hours q ___ hours __ prn pain
Tramadol (Ultram®) __ 50 mg __ 100 mg PO
__ q 4 hours __ q 6 hours __ prn pain
(maximum 400 mg daily)
Other: _____, _____, _____,
_____, _____

Antacid Medications

Aluminum Hydroxide and Magnesium
Hydroxide (Maalox®, Mylanta® ___ 10–20
mL liquid PO pc and qhs (maximum 80 mL
daily), ___ 1–2 tab PO pc and qhs ___ prn
reflux or ___ prn dyspepsia/pain (maximum
16 tablets daily)

Antiemetics

Chlorpromazine (Thorazine®) __ 10 mg PO __
25 mg PO __ q 4 hours __ q 6 hours
__ 25 mg __ 50 mg __ IV __ IM __ q 4 hours __
q 6 hours __ prn nausea/vomiting
Metoclopramide (Reglan®) __ 10 mg __ IV __
IM __ PO __ q 6 hours __ other __ prn
nausea/vomiting
Ondansetron (Zofran®) __ 4 mg __ 8 mg __ IV
__ PO __ q 6 hours ___ other __ prn nausea/
vomiting
Prochlorperazine (Compazine®) __ 5 mg __
10 mg __ IV __ IM __ PO __ q 4 hours __ q
6 hours (maximum dose IV/IM/PO 40 mg
per day) __ 25 mg PR bid __ prn nausea/
vomiting
Promethazine (Phenergan®) __ 12.5 mg __
25 mg __ IV __ IM __ PO __ PR __ q 4 hours
__ q 6 hours ___ prn nausea/vomiting

Trimethobenzamide (Tigan®) __ 200 mg IM
__ 300 mg PO ___ q 6 hours ___ prn nausea/
vomiting

Antireflux (Histamine H2 antagonist) Medications

Famotidine (Pepcid®) __ 20 mg __ 40 mg __
IV __ PO
__ bid ___ qd __ qhs ___prn reflux or
dyspepsia/pain (maximum PO dose 40 mg
bid, maximum IV dose 20 mg bid)

Intravenous Fluids

Saline cap IV ____
Bolus Normal Saline (NS) IV ___ 250 mL ___
500 mL ___ 1,000 mL ____ other,
infuse over ___ minutes ___ hours
Bolus Lactated Ringer's (LR) IV __ 250 mL __
500 mL __ 1,000 mL __ other,
infuse over ___ minutes ___ hours
Maintenance NS at __ mL per hour IV
Maintenance LR at __ mL per hour IV
Maintenance Dextrose 5% in Water (D$_5$W)at __
mL per hour IV
Maintenance Dextrose 5% in ½ Normal Saline
(D$_5$½NS) at __ mL per hour IV
Maintenance Dextrose 5% in Normal Saline
(D$_5$NS) at __ mL per hour IV
Maintenance NS with potassium chloride __
20 mEq or __ 40 mEq per 1 liter bag at mL
per hour IV
Maintenance D$_5$W with potassium chloride __
20 mEq or __ 40 mEq per 1 liter bag at mL
per hour IV
Maintenance D$_5$½NS with potassium chloride
__ 20 mEq or __ 40 mEq per 1 liter bag at __
mL per hour IV
Maintenance D$_5$NS with potassium chloride__
20 mEq or __ 40 mEq per 1 liter bag at __ mL
per hour IV
Other _____ at mL per hour

Education: patient _____ family _____

Abdominal pain _____
Smoking cessation _____
Other _____

Allergic Reaction/Angioedema Order Set

Place in Emergency Department (ED) Observation

Diagnosis *ACUTE ALLERGIC REACTION/ ANGIOEDEMA*, ____, ____

ED Attending _____

Resident (if applicable) _____

Advanced Practice Provider (if applicable) _____

Allergies: Yes _____ No _____

If yes, what _____, _____, _____, _____, _____, _____

Vital Signs

Temperature __ Pulse __ Respiration __ BP__ Pulse oximetry __

__ q 2 hours ___ q 4 hours ___ q 6 hours q ___ hours ___ q shift ___ qd ___ other

Continuous pulse oximetry_____

Cardiac monitoring (telemetry) _____

Other _____

Notify Physician if

Temperature (°C) > 38.0° ___ 38.5° ___ 39° ___ 40° ___ other ___

Systolic blood pressure (mmHg) ≤ 90 ___ ≥ 160 ___ ≥ 180 ___ ≥ 200 ___ other ___

Diastolic blood pressure (mmHg) ≥ 120 ___ other ___

Heart rate ≤ 50 ___ ≥ 120 ___ ≥ 150 ___ ≥ 200 ___ other ___

Oxygen saturation < 90% _____

Any change in mental status _____

Any respiratory distress _____

Any new swelling or increased swelling of the face/neck or any stridor _____

Activity

Up ad lib _____

Assisted _____

Out of bed to chair _____

Bedrest with bathroom privileges _____

Bedrest with bedside commode _____

Bedrest _____

Other _____

Diet

NPO _____

Regular _____

Advance diet as tolerated _____

Clear liquids ____

Dental, mechanical soft _____

Diabetic _____

Formula _____

Full liquids _____

Low cholesterol ____

Pureed _____

Sodium: 1 gram ___ 2 grams ___ unrestricted____

Per feeding tube _____

Other _____

Nursing Interventions

Weight ___ on admission ___ qd ___ prior to discharge ____ other

Height ____

I & Os _____ routine _____ strict _____

Fluid restriction _____ mL/hour _____ mL/ shift ____ mL/24 hour

Fall precautions _____

Seizure precautions _____

Capillary blood glucose __ × 1 ___ q ___ hours ___ before meals and at bedtime

Respiratory Interventions

Oxygen __ liters nasal cannula __ venti mask at ___ liters per minute _____ other

Wean oxygen as tolerated without dyspnea, stridor or oxygen saturation < 90% ____

Peak flow __ on admission ___ prior to discharge ___ pre and post aerosols

Sleep apnea qhs __ CPAP BiPAP settings cm H_2O ___ inspiratory __ expiratory

Emergency airway cart at bedside ____

Cricothyrotomy set at bedside _____

Laboratory Tests

Basic metabolic panel _____

CBC _____ with differential

Cardiac enzymes ___ × 1 ___ q 4 hours × 3 ___ q 4 hours × 4 ____ other

Complete metabolic panel_____

Urinalysis _____ Urine culture _____

Pregnancy test (quantitative blood) ___

Other _____, _____, _____, _____, _____, _____, _____, _____

Radiology Studies

Soft tissue neck (PA and lateral) _____
CXR portable _____
CXR (PA and lateral) _____
CT scan __ of face __ of neck __ other
MRI __ of face __ of neck __ other
Other _____, _____, _____, _____,
        _____ , _____

Cardiac Studies

ECG __ × 1 __ q 4 hours × 3 ___ q 4 hours ×
    4 ___ other ____ with cardiac enzymes
Echocardiogram (transthoracic) __ with
    agitated (bubble) study __ without agitated
    (bubble) study

Consultants

Anesthesiology _____ Notified: Name
        _____ Time _____
Care coordination (Case management)
        _____ Notified: Name _____ Time
    _____
ENT _____ Notified: Name
        _____ Time _____
Social work _____ Notified: Name
        _____ Time _____
Other _____ Notified: Name
        _____ Time _____

Medications for Acute Allergic Reaction/ Angioedema (Adult Dosage)

Diphenhydramine (Benadryl®) __ 25 mg __ 50 mg
    __ other __ IV __ PO __ q 4 hours __ q 6 hours
Famotidine (Pepcid®) __ 20 mg __ other __ IV
    __ PO __ bid __ qd __
Methylprednisolone (Solu-medrol®) __ 125 mg
    __ other __ IV __ qd ___ q 12 hours
Prednisone __ 40 mg ___ 60 mg PO __ q
    12 hours ___ qd
Other _____, _____, _____,
        _____, _____

Inhaled Medications: Aerosols

Albuterol (Proventil®) nebulized solution __
    2.5 mg __ mg aerosol __ × 1 __ q 2 hours __ q
    4 hours __ q 6 hours __ q 8 hours __ other __
    prn wheezing

Ipratropium (Atrovent®) 0.5 mg nebulized
    solution aerosol __ × 1 __ q 2 hours __ q
    4 hours __ q 6 hours __ q 8 hours __ other __
    prn wheezing
Racemic epinephrine (Adrenalin®) 0.5 mL of
    2.25% solution nebulized solution __ × 1 ___
    q 2 hours __ q 4 hours __ q 6 hours __ q
    8 hours __ other __ prn wheezing or stridor

Inhaled Medications: Inhalers

Albuterol (Proventil®) (90 mcg per inhalation)
    metered dose inhaler (MDI) __ puffs __ q
    4 hours __ q 6 hours ___ other ___ prn
    wheezing
Ipratropium (Atrovent®) (7 mcg per
    inhalation) __ puffs __ q 4 hours __ q 6 hours
    __ other ___ prn wheezing
Albuterol 90 mcg and Ipratropium 18 mcg
    (per inhalation) (CombiventRespimat®) __
    puffs __ q 6 hours ___ other __ prn wheezing

Hereditary Angioedema Medications*
Bradykinin B2 Receptor Antagonist

Icatibant (Firazyr®) __ 30 mg SQ __ × 1 ___ q
    6 hours × 3
(maximum up to 3 doses or 90 mg in
    24 hours)

C1 Esterase Inhibitor Concentrate

Berinert® 20 units/kg × ___ kg IV**

Kallikrein Inhibitor

Ecallantide (Kalbitor®) __ 30 mg SQ __ x 1

Intravenous Fluids

Saline cap IV ____
Bolus Normal Saline (NS) IV ___ 250 mL __
    500 mL ___ 1,000 mL ____ other,
    infuse over ___ minutes ___ hours
Bolus Lactated Ringer's (LR) IV __ 250 mL __
    500 mL __ 1,000 mL __ other,
    infuse over ___ minutes ___ hours
Maintenance NS at __ mL per hour IV
Maintenance LR at __ mL per hour IV
Maintenance Dextrose 5% in Water (D_5W) at
    __ mL per hour IV
Maintenance Dextrose 5% in ½ Normal Saline
    (D_5½NS) at __ mL per hour IV

Maintenance Dextrose 5% in Normal Saline (D_5NS) at __ mL per hour IV

Maintenance NS with potassium chloride__ 20 mEq or __ 40 mEq per 1 liter bag at __ mL per hour

Maintenance D_5W with potassium chloride__ 20 mEq or __ 40 mEq per 1 liter bag at __ mL per hour

Maintenance D_5½NS with potassium chloride ___ 20 mEq or __ 40 mEq per 1 liter bag at __ mL per hour IV

Maintenance D_5NS with potassium chloride __ 20 mEq or __ 40 mEq per 1 liter bag at __ mL per hour IV

Other _____ at mL per hour

Education: patient _____ **family** _____

Angioedema _____

Allergic Reaction ____

Asthma/Reactive airway disease _____

EpiPen use _____

Smoking cessation _____

Other _____

* Ordered in conjunction with Department of Allergy and Immunology (Consult should be obtained prior to ordering these drugs)

** Other C1 esterase inhibitors are given for prophylaxis (Cinryze®) 1,000 units IV

Altered Level of Consciousness due to Acute Intoxication Order Set

Place in Emergency Department (ED) Observation

Diagnosis *ALTERED LEVEL OF CONSCIOUSNESS DUE TO ACUTE INTOXICATION,* _____, _____

ED Attending _____

Resident (if applicable) _____

Advanced Practice Provider (if applicable)

_____

Allergies: Yes _____ No _____

If yes, what _____, _____, _____, _____, _____, _____

Vital Signs

Temperature __ Pulse __ Respiration __ BP__
Pulse oximetry __

__ q 2 hours ___ q 4 hours ___ q 6 hours q ___
hours ___ q shift ___ qd ___ other

Cardiac monitoring (telemetry) _____

Neurologic checks ___ q 2 hours __ q 4 hours
__ q 6 hours q __ hours ___ other

Orthostatic vital signs _____

Continuous pulse oximetry_____

Other _____

Notify Physician if

Temperature (°C) > 38.0° ___ 38.5°___ 39° ___
40° ___ other ___

Systolic blood pressure (mmHg) ≤ 90 ___ ≥
160 __ ≥ 180 ___ ≥ 200 __ other _____

Diastolic blood pressure (mmHg) ≥ 120 ____
other _____

Heart rate ≤ 50 ___ ≥ 120 ___ ≥ 150 ___ ≥ 200
____ other

Oxygen saturation < 90% _____

Respiratory rate < 8 per minute or apnea
_____

Any change in mental status _____

Any respiratory distress _____

Activity

Assisted _____

Out of bed to chair _____

Bedrest _____

Bedrest with bedside commode __

Bedrest with bathroom privileges ___

Up ad lib only after fully awake and cleared by
ED attending or advanced practice
provider ___

Other _____

Diet

NPO _____

May have PO intake only after cleared by ED
attending or advanced practice provider ____

Diet after cleared by ED attending or advanced
practice provider:

Regular _____

Advance diet as tolerated _____

Clear liquids ____

Dental, mechanical soft _____

Diabetic _____

Formula _____

Full liquids _____

Low cholesterol ____

Pureed _____

Sodium: 1 gram ___ 2 grams ___
unrestricted ____

Per feeding tube _____

Other _____

Nursing Interventions

Weight ___ on admission ___ qd ___ prior to
discharge ___ other

Height ____

I & Os _____ routine _____ strict _____

Fluid restriction _____ mL/hour _____ mL/
shift _____ mL/24 hour

Fall precautions _____

Seizure precautions _____

Capillary blood glucose __ × 1 __ q __ hours
___ before meals and at bedtime

Respiratory Interventions

Oxygen __ liters nasal cannula __ venti mask at
___ liters per minute _____ other

Wean oxygen as tolerated without dyspnea,
stridor or oxygen saturation < 90% _____

Sleep apnea qhs __ CPAP BiPAP settings cm
H_2O ___ inspiratory __ expiratory

Laboratory Tests

Alcohol level (blood) _____

Arterial blood gas ___ on room air _____ other

Amylase ____ Lipase _____

Basic metabolic panel _____

Carbon monoxide level _____

Cardiac enzymes ___ × 1 ___ q 4 hours × 3 ___ q 4 hours × 4 ____ other

CBC with differential ___

Complete metabolic panel _____

Drug level _____, _____, _____

Ketones in serum _____

Ketones in urine _____

Lactate _____

Liver function tests _____

Magnesium _____

Phosphate _____

Pregnancy test (qualitative urine) _____

Pregnancy test (quantitative blood) _____

Urinalysis _____

Urine culture _____

Toxicology screen urine _____

Toxicology screen blood _____

Venous blood gas _____

Other _____, _____, _____, _____, _____, _____, _____, _____

Radiology Studies

Acute abdominal series ____

CXR portable _____

CXR (PA and lateral) _____

KUB (kidneys, ureters, bladder) _____, _____

CT scan head (without contrast) _____

CT scan spine (without contrast) _____

CT scan _____

Spine films cervical ____ thoracic ____ lumbar ____

Extremity films _____, _____, _____, _____, _____, _____

Other _____, _____, _____, _____, _____, _____

Cardiac Studies

ECG __ × 1 __ q 4 hours × 3 ___ q 4 hours × 4 ___ other ____ with cardiac enzymes

Echocardiogram (transthoracic) __ with agitated (bubble) study __ without agitated (bubble) study

Other _____

Consultants

Care coordination (Case management) _____ Notified: Name _____ Time _____

Psychiatry _____ Notified: Name _____ Time _____

Social work _____ Notified: Name _____ Time _____

Other _____ Notified: Name _____ Time _____

Medications for Altered Level of Consciousness due to Acute Intoxication

Flumazenil (Romazicon®)* for benzodiazepine overdose IV initial dose 0.2 mg, may repeat 0.3 mg at 1 minute if desired LOC is not obtained; repeat doses 0.5 mg at 1-minute intervals (maximum of 4 repeat doses), maximum total cumulative dose 1 mg. If re-sedation occurs, repeat doses may be given at 20-minute intervals at 0.2 mg/min to a maximum of 1 mg total dose and 3 mg in 1 hour (administer the drug IV over 30 seconds) _____

Naloxone (Narcan®) ___ mg IV __ q 4 hours __ q 6 hours _____ other at ___ hours

Naloxone (Narcan®) IV continuous infusion at _____ mg/hour**

Folic acid (Folate) _____ mg PO

Thiamine (Vitamin B1) _____ 100 mg IM ___ PO___

Other _____, _____, _____, _____, _____

Intravenous Fluids

Saline cap IV ____

Bolus Normal Saline (NS) IV ___ 250 mL __ 500 mL ___ 1,000 mL ____ other, infuse over ___ minutes ___ hours

Bolus Lactated Ringer's (LR) IV __ 250 mL __ 500 mL __ 1,000 mL __ other, infuse over ___ minutes ___ hours

Maintenance NS at __ mL per hour IV

Maintenance LR at __ mL per hour IV

Maintenance Dextrose 5% in Water (D_5W) at __ mL per hour IV

Maintenance Dextrose 5% in ½ Normal Saline ($D_5½NS$) at __ mL per hour IV

Maintenance Dextrose 5% in Normal Saline (D_5NS) at __ mL per hour IV

Maintenance NS with potassium chloride __ 20 mEq or __ 40 mEq per 1 liter bag at __ mL per hour

Maintenance D_5W with potassium chloride __ 20 mEq or __ 40 mEq per 1 liter bag at mL per hour IV

Maintenance $D_5\frac{1}{2}$ NS with potassium chloride__ 20 mEq or __ 40 mEq per 1 liter bag at __ mL per hour IV

Maintenance D_5NS with potassium chloride __ 20 mEq or __ 40 mEq per 1 liter bag at __ mL per hour IV

Add IV adult multivitamins to 1 liter __ NS IV _____ to D_5W IV __ to $D_5\frac{1}{2}$ NS __ to D_5NS __ other IV

Other _____ at mL per hour

Education: patient _____ family _____

Alcohol/Drugs cessation _____

Smoking cessation _____

Other _____

* Flumazenil should be used with caution and only when necessary since it has a United States FDA black box warning: benzodiazepine withdrawal may result in seizures. Use with the following precautions:

Seizures may occur more frequently in patients following tricyclic overdose or in patients on benzodiazepines for long-term sedation. Individualize the dose and be prepared to manage seizures. Seizures may also develop in patients with concurrent major sedative-hypnotic drug withdrawal, recent therapy with repeated doses of parenteral benzodiazepines, and/or myoclonic jerking or seizure activity prior to flumazenil administration. Use with caution in patients relying on a benzodiazepine for seizure control.

Considering the many concerns and the black box warning, it may be prudent to avoid use of flumazenil in the observation unit since its use may involve intensive nursing and/or physician care.

** In general, patients on continuous medication infusions may be considered a higher level of care and may be appropriate for "complex" or "extended" observation but not for "simple" observation

LOC = level of consciousness

Asthma -- Acute Exacerbation Order Set

Place in Emergency Department (ED)
  Observation _____
Diagnosis *ASTHMA – ACUTE
  EXACERBATION,* _____, _____,
  _____
ED Attending _____
Resident (if applicable) _____
Advanced Practice Provider (if applicable)
  _____

Allergies: Yes _____ No _____

If yes, what _____, _____, _____, _____,
  _____, _____

Vital Signs

Temperature __ Pulse __ Respiration __ BP__
  Pulse oximetry ____
__ q 2 hours ___ q 4 hours ___ q 6 hours q ___
  hours ___ q shift ___ qd ____ other
Cardiac monitoring (telemetry) _____
Continuous pulse oximetry_____
Other _____

Notify Physician if

Temperature (°C) > 38.0° ___ 38.5°___ 39° ___
  40° ____ other _____
Systolic blood pressure (mmHg) ≤ 90 ___ ≥
  160 __ ≥ 180 ___ ≥ 200 __ other _____
Diastolic blood pressure (mmHg) > 120 ___
  other _____
Heart rate ≤ 50 ___ ≥ 120 __ ≥ 150 ___ ≥
  200 ___ other ____
Any change in mental status _____
Any chest pain _____
Any shortness of breath or respiratory distress
  _____
Oxygen saturation < 90%, worsening dyspnea
  or increasing oxygen requirement ____

Activity

Up ad lib _____
Assisted _____
Out of bed to chair _____
Bedrest with bathroom privileges _____
Bedrest with bedside commode _____
Bedrest _____
Other _____

Diet

NPO _____
Regular _____
Advance diet as tolerated _____
Clear liquids ____
Dental, mechanical soft _____
Diabetic _____
Formula _____
Full liquids _____
Low cholesterol ____
Pureed _____
Sodium: 1 gram ___ 2 grams ___
  unrestricted____
Per feeding tube _____
Other _____

Nursing Interventions

Weight ___ on admission ___ qd ___ prior to
  discharge ____ other
Height ____
I & Os _____ routine _____ strict _____
Fluid restriction ___ mL/hour ___ mL/shift
  ____ mL/24 hour ___ other
Fall precautions _____
Seizure precautions _____
Capillary blood glucose __ × 1 q __ hours __
  before meals and at bedtime

Respiratory Interventions

Oxygen __ liters nasal cannula __ venti mask at
  ___ liters per minute _____ other
Wean oxygen as tolerated without
  dyspnea, stridor or oxygen saturation
  < 90% ____
Peak flow __ on admission ___ prior to
  discharge ___ pre and post aerosols
Sleep apnea qhs __ CPAP BiPAP settings cm
  H_2O ___ inspiratory __ expiratory

Laboratory Tests

CBC _____ with differential
Basic metabolic panel _____
Cardiac enzymes ___ × 1 ___ q 4 hours × 3 ___
  q 4 hours × 4 ____ other _____
Complete metabolic panel _____
Other _____, _____, _____, _____,
  _____, _____, _____, _____
Repeat _____, _____, _____, _____, _____ in
  a.m. ___ in _____ hours

Radiology Studies

CXR portable _____

CXR (PA and lateral) _____

Other _____, _____, _____

If chest pain or worsening shortness of breath or drop in oxygen saturation, portable CXR _____

Cardiac Studies

ECG __ × 1__ q 4 hours × 3 ___ q 4 hours × 4 ___ other ____ with cardiac enzymes

Echocardiogram (transthoracic) __ with agitated (bubble) study __ without agitated (bubble) study

Other _____

If chest pain or worsening shortness of breath, ___ ECG ___cardiac enzymes

Consultants

Care coordinator (Case management) _____ Notified: Name _____ Time _____

Pulmonary _____ Notified: Name _____ Time _____

Social work _____ Notified: Name _____ Time _____

Other _____ Notified: Name _____ Time _____

Asthma Medications (Adult Dosage)

Inhaled Medications: Aerosols

Albuterol (Proventil®) nebulized solution __ 2.5 mg __ other aerosol __ × 1 __ q 2 hours __ q 4 hours __ q 6 hours __ q 8 hours __ prn wheezing __ other

Ipratropium (Atrovent®) 0.5 mg nebulized solution aerosol __ × 1 __ q 2 hours __ q 4 hours __ q 6 hours __ q 8 hours __ prn wheezing __ other

Inhaled Medications: Inhalers

Albuterol (Proventil®) (90 mcg per inhalation) metered dose inhaler (MDI) __ puffs __ q 4 hours __ q 6 hours __ prn wheezing ___ other

Ipratropium (Atrovent®) (17 mcg per inhalation) __ puffs __ q 4 hours __ q 6 hours __ prn wheezing ___ other

Albuterol 90 mcg and Ipratropium 18 mcg (per inhalation) (CombiventRespimat®) __ puffs __ q 6 hours ___ prn wheezing ___ other

Antibiotics – Oral*

Amoxicillin (Amoxil®) __ 250 mg __ 500 mg __ 875 mg PO__ bid ___ tid __ qid __ other

Amoxicillin and Clavulanic Acid, Amoxicillin and Clavulanate (Augmentin®) __ 250 mg ___ 500 mg __ 875 mg PO __ q 8 hours __ q 12 hours __ other

Azithromycin (Zithromax®) __ 500 mg on day 1 followed by 250 mg on subsequent days PO qd __ 500 mg PO qd __ other

Doxycycline (Adoxa®, Doryx®, Vibramycin®) __ 100 mg bid PO __ other

Levofloxacin (Levaquin®) ___ 500 mg ___ 750 mg PO __ qd __ other

Moxifloxacin (Avelox®) __ 400 mg PO qd

Antibiotics – Intravenous*

Ampicillin and Sulbactam (Unasyn®) ___ 1.5 grams __ 3 grams IV ___ q 6 hours __ other

Azithromycin (Zithromax®) __ 500 mg IV __ × 1 __ daily ___ other

Ceftriaxone (Rocephin®) __ 1 gram IV__ × 1 __ other

Doxycycline (Doxy®) ___ 100 mg IV bid __ other

Levofloxacin (Levaquin®) ___ 500 mg ___ 750 mg IV __ qd __ other

Moxifloxacin (Avelox®) __ 400 mg qd IV

Corticosteroids

Methylprednisolone (Solumedrol®) __ 40 mg __ mg IV qd ___ other

Prednisone __ 40 mg PO qd ___ 60 mg PO qd __ other

Other _____, _____, _____, _____, _____

Intravenous Fluids

Saline cap IV _____

Bolus Normal Saline (NS) IV ___ 250 mL __ 500 mL ___ 1,000 mL _____ other, infuse over ___ minutes ___ hours

Bolus Lactated Ringer's (LR) IV __ 250 mL __ 500 mL __ 1,000 mL __ other, infuse over ___ minutes ___ hours

Maintenance NS at __ mL per hour IV

Maintenance LR at __ mL per hour IV

Maintenance Dextrose in Water (D$_5$W) at __ mL per hour IV

Maintenance Dextrose in ½ Normal Saline (D$_5$½NS) at __ mL per hour IV

Maintenance Dextrose 5% in Normal Saline (D$_5$NS) at __ mL per hour IV

Maintenance NS with potassium chloride__ 20 mEq or __ 40 mEq per 1 liter bag at __ mL per hour

Maintenance D$_5$W with potassium chloride__ 20 mEq or __ 40 mEq per 1 liter bag at __ mL per hour

Maintenance D$_5$½NS with potassium chloride __ 20 mEq or __ 40 mEq per 1 liter bag at __ mL per hour IV

Maintenance D$_5$NS with potassium chloride __ 20 mEq or __ 40 mEq per 1 liter bag at __ mL per hour IV

Other _____ at mL per hour

Education: patient _____ family _____

Asthma ____

COPD** ____

Pneumonia/Bronchitis* _____

Smoking cessation _____

Other _____

* Since respiratory infections may trigger an acute asthmatic attack and since bacterial infections including bacterial pneumonia may be an indication for antibiotics, antibiotics are included in the asthma order set.

** Since patients with both asthma and COPD are not unusual, some medications and instructions that relate to COPD are included in the asthma order set.

Atrial Fibrillation Order Set

Place in Emergency Department (ED) Observation _____

Diagnosis *ATRIAL FIBRILLATION,*

_____, _____, _____

ED Attending _____

Resident (if applicable) _____

Advanced Practice Provider (if applicable)

_____

Allergies: Yes _____ No _____

If yes, what _____, _____, _____, _____,

_____, _____

Vital Signs

Temperature __ Pulse __ Respiration __ BP __ Pulse oximetry ____

__ q 2 hours ____ q 4 hours ____ q 6 hours q __ hours ____ q shift ____ qd ____ other

Cardiac monitoring (telemetry) _____

Continuous pulse oximetry _____

Neurologic checks __ q 2 hours ____ q 4 hours ____ q 6 hours ____ q shift ____ qd

Vascular checks __ q 2 hours ____ q 4 hours ____ q 6 hours ____ q shift ____ qd

Other _____

Notify Physician if

Temperature (°C) > 38.0° ____ 38.5° ____ 39° ____ 40° ____ other ____

Systolic blood pressure (mmHg) ≤ 90 ____ ≥ 160 __ ≥ 180 ____ ≥ 200 __ other _____

Diastolic blood pressure (mmHg) > 120 ____ other _____

Heart rate ≤ 50 ____ ≥ 120 __ ≥ 150 ____ ≥ 200 ____ other ____

Oxygen saturation < 90% _____ other _____

Any change in mental status _____

Any shortness of breath or respiratory distress ____

Activity

Up ad lib _____

Assisted _____

Out of bed to chair _____

Bedrest with bathroom privileges _____

Bedrest with bedside commode _____

Bedrest _____

Other _____

Diet

NPO _____

Regular _____

Advance diet as tolerated _____

Clear liquids ____

Dental, mechanical soft _____

Diabetic _____

Formula _____

Full liquids _____

Low cholesterol ____

Low added fat/No added salt _____

Pureed _____

Sodium: 1 gram ___ 2 grams ___ unrestricted ____

Per feeding tube _____
Other _____

Nursing Interventions

Weight ___ on admission ___ qd ___ prior to
discharge ____ other
Height ____
I & Os _____ routine _____ strict _____
Fluid restriction _____ mL/hour _____ mL/
shift ____ mL/24 hour
Fall precautions _____
Seizure precautions _____
Capillary blood glucose __ × 1 q ___ hours
_____ before meals and at bedtime
Defibrillator pads placed on chest _____

Respiratory Interventions

Oxygen __ liters nasal cannula __ venti mask at
___ liters per minute _____ other
Wean oxygen as tolerated without dyspnea,
stridor or oxygen saturation < 90% ____
Peak flow __ on admission ___ prior to
discharge ___ pre and post aerosols
Sleep apnea qhs __ CPAP BiPAP settings cm
H_2O ___ inspiratory __ expiratory

Laboratory Tests

CBC _____ with differential _____
Basic metabolic panel _____
Brain natriuretic peptide (BNP) _____
Complete metabolic panel _____
Cardiac enzymes ___ × 1 ___ q 4 hours × 3 ___
q 4 hours × 4 ____ other
PT ___ INR ____ APTT ____
Other _____, _____, _____, _____,
_____, _____, _____, _____
Repeat _____, _____, _____, _____, _____ in
a.m., in ___ hours q ___ hours

Radiology Studies

CXR portable _____
CXR (PA and lateral) _____
Other _____, _____, _____, _____,
_____, _____

Cardiac Studies

ECG __ × 1__ q 4 hour × 3 ___ q 4 hour X 4
___ other ____ with cardiac enzymes
Echocardiogram (transthoracic) __with
agitated (bubble) study__ without agitated
(bubble) study

Stress Tests/Cardiac Imaging Studies*

Stress Electrocardiogram (treadmill stress test,
exercise tolerance test/ETT) _____
Stress Echocardiogram ____
Pharmacologic Stress Tests
    Coronary Vasodilators:

      Adenosine _____
      Dipyridamole/Persantine _____
      Regadenosine/Lexiscan _____

    Synthetic Catecholamine:

      Dobutamine _____

Myocardial Perfusion Imaging (injection of
radioactive isotopes):
    Nuclear Stress Test

      Thallium-201 _____
      Technetium-99m Sestamibi _____
      Technetium-99 Tetrofosmin _____

Gamma Imaging:

    Single positron emission computed
tomography (SPECT)_____
    Cardiac positron emission tomography (pet)

Stress Cardiovascular Magnetic Resonance
Imaging (CMR) _____
Computed Tomography Coronary
Angiography (CTCA) _____
Other _____

* Not all tests are available at all institutions.
Generally, test availability is limited, depends
on many factors including available expertise
and cost, and is institution specific. This list is
not all inclusive but is intended to list the
stress tests/cardiac imaging discussed in
Chapter 26 Stress Testing.

Consultants

Cardiology _____ Notified:
Name _____ Time _____
Care coordination (Case management)
_____ Notified: Name _____ Time
_____
Electrophysiology service (EPS) ____ Notified:
Name _____ Time _____
Heart failure service _____ Notified:
Name _____ Time _____
Social work _____ Notified: Name
_____ Time _____

Other _____ Notified:
    Name _____ Time _____

Cardiac Medications (Adult Dosage)

Antiplatelet Agent

Aspirin PO qd _____ 81 mg _____ 325 mg

Vitamin K Antagonist

Warfarin (Coumadin®) ___ mg PO __ qd __
qod _____ other

Low Molecular Weight Heparin

Enoxaparin (Lovenox®) ___ mg SQ __ q12
hours __ qd

Rate Controlling Drugs*

Diltiazem (Cardizem®) __ 20 mg IV over 2
minutes, ___

    If heart rate > 110 beats/minute, 15 minutes
later, give diltiazem IV 25 mg over 2
minutes

    Immediate release tab (Cardizem®) __
30 mg __ 60 mg __ other __ mg
PO __ qid __ (usual dose range 120–320
mg daily)

    Extended release tab (Cardizem® LA) ___
180 mg PO daily _____ other
(usual dose range 120–320 mg daily,
maximum dose 360 mg daily)

Metoprolol (Lopressor®) _ 5 mg _ 10 mg IV __
q 6 hours __ q 12 hours _ other q __ hours
___ other

    Immediate release tab (Lopressor®) __
50 mg __ 100 mg __ other __ mg PO __ bid
(usual dose range 50–100 mg daily,
maximum 450 mg daily)

    Extended release tab (Toprol XL®) __ 25 mg
__ 50 mg __ 100 mg __ other __ mg
PO qd (usual dose range 50–100 mg daily,
maximum dose 400 mg daily)

    Other _____, _____, _____, _____,

    _____

* Hold all rate controlling drugs if heart rate <
50 beats/minute or systolic blood pressure <
90 mmHg _____

Intravenous Fluids

Saline cap IV _____

Bolus Normal Saline (NS) IV ___ 250 mL
_____ 500 mL ___ 1,000 mL _____ other,
infuse over ___ minutes ___ hours

Bolus Lactated Ringer's (LR) IV __ 250 mL _ __
500 mL __ 1,000 mL ___ other, infuse over
___ minutes ___ hours

Maintenance NS at __ mL per hour IV

Maintenance LR at __ mL per hour IV

Maintenance Dextrose 5% in Water (D_5W)
_____ at __ mL per hour IV

Maintenance Dextrose 5% in ½ Normal Saline
(D_5½NS) _____ at __ mL per hour IV

Maintenance Dextrose 5% in Normal Saline
(D_5NS) at __ mL per hour IV

Maintenance NS with potassium chloride __
20 mEq or __ 40 mEq per 1 liter bag at __ mL
per hour IV

Maintenance D_5W with potassium chloride __
20 mEq or __ 40 mEq per 1 liter bag at mL
per hour IV

Maintenance D_5½NS with potassium chloride
__ 20 mEq or __ 40 mEq per 1 liter bag at __
mL per hour IV

Maintenance D_5NS with potassium chloride __
20 mEq or __ 40 mEq per 1 liter bag at __ mL
per hour IV

Other maintenance _____ at mL per hour IV

Education: patient _____ family _____

Atrial fibrillation _____

Chest pain _____

Coronary artery disease _____

Smoking cessation _____

Other _____

Back Pain (Acute) Order Set

Place in Emergency Department (ED)
Observation _____

Diagnosis *ACUTE BACK PAIN,* _____,

_____, _____

ED Attending _____

Resident (if applicable) _____

Advanced Practice Provider (if applicable)

_____

Allergies: Yes _____ No _____

If yes, what _____, _____, _____, _____,

_____, _____

Vital Signs

Temperature __ Pulse __ Respiration __ BP __
Pulse oximetry ____

__ q 2 hours ___ q 4 hours ___ q 6 hours q ___
hours ___ q shift ___ qd ____ other Cardiac
monitoring (telemetry) _____

Neurologic checks __ q 2 hours __ q 4 hours __
q 6 hours q __ hours __ q shift __ qd __ other

Vascular checks __ q 2 hours __ q 4 hours __ q
6 hours q __ hours __ q shift __ qd __ other

Continuous pulse oximetry_____

Other _____

Notify Physician if

Temperature (°C) > 38.0° ___ 38.5° ___ 39° ___
40° ____ other _____

Systolic blood pressure (mmHg) ≤ 90 ___ ≥
160 __ ≥ 180 ___ ≥ 200 __ other _____

Diastolic blood pressure (mmHg) ≥ 120 ____
other _____

Heart rate ≤ 50 ___ ≥ 120 __ ≥ 150 ___ ≥
200 ___ other ____

Oxygen saturation < 90% _____ other _____

Any new neurologic symptoms (e.g., weakness,
numbness, tingling) _____

Activity

Up ad lib _____

Assisted _____

Out of bed to chair _____

Bedrest with bathroom privileges _____

Bedrest with bedside commode _____

Bedrest _____

Other _____

Diet

NPO _____

Regular _____

Advance diet as tolerated _____

Clear liquids ____

Dental, mechanical soft _____

Diabetic _____

Formula _____

Full liquids _____

Low added fat/No added salt _____

Low cholesterol ____

Pureed _____

Sodium: 1 gram ___ 2 grams ___
unrestricted____

Per feeding tube _____

Other _____

Nursing Interventions

Weight ___ on admission ___ qd ___ prior to
discharge ____ other

I & Os _____ routine _____ strict _____

Fluid restriction ___ mL/hour ___ mL/shift
____ mL/24 hour ___ other

Fall precautions _____

Seizure precautions _____

Capillary blood glucose __ × 1 q ___ hours
____ before meals and at bedtime

Respiratory Interventions

Oxygen __ liters nasal cannula __ venti mask at
___ liters per minute _____ other

Wean oxygen as tolerated without
dyspnea, stridor or oxygen saturation
< 90% ____

Peak flow __ on admission ___ prior to
discharge ___ pre and post aerosols

Sleep apnea qhs __ CPAP BiPAP settings cm
H_2O ___ inspiratory __ expiratory

Laboratory Tests

CBC _____ with differential

Basic metabolic panel _____

Cardiac enzymes ___ × 1 ___ q 4 hours × 3 ___
q 4 hours × 4 ____ other

Complete metabolic panel _____

C-reactive protein (CRP) _____

Erythrocyte sedimentation rate (ESR)

_____

Lactate _____

Liver function tests _____

Renal function tests (e.g., BUN, creatinine) _____

Urinalysis _____

Urine culture _____

Pregnancy test _____ (qualitative urine) _____ quantitative (blood)

Other _____, _____, _____, _____, _____, _____, _____, _____

Repeat _____, _____, _____, _____, _____ in a.m.___ in _____ hours

Radiology Studies

CXR portable _____

CXR (PA and lateral) _____

Spine x-rays: cervical ___ thoracic ___ lumbar ___

CT scan ___ cervical___ thoracic _____ lumbar ____ other

Ultrasound ____

MRI spine: ___ cervical___ thoracic _____ lumbar ____

Other _____, _____, _____

Cardiac Studies

ECG __ × 1__ q 4 hours × 3 ___ q 4 hours × 4 ___ other ____ with cardiac enzymes

Echocardiogram (transthoracic) __ with agitated (bubble) study __ without agitated (bubble)

Other _____

Consultants

Care coordination (Case management) _____ Notified: Name _____ Time _____

Neurosurgery _____ Notified: Name _____ Time _____

Orthopedics _____ Notified: Name _____ Time _____

Pain management service _____ Notified: Name _____ Time _____

Physical therapy _____ Notified: Name _____ Time _____

Spine service _____ Notified: Name _____ Time _____

Social work _____ Notified: Name _____ Time _____

Other _____ Notified: Name _____ Time _____

Back Pain Medications (Adult Dosage)

Analgesics

Acetaminophen (Paracetamol) (Tylenol®) 325 mg tab __ 1 tab __ 1–2 tabs __ 2 tabs PO __ q 4 hours __ q 6 hours ___ prn pain ___ prn fever (maximum 4 g daily)

____ If unable to take tablet formulation, may give suspension

____ If unable to take PO, may give suppository PR __ 325 mg __ 650 mg __ q 4 hours __ q 6 hours

IV ___ mg __ q 4 hours __ q 6 hours __ prn pain __ prn fever (maximum adult dose: if weight < 50 kg is 15 mg/kg up to 750 mg for a single dose, 75 mg/kg up to 3750 mg for daily dose; if weight > 50 kg is 650 mg q 4 hours or 1000 mg q 6 hours up to 1000 mg for a single dose and 4000 mg for a daily dose)

Acetaminophen-Hydrocodone (Vicodin®) 300 mg/5 mg tabs __ 1 tab __ 1–2 tabs __ 2 tabs PO __ q 4 hours __ q 6 hours ___ prn pain (maximum 4 grams daily based on acetaminophen dose)

Acetaminophen-Oxycodone (Endocet®, Percocet®, Roxicet®) 325 mg/ 5 mg tab __ 1 tab __ 1–2 tabs __ 2 tabs PO q 4 hours __ q 6 hours ___ prn pain (maximum 4 grams daily based on acetaminophen dose)

Hydromorphone (Dilaudid®) __ 0.5 mg __ 1 mg __ 2 mg __ mg __ IV __ q 2 hours __ q 4 hours __ q 6 hours q ___ hours __ prn pain

Ibuprofen (Advil®, Motrin®) __ 400 mg __ 600 mg __ 800 mg PO __ q 4 hours __ q 6 hours __ q 8 hours ___ prn pain

Ketorolac (Toradol®) __ 30 mg IV __ q 6 hours __ prn pain (maximum 120 mg daily)

Morphine __ 0.5 mg __ 1 mg __ 2 mg __ 4 mg __ mg ___ IV q 2 hours __ q 4 hours __ q 6 hours q ___ hours __ prn pain

Tramadol (Ultram®) __ 50 mg __ 100 mg PO __ q 4 hours __ q 6 hours __ prn pain (maximum 400 mg daily)

Other _____, _____, _____, _____, _____

Antiemetics

Chlorpromazine (Thorazine®) __ 10 mg PO __ 25 mg PO __ q 4 hours __ q 6 hours __

25 mg __ 50 mg __ IV __ IM __ q 4 hours __ q 6 hours __ prn nausea/vomiting

Metoclopramide (Reglan®) __10 mg __ IV __ IM __ PO __ q 6 hours __ other __ prn nausea/vomiting

Ondansetron (Zofran®) __ 4 mg __ 8 mg __ IV __ PO __ q 6 hours ___ other __ prn nausea/vomiting

Prochlorperazine (Compazine®) __ 5 mg __ 10 mg __ IV __ IM __ PO __ q 4 hours __ q 6 hours (maximum dose IV/IM/PO 40 mg per day) ___ 25 mg PR bid __ prn nausea/vomiting

Promethazine (Phenergan®) __ 12.5 mg __ 25 mg __ IV__ IM __ PO __ PR __ q4 hours __ q 6 hours ___ prn nausea/vomiting

Trimethobenzamide (Tigan®) __ 200 mg IM __ 300 mg PO ___ q 6 hours ___ prn nausea/vomiting

Intravenous Fluids

Saline cap IV ____

Bolus Normal Saline (NS) IV ___ 250 mL __ 500 mL ___ 1,000 mL ___ other, infuse over ___ minutes ___ hours

Bolus Lactated Ringer's (LR) IV __ 250 mL __ 500 mL __1,000 mL __ other, infuse over ___ minutes ___ hours

Maintenance NS at __ mL per hour IV

Maintenance LR at __ mL per hour IV

Maintenance Dextrose 5% in Water (D_5W) at __ mL per hour IV

Maintenance Dextrose 5% in ½ Normal Saline (D_5½NS) at __ mL per hour IV

Maintenance Dextrose 5% in Normal Saline (D_5NS) at __ mL per hour IV

Maintenance NS with potassium chloride __ 20 mEq or __ 40 mEq per 1 liter bag at __ mL per hour

Maintenance D_5W with potassium chloride__ 20 mEq or __ 40 mEq per 1 liter bag at __ mL per hour

Maintenance D_5½NS with potassium chloride __ 20 mEq or __ 40 mEq per 1 liter bag at __mL per hour IV

Maintenance D_5NS with potassium chloride __ 20 mEq or __ 40 mEq per 1 liter bag at __ mL per hour IV

Other _____ at mL per hour

Education: patient _____ family _____

Back pain ____

Smoking cessation _____

Other _____

Cellulitis Order Set

Place in Emergency Department (ED)
Observation _____
Diagnosis *CELLULITIS,* _____,

_____, _____

ED Attending _____
Resident (if applicable) _____
Advanced Practice Provider (if applicable)

_____

Allergies: Yes _____ No _____

If yes, what _____, _____, _____, _____,

_____, _____

Vital Signs

Temperature __ Pulse __ Respiration __ BP__
Pulse oximetry _____
__ q 2 hours ____ q 4 hours ___ q 6 hours q ___
hours ___ q shift ___ qd ____ other
Cardiac monitoring (telemetry) _____
Continuous pulse oximetry_____
Vascular checks __ q 2 hours ___ q 4 hours ___
q 6 hours q ___ hours __ q shift ___ qd
Other _____

Notify Physician if

Temperature (°C) > 38.0° ____ 38.5°____ 39° ____
40° ____ other ___
Systolic blood pressure (mmHg) ≤ 90 ___ ≥
160 __ ≥ 180 ___ ≥ 200 __ other _____
Diastolic blood pressure (mmHg) > 120 ___
other _____
Heart rate ≤ 50 ___ ≥ 120 __ ≥ 150 ___ ≥
200 ___ other _____
Oxygen saturation < 90% _____ other _____

Activity

Up ad lib _____
Assisted _____
Out of bed to chair _____
Bedrest with bathroom privileges _____
Bedrest with bedside commode _____
Bedrest _____
Other _____

Diet

NPO _____
Regular _____
Advance diet as tolerated _____

Clear liquids _____
Dental, mechanical soft _____
Diabetic _____
Formula _____
Full liquids _____
Low added fat/No added salt _____
Low cholesterol ____
Pureed _____
Sodium: 1 gram ___ 2 grams ___
unrestricted _____
Per feeding tube _____
Other _____

Nursing Interventions

Weight ___ on admission ___ qd ___ prior to
discharge _____ other
Height _____
I & Os _____ routine _____ strict _____
Fluid restriction ___ mL/hour ___ mL/shift
_____ mL/24 hour ___ other
Fall precautions _____
Seizure precautions _____
Capillary blood glucose __ × 1 q ___ hour _____
before meals and at bedtime
Elevate affected extremity _____

Respiratory Interventions

Oxygen __ liters nasal cannula __ venti mask at
___ liters per minute _____ other
Wean oxygen as tolerated without dyspnea,
stridor or oxygen saturation < 90% _____
Peak flow __ on admission ___ prior to
discharge ___ pre and post aerosols
Sleep apnea qhs __ CPAP BiPAP settings cm
H_2O ___ inspiratory __ expiratory

Laboratory Tests

CBC _____ with differential
Basic metabolic panel _____
Blood culture × 1 ___ × 2 ___ other ____
Complete metabolic panel _____
C-reactive protein (CRP) _____
Culture of incision and drainage of
abscess _____
Culture of wound _____
Culture – other _____
Erythrocyte sedimentation rate (ESR) _____
Lactate _____
Liver function tests _____

Pregnancy test _____(qualitative urine)
Pregnancy test (quantitative blood) _____
Renal function test (e.g., BUN, creatinine) _____

Type and Screen _____
Urinalysis _____
Urine culture _____
Other _____, _____, _____, _____,
_____, _____, _____, _____
Repeat _____, _____, _____, _____, _____ in
a.m. ___ in _____ hours q _____ hours

Radiology Studies

Xray _____
Ultrasound ___
CT scan ____
MRI ____
Other ____, _____, _____, _____, _____

Cardiac Tests

ECG __ × 1 __ q 4 hours × 3 ___ q 4 hours ×
4 ___ other ____ with cardiac enzymes
Echocardiogram (transthoracic) __ with
agitated (bubble) study __ without agitated
(bubble) study

Consultants

Care coordination (Case management)
_____ Notified: Name _____
Time _____
Dental _____
Notified: Name _____ Time _____
General surgery _____ Notified:
Name _____ Time _____
Gynecology _____
Notified: Name _____ Time _____
Hand surgery _____ Notified:
Name _____ Time _____
Maxillofacial surgery _____ Notified:
Name _____ Time _____
Orthopedic surgery _____ Notified:
Name _____ Time _____
Otolaryngology _____ Notified:
Name _____ Time _____
Social work _____ Notified:
Name _____ Time _____
Other _____
Notified: Name _____ Time _____

Cellulitis Medications (Adult Dosages)
Antibiotics† Antibiotics – Oral

Amoxicillin and Clavulanic Acid, Amoxicillin
and Clavulanate (Augmentin®)
__ 250 mg ____ 500 mg __ 875 mg PO __ q
8 hours __ q 12 hours __ other
Cephalexin (Keflex®) ___ 500 mg ___ 1,000 mg
PO ___ q 6 hours __ q 8 hours __ q 12 hours
Ciprofloxacin (Cipro®) __ 500 mg bid PO
__ other
Clindamycin* (Cleocin®) ___ 300 mg __
450 mg PO q 6 hours
Doxycycline (Adoxa®, Doryx®, Vibramycin®)
__ 100 mg bid PO __ other
Levofloxacin (Levaquin®) ___ 500 mg ___
750 mg PO qd __ other
Sulfamethoxazole and Trimethoprim
(Bactrim™ DS, Septra® DS) __ 1 tab __
2 tabs PO __ q 12 hours __ q d__ other __
(usual dose 1–2 double strength [DS] tablets
every 12–24 hours where DS =
sulfamethoxazole 800 mg and trimethoprim
[TMP] 180 mg)

Antibiotics – Intravenous

Ampicillin and Sulbactam (Unasyn®) ___ 1.5
grams __ 3 grams IV ___ q 6 hours __ other
Cefazolin (Ancef®) __ 1 gram __ 1.5 grams __
2 grams IV __ q 8 hours __ q 12 hours ___ qd
__ other (usual dose 1–2 grams every 8 hours,
maximum 12 grams daily)
Ciprofloxacin (Cipro®) ___ 400 mg bid IV
___ other
Clindamycin* (Cleocin®) __ 600 mg __ 900 mg
IV__ q 6 hours __ q 8 hours __ __ other
Doxycycline (Doxy®) ___ 100 mg IV bid
__ other
Levofloxacin (Levaquin®) ___ 500 mg ___
750 mg IV qd ___ other

Analgesics

Acetaminophen (Paracetamol) (Tylenol®)
325 mg tab __ 1 tab __ 1–2 tabs __ 2 tabs PO
__ q 4 hours __ q 6 hours ___ prn pain ___
prn fever (maximum 4 g daily)
____ If unable to take tablet formulation, may
give suspension
____ If unable to take PO, may give suppository
PR __ 325 mg __ 650 mg __ q 4 hour __ q 6 hour

IV ___ mg __ q 4 hours __ q 6 hours __ prn pain __ prn fever (maximum adult dose: if weight < 50 kg is 15 mg/kg up to 750 mg for a single dose, 75 mg/kg up to 3750 mg for daily dose; if weight > 50 kg is 650 mg q 4 hours or 1000 mg q 6 hours up to 1000 mg for a single dose and 4000 mg for a daily dose)

Acetaminophen-Hydrocodone (Vicodin®) 300 mg/5 mg tabs __ 1 tab __1–2 tabs __ 2 tabs PO __ q 4 hours __ q 6 hours ___ prn pain (maximum 4 grams daily based on acetaminophen dose)

Acetaminophen-Oxycodone (Endocet®, Percocet®, Roxicet®) 325 mg/5 mg tab __ 1 tab __ 1–2 tabs __ 2 tabs PO q 4 hours __ q 6 hours ___ prn pain (maximum 4 grams daily based on acetaminophen dose)

Hydromorphone (Dilaudid®) __ 0.5 mg __ 1 mg __ 2 mg __ mg __ IV__ q 2 hours __ q 4 hours __ q 6 hours q ___ hours __ prn pain

Ibuprofen (Advil®, Motrin®) __ 400 mg __ 600 mg __ 800 mg PO __ q 4 hours __ q 6 hours __ q 8 hours ___ prn pain

Ketorolac (Toradol®) __ 30 mg IV __ q 6 hours __ prn pain (maximum 120 mg daily)

Morphine __ 0.5 mg __ 1 mg __ 2 mg __ 4 mg __ mg IV __ q 2 hours __ q 4 hours __ q 6 hours q ___ hours __ prn pain

Tramadol (Ultram®) __ 50 mg __ 100 mg PO __ q 4 hours __ q 6 hours __ prn pain (maximum 400 mg daily)

Other _____, _____, _____, _____, _____

Intravenous Fluids

Saline cap IV ____

Bolus Normal Saline (NS) IV ___ 250 mL __ 500 mL ___1,000 mL ____ other, infuse over ___ minutes ___ hours

Bolus Lactated Ringer's (LR) IV __ 250 mL __ 500 mL __ 1,000 mL __ other, infuse over ___ minutes ___ hours

Maintenance NS at __ mL per hour IV

Maintenance LR at __ mL per hour IV

Maintenance Dextrose 5% in Water (D$_5$W) at __ mL per hour IV

Maintenance Dextrose 5% in ½ Normal Saline (D$_5$½NS) at __mL per hour IV

Maintenance Dextrose 5% in Normal Saline (D$_5$NS) at __ mL per hour IV

Maintenance NS with potassium chloride __ 20 mEq or __ 40 mEq per 1 liter bag at __ mL per hour

Maintenance D$_5$W with potassium chloride__ 20 mEq or __ 40 mEq per 1 liter bag at __ mL per hour

Maintenance D$_5$½NS with potassium chloride __ 20 mEq or __ 40 mEq per 1 liter bag at __ mL per hour IV

Maintenance D$_5$NS with potassium chloride __ 20 mEq or __ 40 mEq per 1 liter bag at __ mL per hour IV

Other _____ at mL per hour

Education: patient _____ family _____

Cellulitis _____

Smoking cessation _____

Other _____

*Oral clindamycin is administered in smaller and more frequent doses than IV doses in order to decrease gastrointestinal upset.

† Some antibiotics which are appropriate to treat cellulitis are not included since these drugs do not have an identical oral equivalent (such as vancomycin) and patients in observation are generally given several IV doses of antibiotics, switched to oral medications within 24 hours and sent home on equivalent oral medications. Other antibiotics are not included because these are generally used for complicated and/or severe skin infections or cellulitis and, thus, are not appropriate for observation (e.g., carbapenem therapy).

Chest Pain Order Set

Place in Emergency Department (ED)
Observation _____
Diagnosis **CHEST PAIN,** _____,

_____, _____

ED Attending _____
Resident (if applicable) _____
Advanced Practice Provider (if applicable)

_____

Allergies: Yes _____ No _____

If yes, what _____, _____, _____, _____,

_____, _____

Vital Signs

Temperature __ Pulse __ Respiration __ BP__
Pulse oximetry___
__ q 2 hours ___ q 4 hours ___ q 6 hours ___ q
shift ___ qd ___ other
Cardiac monitoring (telemetry) _____
Continuous pulse oximetry_____
Neurologic checks __ q 2 hours __ q 4 hours __
q 6 hours __ q shift __ qd __ other
Vascular checks __ q 2 hours __ q 4 hours __ q
6 hours __ q shift __ qd __ other

Notify Physician if

Temperature (°C) > 38.0° ___ 38.5°___ 39° ___
40° ____
Systolic blood pressure (mmHg) ≤ 90 __ ≥
160 __ ≥ 180 ___ ≥ 200 __ other _____
Diastolic blood pressure (mmHg) ≥ 120 ____
other _____
Heart rate ≤ 50 ____ ≥ 120 ____ ≥ 150 ____ ≥
200 other ____
Oxygen saturation < 90% _____ other _____
Any chest pain or shortness of breath _____

Activity

Up ad lib _____
Assisted _____
Out of bed to chair _____
Bedrest with bathroom privileges _____
Bedrest with bedside commode _____
Bedrest _____
Other _____

Diet

NPO _____
Regular _____
Advance diet as tolerated _____
Clear liquids ____
Dental, mechanical soft _____
Diabetic _____
Formula_____
Full liquids _____
Low added fat/No added salt _____
Low cholesterol____
Pureed _____
Sodium: 1 gram ___ 2 grams ___
unrestricted ____
Per feeding tube _____
Per specific stress test protocols* _____
Other _____

Nursing Interventions

Weight ___ on admission ___ qd ___ prior to
discharge ____ other
Height ____
I & Os _____ routine _____ strict _____
Fluid restriction _____ mL/hour _____ mL/
shift ____ mL/24 hour
Fall precautions _____
Seizure precautions _____
Capillary blood glucose __ × 1 ____ q hours
____ before meals and at bedtime
If chest pain or shortness of breath or
significant dysrhythmias obtain __ ECG __
cardiac enzymes __ CXR (portable)
If chest pain give nitroglycerin sublingual
0.4 mg X 1 (hold dose if systolic BP <
90 mmHg ___ other __)

Respiratory Interventions

Oxygen __ liters nasal cannula __ venti mask at
___ liters per minute _____ other
Wean oxygen as tolerated without
dyspnea, stridor or oxygen saturation
< 90% ____
Peak flows __ on admission ___ prior to
discharge ____ pre and post aerosols
Sleep apnea qhs __ CPAP BiPAP settings cm
H_2O ___ inspiratory __ expiratory

Laboratory Tests

CBC _____ with differential
Basic metabolic panel _____
Brain natriuretic peptide (BNP) _____
Cardiac enzymes × 1 ___ q 4 hour × 3 ____ q
   4 hour × 4 ___ other ____
Complete metabolic panel _____
D- dimer _____
Lactate _____
Liver function tests _____
Potassium** _____
Pregnancy test (qualitative urine) _____
Pregnancy test (quantitative blood) _____
Renal function tests (e.g., BUN, creatinine)
   _____
Urinalysis _____ Urine culture _____
Other _____, _____, _____, _____,
   _____, _____, _____, _____

Radiology Studies

CXR portable _____
CXR (PA and lateral) _____
Other _____, _____, _____, _____,
   _____ ,_____

Cardiac Studies

ECG ___ × 1 __ q 4 hours × 3 ___ q 4 hours ×
   4 ___ other ____ with cardiac enzymes
Echocardiogram (transthoracic) __ with
   agitated (bubble) study __ without agitated
   (bubble) study

Stress Tests/Cardiac Imaging Studies*

Stress Electrocardiogram (treadmill stress test,
   exercise tolerance test/ETT) ___
Stress Echocardiogram ____
Pharmacologic Stress Tests

   Coronary Vasodilators:

     Adenosine _____
     Dipyridamole/Persantine _____
     Regadenosine/Lexiscan _____

   Synthetic Catecholamine:

     Dobutamine _____

Myocardial Perfusion Imaging (injection of
   radioactive isotopes):

   Nuclear Stress Test

Thallium-201 _____
Technetium-99m Sestamibi _____
Technetium-99 Tetrofosmin _____

Gamma Imaging:

   Single positron emission computed
   tomography (SPECT)_____
   Cardiac positron emission
   tomography (PET)

Stress Cardiovascular Magnetic Resonance
   Imaging (CMR) _____
Computed Tomography Coronary
   Angiography (CTCA) _____
Other _____

* Not all tests are available at all institutions.
   Generally, test availability is limited,
   depends on many factors including available
   expertise and cost, and is institution specific.
   This list is not all inclusive but is intended to
   list the stress tests/cardiac imaging discussed
   in Chapter 26 Stress Testing.

Consultants

Cardiology _____ Notified:
   Name _____ Time _____
Care Coordination (Case management)
   _____ Notified: Name _____ Time
   _____
Heart failure _____ Notified: Name
   _____ Time _____
Social work _____ Notified: Name
   _____ Time _____
Other _____ Notified:
   Name _____ Time _____

Cardiac Medications**

Antiplatelet Agent

Aspirin PO qd ____ 81 mg ____ 325 mg

Antianginal Agent/Vasodilator

Nitroglycerin 0.4 mg SL q 5 minutes x3 prn chest
   pain __ (hold if systolic BP < 90 mmHg) __

Potassium Supplements**

Potassium Chloride __ 20 mEq __ 40 mEq __
   PO __ IV (IV administered per pharmacy/
   nursing protocol)

Intravenous Fluids

Saline cap IV _____

Bolus Normal Saline (NS) IV ____ 250 mL __ 500 mL ____ 1,000 mL ____ other, infuse over ___ minutes ___ hours

Bolus Lactated Ringer's (LR) IV __ 250 mL __ 500 mL __ 1,000 mL __ other, infuse over ___ minutes ___ hours

Maintenance NS at __ mL per hour IV

Maintenance LR at __ mL per hour IV

Maintenance Dextrose 5% in Water (D_5W) at __ mL per hour IV

Maintenance Dextrose 5% in ½ Normal Saline (D_5½NS) at __ mL per hour IV

Maintenance Dextrose 5% Normal Saline (D_5NS) at __ mL per hour IV

Maintenance NS with potassium chloride __ 20 mEq or __ 40 mEq per 1 liter bag at __mL per hour

Maintenance D_5W with potassium chloride__ 20 mEq or __ 40 mEq per 1 liter bag at __ mL per hour

Maintenance D_5½NS with potassium chloride __ 20 mEq or __ 40 mEq per 1 liter bag at __ mL per hour IV

Maintenance D_5NS with potassium chloride __ 20 mEq or __ 40 mEq per 1 liter bag at __ mL per hour IV

Other _____ at mL per hour

Education: patient _____ family

Coronary artery disease _____
COPD _____

Diabetic _____
Heart failure _____
Smoking cessation _____
Other _____

* Modifications in diet or medications as per standing protocols. There are various protocols or prerequisites for the various stress tests. For example, no caffeine is allowed in the diet (such as caffeinated coffee or soft drinks) when patients are placed in the observation unit for a stress test. Certain medications (e.g., beta blockers and nitrates) are held when patients are placed in the observation unit for a stress test.

** Since many patients are on diuretics and often have low potassium, these electrolyte orders for potassium are included in this chest pain and other cardiac protocols. A repeat potassium is usually ordered after supplemental potassium is given for hypokalemia since stress tests may not be done at certain institutions if the potassium is low (e.g., < 3.5 mmol/L).

All patients receiving intravenous electrolyte solutions should have continuous heart rate/ cardiac rhythm monitoring while intravenous electrolyte solutions are infused. Maximum infusion rate for potassium chloride is 10–20 mEq/hour. (See also order set on electrolytes, e.g., hypokalemia.)

See also other cardiac related order sets for additional cardiac medications (e.g., atrial fibrillation, heart failure, hypertensive urgency order sets).

SL = sublingual

Congestive Heart Failure Order Set

Place in Emergency Department (ED)
Observation _____
Diagnosis **CONGESTIVE HEART FAILURE,**

_____, _____, _____
ED Attending _____
Resident (if applicable) _____
Advanced Practice Provider (if applicable)

_____

Allergies: Yes _____ No _____

If yes, what _____,_____,_____,_____,

_____,_____

Vital Signs

Temperature __ Pulse __ Respiration __ BP__
Pulse oximetry ____
__ q 2 hours ___ q 4 hours ___ q 6 hours q ___
hours ___ q shift ___ qd ____ other
Cardiac monitoring (telemetry) _____
Orthostatic vital signs _____
Continuous pulse oximetry_____
Other _____

Notify Physician if

Temperature (°C) > 38.0° ___ 38.5° ___ 39° ___
40° ____ other _____
Systolic blood pressure (mmHg) ≤ 90 ___ ≥
160 __ ≥ 180 ___ ≥ 200 __ other _____
Diastolic blood pressure (mmHg) ≥ 120 ____
other _____
Heart rate ≤ 50 ___ ≥ 120 __ ≥ 150 ___ ≥
200 ___ other ____
Oxygen saturation < 90% _____ other _____
Any change in mental status _____
Any respiratory distress _____

Activity

Up ad lib _____
Assisted _____
Out of bed to chair _____
Bedrest with bathroom privileges _____
Bedrest with bedside commode _____
Bedrest _____
Other _____
Up in chair as tolerated with bedside
commode, advance as tolerated to
ambulating in the observation unit (continue
on telemetry when ambulating) ____

Diet

NPO _____
Dental, mechanical soft _____
Diabetic _____
Formula _____
Low cholesterol____
No added salt/Low added fat _____
Pureed _____
Per feeding tube _____
Other _____

Nursing Interventions

Weight ___ on admission ___ qd ___ prior to
discharge ____ other
Height ____
I & Os _____ routine _____ strict _____
Fall precautions _____
Seizure precautions _____
Capillary blood glucose __ × 1 q ___ hours
____ before meals and at bedtime

Fluid restriction ____ **mL/hour** ____ **mL/shift** _____ **mL/**
24 hours ____ **other**

Fluid restriction: ≤ 1800 mLper 24 hours
and < 1500 mL if serum sodium < 131 mg/
dLdL ___
Monitor urine output ___ Desired is > 0.5 mL/
kg/hour with adequate renal function
(reasonable/normal BUN/creatinine), normal
mentation, and no orthostatic symptoms*

_____

Insert foley catheter prn, especially if heavy
diuresis interferes with sleep ___
Follow potassium nomogram __ (see below)
Follow magnesium nomogram __ (see below)
Follow diuretic (furosemide) protocol __ (see
below)

Respiratory Interventions

Oxygen __ liters nasal cannula __ venti mask at
___ liters per minute _____ other
Wean oxygen as tolerated without dyspnea,
stridor or oxygen saturation < 90% ____
Peak flow __ on admission ___ prior to
discharge ___ pre and post aerosols
Sleep apnea qhs __ CPAP BiPAP settings cm
H_2O ___ inspiratory __ expiratory

Laboratory Tests

CBC _____ with differential

Basic metabolic panel _____
    repeat after treatment _____
Brain natriuretic peptide (BNP) _____
    repeat after treatment _____
Cardiac enzymes __ x 1 __ q 4 hour × 3 __ q
    4 hour × 4 _____*with ECGs*
Complete metabolic panel_____
Lactate __ (if not drawn in emergency
    department), repeat after treatment if
    abnormal___
Liver function tests _____
Magnesium _____ *repeat after treatment* _____
Urinalysis _____ Urine culture _____
Renal function tests (BUN, creatinine)
    _____ *repeat after treatment* _____
Other _____, _____, _____, _____,
    _____, _____, _____, _____
Repeat _____, _____, _____, _____, _____ in
    a.m. ___ in _____ hours
Repeat ___ *BNP,* ___ *renal function tests*
    (BUN, creatinine), ___ *electrolytes (Na, K,*
    Cl, CO2) __ *Magnesium* ___*lactate after*
    therapy/prior to discharge
If there are any new rhythm or conduction
    disturbances, and/or the resting heart rate is
    < 60 beats/minute or > 120 beats/minute,
    then obtain a stat ECG, basic metabolic
    panel, and magnesium level _____
If there is any chest pain, then obtain a stat
    ECG, CXR, and cardiac enzymes _____

Radiology Studies

CXR portable _____ *(if not done in*
    emergency department)
CXR (PA and lateral) _____ *(if not done in*
    emergency department)
Other _____, _____, _____

Cardiac Studies

*ECG X 1*__ *at* __ *hour* ___ *q 4 hour X 3* ___ *q*
    4 hours × 4 __ *other* ___ *with cardiac*
    enzymes
Serial ECGs and cardiac enzymes __ *q 4 hour*
    *X 3*_____ *q 4 hour X 4* ___
Echocardiogram (include ejection fraction) ___
    (if not done within last 12 months)

__ with agitated (bubble) study __ without
    agitated (bubble) study
Other _____

Consultants

Cardiology _____ *Notified:*
    Name _____ *Time* _____
Care coordination (Case management)
    _____ Notified: Name _____
    Time _____
Dietician _____ *Notified:*
    Name _____ *Time* _____
*Heart failure service*_____ *Notified:*
    Name _____ *Time* _____
Social work _____ Notified:
    Name _____ Time _____
Other _____ Notified:
    Name _____ Time _____

*Comment: In many hospitals, cardiology
    may be consulted. But in some larger
    institutions there may be a specialized heart
    failure service, while in other institutions
    internal medicine/family practice may be
    consulted. Initially, we consulted heart
    failure service/cardiology for all heart failure
    patients in the ED observation unit, but after
    a period of time, the ED physicians and
    nurses were comfortable with managing
    these patients so now heart failure service/
    cardiology is generally consulted only for
    those cases that do not respond to the
    protocol and may need inpatient admission.
    All patients are referred to internal
    medicine/family practice and/or cardiology/
    heart failure service after discharge from
    observation.

Cardiac Medications (Adult Dosage)
Diuretics

Intravenous furosemide protocol _____ *(see*
    below)
Furosemide (Lasix®) ___ mg __ IV __ PO __
    once ___ other ____
Torsemide (Demadex®) ___ mg __ IV __ PO
    ___ once ___ other ____

Potassium Nomogram for Congestive Heart Failure in the Observation Unit

Potassium*

Potassium Serum Level mEq/dL	IV Dose	Oral Dose	Recheck Serum Potassium Level
3.7–3.9	20 mEq*	40 mEq*	12 hours or in a.m.
3.4–3.6	20 mEq x 2 doses*	40 mEq x 2 Doses*	6 hours or in a.m.
3.0–3.3	20 mEq x 4 doses*	40 mEq x 3 doses*	4 hours after last dose
< 3.0	20 mEq x 6 doses*	Give IV only	1 hour after last infusion

* Before administering any potassium, check serum creatinine level.

If patient has serum creatinine > 2.5 mg/dL (has renal insufficiency but makes urine, e.g., is not hemodialysis-dependent or anuric) then decrease the potassium dose by half.

Magnesium Nomogram for Congestive Heart Failure in the Observation Unit

Magnesium (Mg)*

Magnesium (Mg) Serum Level mg/dL	IV Dose	Oral Dose	Recheck Serum Magnesium Level
1.9	Give oral dose only	Magnesium oxide (uromag®) 140 mg	In a.m.
1.3–1.8	1 gram magnesium sulfate for every 0.1 mg/dL below 1.9 mg/dL*	Give IV dose only	In a.m.
≤ 1.2	8 grams magnesium sulfate**	Give IV dose only	6 hours after last infusion or in a.m.

* Mix 1 to 2 grams magnesium sulfate in 50 mL of D5W or 0.9% NaCl and infuse 1–2 grams per hour
** Mix 3 to 6 grams of magnesium sulfate in 150 mL of D5W or 0.9% NaCl with an infusion rate no greater than 2 grams per hour.

Intravenous Furosemide Protocol

1. Give IV furosemide dose equivalent to prior outpatient total daily dose (up to 180 mg maximum single dose or 40 mg IV if not on furosemide). Onset of action for IV furosemide is 5 minutes with peak effects in 2–4 hours.
2. Clinical assessment for response to furosemide diuretic: physical exam signs of volume overload such as rales, peripheral edema, JVD and renal function (BUN/creatinine). Desired outcome or goal of therapy: With normal renal function ≥ 500 mL urine output in 2 hours, if renal insufficiency > 250 mL urine output in 2 hours. Net loss of 0.5–1.0 liters of fluid per day, which is equivalent to about 0.5–1.0 kg of body weight
3. Reassess at 3 hours. At 3 hours, double the furosemide dose and give IV if any of the following goals have not been met: 2-hour urine output target has not been met or diuresis targets have not been reached. (see #2)
4. Reassess at 6 hours. If pronounced diuresis (> 2 liters), obtain serum potassium level. If inadequate diuresis, notify MD to reassess for further treatment orders and/or inpatient admission.

Other Cardiac Medications

Aspirin __ 81 mg ___ 325 mg PO qd

Note: for other cardiac medications, see other order sets, such as the hypertension and chest pain order sets.

Other

Acetaminophen (Paracetamol) (Tylenol®) 325 mg tab __ 1 tab __ 1–2 tabs __ 2 tabs PO __ q 4 hours __ q 6 hours ___ prn pain ___ prn fever (maximum 4 g daily)

_____ If unable to take tablet formulation, may give suspension

_____ If unable to take PO, may give suppository PR __325 mg __ 650 mg __ q 4 hours __ q 6 hours

IV ___ mg __ q 4 hours __ q 6 hours __ prn pain __ prn fever (maximum adult dose: if weight < 50 kg is 15 mg/kg up to 750 mg for a single dose, 75 mg/kg up to 3750 mg for daily dose; if weight > 50 kg is 650 mg q 4 hours or 1000 mg q 6 hours up to 1000 mg for a single dose and 4000 mg for a daily dose)

Intravenous Fluids

Saline cap IV _____

Maintenance Dextrose 5% in Water (D_5W) at __ mL per hour IV

Maintenance D_5W with potassium chloride __ 20 mEq or __ 40 mEq per 1 liter bag at __ per hour IV

Maintenance Dextrose 5% in ½ Normal Saline (D_5½NS) at __ mL per hour IV

Maintenance D_5½NS with potassium chloride __ 20 mEq or __ 40 mEq per 1 liter bag at __ mL per hour IV

Other _____ at mL per hour

Education: patient _____ family _____

Heart failure _____ (includes patient video on heart failure, pamphlet on heart failure, etc.)

Dietician _____ (re: low salt foods, no added salt diet, low cholesterol)

Smoking cessation_____

Other _____

See also order set for electrolytes for potassium and magnesium.

Key components of the protocol are in italics and bold to emphasize their importance.

The nomograms for potassium and magnesium and the furosemide protocol are designed to be easy to implement by nursing as a standard order. In general, heart failure patients tend to have long inpatient hospital stays and be difficult to treat. Initially, when starting an observation unit, I recommend starting with common, easy-to-manage diagnoses such as chest pain and later expand the scope of patients placed in the observation unit. Thus, heart failure may not be on the initial list of diagnoses for inclusion in an observation unit. However, with research documenting the success of managing heart failure patients in an observation unit (see Chapter 23 on Heart Failure) and with the focus on readmissions and decreasing inpatient length of stay, it is likely that more complicated patients including those with heart failure will be treated in our Observation Units in the future.

This order set is modified from the work by my colleagues, including Dr. Peacock and others and myself, and employs an aggressive therapeutic regimen using diuretics.[1,2] (See Chapter 23 on heart failure). Recently, there has been discussion regarding the use of low doses of loop diuretics as a strategy for the treatment of heart failure as with the DOSE trial[3] instead of aggressive diuretic therapy as in this protocol. This may be another method for the treatment of heart failure. One benefit of observation unit methodology and protocols is the ability to change and modify protocols to reflect the current standard of care. Although the recommendations for treatment including the drug(s) and their dosages may be changed in the future, other orders (such as strict input and output, the need to replete low levels of potassium and/or magnesium in order to allow for diuretics to be more effective, and the necessity for patient education as a step in patient empowerment) remain essential. As part of their overall framework, observation units with their standardized order sets minimize drug errors, promote patient safety and best practices, and allow for the rapid implementation and standardization of care when new therapeutic regimens occur.

This observation unit protocol is designed for stable patients with acute decompensated heart failure. Unstable patients are not candidates for the observation unit. Treatment of heart failure may differ based upon whether or not there is systolic or diastolic heart failure. In patients with systolic dysfunction, certain medications should not be started or if given should be used with caution in the acute setting, such as ACE inhibitors and beta blockers. For patients with diastolic dysfunction, the key is to treat hypertension and tachycardia. Inotropes are generally not indicated in patients with diastolic dysfunction and preserved systolic function.

In the acute setting, certain treatments are applicable to either systolic or diastolic heart failure. These therapies include diuresis, supplemental oxygen (and assisted ventilation, if needed) and in selected patients, treatment with vasodilators. This is why this protocol focuses on maximizing the use of diuretics and does not include ACE inhibitors or beta blockers, although they can be written in as another order and why the recommendation for an echocardiogram in patients on the order set. As noted previously, critically ill or unstable patients, including those who are intubated on currently on Bipap (or other noninvasive positive pressure ventilation, except for sleep apnea) are not appropriate for the observation unit. (See Administrative Policies Chapter 88 and Clinical Protocols Chapter 82.) However, should they be improved from emergency department therapy and not be on noninvasive positive pressure ventilation or intubated, they may be candidates for observation.

This protocol uses an aggressive approach for achieving a high diuresis rapidly, which has worked well in the past (see Heart Failure Chapter 23). There is some recent literature that suggests another more gradual approach may be effective so we may be adding new protocols or modifying this one in the future.

References

1. Peacock WF, Remer E, Aponte J, et al. Effective observation unit treatment of decompenstated heart failure. *Cong Heart Fail* 2008; 8(2):68–73.

2. Peacok WF, Young J, Collins S, et al. Heart failure observation units: optimizing care. *Ann Emerg Med* 2006; 47(1):22–33.

3. Felker GM, Lee KL, Bull DA, et al. Diuretic strategies in patients with acute decompensated heart failure. *N Engl J Med* 2011; 364:797–805.

Chronic Obstructive Pulmonary Disease (COPD) Acute Exacerbation Order Set

Place in Emergency Department (ED) Observation

Diagnosis *ACUTE EXCERBATION COPD,*

_____, _____, _____

ED Attending _____

Resident (if applicable) _____

Advanced Practice Provider (if applicable)

_____

Allergies: Yes _____ No _____

If yes, what _____, _____, _____, _____,

_____, _____

Vital Signs

Temperature __ Pulse __ Respiration __ BP__ Pulse oximetry __

__ q 2 hours ___ q 4 hours ___ q 6 hours q ___ hours ___ q shift ___ qd ____ other

Cardiac monitoring (telemetry) _____

Continuous pulse oximetry _____

Other _____

Notify Physician if

Temperature (°C) > 38.0° ___ 38.5°___ 39° ___ 40° ____ other ___

Systolic blood pressure (mmHg) ≤ 90 ___ ≥ 160 __ ≥ 180 ___ ≥ 200 __ other _____

Diastolic blood pressure (mmHg) > 120 ___ other _____

Heart rate ≤ 50 ___ ≥ 120 __ ≥ 150 ___ ≥ 200 ___ other _____

Oxygen sat < 90% or worsening dyspnea or increasing oxygen requirement ____

Any new shortness of breath or respiratory distress ____

Any chest pain____

Any change in mental status _____

Activity

Up ad lib _____

Assisted _____

Out of bed to chair _____

Bedrest with bathroom privileges _____

Bedrest with bedside commode _____

Bedrest _____

Other _____

Diet

NPO _____

Regular _____

Advance diet as tolerated _____

Clear liquids ____

Dental, mechanical soft _____

Diabetic _____

Formula_____ per feeding tube _____

Full liquids _____

Low added fat/No added salt _____

Low cholesterol ____

Pureed _____

Sodium: 1 gram ___ 2 grams ___ unrestricted____

Per feeding tube _____

Other _____

Nursing Interventions

Weight ___ on admission ___ qd ___ prior to discharge _____ other

Height ____

I & Os _____ routine _____ strict _____

Fluid restriction _____ mL/hour _____ mL/ shift _____ mL/24 hour

Fall precautions _____

Seizure precautions _____

Capillary blood glucose __ × 1 q ___ hours ___ before meals and at bedtime

Respiratory Interventions

Oxygen __ liters nasal cannula __ venti mask at ___ liters per minute _____ other

Wean oxygen as tolerated without dyspnea or oxygen saturation < 90% _____

Peak flow ___ on admission ___ prior to discharge ___ pre and post aerosols

Sleep apnea qhs __ CPAP BiPAP settings cm H_2O ___ inspiratory __ expiratory

Laboratory Tests

Arterial blood gas ___ on room air ___ on other

Basic metabolic panel _____

Brain natriuretic peptide (BNP) _____

Cardiac enzymes × 1 _____ q 4 hour × 3 _____ q 4 hour × 4 ____ other ____

CBC with differential _____

Complete metabolic panel _____

D-dimer _____

Lactate _____

Urinalysis _____

Urine culture _____

Other _____, _____, _____, _____,

_____, _____, _____, _____

Repeat _____, _____, _____, _____, _____ in
a.m. ___ in _____ hours

Radiology Studies

CXR portable _____

CXR (PA and lateral) _____

Other _____, _____, _____, _____,

_____ ,_____

If chest pain, portable CXR _____ ECG _____
cardiac enzymes _____

Cardiac Studies

ECG __ × 1__ q 4 hours × 3 ___ q 4 hours ×
4 ___ other _____ with cardiac enzymes

Echocardiogram (transthoracic) __ with
agitated (bubble) study __ without agitated
(bubble) study

Consultants

Care coordination (Case management)
_____ Notified: Name _____ Time
_____

Pulmonary _____
Notified: Name _____ Time _____

Social work _____ Notified:
Name _____ Time _____

Other _____
Notified: Name _____ Time _____

COPD Medications (Adult Dosage)

Inhaled Medications: Aerosols

Albuterol (Proventil®) nebulized solution
__2.5 mg __ mg aerosol __ × 1 __ q 2 hours
__ q 4 hours __ q 6 hours ___ q 8 hours __
other __ prn wheezing

Ipratropium (Atrovent®) 0.5 mg nebulized
solution aerosol __ × 1 __ q 2 hours __ q
4 hours __ q 6 hours __ q 8 hours __ other __
prn wheezing

Inhaled Medications: Inhalers*

Albuterol (Proventil®) (90 mcg per inhalation)
metered dose inhaler (MDI) __ puffs __ q
4 hours __ q 6 hours ___ other ___ prn
wheezing

Ipratropium (Atrovent®) (17 mcg per
inhalation) __ puffs __ q 4 hours __ q 6 hours
__ other ___ prn wheezing

Albuterol 90 mcg and Ipratropium 18 mcg (per
inhalation) (Combivent Respimat®) __ puffs
__ q 6 hours ___ other __ prn wheezing

Antibiotics – Oral*

Amoxicillin and Clavulanic acid, Amoxicillin
and Clavulanate (Augmentin®)
__ 250 mg ___ 500 mg __ 875 mg PO__ q
8 hours __ q 12 hours __ other

Azithromycin (Zithromax®) __ 500 mg ×
1 followed by ____ 250 mg qd PO __ other

Amoxicillin (Amoxil®) __ 250 mg __ 500 mg
__ 875 mg PO__ bid ___ tid __ qid __ other

Doxycycline (Adoxa®, Doryx®, Vibramycin®)
__ 100 mg bid PO __ other

Levofloxacin (Levaquin®) ___ 500 mg ___
750 mg PO qd __ other

Antibiotics – Intravenous*

Ampicillin and Sulbactam (Unasyn®) ___ 1.5
grams __ 3 grams IV ___ q 6 hours __ other

Azithromycin (Zithromax®) __ 500 mg (on
day 1) followed by 250 mg IV on subsequent
days __ 250 mg __ 500 mg IV qd for __ days
__ other

Ceftriaxone (Rocephin®) ___ 1 gram × 1
IV__ other

Doxycycline (Doxy®) __ 100 mg bid IV __ other

Levofloxacin (Levaquin®) ___ 500 mg ___
750 mg IV qd __ other

Corticosteroids

Methylprednisolone (Solumedrol®) __ 40 mg
__ mg IV qd___ other

Prednisone __ 40 mg ___ 60 mg PO add __ other

Other: _____, _____, _____,

_____, _____

Intravenous Fluids

Saline cap IV ____

Bolus Normal Saline (NS) IV ___ 250 mL __
500 mL ___1,000 mL ____ other, infuse over
___ minutes ___ hours

Bolus Lactated Ringer's (LR) IV __ 250 mL __
500 mL __1,000 mL __ other, infuse over ___
minutes ___ hours

Maintenance NS at __ mL per hour IV

Maintenance LR at __ mL per hour IV

Maintenance Dextrose 5% in Water (D_5W) at __ mL per hour IV

Maintenance Dexztrose 5% in ½ Normal Saline (D_5½NS) at __ mL per hour IV

Maintenance Dextrose 5% in Normal Saline (D_5NS) at __ mL per hour IV

Maintenance NS with potassium chloride __ 20 mEq or __ 40 mEq per 1 liter bag at __ mL per hour

Maintenance D_5W with potassium chloride__ 20 mEq or __ 40 mEq per 1 liter bag at __ mL per hour

Maintenance D_5½NS with potassium chloride ___ 20 mEq or __ 40 mEq per 1 liter bag at __ mL per hour IV

Maintenance D_5NS with potassium chloride __ 20 mEq or __ 40 mEq per 1 liter bag at __mL per hour IV

Other _____ at mL per hour

Education: patient _____ family _____

Asthma _____

COPD _____

Pneumonia/Acute Bronchitis _____

Smoking cessation _____

Other _____

* Since respiratory infections may trigger an acute exacerbation of COPD and since bacterial infections including bacterial pneumonia are an indication for antibiotics, antibiotics are included in the COPD order set.

Dehydration Order Set

Place in Emergency Department (ED) Observation _____

Diagnosis *DEHYDRATION,* _____,

_____, _____

ED Attending _____

Resident (if applicable) _____

Advanced Practice Provider (if applicable)

_____

Allergies: Yes _____ No _____

If yes, what _____,_____,_____,_____,

_____,_____

Vital Signs

Temperature __ Pulse __ Respiration __ BP__

Pulse oximetry __

__ q 2 hours __ q 4 hours __ q 6 hours q __

hours ___ q shift ___ qd ___ other

Orthostatic vital signs ___

Cardiac monitoring (telemetry) _____

Other _____

Notify Physician if

Temperature (°C) > 38.0° ____ 38.5° ___ 39° ___

40° ____ other _____

Systolic blood pressure (mmHg) ≤ 90 ___ ≥

160 __ ≥ 180 ___ ≥ 200 __ other _____

Diastolic blood pressure (mmHg) ≥ 120 ____

other _____

Heart rate ≤ 50 ___ ≥ 120 __ ≥ 150 ___ ≥

200 ___ other ____

Activity

Up ad lib _____

Assisted _____

Out of bed to chair _____

Bedrest with bathroom privileges _____

Bedrest with bedside commode _____

Bedrest _____

Other _____

Diet

NPO _____

Regular _____

Advance diet as tolerated _____

Clear liquids ____

Dental, mechanical soft _____

Diabetic _____

Formula _____

Full liquids _____

Low added fat/No added salt _____

Low cholesterol ____

Pureed _____

Sodium: 1 gram ___ 2 grams ___

unrestricted ____

Per feeding tube _____

Other _____

Nursing Interventions

Weight ___ on admission ___ qd ___ prior to

discharge ____ other

Height ____

I & Os _____ routine _____ strict _____

Fall precautions _____

Seizure precautions _____

Capillary blood glucose __ × 1 q ___ hours

____ before meals and at bedtime

Respiratory Interventions

Oxygen __ liters nasal cannula __ venti mask at

___ liters per minute _____ other

Wean oxygen as tolerated without dyspnea,

stridor or oxygen saturation < 90% ____

Sleep apnea qhs __ CPAP BiPAP settings cm

H_2O ___ inspiratory __ expiratory

Laboratory Tests

CBC _____ with differential

Amylase ___ Lipase ___

Basic metabolic panel _____

Complete metabolic panel _____

Lactate _____

Liver function tests _____

Pregnancy test (qualitative urine) _____

Pregnancy test (quantitative blood)

_____

Renal function tests (e.g., BUN, creatinine)

_____

Stool for C. diff _____

Stool for ova and parasites _____

Stool for culture and sensitivity _____

Urinalysis _____

Urine culture _____

Other _____, _____, _____, _____,

_____, _____, _____, _____

Repeat _____, _____, _____, _____, _____ in
a.m. ___ in _____ hours

Radiology Studies

Acute abdominal series _____
CXR portable _____
CXR (PA and lateral) _____
Other _____, _____, _____, _____,
_____, _____
CT scan abdomen/pelvis _____ with contrast: __
IV __ po ___ pr ___ CT enterography
Ultrasound Abdomen/Pelvis _____
Ultrasound RUQ _____
MRI _____
Other _____

Cardiac Tests

ECG __ × 1__ q 4 hours × 3 ___ q 4 hours ×
4 ___ other _____ with cardiac enzymes
Echocardiogram (transthoracic) __ with
agitated (bubble) study __ without agitated
(bubble) study

Consultants

Care coordination (Case management)
_____ Notified: Name _____ Time
_____

Gastroenterology _____ Notified:
Name _____ Time _____
General surgery _____ Notified:
Name _____ Time _____
Social work _____
Notified: Name _____ Time _____
Other _____
Notified: Name _____ Time _____

Dehydration (with/without Vomiting/ Diarrhea) Medications (Adult Dosage)

Analgesics

Acetaminophen (Paracetamol) (Tylenol®)
325 mg tab __ 1 tab __ 1–2 tabs __ 2 tabs PO
__ q 4 hours __ q 6 hours ___ prn pain ___
prn fever (maximum 4 g daily)
_____ If unable to take tablet formulation, may
give suspension
_____ If unable to take PO, may give supp PR
__325 mg __ 650 mg __ q 4 hours __ q
6 hours

IV ___ mg __ q 4 hours __ q 6 hours __ prn
pain __ prn fever (maximum adult dose: if
weight < 50 kg is 15 mg/kg up to 750 mg for
a single dose, 75 mg/kg up to 3750 mg for
daily dose; if weight > 50 kg is 650 mg q
4 hours or 1000 mg q 6 hours up to 1000 mg
for a single dose and 4000 mg for a
daily dose)
Acetaminophen-Hydrocodone (Vicodin®) 300
mg/5 mg tab __ 1 tab __ 1–2 tabs __ 2 tabs
PO __ q 4 hours __ q 6 hours ___ prn pain
(maximum 4 grams daily based on
acetaminophen dose)
Acetaminophen-Oxycodone (Endocet®,
Percocet®, Roxicet®) 325 mg/5 mg tab __
1 tab __ 1–2 tabs __ 2 tabs PO q 4 hours __ q
6 hours ___ prn pain (maximum 4 grams
daily based on acetaminophen dose)
Hydromorphone (Dilaudid®) __ 0.5 mg __
1 mg __ 2 mg __ mg __ IV q 2 hours __ q
4 hours __ q 6 hours q ___ hours __ prn pain
Ibuprofen (Advil®, Motrin®) __ 400 mg __
600 mg __ 800 mg PO __ q 4 hours __ q
6 hours __ q 8 hours ___ prn pain
Ketorolac (Toradol®) __ 30 mg IV __ q 6 hours
__ prn pain (maximum 120 mg daily)
Morphine __ 0.5 mg __ 1 mg __ 2 mg __ 4 mg
__ mg IV __ q 2 hours __ q 4 hours __ q
6 hours q ___ hours __ prn pain
Tramadol (Ultram®) __ 50 mg __ 100 mg PO
__ q 4 hours __ q 6 hours __ prn pain
(maximum 400 mg daily)
Other _____, _____, _____,
_____, _____

Antiemetics

Chlorpromazine (Thorazine®) __ 10 mg PO __
25 mg PO __ q 4 hours __ q 6 hours __ 25 mg
__ 50 mg __ IV __IM __ q4 hours __ q
6 hours __ prn nausea/vomiting
Metoclopramide (Reglan®) __10 mg __ IV __
IM __ PO __ q 6 hours __ other __ prn
nausea/vomiting
Ondansetron (Zofran®) __ 4 mg __ 8 mg __IV
__PO __ q 6 hours ___ other __ prn nausea/
vomiting
Prochlorperazine (Compazine®) __ 5 mg __10
mg __ IV __ IM __ PO __ q 4 hours __ q
6 hours (maximum dose IV/IM/PO 40 mg per
day) ____ 25 mg PR bid __ prn nausea/vomiting

Promethazine (Phenergan®) __ 12.5 mg __
25 mg __ IV__ IM __ PO __ PR __
q4 hours __ q 6 hours ___ prn nausea/
vomiting

Trimethobenzamide (Tigan®) __ 200 mg IM __
300 mg PO ___ q 6 hours ___ prn nausea/
vomiting

Intravenous Fluids

Saline cap IV ____

Bolus Normal Saline (NS) IV ___ 250 mL __
500 mL ___ 1,000 mL ____ other, infuse over
___ minutes ___ hours

Bolus Lactated Ringer's (LR) IV __ 250 mL __
500 mL __1,000 mL __ other, infuse over ___
minutes ___ hours

Maintenance NS at __ mL per hour IV

Maintenance LR at __ mL per hour IV

Maintenance Dextrose 5% in Water (D_5W) at
__ mL per hour IV

Maintenance Dextrose 5% ½ Normal Saline
(D_5½NS) at __ mL per hour IV

Maintenance Dextrose 5% in Normal Saline
(D_5NS) at __ mL per hour IV

Maintenance NS with potassium chloride __
20 mEq or __ 40 mEq per 1 liter bag at __ mL
per hour

Maintenance D_5W with potassium chloride__
20 mEq or __ 40 mEq per 1 liter bag at __ mL
per hour

Maintenance D_5½NS with potassium chloride
__ 20 mEq or __ 40 mEq per 1 liter bag at __
mL per hour IV

Maintenance D_5NS with potassium chloride __
20 mEq or __ 40 mEq per 1 liter bag at __ ml
per hour IV

Other _____ at mL per hour

Education: patient _____ family _____

Abdominal pain _____
Dehydration _____
Vomiting/Diarrhea _____
Smoking cessation _____
Other _____

Diabetic Order Set

Insulin

Daily (Basal) Insulin*

Subcutaneous administration	Breakfast (7 a.m.) or Time __ hours	Lunch (12 p. m.) or Time __ hours	Dinner (5 p.m.) or Time __ hours	Bedtime (9 p.m.) or Time __ hours
Glargine (long acting) (Lantus®)	__ units	__ units	__ units	__ units
NPH (intermediate acting) (Humulin®, Novolin®)	__ units	__ units	__ units	__ units
NPH/regular 70/30 (intermediate acting/short acting) (Humulin®, Novolin®)	__ units	__ units	__ units	__ units
Detemir (intermediate to long acting) (Levemir®)	__ units	__ units	__ units	__ units
Other	__ units	__ units	__ units	__ units

Prandial (Meal Time) Insulin*

Subcutaneous Administration	Breakfast (7 a.m.) or Time ____ hours	Lunch (12 p.m.) or Time __ hours	Dinner (5 p.m.) or Time __ hours
Glulisine (rapid acting) (Apidra®) with meal	__ units	__ units	__ units
Regular (short acting) (Humulin®, Novolin®) 30 minutes prior to meal	__ units	__ units	__ units
Other	__ units	__ units	__ units

* The prandial insulin and supplemental insulin can be mixed in the same syringe and given at the same time.

Hyperglycemic Medications: Insulin

Insulin Drip

Regular insulin ___ units/hour IV

Insulin Sliding Scale Coverage ____

If blood glucose is between 150 and 200 mg/dL, give 2 units regular (short acting) insulin SQ

If blood glucose is between 200 and 250 mg/dL, give 4 units regular (short acting) insulin SQ

If blood glucose is between 250 and 300 mg/dL, give 6 units regular (short acting) insulin SQ

If blood glucose is between 300 and 350 mg/dL, give 8 units regular (short acting) insulin SQ

If blood glucose is > 350 mg/dL, give 10 units regular (short acting) insulin SQ and notify MD

Insulin Sliding Scale Coverage (alternate coverage sliding scale)* _____

If blood glucose is between 150 and 200 mg/dL, give __ units regular (short acting) insulin SQ

If blood glucose is between 200 and 250 mg/dL, give __ units regular (short acting) insulin SQ

If blood glucose is between 250 and 300 mg/dL, give __ units regular (short acting) insulin SQ

If blood glucose is between 300 and 350 mg/dL, give __ units regular (short acting) insulin SQ

If blood glucose is > 350 mg/dL, give __ units regular (short acting) insulin SQ and notify MD

* Some physicians may choose an alternative insulin sliding scale coverage. For example, if the patient is thought to be sensitive to insulin, then the sliding scale could be halved so the sliding scale would be 1 unit for a blood glucose between 150 and 200 mg/dL, 2 units for a blood glucose between 200 and 250 mg/dL, 3 units for a blood glucose between 250 and 300 mg/dL, 4 units for a blood glucose between 300 and 350 mg/dL, and 5 units for a blood glucose between 300 and 350 mg/dL. Similarly, if the patient is somewhat resistant to insulin, then the sliding scale could be increased so it would be 1 unit for a blood glucose of 111to 150 mg/dL, 3 units for a blood glucose between 150 and 200 mg/dL, 6 units for a blood glucose between 200 and 250 mg/dL, 9 units for a blood glucose between 250 and 300 mg/dL, 12 units for a blood glucose between 300 and 350 mg/dL, and 15 units for a blood glucose between 300 and 350 mg/dL. (see below)

Insulin Sliding Scale Coverage (alternate coverage sliding scale) (lower dose of insulin)* ____

If blood glucose is between 150 and 200 mg/dL, give 1 units regular (short acting) insulin SQ

If blood glucose is between 200 and 250 mg/dL, give 2 units regular (short acting) insulin SQ

If blood glucose is between 250 and 300 mg/dL, give 3 units regular (short acting) insulin SQ

If blood glucose is between 300 and 350 mg/dL, give 4 units regular (short acting) insulin SQ

If blood glucose is > 350 mg/dL, give 5 units regular (short acting) insulin SQ and notify MD

Insulin Sliding Scale Coverage (alternate coverage sliding scale) (higher dose of insulin)* ____

If blood glucose is between 110 and 250 mg/dL, give 1 units regular (short acting) insulin SQ

If blood glucose is between 150 and 200 mg/dL, give 3 units regular (short acting) insulin SQ

If blood glucose is between 200 and 250 mg/dL, give 6 units regular (short acting) insulin SQ

If blood glucose is between 250 and 300 mg/dL, give 9 units regular (short acting) insulin SQ

If blood glucose is between 300 and 350 mg/dL, give 12 units regular (short acting) insulin SQ

If blood glucose is > 350 mg/dL, give 15 units regular (short acting) insulin SQ and notify MD

Oral Diabetic Medications

Antidiabetic Agents

Biguanide

Metformin (immediate release) (Glucophage®) ____ mg PO __ qd __ bid

Metformin (extended release) (Glucophage XR®) ____ mg PO qd

Sulfonylurea – First Generation

Chlorpropamide (Diabinese®) ____ mg PO ____ qd

Glimepiride (Amaryl®) ____ mg PO ____ qd

Sulfonylurea – Second Generation

Glyburide (Diabeta®, Glynase®, Micronase®) ____ mg PO ____ qd ___bid

Glipizide (Glucotrol®) __ mg PO ____ qd ___bid* (take 30 minutes before meals)

Glipizide (Glucotrol XL®) __ mg PO ____ qd

Combination Biguanide and Sulfonylurea

Glucovance® ____ mg PO ____ qd ____ bid (Note: Glucovance® is equivalent to metformin coadministered with glyburide)

Meglitinides (short acting)

Repaglinide (Prandin®) ____ mg PO (take 15–30 minutes before each meal)

Nateglinide (Starlix®) ____ mg PO (take 15–30 minutes before each meal)

Thiazolidinediones

Pioglitazone (Actos®) (generally preferred over rosiglitazone due to lesser potential risk for cardiovascular events) ____ mg PO ____ qd (may be taken with or without food)

DPP-4 Inhibitors

Sitagliptin (Januvia®) __ mg PO ____ qd (may be taken with or without food)

Alpha-glucosidase inhibitors

Acarbose (Precose®) __ mg PO tid (take with first bite of each main meal)

Sulfonylureas and meglinitides should be administered with food. If qd frequency, take with first meal of the day (breakfast). If bid frequency, take with morning (breakfast) and with evening (dinner) meals. If tid frequency, take with morning (breakfast), afternoon (lunch), and evening (dinner) meals.

Generally, patients are maintained on their usual antidiabetic medications. Prior to starting any additional medications in a patient already on antidiabetic medications, consider a consult with endocrinology or internal medicine or family/general practice.

The different sulfonylureas (first and second generation) are equally effective in lowering blood glucose concentrations, although there are structural characteristics that alter their pharmacokinetics, such as differences in absorption, metabolism, and dose.

Other oral diabetic medications not in the order list and the reason for not including them is noted below:

Sulfonylurea – First Generation: Acetohexamide (Dymelor®) (not available in United States)

Sulfonylurea – Second Generation: Tolazamide (Tolinase®) (not commonly used)

Sulfonylurea – Second Generation: Tolbutamide (Orinase®) (not commonly used)

Glucagon-like peptide 1 Agonists

Exenatide (byetta®) (not commonly used)

Thiazolidinediones: Rosiglitazone (Avandia®) This drug was off the market in the United States, but is currently "available," however, requires completion of a Risk Evaluation and Mitigation Strategy (REMS) by the health care provider.

Gastrointestinal Bleeding Order Set

Place in Emergency Department (ED)
Observation

Diagnosis *GI BLEED*, _____, _____,

_____

ED Attending _____

Resident (if applicable) _____

Advanced Practice Provider (if applicable)

_____

Allergies: Yes _____ No _____

If yes, what _____,_____,_____,_____,

_____,_____

Vital Signs

Temperature __ Pulse __ Respiration __ BP__
Pulse oximetry __

___ q 2 hours ___ q 4 hours ___ q 6 hours q
___ hours ___ q shift ___ qd _____ other

Orthostatic vital signs _____

Cardiac monitoring (telemetry) _____

Continuous pulse oximetry – _____

Other _____

Notify Physician if

Temperature (°C) > 38.0° ___ 38.5°___ 39° ___
40° ____ other ___

Systolic blood pressure (mmHg) ≤ 90 ___ ≥
160 __ ≥ 180 ___ ≥ 200 __ other _____

Diastolic blood pressure (mmHg) > 120 ___
other _____

Heart rate ≤ 50 ___ ≥ 120 __ ≥ 150 ___ ≥
200 ___ other ____

Oxygen saturation < 90% or worsening
dyspnea or increasing oxygen
requirement ____

Any new shortness of breath or respiratory
distress ____

Any chest pain ____

Any change in mental status or syncope or near
syncope _____

Activity

Up ad lib _____

Assisted _____

Out of bed to chair _____

Bedrest with bathroom privileges _____

Bedrest with bedside commode _____

Bedrest _____

Other _____

Diet

NPO _____

Regular _____

Advance diet as tolerated _____

Clear liquids ____

Dental, mechanical soft _____

Diabetic _____

Formula_____ per feeding tube _____

Full liquids _____

Low added fat/No added salt _____

Low cholesterol ____

Pureed _____

Sodium: 1 gram ___ 2 grams ___
unrestricted____

Per feeding tube _____

Other _____

Nursing Interventions

Weight ___ on admission ___ qd ___ prior to
discharge ____ other

Height ____

I & Os _____ routine _____ strict _____

Fluid restriction _____ mL/hour _____ mL/
shift ____ mL/24 hour

Fall precautions _____

Seizure precautions _____

Capillary blood glucose __ × 1 __ q __ hours
____ before meals and at bedtime

Respiratory Interventions

Oxygen __ liters nasal cannula __ venti mask at
___ liters per minute _____ other

Wean oxygen as tolerated without dyspnea or
oxygen saturation < 90% _____

Peak flow ___ on admission ___ prior to
discharge ___ pre and post aerosols

Sleep apnea qhs __ CPAP BiPAP settings cm
H_2O ___ inspiratory __ expiratory

Laboratory Tests

Basic metabolic panel _____

Cardiac enzymes ___ × 1 ____ q 4 hours ×
3____ q 4 hours × 4 _____ other

CBC _____ with differential

Complete metabolic panel _____

Hematocrit/Hemoglobin _____

Lactate _____

PT ____ INR ____ APTT ____

Type and Screen _____

Type and Cross _____ units packed red blood cells

Urinalysis _____ Urine culture _____

Other _____, _____, _____, _____,
_____, _____, _____, _____

Repeat Hematocrit/Hemoglobin one hour post transfusion _____

Serial Hematocrit/Hemoglobin q ___ hour X ___

Radiology Studies

Abdominal series (KUB, upright, CXR)

_____

CXR portable _____

CXR (PA and lateral) _____

KUB _____

Other _____, _____, _____, _____,
_____ , _____

Cardiac Studies

ECG __ × 1 __ q 4 hours × 3 ___ q 4 hours × 4 ___ other _____ with cardiac enzymes

Echocardiogram (transthoracic) __ with agitated (bubble) study __ without agitated (bubble) study

Consultants

Care coordination (Case management) _____ Notified: Name _____ Time _____

Gastroenterology _____ Notified: Name _____ Time _____

General surgery _____ Notified: Name _____ Time _____

Social work _____ Notified: Name _____ Time _____

Other _____ Notified: Name _____ Time _____

GI Medications

Antacids

Aluminum Hydroxide and Magnesium Hydroxide (Mylanta®) ___ 10–20 mL liquid PO qid (maximum 80 mL daily), 1–2 tab PO ___ pc and qhs and ___ prn reflux or _____ prn dyspepsia/pain (maximum 16 tablets daily)

Aluminium Hydroxide/Magnesium Hydroxide/ Simethicone (Maalox®) __ 30 mL PO q 4 hours for reflux or prn pain

Other _____, _____, _____,
_____, _____

Proton Pump Inhibitors

Pantoprazole (Protonix®) __ 40 mg IV __bid __qd __40 mg PO __ bid __ QD __ 80 mg IV bolus followed by 8 mg/hour continuous infusion for 72 hours*

Esomeprazole (Nexium®) __ 40 mg IV __bid __qd __40 mg PO __ bid __ QD __ 80 mg IV bolus followed by 8 mg/hour continuous infusion for 72 hours

Bowel Evacuant for Colonoscopy Prep*

Polyethylene Glycol – electrolyte solution (CoLyte®, GaviLyte®, GoLYTELY®, NuLYTELY®, TriLyte®) 240 mL (8 ounces) PO every 10 minutes up to 4 liters or until rectal effluent is clear ___

Intravenous Fluids

Saline cap IV _____

Bolus Normal Saline (NS) IV ___ 250 mL __ 500 mL ___ 1,000 mL ____ other infuse over ___ minutes ___ hours

Bolus Lactated Ringer's (LR) IV __ 250 mL __ 500 mL __1,000 mL __ other infuse over ____ minutes ___ hours

Maintenance NS at __ mL per hour IV

Maintenance LR at __ mL per hour IV

Maintenance Dextrose 5% in Water (D_5W) at __ mL per hour IV

Maintenance Dextrose 5% in ½ Normal Saline (D_5½NS) at __ mL per hour IV

Maintenance Dextrose 5% in Normal Saline (D_5NS) at __ mL per hour IV

Maintenance NS with potassium chloride __ 20 mEq or __ 40 mEq per 1 liter bag at __mL per hour

Maintenance D_5W with potassium chloride__ 20 mEq or __ 40 mEq per 1 liter bag at __ mL per hour

Maintenance D_5½NS with potassium chloride __ 20 mEq or __ 40 mEq per 1 liter bag at __ mL per hour IV

Maintenance D_5NS with potassium chloride __ 20 mEq or __ 40 mEq per 1 liter bag at __ mL per hour IV

Other _____ at mL per hour

Transfuse**

Transfuse __ units packed red blood cells (Must have consent form signed prior to transfusion)

Recheck hemoglobin/hematocrit ____ 1 hour post transfusion ____ hours post transfusion

GI Diagnostic Procedures

Esophagogastroduodenoscopy (EGD) in a.m.: __ NPO after midnight ____

Colonoscopy in a.m.: ___ bowel prep: ___ NPO after midnight ___

Education: patient _____ family _____

GI bleeding _____

Smoking cessation_____

Other _____

* Sodium phosphate (Fleet® Phospho-soda®) is also used as bowel evacuation but polyethylene glycol may be preferred since there is a risk of phosphate nephropathy with sodium phosphate products so sodium phosphate is not included in this order set.

** See also transfusion order set

Headache Order Set

Place in Emergency Department (ED)
Observation _____

Diagnosis *HEADACHE,* _____,

_____, _____

ED Attending _____

Resident (if applicable) _____

Advanced Practice Provider (if applicable)
_____

Allergies: Yes _____ No _____

If yes, what _____, _____, _____, _____,
_____, _____

Vital Signs

Temperature __ Pulse __ Respiration __ BP__
Pulse oximetry ____

__ q 2 hours ___ q 4 hours ___ q 6 hours q ___
hours ___ q shift ___ qd ____ other

Cardiac monitoring (telemetry) _____

Neurologic Checks __ q 2 hours __ q 4 hours
__ q 6 hours q __hours __ q shift __ qd
__ other

Orthostatic vital signs _____

Continuous pulse oximetry_____

Other _____

Notify Physician if

Temperature (°C) > 38.0° ____ 38.5° ___ 39° ___
40° ____ other _____

Systolic blood pressure (mmHg) ≤ 90 ___ ≥
160 __ ≥ 180 ___ ≥ 200 __ other _____

Diastolic blood pressure (mmHg) ≥ 120 ____
other _____

Heart rate ≤ 50 ___ ≥ 120 __ ≥ 150 ___ ≥
200 ___ other _____

Oxygen saturation < 90% _____ other _____

Any change in mental status _____

Activity

Up ad lib _____

Assisted _____

Out of bed to chair _____

Bedrest with bathroom privileges _____

Bedrest with bedside commode _____

Bedrest _____

Other _____

Diet

NPO _____

Regular _____

Advance diet as tolerated _____

Clear liquids ____

Dental, mechanical soft _____

Diabetic _____

Formula_____

Full liquids _____

Low added fat/No added salt _____

Low cholesterol____

Pureed _____

Sodium: 1 gram ___ 2 grams ___
unrestricted____

Per feeding tube _____

Other _____

Nursing Interventions

Weight ___ on admission ___ qd ___ prior to
discharge ____ other

Height ____

I & Os _____ routine _____ strict _____

Fluid restriction ___ mL/hour ___ mL/shift
____ mL/24 hour ___ other

Fall precautions _____

Seizure precautions _____

Capillary blood glucose __ × 1 q ___ hours ___
before meals and at bedtime

Respiratory Interventions

Oxygen __ liters nasal cannula __ venti mask at
___ liters per minute _____ other

Wean oxygen as tolerated without dyspnea,
stridor or oxygen saturation < 90% ____

Sleep apnea qhs __ CPAP BiPAP settings cm
H_2O ___ inspiratory __ expiratory

Laboratory Tests

CBC _____ with differential

Basic metabolic panel _____

Cardiac enzymes __ × 1 ___ q 4 hours × 3 ___ q
4 hours × 4 _____ other

Complete metabolic panel _____

C-reactive protein ____

Erythrocyte sedimentation test _____

Lactate _____

Liver function tests _____

Urinalysis _____

Pregnancy test _____ (qualitative urine)

Pregnancy test (quantitative blood) _____
Renal function tests (BUN, creatinine) _____
Other _____, _____, _____, _____,
_____, _____, _____, _____
Repeat _____, _____, _____, _____, _____ in
a.m. ___ in _____ hour

Radiology Studies

Computed tomography (CT) brain without
contrast _____
CT brain with contrast if no contrast allergy
and no renal failure (e.g., GFR ≥ 30) ___
Computed tomography angiography (CTA) of
brain with iodinated contrast (ultravist) if no
contrast allergy and no renal failure (e.g.,
GFR ≥ 30) _____
Magnetic resonance imaging (MRI) brain non
contrast ____
Magnetic resonance imaging (MRI) of
brain with contrast (gadolinium) if no
contrast allergy and no renal failure (e.g.,
GFR ≥ 30) ___
Magnetic resonance angiography (MRA) Circle
of Willis (COW) and MRA of Carotids
without contrast (if renal failure) _____
Magnetic resonance angiography (MRA) Circle
of Willis (COW) and MRA of Carotids
without contrast and with contrast
(gadolinium) if no contrast allergy and no
renal failure (e.g., GFR ≥ 30) _____
Carotid Ultrasound ___
Transcranial doppler of brain vessels _____
Other _____

Cardiac Studies

ECG __ × 1 __ q 4 hours × 3 ___ q 4 hours ×
4 ___ other ____ with cardiac enzymes
Echocardiogram (transthoracic) __ with
agitated (bubble) study __ without agitated
(bubble) study

Consultants

Care coordinator (Case management)
_____ Notified: Name _____ Time
_____
Neurology (headache service) _____ Notified:
Name _____ Time _____
Pain management* _____
Notified: Name _____ Time _____

Social work_____
Notified: Name _____ Time _____
Other _____
Notified: Name _____ Time _____

Headache Medications (Adult Dosage)
Antiemetics

Chlorpromazine (Thorazine®) __ 10 mg PO __
25 mg PO __ q 4 hours __ q 6 hours
__ 25 mg __ 50 mg __ IV __ IM __ q 4 hours __
q 6 hours __ prn nausea/vomiting
Metoclopramide (Reglan®) __ 10 mg __ IV __
IM __ PO __ q 6 hours __ other __ prn
nausea/vomiting
Ondansetron (Zofran®) __ 4 mg __ 8 mg __ IV
__ PO __ q 6 hours ___ other __ prn nausea/
vomiting
Prochlorperazine (Compazine®) __ 5 mg __
10 mg __ IV __ IM __ PO __ q 4 hours __ q
6 hours (maximum dose IV/IM/PO 40 mg
per day) ___ 25 mg PR bid __ prn nausea/
vomiting
Promethazine (Phenergan®) __ 12.5 mg __
25 mg __ IV__ IM __ PO __ PR __ q4 hours
__ q 6 hours ___ prn nausea/vomiting
Trimethobenzamide (Tigan®) __ 200 mg IM
__ 300 mg PO ___ q 6 hours ___ prn nausea/
vomiting

Medications for Headache Pain*

Acetaminophen (Paracetamol) (Tylenol®)
325 mg tab __ 1 tab __1–2 tabs __ 2 tabs PO
__ q 4 hours __ q 6 hours ___ prn pain ___
prn fever (maximum 4 g daily)
_____ If unable to take tablet formulation, may
give suspension
_____ If unable to take PO, may give suppository
PR __325 mg __ 650 mg __ q 4 hours __ q
6 hours
IV ___ mg __ q 4 hours __ q 6 hours __ prn
pain __ prn fever (maximum adult dose: if
weight < 50 kg is 15 mg/kg up to 750 mg for
a single dose, 75 mg/kg up to 3750 mg for
daily dose; if weight > 50 kg is 650 mg q
4 hours or 1000 mg q 6 hours up to 1000 mg
for a single dose and 4000 mg for a
daily dose)
Caffeine and Sodium Benzoate ** 500 mg
IV____

Dihydroergotamine*** (D.H.E®, Migranal®)
__ 1 mg __ IV __ SQ ___ prn pain** (may
repeat hourly, maximum 2 mg IV daily, 3 mg
IM or SQ daily)

Diphenhydramine (Benadryl®) __ 25 mg __
50 mg q 6 hours IV___ prn pain

Ketorolac (Toradol®) ___ 30 mg q 6 hours IV
___ prn pain

Magnesium**** __ 2 grams IV prn pain × __
dose(s)

Methylprednisolone (Solu-medrol®) __ 125 mg
IV × 1 ___ prn pain __ other

Valproate (Depacon®, Depakene®,
Depakote®) __ 500 mg q 12 hours X 2 doses
or ___ 1,000 mg IV X 1 ___ prn pain (If
patient is not on valproate)

Intravenous Fluids

Saline cap IV ____

Bolus Normal Saline (NS) IV ___ 250 mL __
500 mL ___1,000 mL ____ other infuse over
___ minutes ___ hours

Bolus Lactated Ringer's (LR) IV __ 250 mL __
500 mL __1,000 mL __ other infuse over ___
minutes ___ hours

Maintenance NS at __ mL per hour IV

Maintenance LR at __ mL per hour IV

Maintenance Dextrose 5% in Water (D_5W) at
__ mL per hour IV

Maintenance Dextrose 5% in ½ Normal Saline
(D_5½NS) at __ mL per hour IV

Maintenance Dextrose 5% in Normal Saline
(D_5NS) at __ mL per hour IV

Maintenance NS with potassium chloride __
20 mEq or __ 40 mEq per 1 liter bag at __mL
per hour

Maintenance D_5W with potassium chloride__
20 mEq or __ 40 mEq per 1 liter bag at __ mL
per hour

Maintenance D_5½NS with potassium chloride
__ 20 mEq or _ 40 mEq per 1 liter bag at __
mL per hour IV

Maintenance D_5NS with potassium chloride __
20 mEq or _ 40 mEq per 1 liter bag at __ mL
per hour IV

Other _____ at mL per hour

Education: patient _____ family _____

Headaches ____

Smoking cessation _____

Other _____

*See also protocol for headache pain.

This is not an all-inclusive list since other
medications including droperidol and
ketamine are being used for the treatment of
headache pain. Opioids are not first-line
therapy for treatment of acute headaches and
are not recommended for several reasons
including the problem of rebound that can
occur with opiate use and concern for opioid
dependence. For patients with shunts (unlike
the headache protocol), sometimes opioids
are used.

** Treatment of post-dural puncture headaches
(e.g., headaches occurring after a lumbar
puncture) may include caffeine/sodium
benzoate IV and/or a blood patch (pain
management or anesthesia consult).
However, there have been shortages of IV
caffeine/sodium benzoate.

*** Can't use dihydroergotamine or imitrex
within 24 hours of each other.
Dihydroergotamine and imitrex are
contraindicated with coronary artery disease,
history of stroke, hemiplegic migraine, poorly
controlled hypertension (systolic blood
pressure > 140 mmHg or diastolic blood
pressure > 90 mm Hg)

**** See also electrolyte order set for
hypomagnesemia.

Headache with a Shunt Order Set

Place in Emergency Department (ED)
Observation _____
Diagnosis **HEADACHE WITH A SHUNT,**
_____, _____, _____
ED Attending _____
Resident (if applicable) _____
Advanced Practice Provider (if applicable)
_____

Allergies: Yes _____ No _____

If yes, what _____, _____, _____, _____,
_____, _____

Vital Signs

Temperature __ Pulse __ Respiration __ BP__
Pulse oximetry ____
__ q 2 hours ___ q 4 hours ___ q 6 hours q ___
hours ___ q shift ___ qd ____ other
Cardiac monitoring (telemetry) _____
Orthostatic vital signs _____
Continuous pulse oximetry_____
Neurologic checks ___ q 2 hours __ q 4 hours
__ q 6 hours q __ hours ___ other
Other _____

Notify Physician if

Temperature (°C) > 38.0° ___ 38.5° ___ 39° ___
40° ____ other _____
Systolic blood pressure (mmHg) ≤ 90 ___ ≥
160 __ ≥ 180 ___ ≥ 200 __ other ____
Diastolic blood pressure (mmHg) ≥ 120 ____
other ____
Heart rate ≤ 50 ___ ≥ 120 __ ≥ 150 ___ ≥
200 ___ other ____
Oxygen saturation < 90% _____ other ____
Any change in mental status _____

Activity

Up ad lib _____
Assisted _____
Out of bed to chair _____
Bedrest with bathroom privileges _____
Bedrest with bedside commode _____
Bedrest _____
Other _____

Diet

NPO _____

Regular _____
Advance diet as tolerated _____
Clear liquids ____
Dental, mechanical soft _____
Diabetic _____
Formula _____
Full liquids _____
Low added fat/No added salt _____
Low cholesterol____
Pureed _____
Sodium: 1 gram ___ 2 grams ___
unrestricted____
Per feeding tube _____
Other _____

Nursing Interventions

Weight ___ on admission ___ qd ___ prior to
discharge ____ other
Height ____
I & Os _____ routine _____ strict _____
Fluid restriction ___ mL/hour ___ mL/shift
____ mL/24 hour ___ other
Fall precautions _____
Seizure precautions _____
Capillary blood glucose __ × 1 q ___ hours ___
before meals and at bedtime

Respiratory Interventions

Oxygen __ liters nasal cannula __ venti mask at
___ liters per minute _____ other
Wean oxygen as tolerated without dyspnea,
stridor or oxygen saturation < 90% ____
Sleep apnea qhs __ CPAP BiPAP settings cm
H$_2$O ___ inspiratory __ expiratory

Laboratory Tests

CBC _____ with differential
Basic metabolic panel _____
Cardiac enzymes __ × 1 ___ q 4 hours × 3 ___
q 4 hours × 4 ___ other
Complete metabolic panel _____
C-reactive protein (CRP) _____
Erythrocyte sedimentation rate (ESR) _____
Lactate ____
Liver function tests ____
Urinalysis _____
Pregnancy test _____ (qualitative urine)
_____ (quantitative blood)
Other ____, ____, ____, ____,
____, ____, ____, ____

Repeat _____, _____, _____, _____, _____ in
a.m. ___ in _____ hours

Cerebrospinal fluid analysis ___ culture ___
gram stain __cell count with differential -___
glucose ___ protein ___ other

Radiology Studies

Shunt series x-rays _____

CT (computed tomography) brain non
contrast _____

CT (computed tomography) brain with
contrast if no contrast allergy and no renal
failure, (e.g., GFR $\geq$ 30) ___

Magnetic resonance imaging (MRI) brain non
contrast _____

Magnetic resonance imaging (MRI) of brain
with contrast (gadolinium) if no contrast
allergy and no renal failure (e.g., GFR
$\geq$ 30) ___

Other _____, _____, _____

Cardiac Studies

ECG __ $\times$ 1__ q 4 hours $\times$ 3 ___ q 4 hours $\times$
4 ___ other _____ with cardiac enzymes

Echocardiogram (transthoracic) __with
agitated (bubble) study__ without agitated
(bubble) study

Consultants

Care coordination (Case management)
_____ Notified: Name _____ Time
_____

Neurology_____
Notified: Name _____ Time _____

Neurosurgery _____ Notified:
Name _____ Time _____

Pain management _____ Notified:
Name _____ Time _____

Social work_____ Notified:
Name _____ Time _____

Other _____
Notified: Name _____ Time _____

Headache with a Shunt Medications (Adult Dosage)

Antiemetics

Chlorpromazine (Thorazine®) __ 10 mg PO __
25 mg PO __ q 4 hours __ q 6 hours
__ 25 mg __ 50 mg __ IV __ q 4 hours __ q
6 hours __ prn nausea/vomiting

Metoclopramide (Reglan®) __10 mg __ IV __
IM __ PO __ q 6 hours __ other __ prn
nausea/vomiting

Ondansetron (Zofran®) __ 4 mg __ 8 mg __ IV
__ PO __ q 6 hours ___ other __ prn nausea/
vomiting ___

Prochlorperazine (Compazine®) __ 5 mg __
10 mg __ IV __ IM __ PO __ q 4 hours __ q
6 hours (maximum dose IV/IM/PO 40 mg
per day) ____ 25 mg PR bid __ prn nausea/
vomiting

Promethazine (Phenergan®) __ 12.5 mg __
25 mg __ IV__ IM __ PO __ PR __ q4 hours
__ q 6 hours ___ prn nausea/vomiting

Trimethobenzamide (Tigan®) __ 200 mg IM
__ 300 mg PO ___ q 6 hours ___ prn nausea/
vomiting

Medications for Headache Pain*

Caffeine and Sodium Benzoate** 500 mg IV_____

Dihydroergotamine*** (D.H.E®, Migranal®)
__ 1 mg __ IV __ SQ ___ prn pain (may
repeat hourly, maximum 2 mg IV daily, 3 mg
IM or SQ daily)

Diphenhydramine (Benadryl®) __ 25 mg __
50 mg q 6 hours IV___ prn pain

Ketorolac (Toradol®) ____ 30 mg q 6 hours IV
___ prn pain

Magnesium**** __ 2 grams IV prn pain $\times$ __
dose(s)

Methylprednisolone (Solu-medrol®) 125 mg
IV X 1 _____ prn pain __ other

Valproate (Depacon®, Depakote®,
Depakene®) __ 500 mg q 12 hours X 2 doses
or ___ 1,000 mg IV X 1 ___ prn pain (If
patient is not on valproate)

Other _____, ____, ____, _____, ____

Analgesics

Acetaminophen (Paracetamol) (Tylenol®)
325 mg tab __ 1 tab __1–2 tabs __ 2 tabs PO
__ q 4 hours __ q 6 hours ___ prn pain ___
prn fever (maximum 4 g daily)

_____ If unable to take tablet formulation, may
give suspension

_____ If unable to take PO, may give suppository
PR __ 325 mg __ 650 mg __ q 4 hours __ q
6 hours

IV ___ mg __ q 4 hours __ q 6 hours __ prn
pain __ prn fever (maximum adult dose: if
weight < 50 kg is 15 mg/kg up to 750 mg for

a single dose, 75 mg/kg up to 3750 mg for daily dose; if weight > 50 kg is 650 mg q 4 hours or 1000 mg q 6 hours up to 1000 mg for a single dose and 4000 mg for a daily dose)

Acetaminophen-Hydrocodone (Vicodin®) 300 mg/5 mg tabs __ 1 tab __ 1–2 tabs __ 2 tabs PO __ q 4 hours __ q 6 hours ___ prn pain (maximum 4 grams daily based on acetaminophen dose)

Acetaminophen-Oxycodone (Endocet®, Percocet®, Roxicet®) 325 mg/ 5 mg tab __ 1 tab __1–2 tabs __ 2 tabs PO q 4 hours __ q 6 hours ___ prn pain (maximum 4 grams daily based on acetaminophen dose)

Hydromorphone (Dilaudid®) __ 0.5 mg __ 1 mg __ 2 mg __ mg __ IV__ q 2 hours __ q 4 hours __ q 6 hours q ___ hours __ prn pain

Ibuprofen (Motrin®, Advil®) __ 400 mg __ 600 mg __ 800 mg PO __ q 4 hours __ q 6 hours __ q 8 hours ___ prn pain

Ketorolac (Toradol®) __ 30 mg IV __ q 6 hours __ prn pain (maximum 120 mg daily)

Morphine __ 0.5 mg __ 1 mg __ 2 mg __ 4 mg __ mg ___ IV __ q 2 hours __ q 4 hours __ q 6 hours q ___ hours __ prn pain

Tramadol (Ultram®) __ 50 mg __ 100 mg PO __ q 4 hours __ q 6 hours __ prn pain (maximum 400 mg daily)

Other _____, _____, _____, _____, _____

Intravenous Fluids

Saline cap IV ____

Bolus Normal Saline (NS) IV ___ 250 mL __ 500 mL ___1,000 mL ____ other infuse over ___ minutes ___ hours

Bolus Lactated Ringer's (LR) IV __ 250 mL __ 500 mL __1,000 mL __ other infuse over ___ minutes ___ hours

Maintenance NS at __ mL per hour IV

Maintenance LR at __ mL per hour IV

Maintenance Dextrose 5% in Water (D$_5$W) at __ mL per hour IV

Maintenance Dextrose 5% in ½ Normal Saline (D$_5$½NS) at __ mL per hour IV

Maintenance Dextrose 5% Normal Saline (D$_5$NS) at __ mL per hour IV

Maintenance NS with potassium chloride __ 20 mEq or __ 40 mEq per 1 liter bag at __mL per hour

Maintenance D$_5$W with potassium chloride__ 20 mEq or __ 40 mEq per 1 liter bag at __ mL per hour

Maintenance D$_5$½NS with potassium chloride __ 20 mEq or __ 40 mEq per 1 liter bag at __ mL per hour IV

Maintenance D$_5$NS with potassium chloride __ 20 mEq or __ 40 mEq per 1 liter bag at __mL per hour IV

Other _____ at mL per hour

Education: patient _____ family _____

Headaches ____

Shunts _____

Smoking cessation _____

Other _____

See also protocol for headache with a shunt protocol.

* Since migraine headaches (and other benign headaches) can occur simultaneously with a shunt headache, the medications administered for migraines and other benign headaches are also included. This is not an all-inclusive list since other medications, including droperidol and ketamine, are being used for the treatment of headache pain.

Opioids are not first-line therapy for treatment of acute headaches and are not recommended for several reasons including the problem of rebound that can occur with opiate use and concern for opioid dependence. For patients with shunts (unlike the headache protocol), sometimes opioids are used.

** Treatment of post-dural puncture headaches (e.g., headaches occurring after a lumbar puncture) may include caffeine/sodium benzoate IV and/or a blood patch (pain management or anesthesia consult). However, there have been shortages of IV caffeine/ sodium benzoate.

*** Can't use dihydroergotamine or imitrex within 24 hours of each other. Dihydroergotamine and imitrex are contraindicated with coronary artery disease, history of stroke, hemiplegic migraine, poorly controlled hypertension (systolic blood pressure > 140 mmHg or diastolic blood pressure > 90 mmHg)

**** See also electrolyte order set for hypomagnesemia.

Hematuria Order Set

Place in Emergency Department (ED)
  Observation _____
Diagnosis *HEMATURIA,* _____,

_____, _____

ED Attending _____
Resident (if applicable) _____
Advanced Practice Provider (if applicable)

_____

Allergies: Yes _____ No _____

if yes, what _____,_____,_____,_____,

_____,_____

Vital Signs

Temperature __ Pulse __ Respiration __ BP__
  Pulse oximetry __
___ q 2 hours ___ q 4 hours ___ q 6 hours q
  ___ hours ___ q shift ___ qd ____ other
Cardiac monitoring (telemetry) _____
Orthostatic vital signs _____
Other _____

Notify Physician if

Temperature (°C) > 38.0° ___ 38.5°___ 39° ___
  40° ____ other _____
Systolic blood pressure (mmHg) ≤ 90 ___ ≥
  160 __ ≥ 180 ___ ≥ 200 __ other _____
Diastolic blood pressure (mmHg) ≥ 120 ____
  other _____
Heart rate ≤ 50 ___ ≥ 120 __ ≥ 150 ___ ≥
  200 ___ other ____
Oxygen saturation < 90% _____ other _____

Activity

Up ad lib _____
Assisted _____
Out of bed to chair _____
Bedrest with bathroom privileges _____
Bedrest with bedside commode _____
Bedrest _____
Other _____

Diet

NPO _____
Regular _____
Advance diet as tolerated _____
Clear liquids ____
Dental, mechanical soft _____

Diabetic _____
Formula _____
Full liquids _____
Low added fat/No added salt _____
Low cholesterol ____
Pureed _____
Sodium: 1 gram ___ 2 grams ___
  unrestricted____
Per feeding tube _____
Other _____

Nursing Interventions

Weight ___ on admission ___ qd ___ prior to
  discharge ____ other
Height ____
I & Os _____ routine _____ strict _____
Fluid restriction _____ mL/hour _____ mL/
  shift ____ mL/24 hour
Fall precautions _____
Seizure precautions _____
Capillary blood glucose __ × 1 q ___ hours
  ____ before meals and at bedtime
Place foley catheter ____ replace foley
  catheter ____
Continuous bladder irrigation with normal
  saline with three-way foley irrigation
  set _____

Respiratory Interventions

Oxygen __ liters nasal cannula __ venti mask at
  ___ liters per minute _____ other
Wean oxygen as tolerated without dyspnea,
  stridor or oxygen saturation < 90% ____
If sleep apnea qhs __ CPAP BiPAP settings cm
  H_2O ___ inspiratory __ expiratory

Laboratory Tests

CBC _____ with differential
Basic metabolic panel _____
Cardiac enzymes __ × 1 ___ q 4 hours × 3 ____
  q 4 hours × 4 ____ other
Complete metabolic panel _____
Lactate _____
Renal function tests (e.g., BUN, creatinine)
  _____
Repeat hematocrit ____ at ____ hours
Type and screen _____
Urinalysis _____ Urine culture _____
Other _____, _____, _____, _____,
  _____, _____, _____, _____

Repeat _____, _____, _____, _____, _____ in
a.m. ___ in _____ hours q ____ hours

Radiology Studies

Acute abdominal series _____
KUB (kidneys, ureters, bladder) X-ray
_____
CXR (PA and lateral) _____
CT scan kidney stone protocol (with contrast)
_____
Ultrasound kidneys _____
MRI _____
Other _____, _____, _____

Cardiac Tests

ECG __ × 1__ q 4 hours × 3 ___ q 4 hours ×
4 ___ other _____ with cardiac enzymes
Echocardiogram (transthoracic) __ with
agitated (bubble) study __ without agitated
(bubble) study

Consultants

Care coordination (Case management)
_____ Notified: Name _____ Time
_____
Urology _____
Notified: Name _____ Time _____
Social work_____ Notified:
Name _____ Time _____
Other _____
Notified: Name _____ Time _____

Hematuria Medications

Analgesics

Acetaminophen (Paracetamol) (Tylenol®)
325 mg tab __ 1 tab __ 1–2 tabs __ 2 tabs PO
__ q 4 hours __ q 6 hours ___ prn pain ___
prn fever (maximum 4 g daily)
_____ If unable to take tablet formulation, may
give suspension
_____ If unable to take PO, may give suppository
PR __325 mg __ 650 mg __ q 4 hours __ q
6 hours
IV ___ mg __ q 4 hours __ q 6 hours __ prn
pain __ prn fever (maximum adult dose: if
weight < 50 kg is 15 mg/kg up to 750 mg for
a single dose, 75 mg/kg up to 3750 mg for
daily dose; if weight > 50 kg is 650 mg q
4 hours or 1000 mg q 6 hours up to 1000 mg

for a single dose and 4000 mg for a
daily dose)
Acetaminophen- Hydrocodone (Vicodin®) 300
mg/5 mg tabs __ 1 tab __ 1–2 tabs __ 2 tabs
PO __ q 4 hours __ q 6 hours ___ prn pain
(maximum 4 grams daily based on
acetaminophen dose)
Acetaminophen-Oxycodone (Endocet®,
Percocet®, Roxicet®) 325 mg/5 mg tab __
1 tab __ 1–2 tabs __ 2 tabs PO __ q 4 hours
__ q 6 hours ___ prn pain (maximum
4 grams daily based on acetaminophen dose)
Hydromorphone (Dilaudid®) __ 0.5 mg __
1 mg __ 2 mg __ mg __ IV __ q 2 hours __ q
4 hours __ q 6 hours q ___ hours __ prn pain
Ibuprofen (Advil®, Motrin®) __ 400 mg __
600 mg __ 800 mg PO __ q 4 hours __ q
6 hours __ q 8 hours ___ prn pain
Ketorolac (Toradol®) __ 30 mg IV __ q 6 hours
__ prn pain (maximum 120 mg daily)
Morphine __ 0.5 mg __ 1 mg __ 2 mg __ 4 mg
__ mg IV __ q 2 hours __ q 4 hours __ q
6 hours q ___ hours __ prn pain
Tramadol (Ultram®) __ 50 mg __ 100 mg PO
__ q 4 hours __ q 6 hours __ prn pain
(maximum 400 mg daily)
Other _____, _____, _____,
_____, _____

Analgesics: Other

Phenazopyridine (Pyridium®) __ 100 mg __
200 mg PO tid after meals for 2 days

Antibiotics*

Antibiotics – Oral

Ciprofloxacin (Cipro®) __ 500 mg PO bid
Cephalexin (Keflex®) __ 500 mg __ 1,000 mg
__ PO q 6 hours __ q 8 hours __ q 12 hours
Levofloxacin (Levaquin®) ___ 250 mg __
500 mg ___ 750 mg PO qd
Nitrofurantoin (Furadantin®, Macrodantin®)
__ 50 mg __ 100 mg PO q 6 hours
Nitrofurantoin dual release capsules
(Macrobid®) __ 100 mg PO every 12 hours
Sulfamethoxazole and Trimethoprim
(Bactrim™ DS, Septra® DS) __1 tab __
2 tabs PO __ q 12 hours __ qd__ (usual dose
1–2 double strength [DS] tablets every 12–24
hours where DS = sulfamethoxazole 800 mg
and trimethoprim [TMP] 180 mg)

Antibiotics – Intravenous

Ampicillin and Sulbactam (Unasyn®) ___ 1.5 grams __ 3 grams IV ___ q 6 hours __ other

Cefazolin (Ancef®) __ 1 gram __ 1.5 grams __ 2 grams IV __ q 8 hours __ q 12 hours ___ qd __ other (usual dose 1–2 grams every 8 hours, maximum 12 grams daily)

Ceftriaxone (Rocephin®) __ 1 gram IV q 24 hours

Ciprofloxacin (Cipro®) ___ 400 mg IV bid ___ other

Gentamicin __ 3 mg/kg __ 5 mg/kg X weight in ___kg IV q 8 hours __ q 24 hours ____other (in underweight and nonobese patients total body weight is commonly used but ideal weight can also be used, in obese patients use ideal body weight)

Levofloxacin (Levaquin®) ___ 500 mg ___ 750 mg IV qd __ other

Antiemetic

Chlorpromazine (Thorazine®) __ 10 mg PO __ 25 mg PO __ q 4 hours __ q 6 hours __ 25 mg __ 50 mg __ IV __ IM __ q4 hours __ q 6 hours __ prn nausea/vomiting

Metoclopramide (Reglan®) __10 mg __ IV __ IM __ PO __ q 6 hours __ other __ prn nausea/vomiting

Ondansetron (Zofran®) __ 4 mg __ 8 mg __IV __PO __ q 6 hours ___ other __ prn nausea/vomiting ___

Prochlorperazine (Compazine®) _5 mg _ 10 mg _ IV _IM _ PO __ q 4 hours __ q 6 hours (maximum dose IV/IM/PO 40 mg per day) ___ 25 mg PR bid __ prn nausea/vomiting

Promethazine (Phenergan®) __12.5 mg __ 25 mg __IV__ IM __ PO __ PR __ q4 hours __ q 6 hours ___ prn nausea/vomiting

Trimethobenzamide (Tigan®) __ 200 mg IM __ 300 mg PO ___ q 6 hours ___ prn nausea/vomiting

Intravenous Fluids

Saline cap IV ____

Bolus Normal Saline (NS) ___ 250 mL __ 500 mL ___1,000 mL ____ mL IV infuse over ___ minutes ___ hours

Bolus Lactated Ringer's (LR) ___ 250 mL __ 500 mL ___1,000 mL ___ mL IV infuse over ___ minutes ___ hours

Maintenance NS at __ mL per hour IV

Maintenance LR at __ mL per hour IV

Maintenance Dextrose 5% in Water (D_5W) at __ mL per hour IV

Maintenance Dextrose 5% in ½ Normal Saline (D_5½NS) at __ mL per hour IV

Maintenance Dextrose 5% Normal Saline (D_5NS) at __ mL per hour IV

Maintenance NS with potassium chloride __ 20 mEq or __ 40 mEq per 1 liter bag at __mL per hour

Maintenance D_5W with potassium chloride__ 20 mEq or __ 40 mEq per 1 liter bag at __ mL per hour

Maintenance D_5½NS with potassium chloride __ 20 mEq or _ 40 mEq per 1 liter bag at __ mL per hour IV

Maintenance D_5NS with potassium chloride __ 20 mEq or __ 40 mEq per 1 liter bag at __ mL per hour IV

Other _____ at mL per hour

Education: patient _____ family _____

Hematuria _____

Cystitis _____

Urinary Tract Infection _____

Smoking cessation_____

Other _____

*Antibiotics may be needed to treat infections that are also present in addition to the hematuria, such as, cystitis or urinary tract infections.

Hyperemesis Gravidarum Order Set

Place in Emergency Department (ED)
Observation _____

Diagnosis *HYPEREMESIS GRAVIDARUM,*

_____, _____, _____

ED Attending _____

Resident (if applicable) _____

Advanced Practice Provider (if applicable)

_____

Allergies: Yes _____ No _____

If yes, what _____,_____,_____,_____,

_____,_____

Vital Signs

Temperature __ Pulse __ Respiration __ BP__
Pulse oximetry ____

__ q 2 hours ___ q 4 hours ___ q 6 hours q ___
hours ___ q shift ___ qd ____ other

Cardiac monitoring (telemetry) _____

Orthostatic vital signs _____

Continuous pulse oximetry_____

Other _____

Notify Physician if

Temperature (°C) > 38.0° ___ 38.5°___ 39° ____
40° ____ other _____

Systolic blood pressure (mmHg) ≤ 90 ___ ≥
160 __ ≥ 180 ___ ≥ 200 __ other _____

Diastolic blood pressure (mmHg) ≥ 120 ____
other _____

Heart rate ≤ 50 ___ ≥ 120 __ ≥ 150 ___ ≥
200 ___ other ____

Oxygen saturation < 90% _____ other _____

Activity

Up ad lib _____

Assisted _____

Out of bed to chair _____

Bedrest with bathroom privileges _____

Bedrest with bedside commode _____

Bedrest _____

Other _____

Diet

Diet: encourage meals/snacks to be eaten slowly
and in small amounts every 1–2 hours to
avoid a full stomach) ___

Diet: encourage frequent small carbohydrate
meals (such as soda crackers or dry
toast) ____

Diet: encourage small amounts of cold, clear
fluids between meals/snacks _____

NPO _____

Regular _____

Advance diet as tolerated _____

Clear liquids ____

Dental, mechanical soft _____

Diabetic _____

Formula _____

Full liquids _____

Low added fat/No added salt _____

Low cholesterol ____

Pureed _____

Sodium: 1 gram ___ 2 grams ___
unrestricted____

Per feeding tube _____

Other _____

Nursing Interventions

Weight ___ on admission ___ qd ___ prior to
discharge ____ other

Height ____

I & Os _____ routine _____ strict _____

Seizure precautions _____

Capillary blood glucose __ × 1 q ___ hours
____ before meals and at bedtime

Respiratory Interventions

Oxygen __ liters nasal cannula __ venti mask at
___ liters per minute _____ other

Wean oxygen as tolerated without dyspnea,
stridor or oxygen saturation < 90% ____

Sleep apnea qhs __ CPAP BiPAP settings cm
H$_2$O ___ inspiratory __ expiratory

Laboratory Tests

CBC _____ with differential

Amylase ___ Lipase___

Basic metabolic panel_____

Cardiac enzymes __ × 1 ___ q 4 hours × 3 ____
q 4 hours × 4 _____ other

Complete metabolic panel_____

Lactate _____

Liver function tests _____

Urinalysis _____ Urine culture _____

Pregnancy test (qualitative urine) _____

Pregnancy test (quantitative blood) _____
Renal function tests (e.g., BUN, creatinine) _____

Type and Screen _____
Other _____, _____, _____, _____,
_____, _____, _____, _____
Repeat _____, _____, _____, _____, _____ in
a.m. ___ in _____ hours

Radiology Studies

Ultrasound Pelvis _____
Other _____, _____, _____

Cardiac Studies

ECG __ × 1__ q 4 hours × 3 ___ q 4 hours ×
4 ___ other ____ with cardiac enzymes
Echocardiogram (transthoracic) __ with
agitated (bubble) study __ without agitated
(bubble) study

Consultants

Care coordination (Case management)
_____ Notified: Name _____ Time
_____
Obstetrics/Gynecology _____ Notified:
Name _____ Time _____
Social work _____ Notified:
Name _____ Time _____
Other _____ Notified:
Name _____ Time _____

Hyperemesis Medications (Adult Dosage)
Medications from ACOG Practice guidelines*
Vitamins

Thiamine (Vitamin B1) ___ 100 mg IV qd
Pyridoxine (Vitamin B6) __ 10 mg __ 25 mg
PO __ q 6 hours __ q 8 hours

Antihistamines (H1 receptor antagonist)

Doxylamine (Aldex AN®, Doxytex®, Nitetime
sleep-aid®, Sleep aid®) __ 12.5 mg PO __ q
6 hours __ q 8 hours
*The order suggested by ACOG in the
2004 guidelines is: vitamin B6, doxylamine,
promethazine; then if no dehydration: any of
the following three medications:
metoclopramide or promethazine or
trimethobenzamide; and if dehydration: IV
fluid replacement and any of the following
three medications: dimenhydrinate,

metoclopramide, or promethazine; and if
still nauseous/vomiting: any of the following
two medications: methylprednisolone
(starting at 16 mg q 8 hours PO or IV for
3 days then taper over 2 weeks to lowest
effective dose) or ondansetron 8 mg q 12
hours IV.
*In the 2015 guidelines by ACOG, "Treatment
of nausea and vomiting of pregnancy with
vitamin B6 or vitamin B6 plus doxylamine is
safe and effective and should be considered
first-line pharmacotherapy." "Medications
for which there are some safety data but no
conclusive evidence of efficacy include
anticholinergics and metoclopramide.
Additionally, evidence is limited on the safety
or efficacy of the 5-hydroxy-tryptamine
3 inhibitors (e.g., ondansetron) for nausea
and vomiting of pregnancy; however, because
of their effectiveness in reducing
chemotherapy-induced emesis, their use
appears to be increasing."

Antiemetics

Chlorpromazine (Thorazine®)* __ 10 mg PO
__ 25 mg PO __ q 4 hours __ q 6 hours __
25 mg __ 50 mg __ IV __ IM __ q 4 hours __
q 6 hours __ prn nausea/vomiting
Dimenhydrinate (Dramamine®, Driminate®,
Motion Sickness®)* __ 50 mg IV ___ q
4 hours ___ q 6 hours
Metoclopramide (Reglan®) __ 5 mg __ 10 mg
__ IV __ IM __ PO __ q 6 hours __ other __
prn nausea/vomiting
Ondasetron (Zofran®) __ 8 mg IV q 12 hours
___ other __ prn nausea/vomiting
(ACOG dose)
Promethazine (Phenergan®)* __ 12.5 mg __
25 mg __IV__ IM __ PO __ PR __ q 4 hours
__ q 6 hours ___ prn nausea/vomiting
Trimethobenzamide (Tigan®)* __ 200 mg IM
__ 300 mg PO __ q 6 hours __ prn nausea/
vomiting
Corticosteroids: Methylprednisolone
(Depomedrol®, Methapred®, Solumedrol®)
** __ 16 mg __ PO __ IV q 8 hours ___ other
* Anticholinergic drugs include
chlorpromazine, dimenhydrinate,
promethazine and tigan. The anticholinergic
drugs, reglan and ondansetron are noted in
the 2015 ACOG guidelines.

**Consultation with obstetrics is recommended when using corticosteroids for hyperemesis gravidarum. "Corticosteroid use for hyperemesis gravidarum should be used with caution and avoided as a first-line agent before 10 weeks of gestation." (2015 ACOG guidelines) In view of the ACOG recommendations, individuals with hyperemesis gravidarum requiring corticosteroid use are probably best managed on an inpatient unit and are not appropriate for the observation unit

See also Chapter 52 on Hyperemesis gravidarum.

Gastrointestinal Medications
Antacids

Aluminum Hydroxide and Magnesium Hydroxide (Mylanta®) ___ 10–20 mL liquid PO qid (maximum 80 mL daily), 1–2 tab PO ___ pc and qhs and ___ prn reflux or ___ prn dyspepsia/pain (maximum 16 tablets daily)

Aluminium Hydroxide/Magnesium Hydroxide/Simethicone (Maalox®) __ 30 mL PO __ q 4 hours for reflux or prn gastrointestinal upset/pain

Histamine H2 Antagonist (for gastroesophageal reflux [GERD] in pregnancy)

Famotidine (Pepcid®) __ 20 mg __IV __ PO __ bid ___ qd
__ 40 mg PO qhs __ prn reflux or ___ prn dyspepsia/pain

Proton Pump Inhibitor (PPI)

Pantoprazole (Protonix®) __ 40 mg IV __ bid __ qd __ 40 mg PO __bid __ qd

Esomeprazole (Nexium®) __ 40 mg IV __ bid __ qd __ 40 mg PO __bid __ qd

Other _____, _____, _____, _____, _____

Intravenous Fluids

Saline cap IV ____

Bolus Normal Saline (NS) IV ___ 250 mL __ 500 mL ___1,000 mL ____ other infuse over ___ minutes ___ hours

Bolus Lactated Ringer's (LR) IV __ 250 mL __ 500 mL __1,000 mL __ other infuse over ___ minutes ___ hours

Maintenance NS at __ mL per hour IV

Maintenance LR at __ mL per hour IV

Maintenance Dextrose 5% in Water (D_5W) at __ mL per hour IV

Maintenance Dextrose 5% in ½ Normal Saline (D_5½NS) at __ mL per hour IV

Maintenance Dextrose 5% in Normal Saline (D_5NS) at __ mL per hour IV

Maintenance NS with potassium chloride __ 20 mEq or __ 40 mEq per 1 liter bag at __mL per hour

Maintenance D_5W with potassium chloride__ 20 mEq or __ 40 mEq per 1 liter bag at __ mL per hour

Maintenance D_5½NS with potassium chloride __ 20 mEq or __ 40 mEq per 1 liter bag at __ mL per hour IV

Maintenance D_5NS with potassium chloride __ 20 mEq or __ 40 mEq per 1 liter bag at __ mL per hour IV

Other _____ at mL per hour

Education: patient _____ family _____

Pregnancy _____
Hyperemesis gravidarum ____
Smoking cessation _____
Other _____

* Recommendations for medications suggested by American College of Obstetrics and Gynecology (ACOG) include some agents generally used for treatment of nausea and vomiting of pregnancy, but not commonly used for other causes of nausea/vomiting unrelated to pregnancy.

References

ACOG Committee on Practice Bulletins. Nausea and Vomiting of Pregnancy. ACOG Practice Bulletin. Clinical Management Guidelines for Obstetrician-Gynecologists (no. 52). *ACOG Practice Bulletin* April 2004; 103(4):803–815.

ACOG Committee on Practice Bulletins. Nausea and Vomiting of Pregnancy. ACOG Practice Bulletin Summary. *Obstetrics & Gynecology* 2015; 126 (3):687–688.53. (Practice Bulletin Summary #153, September 2015).

Hyperglycemia Order Set

Place in Emergency Department (ED)
  Observation _____
Diagnosis *HYPERGLYCEMIA,* _____,

_____, _____

ED Attending _____
Resident (if applicable) _____
Advanced Practice Provider (if applicable)

_____

Allergies: Yes _____ No _____

If yes, what _____,_____,_____,_____,

_____,_____

Vital Signs

Temperature __ Pulse __ Respiration __ BP__
  Pulse oximetry
__ q 2 hours ___ q 4 hours ___ q 6 hours q ___
  hours ___ q shift ___ qd ____ other
Cardiac monitoring (telemetry) _____
Orthostatic vital signs _____
Continuous pulse oximetry _____
Other _____

Notify Physician if

Temperature(°C) > 38.0° ____ 38.5°___ 39° ___
  40° ___ other ___
Systolic blood pressure (mmHg) ≤ 90 ___ ≥
  160 ___ ≥ 180 ___ ≥ 200 ___ other ___
Diastolic blood pressure (mmHg) ≥ 120 _____
  other _____
Heart rate ≤ 50 ___ ≥ 120 ___ 150 ___ ≥
  200 ___ other ___
Blood glucose <60 _____ > 350 _____
Oxygen saturation < 90% _____ other _____
Any change in mental status _____
Any respiratory distress_____

Activity

Up ad lib _____
Assisted _____
Out of bed to chair _____
Bedrest with bathroom privileges _____
Bedrest with bedside commode _____
Bedrest _____
Other _____

Diet

NPO _____

Regular _____
Advance diet as tolerated _____
Clear liquids ____
Dental, mechanical soft _____
Diabetic _____
Formula_____
Full liquids _____
Low added fat/No added salt _____
Low cholesterol ____
Pureed _____
Sodium: 1 gram ___ 2 grams ___
  unrestricted____
Per feeding tube _____
Other _____

Nursing Interventions

Weight ___ on admission ___ qd ___ prior to
  discharge ____ other
Height ____
I & Os _____ routine _____ strict _____
Fluid restriction ___ mL/hour ___ mL/shift
  ____ mL/24 hour ___ other
Fall precautions _____
Seizure precautions _____
Capillary blood glucose __ × 1 q ___ hours ___
  before meals and at bedtime

Respiratory Interventions

Oxygen __ liters nasal cannula __ venti mask at
  ___ liters per minute _____ other
Sleep apnea qhs __ CPAP BiPAP settings cm
  H_2O ___ inspiratory __ expiratory

Laboratory Tests

Arterial blood gas _____
Basic metabolic panel _____
Beta-hydroxybutyrate _____
CBC _____ with differential
Complete metabolic panel _____
Ketones in serum _____
Pregnancy test (qualitative urine) _____
Pregnancy test (quantitative blood)
Renal function tests (BUN, creatinine) _____
Urinalysis _____
Venous blood gas _____
Other _____, _____, _____
Repeat _____, _____, _____, _____, _____ in
  a.m. __ in _____ hours

Radiology Studies

_____, _____, _____

Cardiac Studies

ECG __ × 1__ q 4 hours × 3 ___ q 4 hours × 4 ___ other ____ with cardiac enzymes

Echocardiogram (transthoracic) __ with agitated (bubble) study__ without agitated (bubble) study

Consultants

Care coordination (Case management) _____ Notified: Name _____ Time _____

Endocrinology _____ Notified: Name _____ Time _____

Social work _____ Notified: Name _____ Time _____

Other _____ Notified: Name _____ Time _____

See Diabetic Order Set*

*See also diabetic order set for daily medications and for insulin coverage

Intravenous Fluids

Saline cap IV ____

Bolus Normal Saline (NS) ___ 250 mL __ 500 mL ___1,000 mL ____ mL IV, infuse over ___ minutes ___ hours

Bolus Lactated Ringer's (LR) ___ 250 mL __ 500 mL ___1,000 mL ___ mL IV, infuse over ___ minutes ___ hours

Maintenance NS at __ mL per hour IV

Maintenance LR at __ mL per hour IV

Maintenance Dextrose 5% in Water (D_5W) at __ mL per hour IV

Maintenance Dextrose 5% in ½ Normal Saline (D_5½NS)at __ mL per hour IV

Maintenance Dextrose 5% in Normal Saline (D_5NS) at __ mL per hour IV

Maintenance NS with potassium chloride __ 20 mEq or __ 40 mEq per 1 liter bag at __ mL per hour

Maintenance D_5½NS with potassium chloride __ 20 mEq or __ 40 mEq per 1 liter bag at __ mL per hour IV

Maintenance D_5NS with potassium chloride __ 20 mEq or __ 40 mEq per 1 liter bag at __ mL per hour IV

Other _____ at mL per hour

Education: patient _____ family _____

Diabetic _____

Smoking cessation _____

Other _____

Hypertensive Urgency Order Set

Place in Emergency Department (ED)
Observation _____
Diagnosis **HYPERTENSIVE URGENCY,**

_____, _____, _____

ED Attending _____
Resident (if applicable) _____
Advanced Practice Provider (if applicable)
_____

Allergies: Yes _____ No _____

If yes, what _____,_____,_____,_____,

_____,_____

Vital Signs

Temperature __ Pulse __ Respiration __ BP__
Pulse oximetry ___
___ q 2 hours ___ q 4 hours ___ q 6 hours q
___ hours ___ q shift ___ qd ____ other
Cardiac monitoring (telemetry) _____
Continuous pulse oximetry_____
Other _____

Notify Physician if

Temperature (°C) > 38.0° ___ 38.5°___ 39° ___
40° ____ other _____
Systolic blood pressure (mmHg) ≤ 90 ___ ≥
160 __ ≥ 180 ___ ≥ 200 __ other _____
Diastolic blood pressure (mmHg) ≥ 120 ____
other _____
Heart rate ≤ 50 ___ ≥ 120 __ ≥ 150 ___ ≥
200 ___ other ____
Oxygen saturation < 90% _____ other _____
Any change in mental status _____
Any respiratory distress _____

Activity

Up ad lib _____
Assisted _____
Out of bed to chair _____
Bedrest with bathroom privileges _____
Bedrest with bedside commode _____
Bedrest _____
Other _____

Diet

NPO _____
Regular _____
Advance diet as tolerated _____

Clear liquids ____
Dental, mechanical soft _____
Diabetic _____
Formula _____
Full liquids _____
Low added fat/No added salt _____
Low cholesterol ____
Pureed _____
Sodium: 1 gram ___ 2 grams ___
unrestricted____
Per feeding tube _____
Other _____

Nursing Interventions

Weight ___ on admission ___ qd ___ prior to
discharge ____ other
Height ____
I & Os _____ routine _____ strict _____
Fluid restriction ___ mL/hour ___ mL/shift
____ mL/24 hour ___ other
Fall precautions _____
Seizure precautions _____
Capillary blood glucose __ × 1 q ___ hours
____ before meals and at bedtime

Respiratory Interventions

Oxygen __ liters nasal cannula __ venti mask at
___ liters per minute _____ other
Wean oxygen as tolerated without dyspnea,
stridor or oxygen saturation < 90% ____
Peak flow __ on admission ___ prior to
discharge ___ pre and post aerosols
Sleep apnea qhs __ CPAP BiPAP settings cm
H_2O ___ inspiratory __ expiratory

Laboratory Tests

CBC with differential _____
Basic metabolic panel _____
Brain natriuretic peptide (BNP) _____
Cardiac enzymes __ × 1 ___ q 4 hours × 3 ___ q
4 hours × 4 _____ other
Complete metabolic panel _____
Liver function tests _____
Pregnancy test (qualitative urine) _____
Pregnancy test (quantitative blood) _____
Renal function tests (e.g., BUN, creatinine)

_____
Urinalysis _____ Urine culture _____
Other _____, _____, _____, _____,

_____, _____, _____, _____

Repeat _____, _____, _____, _____, _____ in a.m. ___ in _____ hours

Radiology Studies

CXR portable _____
CXR (PA and lateral) _____
Other _____, _____, _____

Cardiac Studies

ECG __ × 1 __ q 4 hours × 3 ___ q 4 hours × 4 ___ other ____ with cardiac enzymes
Echocardiogram (transthoracic) __ with agitated (bubble) study __ without agitated (bubble) study

Stress Tests/Cardiac Imaging Studies

Stress Electrocardiogram (treadmill stress test, exercise tolerance test/ETT) _____
Stress Echocardiogram ____
Pharmacologic Stress Tests

Coronary Vasodilators:

Adenosine _____
Dipyridamole/Persantine _____
Regadenosine/Lexiscan _____

Synthetic Catecholamine:

Dobutamine _____

Myocardial Perfusion Imaging (injection of radioactive isotopes):

Nuclear Stress Test

Thallium-201 _____
Technetium-99m Sestamibi _____
Technetium-99 Tetrofosmin _____

Gamma Imaging :

Single positron emission computed tomography (SPECT)_____
Cardiac positron emission tomography (pet)

Stress Cardiovascular Magnetic Resonance Imaging (CMR) _____
Computed Tomography Coronary Angiography (CTCA) _____
Other _____

* Not all tests are available at all institutions. Generally, test availability is limited, depends on many factors including available expertise and cost, and is institution specific. This list is not all inclusive but is intended to list the stress tests/cardiac imaging discussed in Chapter 26 Stress Testing.

Consultants

Cardiology _____ Notified:
Name _____ Time _____
Care coordination (Case management)
_____ Notified: Name
_____Time _____
Internal medicine/Family practice ___ Notified:
Name _____ Time _____
Nephrology/Hypertension _____ Notified:
Name _____Time _____
Social work _____ Notified:
Name _____ Time _____
Other _____ Notified:
Name _____ Time _____

Cardiac Medications

Blood Pressure Therapy*

Thiazide Diuretic

Hydrochlorothiazide __ 12.5 mg __ 25 mg __ 50 mg PO qd __ other (usual range 12.5–50 mg daily, maximum 50 mg daily since higher doses show little increase in efficacy but have more electrolyte disturbances)

Vasodilator

Hydralazine (Apresoline®, Hydralazine®) __ 10 mg __ 20 mg __ other __ IV __ qd __ q 4 hours __ q 6 hours (maximum 40 mg IV per dose); __ 10 mg __ 25 mg __ 50 mg __ 100 mg __ PO qid (usual PO dose 25–100 mg/day in 3–4 divided doses, maximum PO 300 mg daily) __ other

Beta blockers (β1-selective)

Metoprolol immediate release (Metoprolol®, Lopressor ®) __ 50 mg __ 100 mg __ 150 mg PO __ bid (100–450 mg daily in 2–3 divided doses, usual range 50–100 mg daily, maximum 450 mg daily) ___ other
Metoprolol (Metoprolol®, Lopressor ®) __ 5 mg __ 10 mg IV __ X 1 __ other
Note: For metoprolol, when switching between oral and intravenous dosage forms, equivalent beta blocking effect is achieved when in 2.5:1 = oral: IV ratio. For example, if started on 5 mg IV q 6 hours (for 20 mg daily IV), then switched to oral, the oral dose would be 25 mg bid PO

immediate release or 50 mg PO qd extended release; since the oral is 2.5 times the IV, it would be 2.5 × 20 (IV total daily dose) = 50 mg total daily oral dose.

Beta blockers (β1-selective) extended release

Metoprolol extended release (Metoprolol ER®, Toprol-XL®) __ 25 mg __ 50 mg __ 100 mg PO qd __ other (usual range 50–100 mg daily, maximum 400 mg daily)

Beta blockers (Beta blocker with alpha-blocking activity)

Labetalol (Normodyne®) __ 10 mg __ 20 mg __ other IV (10 mg/minute is IV push rate, usual dose is 20 mg, maximun 300 mg, may give 40–80 mg at 10 minute intervals) __ 100 mg __ 200 mg __ 300 mg __ 400 mg PO __ bid (usual dose 100–400 mg bid, maximum 2,400 mg daily)

Calcium Channel Blocker

Diltiazem __ 180 mg __ 240 mg __ 300 mg __ 360 mg __ 420 mg PO qd __ other (usual range 180–420 mg/day for all various brands). Maximum per day varies slightly by brand: Cardizem CD® (maximum 480 mg daily), Cardiazem LA (maximum 360 mg daily), Cartia XT® (maximum 480 mg daily), Dilt-CD (maximum 480 mg daily), Dilacor XR® (maximum 480 mg daily), Dilt XR® (maximum 480 mg daily), Dilt XT® (maximum 480 mg daily), Matzim LA (maximum 360 mg daily), Taztia XT® 540 mg/day), Tiazac (maximum 540 mg daily)

Note: When switching between intravenous and oral dosage forms, the oral dose (mg/day) is approximately equal to [rate in mg/hour × 3 + 3] × 10. For example, 3 mg/hour = 120 mg/day, 5 mg/hour = 180 mg/day, 7 mg/hour = 240 mg/day, 11 mg/hour = 360 mg/day.

Angiotensin converting enzyme (ACE) inhibitors

Captopril (Capoten®) __ 12.5 mg __ 25 mg __ 50 mg __ 100 mg PO __ bid __ tid __ other (usual dose 25–100 mg/day in 2 divided doses, maximum dose 450 mg daily)

Alpha2- adrenergic agonist

Clonidine (Catapres®) __ 0.1 mg __ 0.2 mg __ 0.3 mg PO bid __ other

(usual range 0.1–0.8 mg/day in 2 divided doses, maximum 2.4 mg daily)

Angiotensin II receptor blocker (ARBs) (Angiotensin II antagonist)

Losartan (Cozaar®) __ 25 mg __ 50 mg __ 100 mg PO __ bid __ qd
(usual range 25–100 mg daily, initial dose 50 mg daily unless on diuretic or volume depleted then 25 mg daily)

Analgesics

Acetaminophen (Paracetamol) (Tylenol®) 325 mg tab __ 1 tab __ 1–2 tabs __ 2 tabs PO __ q 4 hours __ q 6 hours ___ prn pain ___ prn fever (maximum 4 g daily)
____ If unable to take tablet formulation, may give suspension
____ If unable to take PO, may give suppository PR __325 mg __ 650 mg __ q 4 hours __ q 6 hours
IV ___ mg __ q 4 hours __ q 6 hours __ prn pain __ prn fever (maximum adult dose: if weight < 50 kg is 15 mg/kg up to 750 mg for a single dose, 75 mg/kg up to 3750 mg for daily dose; if weight > 50 kg is 650 mg q 4 hours or 1000 mg q 6 hours up to 1000 mg for a single dose and 4000 mg for a daily dose)

Acetaminophen-Hydrocodone (Vicodin®) 300 mg/5 mg tabs __ 1 tab __ 1–2 tabs __ 2 tabs PO __ q 4 hours __ q 6 hours ___ prn pain (maximum 4 grams daily based on acetaminophen dose)

Acetaminophen-Oxycodone (Percocet®, Roxicet®, Endocet®) 325 mg/ 5 mg tab __ 1 tab __ 1–2 tabs __ 2 tabs PO q 4 hours __ q 6 hours ___ prn pain (maximum 4 grams daily based on acetaminophen dose)

Hydromorphone (Dilaudid®) __ 0.5 mg __ 1 mg __ 2 mg __ mg __ q 2 hours __ q 4 hours __ q 6 hours q ___ hours IV __ prn pain

Ibuprofen (Motrin®, Advil®)__ 400 mg __ 600 mg __ 800 mg PO __ q 4 hours __ q 6 hours __ q 8 hours ___ prn pain (Do not use beyond 31–32 weeks gestation)

Ketorolac (Toradol®) __ 30 mg IV __ q 4 hours __ q 6 hours __ prn pain (maximum 120 mg daily) (Do not use beyond 31–32 weeks gestation)

Morphine __ 0.5 mg __ 1 mg __ 2 mg __ 4 mg
IV ___ q 2 hours __ q 4 hours __ q 6 hours q
___ hours __ prn pain
Tramadol (Ultram®) __ 50 mg __ 100 mg PO
__ q 4 hours __ q 6 hours __ prn pain
(maximum 400 mg daily)

Other Medications

Aspirin _____ 81 mg _____ 325 mg PO qd
Nitroglycerin __ 0.4 mg sl prn chest pain __
once __ q 5 minutes × 3 if BP and HR are
stable (systolic BP > 90, HR > 60) _____ and
notify MD

Intravenous Fluids

Saline cap IV (KVO) _____
Maintenance Normal Saline (NS) at __ mL per
hour IV
Maintenance Lactated Ringer's (LR) at __ mL
per hour IV
Maintenance Dextrose 5% in Water (D_5W) at
__ mL per hour IV
Maintenance Dextrose 5% in ½ Normal Saline
($D_5\frac{1}{2}NS$) at __ mL per hour IV
Maintenance Dextrose 5% in Normal Saline
(D_5NS) at __ mL per hour IV
Maintenance NS with potassium chloride __
20 mEq or _ 40 mEq per 1 liter bag at __mL
per hour
Maintenance D_5W with potassium chloride__
20 mEq or __ 40 mEq per 1 liter bag at __ mL
per hour
Maintenance D_5½ NS with potassium chloride
__ 20 mEq or __ 40 mEq per 1 liter bag at __
mL per hour IV
Maintenance D_5NS with potassium chloride __
20 mEq or __ 40 mEq per 1 liter bag at __ mL
per hour IV
Other _____ at mL per hour

Education: patient _____ family _____

Hypertension _____
Smoking cessation, if applicable _____
Other _____
* Drug doses and indications, when possible,
are based on JNC 7/8 (Seventh Report of the
Joint National Committee on Prevention,
Detection, Evaluation, and Treatment of
High Blood Pressure) Hypertension 2003;
42:1206–1252. Of the diuretics, the thiazide
diuretics are preferred in the treatment of
hypertension based on JNC 7. More recent
JNC 8 guidelines: James PA, Oparil S, Carter
BL, et al. 2014 Evidence-Based Guideline for
the Management of High Blood Pressure in
Adults. JAMA 2014; 311(5): 507–520.
Conversion rates from IV to oral are given
since patients may be given IV
antihypertensives in the emergency
department/observation unit, then switched
to oral and monitored for effectiveness in the
observation unit.
Since patients placed in observation are
considered to be low-risk, stable patients, we
exclude patients on IV continuous infusions
from our observation/clinical decision unit.
Therefore, any patient needing a continuous
infusion to control hypertension – such as
nitroprusside, nicardipine or nitroglycerin or
any other continuous IV infusion – suggests a
critical patient and is not a candidate for the
observation unit. However, if patients improve
after treatment in the emergency department,
and can be switched to IV medications (but not
IV continuous infusions) and oral medications,
they may be placed in observation for further
monitoring and management of blood pressure
and for other reasons including chest pain
"rule out."

Hypoglycemia Order Set

Nursing Orders for Adult Hypoglycemia

1. Assess capillary blood glucose if hypoglycemia is suspected.
2. For a low glucose (e.g., $\leq$ 60 mg/dL) or for a borderline glucose (60–70 mg/dL) in a symptomatic patient (symptoms such as weakness, dizziness, lightheadedness, and/or anxiety), administer treatment for hypoglycemia

   A. For the alert patient who can swallow (e.g., has adequate swallow without risk of aspiration), give the patient 4 ounces (1/2 cup) of juice, or regular (not diet) soda.

   B. For the patient with a decreased level of consciousness who can swallow e.g., has adequate swallow without risk of aspiration, but has a decreased level of consciousness, give 15 gram (half to one tube) of instant glucose gel. Place the instant glucose in the patient's mouth between the gum and cheek. Turn the patient on his/her side to prevent aspiration.

   C. For the patient who is unconscious and unable to swallow or NPO and an IV is in place, give 25 mL (½ ampule) of $D_{50}W$ IV. If an IV is not in place, then give 1 mg glucagon intramuscularly.

3. Notify the physician.
4. Recheck blood glucose in 10–15 minutes.
5. If the blood glucose is still low ($<$ 60 mg/dL or 60–70 mg/dL in a symptomatic patient), then repeat treatment as in step #2 above.
6. If the patient is alert and able to swallow and a meal is greater than 30 minutes from the hypoglycemic episode, provide additional carbohydrate containing food, such as milk or crackers with peanut butter.
7. Document in the medical record: the patient's initial symptoms, if any; the initial and post treatment blood glucose levels; the treatment given; the patient's response to treatment; and the physician or advanced practice provider notified.
8. If there is no IV access, then consider starting an IV in order to obtain IV access in case IV dextrose and/or other IV fluids are needed.

Kidney Stone/Nephroureterolithiasis Order Set

Place in Emergency Department (ED) Observation _____

Diagnosis *KIDNEY STONE/ NEPHROURETEROLITHIASIS*, _____, _____

ED Attending_____
Resident (if applicable)_____
Advanced Practice Provider (if applicable) _____

Allergies: Yes _____ No _____

If yes, what_____,_____,_____,_____, _____,_____

Vital Signs

Temperature__ Pulse __ Respiration __BP__ Pulse oximetry _____
__q 2 hours ___q 4 hours ___q 6 hours q ___ hours ___q shift ___ qd _____ other
Cardiac monitoring (telemetry) _____
Orthostatic vital signs _____
Continuous pulse oximetry _____
Other _____

Notify Physician if

Temperature (°C) > 38.0° ____ 38.5°____ 39° ___40° ____ other _____
Systolic blood pressure (mmHg) ≤ 90 ___ ≥ 160 __ ≥ 180 ___ ≥ 200__ other _____
Diastolic blood pressure (mmHg) ≥ 120 _____ other _____
Heart rate ≤ 50 ___ ≥ 120 __ ≥ 150 ___ ≥ 200___ other _____
Oxygen saturation < 90% _____ other _____
Any change in mental status _____
Any respiratory distress_____

Activity

Up ad lib _____
Assisted _____
Out of bed to chair _____
Bedrest with bathroom privileges _____
Bedrest with bedside commode _____
Bedrest _____
Other _____

Diet

NPO _____
Regular _____
Advance diet as tolerated _____
Clear liquids _____
Dental, mechanical soft _____
Diabetic _____
Formula_____
Full liquids _____
Low added fat/No added salt_____
Low cholesterol_____
Pureed _____
Sodium: 1 gram ___ 2 grams ___ unrestricted_____
Per feeding tube _____
Other _____

Nursing Interventions

Weight ___ on admission ___ qd ___ prior to discharge _____ other
Height _____
I & Os _____ routine _____ strict _____
Fluid restriction ___ mL/hour ___ mL/shift _____ mL/24 hour ___ other
Fall precautions _____
Seizure precautions _____
Capillary blood glucose __ × 1 q___ hours _____ before meals and at bedtime

Respiratory Interventions

Sleep apnea qhs __ CPAP BiPAP settings cm H_2O ___ inspiratory __ expiratory
Other _____

Laboratory Tests

CBC _____ with differential
Basic metabolic panel_____
Complete metabolic panel_____
Pregnancy test (qualitative urine) _____
Pregnancy test (quantitative blood) _____
Renal function tests (e.g., BUN, creatinine) _____
Urinalysis _____ Urine culture _____
Other _____, _____, _____, _____, _____, _____, _____, _____
Repeat _____, _____, _____, _____, _____ in a.m. ___ in _____ hours

Radiology Studies

Acute abdominal series ____

KUB (Kidneys, ureters, bladder) X-ray

_____

CT scan abdomen/pelvis (renal stone protocol) with contrast: _____-

Ultrasound kidneys left ____ right ____ both ____

Other _____, _____, _____

Consultants

Care coordination (Case management) _____ Notified: Name _____ Time _____

Social work_____ Notified: Name_____ Time_____

Urology_____ Notified: Name_____ Time_____

Other _____ Notified: Name _____ Time_____

Medications for Kidney Stone/ Nephroureterolithiasis (Adult Dosage)†

Analgesics

Acetaminophen (Paracetamol) (Tylenol®) 325 mg tab __1 tab __1–2 tabs __ 2 tabs PO __ q 4 hours __ q 6 hours ___ prn pain ___ prn fever (maximum 4 g daily)

____ If unable to take tablet formulation, may give suspension

____ If unable to take PO may give suppository PR __325 mg __ 650 mg __ q 4 hours __ q 6 hours

____ IV ____ mg __ q 4 hours __ q 6 hours __ prn pain __ prn fever (maximum adult dose: if weight < 50 kg is 15 mg/kg up to 750 mg for a single dose, 75 mg/kg up to 3750 mg for daily dose; if weight > 50 kg is 650 mg q 4 hours or 1000 mg q 6 hours up to 1000 mg for a single dose and 4000 mg for a daily dose)

Acetaminophen- Hydrocodone (Vicodin®) 300 mg/5 mg tabs __1 tab __1–2 tabs __ 2 tabs PO __q 4 hours__ q 6 hours ___ prn pain (maximum 4 grams daily based on acetaminophen dose)

Acetaminophen-Oxycodone (Endocet®, Percocet®, Roxicet®) 325 mg/ 5 mg tab __1 tab __1–2 tabs __ 2 tabs PO q 4 hours__ q

6 hours ___ prn pain (maximum 4 grams daily based on acetaminophen dose)

Hydromorphone (Dilaudid®) __ 0.5 mg __ 1 mg __ 2 mg __ mg __ IV __ q 2 hours __ q 4 hours __ q 6 hours q ___ hours __ prn pain

Ibuprofen (Advil®, Motrin®)__ 400 mg __ 600 mg __ 800 mg PO __ q 4 hours __ q 6 hours__ q 8 hours ___ prn pain

Ketorolac (Toradol®) __ 30 mg IV __ q 6 hours _ prn pain (maximum 120 mg daily)

Morphine __ 0.5 mg__ 1 mg __ 2 mg __ 4 mg __ mg ___ IV__ q 2 hours __ q 4 hours __ q 6 hours q ___ hours __ prn pain

Tramadol (Ultram®) __ 50 mg __ 100 mg PO __q 4 hours __ q 6 hours __ prn pain (maximum 400 mg daily)

Other_____, _____, _____, _____, _____

Antiemetics

Chlorpromazine (Thorazine®) __ 10 mg PO __ 25 mg PO __ q 4 hours __q 6 hours __ 25 mg __ 50 mg__ IV __IM __ q 4 hours __ q 6 hours __ prn nausea/vomiting

Metoclopramide (Reglan®) __10 mg __ IV __ IM __ PO __ q 6 hours __ other __ prn nausea/vomiting

Ondansetron (Zofran®) __ 4 mg __ 8 mg __IV __PO __ q 6 hours ___ other __ prn nausea/vomiting ___

Prochlorperazine (Compazine®) _5 mg _ 10 mg _ IV _IM _ PO __ q 4 hours __ q 6 hours (maximum dose IV/IM/PO 40 mg per day) ___ 25 mg PR bid __ prn nausea/ vomiting

Promethazine (Phenergan®) __12.5 mg __ 25 mg __IV__ IM __ PO __ PR __ q 4 hours __ q 6 hours ___ prn nausea/ vomiting

Trimethobenzamide (Tigan®) __ 200 mg IM __ 300 mg PO ___ q 6 hours ___ prn nausea/vomiting

Other

Alpha 1 Blocker

Tamsulosin (Flomax®) __ 0.4 mg PO qd (discontinue after successful expulsion of stone)

Other_____, _____, _____, _____, _____

Intravenous Fluids

Saline cap IV ____

Bolus Normal saline (NS) IV ____ 250 mL ____
500 mL ____1,000 mL ____ other,

infuse over ____ minutes ____ hours

Bolus Lactated Ringer's (LR) IV ____ 250 mL ____
500 mL ____1,000 mL ____ other, infuse over ____
minutes ____ hours

Maintenance NS at ____ mL per hour IV

Maintenance LR at ____ mL per hour IV

Maintenance Dextrose 5% in Water (D_5W) at
____ mL per hour IV

Maintenance Dextrose 5% in ½ Normal Saline
(D_5½NS) at ___mL per hour IV

Maintenance Dextrose 5% in Normal Saline
(D_5NS) at ____ mL per hour IV

Maintenance NS with potassium chloride ___20
mEq or___ 40 mEq per 1 liter bag at ___mL per
hour IV

Maintenance D_5W with potassium chloride
___20 mEq or _ 40 mEq per 1 liter bag at ___
mL per hour IV

Maintenance D_5½NS with potassium chloride
___20 mEq or _ 40 mEq per 1 liter bag at ___
mL per hour IV

Maintenance D_5NS with potassium chloride
___20 mEq or _ 40 mEq per 1 liter bag at ___
mL per hour IV

Other _____ at mL per hour

Education: patient _____ family _____

Kidney stones____

Smoking cessation_____

Other _____

† If antibiotics are needed for a concomitant
pyelonephritis/urinary tract infection, see
also pyelonephritis/urinary tract infection
order set

Overdose – Ingestion – Exposure Order Set

Place in Emergency Department (ED) Observation _____

Diagnosis **OVERDOSE – INGESTION – EXPOSURE** _____, _____

ED Attending_____

Resident (if applicable)_____

Advanced Practice Provider (if applicable)

_____

Allergies: Yes_____ No_____

If yes, what_____, _____, _____, _____,

_____, _____

Vital Signs

Temperature__ Pulse __ Respiration __BP__ Pulse oximetry ____

__q 2 hours ___q 4 hours ___q 6 hours q ___ hours ___q shift ___ qd ____ other

Cardiac monitoring (telemetry) _____

Neurologic checks* _____q 2 hours ___q 4 hours ___q 6 hours q ___ hours ___q shift ___ qd _____ otherOrthostatic vital signs

_____

Continuous pulse oximetry _____

Other _____

Notify Physician if

Temperature (°C) > 38.0° ___ 38.5°___ 39° ___40° ____ other _____

Systolic blood pressure (mmHg) ≤ 90 ___ ≥ 160 __ ≥ 180 ___ ≥ 200__ other _____

Diastolic blood pressure (mmHg) ≥ 120 ____ other _____

Heart rate ≤ 50 ___ ≥ 120 __ ≥ 150 ___ ≥ 200___ other ____

Oxygen saturation < 90 % _____ other _____

Any change in mental status _____

Any respiratory distress_____

Activity

Up ad lib _____

Assisted _____

Out of bed to chair _____

Bedrest with bathroom privileges _____

Bedrest with bedside commode _____

Bedrest _____

Other _____

Diet

NPO _____

Regular _____

Advance diet as tolerated _____

Clear liquids ____

Dental, mechanical soft _____

Diabetic _____

Formula_____

Full liquids _____

Low added fat/No added salt

Low cholesterol____

Pureed _____

Sodium: 1 gram ___ 2 grams ___ unrestricted____

Per feeding tube _____

Other _____

Nursing Interventions

Weight___ on admission ___ qd ___ prior to discharge ____ other

Height ____

I & Os _____ routine _____ strict _____

Fluid restriction ___ mL/hour ___ mL/shift ____ mL/24 hour ___ other

Fall precautions _____

Seizure precautions _____

Capillary blood glucose __ × 1 q___ hours ____ before meals and at bedtime

Respiratory Interventions

Oxygen __ liters nasal cannula __venti mask at ___ liters per minute _____other

Wean oxygen as tolerated without dyspnea, stridor or oxygen saturation < 90% ____

Peak flow __on admission ___ prior to discharge ___ pre and post aerosols

Sleep apnea qhs __ CPAP BiPAP settings cm H_2O ___ inspiratory __ expiratory

Laboratory Tests

Acetaminophen level _____

Ammonia _____

Amylase _____ Lipase _____

Arterial blood gas _____

Basic metabolic panel_____
Blood alcohol level _____
Blood level of _____, _____,

_____, _____
Carbon monoxide level _____
Cardiac enzymes __ × 1 ___ q 4 hours × 3___ q
4 hours × 4_____ other ____
CBC ____ with differential _____
Complete metabolic panel_____
Creatinine phosphokinase (CPK)

_____
Lactate _____
Liver function tests _____
PT___ INR _____ APTT _____
Pregnancy test (qualitative urine) _____
Pregnancy test (quantitative blood) _____
Renal function tests (e.g. BUN, creatinine)
_____

Toxicology: blood toxicology screen†

_____
Toxicology: urine toxicology screen†

_____
Urinalysis _____ Urine culture _____
Venous blood gas _____
Other _____, _____, _____, _____,

_____, _____, _____, _____
Repeat _____, _____, _____, _____, _____ in
am___ in _____ hours
†Urine toxicology screen includes drugs of
abuse such as cocaine, marihuana, opiates,
phencyclidine, and others. Blood toxicology
screen includes "prescribed or over the
counter drugs" such as acetaminophen,
salicyclates and others.

Radiology Studies

Acute abdominal series _____
KUB (Kidneys, ureters, bladder) X-ray

_____
CXR (PA and lateral)_____
CXR (portable) _____
CT scan _____
Ultrasound _____
Other _____, _____, _____

Cardiac Studies

ECG __ × 1__ q 4 hours × 3 ____ q 4 hours ×
4 ____ other _____ with cardiac enzymes
Echocardiogram (transthoracic) __with
agitated (bubble) study__ without agitated
(bubble) study

Consultants

Care coordination (Case management)
_____ Notified: Name ____ Time
Poison control center/toxicologist __ Notified:
Name ____ Time __
Pharmacist _____ Notified:
Name ____ Time __ Psychiatry
_____ Notified: Name
____ Time __
Social work_____ Notified:
Name ____ Time __ Other
_____ Notified:
Name ____ Time __

Medications for Overdose (Adult Dosage)

Antiemetics

Chlorpromazine (Thorazine®) __ 10 mg _
25 mg PO __ q 4 hours __q 6 hours __ 25 mg
__ 50 mg__ IV __IM __ q 4 hour __ q
6 hours __ prn nausea/vomiting
Metoclopramide (Reglan®) __10 mg __ IV __
IM __ PO __ q 6 hours __ other
__ prn nausea/vomiting
Ondansetron (Zofran®) __ 4 mg __ 8 mg __IV
__PO __ q 6 hours ____ other
__ prn nausea/vomiting ____
Prochlorperazine (Compazine®) _5 mg _
10 mg _ IV _IM _ PO __ q 4 hours
__ q 6 hours (maximum dose IV/IM/PO 40 mg
per day) ___ 25 mg PR bid __ prn nausea/
vomiting
Promethazine (Phenergan®) __12.5 mg __
25 mg __IV__ IM __ PO __ PR __ q 4 hours
__ q 6 hours ___ prn nausea/vomiting

Trimethobenzamide (Tigan®) __ 200 mg IM __ 300 mg PO ___ q 6 hours ___ prn nausea/vomiting

Other _____, _____, _____,

_____, _____, _____

Antidotes

(Narcan®)* __ 0.05 mg __ 0.1 mg __ 0.4 mg___ 2 mg ___IV __ may repeat q 2–3 minutes (maximum 10 mg) (if no response after 10 mg, consider other causes of respiratory depression)

Naloxone (Narcan®) IV infusion** __dose in emergency department that achieved desired result as drip rate per hour or ____ two-thirds of initial bolus that achieved the desired effect per hour

Flumazenil (Romazicon®) ***_____

Other antidote(s) _____

Intravenous Fluids

Saline cap IV _____

Bolus Normal Saline (NS) ___ 250 mL __ 500 mL ___1,000 mL ____ mL IV, infuse over ___ minutes ___ hours

Bolus Lactated Ringer's (LR) ___ 250 mL __ 500 mL ___1,000 mL___ mL IV, infuse over ___ minutes ___ hours

Maintenance NS at __ mL per hour IV

Maintenance LRS at __ mL per hour IV

Maintenance Dextrose 5% in Water (D_5W) at __ mL per hour IV

Maintenance Dextrose 5% in ½ Normal Saline ($D_5½NS$) at __ mL per hour IV

Maintenance Dextrose 5% in Normal Saline (D_5NS) at __ mL per hour IV

Maintenance NS with potassium chloride __20 mEq or _ 40 mEq per 1 liter bag at __mL per hour

Maintenance D_5W with potassium chloride __20 mEq or _ 40 mEq per 1 liter bag at __ mL per hour IV

Maintenance $D_5½$ NS with potassium chloride __20 mEq or _ 40 mEq per 1 liter bag at __ mL per hour IV

Maintenance D_5NS with potassium chloride __20 mEq or _ 40 mEq per 1 liter bag at __ mL per hour IV

Other _____ at mL per hour

Education: patient _____ family

_____

Overdose_____

Drug/alcohol abuse, if applicable _____

Smoking Cessation, if applicable _____

Other _____

*Naloxone is used to reverse opioid-induced hypoventilation. Usual starting doses in adults are 0.1 to 0.4 mg IV. Doses of naloxone should be titrated to desired ventilation and conscious state (e.g., adequate respiratory rate, pulse oxygen saturation on room air, and responsiveness to verbal/motor stimuli). Pupil size (e.g., miosis) is not a reliable sign of naloxone's effect. For chronic opioid dependent patients use smaller doses and titrate to effect. Smaller doses in the range of 0.1 to 0.2 mg have been suggested.

For patients with mental status depression but minimal respiratory depression, a very small starting dose, 0.05 mg, has been suggested because higher doses may induce opioid withdrawal. Subsequent doses from 0.05 to 0.4 mg IV may be administered until the desired response is attained.

Naloxone's reversal effect of opioids generally lasts about 20 to 60 minutes; however, the duration of naloxone response is also highly dependent on patient-specific factors including the specific opioid medication and the dose administered. Therefore, patients should be observed for at least 2 to 3 hours following the administration of IV naloxone.

**Various dosing rates have been suggested for naloxone drips. The dose in the emergency department that achieved the desired result can be set as the drip rate per hour. Another method is to use two-thirds of initial bolus that achieved the desired effect per hour.

*** Contraindications to flumazenil use are overdose of unknown agents, seizure disorder, suspected increased intracranial pressure, co-ingestion of seizure-inducing agents, suspected or known physical dependence on benzodiazepines, suspected tricyclic overdose. Because of flumazenil's side effects its use has declined and many clinicians have chosen not to use it. We have opted not to use the drug so the dose is deliberately omitted. Some suggest that a poison control/toxicology consult should be considered prior to administering the drug.

Some would avoid placing emergency department (ED) patients with an overdose in the observation unit since these patients frequently have other co-ingestions and may be uncooperative when the effects of the opiates wears off and may be suicidal. If psychiatric patients are excluded from your observation unit, then intentional self- inflicted overdoses would be excluded from the ED observation unit. However, there may be instances where an overdose/ingestion/exposure may be secondary to accidental ingestion, occupational exposure, etc. and as such, these patients may be appropriate candidates for the ED observation unit.

Pelvic Inflammatory Disease Order Set

Place in Emergency Department (ED)
   Observation _____
Diagnosis *PELVIC INFLAMMATORY
   DISEASE,* _____, _____,

   _____

ED Attending_____
Resident (if applicable)_____
Advanced Practice Provider (if applicable)

   _____

Allergies: Yes_____ No_____

If yes, what_____, _____, _____, _____,

   _____, _____

Vital Signs

Temperature__ Pulse __ Respiration __BP__
   Pulse oximetry _____
__q 2 hours ___q 4 hours ___q 6 hours q ___
   hours ___q shift ___ qd _____ other
Orthostatic vital signs _____
Other _____

Notify Physician if

Temperature (°C) > 38.0° ___ 38.5°___ 39°
   ___40° ____ other _____
Systolic blood pressure (mmHg) ≤ 90 ___ ≥
   160 __ ≥ 180 ___ ≥ 200__ other _____
Diastolic blood pressure (mmHg) ≥ 120 ____
   other _____
Heart rate ≤ 50 ___ ≥ 120 __ ≥ 150 ___ ≥
   200___ other _____

Activity

Up ad lib _____
Assisted _____
Out of bed to chair _____
Bedrest with bathroom privileges _____
Bedrest with bedside commode _____
Bedrest _____
Other _____

Diet

NPO _____
Regular _____
Advance diet as tolerated _____
Clear liquids ____
Dental, mechanical soft _____

Diabetic _____
Formula_____
Full liquids _____
Low added fat/No added salt _____
Low cholesterol____
Pureed _____
Sodium: 1 gram ___ 2 grams ___
   unrestricted____
Per feeding tube _____
Other _____

Nursing Interventions

Weight___ on admission ___ qd ___ prior to
   discharge _____ other
Height ____
I & Os _____ routine _____ strict _____
Fluid restriction ___ mL/hour ___ mL/shift
   _____ mL/24 hour ___ other
Fall precautions _____
Seizure precautions _____
Capillary blood glucose __ × 1 q ___ hours
   _____ before meals and at bedtime

Respiratory Interventions

Oxygen __ liters nasal cannula __venti mask at
   ___ liters per minute _____other
Sleep apnea qhs __ CPAP BiPAP settings cm
   H_2O ___ inspiratory __ expiratory

Laboratory Tests

CBC _____ with differential
Basic metabolic panel_____
Complete metabolic panel_____
Lactate _____
Liver function tests _____
Urinalysis _____ Urine culture _____
Vaginal culture panel (gonococcus, chlamydia,
   gardnerella [bacterial vaginosis],
   trichomonas, fungal [candida])

   _____

Pregnancy test _____(qualitative urine)
   _____Pregnancy test (quantitative blood)
Other _____, _____, _____, _____,

   _____, _____, _____, _____
Repeat _____, _____, _____, _____, _____ in
   a.m.___ in _____ hours

Radiologic Studies

Acute abdominal series ____

KUB (Kidneys, ureters, bladder) X-ray
_____

CT scan abdomen/pelvis ____ with contrast: __ IV __ po, ____

Ultrasound pelvis/abdomen _____

Other _____, _____, _____, _____,
_____ ,_____

Consultants

Care coordination (Case management) _____ Notified: Name ____Time _____

Gynecology _____ Notified: Name____ Time_____

Infectious disease _____ Notified: Name ____Time _____

Social work_____ Notified: Name____ Time_____

Other _____ Notified: Name _____Time_____

Medications for Pelvic Inflammatory Disease (Adult Dosage)

Analgesics

Acetaminophen (Paracetamol) (Tylenol®) 325 mg tab __1 tab __1–2 tabs __ 2 tabs PO __ q 4 hours__ q 6 hours ___ prn pain ___ prn fever (maximum 4 g daily)

_____ If unable to take tablet formulation, may give suspension

_____ If unable to take PO, may give suppository PR __325 mg __ 650 mg __ q 4 hours __ q 6 hours

_____ IV ___ mg __ q 4 hours __ q 6 hours __ prn pain __ prn fever (maximum adult dose: if weight < 50 kg is 15 mg/kg up to 750 mg for a single dose, 75 mg/kg up to 3750 mg for daily dose; if weight > 50 kg is 650 mg q 4 hours or 1000 mg q 6 hours up to 1000 mg for a single dose and 4000 mg for a daily dose)

Acetaminophen- Hydrocodone (Vicodin®) 300 mg/5 mg tabs __1 tab __1–2 tabs __ 2 tabs PO __q 4 hours __ q 6 hours ___ prn pain (maximum 4 grams daily based on acetaminophen dose)

Acetaminophen-Oxycodone (Endocet®, Percocet®, Roxicet®) 325 mg/ 5 mg tab __1 tab __1–2 tabs __ 2 tabs PO q 4 hours __ q

6 hours ___ prn pain (maximum 4 grams daily based on acetaminophen dose)

Hydromorphone (Dilaudid®) __ 0.5 mg __ 1 mg __ 2 mg __ mg __ IV q 2 hours__ q 4 hours __ q 6 hours q ___ hours __ prn pain

Ibuprofen (Advil®, Motrin®)__ 400 mg __ 600 mg __ 800 mg PO __ q 4 hours __ q 6 hours __ q 8 hours ___ prn pain

Ketorolac (Toradol®) __ 30 mg IV __ q 6 hours __ prn pain (maximum 120 mg daily)

Morphine __ 0.5 mg__ 1 mg __ 2 mg __ 4 mg __ mg ___ IV q 2 hours __ q 4 hours __ q 6 hours q ___ hours __ prn pain

Tramadol (Ultram®) __ 50 mg __ 100 mg PO __q 4 hours __ q 6 hours __ prn pain (maximum 400 mg daily)

Other_____, _____, _____, _____, _____

Antibiotics - Recommended Regiment

Mild-moderate

__ (1) Ceftriaxone* (Rocephin®) (third generation cephalosporin) 250 mg IM for 1 dose plus Doxycycline 100 mg PO bid (for 14 days) or

__ (2) Cefoxitin (Mefoxin®) (second generation cephalosporin) 2 grams IM plus Probenecid 1 gram PO for 1 dose plus Doxycycline 100 mg PO bid (for 14 days)

* Preferred since has the best activity against gonococcal infection

Severe

__ (1) Cefoxitin (Mefoxin®) (second-generation cephalosporin) 2 grams IV q 6 hours ___ plus Doxycycline 100 mg PO bid (for 14 days) or

__ (2) Cefotetan (Cefotan®) (second generation cephalosporin) 2 grams IV q 12 hours plus Doxycycline 100 mg PO bid (for 14 days) or

__ (3) Clindamycin (Cleocin®) 900 mg q 8 hours IV plus Gentamicin (Gentamicin) 2 mg/kg × __ kg = mg loading dose followed by 1.5 mg/kg × __ kg = mg q 8 hours or 4.5 mg/ kg Gentamicin × __ kg qd = mg maintenance dose

Alternative Regimens

If penicillin allergy

__ (1) If mild penicillin allergy (rash without signs of IgE-mediated allergy) may give test dose of cephalosporin, if no reaction, may give remainder of cephalosporin dose

__ (2) If severe allergy, Clindamycin (Cleocin®) 900 mg q 8 hours IV plus Gentamicin 2 mg/kg × __ kg = mg loading dose followed by 1.5 mg/kg × __ kg = mg q 8 hours or 4.5 mg/kg Gentamicin × __ kg qd = mg maintenance dose

Optional Additional Anaerobic Coverage for Cephalosporins**

Metronidazole (Flagyl®) ____ 500 mg PO bid (for 14 days)

**Except for Cefotetan and Cefoxitin, which have sufficient anaerobic coverage so no need for addition of Metronidazole

Antiemetics

Chlorpromazine (Thorazine®) __ 10 mg __ 25 mg PO __ q 4 hours __q 6 hours __ 25 mg __ 50 mg__ IV __IM __ q 4 hours __ q 6 hours __ prn nausea/vomiting

Metoclopramide (Reglan®) __10 mg __ IV __ IM __ PO __ q 6 hours __ other __ prn nausea/vomiting

Ondansetron (Zofran®) __ 4 mg __ 8 mg __IV __PO __ q 6 hours ___ other __ prn nausea/vomiting

Prochlorperazine (Compazine®) —5 mg — 10 mg — IV — IM — PO __ q 4 hours __ q 6 hours (maximum dose IV/IM/PO 40 mg per day) ____ 25 mg PR bid __ prn nausea/vomiting

Promethazine (Phenergan®) __12.5 mg __ 25 mg __IV__ IM __ PO __ PR __ q 4 hours __ q 6 hours ___ prn nausea/vomiting

Trimethobenzamide (Tigan®) __ 200 mg IM __ 300 mg PO ___ q 6 hours ___ prn nausea/vomiting

Intravenous Fluids

Saline cap IV ____

Bolus Normal Saline (NS) IV ___ 250 mL __ 500 mL ___1,000 mL ____ other infuse over ___ minutes ___ hours

Bolus Lactated Ringer's (LR) IV __ 250 mL __ 500 mL __1,000 mL __ other infuse over ___ minutes ___ hours

Maintenance NS at __ mL per hour IV

Maintenance LR at __ mL per hour IV

Maintenance Dextrose 5% in Water (D$_5$W) at __ mL per hour IV

Maintenance Dextrose 5% in ½ Normal Saline (D$_5$½NS) at __ mL per hour IV

Maintenance Dextrose 5% in Normal Saline (D$_5$NS) at __ mL per hour IV

Maintenance D$_5$W with potassium chloride __20 mEq or _ 40 mEq per 1 liter bag at __ mL per hour IV

Maintenance D$_5$½NS with potassium chloride __20 mEq or _ 40 mEq per 1 liter bag at__ mL per hour IV

Maintenance D$_5$NS with potassium chloride __20 mEq or _ 40 mEq per 1 liter bag at __ mL per hour IV

Other _____ at mL per hour

Education: patient _____ family _____

Pelvic inflammatory disease____

Smoking cessation_____

Other _____

† Workowski KA, Bolan GA. Sexually transmitted diseases treatment guidelines, 2015. *MMWR Recomm Rep* 2015;64(No. 3): 1–137.

Specific regimens including the 14-day course are listed. There may be other regimens and not all regimens are listed, only the most commonly used regimens. It is anticipated that the initial treatment will begin in the observation unit and then treatment continued as an outpatient with the patient transitioning to oral medications after initial therapy.

Ceftizoxime is not available in the United States so it is not included in the order set. It is suggested as an antibiotic regimen for mild to moderate pelvic inflammatory disease.

Ceftizoxime (Cefizox®) is a third-generation cephalosporin given as a 1 gram IM dose plus Doxycycline 100 mg PO bid (for 14 days) for mild to moderate pelvic inflammatory disease.

Ceftriaxone (Rocephin®) (third-generation cephalosporin) 250 mg IM plus azithromycin (Zithromax®) 1 gram per week (for 2 doses) has been used in the past for mild to moderate pelvic inflammatory disease but the regimen using 1 gram azithromycin is not included in the Centers for Disease Control (CDC) 2015 guidelines because of concerns about the emergence of resistance. The 2-grams azithromycin dose has historically been effective for uncomplicated gonoccocal infection but azithromycin monotherapy is no longer recommended due to concerns over the ease with which Neisseria gonorrhoeae can develop resistance to macrolides and because of documented azithromycin treatment failures.† (CDC 2015 reference)

Fluoroquinolones have been used in the past as an alternative therapy when there is a severe penicillin allergy, but are no longer recommended because of the emergence of resistant Neisseria gonorrohoeae except in limited circumstances.

Pharyngitis/Peritonsilar Abscess Order Set

Place in Emergency Department (ED)
Observation _____
Diagnosis *PHARYNGITIS/PERITONSILAR
ABSCESS,* _____, _____,

_____

ED Attending_____
Resident (if applicable)_____
Advanced Practice Provider (if applicable)

_____

Allergies: Yes_____ No_____

If yes, what_____, _____, _____, _____,

_____, _____

Vital Signs

Temperature__ Pulse __ Respiration __BP__
Pulse oximetry ____
__q 2 hours ___q 4 hours ___q 6 hours ___q
shift q ___ hours ___ qd _____ other
Cardiac monitoring (telemetry) _____
Orthostatic vital signs _____
Continuous pulse oximetry _____
Other _____

Notify Physician if

Temperature (°C) > 38.0° ____ 38.5°___ 39°
___40° ____ other _____
Systolic blood pressure (mmHg) ≤ 90 ___ ≥
160 ___ ≥ 180 ___ ≥ 200__ other _____
Diastolic blood pressure (mmHg) ≥ 120 _____
other _____
Heart rate ≤ 50 ___ ≥ 120 __ ≥ 150 ___ ≥
200___ other ____
Oxygen saturation < 90 % _____ other _____
Any change in mental status _____
Any respiratory distress_____
Any stridor_____

Activity

Up ad lib _____
Assisted _____
Out of bed to chair _____
Bedrest with bathroom privileges _____
Bedrest with bedside commode _____
Bedrest _____
Other _____

Diet

NPO _____
Regular _____
Advance diet as tolerated _____
Clear liquids ____
Dental, mechanical soft _____
Diabetic _____
Formula_____
Full liquids _____
Low added fat/No added salt _____
Low cholesterol____
Pureed _____
Sodium: 1 gram ___ 2 grams ___
unrestricted____
Per feeding tube _____
Other _____

Nursing Interventions

Weight___ on admission ___ qd ___ prior to
discharge _____ other
Height ____
I & Os _____ routine _____ strict _____
Fluid restriction ___ mL/hour ___ mL/shift
____ mL/24 hour ___ other
Fall precautions _____
Seizure precautions _____
Capillary blood glucose __ × 1 q ___ hours
____ before meals and at bedtime
ENT tray at bedside _____
Incision and Drainage tray at bedside (for I and
D of peritonsilar abscess)_____

Respiratory Interventions

Oxygen __ liters nasal cannula __venti mask at
___ liters per minute _____other
Wean oxygen as tolerated without dyspnea,
stridor or oxygen saturation < 90% ____
Humidified oxygen _____

Laboratory Tests

CBC _____ with differential
Basic metabolic panel_____
Blood culture × 1____ × 2 _____
Complete metabolic panel_____
Culture of incision and drainage (I and D) of
abscess _____
Rapid strept __ (If negative, send to clinical
laboratory for routine culture &
sensitivity) ___
Monospot _____

Pregnancy test _____(qualitative urine)

Urinalysis _____

Other _____, _____, _____, _____,

_____, _____, _____, _____

Repeat _____, _____, _____, _____, _____ in a.m.___ in _____ hours

Radiology Studies

Soft tissue neck (PA and lateral) _____

CXR portable ____

CXR: PA and lateral _____

CT neck without contrast ____ with contrast ____

CT face without contrast ___ with contrast _____

Ultrasound neck _____

Ultrasound face ____

MRI neck without contrast ___ with contrast ____

MRI face without contrast ____ with contrast _____

Other _____, _____, _____

Consultants

Care coordination (Case management) _____ Notified: Name_____

Time_____

Otolaryngology (ENT) _____

Notified: Name_____ Time_____

Dentistry _____ Notified:

Name_____ Time_____

Social work _____ Notified:

Name_____ Time_____

Other _____ Notified:

Name_____ Time_____

Acute Pharyngitis Medications (Adult Dosages)

Antibiotics for Group A Streptococcal Pharyngitis† (oral/IM)

Amoxicillin (Amoxil®, Moxatag®) __ 500 mg bid or __ 1000 mg qd PO __ tablet form __ suspension (maximum 1000 mg daily)

Cephalexin (Keflex®) __ 500 mg PO __ q 6 hours __ q 12 hours __ tablet form __ suspension (maximum 500 mg per dose)

Penicillin (Benzathine Penicillin G) (Bicillin®L-A) __ 600,000 units if weight < 27 kg

__ 1.2 million units if weight ≥ 27 kg IM (one dose)

Penicillin V (Pen VK®) __ 250 mg qid or __ 500 mg bid PO __ tablet form __ suspension

If a Penicillin Allergy†

Azithromycin (Zithromax®) ___ 500 mg PO qd __ tablet form __ suspension (maximum 500 mg PO per dose)

Clindamycin* (Cleocin®) ___ 300 mg ___ 450 mg PO __ q 6 hours __ tablet form __ suspension

Clarithromycin (Biaxin®) __ 250 mg PO bid (maximum 250 mg per dose)

Antibiotics for Group A Streptococcal Pharyngitis† (Intravenous)

Ampicillin __ 1 gram __ 2 grams IV __ q 4 hours __ q 6 hours (maximum 2 grams per dose, 12 grams daily)

Ampicillin and Sulbactam (Unasyn®) __ 1.5 grams __ 3.0 grams IV _ q 6 hours _ q 8 hours _ q 12 hours _ qd

Azithromycin (Zithromax®) ___ 500 mg IV qd (maximum 500 mg IV per dose)

Cefazolin (Ancef®) __1 gram __ 2 grams IV __ q 6 hours __ q 8 hours __ q 12 hours ___ qd (usual frequency q 8 hours)

Clindamycin* (Cleocin®) __ 600 mg ___ 900 mg IV __ q 8 hours

Analgesics: Local

Benzocaine Lozenges (Cepacol ®) _ 1–2 lozenges __ q 2 hours __ q 4 hours __ q 6 hours __ q 8 hours _ other __ prn pain

BMX (Benadryl®, Maalox®, viscous lidocaine) ___ 5 mL __ 10 mL PO __ q 4 hours __ q 6 hours ___ prn pain (swirl, and swish in mouth then swallow)

2% viscous lidocaine ___ 5 mL __ 10 mL PO __ prn pain (swirl and swish in mouth then swallow)

Throat spray (Chloraseptic®) spray throat _ q 2 hours _ q 4 hours_ q 6 hours _ prn pain

Analgesics: Systemic

Acetaminophen (Paracetamol) (Tylenol®) 325 mg tab __1 tab __1–2 tabs __ 2 tabs PO __ q 4 hours__ q 6 hours ___ prn pain ___ prn fever (maximum 4 g daily)

____ If unable to take tablet formulation, may give suspension

____ If unable to take PO, may give suppository PR __325 mg __ 650 mg __ q 4 hour __ q 6 hour

____ IV ___ mg __ q 4 hours __ q 6 hours __ prn pain __ prn fever (maximum adult dose: if weight < 50 kg is 15 mg/kg up to 750 mg for a single dose, 75 mg/kg up to 3750 mg for daily dose; if weight > 50 kg is 650 mg q 4 hours or 1000 mg q 6 hours up to 1000 mg for a single dose and 4000 mg for a daily dose)

Acetaminophen-Hydrocodone (Vicodin®) 300 mg/5 mg tabs __1 tab __1–2 tabs __ 2 tabs PO __q 4 hours__ q 6 hours ___ prn pain (maximum 4 grams daily based on acetaminophen dose)

Acetaminophen-Oxycodone (Endocet®, Percocet®, Roxicet®) 325 mg/ 5 mg tab __1 tab __1–2 tabs __ 2 tabs PO q 4 hours__ q 6 hours ___ prn pain (maximum 4 grams daily based on acetaminophen dose)

Hydromorphone (Dilaudid®) __ 0.5 mg __ 1 mg __ 2 mg __ mg __ IV __ q 2 hours__ q 4 hours __ q 6 hours q ___ hours __ prn pain

Ibuprofen (Advil®, Motrin®)__ 400 mg __ 600 mg __ 800 mg PO __ q 4 hours __ q 6 hours __ q 8 hours ___ prn pain

Ketorolac (Toradol®) __ 30 mg IV __ q 6 hours _ prn pain (maximum 120 mg daily)

Morphine __ 0.5 mg__ 1 mg __ 2 mg __ 4 mg __ mg ___ IV __ q 2 hours __ q 4 hours__ q 6 hours q ___ hours __ prn pain

Tramadol (Ultram®) __ 50 mg __ 100 mg PO __q 4 hours __ q 6 hours __ prn pain (maximum 400 mg daily)

Other_____, _____, _____, _____, _____

Glucocorticoids†

Dexamethasone (Decadron®) __ 10 mg __IV __ PO __ tablet form __ solution __ qd __ bid

Prednisone __ 60 mg PO qd __ tabletl form __ solution

Intravenous Fluids

Saline cap IV ____

Bolus Normal Saline (NS) ___ 250 mL __ 500 mL ___1,000 mL ____ mL IV, infuse over ___ minutes ___ hours

Bolus Lactated Ringer's (LR) ___ 250 mL __ 500 mL ___1,000 mL___ mL IV, infuse over ___ minutes ___ hours

Maintenance NS at __ mL per hour IV

Maintenance LRS at __ mL per hour IV

Maintenance Dextrose 5% in Water (D_5W) at __ mL per hour IV

Maintenance Dextrose 5% in ½ Normal Saline (D_5½NS) at __ mL per hour IV

Maintenance Dextrose 5% in Normal Saline (D_5NS) at __ mL per hour IV

Maintenance NS with potassium chloride __20 mEq or _ 40 mEq per 1 liter bag at __mL per hour

Maintenance D_5W with potassium chloride __20 mEq or _ 40 mEq per 1 liter bag at __ mL per hour IV

Maintenance D_5½NS with potassium chloride __20 mEq or _ 40 mEq per 1 liter bag at __ mL per hour IV

Maintenance D_5NS with potassium chloride __20 mEq or _ 40 mEq per 1 liter bag at __ mL per hour IV

Other _____ at mL per hour

Education: patient _____ family _____

Pharyngitis/peritonsilar abscess ____

Smoking cessation_____

Other _____

*Oral clindamycin is administered in smaller and more frequent doses than IV doses in order to decrease gastrointestinal upset.

Cefadroxil (Duricef®, Ultracef®) is no longer on the market so would delete this as an option unless it becomes available again.

The option for tablet or capsule or suspension is listed for oral medications when available since there may be significant pain with swallowing and liquid forms may be easier for the patient to swallow. Systemic pain medications, most commonly, acetaminophen and non-steroidal anti-inflammatory drugs (NSAIDS), have been shown to decrease sore throat pain. Aspirin has also been shown to decrease the sore throat pain but because of the association with Reyes syndrome in children is not indicated in this age group.

† The oral antibiotic recommendations are for acute group A streptococcal pharyngitis from the Clinical Practice Guideline from the Infectious Disease Society of America (IDSA). They do not discuss IV antibiotics but some patients are unable to take oral antibiotics initially so they may be started on an IV antibiotic then switched to an oral antibiotic and discharged home to complete a full course of antibiotics.

The IDSA did not recommend corticosteroids. However, although controversial, based on some studies including a Cochrane review, there is data that corticosteroids can decrease the duration of throat pain, but their use is generally limited to those with severe pain and/or those with inability to swallow. This tends to be the patient population that is appropriate for placement in the observation clinical decision unit.

References

1. Shulman ST, Bisno AL, Clegg HW, et al. Clinical practice guideline for the diagnosis and management of group A streptococcal pharyngitis 2012 update by the Infectious Diseases Society of America. *CID* 2012; 55(10):E86-102.

2. Hayward G, Thompson MJ, Perera R, et al. Corticosteroids as stand alone or add-on-treatment for sore throat. *Cochrane Database Syst Rev* 2012; 10:CD008268.

Pneumonia/Acute Bronchitis Order Set

Place in Emergency Department (ED)
Observation _____
Diagnosis *PNEUMONIA/ACUTE
BRONCHITIS*_____, _____, _____
ED Attending_____
Resident (if applicable)_____
Advanced Practice Provider(if applicable)

_____

Allergies: Yes_____ No_____

If yes, what_____,_____,_____,_____,

_____,_____

Vital Signs

Temperature__ Pulse __ Respiration __BP__
Pulse oximetry _____
__q 2 hours ___q 4 hours ___q 6 hours q ___
hours ___q shift ___ qd _____ other
Cardiac monitoring (telemetry) _____
Orthostatic vital signs _____
Continous pulse oximetry _____
Other _____

Notify Physician if

Temperature (°C) > 38.0° ___ 38.5°___ 39°
___40° _____ other _____
Systolic blood pressure (mmHg) ≤ 90 ___ ≥
160 __ ≥ 180 ___ ≥ 200__ other _____
Diastolic blood pressure (mmHg) ≥ 120 ____
other _____
Heart rate ≤ 50 ___ ≥ 120 __ ≥ 150 ___ ≥
200___ other _____
Oxygen saturation < 90% _____ other _____
Any change in mental status _____
Any respiratory distress _____

Activity

Up ad lib _____
Assisted _____
Out of bed to chair _____
Bedrest with bathroom privileges _____
Bedrest with bedside commode _____
Bedrest _____
Other _____

Diet

NPO _____
Regular _____
Advance diet as tolerated _____
Clear liquids ____
Dental, mechanical soft _____
Diabetic _____
Formula_____
Full liquids _____
Low added fat/No added salt ____
Low cholesterol_____
Pureed _____
Sodium: 1 gram ___ 2 grams ___
unrestricted_____
Per feeding tube _____
Other _____

Nursing Interventions

Weight___ on admission ___ qd ___ prior to
discharge _____ other
Height _____
I & Os _____ routine _____ strict _____
Fluid restriction ___ mL/hour ___ mL/shift
_____ mL/24 hour ___ other
Fall precautions _____
Seizure precautions _____
Capillary blood glucose __ × 1 q__ hours ____
before meals and at bedtime

Respiratory Interventions

Oxygen __ liters nasal cannula __venti mask at
___ liters per minute _____other
Wean oxygen as tolerated without dyspnea,
stridor or oxygen saturation < 90% ____
Peak flow __on admission ___ prior to
discharge ___ pre and post aerosols
Sleep apnea qhs __ CPAP BiPAP settings cm
H₂O ___ inspiratory __ expiratory

Laboratory Tests

Arterial blood gas (ABG)_____
CBC _____ with differential
Basic metabolic panel_____
Cardiac enzymes __ × 1 ___ q 4 hours × 3 ___ q
4 hours × 4 _____ other
Complete metabolic panel_____
Lactate _____
Liver function tests _____

Urinalysis _____ Urine culture _____
Pregnancy test (qualitative urine) _____
Pregnancy test (quantitative blood) _____
Renal function tests (e.g. BUN, creatinine)

_____

Other _____, _____, _____, _____,

_____, _____, _____, _____

Repeat _____, _____, _____, _____, _____ in
a.m.____ in _____ hours

Radiology Studies

CXR (PA and lateral) _____
CT scan chest without contrast _____ with
contrast _____
Ultrasound _____
MRI _____
Other _____, _____, _____

Cardiac Studies

ECG __ × 1__ q 4 hours × 3 ___ q 4 hours ×
4 ___ other _____ with cardiac enzymes
Echocardiogram (transthoracic) __with
agitated (bubble) study__ without agitated
(bubble) study

Consultants

Care coordination (Case management)
_____ Notified: Name _____
Time ____
Internal medicine/Family practice ___ Notified:
Name _____ Time ___ Pulmonary
_____ Notified:
Name_____ Time_____
Social work_____ Notified:
Name_____ Time_____
Other _____ Notified:
Name_____ Time_____

Medications for Pneumonia (Adult Dosage)

Antibiotic Regimens for Non-Intensive Care Unit Inpatients with Community Acquired Pneumonia†

Ceftriaxone plus Azithromycin __
Ampicillin and Sulbactam plus
Azithromycin ___
Respiratory Fluoroquinolone ___
(See doses below for the antibiotic regimens)

Antibiotics – Oral

Azithromycin (Zithromax®) __ 500 mg × 1
followed by 250 mg qd __ 500 mg PO qd
__other
Levofloxacin (Levaquin®) ___ 500 mg ___
750 mg PO __ qd __ other
Moxifloxacin (Avelox®) __ 400 mg PO qd

Antibiotics – Intravenous

Ampicillin and Sulbactam (Unasyn®) ___ 1.5
grams __ 3 grams IV __ q 6 hours __ other
Azithromycin (Zithromax®) __ 500 mg IV __
× 1 __ qd
Ceftriaxone (Rocephin®) __ 1 gram IV × 1 __
qd __other
Levofloxacin (Levaquin®) ___ 500 mg ___
750 mg IV __ qd __ other
Moxifloxacin (Avelox®) __ 400 mg qd IV

Inhaled Medications: Aerosols

Albuterol (Proventil®) nebulized solution __
2.5 mg __ 5.0 mg aerosol __ × 1 __ q 2 hours
__ q 4 hours __ q 6 hours __ q 8 hours __ prn
wheezing __ other
Ipratropium (Atrovent®) 0.5 mg nebulized
solution aerosol __ × 1__ q 2 hours __ q
4 hours __ q 6 hours __ q 8 hours __ prn
wheezing __ other

Inhaled Medications: Inhalers

Albuterol (Proventil®) (90 mcg per inhalation)
metered dose inhaler (MDI) __ puffs __ q
4 hours __ q 6 hours __ prn wheezing
___ other
Ipratropium (Atrovent®) (17 mcg per
inhalation) __ puffs __ q 4 hours __ q 6 hours
__ prn wheezing ___other
Albuterol 90 mcg and Ipratropium 18 mcg (per
inhalation) (Combivent®, Duoneb®,
Respimat®) __ puffs ___ qid __ q 6 hours
___ prn wheezing ___other

Corticosteroids

Methylprednisolone (Depomedrol®,
Methapred®, Medrol®, Solumedrol®) __
40 mg __ mg IV qd___ other
Prednisone __ 40 mg PO qd ___ 60 mg PO qd
__ other

Analgesics

Acetaminophen (Paracetamol) (Tylenol®)
325 mg tab __1 tab __1–2 tabs __ 2 tabs PO
__ q 4 hours__ q 6 hours ___ prn pain ___
prn fever (maximum 4 g daily)

____ If unable to take tablet formulation, may
give suspension

____ If unable to take PO, may give suppository
PR __325 mg __ 650 mg __ q 4 hours __ q
6 hours

____ IV ___ mg __ q 4 hours __ q 6 hours __ prn
pain __ prn fever (maximum adult dose: if
weight < 50 kg is 15 mg/kg up to 750 mg for a
single dose, 75 mg/kg up to 3750 mg for daily
dose; if weight > 50 kg is 650 mg q 4 hours or
1000 mg q 6 hours up to 1000 mg for a single
dose and 4000 mg for a daily dose)

Acetaminophen- Hydrocodone (Vicodin®) 300
mg/5 mg tabs __1 tab __1–2 tabs __ 2 tabs
PO __q 4 hours__ q 6 hours ___ prn pain
(maximum 4 grams daily based on
acetaminophen dose)

Acetaminophen-Oxycodone (Endocet®,
Percocet®, Roxicet®) 325 mg/ 5 mg tab __1
tab __1–2 tabs __ 2 tabs PO q 4 hours__ q
6 hours ___ prn pain (maximum 4 grams
daily based on acetaminophen dose)

Hydromorphone (Dilaudid®) __ 0.5 mg __
1 mg __ 2 mg __ mg __ IV __ q 2 hours __ q
4 hours __ q 6 hours q ___ hours __ prn pain

Ibuprofen (Advil®, Motrin®)__ 400 mg __
600 mg __ 800 mg PO __ q 4 hours __ q
6 hours__ q 8 hours ___ prn pain

Ketorolac (Toradol®) __ 30 mg IV __ q 6 hours
_ prn pain (maximum 120 mg daily)

Morphine __ 0.5 mg__ 1 mg __ 2 mg __ 4 mg
__ mg ___ IV __ q 2 hours __ q 4 hours __ q
6 hours q ___ hours__ prn pain

Tramadol (Ultram®) __ 50 mg __ 100 mg PO
__q 4 hours __ q 6 hours __ prn pain
(maximum 400 mg daily)

Intravenous Fluids

IV (KVO) ____

Bolus Normal Saline (NS) IV ___ 250 mL __
500 mL ___1,000 mL ____ other, infuse over
___ minutes ___ hours

Bolus Lactated Ringer's (LR) IV __ 250 mL __
500 mL __1,000 mL __ other, infuse over ___
minutes ___ hours

Maintenance NS at __ mL per hour IV

Maintenance LRS at __ mL per hour IV

Maintenance Dextrose 5% in Water (D$_5$W) at
__ mL per hour IV

Maintenance Dextrose 5% in ½ Normal Saline
(D$_5$½NS) at __ mL per hour IV

Maintenance Dextrose 5% in Normal Saline
(D$_5$NS) at __ mL per hour IV

Maintenance NS with potassium chloride __20
mEq or__ 40 mEq per 1 liter bag at __mL
per hour

Maintenance D$_5$W with potassium
chloride__20 mEq or _ 40 mEq per 1 liter bag
at __ mL per hour IV

Maintenance D$_5$½NS with potassium chloride
__20 mEq or _ 40 mEq per 1 liter bag at __
mL per hour IV

Maintenance D$_5$NS with potassium chloride
__20 mEq or _ 40 mEq per 1 liter bag at __
mL per hour IV

Other _____ at mL per hour

Education: patient _____ family _____

Pneumonia ____
Acute Bronchitis _____
Asthma _____
COPD _____
Smoking cessation_____
Other _____

There are multiple scoring systems for pneumonia including the PSI (Pneumonia Severity
Index)/PORT (Pneumonia Patient Outcomes
Research Team), and CURB-65 scores. These
could be incorporated into the inclusion and
exclusion criteria or a clinical based system (see
our protocol for pneumonia) for determining the
appropriate patients for observation.

Outpatient therapy is not included since
patients well enough to be treated as outpatients
would be discharged from the emergency department and receive outpatient oral therapy. Therapy
for critically ill patients (e.g. patients in the intensive care unit) are also not included since observation unit patients should not be critically ill.

† The regimens listed are based on Infectious
Diseases Society of America (IDSA) guidelines
recommended regimens for inpatients. There are
also various practice guidelines including British
Thoracic Society (BTS), Canadian Infectious Disease Society (CIDS) and consensus guidelines

from Infectious Diseases Society of America (IDSA) and the American Thoracic Society (ATS). The guidelines clearly state that objective criteria should be used as an adjunct to, but *not* a replacement for, physician decision making.

References

Fine MJ, Auble TE, Yealy DM, et al. A prediction rule to indentify low-risk patients with community-acquired pneumonia. *N Engl J Med* 1997; 23:336 (4):243–250. (PSI/PORT score)

Lim WS, van der Eerden MM, Laing R, et al. Defining community acquired pneumonia severity on presentation to hospital: an international derivation and validation study. *Thorax* 2003; 58: 377-382. (CURB-65)

Mandel LA. Severe community-acquired pneumonia (CAP) and the Infectious Diseases Society of America/American Thoracic Society CAP guidelines prediction rule: validated or not. *Clin Inf Dis* 2009; 48: 386-388. (BTS)

Charles PG, Wolfe R, Whitby M, et al. SMART-COP: a tool for predicting the need for intensive respiratory or vasopressor support in community-acquired pneumonia. *Clin Infect Dis* 2008: 47: 375–384. (CIDS)

Chalmers JD, Singanayagam A, Hill AT. Predicting the need for mechanical ventilation and/or inotropic support for young adults admitted to the hospital with community-acquired pneumonia. *Clin Infect Dis* 2008; 47: 1571–1574. (IDSA/ATS)

Pyelonephritis/Urinary Tract Infection Order Set

Place in Emergency Department (ED)
Observation _____
Diagnosis *PYELONEPHRITIS/URINARY TRACT INFECTION*_____, _____
ED Attending_____
Resident (if applicable)_____
Advanced Practice Provider (if applicable)
_____

Allergies: Yes_____ No_____

If yes, what_____,_____,_____,_____,
_____,_____

Vital Signs

Temperature__ Pulse __ Respiration __BP__
Pulse oximetry ____
__q 2 hours ___q 4 hours ___q 6 hours q ___
hours ___q shift ___ qd ____ other
Cardiac monitoring (telemetry) _____
Orthostatic vital signs _____
Continuous pulse oximetry _____
Other _____

Notify Physician if

Temperature (°C) > 38.0° ___ 38.5°___ 39°
___40° ____ other _____
Systolic blood pressure (mmHg) ≤ 90 ___ ≥
160 __ ≥ 180 ___ ≥ 200__ other _____
Diastolic blood pressure (mmHg) ≥ 120 ____
other _____
Heart rate ≤ 50 ___ ≥ 120 __ ≥ 150 ___ ≥
200___ other ____
Oxygen saturation < 90 % _____ other _____
Any change in mental status _____
Any respiratory distress_____

Activity

Up ad lib _____
Assisted _____
Out of bed to chair _____
Bedrest with bathroom privileges _____
Bedrest with bedside commode _____
Bedrest _____
Other _____

Diet

NPO _____

Regular _____
Advance diet as tolerated _____
Clear liquids ____
Dental, mechanical soft _____
Diabetic _____
Formula_____
Full liquids _____
Low added fat/No added salt ____
Low cholesterol____
Pureed _____
Sodium: 1 gram ___ 2 grams ___
unrestricted____
Per feeding tube _____
Other _____

Nursing Interventions

Weight___ on admission ___ qd ___ prior to
discharge ____ other
Height ____
I & Os _____ routine _____ strict _____
Fluid restriction ___ mL/hour ___ mL/shift
____ mL/24 hour ___ other
Fall precautions _____
Seizure precautions _____
Capillary blood glucose __ × 1 q ___ hours
____ before meals and at bedtime

Respiratory Interventions

If sleep apnea __ CPAP BiPAP settings cm
H_2O ___ inspiratory __ expiratory ___ qhs

Laboratory Tests

CBC _____ with differential
Basic metabolic panel_____
Cardiac enzymes __ × 1 ___ q 4 hours × 3 ____
q 4 hours × 4 ___ other
Complete metabolic panel_____
Lactate _____
Liver function tests _____
Urinalysis _____ Urine culture _____
Pregnancy test _____(qualitative urine)
_____
Pregnancy test (quantitative blood) _____
Renal function tests (e.g. BUN, creatinine)
_____
Other _____, _____, _____, _____,
_____, _____, _____, _____
Repeat _____, _____, _____, _____, _____ in
a.m.___ in _____ hours q____ hours

Radiology Studies

Acute abdominal series _____

CXR portable_____

CXR (PA and lateral) _____

KUB (Kidneys, ureters, bladder) _____

CT scan abdomen/pelvis _____ with contrast: __
   IV __ po ___ pr

CT scan kidney stone protocol _____

Ultrasound Kidneys _____

MRI _____

Other _____, _____, _____

Cardiac Studies

ECG __ × 1__ q 4 hours × 3 ___ q 4 hours ×
   4 ___ other _____ with cardiac enzymes

Echocardiogram (transthoracic) __with
   agitated (bubble) study__ without agitated
   (bubble) study

Consultants

Care coordination (Case management)
   _____ Notified: Name ___
   Time _____

Urology _____ Notified:
   Name___ Time_____

Social work_____ Notified:
   Name___ Time_____

Other _____ Notified:
   Name ___ Time_____

Medications for Pyelonephritis/Urinary Tract Infections (Adult Dosage)†

Medications: Antibiotics - Oral

Ciprofloxacin (Cipro®) __ 500 mg PO bid$

Cephalexin (Keflex®) __500 mg __1000 mg
   PO__ q 6 hours __ q 8 hours __ q 12 hours

Levofloxacin (Levaquin®) ___ 500 mg ___
   750 mg PO qd

Sulfamethoxazole and Trimethoprim
   (Bactrim™ DS, Septra® DS) __1 tab __
   2 tabs PO __ q 12 hour__ q d__ other __
   (usual dose 1–2 double strength [DS] tablets
   every 12–24 hours) where DS =
   sulfamethoxazole 800 mg and trimethoprim
   [TMP] 180 mg)

Medications: Antibiotics - Intravenous

Ceftriaxone (Rocephin®) __ 1 gram IV qd

Ciprofloxacin (Cipro®) ___ 400 mg IV bid$

Gentamicin* __ 1 mg/kg X weight in ___kg IV__
   q 8 hours __ q 12 hours __ qd (in underweight
   and nonobese patients total body weight is
   commonly used but ideal weight can also be
   used, in obese patients use ideal body weight)

Other _____

Analgesics

Acetaminophen (Paracetamol) (Tylenol®)
   325 mg tab __1 tab __1–2 tabs __ 2 tabs PO
   __ q 4 hours __ q 6 hours ___ prn pain __
   prn fever (maximum 4 g daily)

_____ If unable to take tablet formulation, may
   give suspension

_____ If unable to take PO, may give suppository
   PR __325 mg __ 650 mg __ q 4 hours __ q
   6 hours

____IV ___ mg __ q 4 hours __ q 6 hours __
   prn pain __ prn fever (maximum adult dose
   if weight < 50 kg is 15 mg/kg up to 750 mg
   for a single dose, 75 mg/kg up to 3750 mg for
   daily dose; if weight > 50 kg is 650 mg q
   4 hours or 1000 mg q 6 hours up to 1000 mg
   for a single dose and 4000 mg for a
   daily dose)

Acetaminophen-Hydrocodone (Vicodin®) 300
   mg/5 mg tabs __1 tab __1–2 tabs __ 2 tabs
   PO __q 4 hours __ q 6 hours ___ prn pain
   (maximum 4 grams daily based on
   acetaminophen dose)

Acetaminophen-Oxycodone (Endocet®,
   Percocet®, Roxicet®) 325 mg/5 mg tab __1
   tab __1–2 tabs __ 2 tabs PO q 4 hours __ q
   6 hours ___ prn pain (maximum 4 grams
   daily based on acetaminophen dose)

Hydromorphone (Dilaudid®) __ 0.5 mg __
   1 mg __ 2 mg __ mg __ IV __ q 2 hours __
   4 hours __ q 6 hours q ___ hours __ prn pain

Ibuprofen (Advil®, Motrin®)__ 400 mg __
   600 mg __ 800 mg PO __ q 4 hours __ q
   6 hours__ q 8 hours ___ prn pain

Ketorolac (Toradol®) __ 30 mg IV __ q 6 hour
   _ prn pain (maximum 120 mg daily)

Morphine __ 0.5 mg__ 1 mg __ 2 mg __ 4 mg
   __ mg ___ IV __ q 2 hours __ q 4 hours __
   6 hours q ___ hours __ prn pain

Tramadol (Ultram®) __ 50 mg __ 100 mg PO
   __q 4 hours __ q 6 hours __ prn pain
   (maximum 400 mg daily)

Other_____, _____, _____

   _____, _____

Antiemetics

Chlorpromazine (Thorazine®) __ 10 mg PO __
25 mg PO __ q 4 hours __q 6 hours __ 25 mg
__ 50 mg __ IV __ IM __ q4 hours __ q
6 hours __ prn nausea/vomiting

Metoclopramide (Reglan®) __10 mg __ IV __
IM __ PO __ q 6 hours __ other __ prn
nausea/vomiting

Ondansetron (Zofran®) __ 4 mg __ 8 mg __IV
__PO __ q 6 hours ___ other __ prn nausea/
vomiting ___

Prochlorperazine (Compazine®) _5 mg _
10 mg _ IV _IM _ PO __ q 4 hours __ q
6 hours (maximum dose IV/IM/PO 40 mg
per day) ___ 25 mg PR bid __ prn nausea/
vomiting

Promethazine (Phenergan®) __12.5 mg __
25 mg __IV__ IM __ PO __ PR __ q
4 hours__ q 6 hours ___ prn
nausea/vomiting

Trimethobenzamide (Tigan®) __ 200 mg IM
__ 300 mg PO ___ q 6 hours ___ prn nausea/
vomiting

Intravenous Fluids

Saline cap IV ____

Bolus Normal Saline (NS) IV ___ 250 mL __
500 mL ___1,000 mL ____ ml
___ other infuse over ___ minutes ___ hours

Bolus Lactated Ringer's (LR) IV ___ 250 mL __
500 mL ___1,000 mL ___ other infuse over
___ minutes ___ hours

Maintenance NS at __ mL per hour IV

Maintenance LRS at __ mL per hour IV

Maintenance Dextrose 5% in Water (D_5W) at
__ mL per hour IV

Maintenance Dextrose 5% in ½ Normal Saline
(D_5½NS) at __ mL per hour IV

Maintenance Dextrose 5%in Normal Saline
(D_5NS) at __ mL per hour IVMaintenance
NS with potassium chloride __20 mEq or _
40 mEq per 1 liter bag at __mL per hour

Maintenance D_5W with potassium chloride
__20 mEq or _ 40 mEq per 1 liter bag at __
mL per hour IV

Maintenance D_5½NS with potassium chloride
__20 mEq or _ 40 mEq per 1 liter bag at __
mL per hour IV

Maintenance D_5NS with potassium chloride
__20 mEq or _ 40 mEq per 1 liter bag at __
mL per hour IVOther _____ at mL per hour

Education: patient _____ family _____

Pyelonephritis/Urinary tract infections
_____

Smoking Cessation, if applicable _____
Other _____

† based on Infectious Disease Society of
America (IDSA) guidelines

* Lower doses of aminoglycosides (e.g.
gentamicin at 1mg/kg) can be used for
pyelonephritis since the aminoglycosides
concentrate in the urine.

Nitrofurantoin (furadantin®, macrobid®,
macrodantoin®) can be given for an
uncomplicated urinary tract infection (UTI)
in younger patients with normal renal
function, but is not recommended for
pyelonephritis. The dose is macrobid®
100 mg bid PO or macrodantoin® 50–100
mg q 6 hours PO for a urinary tract infection.

§The FDA and IDSA no longer recommend
fluoroquinolones as first-line therapy for
uncomplicated UTI due to the risk of
disabling and potentially permanent serious
adverse effects.

Seizures Order Set

Place in Emergency Department (ED)
Observation _____
Diagnosis *SEIZURES*, _____,

_____, _____

ED Attending_____
Resident (if applicable)_____
Advanced Practice Provider(if applicable)

_____

Allergies: Yes_____ No_____

If yes, what_____,_____,_____,_____,

_____,_____

Vital Signs

Temperature__ Pulse __ Respiration __BP__
Pulse oximetry ____
__q 2 hours ___q 4 hours ___q 6 hours q ___
hours ___q shift ___ qd ____ other
Cardiac monitoring (telemetry) _____
Orthostatic vital signs _____
Continuous pulse oximetry _____
Neurologic checks‡ __q 2 hours __q 4 hours
__q 6 hours q _ hours _q shift __ qd __other
Other _____
‡ Neurologic checks done by nursing may
include level of consciousness, orientation,
follows commands, hearing, sight, behavior,
GCS (Glasgow Coma Scale) including eyes
open, best verbal response and best motor
response, motor strength: right/left arms and
legs, pupils (right/left size, reaction),
musculoskeletal assessment (range of motion,
weakness, paralysis, atrophy, movement) and
gait. See also nursing chapter for neurologic
and other nursing assessments.

Notify Physician if

Temperature (°C) > 38.0° ____ 38.5°____ 39°
___40° ____ other _____
Systolic blood pressure (mmHg) ≤ 90 ___ ≥
160 __ ≥ 180 ___ ≥ 200__ other _____
Diastolic blood pressure (mmHg) ≥ 120 _____
other _____
Heart rate ≤ 50 ___ ≥ 120 __ ≥ 150 ___ ≥
200___ other ____
Oxygen saturation < 90 % _____ other _____
Any change in mental status _____
Any respiratory distress_____

Activity

Up ad lib _____
Assisted _____
Out of bed to chair _____
Bedrest with bathroom privileges _____
Bedrest with bedside commode _____
Bedrest _____
Other _____

Diet

NPO _____
Regular _____
Advance diet as tolerated _____
Clear liquids ____
Dental, mechanical soft _____
Diabetic _____
Formula_____
Full liquids _____
Low added fat/No added salt ____
Low cholesterol____
Pureed _____
Sodium: 1 gram ___ 2 grams ___
unrestricted____
Per feeding tube _____
Other _____

Nursing Interventions

Weight___ on admission ___ qd ___ prior to
discharge _____ other
Height ____
I & Os _____ routine _____ strict _____
Fluid restriction ___ mL/hour ___ mL/shift
____ mL/24 hour ___ other
Fall precautions _____
Seizure precautions _____
Capillary blood glucose __ × 1 q ___ hours
_____ before meals and at bedtime

Respiratory Interventions

Oxygen __ liters nasal cannula __venti mask at
___ liters per minute _____other
Sleep apnea qhs __ CPAP BiPAP settings cm
H₂O ___ inspiratory __ expiratory

Laboratory Tests

Anticonvulsant drug level: phenytoin___
phenobarbitol ___ carbamazepine __valproic
acid ___
other _____, _____, _____

CBC _____ with differential
Basic metabolic panel_____
Cardiac enzymes __ × 1___ q 4 hours × 3 ____
   q 4 hours × 4 ____ other
Complete metabolic panel_____
Lactate _____
Liver function tests _____
Magnesium _____
Pregnancy test (qualitative urine) _____
Pregnancy test (quantitative blood) _____
Renal function tests (e.g. BUN, creatinine)
_____

Toxicology: urine drug screen
_____

Toxicology: blood drug screen
_____

Urinalysis _____ Urine culture _____
Other _____, _____, _____, _____,
   _____, _____, _____, _____
Repeat _____, _____, _____, _____, _____ in
   a.m.___ in _____ hours

Radiology Studies

CXR portable_____
CXR (PA and lateral) _____
CT (computed tomogtraphy) brain noncontrast
_____
CT (computed tomogtraphy) brain with
   iodinated contrast (ultravist) if no allergy and
   no renal failure (e.g. GFR ≥ 30)____
CTA (computed tomogtraphy angiography)
   brain (include neck vessels) with iodinated
   contrast if no allergy and no renal failure (e.g.
   GFR ≥ 30)____
MRI (magnetic resonance imaging) brain
   noncontrast_____
MRI (magnetic resonance imaging) brain with
   contrast (gadolinium) if no allergy and no
   renal failure (e.g. GFR ≥ 30) _____
Magnetic resonance angiography (MRA) Circle
   of Willis (COW) and MRA of Carotids
   without contrast and with contrast
   (gadolinium) if no allergy and no renal
   failure, e.g. GFR ≥ 30 _____
Magnetic resonance venography (MRV) brain
   with contrast (gadolinium) if no allergy and
   no renal failure (e.g. GFR ≥ 30)
   _____Ultrasound Carotid ___
Other _____

Cardiac Studies

ECG __ × 1__ q 4 hours × 3 ___ q 4 hours ×
   4 ___ other ____ with cardiac enzymes
Echocardiogram (transthoracic) __with agitated
   (bubble) study__ without agitated
   (bubble) study

Consultants

Care coordination (Case management)
   _____ Notified: Name_____
   Time_____
Neurosurgery _____ Notified:
   Name_____ Time_____
Neurology _____ Notified:
   Name_____ Time_____
Social work_____ Notified: Name
   _____ Time_____
Other _____ Notified: Name
   _____ Time_____

Anticonvulsant Medications (Adult Doses)†

Oral Loading Dose

Phenytoin* (Dilantin®) _ 15 mg × __ weight
   (kg) or__ 20 mg/kg × weight (kg)
   administered in 3 divided doses __ q 2 hours
   __ q 4 hours PO (maximum single PO dose
   300–400 mg) (given q 2–4 hours to maximize
   absorption pharmacokinetics and to decrease
   gastrointestinal side effects)
Levetiracetan (Keppra®) 500 mg bid PO (may
   increase every 2 weeks by 500 mg/dose to the
   recommended dose of 1,500 mg bid PO)

Intravenous Loading Dose

Fosphenytoin* (Cerebyx®) __ 15 mg PEs/kg ×
   __ weight (kg) __ 20 mg PEs/kg × __ weight
   (kg) IV (maximum infusion rate 100–150 PE/
   min where PEs = phenytoin equivalents)
Levetiracetan (Keppra®) __ 500 mg bid IV
(note: higher IV loading doses in the range of
   1,000 to 3,000 mg administered over
   15 minutes are given for status epilepticus,
   but this is an off-label use and status
   epilepticus is not usually an appropriate
   diagnosis for the observation unit)
Phenobarbital __ 20 mg/kg IV at an infusion
   rate of 50 mg/min
(note: loading doses of fosphenytoin and
   levetiracetan are administered more

frequently than loading dose of phenobarbital; loading doses of phenobarbital are administered more often for pediatric than adult patients)

Intravenous Anticonvulsants

Lorazepam (Ativan®) __0.5 mg __ 1 mg ___ 2 mg IV __ other for breakthrough seizure (0.05 mg/kg up to maximum of 4 mg, given as slow IV push, maximum rate 2 mg/minute to avoid respiratory depression)

Diazepam (Valium®) __ 5 mg __ 10 mg IV (up to 0.15 mg/kg) (generally only used if lorazepam is unavailable because of its longer half-life, given as slow IV push to avoid respiratory depression)

Other _____, _____, _____

Anticonvulsants – Oral Maintenance Medications (if already on the medication)

Carbamazepine**†† (Tegretol®) __ 400 mg per day __ 600 mg per day __ 800 mg per day __ 1200 mg per day PO given in 2 divided doses or bid if in__ tablet form and 4 divided doses if in suspension form (100 mg/5 ml) (initial dose 400 mg per day in 2 divided doses, usual dose 800–1200 mg daily in divided doses, maximum dose 1600 mg per day, although some patients have required up to 2400 mg per day)

Gabapentin†† (Neurontin®) __ 300 mg __ 600 mg __ 900 mg PO tid (initial dose 300 mg tid if patients have normal renal function, some patients have required up to 3600 mg per day)

Lamotrigine***†† (Lamictal®) ___ mg bid PO (usual dose 25–500 mg/day in 2 divided doses, maximum dose 700 mg per day)

Levetiracetam (Keppra®) ___ mg bid PO (usual dose 1000–3000 mg per day in 2 divided doses, maximum dose 3000 mg per day)

Oxcarbazepine†† (Trileptal®) ___ mg PO bid (usual dose 600–1200 mg per day in 2 divided doses, maximum dose 2400 mg per day)

Phenobarbital __ mg PO __ bid __ tid (usual dose 150–300 mg per day in 2 or 3 divided doses)

Phenytoin (Dilantin®) ___ mg PO tid (usual dose 300–600 mg per day in 3 divided doses)

Primidone (Mysoline®) ___ mg PO __ tid __ qid (usual dose 750–1500 mg per day in divided doses 3 or 4 times a day, maximum dose 2000 mg per day)

Topiramate†† (Topiramax®) __ mg PO bid (initial dose 25 mg bid with slow titration upward to decrease risk of adverse CNS side effects, usual dose 200–400 mg/day in 2 divided doses, maximum 200 mg per day)

Valproic acid (Valproate Sodium) (Depacon®, Depakene®, Depakote®) __ mg PO __ bid __ tid (usual dose 15–60 mg/kg/day in 2 or 3 divided doses)

Other ____, ____, ____, ____

Intravenous Fluids

Saline lock IV ____

Maintenance Normal Saline (NS) at __ mL per hour IV

Maintenance Lactated Ringer's (LR) at __ mL per hour IV

Maintenance Dextrose 5% in Water (D_5W) _____ at __ mL per hour IV

Maintenance Dextrose 5% in ½ Normal Saline (D_5½NS) _____ at __ mL per hour IV

Maintenance Dextrose in Normal Saline (D_5NS) at __ mL per hour IV

Maintenance NS with potassium chloride __20 mEq or __ 40 mEq per 1 liter bag at __ mL per hour IV

Maintenance D_5W with potassium chloride __20 mEq or _ 40 mEq per 1 liter bag

Maintenance D_5½NS with potassium chloride __20 mEq or _ 40 mEq per 1 liter bag at __ mL per hour IV

Maintenance D_5NS with potassium chloride __20 mEq or _ 40 mEq per 1 liter bag at __ per hour IV

Other maintenance _____at mL/hour IV

Education: patient _____ family _____

Seizures _____

Smoking cessation_____, if indicated

Other _____

† Medications for status epilepticus are not listed since these are higher acuity patients who should be inpatients and are not observation unit candidates. Most of the common (but not all) oral anticonvulsant medications are listed.

Patients receiving anticonvulsant therapy may also need diagnostic evaluation for their seizures.

Many of the anticonvulsants have significant side effects and associated toxicity, which may be somewhat less of a risk if doses are adjusted gradually and carefully monitored. Therefore, initiating and/or titrating and adjusting anticonvulsants is usually done in conjunction with the neurology service and a neurology consult is generally obtained prior to beginning new anticonvulsants or adjusting current anticonvulsants.

It may be reasonable to place patients who have been noncompliant in the observation unit who may need only to be given their medications and observed for seizure activity and do not need any significant adjustments in their anticonvulsants. However, patients with significant breakthrough seizures whose seizures are difficult to manage and/or on maximum doses of their anticonvulsants (see above maintenance doses in order sets) and who may need significant adjustments in their medications and/or new anticonvulsants with serious side effects/toxicities may better be served on an inpatient neurology service.

†† Medications not usually given in loading dose.

* Phenytoin IV is not listed for several reasons. Phenytoin IV is associated with cardiovascular dysrhythmias so cardiac monitoring should be done when it is given IV. Fosphenytoin IV is preferred over phenytoin IV since phenytoin is a vesicant and can cause significant local tissue injury if extravasation occurs. IM and subcutaneous phenytoin should be avoided because of the possibility of local tissue damage from the high pH. Phenytoin IV also has a greater potential to cause hypotension during administration than fosphenytoin IV. Phenytoin has a United States boxed warning.

** Carbamazepine is usually not given in "loading" doses. There is a strong association between the risk of Stevens-Johnson syndrome/ toxic epidermal necrolysis (TENS) and the HLA-B1502 allele. Carbamazepine has a United States boxed warning for serious dermatologic side effects, including TENS and Stevens-Johnson syndrome, and hematologic reactions: aplastic anemia and agranulocytosis.

*** Lamotrigine requires very slow titration to limit the risk of potentially life-threatening dermatological hypersensitivity reactions. Therefore, we do not recommend starting or adjusting the lamotrigine dose in the observation unit. The incidence of serious rashes is higher in pediatric patients than in adults, may be increased by co-administration with valproic acid, higher than recommended starting doses and exceeding recommended dose titration. Lamotrigine has a United States boxed warning for serious dermatologic reactions, including Stevens-Johnson syndrome.

Sickle Cell Disease Order Set

Place in Emergency Department (ED) Observation _____
Diagnosis *SICKLE CELL DISEASE,*

_____, _____, _____

ED Attending_____
Resident (if applicable)_____
Advanced Practice Provider (if applicable)

_____

Allergies: Yes_____ No_____

If yes, what_____, _____, _____, _____,

_____, _____

Vital Signs

Temperature__ Pulse __ Respiration __BP__
Pulse oximetry ____
__q 2 hours ___q 4 hours ___q 6 hours q ___
hours ___q shift ___ qd ____ other
Cardiac monitoring (telemetry) _____
Orthostatic vital signs _____
Continuous pulse oximetry _____
Other _____

Notify Physician if

Temperature (°C) > 38.0° ___ 38.5°___ 39°
___40° ____ other _____
Systolic blood pressure (mmHg) ≤ 90 ___ ≥
160 __ ≥ 180 ___ ≥ 200__ other _____
Diastolic blood pressure (mmHg) ≥ 120 ____
other _____
Heart rate ≤ 50 ___ ≥ 120 __ ≥ 150 ___ ≥
200___ other ____
Respiratory rate < 12 / minute ____
Oxygen saturation < 90% _____ other _____
Any change in mental status _____
Any respiratory distress or hypoventilation

_____

Activity

Up ad lib _____
Assisted _____
Out of bed to chair _____
Bedrest with bathroom privileges _____
Bedrest with bedside commode _____
Bedrest _____
Other _____

Diet

NPO _____
Regular _____
Advance diet as tolerated _____
Clear liquids ____
Dental, mechanical soft _____
Diabetic _____
Formula_____
Full liquids _____
Low added fat/No added salt ____
Low cholesterol____
Pureed _____
Sodium: 1 gram ___ 2 grams ___
unrestricted____
Per feeding tube _____
Other _____

Nursing Interventions

Weight___ on admission ___ qd ___ prior to
discharge ____ other
Height ____
I & Os _____ routine _____ strict _____
Fluid restriction ___ mL/hour ___ mL/shift
____ mL/24 hour ___ other
Fall precautions _____
Seizure precautions _____
Capillary blood glucose __ × 1 q___
hours_____ before meals and at bedtime
Document respiratory rate, pulse oximetry,
somnolence/sedation scale‡ and pain scale
every 4 hours at a minimum and with every
opioid dose ___
‡ On arrival in observation unit, reassess pain
levels and sedation q 30 minutes x 4

Respiratory Interventions

Oxygen __ liters nasal cannula __venti mask at
___ liters per minute _____other
Sleep apnea qhs __ CPAP BiPAP settings cm
H_2O ___ inspiratory __ expiratory

Laboratory Tests

CBC _____ with differential
Amylase ___ Lipase___
Basic metabolic panel_____
Cardiac enzymes __ × 1___ q 4 hours × 3 ___ q
4 hours × 4 ___ other
Complete metabolic panel_____
Hemoglobin/hematocrit _____

Lactate _____
Liver function tests _____
Urinalysis _____ Urine culture _____
Pregnancy test (qualitative urine) ____
 Pregnancy test (quantitative blood) _____
Reticulocyte count _____
Type and screen ___
Type and cross ____ units packed red blood
 cells (PRBCs)
Other _____, _____, _____, _____,
 _____, _____, _____, _____
Repeat ___ hemoglobin/hematocrit ___ CBC
 __ 1 hour post transfusion of PRBCs __ other
Repeat _____, _____, _____, _____, _____ in
 a.m.___ in _____ hours q____

Radiology Studies

Acute abdominal series ____
CXR portable_____
CXR (PA and lateral) _____
KUB (Kidneys, ureters, bladder) _____
CT scan _____
Ultrasound ____
MRI _____
Other _____, _____, _____

Cardiac Studies

ECG __ × 1__ q 4 hours × 3 ___ q 4 hours ×
 4 ___ other ____ with cardiac enzymes
Echocardiogram (transthoracic) __with
 agitated (bubble) study__ without agitated
 (bubble) study

Consultants

Care coordination (Case management)
 _____ Notified: Name_____
 Time____
Hematology _____ Notified:
 Name_____ Time____
Social work_____ Notified:
 Name_____ Time____
Other _____ Notified:
 Name _____ Time____

Sickle Cell Disease - Acute Pain Crisis Medications (Adult Dosage)
Routine Daily Medications*

Folic acid (Folate) __ 1 mg PO qd
Hydroxyurea (Droxia®) __ 500 mg PO qd

Antiemetics

Chlorpromazine (Thorazine®) __ 10 mg PO __
 25 mg PO __ q 4 hours __q 6 hours
 __ 25 mg __ 50 mg__ IV __IM __ q 4 hours __
 q 6 hours __ prn nausea/vomiting
Metoclopramide (Reglan®) __10 mg __ IV __
 IM __ PO __ q 6 hours __ other __ prn
 nausea/vomiting
Ondansetron (Zofran®) __ 4 mg __ 8 mg __IV
 __PO __ q 6 hours ___ other __ prn nausea/
 vomiting ___
Prochlorperazine (Compazine®) _5 mg _
 10 mg _ IV _IM _ PO __ q 4 hours __ q
 6 hours (maximum dose IV/IM/PO 40 mg
 per day) ___ 25 mg PR bid __ prn nausea/
 vomiting
Promethazine (Phenergan®) __12.5 mg __
 25 mg __IV__ IM __ PO __ PR __ q 4 hours
 __ q 6 hours ___ prn nausea/vomiting
Trimethobenzamide (Tigan®) __ 200 mg IM
 __ 300 mg PO ___ q 6 hours __ prn nausea/
 vomiting

Analgesics: Oral Medications

Acetaminophen (Paracetamol) (Tylenol®)
 325 mg tab __1 tab __1–2 tabs __ 2 tabs PO
 __ q 4 hours__ q 6 hours ___ prn pain ___
 prn fever (maximum 4 g daily)
 ____ If unable to take tablet formulation, may
 give suspension
 ____ If unable to take PO, may give suppository
 PR __325 mg __ 650 mg __ q 4 hours __ q
 6 hours
 ____ IV ___ mg __ q 4 hours __ q 6 hours __
 prn pain __ prn fever (maximum adult dose:
 if weight < 50 kg is 15 mg/kg up to 750 mg
 for a single dose, 75 mg/kg up to 3750 mg for
 daily dose; if weight > 50 kg is 650 mg q
 4 hours or 1000 mg q 6 hours up to 1000 mg
 for a single dose and 4000 mg for a
 daily dose)
Acetaminophen- Hydrocodone (Vicodin®) 300
 mg/5 mg tabs __1 tab __1–2 tabs __ 2 tabs
 PO __q 4 hours__ q 6 hours ___ prn pain
 (maximum 4 grams daily based on
 acetaminophen dose)
Acetaminophen-Oxycodone (Endocet®,
 Percocet®, Roxicet®) 325 mg/ 5 mg tab __1
 tab __1–2 tabs __ 2 tabs PO q 4 hours __ q

6 hours ___ prn pain (maximum 4 grams daily based on acetaminophen dose)

Ibuprofen (Advil®, Motrin®)__ 400 mg __ 600 mg __ 800 mg PO __ q 4 hours __ q 6 hours __ q 8 hours ___ prn pain

Tramadol (Ultram®) __ 50 mg __ 100 mg PO __q 4 hours __ q 6 hours __ prn pain (maximum 400 mg daily)

Analgesics: Intravenous Medications

Fentanyl** ___ micrograms __ IV __ IM (usual dose 25–75 micrograms per dose)

Hydromorphone (Dilaudid®) __ 0.5 mg __ 1 mg __ 2 mg __ mg __ IV __ q 2 hours __ q 4 hours __ q 6 hours q ___ hours __ prn pain __ other

Ketorolac (Toradol®) __ 30 mg IV __ q 6 hours _ prn pain (maximum 120 mg daily)

Morphine __ 0.5 mg__ 1 mg __ 2 mg __ 4 mg __ mg ___ IV__ q 2 hours __ q 4 hours __ q 6 hours q ___ hours __ prn pain ___ other

Other Medications

Diphenhydramine (Benadryl®) *** __ 25 mg __ 50 mg __ q 4 hours __q 6 hours PO prn for documented rash and/or itching

* Sickle cell patients are commonly on folic acid and hydroxyurea as a daily or routine medication. Hydroxyurea and folic acid are not indicated for the treatment of acute sickle cell crisis. Hydroxyurea requires CBC monitoring when initiating therapy and patient follow-up so we would not recommend initiating hydroxyurea therapy in the observation unit. If the patient is on the medication, then it may be continued.

** Fentanyl generally used only if patient has an allergy or intolerance to morphine or hydromorphone.

*** Diphenhydramine (Benadryl®) is not routinely given IV except for documented acute allergic reaction (such as significant rash or urticaria) because of potential for abuse with IV route of administration.

Patient controlled analgesia (PCA)†

Morphine 2 mg/ml IV PCA _____

Fentanyl 20 mcg/ml IV PCA ____

Hydromorphone 0.5 mg/ml in normal saline IV PCA ____

Basal rate (while sleeping and/or 11 p.m. to 6 a.m.) ___ mg/hour

Demand bolus dose _____

Bolus interval _____

Intravenous Fluids

Saline cap IV ____

Bolus Normal Saline (NS) IV ___ 250 mL __ 500 mL ___1,000 mL ____ other infuse over ___ minutes ___ hours

Bolus Lactated Ringer's (LR) IV __ 250 mL __ 500 mL __1,000 mL __ other, infuse over __ minutes ___ hours

Maintenance NS at __ mL per hour IV

Maintenance LR at __ mL per hour IV

Maintenance D_5W at __ mL per hour IV

Maintenance $D_5\frac{1}{2}NS$ at __ mL per hour IV

Maintenance D_5NS at __ mL per hour IV

Maintenance NS with potassium chloride __20 mEq or__ 40 mEq per 1 liter bag at __mL per hour

Maintenance D_5W with potassium chloride __20 mEq or _ 40 mEq per 1 liter bag at __ mL per hour IV

Maintenance $D_5\frac{1}{2}NS$ with potassium chloride __20 mEq or _ 40 mEq per 1 liter bag at __ mL per hour IV

Maintenance D_5NS with potassium chloride __20 meq or _ 40 meq per 1 liter bag at __ mL per hour IV

Other _____ at mL per hour

Education: patient _____ family _____

Sickle cell disease____

Smoking cessation, if applicable _____

‡ Somnolence/Sedation Scale

1 = Wide awake

2 = Drowsy

3 = Dozing intermittently

4 = Awakens when aroused to verbal or mild tactile stimuli

5 = Not arousable to verbal or mild tactile stimuli

Because of the possibility of hypoventilation/apnea with the high doses of opioids administered to these patients, several precautions can be taken including the use of somnolence/sedation scales in addition to pain scales. Specific orders on the order set can be included, such as notify physician for respiratory rate < 10/minute, pulse oxygen saturation $< 90\%$, any change in mental status, any respiratory distress or hypoventilation, and/or somnolence/sedation scale of 5.

†PCA pumps are not generally used in the observation unit. However, with the impetus for increasing the types and severity of patients placed in the observation unit, the use of PCA pumps has been suggested for sickle cell patients. Future research is needed on the topic of the observation unit management of sickle cell patients.

Syncope/Near-Syncope/Presyncope Order Set

Place in Emergency Department (ED)
Observation _____
Diagnosis **SYNCOPE**, _____, _____,
_____
ED Attending_____
Resident (if applicable)_____
Advanced Practice Provider (if applicable)
_____

Allergies: Yes_____ No_____

If yes, what_____, _____, _____, _____,
_____, _____

Vital Signs

Temperature__ Pulse __ Respiration __BP__
Pulse oximetry ____
__q 2 hours ___q 4 hours ___q 6 hours q ___
hours ___q shift ___ qd ____ other
Cardiac monitoring (telemetry) _____
Orthostatic vital signs _____
Continuous pulse oximetry _____
Other _____

Notify Physician if

Temperature (°C) > 38.0° ___ 38.5°___ 39°
___40° ____ other _____
Systolic blood pressure (mmHg) ≤ 90 ___ ≥
160 __ ≥ 180 ___ ≥ 200__ other _____
Diastolic blood pressure (mmhg) ≥ 120 ____
other _____
Heart rate ≤ 50 ___ ≥ 120 __ ≥ 150 ___ ≥
200___ other ____
Oxygen saturation < 90 % _____ other _____
Any change in mental status _____
Any respiratory distress_____

Activity

Up ad lib _____
Assisted _____
Out of bed to chair _____
Bedrest with bathroom privileges _____
Bedrest with bedside commode _____
Bedrest _____
Other _____

Diet

NPO _____
Regular _____
Advance diet as tolerated _____
Clear liquids ____
Dental, mechanical soft _____
Diabetic _____
Formula_____
Full liquids _____
Low added fat/No added salt ____
Low cholesterol____
Pureed _____
Sodium: 1 gram ___ 2 grams ___
unrestricted____
Per feeding tube _____
Other _____

Nursing Interventions

Weight___ on admission ___ qd ___ prior to
discharge _____ other
Height ____
I & Os _____ routine _____ strict _____
Fluid restriction ___ mL/hour ___ mL/shift
____ mL/24 hour ___ other
Fall precautions _____
Seizure precautions _____
Capillary blood glucose __ × 1 q ___ hours
____ before meals and at bedtime

Respiratory Interventions

Oxygen __ liters nasal cannula __venti mask at
___ liters per minute _____other
Sleep apnea qhs __ CPAP BiPAP settings cm
H_2O ___ inspiratory __ expiratory

Laboratory Tests

CBC with differential __
Basic metabolic panel_____
Blood alcohol level _____
Brain natriuretic peptide (BNP) _____
Calcium _____
Cardiac enzymes __ × 1 ___ q 4 hours × 3 ___
q 4 hours × 4 ___ other
Complete metabolic panel_____
Fasting blood sugar in a.m. _____
Lipid panel, fasting _____
Hematocrit/Hemoglobin __ × 1 __ q 4 hours __
q 6 hours ___ other
Hemoglobin A1C_____

Lactate _____

Liver function tests _____

Magnesium _____

Pregnancy test _____(qualitative urine)
_____ (quantitative blood) _____

Renal function tests (BUN, creatinine) _____

Toxicology screen (urine) _____

Toxicology screen (blood) _____

Type and Screen _____

Urinalysis _____ Urine culture _____

Other _____, _____, _____, _____,
_____, _____, _____, _____

Repeat _____, _____, _____, _____, _____ in
a.m.___ in _____ hours q____ hours x ___

Radiology Studies

CXR portable_____

CXR (PA and lateral) _____

CT Chest (rule out pulmonary emboli) ____

CT scan of _____ without contrast ____ with
contrast: __ IV __ PO ___ PR ___

Ultrasound of _____

MRI of _____

Ventilation/perfusion scan (rule out pulmonary
emboli) _____

Other _____, _____, _____

Cardiac Studies

ECG __ × 1__ q 4 hours × 3 ___ q 4 hours ×
4 ___ other _____ with cardiac enzymes

Echocardiogram (transthoracic) __with
agitated (bubble) study__ without agitated
(bubble) study

Tilt Test _____

Stress test _____ (see chest pain order
set for specific stress tests)

Holter monitor at discharge _____

30-day (King of Hearts) monitor at discharge

_____

Other _____

Other Tests

EEG _____

Esophagogastroduodenoscopy in a.m. (NPO
after midnight) _____

Colonoscopy in a.m. (NPO after midnight)
_____ with bowel prep ___

Consultants

Care coordination (Case management)
_____ Notified: Name _____
Time ____

Cardiology _____Notified:
Name_____ Time____

Neurology _____ Notified:
Name_____ Time____

Social work_____ Notified:
Name_____ Time_____

Other _____Notified:
Name _____ Time____

Syncope Intravenous Fluids (Adults)

Saline cap IV ____

Bolus Normal Saline (NS) IV ___ 250 mL __
500 mL ___1,000 mL ____ other
infuse over ___ minutes ___ hours

Bolus Lactated Ringer's (LR) IV __ 250 mL __
500 mL __1,000 mL __ other
infuse over ___ minutes ___ hours

Maintenance NS at __ mL per hour IV

Maintenance LR at __ mL per hour IV

Maintenance Dextrose 5% in Water (D_5W) at
__ mL per hour IV

Maintenance Dextrose 5% in ½ Normal Saline
(D_5½NS) at __ mL per hour IV

Maintenance Dextrose 5% in Normal Saline
(D_5NS) at __ mL per hour IVMaintenance
NS with potassium chloride __20 mEq or__
40 mEq per 1 liter bag at __mL per hour

Maintenance D_5W with potassium chloride
__20 mEq or _ 40 mEq per 1 liter bag at __
mL per hour IV

Maintenance D_5½NS with potassium chloride
__20 mEq or _ 40 mEq per 1 liter bag at __
mL per hour IV

Maintenance D_5NS with potassium chloride
__20 mEq or _ 40 mEq per 1 liter bag at __
mL per hour IV

Other _____ at mL per hour

Education: patient _____ family _____

Syncope____

Smoking cessation_____

Other _____

Transfusion Order Set

Place in Emergency Department (ED)
  Observation _____
Diagnosis *ANEMIA (FOR TRANSFUSION)*,
_____, _____, _____
ED Attending_____
Resident (if applicable)_____
Advanced Practice Provider (if applicable)
  _____

Allergies: Yes_____ No_____

If yes, what_____, _____, _____, _____,
  _____, _____

Vital Signs

Temperature__ Pulse __ Respiration __BP__
  Pulse oximetry
__ q 2 hours ___q 4 hours ___q 6 hours q ___
  hours ___q shift ___ qd ____ other
Cardiac monitoring (telemetry) _____
Other _____

Notify Physician if:

Temperature (°C) > 38.0° ___ 38.5°___ 39°
  ___40° ____ other _____
Systolic blood pressure (mmHg) ≤ 90 ___ ≥
  160 __ ≥ 180 ___ ≥ 200__ other _____
Diastolic blood pressure (mmHg) ≥ 120 _____
  other _____
Heart rate ≤ 50 ___ ≥ 120 __ ≥ 150 ___ ≥
  200___ other _____
Oxygen saturation < 90% _____ other _____
Any change in mental status _____
Any respiratory distress_____

Activity

Up ad lib _____
Assisted _____
Out of bed to chair _____
Bedrest with bathroom privileges _____
Bedrest with bedside commode _____
Bedrest _____
Other _____

Diet

NPO _____
Regular _____
Advance diet as tolerated _____
Clear liquids ____

Dental, mechanical soft _____
Diabetic _____
Formula_____
Full liquids _____
Low added fat/No added salt ____
Low cholesterol____
Pureed _____
Sodium: 1 gram ___ 2 grams ___
  unrestricted____
Per feeding tube _____
Other _____

Nursing Interventions

Weight___ on admission ___ qd ___ prior to
  discharge ____ other
Height ____
I & Os _____ routine _____ strict _____
Fluid restriction _____ mL/hour _____ mL/
  shift _____ mL/24 hour
Fall precautions _____
Seizure precautions _____
Capillary blood glucose __ × 1 q ___ hours
  _____ before meals and at bedtime
Hemoccult all stools ____

Respiratory Interventions

Oxygen __ liters nasal cannula __venti mask at
  ___ liters per minute _____other
Sleep apnea qhs __ CPAP BiPAP settings cm
  H_2O ___ inspiratory __ expiratory

Laboratory Tests*

CBC _____ with differential
Basic metabolic panel_____
Cardiac enzymes __ × 1 ___ q 4 hours × 3 ___ q
  4 hours × 4 __ other
Complete metabolic panel_____
Hematocrit/hemoglobin _____ Serial
  hematocrit/hemoglobin ___ q 4 hours
  ___ other
Lactate _____
Liver function tests _____
Urinalysis _____
Pregnancy test _____(qualitative urine)
  _____Pregnancy test (quantitative blood)
Repeat hematocrit/hemoglobin ____hour(s)
  post transfusion ___ in a.m
Serum iron level ____
Total iron binding capacity (TIBC) ____
Folate ____ Ferritin level _____

B12 level _____
Reticulocyte count _____ Hemoglobin
   electrophoresis _____
Smear to pathology lab for review _____
Other _____, _____, _____, _____,
   _____, _____, _____, _____
* Specialized tests for diagnostic evaluation of
   anemia should be drawn prior to any blood
   transfusion, if indicated

Radiologic Studies

CXR portable_____
CXR (PA and lateral) _____
CT scan _____
Ultrasound _____
MRI _____
Other _____, _____, _____

Cardiac Studies

ECG __ × 1__ q 4 hours × 3 ___ q 4 hours ×
   4 ___ other ____ with cardiac enzymes
Echocardiogram (transthoracic) __with
   agitated (bubble) study__ without agitated
   (bubble) study

Consultants

Care coordination (Case management)
   _____Notified: Name _____ Time _____
Hematology _____ Notified:
   Name_____ Time _____
Social work_____ Notified:
   Name_____ Time_____
Other _____Notified: Name
   _____ Time_____

Transfusion

Procedure (transfusion) explained _____
   Consent signed _____
Transfuse Packed Red Blood Cells (PRBCs)
   _____units IV over _____ hours

Premedication prior to transfusion (only if indicated, such as prior transfusion reaction)

Diphenhydramine (Benadryl®) ____ 25 mg
   ____ 50 mg __ PO __ IV prior to transfusion
Prednisone __ 40 mg PO ___ 60 mg PO prior
   to transfusion

If any transfusion reaction

Immediately stop transfusion _____
Notify attending physician _____
Notify blood bank _____
Send PRBC unit with identifying tag to blood
   bank ___
Draw extra tubes of blood and send to blood
   bank _____

Intravenous Fluids

Saline cap IV _____
Bolus Normal Saline (NS) IV ___ 250 mL __
   500 mL ___1,000 mL _____ mL infuse over
   ___ minutes ___ hours
Bolus Lactated Ringer's (LR) IV ___ 250 mL __
   500 mL ___1,000 mL___ infuse over ___
   minutes ___ hours
Maintenance NS at __ mL per hour IV
Maintenance LR at __ mL per hour IV
Maintenance Dextrose 5% in Water (D_5W) at
   __ mL per hour IV
Maintenance Dextrose 5% ½ Normal Saline
   (D_5½NS) at __ mL per hour IV
Maintenance Dextrose 5% Normal Saline
   (D_5NS) at __ mL per hour IV
at __ mL per hour IV
Maintenance NS with potassium chloride __20
   mEq or _ 40 mEq per 1 liter bag at__mL
   per hour
Maintenance D_5W with potassium chloride
   __20 mEq or _ 40 mEq per 1 liter bag at__mL
   per hour
Maintenance D_5½NS with potassium chloride
   __20 mEq or _ 40 mEq per 1 liter bag at __
   mL per hour IV
Maintenance D_5NS with potassium chloride
   __20 mEq or _ 40 mEq per 1 liter bag
Other _____ at mL per hour

Education: patient _____ family _____

Transfusion _____
Anemia _____
Smoking cessation_____
Other _____

Transient Ischemic Attack (TIA) Order Set

ABCD² Score* _____

If ABCD² score ≥ 3 admit to inpatient neurology service _____

If ABCD² score ≤ 2 place in Emergency Department (ED) Observation _____

Place in Emergency Department (ED) Observation _____

Diagnosis *TRANSIENT ISCHEMIC ATTACK,*

_____, _____, _____

ED Attending_____

Resident (if applicable)_____

Advanced Practice Provider(if applicable)

_____

Allergies: Yes_____ No_____

If yes, what_____, _____, _____, _____,

_____, _____

Vital Signs

Temperature__ Pulse __ Respiration __BP__ Pulse oximetry ____

__q 2 hours × 4 then q 4 hours if stable

Neurologic checks q 2 hours × 4 then q 4 hours if stable _____

Cardiac monitoring (telemetry) _____

Orthostatic vital signs _____

Continous pulse oximetry _____

Other _____

Notify Physician if:

Temperature (°C) > 38.0° ____ 38.5°____ 39° ____40° ____ other _____

Heart rate ≤ 50 ___ ≥ 120 __ ≥ 150 ___ ≥ 200___ other ____

Oxygen saturation < 90% _____ other _____

Any change in mental status _____

Any respiratory distress_____

Any chest pain _____

Systolic blood pressure (mmHg) ___≥ 160 __ ≥ 180 ___ other

Diastolic blood pressure (mmHg) ___> 100 ___> 120 ___ other

Activity**

Up ad lib _____

Assisted _____

Other _____

Diet**

Dysphagia screen prior to any PO intake _____

NPO _____

Regular _____

Advance diet as tolerated _____

Clear liquids ____

Dental, mechanical soft _____

Diabetic _____

Formula_____

Full liquids _____

Low added fat/No added salt _____

Low cholesterol____

Pureed _____

Sodium: restricted____ 1 gram ___ other ____

Per feeding tube _____

Other _____

Nursing Interventions

Weight___ on admission ___ qd ___ prior to discharge _____ other

Height ____

I & Os _____ routine _____ strict _____

Fluid restriction ___ mL/hour ___ mL/shift _____ mL/24 hour ___ other

Fall precautions _____

Seizure precautions _____

Capillary blood glucose __ × 1 q ___ hours ____ before meals and at bedtime __ other

Notify Physician if

Any new or worsening neurologic symptoms (including but not limited to: confusion or change in mental status, weakness, numbness, paresthesias, difficulty talking, facial droop) _____

Respiratory Interventions ____

Maintain oxygen saturation ≥ 92% _____

If administering supplemental oxygen, then place oxygen __ liters nasal cannula ___other

Sleep apnea qhs __ CPAP BiPAP settings cm H_2O ____ inspiratory __ expiratory

Laboratory Tests

CBC with differential ___ with platelets ____

Basic metabolic panel_____

Cardiac enzymes __ × 1 ___ q 4 hours × 3 ____ q 4 hours × 4 ____ other ____

Complete metabolic panel_____

(Total) Creatinine phosphokinase (total CPK)

_____

Fasting lipids _____

Hemoglobin A1C (recommended even if patient is not a known diabetic) _____

Hypercoagulation panel _____ (consider in patients < 60 years of age) ***

Lactate _____

Liver function tests _____

Urinalysis _____ Urine culture _____

Pregnancy test (qualitative urine) _____

Pregnancy test (quantitative blood) _____

PT/INR ____ PTT _____

Renal function tests (e.g. BUN, creatinine) _____

Type and Screen _____

Other _____, _____, _____, _____,

_____, _____, _____, _____

Repeat _____, _____, _____, _____, _____ in a.m.___ in _____ hours

Radiology Studies

CXR portable_____

CXR (PA and lateral) _____

CT (computed tomography) scan of brain without contrast if not done in ED _____

CTA (computed tomography angiography) of brain with and without contrast (ultravist) if no contrast allergy and no renal failure (e.g. GFR ≥ 30) _____

MRI (Magnetic resonance imaging) of brain without contrast _____

MRI (Magnetic resonance imaging) of brain with and without contrast (gadolinium) if no allergy and no renal failure (e.g. GFR ≥ 30) _____

MRA (Magnetic resonance angiography) Circle of Willis and of Carotids without contrast (if renal failure) _____

MRA (Magnetic resonance angiography) Circle of Willis and of Carotids with and without contrast (gadolinium) if no allergy and no renal failure (e.g. GFR ≥ 30) _____

MRV (magnetic resonance venography) ___ without contrast (if renal failure)

MRV (magnetic resonance venography) ___with contrast

Ultrasound of carotids _____

Transcranial doppler of brain vessels _____

Note: For evaluation of recurrent TIAs, the radiology diagnostic study of choice is MRA with and without contrast, and if MRA can't be done, a CTA with and without contrast is the next choice.

Cardiac Studies

ECG __ × 1__ q 4 hours × 3 ___ q 4 hours × 4 ___ other ____ with cardiac enzymes

Echocardiogram (transthoracic) __with agitated (bubble) study__ without agitated (bubble) study

Consultants

Care coordination (Case management) _____ Notified: Name _____ Time ____

Cardiology _____ Notified: Name_____ Time____

Internal medicine/Family practice __ Notified: Name__Time____

Neurology _____ Notified: Name_____ Time____

Physical therapy _____ Notified: Name_____ Time____

Social work_____ Notified: Name_____ Time____

Other _____ Notified: Name _____ Time_____

Medications for Transient Ischemic Attack (Adult Dosage)

Antiplatelet Agent

Aspirin PO 325 mg qd (if patient passes dysphagia screening and has no allergy or contraindication) _____

Aspirin PR 300 mg suppository qd if patient fails dysphagia screening and has no allergy or contraindication) _____

Analgesics

Acetaminophen (Paracetamol) (Tylenol®) 325 mg tab __1 tab __1–2 tabs __ 2 tabs PO __ q 4 hours __ q 6 hours ___ prn pain ___ prn fever (maximum 4 g daily)

____ If unable to take pill form, may give liquid equivalent

____ If unable to take PO, may give suppository PR __325 mg __ 650 mg __ q 4 hours __ q 6 hours

____ IV ___ mg ___ q 4 hours __ q 6 hours __ prn pain __ prn fever (maximum adult dose: if weight < 50 kg is 15 mg/kg up to 750 mg for a

single dose, 75 mg/kg up to 3750 mg for daily
dose; if weight > 50 kg is 650 mg q 4 hours or
1000 mg q 6 hours up to 1000 mg for a single
dose and 4000 mg for a daily dose)

Other _____

Intravenous Fluids

Saline lock IV _____

Maintenance Normal Saline (NS) at __ mL per
hour IV

Maintenance Lactated Ringer's (LR) at __ mL
per hour IV

Maintenance Dextrose 5% in Water (D_5W) at
__ mL per hour IV

Maintenance Dextrose 5% in ½ Normal Saline
($D_5\frac{1}{2}NS$) at __ mL per hour IV

Maintenance Dextrose 5% in Normal Saline
(D_5NS) at __ mL per hour IV

Maintenance NS with potassium chloride __20
mEq or__ 40 mEq per 1 liter bag at __mL
per hour

Maintenance D_5W with potassium chloride
__20 mEq or _ 40 mEq per 1 liter bag at __
mL per hour IV

Maintenance $D_5\frac{1}{2}NS$ with potassium chloride
__20 mEq or _ 40 mEq per 1 liter bag at __
mL per hour IV

Maintenance Dextrose in Normal Saline (D_5NS)
with potassium chloride __20 mEq or __
40 mEq per 1 liter bag at __ mL per hour IV

Other _____ at mL per hour

Education: patient _____ family _____

Stroke/TIA_____

Smoking cessation_____

Other _____

* $ABCD^2$ Scoring system

Reference

Johnson SC, Rothwell PM, Nguyen-Huynh MN, et al.
Validation and refinement of scores to predict very
early stroke risk after transient ischaemic attack.
Lancet 2007; 369: 283–292.

** Activity depends upon clinical situation.
Consider physical therapy as indicated.
Encourage ambulation whenever possible.
A swallowing screen can be done on patients prior
to PO intake. The option for unlimited sodium in
the diet can be deleted to promote a decreased
sodium intake as part of control for hypertension.
Check for diabetes and hypercholesterolemia, and
counsel for smoking cessation, which are treatable
risk factors for stroke and TIA. Consider consult
with internal medicine/family practice regarding
initiation of treatment for diabetes and
hypercholesterolemia. Neurology consult is
recommended for patients with TIA and stroke.
The TIA order set can be customized from our
template by stressing certain key factors.
*** Consider hypercoagulation panel if patient has
strong family history of clotting disorders (such as deep
vein thrombosis [DVT] or pulmonary emboli [PE])
and/or is young and has no risk factors for DVT yet has
a DVT or PE. The coagulation panel includes such tests
as protein S, protein C, antithrombin III, and factor
VIII; and is a screen for inherited clotting disorders. It
is expensive and thus, should be done only when there
is a suspicion for an inherited disorder being present.

	Age	Blood Pressure	Clinical Features	Duration	Diabetes
$ABCD^2$ score					
0 points	< 60 years	Normal	other than those specified	< 10 minutes	no diabetes
1 points	≥ 60 years	raised (blood pressure ≥ 140/90)	speech disturbance without weakness	10 to 59 minutes	diabetes present
2 points			unilateral (one-sided) weakness	≥ 60 minutes	

Vaginal Bleeding Order Set

Place in Emergency Department (ED)
Observation _____
Diagnosis **_VAGINAL BLEEDING,_** _____,

_____, _____

ED Attending_____
Resident (if applicable)_____
Advanced Practice Provider (if applicable)

_____

Allergies: Yes_____ No_____

If yes, what_____, _____, _____, _____,

_____, _____

Vital Signs

Temperature__ Pulse __ Respiration __BP__
Pulse oximetry ____
__q 2 hours ___q 4 hours ___q 6 hours q ___
hours ___q shift ___ qd ____ other
Cardiac monitoring (telemetry) _____
Orthostatic vital signs _____
Continuous pulse oximetry _____
Other _____

Notify Physician if

Temperature (°C) > 38.0° ___ 38.5°___ 39°
___40° ____ other _____
Systolic blood pressure (mmHg) ≤ 90 ___ ≥
160 __ ≥ 180 ___ ≥ 200__ other _____
Diastolic blood pressure (mmHg) ≥ 120 ____
other _____
Heart rate ≤ 50 ___ ≥ 120 __ ≥ 150 ___ ≥
200___ other ____
Oxygen saturation < 90 % _____ other _____
Any change in mental status _____
Any respiratory distress_____

Activity

Up ad lib _____
Assisted _____
Out of bed to chair _____
Bedrest with bathroom privileges _____
Bedrest with bedside commode _____
Bedrest _____
Other _____

Diet

NPO _____
Regular _____

Advance diet as tolerated _____
Clear liquids ____
Dental, mechanical soft _____
Diabetic _____
Formula_____
Full liquids _____
Low added fat/No added salt _____
Low cholesterol____
Pureed _____
Sodium: 1 gram ___ 2 grams ___
unrestricted____
Per feeding tube _____
Other _____

Nursing Interventions

Weight___ on admission ___ qd ___ prior to
discharge ____ other
Height ____
I & Os _____ routine _____ strict _____
Fall precautions _____
Seizure precautions _____
Capillary blood glucose __ × 1 q___ hours ___
before meals and at bedtime

Respiratory Interventions

Oxygen __ liters nasal cannula __venti mask at
___ liters per minute _____other
Sleep apnea qhs __ CPAP BiPAP settings cm
H_2O ___ inspiratory __ expiratory

Laboratory Tests

CBC _____ with differential
Basic metabolic panel_____
Complete metabolic panel_____
Hematocrit/hemoglobin ____
Lactate _____
Liver function tests _____
Urinalysis _____ Urine culture _____
Pregnancy test (qualitative urine) _____
Pregnancy test (quantitative blood) _____
Renal function tests (e.g. BUN, creatinine)

_____

Type and Screen _____ Type and Cross ___
units packed red blood cells _____
Other _____, _____, _____, _____,

_____, _____, _____, _____

Repeat _____, _____, _____, _____, _____ in
a.m. in ___ hours

Hematocrit/hemoglobin ____hour(s) post transfusion ___ in a.m.

Radiology Studies

CT scan abdomen/pelvis ____ with contrast: __ IV __ PO ___

Ultrasound abdomen _____ pelvis _____

MRI abdomen _____ pelvis _____

Other _____, _____, _____

Consultants

Care coordination (Case management) _____ Notified: Name _____ Time _____

Obstetrics/Gynecology ___ Notified: Name_____ Time____

Social work_____ Notified: Name_____ Time____

Other _____ Notified: Name _____ Time____

Transfusion

Transfusion

Procedure explained _____ Consent signed _____

Transfuse Packed Red Blood Cells (PRBCs) _____units IV over _____ hours

Premedication prior to transfusion (only if indicated, such as prior transfusion reaction)

Diphenhydramine (Benadryl®) ____ 25 mg ____ 50 mg __ PO __ IV prior to transfusion

Prednisone __ 40 mg PO ___ 60 mg PO prior to transfusion __ other

If any transfusion reaction

Immediately stop transfusion ____

Notify attending physician _____

Notify blood bank _____

Send PRBC unit with identifying tag to blood bank ___

Draw extra tubes of blood and send to blood bank ____

Intravenous Fluids

Saline cap IV ____

Bolus Normal Saline (NS) IV ___ 250 mL __ 500 mL ___1,000 mL ____ mL infuse over ___ minutes ___ hours

Bolus Lactated Ringer's (LR) IV ___ 250 mL __ 500 mL ___1,000 mL___ infuse over ___ minutes ___ hours

Maintenance NS at __ mL per hour IV

Maintenance LRS at __ mL per hour IV

Maintenance NS with potassium __20 meq or _ 40 meq per 1 liter bag at __mL per hour

Maintenance Dextrose 5% in Water (D_5W) at __ mL per hour IV

Maintenance Dextrose 5% ½ Normal Saline ($D_5\frac{1}{2}NS$) at __ mL per hour IV

Maintenance Dextrose 5% in Normal Saline (D_5NS) at __ mL per hour IV

Maintenance D_5NS with potassium chloride __20 mEq or _ 40 mEq per 1 liter bag at __ mL per hour IV

Maintenance $D_5\frac{1}{2}NS$ with potassium chloride __20 mEq or _ 40 mEq per 1 liter bag at __ mL per hour IV

Other _____ at mL per hour

Education: patient _____ family _____

Vaginal Bleeding _____

Anemia _____

Smoking cessation_____

Other _____

See also transfusion order set

Vertigo/Dizziness Order Set

Place in Emergency Department (ED)
Observation _____
Diagnosis **VERTIGO/DIZZINESS,** _____,
_____, _____

ED Attending_____
Resident (if applicable)_____
Advanced Practice Provider (if applicable)
_____

Allergies: Yes_____ No_____

If yes, what_____,_____,_____,_____,
_____,_____

Vital Signs

Temperature__ Pulse __ Respiration __BP__
Pulse oximetry ____
__q 2 hours ___q 4 hours ___q 6 hours q ___
hours ___q shift ___ qd ____ other
Cardiac monitoring (telemetry) _____
Orthostatic vital signs _____
Continuous Pulse oximetry _____
Other _____

Notify Physician if

Temperature (°C) > 38.0° ___ 38.5°___ 39°
___40° ____ other _____
Systolic blood pressure (mmHg) ≤ 90 ___ ≥
160 __ ≥ 180 ___ ≥ 200__ other _____
Diastolic blood pressure (mmHg) ≥ 120 _____
other _____
Heart rate ≤ 50 ___ ≥ 120 __ ≥ 150 ___ ≥
200___ other ____
Oxygen saturation < 90% _____ other _____
Any change in mental status _____
Any respiratory distress_____

Activity

Up ad lib _____
Assisted _____
Out of bed to chair _____
Bedrest with bathroom privileges _____
Bedrest with bedside commode _____
Bedrest _____
Other _____

Diet

NPO _____
Regular _____

Advance diet as tolerated _____
Clear liquids ____
Dental, mechanical soft _____
Diabetic _____
Formula_____
Full liquids _____
Low added fat/No added salt
Low cholesterol____
Pureed _____
Sodium: 1 gram ___ 2 grams ___
unrestricted____
Per feeding tube _____
Other _____

Nursing Interventions

Weight___ on admission ___ qd ___ prior to
discharge ____ other
Height ____
I & Os _____ routine _____ strict _____
Fluid restriction ___ mL/hour ___ mL/shift
____ mL/24 hour ___ other
Fall precautions _____
Seizure precautions _____
Capillary blood glucose __ × 1 q ___ hours
____ before meals and at bedtime

Respiratory Interventions

Oxygen __ liters nasal cannula __venti mask at
___ liters per minute _____other
Sleep apnea qhs __ CPAP BiPAP settings cm
H_2O ___ inspiratory __ expiratory

Laboratory Tests

CBC _____ with differential
Basic metabolic panel_____
Cardiac enzymes ___ × 1 ___ q 4 hours × 3 ___
q 4 hours × 4 ____ other
Complete metabolic panel_____
Lactate _____
Liver function tests _____
Urinalysis _____ Urine culture _____
Pregnancy test (qualitative urine) _____
Pregnancy test (quantitative blood) _____
Renal function tests (e.g. BUN, creatinine)
_____

Other _____, _____, _____, _____,
_____, _____, _____, _____
Repeat _____, _____, _____, _____, _____ in
a.m.___ in _____ hours

Radiology Studies

CXR portable_____

CXR (PA and lateral) _____

CT scan: head without contrast __

MRI head without contrast _____

Ultrasound _____

Other _____, _____, _____

Cardiac Studies

ECG __ × 1__ q 4 hours × 3 ___ q 4 hours × 4 ___ other ____ with cardiac enzymes

Echocardiogram (transthoracic) __with agitated (bubble) study__ without agitated (bubble) study

Consultants

Care coordination (Case management) _____ Notified: Name_____ Time____

Neurology _____ Notified: Name_____ Time____

Otolaryngology (ENT) _____ Notified: Name_____ Time____

Neuro-otolaryngology for vestibular rehabilitation (physical therapy) Notified: Name_____ Time_____

Social work_____ Notified: Name_____ Time____

Other _____ Notified: Name _____ Time____

Vertigo Medications (Adult Dosage)

Medications for Suppression of Vestibular Symptoms: Antihistamines*

Dimenhydrinate (Dramamine®) __ 50 mg __ 100 mg __ q 4 hours __ q 6 hours __ PO __IV __IM __ prn vertigo (maximum 400 mg daily)

Diphenhydramine (Benadryl®) __ 25 mg __ 50 mg __ q 4 hours __ q 6 hours __ PO __ IV __ IM__ prn vertigo (maximum 400 mg daily)

Meclizine (Antivert®)__ 25 mg __ 50 mg __q 4 hours __ q 6 hours __ prn vertigo

*Antihistamines are the drugs of choice in most patients.

Medications for Suppression of Vestibular Symptoms: Antiemetics

Metoclopramide (Reglan®) __10 mg __ IV __ IM __ PO __ q 6 hours __ prn nausea/vomiting

Ondansetron (Zofran®) __ 4 mg __ 8 mg __IV __PO __ q 6 hour __ prn nausea/vomiting

Prochlorperazine (Compazine®) _5 mg _ 10 mg _ IV _IM _ PO __ q 4 hours __ q 6 hours (maximum 40 mg daily) 25 mg ___ PR bid __ prn nausea/vomiting

Promethazine (Phenergan®) __12.5 mg __ 25 mg __IV__ IM __ PO __ PR __ q4 hours __ q 6 hours ___ prn nausea/vomiting

Medications for Suppression of Vestibular Symptoms: Benzodiazepines

Alprazolam (Xanax®) __ 0.5 mg immediate release PO __q 8 hours __ prn vertigo

Clonazepam (Klonopin®) __ 0.25 mg __ 0.5 mg __PO q 8 hours __ prn vertigo

Diazepam (Valium®, Diastat®) __ 5 mg PO __ 10 mg PO __ q 12 hours __ 0.5 __ 1.0 mg IV __ q 12 hours __ prn vertigo

Lorazepam (Ativan®) __ 1 mg __ 2 mg PO __ q 8 hours ___0.5 mg IV q 8 hours __ prn vertigo

Other

Acetaminophen (Paracetamol) (Tylenol®) 325 mg tab __1 tab __1–2 tabs __ 2 tabs PO __ q 4 hours__ q 6 hours ___ prn pain ___ prn fever (maximum 4 g daily)

____ If unable to take tablet formulation, may give suspension

____ If unable to take PO, may give suppository PR __325 mg __ 650 mg __ q 4 hour __ q 6 hour

____ IV ___ mg __ q 4 hours __ q 6 hours __ prn pain __ prn fever (maximum adult dose: if weight < 50 kg is 15 mg/kg up to 750 mg for a single dose, 75 mg/kg up to 3750 mg for daily dose; if weight > 50 kg is 650 mg q 4 hours or 1000 mg q 6 hours up to 1000 mg for a single dose and 4000 mg for a daily dose)

Other_____, _____, _____, _____, _____

Intravenous Fluids

Saline cap IV ____

Bolus Normal Saline (NS) IV ___ 250 mL __ 500 mL ___1,000 mL _____ other, infuse over ___ minutes ___ hours

Bolus Lactated Ringer's (LR) IV __ 250 mL __ 500 mL __1,000 mL __ other, infuse over ___ minutes ___ hours

Maintenance NS at __ mL per hour IV

Maintenance LR at __ mL per hour IV

Maintenance Dextrose 5% in Water (D_5W) at __ mL per hour IV

Maintenance Dextrose 5% in ½ Normal Saline ($D_5½NS$) at __ mL per hour IV

Maintenance Dextrose 5% in Normal Saline (D_5NS) at __ mL per hour IV

Maintenance NS with potassium chloride __20 mEq or__ 40 mEq per 1 liter bag at __mL per hour

Maintenance D_5W with potassium chloride __20 mEq or _ 40 mEq per 1 liter bag

Maintenance $D_5½NS$ with potassium chloride __20 mEq or__ 40 mEq per 1 liter bag at __mL per hour

Maintenance D_5NS with potassium chloride __20 mEq or _ 40 mEq per 1 liter bag at __ mL per hour IV

Other _____ at mL per hour

Education: patient _____ family _____

Vertigo ____

Smoking cessation_____

Other _____

Venous Thromboembolic Disease (VTE)/Deep Vein Thrombosis (DVT) Order Set

Place in Emergency Department (ED) Observation _____

Diagnosis *VENOUS THROMBOEMBOLIC DISEASE/DEEP VEIN THROMBOSIS,*

_____, _____

ED Attending_____

Resident (if applicable)_____

Advanced Practice Provider(if applicable)

_____

Allergies: Yes_____ No_____

if yes, what_____,_____,_____,_____,

_____,_____

Vital Signs

Temperature__ Pulse __ Respiration __BP__ Pulse oximetry ____

__q 2 hours ___q 4 hours ___q 6 hours q ___ hours ___q shift ___ qd ____ other

Cardiac monitoring (telemetry) _____

Continuous pulse oximetry _____

Vascular checks __q 2 hours __q 4 hours __q 6 hours q __hours __q shift __ qd __other

Other _____

Notify Physician if

Temperature (°C) > 38.0° ___ 38.5°___ 39° ___40° ____ other _____

Systolic blood pressure systolic (mmHg) ≤ 90 ___ ≥ 160 __ ≥ 180 ___ ≥ 200__ other _____

Diastolic blood pressure (mmHg) ≥ 120 ____ other _____

Heart rate ≤ 50 ___ ≥ 120 __ ≥ 150 ___ ≥ 200___ other ____

Oxygen saturation < 90% _____ other _____

Activity

Up ad lib _____

Assisted _____

Out of bed to chair _____

Bedrest with bathroom privileges _____

Bedrest with bedside commode _____

Bedrest _____

Other _____

Diet

NPO _____

Regular _____

Advance diet as tolerated _____

Clear liquids ____

Dental, mechanical soft _____

Diabetic _____

Formula_____

Full liquids _____

Low added fat/No added salt ____

Low cholesterol____

Pureed _____

Sodium: 1 gram ___ 2 grams ___ unrestricted____

Per feeding tube _____

Other _____

Nursing Interventions

Weight___ on admission ___ qd ___ prior to discharge ____ other

Height ____

I & Os ____ routine _____ strict ____

Fluid restriction ___ mL/hour ___ mL/shift ____ mL/24 hour ___ other

Fall precautions _____

Seizure precautions _____

Capillary blood glucose __ × 1 q ___ hours ___ before meals and at bedtime

Compression stockings _____

Elevate the extremity ___ right ___ left __ upper extremity ___ lower extremity

Respiratory Interventions

Oxygen __ liters nasal cannula __ venti mask at ___ liters per minute _____other

Sleep apnea qhs __ CPAP BiPAP settings cm H_2O ___ inspiratory __ expiratory

Laboratory Tests

CBC _____ with differential

Basic metabolic panel_____

Cardiac enzymes X 1 ___ q 4 hours × 3 ____ q 4 hours × 4 ____ other

Complete metabolic panel_____

Hypercoagulation Panel*____

Lactate ____

Liver function tests ____

PT ___ INR ___

APTT _____

Renal function tests (BUN, creatinine) _____
Urinalysis _____
Pregnancy test - qualitative urine _____
Other _____, _____, _____, _____,

_____, _____, _____, _____
Repeat _____, _____, _____, _____, _____ in
a.m.___ in _____ hours

Radiologic Studies

CXR portable_____
CXR (PA and lateral) _____
CT chest (PE protocol) _____
V/Q scan of chest _____
Ultrasound for DVT ___right ___ left ___
upper ___ lower extremities
Other _____, _____, _____

Cardiac Studies

ECG __ × 1__ q 4 hours × 3 ___ q 4 hours ×
4 ___ other ____ with cardiac enzymes
Echocardiogram (transthoracic) __with
agitated (bubble) study__ without agitated
(bubble) study

Consultants

Care coordination (Case management)
_____ Notified: Name_____
Time_____
Vascular medicine _____ Notified:
Name_____ Time_____
Vascular surgery _____ Notified:
Name_____ Time_____
Social work_____ Notified:
Name_____ Time_____
Other _____ Notified:
Name _____ Time_____

Deep Vein Thrombosis Medications†

Vitamin K Antagonist

Warfarin (Coumadin®) ___ mg PO qd

Low Molecular Weight Heparins

Enoxaparin (Lovenox®) _____ 1 mg/kg/dose ×
___ weight (kg) q 12 hours SQ
Tinzaparin (Innohep®) __ 175 units/kg ×
___weight (kg) qd SQ (maximum 18,000
anti-Xa units/day)
Dalteparin (Fragmin) _____ 200 units/kg × ___
weight (kg) qd SQ

Factor Xa inhibitor

Fondaparinux (Arixtra®) _ 5 mg if < 50 kg _
7.5 mg if 50–100 kg _10mg if >100 kg __ qd
SC

Analgesics

Acetaminophen (Paracetamol) (Tylenol®)
325 mg tab __1 tab __1–2 tabs __ 2 tabs PO
__ q 4 hours__ q 6 hours ___ prn pain ___
prn fever (maximum dose 4 grams per day)
____ If unable to take tablet formulation, may
give suspension
____ If unable to take PO, may give suppository
PR __325 mg __ 650 mg __ q 4 hours __ q
6 hours
____IV ___ mg __ q 4 hours __ q 6 hours __
prn pain __ prn fever (maximum adult dose:
if weight < 50 kg is 15 mg/kg up to 750 mg
for a single dose, 75 mg/kg up to 3750 mg for
daily dose; if weight > 50 kg is 650 mg q
4 hours or 1000 mg q 6 hours up to 1000 mg
for a single dose and 4000 mg for a
daily dose)
Acetaminophen- Hydrocodone (Vicodin®) 300
mg/5 mg tabs __1 tab __1–2 tabs __ 2 tabs
PO __q 4 hours__ q 6 hours ___ prn pain
(maximum dose 4 grams per day based on
acetaminophen dose)
Acetaminophen-Oxycodone (Endocet®,
Percocet®, Roxicet®) 325 mg/ 5 mg tab __1
tab __1–2 tabs __ 2 tabs PO q 4 hours__ q
6 hours ___ prn pain (maximum dose
4 grams per day based on
acetaminophen dose)
Hydromorphone (Dilaudid®) __ 0.5 mg __
1 mg __ 2 mg __ mg IV __ q 2 hours __ q
4 hours __ q 6 hours q __ hours__ prn pain
Ibuprofen (Advil®, Motrin®)__ 400 mg __
600 mg __ 800 mg PO __ q 4 hours __ q
6 hours __ q 8 hours___ prn pain
Ketorolac (Toradol®) __ 30 mg IV __ q 6 hours
_ prn pain (maximum dose: 120 mg per day)
Morphine __ 0.5 mg__ 1 mg __ 2 mg __ 4 mg
___ mg IV __ q 2 hours __ q 4 hours __ q
6 hours q ___ hours __ prn pain
Tramadol (Ultram®) __ 50 mg __ 100 mg PO
__q 4 hours __ q 6 hours __ prn pain
(maximum dose 400 mg per day)
Other_____, _____, _____,
_____, _____

Intravenous Fluids

Saline cap IV ____

Bolus Normal Saline (NS) IV ___ 250 mL __ 500 mL ___1,000 mL ____ other, infuse over ___ minutes ___ hours

Bolus Lactated Ringer's (LR) IV __ 250 mL __ 500 mL __1,000 mL __ othernfuse over ____ minutes ___ hours

Maintenance NS at __ mL per hour IV

Maintenance LR at __ mL per hour IV

Maintenance Dextrose 5% in Water (D_5W) at __ mL per hour IV

Maintenance Dextrose 5% ½ Normal Saline (D_5½NS) at __ mL per hour IV

Maintenance Dextrose 5% in Normal Saline (D_5NS) at __ mL per hour IV

Maintenance NS with potassium chloride __20 mEq or _ 40 mEq per 1 liter bag at __ mL per hour IV

Maintenance D_5W with potassium chloride __20 mEq or _ 40 mEq per 1 liter bag at __ mL per hour IV

Maintenance D_5½NS with potassium chloride __20 mEq or _ 40 mEq per 1 liter bag at __ mL per hour IV

Maintenance D_5NS with potassium chloride __20 mEq or _ 40 mEq per 1 liter bag at __ mL per hour IV

Other _____ at mL per hour

Education: patient _____ family _____

Deep Vein Thrombosis___

Smoking cessation_____

Other _____

* Consider hypercoagulation panel if patient has strong family history of clotting disorders (such as deep vein thrombosis [DVT] or pulmonary emboli [PE]) and/or is young and has no risk factors for DVT yet has a DVT or PE. The coagulation panel includes such tests as protein S, protein C, antithrombin III, and factor VIII; and is a screen for inherited clotting disorders. It is expensive and thus, should be done only when there is a suspicion for an inherited disorder being present.

† Multiple terms are in use for the anticoagulants. Initially, "NOAC" has been used for "novel oral anticoagulant" or "new (er) oral anticoagulant". These drugs are also referred to as "non-vitamin K antagonist oral anticoagulant". They are also referred to as "TSOACs" or "target-specific oral anticoagulants" since these medications are oral agents that inhibit a specific enzyme in the coagulation cascade and with usage, the NOACs are no longer "new" or "novel". Other terms include DOACs or direct oral anticoagulants, and ODIs or oral direct inhibitors. We anticipate that in the near future, there will be other anticoagulants both oral and parenteral available for use.

Currently, there are no antidotes or specific reversal agents for these TSOACs available for clinical use with the exception of idarucizamab for reversal of dabigatran. However, there is research in this area and clinical trials of specific reversal agents are underway so it is likely that in the future, we will be adding additional reversal agents to our order sets.

This is not intended to be an all-inclusive list. Three low molecular weight heparins

(LMWH): enoxaparin, dalteparin and tinzaparin and a closely related synthetic pentasaccharide, fondaparinux, are approved for clinical use in the United States. There are multiple other anticoagulants and/or low molecular weight heparins (LMWH) available outside the United States and/or in clinical trials.

Antithrombotic agents include antiplatelet agents, such as aspirin and clopidogrel; and anticoagulants. Anticoagulants work by inhibiting a step or multiple steps in the coagulation cascade. Anticoagulants have various mechanisms of action: antagonism of vitamin-K dependent factors via prevention of liver synthesis of the vitamin K dependent factors or altering the calcium-binding properties of the vitamin-K dependent factors; binding to antithrombin causing indirect inhibition, or inhibition of enzymes causing direct inhibition. Currently available agents include unfractionated heparin, low molecular weight heparins (LMWH), fondaparinux, direct thrombin inhibitors (DTIs) (parenteral: bivalirudin, argatroban, desirudin; and oral: dabigatran), and direct factor Xa inhibitors: rivaroxaban, apixaban, edoxaban, plus other agents in development.

Adult Order Sets
Electrolyte Abnormalities

Sharon E. Mace, MD, FACEP, FAAP
Matthew J. Campbell, PharmD, BCPS, BCCCP

Hypocalcemia Order Set

Place in emergency department (ED)
  Observation _____
Diagnosis **HYPOCALCEMIA**, _____,

_____, _____
ED Attending _____
Resident (if applicable) _____
Advanced Practice Provider (if applicable)

_____

Allergies: Yes _____ No _____

If yes, what _____, _____, _____, _____,

_____, _____

Vital Signs

Temperature __ Pulse __ Respiration __ BP__
  Pulse oximetry ____
__ q 2 hours ___ q 4 hours ___ q 6 hours q ___
  hours ___ q shift ___ qd ____ other
Cardiac monitoring (telemetry)* _____
Orthostatic vital signs _____
Continuous pulse oximetry _____
Other _____

Notify Physician if

Temperature (°C) > 38.0° ___ 38.5°___ 39° ___
  40° ____ other _____
Systolic blood pressure (mm Hg) ≤ 90 ___ ≥
  160 __ ≥ 180 ___ ≥ 200 __ other _____
Diastolic blood pressure (mm Hg) ≥ 120 ____
  other _____
Heart rate ≤ 50 ___ ≥ 120 __ ≥ 150 ___ ≥
  200 ___ other ____
Oxygen saturation < 90% _____ other _____
Any change in mental status _____
Any respiratory distress _____

Activity

Up ad lib _____

Assisted _____
Out of bed to chair _____
Bedrest with bathroom privileges _____
Bedrest with bedside commode _____
Bedrest _____
Other _____

Diet

NPO _____
Regular _____
Advance diet as tolerated _____
Clear liquids ____
Dental, mechanical soft _____
Diabetic _____
Formula _____
Full liquids _____
Low added fat/No added salt _____
Low cholesterol ____
Pureed _____
Sodium: 1 gram ___ 2 gram ___
  unrestricted____
Per feeding tube _____
Other _____

Nursing Interventions

Weight ___ on admission ___ qd ___ prior to
  discharge ____ other
Height ____
I & Os _____ routine _____ strict _____
Fluid restriction ___ mL/hour ___ mL/shift
  ____ mL/24 hour ___ other
Fall precautions _____
Seizure precautions _____
Capillary blood glucose __ × 1 q __ hours
  ____ before meals and at bedtime

Respiratory Interventions

Oxygen __ liters nasal cannula __ venti mask at
  ___ liters per minute _____ other

For sleep apnea qhs ___ CPAP ___ BiPAP settings cm H_2O ___ inspiratory ___ expiratory

Laboratory Tests

CBC _____ with differential

Amylase ___ Lipase ___

Basic metabolic panel _____

Blood alcohol level ____

Calcium (total) _____ Calcium (ionized) _____

Cardiac enzymes ___ × 1 ___ q 4 hours × 3 ___ q 4 hours × 4 ___ other

Complete metabolic panel _____

Lactate _____

Liver function tests _____

Magnesium _____

Phosphorus _____

Potassium _____

Pregnancy test (qualitative urine) _____
Pregnancy test (quantitative blood) _____

Renal function tests: ___ BUN ___ creatinine

Toxicology: blood drug screen ____ urine drug screen ____ drug level for ___

Urinalysis _____ Urine culture _____

Other _____, _____, _____, _____,
_____, _____, _____, _____

Repeat _____, _____, _____ in a.m. ___ in ___ hours, q ___ hours × ___

Radiology Studies

CXR portable _____

CXR (PA and lateral) _____

Other ____

Cardiac Studies

ECG ___ × 1___ q 4 hours × 3 ___ q 4 hours × 4 ___ other ____ with cardiac enzymes

Echocardiogram (transthoracic) ___ with agitated (bubble) study ___ without agitated (bubble) study

Consultants

Care coordination (Case management) _____ Notified: Name ___ Time ___

Endocrinology _____ Notified: Name ___ Time ___

Internal medicine/family practice ___ Notified: Name ___ Time ___

Nephrology _____ Notified: Name ___ Time ___

Social work _____ Notified:
Name ____ Time __
Other _____ Notified:
Name ____ Time __

Education: patient _____ family _____

Dehydration _____

Hypocalcemia _____

Smoking cessation _____

Other _____

Electrolyte Replacement (Adult Dosage)*

Hypocalcemia Intravenous Fluids**

Calcium Gluconate 1 g /100 mL NS IV infused over 1 hour × _____ doses

Calcium Gluconate 2 g /100 mL NS IV infused over 2 hours × _____ doses

*All patients receiving intravenous electrolyte solutions should have continuous heart rate/ cardiac rhythm monitoring while intravenous electrolyte solutions are infused

** Maximum infusion rate is 1 gram Calcium Gluconate per hour

Note: Administration of Calcium Chloride is via a *central line* except in emergency situations so Calcium Gluconate is the IV solution of choice instead of Calcium Chloride since a peripheral IV can be used.

Hypocalcemia Oral Replacement Medications

Calcium Carbonate 1250 mg tablet (Os-cal 500®) PO _____ 1 tablet every _____ hours

Calcium Carbonate 500 mg chewable tablets (Tums®) PO _____ 1 tablet _____ 2 tablets every _____ hours

Laboratory Studies

Recheck ___ calcium ___ ionized calcium ___ hours after IV infusion or PO administration

Recheck ___ sodium ___ potassium ___ magnesium ___ phosphate ___ basic metabolic panel ___ hours after IV infusion or PO administration

Intravenous (IV) Fluids Order Set

Saline cap IV ____

Bolus Normal Saline (NS) IV ___ 250 mL _____ 500 mL ___ 1,000 mL ____ other, infuse over ___ minutes ___ hours

Bolus Lactated Ringer's (LR) IV __ 250 mL __ 500 mL __ 1,000 mL ___ other, infuse over ___ minutes ___ hours

Maintenance NS at __ mL per hour IV

Maintenance LR at __ mL per hour IV

Maintenance Dextrose 5% in Water (D_5W) _____ at __ mL per hour IV

Maintenance Dextrose 5% in ½ Normal Saline (D_5½NS) ____ at __ mL per hour IV

Maintenance Dextrose 5% in Normal Saline (D_5NS) at __ mL per hour IV

Other maintenance ____ at mL per hour IV

Hypokalemia Order Set

Place in ED Observation _____

Diagnosis *HYPOKALEMIA*, _____,

_____, _____

ED Attending _____

Resident (if applicable) _____

Advanced Practice Provider (if applicable)

_____

Allergies: Yes _____ No _____

If yes, what _____,_____,_____,_____,

_____,_____

Vital Signs

Temperature __ Pulse __ Respiration __ BP__ Pulse oximetry ____

__ q 2 hours ___ q 4 hours ___ q 6 hours q ___ hours ___ q shift ___ qd ____ other

Cardiac monitoring (telemetry)* _____

Orthostatic vital signs _____

Continuous pulse oximetry _____

Other _____

Notify Physician if

Temperature (°C) > 38.0° ___ 38.5°___ 39° ___ 40° ____ other _____

Systolic blood pressure (mmHg) ≤ 90 ___ ≥ 160 __ ≥ 180 ___ ≥ 200 __ other _____

Diastolic blood pressure (mmHg) ≥ 120 ____ other _____

Heart rate ≤ 50 ___ ≥ 120 __ ≥ 150 ___ ≥ 200 ___ other ____

Oxygen saturation < 90% _____ other _____

Any change in mental status _____

Any respiratory distress _____

Activity

Up ad lib _____

Assisted _____

Out of bed to chair _____

Bedrest with bathroom privileges _____

Bedrest with bedside commode _____

Bedrest _____

Other _____

Diet

NPO _____

Regular _____

Advance diet as tolerated _____

Clear liquids ____

Dental, mechanical soft _____

Diabetic _____

Formula_____

Full liquids _____

Low added fat/No added salt _____

Low cholesterol _____

Pureed _____

Sodium: 1 gram ___ 2 gram ___ unrestricted____

Per feeding tube _____

Other _____

Nursing Interventions

Weight ___ on admission ___ qd ___ prior to discharge ____ other

Height ____

I & Os _____ routine _____ strict _____

Fluid restriction ___ mL/hour ___ mL/shift ____ mL/24 hour ___ other

Fall precautions _____

Seizure precautions _____

Capillary blood glucose __ × 1 q ___ hours ___ before meals and at bedtime

Respiratory Interventions

Oxygen __ liters nasal cannula __ venti mask at ___ liters per minute _____ other

For sleep apnea qhs __ CPAP ___ BiPAP settings cm H2O ___ inspiratory __ expiratory

Laboratory Tests

CBC _____ with differential

Amylase ___ Lipase___

Basic metabolic panel _____

Blood alcohol level ____
Calcium (total) _____ Calcium (ionized) _____

Cardiac enzymes __ × 1 ___ q 4 hours × 3 __ q 4 hours × 4 __ other
Complete metabolic panel _____
Lactate _____
Liver function tests _____
Magnesium _____
Phosphorus _____
Potassium _____
Pregnancy test (qualitative urine) _____
   Pregnancy test (quantitative blood) _____
Toxicology: blood drug screen ____ urine drug screen ____ drug level for ___
Urinalysis _____ Urine culture _____
Other _____, _____, _____, _____, _____, _____, _____, _____
Repeat _____, _____, _____, _____ in a.m. ___ in ___ hours, q ____ hours × __

Radiology Studies

CXR portable _____
CXR (PA and lateral) _____
Other ___

Cardiac Studies

ECG __ × 1 __ q 4 hours × 3 ___ q 4 hours × 4 ___ other ____ with cardiac enzymes
Echocardiogram (transthoracic) __ with agitated (bubble) study __ without agitated (bubble) study

Consultants

Care coordination (Case management) _____ Notified: Name ___ Time ___
Endocrinology _____ Notified: Name ___ Time ___
Internal medicine/family practice ___ Notified: Name ____ Time ___
Nephrology _____ Notified: Name ____ Time ____
Social work_____ Notified: Name ____ Time ____
Other _____ Notified: Name ____ Time ____

Education: patient _____ family _____

Dehydration _____
Hypokalemia _____

Smoking cessation _____
Other _____

Electrolyte Replacement (Adult Dosage)*
Hypokalemia Intravenous Fluids**

Potassium Chloride 10 mEq/100 mL IV infused over 1 hour × _____ doses
Potassium Chloride 20 mEq/100 mL IV infused over 1 hour × _____ doses
*All patients receiving intravenous electrolyte solutions should have
continuous heart rate/cardiac rhythm monitoring while intravenous electrolyte solutions are infused.
** Maximum infusion rate for potassium chloride is 10–20 mEq/hour.

Hypokalemia Oral Replacement Medications

Potassium Chloride 20 mEq SR tablets (K-dur®) PO __ 1 tablet __ 2 tablets every __ hours × __ doses
Potassium Chloride 20 mEq/15 mL oral solution PO __ 15 mL __ 30 mL every __ hours × ___ doses

Laboratory Studies

Recheck __ potassium __ hours after IV infusion or PO administration
Recheck __ sodium __ magnesium __ calcium __ phosphate __ basic metabolic panel __ hours after IV infusion or PO administration

Intravenous (IV) Fluids Order Set

Saline cap IV ____
Bolus Normal Saline (NS) IV ___ 250 mL _____ 500 mL ___ 1,000 mL ____ other, infuse over ___ minutes ___ hours
Bolus Lactated Ringer's (LR) IV __ 250 mL __ __ 500 mL __ 1,000 mL ___ other, infuse over ___ minutes ___ hours
Maintenance NS at __ mL per hour IV
Maintenance LR at __ mL per hour IV
Maintenance Dextrose 5% in Water (D_5W) _____ at __ mL per hour IV
Maintenance Dextrose 5% in ½ Normal Saline (D_5½NS) ____ at __ mL per hour IV
Maintenance Dextrose 5% in Normal Saline (D_5NS) at __ mL per hour IV
Other maintenance _____ at mL per hour IV

Hypomagnesemia Order Set

Place in ED Observation _____

Diagnosis *HYPOMAGNESEMIA,* _____,

_____, _____

ED Attending _____

Resident (if applicable) _____

Advanced Practice Provider (if applicable)

_____

Allergies: Yes _____ No _____

If yes, what _____, _____, _____, _____,

_____, _____

Vital Signs

Temperature __ Pulse __ Respiration __ BP__
Pulse oximetry ____

__ q 2 hours ___ q 4 hours ___ q 6 hours q ___
hours ___ q shift ___ qd ____ other

Cardiac monitoring (telemetry)* _____

Orthostatic vital signs _____

Continuous pulse oximetry _____

Other _____

Notify Physician if

Temperature (°C) > 38.0° ____ 38.5°___ 39° ___
40° ____ other _____

Systolic blood pressure (mm Hg) ≤ 90 ___ ≥
160 ___ ≥ 180 ___ ≥ 200 __ other _____

Diastolic blood pressure (mm Hg) ≥ 120 ____
other _____

Heart rate ≤ 50 ___ ≥ 120 __ ≥ 150 ___ ≥
200 ___ other ____

Oxygen saturation < 90% _____ other _____

Any change in mental status _____

Any respiratory distress _____

Activity

Up ad lib _____

Assisted _____

Out of bed to chair _____

Bedrest with bathroom privileges _____

Bedrest with bedside commode _____

Bedrest _____

Other _____

Diet

NPO _____

Regular _____

Advance diet as tolerated _____

Clear liquids ____

Dental, mechanical soft _____

Diabetic _____

Formula _____

Full liquids _____

Low added fat/No added salt _____

Low cholesterol ____

Pureed _____

Sodium: 1 gram ___ 2 gram ___
unrestricted____

Per feeding tube _____

Other _____

Nursing Interventions

Weight ___ on admission ___ qd ___ prior to
discharge ____ other

Height ____

I & Os _____ routine _____ strict _____

Fluid restriction ___ mL/hour ___ mL/shift
____ mL/24 hour ___ other

Fall precautions _____

Seizure precautions _____

Capillary blood glucose __ × 1 q ___ hours
_____ before meals and at bedtime

Respiratory Interventions

Oxygen __ liters nasal cannula __ venti mask at
___ liters per minute _____ other

For sleep apnea qhs __ CPAP ___ BiPAP
settings cm H_2O ___ inspiratory __
expiratory

Laboratory Tests

CBC _____ with differential

Amylase ___ Lipase___

Basic metabolic panel _____

Blood alcohol level ____

Calcium (total) _____ Calcium (ionized) _____

Cardiac enzymes __ × 1 ___ q 4 hours × 3 __ q
4 hours × 4 __ other

Complete metabolic panel_____

Lactate _____

Liver function tests _____

Magnesium _____

Phosphorus _____

Potassium _____

Pregnancy test (qualitative urine) _____
Pregnancy test (quantitative blood) _____

Toxicology: blood drug screen ____ urine drug screen ____ drug level for ___

Urinalysis _____ Urine culture _____

Other _____, _____, _____, _____, _____, _____, _____, _____

Repeat _____, _____, _____ in a.m. ___ in ___ hours, q ___ hours × ___

Radiology Studies

CXR portable _____

CXR (PA and lateral) _____

Other ____

Cardiac Studies

ECG __ × 1__ q 4 hours × 3 ___ q 4 hours × 4 ___ other _____ with cardiac enzymes

Echocardiogram (transthoracic) __ with agitated (bubble) study __ without agitated (bubble) study

Consultants

Care coordination (Case management)_____ Notified: Name ___ Time ___

Endocrinology _____ Notified: Name ___ Time ___ ___

Internal medicine/family practice ___ Notified: Name ____ Time ___

Nephrology _____ Notified: Name ____ Time ___

Social work _____ Notified: Name ____ Time ___

Other _____ Notified: Name ____ Time ___

Education: patient _____ family _____

Dehydration _____

Hypomagnesemia _____

Smoking cessation _____

Other _____

Electrolyte Replacement (Adult Dosage)*

Hypomagnesemia Intravenous Fluids**

Magnesium Sulfate 1 gram/100 mL D_5W IV infused over 1 hour × _____ doses

Magnesium Sulfate 2 gram/100 mL D_5W IV infused over 1 hour × _____ doses

*All patients receiving intravenous electrolyte solutions should be have continuous heart rate/cardiac rhythm monitoring while intravenous electrolyte solutions are infused

** Maximum infusion rate is 1 gram magnesium sulfate per hour

Hypomagnesemia Oral Replacement Medications

Magnesium Oxide 400 mg tablet (Mag-ox®) PO __ 1 tab __ 2 tab every__ hours × __ doses

Magnesium Chloride 64 mg tablet (Slow-mag®) PO __ 1 tab __ 2 tab every ___ hours × __ doses

Laboratory Studies

Recheck __ magnesium __ hours after IV infusion or PO administration

Recheck __ sodium __ potassium __ calcium __ phosphate __ basic metabolic panel __ hours after IV infusion or PO administration

Intravenous (IV) Fluids Order Set

Saline cap IV ____

Bolus Normal Saline (NS) IV ___ 250 mL _____ 500 mL ___ 1,000 mL _____ other, infuse over ___ minutes ___ hours

Bolus Lactated Ringer's (LR) IV __ 250 mL __ __ 500 mL __ 1,000 mL ___ other, infuse over ___ minutes ___ hours

Maintenance NS at __ mL per hour IV

Maintenance LR at __ mL per hour IV

Maintenance Dextrose 5% in Water (D5W) _____ at __ mL per hour IV

Maintenance Dextrose 5% in ½ Normal Saline (D5½NS) ____ at __ mL per hour IV

Maintenance Dextrose 5% in Normal Saline (D5NS) at __ mL per hour IV

Other maintenance ____ at mL per hour IV

Hypophosphatemia Order Set

Place in ED Observation _____

Diagnosis *HYPOPHOSPATEMIA*, _____, _____, _____

ED Attending _____

Resident (if applicable) _____

Advanced Practice Provider (if applicable) _____

Allergies: Yes _____ No _____

If yes, what _____, _____, _____, _____, _____, _____

Vital Signs

Temperature __ Pulse __ Respiration __ BP__
Pulse oximetry ____
__ q 2 hours ___ q 4 hours ___ q 6 hours q ___
hours ___ q shift ___ qd ____ other
Cardiac monitoring (telemetry)* _____
Orthostatic vital signs _____
Continuous pulse oximetry _____
Other _____

Notify Physician if

Temperature (°C) > 38.0° ___ 38.5°___ 39° ___
40° ____ other _____
Systolic blood pressure (mm Hg) ≤ 90 ___ ≥
160 __ ≥ 180 ___ ≥ 200 __ other _____
Diastolic blood pressure (mm Hg) ≥ 120 ____
other _____
Heart rate ≤ 50 ___ ≥ 120 __ ≥ 150 ___ ≥
200 ___ other ____
Oxygen saturation < 90% _____
other _____
Any change in mental status _____
Any respiratory distress _____

Activity

Up ad lib _____
Assisted _____
Out of bed to chair _____
Bedrest with bathroom privileges _____
Bedrest with bedside commode _____
Bedrest _____
Other _____

Diet

NPO _____
Regular _____
Advance diet as tolerated _____
Clear liquids ____
Dental, mechanical soft _____
Diabetic _____
Formula _____
Full liquids _____
Low added fat/No added salt _____
Low cholesterol ____
Pureed _____
Sodium: 1 gram ___ 2 gram ___
unrestricted____
Per feeding tube _____
Other _____

Nursing Interventions

Weight ___ on admission ___ qd ___ prior to
discharge ____ other
Height ____
I & Os _____ routine _____ strict _____
Fluid restriction ___ mL/hour ___ mL/shift
____ mL/24 hour ___ other
Fall precautions _____
Seizure precautions _____
Capillary blood glucose __ × 1 q ___ hours
_____ before meals and at bedtime

Respiratory Interventions

Oxygen __ liters nasal cannula __ venti mask at
___ liters per minute _____ other
For sleep apnea qhs ___ CPAP ___ BiPAP
settings cm H_2O ___ inspiratory __
expiratory

Laboratory Tests

CBC _____ with differential
Amylase ___ Lipase___
Basic metabolic panel _____
Blood alcohol level ____
Calcium (total) _____ Calcium (ionized)
_____
Cardiac enzymes __ × 1 ___ q 4 hours × 3 __ q
4 hours × 4 ___ other
Complete metabolic panel _____
Lactate _____
Liver function tests _____
Magnesium _____
Phosphorus _____
Potassium _____
Pregnancy test (qualitative urine) _____
Pregnancy test (quantitative blood)
_____
Toxicology: blood drug screen ____ urine drug
screen _____ drug level for ___
Urinalysis _____ Urine culture _____
Other _____, _____, _____, _____,
_____, _____, _____, _____
Repeat _____, _____, _____, _____, _____ in a.
m. ___ in ___ hours

Radiology Studies

CXR portable _____
CXR (PA and lateral) _____
Other ____

Cardiac Studies

ECG __ × 1__ q 4 hours × 3 ___ q 4 hours × 4 ___ other ____ with cardiac enzymes

Echocardiogram (transthoracic) __ with agitated (bubble) study __ without agitated (bubble) study

Consultants

Care coordination (Case management)_____
Notified: Name ___ Time ___

Endocrinology _____ Notified:
Name ___ Time ___

Internal medicine/family practice ___ Notified:
Name ____ Time ___

Nephrology _____ Notified:
Name ____ Time ____

Social work _____ Notified:
Name ____ Time ____

Other _____ Notified:
Name ____ Time _____

Education: patient _____ family _____

Dehydration _____
Hypophosphatemia _____
Smoking cessation _____
Other _____

Electrolyte Replacement (Adult Dosage)*

Hypophosphatemia Intravenous Fluids**

Sodium Phosphates 15 mmol /250 mL NS IV infused over 4–6 hours × 1 dose ____ (contains 4 mEq of sodium for each 3 mmol of phosphorus)

Sodium Phosphates 30 mmol /250 mL NS IV infused over 4–6 hours × 1 dose ____ (contains 4 mEq of sodium for each 3 mmol of phosphorus)

Potassium Phosphates 15 mmol/250 mL NS IV infused over 4–6 hours × 1 dose _____ (contains 4.4 mEq of potassium for each 3 mmol of phosphorus)

Potassium Phosphates 30 mmol/250 mL NS IV infused over 4–6 hours × 1 dose _____

(contains 4.4 mEq of potassium for each 3 mmol of phosphorus)

*All patients receiving intravenous electrolyte solutions should have continuous heart rate/cardiac rhythm monitoring while intravenous electrolyte solutions are infused.

** All phosphate solutions must be infused over 4–6 hours.

Hypophosphatemia Oral Replacement Medications

K-phos® neutral tablets (Potassium and Sodium Phosphates) PO____ 250 mg ____ 500 mg every ____ hours × ____ doses (each 250 mg tab contains 8 mmol of phosphorus)

Neutra-phos® packets (Potassium and Sodium Phosphates) PO____ 1 packet ____

2 packets every ____ hours × ____ doses (each packet contains 8 mmol of phosphorus)

Laboratory Studies

Recheck __ phosphate __ hours after IV infusion or PO administration

Recheck __ sodium __ potassium __ calcium __ magnesium __ basic metabolic panel __ hours after IV infusion or PO administration

Intravenous (IV) Fluids Order Set

Saline cap IV ____

Bolus Normal Saline (NS) IV ___ 250 mL ____ 500 mL ___ 1,000 mL ____ other, infuse over ___ minutes ___ hours

Bolus Lactated Ringer's (LR) IV __ 250 mL _ __ 500 mL __ 1,000 mL ___ other, infuse over ___ minutes ___ hours

Maintenance NS at __ mL per hour IV

Maintenance LR at __ mL per hour IV

Maintenance Dextrose 5% in Water (D_5W) ____ at __ mL per hour IV

Maintenance Dextrose 5% in ½ Normal Saline (D_5½NS) ____ at __ mL per hour IV

Maintenance Dextrose 5% in Normal Saline (D_5NS) at __ mL per hour IV

Other maintenance ____ at mL per hour IV

Chapter

91

Adult Order Sets
Trauma

Sharon E. Mace, MD, FACEP, FAAP

Abdominal Trauma Order Set

Place in Emergency Department (ED)
Observation _____
Diagnosis ***ABDOMINAL TRAUMA,***

_____, _____, _____

ED Attending _____
Resident (if applicable) _____
Advanced Practice Provider (if applicable)

_____

Allergies: Yes _____ No _____

If yes, what _____, _____, _____, _____,

_____, _____

Vital Signs

Temperature __ Pulse __ Respiration __ BP__
Pulse oximetry _____
__ q 2 hours ___ q 4 hours ___ q 6 hours q ___
hours ___ q shift ___ qd
____ other
Cardiac monitoring (telemetry) _____
Neurologic checks __ q 2 hours __ q 4 hours __
q 6 hours q __hours __ q shift __ qd __ other
Orthostatic vital signs _____
Continuous pulse oximetry _____
Vascular checks __ q 2 hours __ q 4 hours __
q 6 hours q __hours __ q shift __ qd __ other
Other _____

Activity

Cervical spine immobilization ___
Up ad lib _____
Assisted _____
Out of bed to chair _____
Bedrest with bathroom privileges _____
Bedrest with bedside commode _____
Bedrest _____
Other _____

Diet

NPO _____
Regular _____
Advance diet as tolerated _____
Clear liquids ____
Dental, mechanical soft _____
Diabetic _____
Formula_____
Full liquids _____
Low added fat/No added salt _____
Low cholesterol ____
Pureed _____
Sodium: 1 gram ___ 2 gram ___
unrestricted____
Per feeding tube _____
Other _____

Nursing Interventions

Weight ___ on admission ___ qd ___ prior to
discharge ____ other
Height ____
I & Os _____ routine _____ strict _____
Fluid restriction ___ mL/hour ___ mL/shift
____ mL/24 hour ___ other
Fall precautions _____
Seizure precautions _____
Capillary blood glucose __ × 1 q ___ hours ___
before meals and at bedtime
Foley catheter ___ Straight cath for urine

_____

Nasogastric tube placement ____ to intermittent
suction ___ to continuous suction
Elevate head of bed to 30 ° ____

Respiratory Interventions

Oxygen __ liters nasal cannula __ venti mask at
___ liters per minute _____ other
Wean oxygen as tolerated without dyspnea,
stridor or oxygen saturation < 90% ____

Peak flow __ on admission ___ prior to discharge ___ pre and post aerosols

Sleep apnea qhs __ CPAP BiPAP settings cm H2O ___ inspiratory __ expiratory

Incentive spirometry __ q 2 hours __ q 4 hours __ q 6 hours q __ hours __ q shift __ qd __ other

Laboratory Tests

Amylase ___ Lipase ___

Arterial blood gas ___ on room air ___ on other FiO2 ____

Basic metabolic panel _____

Blood alcohol level ____

Cardiac enzymes __ × 1, ___ q 4 hours × 3, __ q 4 hours × 4, __ other

CBC _____ with differential, ___ repeat in a. m., q ___ hours × ___

Complete metabolic panel _____

Creatinine phosphokinase (total) (total CPK) __ × 1, __ repeat in a.m., q __ hours × ___

CK-MB (creatinine kinase – myocardial band) ___ repeat in a.m., q ___ hours × ___

Hemoglobin/hematocrit _____ repeat in a.m., q ___ hours × ___

Lactate _____ repeat in a.m., q ___ hours × ___

Liver function tests _____

Pregnancy test (qualitative urine) _____ Pregnancy test (quantitative blood) _____

Toxicology: blood drug screen ____ urine drug screen ____ drug level for ___

Troponin _____ × 1, ___ repeat in a.m., q ___ hours × ____

Type and screen _____

Urinalysis _____ Urine culture _____

Other _____, _____, _____, _____, _____, _____, _____, _____

Repeat _____, _____, _____ in a.m. ___ in ___ hours, q _____ hours × ___

Radiology Studies

Acute abdominal series ____

CXR portable _____

CXR (PA and lateral) _____

KUB (Kidneys, ureters, bladder) X-ray _____

Spine X-rays: cervical ___ thoracic __ lumbar ____

CT scan abdomen/pelvis ____ with contrast: __ IV __ po ___ pr ___

CT scan chest _____ with IV contrast __

MRI _____

Ultrasound RUQ _____

Ultrasound Pelvis _____

Ultrasound (FAST) exam _____

Other _____, _____, _____

Repeat _____, _____, _____

Cardiac Studies

ECG __ × 1__ q 4 hours × 3 ___ q 4 hours × 4 ___ other _____ with cardiac enzymes

Echocardiogram (transthoracic) __ with agitated (bubble) study __ without agitated (bubble) study

Consultants

Care coordination (Case management) _____Notified: Name _____ Time ____

Trauma/General surgery _____ Notified: Name _____ Time ____

Social work _____ Notified: Name _____ Time ____

Other _____ Notified: Name _____ Time _____

Medications for Abdominal Trauma (Adult Dosage)

Analgesics

Acetaminophen (Paracetamol) (Tylenol®) 325 mg tab __ 1 tab __ 1–2 tabs __ 2 tabs PO __ q 4 hours __ q 6 hours ___ prn pain __ prn fever (maximum 4 g daily)

____ If unable to take tablet formulation, may give suspension

____ If unable to take PO, may give suppository PR __325 mg __ 650 mg __ q 4 hours __ q 6 hours

____ IV ___ mg __ q 4 hours __ q 6 hours __ prn pain __ prn fever (maximum adult dose: if weight < 50 kg is 15 mg/kg up to 750 mg for a single dose, 75 mg/kg up to 3750 mg for daily dose; if weight > 50 kg is 650 mg q 4 hours or 1000 mg q 6 hours up to 1000 mg for a single dose and 4000 mg for a daily dose)

Acetaminophen-Hydrocodone (Vicodin®) 300 mg/5 mg tabs __ 1 tab __ 1-2 tabs __ 2 tabs PO __ q 4 hours __ q 6 hours ___ prn pain (maximum 4 grams daily based on acetaminophen dose)

Acetaminophen-Oxycodone (Endocet®, Percocet®, Roxicet®) 325 mg/5 mg tab __ 1 tab __1–2 tabs __ 2 tabs PO __ q 4 hours __ q 6 hours ____ prn pain (maximum 4 grams daily based on acetaminophen dose)

Hydromorphone (Dilaudid®) __ 0.5 mg __ 1 mg __ 2 mg __ mg __ IV __ q 2 hours __ q 4 hours __ q 6 hours q ___ hours __ prn pain

Ibuprofen (Advil®, Motrin®) __ 400 mg __ 600 mg __ 800 mg PO __ q 4 hours __ q 6 hours __ q 8 hours ___ prn pain

Ketorolac (Toradol®) __ 30 mg IV __ q 6 hours __ prn pain (maximum 120 mg daily)

Morphine __ 0.5 mg __ 1 mg __ 2 mg __ 4 mg __ mg ___ IV __ q 2 hours __ q 4 hours __ q 6 hours q ___ hours __ prn pain

Tramadol (Ultram®) __ 50 mg __ 100 mg PO __ q 4 hours __ q 6 hours __ prn pain (maximum 400 mg daily)

Other _____, _____, _____, _____, _____

Antiemetics

Chlorpromazine (Thorazine®) __ 10 mg PO __ 25 mg PO __ q 4 hours __ q 6 hours __ 25 mg __ 50 mg __ IV __ IM __ q 4 hours __ q 6 hours __ prn nausea/vomiting

Metoclopramide (Reglan®) __10 mg __ IV __ IM __ PO __ q 6 hours __ other __ prn nausea/vomiting

Ondansetron (Zofran®) __ 4 mg __ 8 mg __ IV __ PO __ q 6 hours ___ other __ prn nausea/vomiting ___

Prochlorperazine (Compazine®) __ 5 mg __ 10 mg __ IV __ IM __ PO __ q 4 hours __ q 6 hours (maximum dose IV/IM/PO 40 mg per day) ___ 25 mg PR bid __ prn nausea/vomiting

Promethazine (Phenergan®) __ 12.5 mg __ 25 mg __ IV__ IM __ PO __ PR __ q 4 hours __ q 6 hours ___ prn nausea/vomiting

Trimethobenzamide (Tigan®) __ 200 mg IM __ 300 mg PO ___ q 6 hours ___ prn nausea/vomiting

Intravenous Fluids

Saline cap IV ____

Bolus Normal Saline (NS) IV ___ 250 mL __ 500 mL ___ 1,000 mL ____ other, infuse over ___ minutes

Bolus Lactated Ringer's (LR) IV __ 250 mL __ 500 mL __ 1,000 mL __ other, infuse over ___ minutes

Maintenance NS at __ mL per hour IV

Maintenance LR at __ mL per hour IV

Maintenance Dextrose 5% in Water (D$_5$W) at __ mL per hour IV

Maintenance Dextrose 5% in ½ Normal Saline (D$_5$½NS) at __ mL per hour IV

Maintenance Dextrose 5% in Normal Saline (D$_5$NS) at __ mL per hour IV

Other _____ at mL per hour

Education: patient _____ family _____

Abdominal trauma____

Smoking cessation_____

Other _____

Incentive spirometry, treatment of pain, evaluation to rule out other injuries and to monitor for associated injuries, obtaining additional tests (laboratory and radiology), administering IV fluids, repeating the examination and studies, such as FAST exam, (initial FAST exam is usually done in the emergency department), obtaining consults, etc. can be part of the management. Trauma order sets and protocols, like most protocols and order sets, should be done with the concurrence of the respective service/subspecialty, in this case with the trauma service/general surgeons.

Isolated Chest Injury/ Rib Fracture Order Set

Place in Emergency Department (ED) Observation _____
Diagnosis *ISOLATED CHEST INJURY/RIB FRACTURE* _____, _____, _____
ED Attending _____
Resident (if applicable) _____
Advanced Practice Provider (if applicable) _____

Allergies: Yes _____ No _____

If yes, what _____, _____, _____, _____, _____, _____

Vital Signs

Temperature __ Pulse __ Respiration __ BP__ Pulse oximetry ____
__ q 2 hours ____ q 4 hours ____ q 6 hours q __ hours ____ q shift ____ qd ____ other
Cardiac monitoring (telemetry) _____
Neurologic checks __ q 2 hours __ q 4 hours __ q 6 hours q __hours __ q shift __ qd __ others
Orthostatic vital signs _____
Continous pulse oximetry _____
Vascular checks __ q 2 hours __ q 4 hours __ q 6 hours q __hours __ q shift __ qd __ other
Other _____

Notify Physician if

Temperature (°C) > 38.0° ___ 38.5°___ 39° ___ 40° ____ other _____
Systolic blood pressure (mmHg) ≤ 90 ___ ≥ 160 __ ≥ 180 ___ ≥ 200 __ other ____
Diastolic blood pressure (mmHg) ≥ 120 ____ other ____
Heart rate ≤ 50 ___ ≥ 120 __ ≥ 150 ___ ≥ 200 ___ other ____
Oxygen saturation < 90% _____ other ____
Any change in mental status _____
Any respiratory distress _____

Activity

Cervical spine immobilization ___
Up ad lib _____
Assisted _____
Out of bed to chair _____
Bedrest with bathroom privileges _____
Bedrest with bedside commode _____
Bedrest _____
Other _____

Diet

NPO _____
Regular _____
Advance diet as tolerated _____
Clear liquids ____
Dental, mechanical soft _____
Diabetic _____
Formula _____
Full liquids _____
Low added fat/No added salt _____
Low cholesterol ____
Pureed _____
Sodium: 1 gram ___ 2 gram ___ unrestricted ____
Per feeding tube _____
Other _____

Nursing Interventions

Weight ___ on admission ___ qd ___ prior to discharge ____ other
Height ____
I & Os _____ routine _____ strict ____
Fluid restriction ___ mL/hour ___ mL/shift ____ mL/24 hour ___ other
Fall precautions _____
Seizure precautions _____
Capillary blood glucose __ × 1 q __ hours ____ before meals and at bedtime
Elevate head of bed at 30° _____

Respiratory Interventions

Oxygen __ liters nasal cannula __ venti mask at ___ liters per minute _____ other
Wean oxygen as tolerated without dyspnea, stridor or oxygen saturation < 90% ____
Peak flow __ on admission ___ prior to discharge ___ pre and post aerosols
Sleep apnea qhs __ CPAP BiPAP settings cm H_2O ____ inspiratory __ expiratory
Incentive spirometry __ q 2 hours __ q 4 hours __ q 6 hours q __ hours __ q shift __ qd __ other ___

Laboratory Tests

Amylase ___ Lipase___

Arterial blood gas ___ on room air ___ on other FiO2 ____

Basic metabolic panel _____

Blood alcohol level ____

Cardiac enzymes __ × 1, ___ q 4 hours × 3, __ q 4 hours × 4, __ other

CBC _____ with differential, ___ repeat in a. m., q ___ hours × ___

Complete metabolic panel _____

Creatinine phosphokinase (total) (total CPK) __ × 1, __ repeat in a.m., q __ hours × ____

CK-MB (creatinine kinase – myocardial band) ___ × 1, repeat in a.m., q ___ hours × ____

Hemoglobin/hematocrit __ × 1, ____ repeat in a.m., q ___ hours × ____

Lactate __ × 1, ___ repeat in a.m., q ___ hours × ___

Liver function tests _____

Pregnancy test (qualitative urine) _____ Pregnancy test (quantitative blood) _____

Toxicology: blood drug screen ____ urine drug screen ____ drug level for ____

Troponin __ × 1, _____ repeat in a.m., q ___ hours × ___

Type and screen _____

Urinalysis _____ Urine culture _____

Other _____, _____, _____, _____, _____, _____, _____, _____

Repeat _____, _____, _____ in a.m., repeat ___ in ___ hours, q ___ hours × ____

Radiology Studies

Acute abdominal series ____

CXR portable _____

CXR (PA and lateral) _____

Spine X-rays: cervical ___ thoracic __ lumbar ____

CT scan chest _____ with IV contrast __

CT scan abdomen/pelvis ____ with contrast: __ IV __ po ___ pr ___

MRI _____

Ultrasound (FAST exam) _____

Ultrasound _____

Other _____, _____, _____

Repeat CXR (portable) ___ CXR (PA and lateral) ___ Other ____

Cardiac Studies

ECG __ × 1,__ q 4 hours × 3, ___ q 4 hours × 4, ___ other, ____ with cardiac enzymes

Echocardiogram (transthoracic) __ with agitated (bubble) study__ without agitated (bubble) study

Consultants

Care coordination (Case management)_____ Notified: Name _____ Time ___

Trauma/General surgery _____ Notified: Name _____ Time _____

Cardiology _____ Notified: Name _____ Time _____

Cardiothoracic Surgery _____ Notified: Name _____ Time ____

Social work _____ Notified: Name _____ Time ____

Other _____ Notified: Name _____ Time ____

Medications for Isolated Chest Trauma/Rib Fracture (Adult Dosage)

Analgesics

Acetaminophen* (Paracetamol) (Tylenol®) 325 mg tab __1 tab __1–2 tabs __ 2 tabs PO __ q 4 hours __ q 6 hours ___ prn pain ___ prn fever (maximum 4 g daily)

____ If unable to take tablet formulation, may give suspension

____ If unable to take PO, may give suppository PR __ 325 mg __ 650 mg __ q 4 hours __ q 6 hours

____ IV ___ mg __ q 4 hours __ q 6 hours __ prn pain __ prn fever (maximum adult dose: if weight < 50 kg is 15 mg/kg up to 750 mg for a single dose, 75 mg/kg up to 3750 mg for daily dose; if weight > 50 kg is 650 mg q 4 hours or 1000 mg q 6 hours up to 1000 mg for a single dose and 4000 mg for a daily dose)

Acetaminophen-Hydrocodone (Vicodin®) 300 mg/5 mg tabs __1 tab __1–2 tabs __ 2 tabs PO __ q 4 hours __ q 6 hours ___ prn pain (maximum 4 grams daily based on acetaminophen dose)

Acetaminophen-Oxycodone (Endocet®, Percocet®, Roxicet®) 325 mg/5 mg tab __ 1 tab __1–2 tabs __ 2 tabs PO __ q 4 hours __ q 6 hours ___ prn pain (maximum 4 grams daily based on acetaminophen dose)

Hydromorphone (Dilaudid®) __ 0.5 mg __ 1 mg __ 2 mg __ mg __ IV __ q 2 hours __ q 4 hours __ q 6 hours q ___ hours __ prn pain

Ibuprofen (Advil®, Motrin®) __ 400 mg __ 600 mg __ 800 mg PO __ q 4 hours __ q 6 hours __ q 8 hours ___ prn pain

Ketorolac (Toradol®) __ 30 mg IV __ q 6 hours __ prn pain (maximum 120 mg daily)

Morphine __ 0.5 mg __ 1 mg __ 2 mg __ 4 mg __ mg ___ IV __ q 2 hours __ q 4 hours __ q 6 hours q ___ hours __ prn pain

Tramadol (Ultram®) __ 50 mg __ 100 mg PO __ q 4 hours __ q 6 hours __ prn pain (maximum 400 mg daily)

Other _____, _____, _____, _____, _____

Antiemetics

Chlorpromazine (Thorazine®) __ 10 mg PO __ 25 mg PO __ q 4 hours __ q 6 hours __ 25 mg __ 50 mg __ IV __ IM __ q 4 hours __ q 6 hours __ prn nausea/vomiting

Metoclopramide (Reglan®) __ 10 mg __ IV __ IM __ PO __ q 6 hours __ other __ prn nausea/vomiting

Ondansetron (Zofran®) __ 4 mg __ 8 mg __IV __PO __ q 6 hours ___ other __ prn nausea/vomiting ___

Prochlorperazine (Compazine®) __ 5 mg __ 10 mg __ IV __ IM __ PO __ q 4 hours __ q 6 hours (maximum dose IV/IM/PO 40 mg per day) ___ 25 mg PR bid __ prn nausea/vomiting

Promethazine (Phenergan®) __ 12.5 mg __ 25 mg __ IV__ IM __ PO __ PR __ q 4 hours __ q 6 hours ___ prn nausea/vomiting

Trimethobenzamide (Tigan®) __ 200 mg IM __ 300 mg PO ___ q 6 hours ___ prn nausea/vomiting

Intravenous Fluids

Saline cap IV ____

Bolus Normal Saline (NS) IV ___ 250 mL __ 500 mL ___ 1,000 mL ____ other, infuse over ___ minutes

Bolus Lactated Ringer's (LR) IV __ 250 mL __ 500 mL __ 1,000 mL __ other, infuse over ___ minutes

Maintenance NS at __ mL per hour IV

Maintenance LR at __ mL per hour IV

Maintenance Dextrose 5% in Water (D_5W) at __ mL per hour IV

Maintenance Dextrose 5% in ½ Normal Saline ($D_5½NS$) at __ mL per hour IV

Maintenance Dextrose 5% in Normal Saline (D_5NS) at __ mL per hour IV

Other _____ at mL per hour

Education: patient _____ family _____

Rib fractures ____

Smoking cessation _____

Other _____

Incentive spirometry, treatment of pain, evaluation to rule out other injuries and to monitor for associated injuries, obtaining additional tests (laboratory, cardiac [such as: cardiac enzymes, ECGs, echocardiogram] and radiology), consults, administering IV fluids, etc. can be part of the management of isolated chest trauma/rib fractures. Trauma order sets and protocols, like most protocols and order sets, should be done with the concurrence of the respective service/subspecialty, in this case with the trauma service/general surgeons.

Extremity Trauma Order Set

Place in Emergency Department (ED)
Observation _____
Diagnosis *EXTREMITY TRAUMA,*

_____, _____, _____

ED Attending _____
Resident (if applicable) _____
Advanced Practice Provider (if applicable)

_____

Allergies: Yes _____ No _____

If yes, what _____,_____,_____,_____,

_____,_____

Vital Signs

Temperature __ Pulse __ Respiration __ BP__
Pulse oximetry ____
__ q 2 hours ___ q 4 hours ___ q 6 hours q ___
hours ___ q shift ___ qd ____ other
Cardiac monitoring (telemetry) _____
Neurologic checks __ q 2 hours __ q 4 hours __
q 6 hours q __hours __ q shift __ qd __ other
Orthostatic vital signs _____
Continuous pulse oximetry _____
Vascular checks __ q 2 hours __ q 4 hours __
q 6 hours q __ hours __ q shift __ qd __ other
Other _____

Notify Physician if

Temperature (°C) > 38.0° ____ 38.5°____ 39° ____
40° ____ other _____
Systolic blood pressure (mmHg) ≤ 90 ___
≥ 160 __ ≥ 180 ___ ≥ 200 __ other _____
Diastolic blood pressure (mmHg) ≥ 120 _____
other _____
Heart rate ≤ 50 ___ ≥ 120 __ ≥ 150 ___
≥ 200 ___ other ____
Oxygen saturation < 90% _____ other _____
Any change in mental status _____
Any respiratory distress _____
Any new or worsening change in extremity (such
as color: pale or cyanotic, decreased capillary
fill, diminished or absent pulses, increased
pain, numbness or paresthesias) ____

Activity

Cervical spine immobilization ___
Up ad lib _____
Assisted _____

Out of bed to chair _____
Bedrest with bathroom privileges _____
Bedrest with bedside commode _____
Bedrest _____
Other _____

Diet

NPO _____
Regular _____
Advance diet as tolerated _____
Clear liquids ____
Dental, mechanical soft _____
Diabetic _____
Formula _____
Full liquids _____
Low added fat/No added salt _____
Low cholesterol ____
Pureed _____
Sodium: 1 gram ___ 2 gram ___
unrestricted____
Per feeding tube _____
Other _____

Nursing Interventions

Weight ___ on admission ___ qd ___ prior to
discharge _____ other
Height ____
I & Os _____ routine _____ strict _____
Fluid restriction ___ mL/hour ___ mL/shift
____ mL/24 hour ___ other
Fall precautions _____
Seizure precautions _____
Capillary blood glucose __ × 1 q ___ hours
____ before meals and at bedtime
Measure circumference of extremity _____
q ___ hours
Measurement of tissue pressure for
compartment syndrome _____
Wound care with dressing changes _____
Elevation of extremity _____

Respiratory Interventions

Oxygen __ liters nasal cannula __
venti mask at ___ liters per minute
_____ other
Wean oxygen as tolerated without dyspnea,
stridor or oxygen saturation < 90% ____
Peak flow __ on admission ___ prior to
discharge ___ pre and post aerosols

Sleep apnea qhs __ CPAP BiPAP settings cm
  H_2O ___ inspiratory __ expiratory
Incentive spirometry __ q 2 hours __ q 4 hours __
  q 6 hours q __ hours __ q shift __ qd __ other

Laboratory Tests

Amylase ___ Lipase ___
Arterial blood gas ___ on room air ___ on
  other FiO2 ____
Basic metabolic panel _____
Blood alcohol level ____
Cardiac enzymes __ × 1, ___ q 4 hours × 3, __
  q 4 hours × 4, __ other
CBC ___ with differential, ___ repeat in a.m.,
  q __ hours × ___
Complete metabolic panel _____
Creatinine phosphokinase (total) (total CPK)
  __ × 1, __ repeat in a.m.,
q ___ hours × ___
CK-MB (creatinine kinase – myocardial band)
  __ × 1, q ___ hours × ___
Hemoglobin/hematocrit __ × 1, ____ repeat in
  a.m., q ___ hours × ___
Lactate __ × 1, ____ repeat in a.m., q ___ hours
  × ___
Liver function tests _____
Pregnancy test (qualitative urine) _____
  Pregnancy test (quantitative blood) _____
Toxicology: blood drug screen ____ urine drug
  screen ____ drug level for ___
Troponin __ × 1, ____ repeat in a.m., q ___
  hours × ___
Type and screen _____
Urinalysis _____ Urine culture _____
Other _____, _____, _____, _____,
  _____, _____, _____, _____
Repeat _____, _____, _____ in a.m., repeat
  ___, ___, ___ q ___ hours × ___

Radiology Studies

Extremity X-rays: _____, _____, _____, _____
CT scan
MRI _____
Ultrasound _____
Repeat ____
Other _____, _____, _____

Cardiac Studies

ECG __ × 1 __ q 4 hours × 3 ___ q 4 hours ×
  4 ___ other ____ with cardiac enzymes

Echocardiogram (transthoracic) __ with
  agitated (bubble) study__ without agitated
  (bubble) study

Consultants

Care coordination (Case management)
  _____ Notified: Name _____
  Time ____
Hand surgery _____ Notified:
  Name _____ Time ___
Orthopedic _____ Notified:
  Name _____ Time ____
Plastic surgery _____ Notified:
  Name _____ Time ___
Social work _____ Notified:
  Name _____ Time ____
Trauma/General Surgery _____ Notified:
  Name _____ Time ___
Other _____ Notified:
  Name _____ Time ____

Medications for Extremity Trauma (Adult Dosage)

Analgesics

Acetaminophen (Paracetamol) (Tylenol®)
  325 mg tab __ 1 tab __ 1–2 tabs __ 2 tabs PO
  __ q 4 hours __ q 6 hours ___ prn pain ___
  prn fever (maximum 4 g daily)
____ If unable to take tablet formulation, may
  give suspension
____ If unable to take PO, may give suppository
  PR __325 mg __ 650 mg __ q 4 hours __ q
  6 hours
____IV ___ mg __ q 4 hours __ q 6 hours __ prn
  pain __ prn fever (maximum adult dose: if
  weight < 50 kg is 15 mg/kg up to 750 mg for a
  single dose, 75 mg/kg up to 3750 mg for daily
  dose; if weight > 50 kg is 650 mg q 4 hours or
  1000 mg q 6 hours up to 1000 mg for a single
  dose and 4000 mg for a daily dose)
Acetaminophen-Hydrocodone (Vicodin®) 300
  mg/5 mg tabs __ 1 tab __ 1–2 tabs __ 2 tabs
  PO __ q 4 hours __ q 6 hours ___ prn pain
  (maximum 4 grams daily based on
  acetaminophen dose)
Acetaminophen-Oxycodone (Endocet®,
  Percocet®, Roxicet®) 325 mg/5 mg tab __
  1 tab __1–2 tabs __ 2 tabs PO __ q 4 hours __
  q 6 hours ___ prn pain (maximum 4 grams
  daily based on acetaminophen dose)

Hydromorphone (Dilaudid®) __ 0.5 mg __ 1 mg __ 2 mg __ mg __ IV __ q 2 hours __ q 4 hours __ q 6 hours q ___ hours __ prn pain

Ibuprofen (Advil®, Motrin®) __ 400 mg __ 600 mg __ 800 mg PO __ q 4 hours __ q 6 hours __ q 8 hours ___ prn pain

Ketorolac (Toradol®) __ 30 mg IV __ q 6 hours __ prn pain (maximum 120 mg daily)

Morphine __ 0.5 mg __ 1 mg __ 2 mg __ 4 mg __ mg ___ IV __ q 2 hours __ q 4 hours __ q 6 hours q ___ hours __ prn pain

Tramadol (Ultram®) __ 50 mg __ 100 mg PO __ q 4 hours __ q 6 hours __ prn pain (maximum 400 mg daily)

Other _____, _____, _____, _____, _____.

Antiemetics

Chlorpromazine (Thorazine®) __ 10 mg PO __ 25 mg PO __ q 4 hours __ q 6 hours __ 25 mg __ 50 mg __ IV __IM __ q 4 hours __ q 6 hours __ prn nausea/vomiting

Metoclopramide (Reglan®) __10 mg __ IV __ IM __ PO __ q 6 hours __ other __ prn nausea/vomiting

Ondansetron (Zofran®) __ 4 mg __ 8 mg __ IV __ PO __ q 6 hours ___ other __ prn nausea/vomiting

Prochlorperazine (Compazine®) __5 mg __ 10 mg __ IV __ IM __ PO __ q 4 hours ___ q 6 hours (maximum dose IV/IM/PO 40 mg per day) ___ 25 mg PR bid ___ prn nausea/vomiting

Promethazine (Phenergan®) __ 12.5 mg __ 25 mg __ IV__ IM __ PO __ PR __ q 4 hours ___ q 6 hours ___ prn nausea/vomiting

Trimethobenzamide (Tigan®) __ 200 mg IM __ 300 mg PO ___ q 6 hours ___ prn nausea/vomiting

Antibiotics: Oral and Intravenous Antibiotics – Oral

Amoxicillin and Clavulanic Acid (Amoxicillin and Clavulanate) (Augmentin®) __ 250 mg ___ 500 mg __ 875 mg PO __ q 8 hours __ q 12 hours __ other

Ciprofloxacin (Cipro®) __ 500 mg PO bid __ other

Clindamycin* (Cleocin®) __ 300 mg __ 450 mg PO __ q 6 hours

Doxycycline (Adoxa®, Doryx®, Doxy 100®, Vibramycin®) __ 100 mg PO bid __ other

Levofloxacin (Levaquin®) ___ 500 mg ___ 750 mg PO qd__ other

Sulfamethoxazole and Trimethoprim (Bactrim DS®, Septra® DS) __ 1 tab __ 2 tabs PO __ q 12 hours __ q d __ other __ (usual dose 1–2 double strength [DS] tablets every 12–24 hours) where DS = sulfamethoxazole 800 mg and trimethoprim [TMP] = 180 mg

Antibiotics – Intravenous

Ampicillin and Sulbactam (Unasyn®) ___ 1.5 grams __ 3 grams ___ IV q 6 hours __ other

Cefazolin (Ancef®) __ 1 gram __ 2 grams IV __ q 4 hours __ q 6 hours __ q 8 hours __ q 12 hours ___ qd ___ other (usual dose 1–2 grams every 8 hours, maximum 12 grams per day)

Ciprofloxacin (Cipro®) ___ 400 mg IV bid ___ other

Clindamycin* (Cleocin®) ___ 600 mg __ 900 mg IV __ q 8 hours

Doxycycline (Doxy®) ___ 100 mg IV bid __ other

Levofloxacin (Levaquin®) ___ 500 mg ___ 750 mg IV qd __ other

Penicillin G (parenteral) (Pfizerpen-G®) ___ million units IV __ q 4 hours __ q 6 hours __ other

Sulfamethoxazole and Trimethoprim (Bactrim™ DS, Septra® DS) __ 1 tab __ 2 tabs PO __ q 12 hours __ q d __ other __ (usual dose 1–2 double strength [DS] tablets every 12–24 hours where DS = sulfamethoxazole 800 mg and trimethoprim [TMP] 180 mg)

Intravenous Fluids

Saline cap IV ____

Bolus Normal Saline (NS) IV ___ 250 mL __ 500 mL ___ 1,000 mL ___ other, infuse over ___ minutes

Bolus Lactated Ringer's (LR) IV __ 250 mL __ 500 mL __ 1,000 mL __ other, infuse over ___ minutes

Maintenance NS at __ mL per hour IV

Maintenance LR at __ mL per hour IV

Maintenance Dextrose 5% in Water (D_5W) at __ mL per hour IV

Maintenance Dextrose 5% in ½ Normal Saline (D_5½NS) at __ mL per hour IV

Maintenance Dextrose 5% in Normal Saline
(D$_5$NS) at __ mL per hour IV
Other _____ at mL per hour

Education: patient _____ family _____

Casts/splints/crutches _____
Extremity injuries ____

Wound Care/lacerations/sutures _____
Smoking cessation _____
Other _____

* Oral clindamycin is administered in
smaller and more frequent doses than IV
doses in order to decrease gastrointestinal
upset.

General Trauma Order Set

Place in Emergency Department (ED)
  Observation _____
Diagnosis **GENERAL TRAUMA,** _____,

_____, _____

ED Attending _____
Resident (if applicable) _____
Advanced Practice Provider (if applicable)

  _____

Allergies: Yes _____ No _____

If yes, what _____,_____,_____,_____,

  _____,_____

Vital Signs

Temperature __ Pulse __ Respiration __ BP__
  Pulse oximetry ____
__ q 2 hours ___ q 4 hours ___ q 6 hours q ___
  hours ___ q shift ___ qd ____ other
Cardiac monitoring (telemetry) _____
Neurologic checks __ q 2 hours __ q 4 hours
  __ q 6 hours q __hours __ q shift __ qd __ other
Orthostatic vital signs _____
Continuous pulse oximetry _____
Vascular checks __ q 2 hours __ q 4 hours __
  q 6 hours q __hours __ q shift __ qd __ other
Other _____

Notify Physician if

Temperature (°C) > 38.0° ___ 38.5°___ 39° ___
  40° ____ other _____
Systolic blood pressure (mmHg) ≤ 90 ___
  ≥ 160 __ ≥ 180 ___ ≥ 200 __ other _____
Diastolic blood pressure (mmHg) ≥ 120 ____
  other _____
Heart rate ≤ 50 ___ ≥ 120 __ ≥ 150 ___
  ≥ 200 ___ other ____
Oxygen saturation < 90% _____ other _____
Any change in mental status _____
Any respiratory distress _____
Any new or worsening change in extremity (such
  as color: pale or cyanotic, decreased capillary
  fill, diminished or absent pulses, increased
  pain, numbness or paresthesias) ____

Activity

Cervical spine immobilization ___
Up ad lib _____

Assisted _____
Out of bed to chair _____
Bedrest with bathroom privileges _____
Bedrest with bedside commode _____
Bedrest _____
Other _____

Diet

NPO _____
Regular _____
Advance diet as tolerated _____
Clear liquids ____
Dental, mechanical soft _____
Diabetic _____
Formula _____
Full liquids _____
Low added fat/No added salt _____
Low cholesterol ____
Pureed _____
Sodium: 1 gram ___ 2 gram ___
  unrestricted____
Per feeding tube _____
Other _____

Nursing Interventions

Weight ___ on admission ___ qd ___ prior to
  discharge ____ other
Height ____
I & Os _____ routine _____ strict _____
Fluid restriction ___ mL/hour ___ mL/shift
  ____ mL/24 hour ___ other
Fall precautions _____
Seizure precautions _____
Capillary blood glucose __ × 1 q ___ hours
  ____ before meals and at bedtime
Measure circumference of extremity __ × 1 q
  ___ hours × ___
Measurement of tissue pressure of extremity for
  compartment syndrome _____
Wound care with dressing changes _____
Elevation of extremity _____
Nasogastric tube placement ____ to
  intermittent suction ___ to continuous
  suction
Foley catheter ____ Straight cath for urine

  _____
Elevate head of bed to 30° ____
Seizure precautions _____

Respiratory Interventions

Oxygen __ liters nasal cannula __ venti mask at ___ liters per minute _____ other

Wean oxygen as tolerated without dyspnea, stridor or oxygen saturation < 90% ____

Peak flow __ on admission ___ prior to discharge ___ pre and post aerosols

Sleep apnea qhs __ CPAP BiPAP settings cm H_2O ___ inspiratory __ expiratory

Incentive spirometry __ q 2 hours __ q 4 hours __ q 6 hours q __ hours __ q shift __ qd __ other

Laboratory Tests

Amylase ___ Lipase___

Arterial blood gas ___ on room air ___ on other FiO_2 ____

Basic metabolic panel _____

Blood alcohol level ____

Cardiac enzymes __ × 1, ___ q 4 hours × 3, __ q 4 hours × 4, __ other

CBC ___ with differential, repeat in a.m., q ___ hours × ___

Complete metabolic panel _____

Creatinine phosphokinase (total) (total CPK) __ × 1, __ repeat in a.m., q __ hours × __

CK-MB (creatinine kinase – myocardial band) __ × 1, __ repeat in a.m. q __ hours × __

Hemoglobin/hematocrit __ × 1 __ repeat in a. m., q __ hours × __

Lactate ___ × 1, __ repeat in a.m., q __ hours × __

Liver function tests _____

Pregnancy test (qualitative urine) _____
Pregnancy test (quantitative blood) _____

Toxicology: blood drug screen ____ urine drug screen ____ drug level for ___, ___

Troponin___ × 1, __ repeat in a.m., q __ hours × __

Type and screen _____

Urinalysis _____ Urine culture _____

Other _____, _____, _____, _____, _____, _____, _____, _____

Repeat _____, _____, _____ in a.m. ___ in ___ hours, q ___ hours × ___

Radiology Studies

Acute abdominal series ____
CXR portable _____

CXR (PA and lateral) _____
Extremity films ____, ____, ____, ____, ____, ____

KUB (Kidneys, ureters, bladder) X-ray _____

Spine X-rays: cervical ___ thoracic __ lumbar ____

CT scan without contrast: head ___ neck ___ chest ___ abdomen ___ spine ___ other ___

CT scan with IV contrast: head ___ neck ___ chest ___ abdomen ___ spine ___ other ___

MRI without contrast: head __ neck ___ chest ___ abdomen ___ spine ___ other ___

MRI with contrast: head ___ neck ___ chest ___ abdomen ___ spine ___ other ___

Ultrasound (FAST exam) _____
Ultrasound RUQ _____
Ultrasound Pelvis _____
Ultrasound carotids _____
Ultrasound _____
Other _____, _____, _____
Repeat _____, _____, _____

Cardiac Studies

ECG __ × 1 __ q 4 hours × 3 ___ q 4 hours × 4 ___ other ____ with cardiac enzymes

Echocardiogram (transthoracic) __ with agitated (bubble) study __ without agitated (bubble) study

Consultants

Care coordination (Case management)_____ Notified: Name _____ Time ____

Trauma/General surgery _____ Notified: Name _____ Time ____

Social work _____ Notified: Name _____ Time ____

Other _____ Notified: Name _____ Time ____

Medications for General Trauma (Adult Dosage)

Analgesics

Acetaminophen (Paracetamol) (Tylenol®) 325 mg tab __ 1 tab __ 1–2 tabs __ 2 tabs PO __ q 4 hours __ q 6 hours ___ prn pain ___ prn fever (maximum 4 g daily)
____ If unable to take tablet formulation, may give suspension

____ If unable to take PO, may give suppository PR __ 325 mg __ 650 mg __ q 4 hours __ q 6 hours

____ IV ___ mg __ q 4 hours __ q 6 hours __ prn pain __ prn fever (maximum adult dose: if weight < 50 kg is 15 mg/kg up to 750 mg for a single dose, 75 mg/kg up to 3750 mg for daily dose; if weight > 50 kg is 650 mg q 4 hours or 1000 mg q 6 hours up to 1000 mg for a single dose and 4000 mg for a daily dose)

Acetaminophen-Hydrocodone (Vicodin®) 300 mg/5 mg tabs __1 tab __1–2 tabs __ 2 tabs PO __ q 4 hours __ q 6 hours ___ prn pain (maximum 4 grams daily based on acetaminophen dose)

Acetaminophen-Oxycodone (Endocet®, Percocet®, Roxicet®) 325 mg/ 5 mg tab __ 1 tab __1–2 tabs __ 2 tabs PO __ q 4 hours __ q 6 hours ___ prn pain (maximum 4 grams daily based on acetaminophen dose)

____IV ___ mg __ q 4 hours __ q 6 hours __ prn pain __ prn fever (maximum adult dose: if weight < 50 kg is 15 mg/kg up to 750 mg for a single dose, 75 mg/kg up to 3750 mg for daily dose; if weight > 50 kg is 650 mg q 4 hours or 1000 mg q 6 hours up to 1000 mg for a single dose and 4000 mg for a daily dose)

Hydromorphone (Dilaudid®) __ 0.5 mg __ 1 mg __ 2 mg __ mg __ IV __ q 2 hours __ q 4 hours __ q 6 hours q ___ hours __ prn pain

Ibuprofen (Advil®, Motrin®) __ 400 mg __ 600 mg __ 800 mg PO __ q 4 hours __ q 6 hours __ q 8 hours ___ prn pain

Ketorolac (Toradol®) __ 30 mg IV __ q 6 hours __ prn pain (maximum 120 mg daily)

Morphine __ 0.5 mg __ 1 mg __ 2 mg __ 4 mg __ mg ___ IV __ q 2 hours __ q 4 hours __ q 6 hours q ___ hours __ prn pain

Tramadol (Ultram®) __ 50 mg __ 100 mg PO __ q 4 hours __ q 6 hours __ prn pain (maximum 400 mg daily)

Other _____, _____, _____, _____, _____

Antiemetics

Chlorpromazine (Thorazine®) __ 10 mg PO __ 25 mg PO __ q 4 hours __ q 6 hours __ 25 mg __ 50 mg __ IV __IM __ q 4 hours __ q 6 hours __ prn nausea/vomiting

Metoclopramide (Reglan®) __10 mg __ IV __ IM __ PO __ q 6 hours __ other __ prn nausea/vomiting

Ondansetron (Zofran®) __ 4 mg __ 8 mg __IV __PO __ q 6 hours ___ other __ prn nausea/vomiting

Prochlorperazine (Compazine®) __ 5 mg __ 10 mg __ IV __ IM __ PO __ q 4 hours __ q 6 hours (maximum dose IV/IM/PO 40 mg per day) ____ 25 mg PR bid __ prn nausea/vomiting

Promethazine (Phenergan®) __ 12.5 mg __ 25 mg __IV__ IM __ PO __ PR __ q 4 hours __ q 6 hours ___ prn nausea/vomiting

Trimethobenzamide (Tigan®) __ 200 mg IM __ 300 mg PO ___ q 6 hours ___ prn nausea/vomiting

Intravenous Fluids

Saline cap IV ____

Bolus Normal Saline (NS) IV ___ 250 mL __ 500 mL ____ 1,000 mL ____ other, infuse over ___ minutes

Bolus Lactated Ringer's (LR) IV __ 250 mL __ 500 mL __ 1,000 mL __ other, infuse over ___ minutes

Maintenance NS at __ mL per hour IV

Maintenance LR at __ mL per hour IV

Maintenance Dextrose 5% in Water (D5W) at __ mL per hour IV

Maintenance Dextrose 5% in ½ Normal Saline (D5½NS) at __ mL per hour IV

Maintenance Dextrose 5% in Normal Saline (D5NS) at __ mL per hour IV

Other _____ at mL per hour

Education: patient _____ family _____

General trauma ___

Smoking cessation _____

Other _____

Obtaining consults, treatment of symptoms such as pain and nausea, incentive spirometry, evaluation to rule out other injuries and to monitor for associated injuries, obtaining additional tests (laboratory and radiology), administering IV fluids, repeating the examination and studies, etc. can be part of the management of general trauma. Trauma order sets and protocols, like most protocols and order sets, should be done with the concurrence of the respective service/subspecialty, in this case with the trauma service/general surgeons.

Head Injury (Blunt Head Trauma) Order Set

Place in Emergency Department (ED)
Observation _____
Diagnosis **HEAD TRAUMA,** _____,

_____, _____
ED Attending _____
Resident (if applicable) _____
Advanced Practice Provider (if applicable)

_____

Allergies: Yes _____ No _____

If yes, what _____,_____,_____,_____,

_____,_____

Vital Signs

Temperature __ Pulse __ Respiration __ BP__
Pulse oximetry ____
__ q 2 hours ___ q 4 hours ___ q 6 hours q ___
hours ___ q shift ___ qd ____ other
Cardiac monitoring (telemetry) _____
Orthostatic vital signs _____
Continuous pulse oximetry _____
*Neurologic checks __ q 2 hours __ q 4 hours __
q 6 hours q __ hours __ q shift __ qd __ other*
Other _____

Notify Physician if

Temperature (°C) > 38.0° ___ 38.5°___ 39° ___
40° ____ other _____
Systolic blood pressure (mmHg) ≤ 90 ___
≥ 160 __ ≥ 180 ___ ≥ 200 __ other _____
Diastolic blood pressure (mmHg) ≥ 120 ____
other _____
Heart rate ≤ 50 ___ ≥ 120 __ ≥ 150 ___
≥ 200 ___ other ____
Pulse oxygen saturation < 90% _____
other _____
Any change in mental status _____
Any respiratory distress _____

Activity

Cervical spine immobilization until radiology
studies completed and with negative report
for acute injury ___
Up ad lib _____
Assisted _____
Out of bed to chair _____

Bedrest with bathroom privileges _____
Bedrest with bedside commode _____
Bedrest _____
Other _____

Diet

NPO _____
Regular _____
Advance diet as tolerated _____
Clear liquids ____
Dental, mechanical soft _____
Diabetic _____
Formula_____
Full liquids _____
Low added fat/No added salt _____
Low cholesterol ____
Pureed _____
Sodium: 1 gram ___ 2 gram ___
unrestricted ____
Per feeding tube _____
Other _____

Nursing Interventions

Weight ___ on admission ___ qd ___ prior to
discharge ____ other
Height ____
I & Os _____ routine _____ strict _____
Fluid restriction ___ mL/hour ___ mL/shift
____ mL/24 hour ___ other
Fall precautions _____
Capillary blood glucose __ × 1 q ___ hours
____ before meals and at bedtime
Foley catheter ___ Straight cath for urine

_____
Seizure precautions _____
Elevate head of bed at 30° _____

Respiratory Interventions

Oxygen __ liters nasal cannula __ venti mask at
___ liters per minute _____ other
Wean oxygen as tolerated without dyspnea,
stridor or oxygen saturation < 90% ____
Peak flow __ on admission ___ prior to
discharge ___ pre and post aerosols
Sleep apnea qhs __ CPAP BiPAP settings cm
H₂O ___ inspiratory __ expiratory
Incentive spirometry __ q 2 hours __ q 4 hours
__ q 6 hours q __ hours __ q shift __ qd
__ other

Laboratory Tests

Amylase ___ Lipase___

Arterial blood gas ___ on room air ___ on other FiO2 ____

Basic metabolic panel _____

Blood alcohol level ____

Cardiac enzymes __ × 1, ___ q 4 hours × 3, __ q 4 hours × 4, __ other

CBC ____with differential, repeat in a.m., q ___ hours × ____

Complete metabolic panel _____

Creatinine phosphokinase (total) (total CPK) __ × 1, __ repeat in a.m.

q __ hours × __

CK-MB (creatinine kinase – myocardial band) __ × 1, __ repeat in a.m.

q __ hours × __

Hemoglobin/hematocrit __ × 1 __ repeat in a. m., q __ hours × __

Lactate ___ × 1, __ repeat in a.m., q __ hours × __

Liver function tests _____

Pregnancy test (qualitative urine) _____
Pregnancy test (quantitative blood) _____

Toxicology: blood drug screen ____ urine drug screen ____ drug level for ___

Troponin___ × 1, __ repeat in a.m., q __ hours × __

Type and screen _____

Urinalysis _____ Urine culture _____

Other _____, _____, _____, _____,
_____, _____, _____, _____

Repeat _____, _____, _____ in a.m. ___ in ___ hours, q ___ hours × ___

Radiology Studies

CXR portable _____

CXR (PA and lateral) _____

Spine X-rays: cervical ___ thoracic __ lumbar ____

CT scan head without contrast _____with IV contrast _____

CT scan neck without contrast ____ with contrast ____

MRI brain _____

MRI cervical spine _____

MRA brain _____

Ultrasound (FAST exam) _____

Ultrasound carotids _____
Ultrasound _____
Other _____, _____, _____

Cardiac Studies

ECG __ × 1__ q 4 hours × 3 ___ q 4 hours × 4 ___ other ____ with cardiac enzymes

Echocardiogram (transthoracic) __ with agitated (bubble) study __ without agitated (bubble) study

Consultants

Care coordination (Case management) ____
Notified: Name_____ Time ___

Neurosurgery_____ Notified:
Name _____ Time ___

Neurology _____ Notified:
Name _____ Time ___

Orthopedics _____ Notified:
Name _____ Time ___

Spine surgery _____ Notified:
Name _____ Time ___

Social work_____ Notified:
Name _____ Time ___

Trauma/General surgery _____ Notified:
Name _____ Time ___

Other _____ Notified:
Name _____ Time ___

Medications for Head /Spine Injury (Adult Dosage)

Analgesics*

Acetaminophen (Paracetamol) (Tylenol®)
325 mg tab __ 1 tab __ 1–2 tabs __ 2 tabs PO __ q 4 hours __ q 6 hours ___ prn pain ___ prn fever (maximum 4 g daily)

____ If unable to take tablet formulation, may give suspension

____ If unable to take PO, may give suppository PR __325 mg __ 650 mg __ q 4 hours __ q 6 hours

____ IV ___ mg __ q 4 hours __ q 6 hours __ prn pain __ prn fever (maximum adult dose: if weight < 50 kg is 15 mg/kg up to 750 mg for a single dose, 75 mg/kg up to 3750 mg for daily dose; if weight > 50 kg is 650 mg q 4 hours or 1000 mg q 6 hours up to 1000 mg for a single dose and 4000 mg for a daily dose)

Acetaminophen-Hydrocodone (Vicodin®) 300 mg/5 mg tabs __ 1 tab __ 1–2 tabs __ 2 tabs PO __ q 4 hours __ q 6 hours ___ prn pain (maximum 4 grams daily based on acetaminophen dose)

Acetaminophen-Oxycodone (Endocet®, Percocet®, Roxicet®) 325 mg/ 5 mg tab __ 1 tab __ 1–2 tabs __ 2 tabs PO __ q 4 hours __ q 6 hours ___ prn pain (maximum 4 grams daily based on acetaminophen dose)

Hydromorphone (Dilaudid®) __ 0.5 mg __ 1 mg __ 2 mg __ mg __ IV __ q 2 hours __ q 4 hours __ q 6 hours q ___ hours __ prn pain

Ibuprofen (Advil®, Motrin®) __ 400 mg __ 600 mg __ 800 mg PO __ q 4 hours __ q 6 hours __ q 8 hours ___ prn pain

Ketorolac (Toradol®) __ 30 mg IV __ q 6 hours __ prn pain (maximum 120 mg daily)

Morphine __ 0.5 mg __ 1 mg __ 2 mg __ 4 mg __ mg ___ IV __ q 2 hours __ q 4 hours __ q 6 hours q ___ hours __ prn pain

Tramadol (Ultram®) __ 50 mg __ 100 mg PO __ q 4 hours __ q 6 hours __ prn pain (maximum 400 mg daily)

Other _____, _____, _____, _____, _____

* Analgesics may be limited to nonopioid analgesics or held initially until neurologic evaluation is done depending on the clinical scenario.

Antiemetics

Chlorpromazine (Thorazine®) __ 10 mg PO __ 25 mg PO __ q 4 hours __ q 6 hours __ 25 mg __ 50 mg __ IV __ IM __ q 4 hours __ q 6 hours __ prn nausea/vomiting

Metoclopramide (Reglan®) __ 10 mg __ IV __ IM __ PO __ q 6 hours __ other __ prn nausea/vomiting

Ondansetron (Zofran®) __ 4 mg __ 8 mg __ IV __ PO __ q 6 hours ___ other __ prn nausea/vomiting

Prochlorperazine (Compazine®) __ 5 mg __ 10 mg __ IV __ IM __ PO __ q 4 hours __ q 6 hours (maximum dose IV/IM/PO 40 mg per day) ___ 25 mg PR bid __ prn nausea/vomiting

Promethazine (Phenergan®) __ 12.5 mg __ 25 mg __ IV __ IM __ PO __ PR __ q 4 hours __ q 6 hours ___ prn nausea/vomiting

Trimethobenzamide (Tigan®) __ 200 mg IM __ 300 mg PO ___ q 6 hours ___ prn nausea/vomiting

Intravenous Fluids**

Saline cap IV _____

Bolus Normal Saline (NS) IV ___ 250 mL __ 500 mL ___ 1,000 mL _____ other, infuse over ___ minutes

Bolus Lactated Ringer's (LR) IV __ 250 mL __ 500 mL __ 1,000 mL __ other, infuse over ___ minutes

Maintenance NS at __ mL per hour IV

Maintenance LR at __ mL per hour IV

Maintenance Dextrose 5% in Water (D5W) at __ mL per hour IV

Maintenance Dextrose 5% in ½ Normal Saline (D5½NS) at __ mL per hour IV

Maintenance Dextrose 5% in Normal Saline (D5NS) at __ mL per hour IV

Other _____ at mL per hour

**Fluids may be limited at least initially until neurologic evaluation is done depending on the clinical scenario due to concern over excessive fluid administration in a head injured patient.

Education: patient _____ family _____

Head injury _____

Postconcussive syndrome _____

Smoking cessation _____

Other _____

Treatment of a postconcussive syndrome with antiemetics, analgesics, judicious use of IV fluids, monitoring for other serious injuries, and obtaining additional testing may be useful in the treatment of patients with postconcussive syndrome or a mild blunt head injury patient. The head injury protocol and order set should be done with the concurrence of the appropriate service, in this case, neurosurgery and neurology.

Adult Order Sets

Intravenous Fluids, Laboratory, Radiology, and Special Studies

Sharon E. Mace, MD, FACEP, FAAP
Matthew J. Campbell, PharmD, BCPS, BCCCP

Intravenous (IV) Fluids Order Set

Weight (in kg) _____
Normal Saline (NS) _____
Lactated Ringer's (LR) _____
Dextrose 5% in Water (D_5W) _____
Dextrose 5% in ½ Normal Saline
   (D_5½NS) ____
Dextrose 5% in Normal Saline (D_5NS) ____
NS bolus IV ___ mL ___ 250 mL____500 mL
   ____ 1,000 mL ____ 20 mL/kg
infuse over __ minutes ___ hours
LR bolus IV ___ mL ___ 250 mL ____ 500 mL
   ____ 1,000 mL ____ 20 mL/kg
infuse over ___minutes ___ hours
Maintenance NS at _____ mL/hour IV

Maintenance D_5 W at _____ mL/hour IV
Maintenance D_5 ½ NS at ____ mL/hour IV
Maintenance D_5 NS at _____ mL/hour IV
Maintenance NS with potassium chloride __
   20 mEq or 40 mEq per 1liter bag at _____
   mL/hour IV
Maintenance D_5 W with potassium chloride __
   20 mEq or 40 mEq per 1 liter bag at _____
   mL/hour IV
Maintenance D_5 ½ NS with potassium chloride
   __ 20 mEq or 40 mEq per 1 liter bag at
   _____ mL/hour IV
Maintenance D_5 NS with potassium chloride __
   20 mEq or 40 mEq per 1 liter bag at _____
   mL/hour IV
Other _____at mL/hour IV

Laboratory Tests Order Set

Amylase ___

Arterial blood gas ___ on room air _____ other FiO2

Basic metabolic panel _____

Blood alcohol level _____

Blood urea nitrogen (BUN) _____

Brain natriuretic peptide (BNP) _____

Calcium ____ total ___ ionized _____

Carbon monoxide _____

Cardiac enzymes __ × 1 __ q 4 hours × 3 __ q 4 hours × 4 __ other __ with ECGs

CBC with differential _____

Chloride _____

Complete metabolic panel _____

C-reactive protein (CRP) _____

Creatinine _____

Creatinine phosphokinase (CPK) _____

Creatine kinase (CK-MB) _____

D-dimer _____

Drug level _____, _____, _____

Erythrocyte sedimentation rate (ESR)

_____

Fasting lipid panel _____

Glucose _____

Hemoglobin/Hematocrit _____

Influenza studies (influenza A and B) (by nasal swab) _____

Lactate _____

Lipase___

Liver function tests _____

Magnesium _____

Monospot _____

Phosphorus _____

Potassium _____

Pregnancy test (qualitative urine) _____

Pregnancy test (quantitative blood) _____

Rapid Strep (throat swab) ____

Renal function tests (e.g., BUN, creatinine)

_____

Respiratory antigen panel (by nasal swab) _____

Respiratory syncytial virus (RSV) (by nasal swab) ____

Sodium _____

Toxicology screen blood _____

Toxicology screen urine _____

Troponin __ × 1 __ q 4 hours × 3 __ q 4 hours × 4 __ other __ with ECGs __

TSH (thyroid stimulating hormone) ___ Thyroid function tests (T3, T4, TSH) ____

Type and Cross ____ units PRBCs (packed red blood cells)

Type and Screen _____

Urinalysis _____

Venous blood gas _____

Cultures

Blood culture (peripheral) × ___ from central line × ___

Throat culture ____

Urine culture _____

Wound culture _____ site _____

Gonorrhea _____ Chlamydia _____ site _____

Fungal (Candida, KOH) ____ site ____

Trichomonas _____ site _____

Other _____, _____, _____, _____, _____, _____, _____, _____

Repeat _____, _____, _____ in a.m. ___ in____ hours

Radiology Tests Order Set

Plain X-rays

Acute abdominal series ____

CXR portable _____

CXR (PA and lateral) _____

Extremity x-rays _____ Right ___ Left ____

KUB (Kidneys, ureters, bladder) x-ray _____

Spine x-rays ___ cervical ___ thoracic ___ lumbar

Other _____, _____, _____

CT (Computed Tomography) Scan

CT abdomen/pelvis ____ without contrast ____ with contrast ___ IV ___ PO ___ PR

CT brain _____ without contrast ____ with contrast

CT chest _____ without contrast ____ with contrast

CT kidneys ____ without contrast ____ with contrast

CT enterography _____

CT _____

CTA (computed tomography angiography) of brain with and without contrast (ultravist) if no contrast allergy and no renal failure (e.g., GFR $\geq$ 30) _____

CTA _____

Other _____, _____, _____

Ultrasound

Ultrasound Abdomen (right upper quadrant) _____

Ultrasound Carotids _____

Ultrasound Extremity (rule out deep vein thrombosis) __ Upper __ Lower __ Right __ Left

Ultrasound Pelvis _____

Ultrasound _____

Other _____, _____, _____

MRI (Magnetic Resonance Imaging)

MRI (Magnetic resonance imaging) of brain without contrast _____

MRI (Magnetic resonance imaging) of brain with and without contrast (gadolinium) if no allergy and no renal failure (e.g., GFR $\geq$30) _____

MRA (Magnetic resonance angiography) Circle of Willis and of Carotids without contrast (if renal failure) _____

MRA (Magnetic resonance angiography) Circle of Willis and of Carotids with and without contrast (gadolinium) if no allergy and no renal failure (e.g., GFR $\geq$30) _____

MRA _____

MRI _____

Other _____, _____, _____

Other Studies

Cholescintigraphy (hepatic iminodiacetic acid [HIDA] scan) _____

Injection for feeding tube placement ____

Transcranial doppler of brain vessels _____

Other _____, _____, _____

Special Studies Order Set

Cardiac Studies

ECG _____ at _____ hours

Serial ECGs _____ q 4 hours × 3 _____ q 4 hours × 4 _____ other _____ with cardiac enzymes _____

Echocardiogram (transthoracic) __ with agitated (bubble) study ___ without agitated (bubble) study

Stress Tests/Cardiac Imaging Studies

Stress Electrocardiogram (treadmill stress test, exercise tolerance test/ETT) ___

Stress Echocardiogram _____

Pharmacologic Stress Tests

   Coronary Vasodilators:

      Adenosine _____
      Dipyridamole/Persantine _____
      Regadenosine/Lexiscan _____

   Synthetic Catecholamine:

      Dobutamine _____

Myocardial Perfusion Imaging (injection of radioactive isotopes):

   Nuclear Stress Test

      Thallium-201 _____
      Technetium-99m Sestamibi _____
      Technetium-99 Tetrofosmin _____

Gamma Imaging:

   Single positron emission computed tomography (SPECT) _____

Cardiac positron emission tomography (PET)

Stress Cardiovascular Magnetic Resonance Imaging (CMR) _____

Computed Tomography Coronary Angiography (CTCA) _____

Other _____

* Not all tests are available at all institutions. Generally, test availability is limited, depends on many factors including available expertise and cost, and is institution specific. Selection of the appropriate stress test depends on many factors, including the patient and the availability of a particular test at a given institution. This list is not all inclusive but is intended to list the stress tests/cardiac imaging discussed in Chapter 26 Stress Testing.

Gastrointestinal Studies

Esophagogastroduodenoscopy (EGD) _____ NPO after midnight _____

Colonoscopy in a.m. _____ NPO after midnight _____ Bowel prep _____

Neurologic Studies

Electroencephalogram (EEG) _____

Pulmonary Studies

Pulmonary function tests _____

Other

_____

Adult Order Sets
Medications

93

Sharon E. Mace, MD, FACEP, FAAP
Matthew J. Campbell, PharmD, BCPS, BCCCP

Drug, Dose, Route, Frequency, Indication, Formulation

Analgesics/Antipyretics

Acetaminophen (Paracetamol) (Tylenol®)

__ mg PO administered as __ 325 mg tablets or __ 500 mg tablets or __ solution/suspension __ q 4 hours __ q 6 hours __ q 8 hours __ other ____ prn pain ___ prn fever (temperature > 100.5°F)

__ mg suppository PR __ q 4 hours __ q 6 hours __ q 8 hours __ other ____ PRN pain ___ PRN fever (temperature > 100.5°F)

Dosage: immediate release: regular strength 650 mg PO every 4–6 hours, extra strength 1,000 mg PO every 6 hours, rectal: 650 mg PR every 4–6 hours

Maximum: in 24 hours: regular strength 3250 mg PO, extra strength 3,000 mg PO, rectal 3,900 mg PR, if under health care provider supervision, oral doses up to 4,000 mg/24 hours may be given

Formulations: oral solution or suspension: 160 mg/5 mL, 500 mg/5 mL; tablet or gelcap in 325 mg or 500 mg, chewable or oral disintegrating in 80 mg, rectal suppository in 120 mg or 325 mg or 650 mg

Comments: Health care professionals may prescribe or recommend up to 4 grams per day but are advised to use their own discretion and clinical judgment.

Over the counter (OTC) dosing may differ by product and manufacturer.

___ mg IV __ q 4 hours __ q 6 hours __ prn pain __ prn fever (temperature > 100.5°F)

Maximum adult IV dose: if weight < 50 kg is 15 mg/kg up to 750 mg for a single dose, 75 mg/kg up to 3750 mg for daily dose; if weight > 50 kg is 650 mg q 4 hours or 1000 mg q

6 hours up to 1000 mg for a single dose and 4000 mg for a daily dose.

Aspirin (Acetylsalicylic Acid)

__ 81 mg __ 325 mg __ 650 mg __ mg PO administered as __ chewable tablets or __ tablets/caplets __ q 4 hours __ q 6 hours __ q 8 hours __ qd ___ other __ prn pain ___ prn fever (temperature > 100.5°F)

__ mg suppository PR __ q 4 hours __ q 6 hours __ q 8 hours __ qd ___ other __ prn pain __ prn fever (temperature > 100.5°F)

Dosage: when used for antipyretic or analgesic: 325–650 mg PO every 4–6 hours, 300–600 mg PR every 4–6 hours

Maximum: 4 grams in 24 hours

Formulations: tablets or caplets: 81 mg or 325 mg or 650 mg, chewable tablet 81 mg, suppository 300 mg or 600 mg

Comments: Higher doses may be administered when used as anti-inflammatory but patients needing the higher anti-inflammatory doses are not likely to be good candidates for the observation unit

Avoid with Reyes syndrome, "*Do not use aspirin in children < 12 years and adolescents who have or who are recovering from chickenpox or flu symptoms due to the association with Reye's syndrome.*"

Fentanyl (Duragesic®)

__ mcg __ IV __ IM __ q 2 hours __ q 4 hours __ q 6 hours __ q 8 hours __ other __ prn pain

Transdermal patch __ 12.5 mcg/hour __ 25 mcg/hour __ 50 mcg/hour __ 75 mcg/hour __ 100 mcg/hour, apply to skin __ q 72 hours __ other

Dosage: intermittent IV/ IM 25–35 mcg by slow IV administration or IM, or 0.35–0.5 mcg/kg every 30–60 minutes. If severe pain persists and there are no or minimal adverse events at the expected peak effect (e.g. 5 minutes after IV administration), then the dose may be repeated.

Maximum: varies, may cause respiratory depression and CNS depression so dose should be titrated and used with caution

Formulations: transdermal __ 12.5 mcg/hour __ 25 mcg/hour __ 50 mcg/hour __ 75 mcg/ hour __ 100 mcg/hour

Comments: Opioid-tolerant patients may need higher doses.

Transdermal patch dosages listed since patients already on these medications may be placed in the observation unit. Oral forms are also available but have slower onset than parenteral and so may not be as desirable for acute pain and other oral opioids are more commonly used.

Continuous infusions may be administered including patient-controlled analgesia (PCA) but these patients tend not to be placed in the observation unit.

Transmucosal (buccal, sublingual, and nasal forms) available but have variable absorption so they are not listed.

Hydrocodone and Acetaminophen (Lorcet®, Vicodin®)

__ 5 mg __ 10 mg __ mg (based on hydrocodone component) PO administered as __ tablets ___ solution/elixir __ q 4 hours __ q 6 hours __ other ___ prn pain

Dosage: If opioid naïve usual initial dose is 5–10 mg of hydrocodone component 4 times a day

Maximum: acetaminophen dose 4 grams in 24 hours (see also acetaminophen)

Formulations: solution = hydrocodone 7.5 mg/ acetaminophen 325 mg per 15 mL, tablet = hydrocodone 5 mg/acetaminophen 325 mg

Comments: Opioid tolerant patients may need higher doses

Hydromorphone (Dilaudid®)

___ mg __ IV or __ PO administered as __ tablet __ oral liquid __ q 2 hours __ q 4 hours __ q 6 hours __ q 8 hours __ other __ prn pain

Dosage: for acute pain: PO initial dose if opioid naïve: 2–4 mg every 4–6 hours, 4–8 mg if severe pain per American Pain Society (APS) recommendation; IV initial dose 0.2–1 mg every 2–3 hours

Maximum: varies, depends on opioid naïve or opioid tolerant

Formulations: oral liquid: 1 mg/mL; tablets: 2 mg, 4 mg,

Comments: May cause respiratory depression and CNS depression so the dose should be individualized, titrated, and used with caution. Lower doses may be administered in elderly or debilitated patients, while patients with prior opioid exposure or opioid-tolerant patients may need higher doses. Continuous infusions may be administered including patient-controlled analgesia (PCA) but these patients tend not to be placed in the observation unit.

IM has variable absorption and is not recommended.

Oral and parenteral forms are not equivalent. Parenteral forms may be up to 5 times more potent than PO forms. When administered parenterally, one-fifth of the oral dose will provide similar analgesia.

Ibuprofen (Advil®, Motrin®)

__ 200 mg __ 400 mg __ 600 mg __ 800 mg __ mg __PO __ q 4 hours __ q 6 hours __ q 8 hours

__ other administered as __ tablets __ suspension __ prn pain ___ prn fever (temperature > 100.5°F)

Dosage: for analgesia/pain/fever/dysmenorrhea: 200–400 mg/dose PO every 4–6 hours, for inflammatory disease/pericarditis: 400–800 mg PO every 6–8 hours

Maximum: for analgesia/pain/fever/ dysmenorrhea: 1.2 g per day (with physician supervision ≤ 2.4 g PO per day), for inflammatory disease/pericarditis: 3.2 g PO per day (with physician supervision)

Formulation: oral suspension = 100 mg/5 mL, tablets in 100 mg, 200 mg, 400 mg, 600mg or 800 mg, chewable tablets 50 mg or 100 mg

Comments: Patients should be well hydrated prior to administration.

Morphine (Duramorph®, Kadian®, MS Contin®)

__ mg __ IV __ or __ PO administered as __ tablet __ extended release tablet __ oral liquid __ q 2 hours __ q 4 hours __ q 6 hours __ q 8 hours __ other __ prn pain

Dosage: for acute pain: 10–30 mg PO every 4 hours, if opioid naïve 5–10 mg IM every

4 hours (usual 5–15 mg IM every 4 hours), if opioid naïve 2.5–5 mg IV every 3–4 hours (patients with prior opioid exposure may require higher doses)

Maximum: varies, depends on opioid naïve or opioid tolerant

Formulations: morphine oral solution = 10 mg/ 5 mL, tablets in 15 mg, 30 mg; extended release tablets: 15 mg, 30 mg, 60 mg, 100 mg

Comments: **IM is no longer recommended because of painful administration, variable absorption, and lag time to peak effect.**

Repeated SQ causes local pain, irritation, and induration.

Continuous infusions may be administered including patient-controlled analgesia (PCA) but these patients tend not to be placed in the observation unit.

Oxycodone and Acetaminophen (Endocet®, Percocet®, Roxicet®)

__ mg PO administered as tablet __ or __ oral solution __ q 2 hours __ q 4 hours __ q 6 hours __ q 8 hours __ other __ prn pain

Dosage: immediate release: 2.5–10 mg PO every 6 hours per manufacturer's labeling, 10–20 mg PO every 4–6 hours for moderate pain per American Pain Society (APS) 2008 recommendations

Maximum: 4 grams per 24 hours based on acetaminophen component

Formulations: Roxicet® solution = oxycodone 5 mg and acetaminophen 325 mg/5 mL, Endocet® 5/325, Percocet® 5/325, Roxicet ® 5/325 tablets: 5/325 = 5 mg oxycodone/325 acetaminophen

Comments: Dosage varies based on opioid naïve or opioid tolerant and on specific recommendations (manufacturer or APS and others)

Toradol (Ketorolac®)

__ IV __ IM __ 30 mg __ q 6 hours __ q 8 hours __ other __ prn pain

Dosage: 30 mg every 6 hours

Maximum: 30 mg per dose and 120 mg per day IV/IM

Comments: Therapy should not exceed 5 days. Oral formulations are available but are not recommended and other alternative PO

NSAIDs are recommended in pediatric and adult patients

Tramadol (Ultram®, Synapryn®)

__ 50 mg __ 100 mg PO administered as __ tablets __ or __ suspension __ q 4 hours __ q 6 hours __ other ___ prn pain

Dosage: 50–100 mg PO every 4–6 hours

Maximum: 400 mg PO per day

Formulations: tablets 50 mg; suspension 10 mg/ mL, extended release 24-hour tablets or capsules: 100 mg, 200 mg, 300 mg

Antibiotics

Amoxicillin (Amoxil®, Moxatag®)

__ 250 mg ___ 500 mg ___ 875 mg PO administered as ___capsules/tablets or ___ suspension __ q 8 hours ___ q 12 hours __ other

Dosage: 250–500 mg q 8 hours or 500–875 mg every 12 hours

Maximum: single dose 1000 mg PO, daily dose 2,000–4,000 mg PO per day depending on indication

Formulations: suspensions: 125 mg/5 mL, 250 mg/5mL, 200 mg/5 mL, 400 mg/5 mL; capsules 250 mg, 500 mg, tablets: 500 mg, 875 mg

Amoxicillin and Clavulanic Acid (Amoxicillin and Clavulanate) (Augmentin®)

__ 250 mg ___ 500 mg __ 875 mg __ other __ PO __ q 8 hours __ q 12 hours administered as ___capsules or tablet ___suspension

Dosage: 250–500 mg PO q 8 hours or 500–875 mg every 12 hours

Maximum: same maximums as for amoxicillin

Formulations: suspensions: 125 mg/ 5 mL, 200 mg/5 mL, 250mg/5 mL, 400 mg/5 mL, 600 mg/5 mL; tablets: 250 mg, 500 mg, 875 mg

Comments: Dose is based on the amoxicillin component. Suspension formulations are not interchangeable as the clavulanate content varies.

Ampicillin and Sulbactam (Unasyn®)

__ 1.5 grams __ 3 grams __ other __ IV __ IM __ q 6 hours __ q 8 hours __ qd

Dosage: 1.5–3 grams IV/IM every 6 hours

Maximum: 12 grams ampicillin and sulbactam IV/IM in 24 hours

Azithromycin (Zithromax®)

__ 250 mg ___ 500 mg ___ 1 gram __ PO administered as __ tablet or ___ suspension or __ 400 mg __ other __ IV __ once __ qd __ other

Dosage: for pneumonia (community acquired) and for acute bacterial pharyngitis (including susceptible group A streptococci) in penicillin allergic patients: PO 500 mg on day one then 250 mg on days 2/3/4/5, for uncomplicated gonococcal infection 1 gram single dose PO with IM ceftriaxone; for bacterial sinusitis: 500 mg daily for 3 days

Maximum: for pneumonia, pharyngitis, sinusitis: 500 mg per day

Formulations: oral suspensions: 100 mg/5 mL, 200 mg/5 mL, tablets: 250 mg, 500 mg

Cefazolin (Ancef®, Kefzol®)

__ 1 gram __ 2 grams __ grams __ IV __ IM ___ q 6 hours __ q 8 hours

Dosage: usual 1–2 grams IV or IM every 8 hours

Maximum: 12 grams daily IV or IM

Ceftriaxone (Rocephin®)

IV __ 1 gram __ 2 grams __ other __ q 12 hours __ qd, __ 250 mg IM once

Dosage: usual 1–2 gram IV every 12–24 hours; for uncomplicated gonococcal infection: 250 mg IM once with oral azithromycin (first choice) or oral doxycycline (second choice)

Maximum: 2 grams per dose

Comments: Higher doses of 100 mg/kg/day up to 4 grams per day for meningitis/other CNS infections

Cephalexin (Keflex®)

___ 250 mg __ 500 mg __ 1,000 mg ___ mg PO administered as ___ tablet/capsule or ___ suspension __ q 6 hours __ q 12 hours

Dosage: 1–4 grams PO per day divided into 4 doses

Maximum 4 grams per day

Formulations: suspensions: 125 mg/5 mL, 250 mg/5 mL; tablets/capsules: 250 mg, 500 mg

Ciprofloxacin (Cipro®)

__ 400 mg IV or ___ 500 mg PO administered as __ tablet or __ oral suspension __ q 12 hours __ other

Dosage: PO 500 mg or IV 400 mg every 12 hours for most indications. Recent FDA

black box warning and advisory for fluoroquinolones. Don't use fluoroquinolones for sinusitis, bronchitis, or cystitis if other options are available. Fluoroquinolones are no longer recommended for treating STD in United States due to resistance.

Maximum: depends on indication

Formulations: oral suspension: 250 mg/5 mL, 500 mg/5 mL; tablets: 250 mg, 500 mg

Clindamycin (Cleocin®)

__ 300 mg __ 450 mg PO q 6 hours administered as __ capsules or __ oral solution ___ other or __ 600 mg __ 900 mg IV__ q 6 hours __ q 8 hours __ other

Dosage: dose 150–450 mg per dose PO every 6–8 hours, 1,200–2,700 mg IV per day in 2–4 divided doses

Maximum: 1800 mg per day PO, 4800 mg IV/ per day

Formulations: oral solution 75 mg/5 mL; capsules: 75 mg, 150 mg, 300 mg

Comments: Oral clindamycin is administered in smaller and more frequent doses than IV doses in order to decrease gastrointestinal upset.

Doxycycline (Adoxa®, Doryx®, Vibramycin®)

__ 50 mg __ 100 mg __ other PO as __ tablets/ capsules or __ oral suspension or syrup __ bid __ qd

Dosage: 100–200 mg per day in 1–2 divided doses, usually 100 mg bid

Maximum: 100 mg per dose, 200 mg per day

Formulations: oral suspension 25 mg/mL, oral syrup 50 mg/5 mL, capsules/tablets: 50 mg, 100 mg

Levofloxacin (Levaquin®)

__ 500 mg __ 750 mg __ IV __ PO administered as __ tablets or __ oral solution __ qd __ other

Dosage: 500–750 mg daily for most indications (such as pneumonia, chronic bronchitis, skin/ skin structure infections)

Maximum: 750 mg daily

Formulations: oral solution: 25 mg/mL; tablets: 250 mg, 500 mg, 750 mg

Moxifloxacin (Avelox®)

__ 400 mg ___ IV __ PO (tablets) qd ___ other

Dosage: 400 mg PO or IV daily

Maximum: 400 mg
Formulations: tablets: 400 mg

Penicillin G Benzathine (Bicillin L-A®)

__ 1.2 million units IM once ___ other ___
Dosage: usual dose for group A streptococcal infections: 1.2 million units IM × 1
Maximum: single dose 2.4 million units
Comments: Used for treatment of streptococcal infections
Only for IM injection, not for IV use

Penicillin G (Benzathine and Procaine) (Bicillin C-R®)

__ 2.4 million units IM once ___ other
Dosage: usual dose for group A streptococcal infections: 2.4 million U/dose IM × 1
Maximum: 2.4 million units
Comments: Used for treatment of streptococcal infections and primary prevention of rheumatic fever. Contains penicillin G benzocaine and penicillin G procaine
Only for IM injection, not for IV use

Penicillin V Potassium (Veetids®)

__ 250 mg __ 500 mg PO administered as __ tablets or __ solution __ q 6 hours __ q 8 hours __ other
Dosage: 250–500 mg/dose q 6–8 hours
Maximum: 4 grams per day
Formulations: oral solutions: 125 mg/5 mL, 250 mg/5 mL; tablets: 250 mg, 500 mg

Piperacillin/Tazobactam (Zosyn®)

___ 3.375 g IV ___ q 4 hours __ q 6 hours __ q 8 hours ___ other
Dosage: 3.375 grams per dose every 6 hours
Maximum: 18 grams per day

Sulfamethoxazole and Trimethoprim (SMX-TMP, Co-trimoxazole) (Bactrim DS®, Septra DS®)

__ 1 tab __ 2 tabs or ___ mg of suspension PO __ q 12 hours __ q d __ other __ (usual dose 1–2 double strength [DS] tablets every 12–24 hours) where DS = sulfamethoxazole 800 mg and trimethoprim [TMP] 180 mg)
Dosage: PO: 1–2 DS tablets every 12–24 hours, IV: 8–20 mg TMP/kg/day every 6–12 hours
Maximum: up to 20 mg TMP/kg/day in divided doses
Formulations: oral suspension: SMX 200 mg and TMP 40 mg/ 5 mL, tablet: SMX 400 mg

and TMP 80 mg; double strength [DS] tablet = SMX 800 mg and TMP 160 mg,
Comments: Once a day oral dosing is usually for prophylaxis of urinary tract infection.

Antiemetics

Hydroxyzine (Vistaril®)

__ 25 mg __ 50 mg PO __ q 6 hours __ other ___ prn pruritus ___ prn anxiety
__ 25 mg __ 50 mg IM q 6 hours __ other __ prn nausea/vomiting
Dosage: for pruritus: 25 mg PO tid or qid, for anxiety 50–100 mg PO qid (start with lower 50 mg dose), for antiemetic: 25–100 mg/ dose IM
Maximum: single dose maximum 100 mg IM, maximum 600 mg per day IM
Comments: Oral formulations are available but antiemetic indication only lists IM dosing.
IV administration is not recommended

Metoclopramide (Reglan®)

__ 5 mg __ 10 mg __ IV __ IM __ PO administered as __ tablets __ ODT __ oral syrup __ q 6 hours __ other __ prn reflux/GI dysmotility __ prn nausea/vomiting
Dosage: usual dose for reflux/GI dysmotility or nausea/vomiting
10 mg/dose every 6 hours IV/PO/IM
Maximum: 5 doses per day
Formulations: oral syrup 5 mg/5 mL, tablets: 5 mg, 10 mg; oral disintegrating tablet: 5 mg

Ondansetron (Zofran®)

___ 4 mg __ 8 mg __ IV __ PO administered as __ ODT or __ oral solution
__ q 6 hours __ q 8 hours ___ other __ prn nausea/vomiting
Dosage: usual single dose 4–8 mg PO, 4 mg IV
Maximum: single dose 16 mg
Formulations: oral solution = 4 mg/5 mL, oral disintegrating tablet: 4 mg, 8 mg
Comments: **Avoid single dose > 16 mg due to possible QT prolongation**

Prochlorperazine (Compazine®)

__ 5 mg __ 10 mg __ IV __ IM __ PO (tablets) __ q 6 hours __ q 8 hours __ other
25 mg PR bid ___ prn nausea/vomiting

Dosage: PO/IV/IM: 5–10 mg/dose, PR: 25 mg bid

Maximum: single dose IV 10 mg, PO/IV/IM 40 mg per day

Formulations: tablets: 5 mg, 10 mg; rectal suppository: 25 mg

Comments: PR dosing indication is listed for adults, but no PR dosing indication is listed for children

Promethazine (Phenergan®)

___ 12.5 mg __ 25 mg ___ IM __ PO administered as __ tablets or __ oral syrup __ suppository PR __ q 4 hours __ q 6 hours __ other __ prn nausea/vomiting

Dosage: usual dose PO/IM/PR: 12.5–25 mg/dose every 4–6 hours

Maximum: 25 mg/dose

Formulations: oral syrup/solution 6.25 mg/5 mL, tablets: 12.5 mg, 25 mg, 50 mg; rectal suppository: 12.5 mg, 25 mg, 50 mg

Comments: **IV is not recommended due to risk of severe tissue injury. Avoid SQ or intra-arterial due to severe local reaction.**

Avoid age < 2 years due to risk of respiratory depression.

Trimethobenzamide (Tigan®)

__ 300 mg PO __ q 6 hours __ q 8 hours __ other __ prn nausea/vomiting

__ 200 mg IM __ q 6 hours __ q 8 hours __ other __ prn nausea/vomiting

Dosage: 300 mg/dose PO q 6–8 hours, 200 mg IM tid or qid

Maximum: single dose: 300 mg PO, 200 mg IM

Formulations: capsule 300 mg

Comments: **IV is not recommended. IM is not recommended in children. PR is no longer available.**

Antitussives* and Oral Topical Solutions

Promethazine and Codeine (Phenergan® with Codeine)

__ 5 mL PO __ q 4 hours ___ q 6 hours __ other __ prn cough

Dosage: 5 mL every 4–6 hours

Maximum: 30 mL in 24 hours

Formulations: 6.25 mg promethazine/10 mg codeine/per 5 mL

Guaifenesin (Robitussin Chest Congestion®, Mucinex®, Good Sense Mucus Relief®)

__ 200 mg __ 400 mg PO __ q 4 hours administered as ___ oral liquid/solution/syrup or ___ tablet

__ 600 mg __ 1200 mg PO extended release tablets q 12 hours __ prn cough

Dosage: 200–400 mg every 4 hours, extended release tablets 600–1200 mg every 12 hours

Maximum: 2.4 grams per day

Formulations: oral liquid/solution/syrup: 100 mg/5 mL, tablets: 200 mg, 400 mg, extended release tablet (12 hour): 600 mg, 1200 mg

Guaifenesin and Codeine Robitussin AC

__ mL oral solution/syrup or __ tablets __ capsules PO ___ q 4 hours __ q 6 hours __ other __ prn cough

Dosage: tablets: 1 tablet every 4–6 hours, 2 capsules every 4 hours, liquid/solution/syrup (100 mg guaifenesin/10 mg codeine) 10 mL every 4 hours

Maximum: maximum in 24 hours: tablets: 6, capsules: 12, liquid (100–200 mg guaifenesin/10 mg codeine): 60 mL

Formulations: liquid/solution/syrup: 100 mg guaifenesin and 10 mg codeine/ 5 mL, tablets: 400 mg guaifenesin and 10 mg codeine, 400 mg guaifenesin and 20 mg codeine; oral capsules: guaifenesin 200 mg and 9 mg codeine

Guaifenesin and Dextromethorphan (Cheracol D®, Coricidin HBP®, Mucinex DM®, Robitussin DM®)

___ 5 mL __ 10 mL __15 mL __ 1 tablet __ 1–2 tablets ___ 2 tablets PO __ q 4 hours __ q 6 hours __ q 12 hours __ other ___ prn cough

Dosage: guaifenesin 200–400 mg and dextromethorphan 10–20 mg q 4–6 hours cough

Maximum: guaifenesin 2400 mg and dextromethorphan 120 mg per day

Formulations: oral liquid/syrup: guaifenesin 100 mg and dextromethorphan 10 mg/5 mL, oral capsule: guaifenesin 200 mg and dextromethorphan 10 mg, oral caplet: guaifenesin 400 mg and dextromethorphan 20 mg, tablets: guaifenesin 1,000 mg and dextromethorphan 60 mg, extended release: guaifenesin 600 mg and dextromethorphan 30 mg, guaifenesin 1200 mg and dextromethorphan 60 mg

Hydrocodone and Homatropine (Hycodan®)

PO administered as __ mL syrup __ 1 tab __ q 4 hours __ q 6 hours prn cough

Dosage: 1 tablet or 5 mL every 4–6 hours prn

Maximum: 6 tablets or 30 mL in 24 hours

Formulation: oral syrup: hydrocodone 5 mg and homatropine 1.5 mg/mL, tablet: hydrocodone 5 mg and homatropine 1.5 mg

Lidocaine (Xylocaine®) viscous 2% (oral topical solution)

PO solution __ 5 mL __ 10 mL __ 15 mL __ q 4 hours __ q 6 hours q ___ hours (swish in mouth or gargled then spit out)

Dosage: 15 mL swished in mouth or gargled and spit out, frequency q 3 hours or greater

Maximum: frequency: no greater than every 3 hours; per dose: 300 mg or 4.5 mg/kg, 8 doses per 24 hours

Formulations: solution, viscous 2% = 20 mg/mL

* There are many different formulations and strengths for the various antitussives depending on the manufacturer so it is important to verify specific formulations before prescribing

Anxiolytics/Medications for Sleep**

Benzodiazepine Hypnotics

Lorazepam (Ativan®)

__ 0.5 mg ___1 mg __ 2 mg __ other ___ qhs __ IV__ PO administered as __ tablet or __ oral solution __ q 4 hours ___ q 6 hours __ q 12 hours __ other ___ prn sleep ___ prn anxiety

Dosage: 2 mg PO, 1 mg IV

Maximum: single dose 2 mg

Formulations: oral solution: 2 mg/mL, tablets: 0.5 mg, 1 mg

Comments: Use lower dose 0.5 mg IV and 1 mg PO in elderly or debilitated. Administered qhs for sleep. Other dosage administration schedules including qhs are used for treatment of anxiety.

Temazepam (Restoril®)

__ 7.5 mg __ 15 mg __ 30 mg __ other PO qhs

Dosage: 15–30 mg PO qhs

Maximum: 30 mg daily

Formulations: capsule: 7.5 mg, 15 mg, 22.5 mg, 30 mg

Comments: In elderly or debilitated start with 7.5 mg

Triazolam (Halcion®)

___ 0.125 mg ___ 0.25 mg PO qhs

Dosage: 0.25 mg qhs

Maximum: 0.5 mg daily

Formulations: 0.125 mg, 0.25 mg

Comments: In elderly or debilitated start with 0.125 mg

Nonbenzodiazepine Hypnotics

Zolpidem (Ambien®)

__ 5 mg __ 10 mg PO administered as __ tablets __ sublingual tablets __ spray or __ oral solution qhs __ other

Dosage: immediate release tablet/spray: females 5 mg, males: 5–10 mg, extended release tablet: females 6.25 mg, males: 6.25–12.5 mg

Maximum: immediate release tablets/spray or sublingual tablets: 10 mg daily, extended release tablets: 12.5 mg daily

Formulations: oral solution 5 mg/7.7 mL; tablets: 5 mg, 10 mg; sublingual tablets: 1.75 mg, 3.5 mg, 5 mg, 10 mg; extended or controlled release tablets: 6.25 mg, 12.5 mg

Comments: Use 5 mg of immediate release tablet/spray or 6.25 mg of extended release tablet in debilitated or elderly as well as in females.

Eszopiclone (Lunesta®)

__ 1 mg __ 2 mg __ 3 mg PO qhs

Dosage: single dose 2 mg

Maximum: 2 mg

Formulations: tablets: 1 mg, 2 mg, 3 mg

Comments: Start with 1 mg in elderly or debilitated. Use lowest effective dose.

Other Hypnotics

Diphenhydramine (Benadryl®)

__ 25 mg ___ 50 mg __ IV __ PO administered as __ capsule __ oral elixir qhs

Dosage: 25 mg or 50 mg qhs

Maximum: single dose 50 mg

Formulations: oral elixir: 12.5 mg/5 mL, 25 mg/10 mL; capsule: 25 mg, 50 mg

Comments: Not recommended in elderly because it is a potent anticholinergic and has increased risk of side effects in this age group.

May cause paradoxical excitation especially in pediatric patients.

** In general, use lower doses in the elderly or the debilitated.

Allergy Medications

Cetirizine (Zyrtec®)

__ 2.5 mg __ 5 mg __ 10 mg __ PO administered as __ tablets __ oral solution daily

Dosage: 5–10 mg daily

Maximum: 10 mg per dose

Formulations: oral solution: 5 mg/5 mL; tablet: 5 mg, 10 mg; chewable tablet: 5 mg, 10 mg

Diphenhydramine (Benadryl®)

__ 25 mg ___ 50 mg __ IV __ PO administered as __ capsules __ oral elixir q 6 hours ___ other __ prn itching/allergy

Dosage: 25–50 mg per dose PO/IM/IV

Maximum: single dose 100 mg, PO 300 mg per day, IM/IV 400 mg per day

Formulations: oral elixir: 12.5 mg/5 mL, 25 mg/10 mL; capsule: 25 mg, 50 mg

Loratadine (Claritin®)

___ 5 mg __ 10 mg PO daily administered as __ capsule/tablet __ chewable tablet __ solution/syrup __ oral concentrate

Dosage: 10 mg daily

Maximum: 10 mg daily

Formulations: oral solution/syrup: 5mg/5 mL; oral concentrate 1mg/mL, capsule/tablet/ODT tablet 10 mg, oral chewable tablet: 5 mg

Asthma/COPD Medications (Adult Dosage)

Inhaled Medications: Aerosols

Albuterol Nebulization (Proair®, Proventil®, Ventolin®)

__ 2.5 mg/dose __ 5.0 mg/dose × 1 __ q 4 hours __ q 6 hours __ every 20 minutes × 3 __ other ___ continuous nebulization __ 10 mg/hour __15 mg/hour ___ other __ prn wheezing

Dosage: usual dose: 2.5–5 mg/dose, continuous nebulization is 10–15 mg/hour

Maximum: minimum single dose 2.5 mg, maximum single dose 5.0 mg

Formulation: solution for inhalation: 2.5 mg/0.5 mL, 2.5 mg/3 mL

Comments: Doses recommended by National Heart Lung and Blood Institute (NHLBI) Expert Panel Report (EPR) – 3

Ipratropium Nebulization (Atrovent®)

___ 0.5 mg/dose __ q 6 hours __ q 8 hours __ other __ prn wheezing

Dosage: usual dose: infants/children up to 12 years: 0.25–0.5 mg/dose, adults 0.5 mg/dose

Maximum: single dose: 500 mcg (2.5 mL)

Formulation: solution for inhalation: 500 mcg (2.5 mL of 0.02% solution)

Comments: Doses recommended by National Heart Lung and Blood Institute (NHLBI) Expert Panel Report (EPR) – 3

Inhaled Medications: Inhalers

Albuterol (Proventil®, Ventolin®) Inhaler (MDI with spacer)

__ 1–2 puffs (90–180 mcg) __ q 4 hours __ q 6 hours __ other ___ prn wheezing

Dosage: usual dose: child and adult 1–2 puffs [90–180 mcg] q 4–6 hours

Maximum: 8 puffs per 24 hours

Formulation: 90 mcg/actuation

Ipratropium (Atrovent®) Inhaler

__ 1–2 puffs __ 2–3 puffs every 6 hours __ other __ prn wheezing

Dosage: usual dose: child < 12 years 1–2 puffs, ≥ 12 years and adult 2–3 puffs every 6 hours

Maximum: 12 puffs per 24 hours

Formulation: 17 mcg/actuation

Cardiac Medications/Antihypertensives

Diltiazem (Cardizem®, Cardizem CD®, Cardizem LA®, Cartia XT®, Dilacor XR®, Dilt-CD®, Dilt- XR®, Diltiazem HCl CD®, Matzim LA®, TaztiaXT®, Tiazac)

__ 120 mg __ 180 mg __ 240 mg __ 300mg __ 360 mg __ 420 mg extended release tablets/capsules PO __ qd __ other

Dosage: PO *for hypertension*: once daily extended release tablet (Cardizem LA®) initial dosing 180–240 mg once daily, usual dose 240–360 mg daily; extended release capsule (once daily dosing) (Cardizem CD®, Dilacor XR®) initial 180–240 mg once daily, usual 240–360 mg once daily; PO *for atrial fibrillation*: extended release capsule or tablet: usual dose: 120–360 mg once daily

Maximum: depends on indications and specific drug: PO *for hypertension:* once daily extended release capsule 480 mg (Cardizem CD®, Cartia XT, Dilt-CD), 540 mg (Dilacor XR®, Diltia XT, Dilt-XR, Tiazac XT®)

Formulations: extended 24-hour release tablets or 24-hour extended release capsules: 120 mg, 180 mg, 240 mg, 300 mg, 360 mg, 420 mg

Comments: The IV forms are not listed since they are used for atrial fibrillation with rapid ventricular response, and these patients are not usually treated in the observation unit. Doses for angina differ from the doses for hypertension. In general, patients with acute angina are not generally placed in the observation unit so doses for immediate release (which has an indication for angina) and the angina doses are not listed. The 12-hour extended release capsules/tablets are not listed since once-a-day dosing is more convenient and has greater compliance.

Hydralazine (Apresoline®)

__ 10 mg __ 25 mg __ 50 mg __ other __ PO q 6 hours __ 5 mg __ 10 mg __ 20 mg __ other __ mg IV × 1 ___ other

Dosages: PO initially 10 mg qid with increase to 25 mg during first week, further increase to 50 mg qid, IV: 10–20 mg for hypertensive emergencies

Maximum: PO 300 mg daily in divided doses

Formulations: tablets: 10 mg, 25 mg, 50 mg, 100 mg

Comments: IV may have unpredictable and prolonged antihypertensive effects and is an unlabeled dose but is used for hypertensive emergencies.

Metoprolol (Lopressor®, Toprol®)†

__ 50 mg __ 100 mg __ mg __ other PO immediate release tab (Lopressor®) __ bid
__ 25 mg __ 50 mg __ 100 mg __ mg __ other PO extended release tab (Toprol®) qd
___ 5 mg __ 10 mg IV __ × 1 __ q 6 hours __ q 12 hours q __ hours __ other

† Hold all rate controlling drugs if heart rate < 50 beats/minute or systolic BP < 90 mmHg

_____

Dosages: PO for hypertension: immediate release: initially 50 mg twice daily, usual dose range 50–100 mg daily, extended release

initially 25 to 100 mg once daily, usual dose range 50–100 mg daily

Maximum: PO for hypertension: immediate release 450 mg daily dose, extended release 400 mg daily

Formulations: tablets: 25 mg, 50 mg, 100 mg: extended release 24-hour tablets: 25 mg, 50 mg, 100 mg, 200 mg

Comments: Doses for angina and myocardial infarction are not listed since these patients are not generally placed in the observation unit.

Diuretics

Furosemide (Lasix®)

__ mg __ IV or __ PO administered as __ tablet ___ solution __ bid __ qd

Dosage: for hypertension 40 mg PO bid; for heart failure initially 20–80 mg PO per dose, double the dose or increase by 20–40 mg per dose if inadequate response. IV: initially 20–40 mg, double the dose or increase by 20–40 mg per dose if inadequate response.

Maximum: 600 mg PO daily, 200 mg IV daily

Formulations: oral solution: 10 mg/mL, 40 mg/5 mL; tablets: 20 mg, 40 mg, 80 mg

Comments: American Heart Association heart failure guidelines recommend PO initially 20–40 mg qd or bid up to a maximum of 600 mg daily

Hydrochlorothiazide (Microzide®)

__ 12.5 mg __ 25 mg __ 50 mg PO __ bid __ qd

Dosage: for hypertension: initially 12.5 to 25 mg daily, up to 50 mg daily in 1–2 divided doses; for edema: 25–100 mg daily in 1–2 divided doses

Maximum: 50 mg daily

Formulations: tablets: 12.5 mg, 25 mg, 50 mg; capsules: 12.5 mg

Comments: Doses higher than 50 mg daily do not result in a greater diuretic response and are associated with greater incidence of electrolyte abnormalities and is not recommended.

Statins

Atorvastatin (Lipitor®)

__ 20 mg __ 40 mg __ 80 mg PO qd
Dosage: 10–80 mg daily
Maximum: 80 mg daily

Formulations: tablets: 10 mg, 20 mg, 40 mg, 80 mg

Lovastatin (Mevacor®)

__ 20 mg __ 40 mg __ 80 mg immediate release tablets PO taken with evening meal

__ 20 mg __ 40 mg __ 60 mg PO extended release tablets qhs

Dosage: for immediate release 20–80 mg taken with evening meal; for extended release: 20 mg, 40 mg, or 60 mg taken at bedtime

Maximum: immediate release: 80 mg daily, extended release 60 mg daily

Formulations: tablets: 10 mg, 20 mg, 40 mg; extended release 24-hour tablets: 20 mg, 40 mg, 60 mg

Rosuvastatin (Crestor®)

__ 10 mg __ 20 mg __ 40 mg PO qd

Dosage: 10–40mg once daily

Maximum: 40 mg daily

Formulations: tablets: 5 mg, 10 mg, 20 mg, 40 mg

Simvastatin (Zocor®)

__ 5 mg __ 10 mg __ 20 mg __ 40 mg PO qhs

Dosage: doses from 5–40 mg daily

Maximum: 40 mg daily

Formulations: tablets: 5 mg, 10 mg, 20 mg, 40 mg, 80 mg (do not use 80 mg tablets, see comments)

Comments: The risk of myopathy is increased with higher doses (80 mg) so doses > 40 mg of simvastatin should be avoided.

Steroids

Prednisone† (Deltasone®, Liquid Pred®, Orasone®)

__ 40 mg __ 60 mg PO __ qd __ bid __ other

Dosage: 40–80 mg per day, in 1–2 divided doses

Maximum: 80 mg per day

Formulations: oral solution 5 mg/5 mL, tablets: 1 mg, 2.5 mg, 5 mg, 10 mg, 20 mg, 50 mg

Comments: Greater patient compliance is more likely with once a day vs. bid dosing

Prednisolone† (Oraped®, Prelone®, Pediapred®, Veripred®)

__ 40 mg __ 60 mg PO __ qd __ bid__ other

Dosage: 40–80 mg per day

Maximum: 80 mg per day

Formulations: oral solutions: Pediapred® 5 mg/5 mL, Orapred® 15 mg/5 mL, Veripred® 20 mg/ 5mL: oral syrup: Prelone® 15mg/5 mL, tab = 5 mg

Comments: Dosing for prednisone and prednisolone is the same. Greater patient compliance is more likely with once a day vs. bid dosing.

Methylprednisolone‡ (Medrol®, Medrol Dose Pack®, Solu-medrol®)

__ mg __ PO __ IV __ IM __ every 12 hours __ daily __ other ___

Dosage: 40–60 mg/day; in 1–2 divided doses per day PO/IV/IM, in adults initial higher dose sometimes used__ 125 mg × 1 followed by 40–60 mg every 6 hours

Maximum: initial dose 125 mg, subsequent doses: 60 mg per dose

Formulations: tablets: 2 mg, 4 mg, 8 mg

‡ Doses generally used for asthma. Much higher doses used in some specific disorders such as exacerbation of multiple sclerosis or for cerebral edema

†National Heart, Lung, and Blood Institute (NHBLI) Expert Panel Report (EPR) 3 guidelines for the diagnosis and treatment of asthma recommends prednisone or prednisolone 1–2 mg/kg/day for pediatrics, for adults 40–80 mg/day in 1–2 divided doses. Commonly, once-a-day dosing is used due for better compliance and the lower total daily dose of 40 or 60 mg maximum is used.

Medications for DEEP VEIN THROMBOSIS***††

Vitamin K Antagonist

Warfarin (Coumadin®)

___ mg PO __ qd __ qod __ other

Dosage: Initially 2–5 mg once daily for healthy individual. Initial dosing must be individualized.

Maximum: Dosage must be adjusted according to the INR.

Comments: In patients with acute venous thromboembolism (VTE), initiation of warfarin may begin on the first or second day of low molecular weight heparin or unfractionated heparin therapy.

Initial dose in geriatric patients is ≤ 5 mg po.

Lower starting doses are used in patients with significant comorbidities (such as heart failure or hepatic impairment). Patients with significant comorbidities are not usually placed in the observation unit with VTE.

Low Molecular Weight Heparins

Dalteparin (Fragmin®)††

___ 200 units/kg × ___ weight (kg) SQ qd

Dosage: for DVT (with or without PE) ††: 200 units/kg SC daily or 100 units/kg bid

Maximum: 18,000 units/day

Comment: Once-a-day dosing is preferred.

††Unlabeled use in United States.

Enoxaparin (Lovenox®)

___ 1 mg/kg/dose × ___ weight (kg) q 12 hours SQ

Dosage: for DVT treatment (without PE) ††: 1 mg/kg/dose every 12 hours

Maximum: single dose 1mg/kg

Comments: Weight-based doses are generally rounded to the nearest 10 mg for doses ≤ 100 mg and rounded to the nearest graduation mark on the prefilled syringe for doses > 100 mg

Tinzaparin (Innohep®)

___ 175 units/kg × ___weight (kg) SQ qd

Dosage: for DVT treatment (without PE) †† 175 anti-Xa units/kg once daily SC

Maximum: 18,000 anti-Xa units/day

Comments: 1 mg of tinzaparin equals 70–120 units of anti-Xa activity.

Factor Xa inhibitor

Fondaparinux (Arixtra®)

___ 5 mg if < 50 kg, ___ 7.5 mg if 50–100 kg, ___ 10mg if ≥100 kg SQ qd

Dosage: for acute DVT/PE treatment†: 5 mg if < 50 kg, 7.5 mg if 50–100 kg, 10mg if ≥100 kg daily administered SQ

Maximum: 10 mg daily

Comments: Warfarin is started on the first or second treatment day and fondaparinux is continued until the INR is ≥ 2 for at least 24 hours (usually 5–7 days)

††There are other indications including DVT prophylaxis prior to surgery but these patients are generally inpatients.

*** There are many new anticoagulants as well as additional new indications for the various drugs in this class of medications. There is much discussion regarding treatment of uncomplicated VTE in the observation unit (See chapter 31) so these drugs are included. There are many terms for these drugs including novel or newer or "non-vitamin K oral anticoagulants" (NOACs), target specific oral anticoagulants (TSOACs), "direct oral Anticoagulants" (DOACs), and oral direct inhibitors ("ODIs").

Heparin

___ bolus of ___ units/kg IV then maintenance infusion at ___ units/kg/hour IV

Dosage: usual VTE dose is 80 units/kg IV bolus followed by 18 mg/kg/hour‡‡

Comment: Warfarin is started on the first or second treatment day and the heparin is continued until the INR is ≥ 2 for at least 24 hours (usually 5–7 days). This is an unlabeled usage.

‡‡ From: "Executive summary: antithrombotic therapy and prevention of thrombosis" 9th ed., American College of Chest Physicians Evidenced Based Clinical Practice Guidelines. Chest 2012; 141 (2 suppl):7-47.

VTE = venous thromboembolism

DVT = deep vein thrombosis

Medications for Headache Pain (Abortive Medications for Acute Attack)△

Acetaminophen (Paracetamol) (Tylenol®)

325 mg tab ___ 1 tab ___ 1–2 tabs ___ 2 tabs PO ___ q 4 hours ___ q 6 hours ___ prn pain ___ prn fever (maximum 4 g daily)

____ If unable to take tablet formulation, may give suspension

____ If unable to take PO, may give suppository PR ___325 mg ___ 650 mg ___ q 4 hours ___ q 6 hours

Dosage: regular strength: 650 mg every 4–6 hours, extra-strength: 1,000 mg every 6 hours, rectal 650 mg every 6 hours

Maximum: 4,000 mg per day.

Formulations: oral solution or suspension = 160 mg/5 mL, tablet or gelcap in 325 mg or 500 mg, chewable or oral disintegrating in 80 mg, rectal suppository in 120 mg or 325 mg or 650 mg

Comments: Over the counter (OTC) dosing may differ by product and manufacturer. For children > 12 years and adults OTC dosages are: regular strength 650 mg every 4–6 hours with maximum daily dose of 3,250 mg daily; extra strength: 1,000 mg every 6 hours with a maximum daily dose of 3,000 mg; and rectal: 650 mg every 4–6 hours with a maximum daily dose of 3,900 mg.

IV ___ mg ___ q 4 hours ___ q 6 hours ___ prn pain ___ prn fever (maximum adult dose: if weight < 50 kg is 15 mg/kg up to 750 mg for a single dose, 75 mg/kg up to 3750 mg for daily dose; if weight > 50 kg is 650 mg q 4 hours or 1000 mg q 6 hours up to 1000 mg for a single dose and 4000 mg for a daily dose)

Dihydroergotamine△△ (D.H.E®, Migranal®)

___1 mg ___ IV ___ IM ___ SQ ___ prn pain
___ may repeat q hourly if headache still present × 1 IV (up to total of 2 doses, 1 hour apart) or × 2 if SQ or IM (up to total of 3 doses, each 1 hour after the last dose)

IN ___ 1 mg ___ prn pain ___ may repeat after 15 minutes if headache still present

Dosage: 1 mg IV/IM/SQ, may repeat hourly (× 1 for IV up to 2 mg/day, × 2 for IM/SQ up to 3 mg/day); 1 mg IN, may repeat after 15 minutes if headache still present up to 2 mg/day

Maximum: IV: 2 mg IV daily, 6 mg/ week; IM/SQ 3 mg daily, 6 mg/week; IN: 3 mg (6 sprays)/day, 4 mg (8 sprays)/week

Formulations: solution (as injection): 1 mg/mL; nasal: 4 mg/mL

Comment: IN is administered as 0.5 mg in each nostril for 1 mg dose

IN = intranasal

Diphenhydramine (Benadryl®)

___ 25 mg ___ 50 mg ___ IV ___ IM ___ PO administered as ___capsule ___ elixir ___ every 6 hours ___ other ___ prn headache

Dosage: 25–50 mg per dose PO/IM/IV

Maximum: single dose 100 mg, PO 300 mg per day, IV/IM 400 mg per day

Formulations: oral elixir: 12.5 mg/5 mL, 25 mg/ 10 mL; capsule: 25 mg, 50 mg

Toradol (Ketorolac®)

___ 30 mg ___ IV ___IM ___ q 6 hours ___ q 8 hours ___ other ___ prn pain

Dosage: 30 mg every 6 hours

Maximum: 30 mg per dose and 120 mg per day IV/IM

Comments: Therapy should not exceed 5 days. Oral formulations are available but are not recommended and other alternative PO NSAIDs are recommended in pediatric and adult patients

Magnesium (PO forms: Mag-200®, Mag-Ox®, Uro-mag®)

___ mg PO ___ q 6 hours ___ qd ___ other ___ 2 grams × 1 IV ___ prn pain

Dosage: Magnesium sulfate 2 grams IV

Maximum: Magnesium sulfate single dose IV 2 grams, infusion rate is 1 gram/hour; tablets: 8/day

Formulations: PO (magnesium oxide): tablets: 200 mg, 250 mg, 400 mg, 420 mg; capsules 140 mg

Comments: For the IV infusion, place the patient on a monitor. Magnesium administered for headache is similar to the use of magnesium for asthma. See also electrolyte-hypomagnesemia order set.

Methylprednisolone (Solumedrol®)

___ 60 mg ___ 125 mg IV × 1 ___ other ___ prn pain

Dosage: sometimes higher dose (125 mg) is used initially followed by 40– 60 mg every 6 hours or 60 mg every 6 hours

Maximum: initial dose 125 mg, subsequent doses: 60 mg per dose

Sumatriptan△△ (Imitrex®)

___ 50 mg PO administered as ___ tablets ___ solution ___ may repeat in 2 hours if headache persists; ___ 6 mg SQ × 1, ___ 20 mg IN × 1

Dosage: 50 mg PO × 1, may repeat in 2 hours if headache persists, IN: 5 mg, 10 mg or 20 mg, may repeat in 2 hours if headache persists

Maximum: PO 200 mg daily; IN: 40 mg daily; SQ 12 mg daily

Formulations: tablets: 25 mg, 50 mg, 100 mg: subcutaneous: 6 mg/0.5 mL, intranasal: 5 mg/ actuation, 20 mg/actuation

Comments: For the oral route, 50 mg and 100 mg are more effective than 25 mg. The 100 mg dose has more side effects than the 50 mg dose so the 50 mg dose for PO is recommended.

For the SQ route, if the first 6 mg has not been effective, a second dose SQ is not likely to be effective and thus, is not recommended. For the IN route, an initial dose of 20 mg is more effective than 5 mg or 10 mg, so the initial dose of 20 mg IN is recommended. Since these patients are usually nauseous and/or vomiting, we tend not to use the oral route. The nasal route of administration is a less commonly used option since absorption may be more variable.

Valproate (Depacon®, Depakene®, Depakote®)

__ 500 mg IV q 12 hours or ___1,000 mg qd ___ prn pain

Dosage: 500 mg IV q12 hours or 1,000 mg daily

Maximum: 1000 mg daily

Comments: Oral forms are also available but generally patients placed in the observation unit have nausea/vomiting, have failed initial emergency department therapy, and have a severe enough headache that they will need IV therapy.

⌂ See also protocol for headache pain. For patients with shunts (unlike the headache protocol), sometimes opioids are used.

Consider giving IV fluids such as normal saline since patients are often dehydrated from nausea/vomiting and poor po intake; and giving antiemetics to treat nausea/vomiting.

Opioids are not first-line therapy for treatment of acute headaches and are not recommended for several reasons including the problem of rebound that can occur with opiate use and concern for addiction.

Treatment of post-dural puncture headaches (e.g., headaches occurring after a lumbar puncture) may include caffeine with sodium benzoate IV and/or a blood patch (pain management or anesthesia consult). However, caffeine IV is no longer available so this option was not included.

Some of these medications are used for other indications, such as treatment of seizures, in addition to treatment of headaches. Other medications such as droperidol and low dose ketamine have also been used and recommended by some clinicians.

Oral forms of some of these medications are also available but generally patients placed in the observation unit have nausea/vomiting, have failed initial emergency department therapy, and have a severe enough headache that they will need IV therapy. Thus, for some of these headache medications, we have omitted the non-parenteral forms of the drug.

⌂⌂ Cannot use dihydroergotamine or sumatriptan within 24 hours of each other.

Dihydroergotamine and sumatriptan are contraindicated with coronary artery disease, history of stroke, hemiplegic migraine, and poorly controlled hypertension (systolic blood pressure > 140 mmHg or diastolic blood pressure > 90 mmHg).

Gastrointestinal (GI) Medications

Gastric Acid Proton Pump Inhibitors

Lansoprazole (Prevacid®)

___ 15 mg ___ 30 mg PO administered as ___ suspension ___ ODT

Dosage: for gastroesophageal reflux or duodenal ulcer: 15 mg daily; for erosive esophagitis: 30 mg daily

Maximum: usual single dose 30 mg; for hypersecretory conditions, single dose up to up to 60 mg

Formulations: oral suspension: 3 mg/mL; ODT tablets (oral disintegrating tablets): 15 mg, 30 mg, delayed release capsules: 15 mg, 30 mg

Comments: Used with the co-administration of antibiotics for the eradication of *Helicobacter pylori*.

Omeprazole (Prilosec®)

__ 20 mg __ 40 mg __ mg __ PO administered as __ capsule __ suspension __ qd __ bid

Dosage: 20–40 mg/day in 1–2 divided doses

Maximum: usual single dose 40 mg

Formulations: oral suspension 2 mg/mL; delayed release capsules: 10 mg, 20 mg, 40 mg

Comments: Used with the co-administration of antibiotics for the eradication of *Helicobacter pylori*

Pantoprazole (**Protonix**®)

__ 40 mg PO __ other administered as __ tablet __ oral pack qd

Dosage: for gastroesophageal reflux, erosive esophagitis, peptic ulcer disease: 40 mg daily

Maximum: usual single dose 40 mg

Formulations: tablets: 20 mg, 40 mg; oral pack: 40 mg

Comments: Used with the co-administration of antibiotics for the eradication of *Helicobacter pylori* (unlabeled use in the United States).

Histamine-2-Receptor Antagonists

Famotidine (**Pepcid**®)

__ mg __ IV __ PO administered as __ capsule __ suspension __ bid ___ qd

Dosage: for gastrointestinal reflux: PO 20 mg bid; for ulcers: 40 mg qhs; for esophagitis: 20 mg bid or 40 mg bid

Maximum: single dose 40 mg PO or 20 mg IV

Formulations: oral suspension: 40 mg/5 mL, tablet: 10 mg, 20 mg, 40 mg

Antacids

Aluminum Hydroxide (**Amphogel**®)

__ 600 mg __ 1200 mg PO administer 1–3 hours after meals

Dosage: for hyperacidity: 600–1200 mg taken between meals and qhs

Maximum: 3,840 mg in 24 hours

Formulations: suspension 300 mg/5 mL

Comments: When given for an antacid, take 1–3 hours after a meal. Also given for hyperphosphatemia but these doses are not listed since patients with severe electrolyte abnormalities are not generally placed in the observation unit.

Aluminum Hydroxide, Magnesium Hydroxide, and Simethicone (**Maalox Advanced Regular Strength**®, **Mylanta Classic Regular Strength**®)

__ 10 mL __ 20 mL oral liquid or __ 2 tab __ 4 tab PO __ once __ q 4 hours __ q 6 hours ____ prn GI upset (take between meals and qhs)

Dosage: 10–20 mL or 2–4 tablets every 4–6 hours

Maximum: not listed

Formulations: oral liquid: aluminum hydroxide 200 mg, magnesium hydroxide 200 mg, and simethicone 20 mg per 5 mL; chewable tablets: aluminum hydroxide 200mg, magnesium hydroxide 200 mg, and simethicone 25 mg

Comments: Administer 1–3 hours after a meal and 1–2 hours apart from oral medications.

Antacid/Laxative

Magnesium Hydroxide (**Milk of Magnesia**®)

__ 5–15 mL oral suspension __ 2–4 tabs PO ___ once __ 4 times a day ___ prn GI upset

Dosage: 5–15 mL or 2–4 tablets every 4 hours up to 4 times a day

Maximum: 16 tabs daily

Formulations: oral suspension 400 mg/5 mL, oral chewable tablets: tablets: 400 mg

Laxatives

Bisacodyl (**Ducolax**®)

__ 5 mg __ 15 mg PO (tablets) __ once __ other

Dosage: 5–15 mg PO, up to 30 mg for bowel evacuation

Formulations: tablets: 5 mg

Docusate (**Colace**®)

___ mg PO administered as __ capsule/tablet or __ syrup/liquid __ once ___ q 12 hours

Dosage: PO 50–500 mg/day in 1–4 divided doses

Formulations: oral capsules (as sodium): 50 mg, 100 mg, 250 mg; oral capsules (as calcium): 240 mg; oral tablets: 100 mg; oral syrup: 60 mg/15 mL; oral liquid: 50 mg/5 mL

Magnesium Citrate (**Citroma**®)

PO administered as __ tablets __ oral solution __ 195 mL ____ 300 mL once __ other

Dosage: 195–300 mL given once or in divided doses

Maximum: 300 mL/day

Formulations: oral solution: 1.75 g magnesium citrate/30 mL

Polyethylene Glycol (**Miralax**®)

__ 17 grams PO __ × 1 __ daily

Dosage: 17 grams daily

Maximum: dose 17 grams/day

Formulations: 17 grams powder dissolved in 8 ounces clear liquid

Comments: Do not use for more than 1 week

Enemas

Docusate (DucoSol®, Vacuant Mini-enema®) __ 283 mg PR once

Bisacodyl (Fleet®) __ 10 mg PR once

Soap suds enema __ PR once

Cotton seed enema __ PR once

GI Preparations for Colonoscopy

Polyethylene Glycol-electrolyte Solution (GoLytely®)

__ 240 mL q 10 minutes up to 4 liters PO or until rectal effluent is clear

Dosage: 240 mL (8 ounces)

Maximum: 4 liters PO

Formulations: PEG-3350 17.6 mmol/L, sodium 125 mmol/L, sulfate 40 mmol/L, chloride 35 mmol/L, bicarbonate 20 mmol/L, and potassium 10 mmol/L when dissolved in sufficient water to yield total volume of 4 L

Comments: Rehydrate before and after colonoscopy

Radiology Studies for Patients with Contrast Allergy: Prestudy Orders

Administer 13 hours prior to the study prednisone 50 mg PO, administer 7 hours prior to the study prednisone 50 mg PO, and administer 1 hour prior to the study prednisone 50 mg PO and diphenhydramine 50 mg PO _____

Other

Smoking Cessation

For smokers: Nicotine (Nicoderm®) patch __ 7 mg __ 14 mg __ 21 mg qd

Comments

* This is not an all-inclusive list but gives some of the more commonly used medications and routes of administration and frequently used brand names in the United States.

Dosing is for adults and does not include dosing for geriatric or pediatric age groups or for renal or hepatic impairment. The oral forms for tablets/capsules and liquid forms are both listed since some adult patients prefer liquid forms (such as patients with pharyngitis).

The formulations (e.g., oral, rectal, some subcutaneous) are listed since the health care provider may be starting a medication in the observation unit and then be writing a prescription for continuing the medication when the patient is discharged. Preparations and formulations vary greatly between manufacturers and specific institutions.

This list and any other medication list or medications mentioned throughout this textbook does not imply endorsement of any given medication or product.

These order sets are designed to serve as a guide for therapeutic decisions by including the usual suggested dose range. Patient-specific factors should always be taken into account in addition to the most current medical literature, drug information, and standards of practice to individualize therapy for a given patient.

Chapter

94

Adult Order Sets
Generic or General Order Set

Sharon E. Mace, MD, FACEP, FAAP

Adult Generic (General) Order Set

Place in Emergency Department (ED)
   Observation _____
Diagnosis _____, _____,

   _____

ED Attending _____
Resident (if applicable) _____
Advanced Practice Provider (if applicable)

   _____

Allergies: Yes _____ No _____

If yes, what _____,_____,_____,_____,

   _____,_____

Vital Signs

Temperature __ Pulse __ Respiration __ BP__
   Pulse oximetry ____
__ q 2 hours ___ q 4 hours ___ q 6 hours q ___
   hours ___ q shift ___ qd ____ other
Cardiac monitoring (telemetry) _____
Orthostatic vital signs _____
Continuous pulse oximetry _____
Neurologic checks __ q 2 hours __ q 4 hours __
   q 6 hours q __ hours __ q shift __ qd __ other
Vascular checks __ q 2 hours __ q 4 hours __
   q 6 hours q __hours __ q shift __ qd __ other
Other _____

Notify Physician if

Temperature (°C) > 38.0° ___ 38.5°___ 39° ___
   40° ____ other _____
Systolic blood pressure (mmHg) ≤ 90 ___
   ≥ 160 __ ≥ 180 ___ ≥ 200 __ other _____
Diastolic blood pressure (mmHg) ≥ 120 ____
   other _____
Heart rate ≤ 50 ___ ≥ 120 __ ≥ 150 ___ ≥
   200 ___ other _____
Oxygen saturation < 90% _____ other _____
Any change in mental status _____

Any respiratory distress _____
Any new or worsening change in extremity (such
   as color: pale or cyanotic, decreased capillary
   fill, diminished or absent pulses, increased
   pain, numbness or paresthesias) ____

Activity

Up ad lib _____
Assisted _____
Out of bed to chair _____
Bedrest with bathroom privileges _____
Bedrest with bedside commode _____
Bedrest _____
Other _____

Diet

NPO _____
Regular _____
Advance diet as tolerated _____
Clear liquids ____
Dental, mechanical soft _____
Diabetic _____
Formula _____
Full liquids _____
Low added fat/No added salt _____
Low cholesterol ____
Pureed _____
Sodium: 1 gram ___ 2 gram ___
   unrestricted____
Per feeding tube _____
Other _____

Nursing Interventions

Weight ___ on admission ___ qd ___ prior to
   discharge ____ other
Height ____
I & Os _____ routine _____ strict _____
Fluid restriction ___ mL/hours ___ mL/shift
   ____ mL/24 hours ___ other
Fall precautions _____

Seizure precautions _____

Capillary blood glucose ___ × 1 q ___ hours ___ before meals and at bedtime

Foley catheter ___ Straight cath for urine

_____

Elevation of extremity _____

Elevate head of bed at 30° _____

Wound Care

Dressing change q ___ hours ___ qd Wet-to-dry dressing q ___ hours ___ qd

Packing change in __ hours __ qd Packing removal in _____ hours

Respiratory Interventions

Oxygen __ liters nasal cannula __ venti mask at ___ liters per minute _____ other

Wean oxygen as tolerated without dyspnea, stridor or oxygen saturation < 90% ____

Peak flow __ on admission ___ prior to discharge ___ pre and post aerosols

Sleep apnea qhs __ CPAP BiPAP settings cm H_2O ___ inspiratory __ expiratory

Incentive spirometry __ q 2 hours __ q 4 hours __ q 6 hours q __ hours __ q shift __ qd __ other

Laboratory Tests

Amylase ___

Arterial blood gas ___ on room air ___ on other FiO2 ____

Basic metabolic panel _____

Blood alcohol level ____

Blood culture x ___

Brain natriuretic peptide (BNP) _____ repeat after treatment _____

Calcium ____ total ___ ionized

Carbon monoxide _____

Cardiac enzymes __ × 1 __ q 4 hours × 3 __ q 4 hours × 4 __ other __ with ECGs

CBC _____ with differential

Complete metabolic panel _____

C-reactive protein (CRP) _____

Creatinine phosphokinase (total) (total CPK) __ × 1 __ repeat in a.m., repeat q __ hours × __

CK-MB (creatinine kinase – myocardial band) __ × 1 __ q 4 hours × 3 __ q 4 hours × 4 __ other __ with ECGs

D-dimer _____

Drug level _____, _____, _____

Erythrocyte sedimentation rate (ESR)

_____

Fasting lipid panel ___

Glucose _____

Hemoglobin/hematocrit _____ Repeat hemoglobin/hematocrit in a.m. ___ at ___ hours

Influenza studies (influenza A and B) (by nasal swab) _____

Lactate _____

Lipase ___

Liver function tests _____

Magnesium ____

Monospot ___

Phosphorus ___

Pregnancy test (qualitative urine) _____

Pregnancy test (quantitative blood) _____

Rapid Strept ___

Renal function tests (BUN, creatinine) _____

Respiratory antigen panel (by nasal swab) ___

Respiratory syncytial virus (RSV) swab (by nasal swab) ___

Throat culture ___

Toxicology: blood drug screen ____

Toxicology: urine drug screen ____

Troponin __ × 1 __ q 4 hours × 3 __ q 4 hours × 4 __ other __ with ECGs

TSH (thyroid stimulating hormone) ___

Thyroid function tests (T3, T4, TSH) ____

Type and cross for __ units packed red blood cells

Type and Screen _____

Urinalysis _____

Urine culture _____

Venous blood gas ____

Cultures:

Blood culture ___ peripheral × ___, from central line ___ × ___

Urine culture _____

Wound culture _____ site _____

Gonorrhea_____ site

Chlamydia _____ site _____

Trichomonas _____ site _____

Fungal (Candida, KOH) ____ site ____

Other _____, _____, _____,

_____, _____

Repeat _____, _____, _____ in a.m. ___ in _____ hours

Radiology Studies

Plain X-rays

Acute abdominal series ____

CXR portable_____

CXR (PA and lateral) _____

Extremity x-rays _____right ___ left ____

KUB (Kidneys, ureters, bladder) x-ray

_____

Spine x-rays: Cervical ___ Thoracic ___ Lumbar ____

Soft tissue neck (PA and lateral) _____

Other _____, _____, _____

CT (Computed Tomography) Scans

CT abdomen/pelvis ____ without contrast ____ with contrast ___ IV ___ PO ___ PR

CT abdomen, renal stone protocol ____

CT brain _____ without contrast ____ with contrast

CT chest _____ without contrast ____ with contrast

CT face ____ without contrast ____ with contrast

CT neck ___ without contrast ____ with contrast

CT kidneys _____ without contrast ____ with contrast

CT enterography _____

CTA (computed tomography angiography) of brain with and without contrast (ultravist) if no contrast allergy and no renal failure (e.g., GFR ≥ 30) _____

CTA _____

Other _____, _____, _____

Ultrasound

Ultrasound abdomen (right upper quadrant)

_____

Ultrasound carotids: right __ left __ bilateral ____

Ultrasound extremity (rule out deep vein thrombosis) __ Upper __ Lower __ Right __ Left

Ultrasound kidneys ____

Ultrasound pelvis _____

Ultrasound _____

MRI (Magnetic Resonance Imaging)

MRI (Magnetic resonance imaging) of brain without contrast _____

MRI (Magnetic resonance imaging) of brain with and without contrast (gadolinium) if no allergy and no renal failure (e.g., GFR ≥30)

_____

MRA (Magnetic resonance angiography) Circle of Willis and of Carotids without contrast (if renal failure) _____

MRA (Magnetic resonance angiography) Circle of Willis and of Carotids with and without contrast (gadolinium) if no allergy and no renal failure (e.g., GFR ≥30) _____

MRI chest ___

MRI abdomen ___

MRI extremity ___

MRI spine: cervial __ thoracic __ lumbar __

MRI _____

MRA ____

Other Radiology Studies

Cholescintigraphy (hepatic iminodiacetic acid [HIDA] scan) _____

Transcranial doppler of brain vessels _____

Other _____, _____, _____

Interventional Radiology Procedures

Lumbar puncture under fluoroscopy

_____

Line placement _____

Feeding tube placement _____

Allergy Pretreatment for CT scans if contrast given: for contrast allergy

Administer 13 hours prior to the study: prednisone 50 mg PO, administer 7 hours prior to the study: prednisone 50 mg PO, and administer 1 hours prior to the study: prednisone 50 mg PO and diphenhydramine 50 mg PO _____

Cardiac Studies

Serial ECGs __ × 1 __ q 4 hours × 3 __ q 4 hours × 4 __ other ___ with cardiac enzymes

Echocardiogram (transthoracic) __ with agitated (bubble) study ___ without agitated (bubble)

Stress Tests/Cardiac Imaging Studies

Stress Electrocardiogram (treadmill stress test, exercise tolerance test/ETT) ___

Stress Echocardiogram ____

Pharmacologic Stress Tests

Coronary Vasodilators:

Adenosine _____
Dipyridamole/Persantine _____
Regadenosine/Lexiscan _____

Synthetic Catecholamine:

Dobutamine _____

Myocardial Perfusion Imaging (injection of radioactive isotopes):

Nuclear Stress Test

Thallium-201 _____
Technetium-99m Sestamibi _____
Technetium-99 Tetrofosmin _____

Gamma Imaging:

Single positron emission computed tomography (SPECT)_____
Cardiac positron emission tomography (PET)

Stress Cardiovascular Magnetic Resonance Imaging (CMR) _____
Computed Tomography Coronary Angiography (CTCA) _____
Other _____

* Not all tests are available at all institutions. Generally, test availability is limited, depends on many factors including available expertise and cost, and is institution specific. This list is not all inclusive but is intended to list the stress tests/cardiac imaging discussed in chapter 26 Stress Testing.

Gastrointestinal Studies

Esophagogastroduodenoscopy (EGD) _____
NPO after midnight _____
Colonoscopy in a.m. _____ NPO after midnight _____ Bowel prep _____

Neurologic Studies

Electroencephalogram (EEG) _____

Pulmonary Studies

Pulmonary function tests _____
OTHER _____, _____, _____

Consultants

Cardiology _____ Notified:
Name _____ Time _____
Care coordination (Case manager)_____
Notified: Name _____ Time _____

Colorectal surgery _____ Notified:
Name _____ Time _____
Dentistry _____ Notified:
Name _____ Time _____
Dermatology _____ Notified:
Name _____ Time _____
Dietician _____ Notified:
Name _____ Time _____
Endocrinology _____ Notified:
Name _____ Time _____
Family practice _____ Notified:
Name _____ Time _____
Gastroenterology _____Notified:
Name _____ Time _____
General surgery _____Notified:
Name _____ Time _____
Hand surgery _____Notified:
Name _____ Time _____
Heart failure _____ Notified:
Name _____ Time _____
Internal medicine _____ Notified:
Name _____ Time _____
Nephrology _____Notified:
Name _____ Time _____
Neurology _____Notified:
Name _____ Time _____
Neurosurgery _____ Notified:
Name _____ Time _____
Orthopedics _____ Notified:
Name _____ Time _____
PICC line _____Notified:
Name _____ Time _____
Psychiatry _____Notified:
Name _____ Time _____
Pulmonary _____ Notified:
Name _____ Time _____
Radiology _____ Notified:
Name _____ Time _____
Rheumatology _____ Notified:
Name _____ Time _____
Social work _____ Notified:
Name _____ Time _____
Urology _____ Notified:
Name _____ Time _____
Other _____ Notified:
Name _____ Time _____

Education: **patient** _____ **family** _____

Smoking cessation _____
Other _____

Chapter

95

Pediatric Order Sets
Medications

Sharon E. Mace, MD, FACEP, FAAP
Matthew J. Campbell, PharmD, BCPS, BCCCP

Drug, Dose, Route, Frequency, Indication, Formulation

PATIENT WEIGHT (kg) ____

Analgesics/Antipyretics
Acetaminophen (Paracetamol) (Tylenol®)

__ 10 mg/kg/dose __ 15 mg/kg/dose ____mg PO ____ other administered as ___ solution/ suspension ___ tablets/gelcaps ___ chewable/ oral disintegrating tablets __ PR suppository __ q 4 hours __ q 6 hours __ q 8 hours ___ prn pain ___ prn fever (temperature ≥ 38°C or 100.4°F)

Dosage: child/infants usual dose 10–15 mg/kg/ dose, children 6–11 years: 325 mg every 4–6 hours, children ≥ 12 years/adolescents: refer to adult dosing, adults: regular strength: 650 mg every 4–6 hours, extra-strength: 1,000 mg every 6 hours, rectal 650 mg every 6 hours

Maximum: children: single dose 15 mg/kg; daily dose: lesser of 75 mg/kg/day or 4,000 mg per day; no greater than 5 doses in 24 hours; adults: 4,000 mg per day.

Formulations: oral solution or suspension: 160 mg/5 mL, 500 mg/5 mL; tablets/gelcaps: 325 mg, 500 mg, chewable or oral disintegrating tablets (ODT) 80 mg, rectal suppositories: 120 mg, 325 mg, 650 mg

Comments: Over the counter (OTC) dosing may differ by product and manufacturer. For children > 12 years and adults OTC dosages are regular strength 650 mg every 4–6 hours with maximum daily dose of 3,250 mg daily; extra strength: 1,000 mg every 6 hours with a maximum daily dose of 3,000 mg; rectal: 650 mg every 4–6 hours with a maximum daily dose of 3,900 mg.

IV ___ mg __ q 4 hours __ q 6 hours ___ prn pain ___ prn fever (maximum dose: if weight < 50 kg is 15 mg/ kg up to 750 mg for a single dose, 75 mg/kg up to 3750 mg for daily dose; if weight > 50 kg is 650 mg q 4hours or 1000 mg q 6 hours up to 1000 mg for a single dose and 4000 mg for daily dose)

Aspirin (Acetylsalicylic Acid)

__ 10 mg/kg/dose __ 15 mg/kg/dose __ 81 mg __ 325 mg __ 650 mg __ other __ PO administered as __ tablets/caplets __ chewable tablets __PR __ q 4 hours __ q 6 hours __ q 8 hours __ daily __ other ___prn pain ___ prn fever (temperature ≥ 38°C or 100.4°F) ___ other

Dosage: usual dose when used as for antipyretic or analgesic: weight < 50 kg: 10–15 mg/kg/ dose every 4–6 hours, for children ≥ 12 years old and adolescents ≥ 50 kg: 325–650 mg every 4–6 hours

Maximum: for weight < 50 kg: maximum dose is lesser of either 120 mg/kg/day or 4,000 milligrams per day, for age ≥ 12 and adolescents weighing ≥ 50 kg: maximum is 4,000 mg per day

Formulations: tablets/caplets: 81 mg, 325 mg, 650 mg; chewable tablets: 81 mg; suppositories: 300 mg or 600 mg

Comments: Higher doses may be required for more potent anti-inflammatory properties, but patients needing the higher anti-inflammatory doses are not likely to be good candidates for the observation unit

Avoid with Reyes syndrome, "***Do not use aspirin in children < 12 years and adolescents who have or who are recovering from chickenpox or flu symptoms due to the association with Reye's syndrome.***"

Fentanyl (Duragesic®)

__ 0.5 mcg/kg/dose __ 1 mcg/kg/dose __ 2 mcg/kg/dose __ other __ IV __ IM __ q 2 hours __ q 4 hours __ other _ prn pain

Dosage: age $\geq$ 2 years, usual dose for pain 1–2 mcg/kg/dose. Weight based pediatric doses shouldn't exceed typical adult doses.

Maximum: not established, but may cause respiratory depression and CNS depression so dose should be titrated and used with caution

Formulations: Transdermal patches available in various mcg/hour but pediatric patients on such chronic pain medications are generally not candidates for the observation unit.

Transmucosal (buccal, sublingual, and nasal forms) available but have variable absorption so they are not listed. Oral forms are also available but have slower onset than parenteral and so may not be as desirable for acute pain and other oral opioids are more commonly used.

Comments: Opioid-tolerant patients may need higher doses. Single IV doses have a duration of about 30–60 minutes, while single IM doses have a duration of 1–2 hours.

Continuous infusions may be administered including patient controlled analgesia (PCA) but these pediatric patients tend not to be placed in the observation unit.

Hydrocodone and Acetaminophen (Lorcet®, Vicodin®)

__ 0.1 mg/kg/dose __ 0.2 mg/kg/dose __ mg (based on hydrocodone component) PO administered as __ solution __ tablets __ q 4 hours __ q 6 hours __ other __ prn pain

Dosage: usual dose is 0.1- 0.2 mg/kg/dose every 4–6 hours

Maximum: no more than 6 doses per day or the recommended maximum acetaminophen dose; weight $\geq$ 50 kg, refer to adult dose

Formulations: oral solution: hydrocodone 7.5 mg/acetaminophen 325 mg per 15 mL, tablets: hydrocodone 5 mg/acetaminophen 325 mg

Hydromorphone (Dilaudid®)

___ mg/kg/dose ___ mg __ IV __ PO administered as __ liquid __ tablets __ q 2 hours ___ q 4 hours __ q 6 hours __ q 8 hours __ other ___ prn pain

Dosage: usual dose child: IV 0.015 mg/kg/dose, PO 0.03–0.08 mg/kg/dose, every 4–6 hours; usual adolescent or adult dose: for opioid naïve patients IV/SQ: 0.2–0.6 mg/dose, PO 1–4 mg/dose, every 4–6 hours; > 50 kg refer to adult dose

Maximum: varies, depends on opioid naïve or opioid tolerant

Formulations: oral liquid: 1 mg/mL; tablets: 2 mg, 4 mg

Comments: IM has variable absorption and is not recommended.

Opioid-tolerant patients may need higher doses.

May cause respiratory depression and CNS depression so dose should be individualized, titrated, and used with caution.

Continuous infusions may be administered including patient controlled analgesia (PCA) but these patients tend not to be placed in the observation unit.

Ibuprofen (Advil®, Motrin®)

__ 200 mg __ 400 mg __ 600 mg __ 800 mg __ other PO __ q 6 hours __ q 8 hours __ other administered as __ suspension __ tablets __ chewable tablets __ prn pain ___prn fever (temperature $\geq$ 38°C or 100.4°F)

Dosage: age 6 months to 12 years: usual dose 5–10 mg/kg/dose every 6–8 hours as analgesic/antipyretic; age $\geq$ 12 years: use adult dose, usual adult dose 400–600 mg every 4–6 hours, 800 mg every 8 hours, 400–800 mg per dose

Maximum: for children < 12 years of age: single dose is 400 mg, 40 mg/kg per day up to 1,200 mg per day; for adults 3,200 mg per day

Formulation: oral suspension: 100 mg/5 mL, tablets: 100 mg, 200 mg, 400 mg, 600mg, 800 mg; chewable tablets: 50 mg, 100 mg

Comments: Patients should be well hydrated prior to administration.

Morphine (Duramorph®, Kadian®, MS Contin®)

__ mg/kg/dose __ mg __ IV __ PO administered as __ solution __ tablets __ extended release tablets __ q 2 hours __ q 3 hours __ q 4 hours __ qd __ other __ prn pain

Dosage: child/infant < 50 kg: usual dose PO 0.2–0.5 mg/kg/dose every 3–4 hours or IV 0.05–0.2 mg/kg/dose every 2–4 hours prn pain, for severe pain the higher dose is recommended

Maximum: initial maximum PO dose 15–20 mg, maximum IV doses for infants 2 mg/dose, for ages 1–6 years 4 mg/dose, for ages 7–12 years 8 mg/dose, adolescents and adults 10 mg/dose

Formulations: morphine oral solution: 10 mg/5 mL, tablets: 15 mg, 30 mg; extended release tablets: 15 mg, 30 mg, 60 mg, 100 mg

Comments: **IM is no longer recommended because of painful administration, variable absorption, and lag time to peak effect.**

Repeated SQ causes local pain, irritation, and induration.

Continuous infusions may be administered including patient-controlled analgesia (PCA) but these patients tend not to be placed in the observation unit.

Oxycodone and Acetaminophen (Endocet®, Percocet ®, Roxicet®)

__ 0.1 mg/kg/dose __ 0.2 mg/kg/dose (based on oxycodone component) __ other PO administered as __ solution __ tablets (5 mg oxycodone/325 mg acetaminophen) __ other __ q 4 hours __ q 6 hours __ other ___ prn pain

Dosage: initial dose is based on the oxycodone content, usual dose 0.1–0.2 mg/kg/dose every 4–6 hours; q 6 hours is the manufacturer's recommendation

Maximum: maximum initial oxycodone dose is 5 mg/dose, maximum daily dose is based on the acetaminophen content, see also recommendations for acetaminophen as above

Formulations: Roxicet solution: oxycodone 5 mg and acetaminophen 325 mg/ 5 mL, tablets: Roxicet 5 = 5 mg oxycodone/325 acetaminophen

Ketorolac (Toradol®)

__ 0.5 mg/kg/dose __ 30 mg __ other __ IV __ IM __ q 6 hours __ q 8 hours __ other __ prn pain

Dosage: usual IV dose: child 0.5 mg/kg/dose, child > 50 kg and adult 30 mg per dose

Maximum: for children > 16 years and > 50 kg and adults: 30 mg per dose and 120 mg per day IV/IM, not to exceed 5 days

Comments: Therapy should not exceed 5 days. Oral formulations are available but are not recommended and other alternative PO NSAIDs are recommended in pediatric and adult patients.

Tramadol (Synapryn®, Ultram®)

__ 1 mg/kg/dose __ 2 mg/kg/dose __ 50 mg __ 100 mg __ other PO administered as __

suspension __ tablets __ extended release tablets/capsules __ q 4 hours __ q 6 hours __ other ___ prn pain

Dosage: usual dose: child 1–2 mg/kg/dose; adult: 50–100 mg/dose every 4–6 hours

Maximum: 400 mg per day (pediatric and adult)

Formulations: oral suspension 10 mg/mL; tablets 50 mg; extended release 24-hour tablets or capsules: 100 mg, 200 mg, 300 mg

Comments: Tramadol is not Food and Drug Administration (FDA) approved for use in children, although there is data showing "off-label" use in children. The FDA is currently further evaluating the use of tramadol in pediatric patients < 17 years old and encouraging providers to consider alternative analgesic therapy. Ultrarapid metabolizers of CYP2D6 may generate more active opioid metabolites which potentially increases the risk of adverse events. In view of this information, it is probably best to use other opioids in the pediatric population.

Antibiotics

Amoxicillin (Amoxil®, Moxatag®)

__ mg/kg/dose __ 250 mg __ 500 mg ___ 875 mg __ other __ q 8 hours ___ q 12 hours PO administered as ___ suspension ___ capsules/tablets

Dosage: child > 3 months standard dose 25–50 mg/kg/24 hour, high dose 80–90 mg/kg/day divided into 2–3 doses; usual adult dose: 250–500 mg q 8 hours or 500–875 mg every 12 hours

Maximum: single dose 875 mg, daily dose 2,000–4,000 mg per day depending on indication

Formulations: oral suspensions: 125 mg/5 mL, 250 mg/5mL, 200 mg/5 mL, 400 mg/5 mL; capsules 250 mg, 500 mg, tablets: 500 mg, 875 mg

Amoxicillin and Clavulanic Acid (Amoxicillin and Clavulanate) (Augmentin®)

__ mg/kg/dose __ 250 mg __ 500 mg ___ 875 mg ___ other PO administered as __ suspension __ tablets __ q 8 hours __ q 12 hours

Dosage: usual dose 20–40 mg/kg/day divided into 2 doses given every 12 hours or high dose is 80-90 mg/kg/day in 2 divided doses given every 12 hours

Maximum: same maximums as for amoxicillin

Formulations: oral suspensions: 125 mg/ 5 mL, 200 mg/5 mL, 250mg/5 mL, 400 mg/5 mL, 600 mg/5 mL; tablets: 250 mg, 500 mg, 875 mg

Comments: Dose is based on the amoxicillin component; not all suspension formulations are interchangeable due to variable concentrations of the clavulanic acid

Ampicillin

__ mg/kg/dose __ mg __ IV__ IM __ PO administered as __ suspension __ capsules q 6 hours

Dosage: child/infant usual dose PO 50–100 mg/ kg/day every 6 hours, IM/IV 100–400 mg/kg/ day given every 6 hours

Maximum: 2–4 grams PO per day, IV 400 mg/ kg/day up to 12 grams IM/IV per day

Formulations: oral suspension 125 mg/5 mL, 250 mg/5 mL; oral capsules: 250 mg, 500 mg

Ampicillin and Sulbactam (Unasyn®)

__ mg/kg/dose __ mg __ IV __ IM q 6 hours ___ other

Dosage: usual dose child/infant (age > 1 month) IM/IV 100–200 mg/kg/day divided into 4 doses given every 6 hours

Maximum: 8 grams ampicillin per 24 hours or 12 grams ampicillin and sulbactam per 24 hours

Azithromycin (Zithromax®)

__ mg/kg/dose __ mg __ IV__ PO administered as __ suspension __ tablets daily or

__ mg/kg/dose __ mg __ IV __PO administered as __ suspension __ tablets on day 1 and __ mg/kg __ mg on days 2–5; for adolescents and adults: __ 500 mg on day 1 then 250 mg on days 2–5 __ IV __ PO administered as __ suspension __ tablets; __ 500 mg days 1–3 __ IV or __ PO administered as __ suspension __ tablets; __ other

Dosage: usual dose 5–10 mg/kg/day depending on 1, 3, or 5 day regimen

Maximum: dose for one day 500 mg

Formulations: oral suspensions: 100 mg/5 mL, 200 mg/5 mL; tablets: 250 mg, 500 mg

Cefazolin (Ancef®, Kefzol®)

Child/infant > 1 month __ mg/kg/dose __ mg __IV __IM q 8 hours

Adolescents/adults __ milligrams/dose __ IV __ IM __ q 6 hours __ q 8 hours

Dosage: usual child/infant dose 50–100 mg/ day divided into 3 doses, usual adult dose 2–6 grams per day divided into 3 or 4 doses

Maximum: 6 grams per day; up to 12 grams per day in adults

Ceftriaxone (Rocephin®)

Child/infant __ mg/kg/dose __ mg __ IV __ IM __ qd __ q 12 hours

Adolescent/adult __ 1 gram/dose __ 2 grams/ dose __ other __ IV __ IM __ qd __ q 12 hours; for gonococcal cervicitis __ 125 mg IM × 1 __ 250 mg IM × 1

Dosage: usual dose for child/infant 50–100 mg/ kg/day divided into 1–2 doses, usual dose for adolescent/adult 1–2 grams/dose; for gonococcal cervicitis, one IM dose of 125 mg if weight < 45 kg, 250 mg if weight > 45 kg

Maximum: child/infant: usual maximum 2 grams per day, for adolescent/adult: maximum 2 grams per dose

Comments: Higher doses of 100 mg/kg/day up to 4 grams per day for meningitis/other CNS infections

Cephalexin (Keflex®)

__ mg/kg/dose __ mg PO administered as __ suspension __ tablets/capsules

__ q 6 hours __ q 12 hours

Dosage: usual infant/child dose 25–100 mg/kg/ dose divided into 2 or 4 doses, adult dose 1–4 grams per day divided into 4 doses

Maximum: 4 grams per day

Formulations: oral suspensions: 125 mg/5 mL, 250 mg/5 mL; tablets/capsules: 250 mg, 500 mg

Clindamycin (Cleocin®)

__ mg/kg/dose ___ mg/dose __ IV __ PO administered as __ solution __ capsules

__ q 6 hours __ q 8 hours

Dosage: usual dose child: 10–40 mg/kg/day PO or 20–40 mg/kg/day IV in 3–4 divided doses; usual adult dose 150–450 mg per dose PO every 6–8 hours, 1,200–2,700 mg IV per day in 2–4 divided doses

Maximum: child: 1,800 mg per day PO; 2,700 mg per day IV; adult: 1,800 mg per day PO, 4,800 mg IV/IM per day

Formulations: oral solution 75 mg/5 mL; capsules: 75 mg, 150 mg, 300 mg

Comments: Oral clindamycin is administered in smaller and more frequent doses than IV doses in order to decrease gastrointestinal upset

Penicillin G Benzathine (Bicillin L-A®)

__ 600,000 units __ 1.2 million units ___ 2.4 million units __ IM once

Dosage: usual dose for group A streptococcal infections: child: weight ≤ 27 kg is 600,000 U/dose IM × 1 and weight > 27 kg and adults 1.2 million units IM × 1

Maximum: single dose 2.4 million units

Comments: Used for treatment of streptococcal infections

Only for IM injection, not for IV use

Penicillin G (Benzathine and Procaine) (Bicillin C-R®)

__ 600,000 units __ 1.2 million units ___ 2.4 million units IM once

Dosage: usual dose for group A streptococcal infections: child: weight < 14 kg is 600,000 U/dose IM × 1, weight 14–27 kg: 900,000 to 1.2 million units IM × 1, weight ≥ 27 kg and adults is 2.4 million U/dose IM × 1; for primary prevention of rheumatic fever in children 6 months to 12 years: 1.2 million units IM × 1

Maximum: 1.2 million units for primary prevention dose, 2.4 million units for acute group A streptococcal infections

Comments: Used for treatment of streptococcal infections and primary prevention of rheumatic fever

Only for IM injection, not for IV use

Penicillin V Potassium (Veetids®)

___ mg/dose __ 250 mg __ 500 mg PO administered as __ solution __ tablets
__ q 6 hours __ q 8 hours __ other

Dosage: usual dose: child 25–50 mg/kg/day in 3–4 divided dose, adult 250–500 mg/dose q 6–8 hours

Maximum: child: 2 grams per day, adult; adult: 3 grams per day

Formulations: oral solutions: 125 mg/5 mL, 250 mg/5 mL; tablets: 250 mg, 500 mg

Piperacillin/Tazobactam (Zosyn®)

__ mg/kg/dose ___ 2.25 grams ___ 3.375 g __ other __ IV __ q 6 hours __ q 8 hours

Dosage: usual dose: infant > 9 months and child: 100 mg piperacillin/kg/dose every 8 hours, pediatric patients > 40 kg and adults 3.375 grams per dose every 6 hours

Maximum: 16 grams per day

Sulfamethoxazole and Trimethoprim (SMX-TMP, Co-trimoxazole®) (Bactrim DS®, Septra DS®)

__ mg/kg/dose __ mg __ other PO administered as __ suspension __ 1 tab __ 1 DS tab __ q 12 hours __ qd

Dosage: usual dose: child 8–12 mg/kg/day, adult 160–320 mg TMP/dose (dose based on TMP component)

Maximum: up to 20 mg TMP/kg/day in divided doses for more severe infections

Formulations: oral suspension: SMX 200 mg and TMP 40 mg/5 mL, tablets: SMX 400 mg and TMP 80 mg; double strength (DS) tablets = SMX 800 mg and TMP 160 mg

Comments: Once a day is usually for prophylaxis for urinary tract infection.

Drug not recommended for age < 2 months

Antiemetics
Hydroxyzine (Vistaril®)

__ mg/kg/dose __ 12.5 mg __ 25 mg __ 50 mg __ other __ IM __ q 6 hours __ q 8 hours ___ other __ prn pruritis __ prn anxiety __ prn nausea/vomiting

Dosage: for antiemetic: IM dose: usual child dose 1.1 mg/kg/dose; usual adult dose: 25–50 mg/dose, every 4–6 hours; for pruritus/anxiety: child < 6 years: 50 mg daily in 4 divided doses as needed; ≥ 6 years: 50–100 mg daily in 4 divided doses as needed; adult: 25 mg PO tid or qid

Maximum: single IM dose maximum 100 mg

Comments: Oral formulations are available but antiemetic indication only lists IM dosing.

IV administration is not recommended

Ondansetron (Zofran®)

__ 0.1 mg/kg/dose __ 0.15 mg/kg/dose __4 mg __ 8 mg __ other ___ IV __ PO administered as oral solution __ as ODT __ q 6 hours __ prn nausea/vomiting

Dosage: usual dose PO for gastroenteritis: child weight 8–15 kg 2 mg/dose, 16 to 30 kg 4 mg/dose, > 30 kg 4–8 mg; adult 4–8 mg; usual IV dose: child 0.1–0.15 mg/kg/dose; adult:4 mg/dose

Maximum: child: single dose 4 mg

Formulations: oral solution = 4 mg/5 mL, oral disintegrating tablets: 4 mg, 8 mg

Comments: **Avoid single dose > 16 mg due to possible QT prolongation**

Prochlorperazine (Compazine®)

__ mg/kg/dose __ 2.5 mg __ 5 mg __ 10 mg __ other __ IV__ IM __ PO __ q 6 hours __ q 8 hours ___ other __ prn nausea/vomiting

Dosage: usual PO dose: child age ≥ 2 years and ≥ 9 kg; by weight 9–13 kg 2.5 mg per dose every 12–24 hours, > 13–18 kg: 2.5 mg every 8–12 hours, > 18–39 kg: 2.5 mg PO every 8 hours or 5 mg every 12 hours; > 39 kg and adults 5–10 mg every 6–8 hours, usual child IM or IV dose: 0.1–0.15 mg/kg/dose every 6 or 8 hours; usual adult dose: PO/IV/IM is 5–10 mg/dose; usual adult dose PR: 25 mg bid

Maximum: child ≥ 2 years and weight ≥ 9 kg: daily dosing PO/PR maximum for 9–13 kg = 7.5 mg, > 13 kg is 10 mg, >18–39 kg is 15 mg > 39 kg is 40 mg; child maximum single IV dose = 10 mg, adult maximum for PO/IV/IM is 40 mg per day

Formulations: tablets: 5 mg, 10 mg; rectal suppository: 25 mg

Comments: PR dosing indication is listed for adults, but no PR dosing indication is listed for children

Promethazine (Phenergan®)

__ mg/kg/dose ___ 12.5 mg __ 25 mg __ other ___ IM __PR __ PO administered as __ syrup __ tablets __ q 4 hours __ q 6 hours __ q 8 hours ___ prn nausea/vomiting

Dosage: usual dose PO/IM/PR: child ≥ 2 years 0.25–1 mg/kg/dose every 4–6 hours, adult 12.5–25 mg/dose, every 4–6 hours

Maximum: 25 mg/dose

Formulations: oral syrup 6.25 mg/mL, tablets 12.5 mg, 25 mg; rectal suppositories 12.5 mg, 25 mg

Comments: **Avoid age < 2 years due to risk of respiratory depression. IV is not recommended**

due to risk of severe tissue injury. Avoid SQ or intra-arterial due to severe local reaction.

Trimethobenzamide (Tigan®)

__ mg/kg/dose __ 100mg __ 200 mg __ 300 mg __ other PO __ q 6 hours __ q 8 hours __ other ___ prn nausea/vomiting

Dosage: usual dose PO: child 15–20 mg/kg/day in 3–4 divided doses or by weight < 14 kg 100 mg/dose, 14–40 kg 100–200 mg/dose, > 40 kg and adult 300 mg/dose q 6–8 hour __ prn nausea/vomiting

Maximum: not listed

Formulations: capsules 300 mg, IM solution is available but not recommended in children

Comments: **IV is not recommended. IM is not recommended in children. PR is no longer available.**

Anxiolytics/Sleeping Pills

Lorazepam (Ativan®)

__ mg/kg/dose ___0.5 mg ___1 mg __ 2 mg __ other __ IV __ PO administered as __ solution __ tablets __ q 4 hours ___ q 6 hours ___ q 12 hours ___ qhs __ other ___ prn anxiety ___prn sleep

Dosage: usual PO/IV dose: child: 0.05 mg/kg/dose, adult: 2 mg PO, 1 mg IV with lower dose 0.5 mg IV, 1 mg PO in elderly or debilitated

Maximum: child: single dose 2 mg

Formulations: oral solution: 2 mg/mL, tablets: 0.5 mg, 1 mg, 2 mg

Allergy Medications

Cetirizine (Zyrtec®)

__ 2.5 mg daily __ 5 mg daily __ 10 mg PO administered as __ solution __ tablets __ chewable tablets qd

Dosage: age 6–12 months: 2.5 mg PO daily; 12 months to < 5 years: 2.5 mg daily, may increase to 2.5 mg every 12 hours; > 6 years and adults: 5–10 mg daily

Maximum: 10 mg per dose

Formulations: oral solution: 5 mg/5 mL; tablets: 5 mg, 10 mg; chewable tablets: 5 mg, 10 mg

Diphenhydramine (Benadryl®)

___ mg/kg/dose __ 25 mg ___ 50 mg __ IV __ PO administered as __ elixir __ capsules

__ every 6 hours __ qhs __ other __ prn itching

Dosage: allergic reaction usual dose PO/IM/IV: child 5 mg/kg/day in divided doses every 6–8 hours, > 12 years and adult 25–50 mg per dose; anaphylaxis (adjunct with epinephrine) PO/IM/IV 1–2 mg/kg/dose with 50 mg single dose maximum

Maximum: for allergic reaction: PO by age: < 6 years: 37.5 mg per day, 6–11 years 150 mg per day, > 12 years and adult: 300 mg per day; IM/IV: infants/children/adolescents: 300 mg daily; adult: single dose 100 mg, 400 mg per day

Formulations: oral elixir: 12.5 mg/5 mL, 25 mg/10 mL; capsules: 25 mg, 50 mg

Loratadine (Claritin®)

____ 5 mg __ 10 mg PO administered as __ solution/syrup __ oral concentrate __ capsules/tablets __ chewable tablets qd

Dosage: usual child dose: age 2–5 years 5 mg daily, ≥ 6 years and adult: 10 mg daily

Maximum: child: 5 mg daily, adult: 10 mg daily

Formulations: oral solution/syrup: 5mg/5 mL; oral concentrate 1mg/mL, capsule/tablet/ODT tablet 10 mg, oral chewable tablet: 5 mg

Steroids

Dexamethasone (Decadron®)

____ 0.02 mg/kg/day __ 0.3 mg/kg/day ____ mg/kg/day __ mg __ IV __ IM __PO administered as __ elixir/solution __ oral concentrate __ tablets __ qd

q __ hours __ other

Dosage: anti-inflammatory/immunosuppressant: 0.02–0.3 mg/kg/day, croup: 0.6 mg/kg × 1

Maximum: croup: 16–20 mg single dose

Formulations: oral elixir/solution: 0.5 mg/5 mL, oral concentrate 1 mg/mL, tablets: 0.5 mg, 0.75 mg, 1 mg, 1.5 mg, 2 mg, 4 mg, 6 mg

Comment: Recent studies have shown doses as low as 0.15 mg/kg may be effective with croup. Higher doses (1–2 mg/kg) are used for cerebral edema.

Prednisone† (Deltasone®, Liquid Pred®, Orasone®)

__ mg/kg/dose __ mg __ 40 mg __ 60 mg PO administered as __ solution __ tablets __ qd q __hours __ other

Dosage: usual dose: child 1–2 mg/kg/day, adult 40–80 mg per day, in 1–2 divided doses for pediatric and adult patients

Maximum: adults: 80 mg per day

Formulations: oral solution 5 mg/5 mL, tablets: 1 mg, 2.5 mg, 5 mg, 10 mg, 20 mg, 50 mg

Comments: Greater patient compliance is more likely with once-a-day vs. twice-daily dosing

Prednisolone† (Orapred®, Pediapred®, Prelone®, Veripred®)

__ mg/kg/dose ____ mg __ 40 mg __ 60 mg __ other PO administered as __ solution __ syrup __ tablets __ qd __ q 12 hours __ other

Dosage: usual dose: child 1–2 mg/kg/day, adult 40–80 mg per day, in 1–2 divided doses for pediatric and adult patients

Maximum: adults: 80 mg per day

Formulations: oral solutions: Pediapred® 5 mg/5 mL, Orapred® 15 mg/5 mL, Veripred® 20 mg/5mL: oral syrup: Prelone® 15mg/5 mL, tab = 5 mg

Comments: Dosing for prednisone and prednisolone is the same. Greater patient compliance is more likely with once-a-day vs. twice-daily dosing.

Methylprednisolone† (Medrol®, Medrol Dose Pack®, Solumedrol®)

__ mg/kg/dose __ mg __ every 12 hours __ daily __ other __ PO __ IV __ IM

Dosage: usual dose: child ≤ 12 years 1–2 mg/kg/day; child > 12 years and adult 40–60 mg/day; in 1–2 divided doses per day PO/IV/IM, in adults initial higher dose sometimes used __ 125 mg × 1 followed by 40–60 mg every 6 hours

Maximum: adults: initial dose 125 mg, subsequent doses: 80 mg per dose

Formulations: tablets: 2 mg, 4 mg, 8 mg

† Doses generally used for asthma. Much higher doses used in some specific disorders such as exacerbation of multiple sclerosis or for cerebral edema.

National Heart, Lung, and Blood Institute (NHBLI) Expert Panel Report (EPR) 3 guidelines for the diagnosis and treatment of asthma recommends prednisone or prednisolone 1–2 mg/kg/day for pediatrics, for adults 40–80 mg/day in 1–2 divided doses. Commonly, once-a-day dosing is used due for better compliance and the lower total daily dose of 40 or 60 mg maximum is used.

Asthma Medications

Nebulized Medications

Albuterol Nebulization (Proair®, Proventil®, Ventolin®)

__ mg/kg/dose __ 2.5 mg/dose __ 5.0 mg/dose __ × 1 __ q 20 minutes × 3__ q 4 hours __ q 6 hours ___ continuous nebulization __ 10 mg/ hour __15 mg/hour ___ other prn wheezing

Dosage: usual dose: infants/children up to 12 years 0.15 mg/kg/dose, adults 2.5–5 mg/ dose, continuous nebulization is 10–15 mg/ hour

Maximum: minimum single dose = 2.5 mg, maximum single dose = 5 mg

Formulation: solution for inhalation: 0.63 mg/3 mL, 1.25 mg/3 mL, 2.5 mg/3 mL

Comments: Doses recommended by National Heart Lung and Blood Institute (NHLBI) Expert Report Panel (EPR) – 3

Ipratropium Nebulization (Atrovent®)

__ 0.25 mg/dose ___ 0.5 mg/dose __ q 6 hours __ q 8 hours __ other __ prn wheezing

Dosage: usual dose: infants/children up to 12 years: 0.25–0.5 mg/dose, adults 0.5 mg/dose

Maximum: single dose: 0.5 mg (2.5 mL)

Formulation: solution for inhalation: 500 mcg (2.5 mL of 0.02% solution)

Comments: Doses recommended by National Heart Lung and Blood Institute (NHLBI) Expert Report Panel (EPR) – 3

Inhalers

Albuterol (Proventil®, Ventolin®) (MDI with spacer)

__ 1–2 puffs (90–180 mcg) __ q 4 hours __ q 6 hours __ other __ prn wheezing

Dosage: usual dose: child and adult 1–2 puffs [90–180 mcg] q 4–6 hours

Maximum: 8 puffs in a single dose for acute exacerbations

Formulation: 90 mcg/actuation

Ipratropium (Atrovent®)

__ 1–2 puffs __ 2–3 puffs q 6 hours __ other __ prn wheezing

Dosage: usual dose: child < 12 years 1–2 puffs, ≥ 12 years and adult 2–3 puffs, every 6 hours

Maximum: 8 puffs in a single dose for acute exacerbations

Formulation: 17 mcg/actuation

Cardiac

Furosemide (Lasix®)

___ mg ___ IV ___ PO administered as __ solution __ tablets q __ hours __ qd

Dosage: usual initial dose: child/infant PO 2 mg/kg/dose daily IV: 1–2 mg/kg/dose every 6–12 hours

Maximum: single dose PO 6 mg/kg; adults: IV: 200 mg daily, oral 600 mg daily

Formulations: oral solution: 10 mg/mL, 40 mg/5 mL; tablets: 20 mg, 40 mg, 80 mg

Gastrointestinal Drugs

Gastric Acid Proton Pump Inhibitors

Lansoprazole (Prevacid®)

___ 15 mg ___ 30 mg PO administered as ___ suspension ___ ODT ___ delayed release capsules qd

Dosage: usual dose: children 1–11 years old 15-30 mg once a day for gastroesophageal reflux disease (GERD), esophagitis or ulcer

Maximum: single dose 30 mg

Formulations: oral suspension: 3 mg/mL; ODT tablets (oral disintegrating tablets): 15 mg, 30 mg, delayed release capsules: 15 mg, 30 mg

Comments: Ineffective for treatment of symptomatic GERD in infants ages 1 to 11 months of age. Also used with the co-administration of antibiotics for the eradication of *Helicobacter pylori*.

Omeprazole (Prilosec®)

__ mg PO administered as __ suspension __ delayed release capsules __ bid __ qd

Dosage: usual PO dose: weight 5–10 kg: 5 mg daily, weight 10 to < 20 kg: 10 mg daily, weight > 20 kg: 20 mg daily, adult 20–40 mg/ day in 1–2 divided doses

Maximum: not listed

Formulations: oral suspension 2 mg/mL; delayed release capsules: 10 mg, 20 mg, 40 mg

Comments: Used with the co-administration of antibiotics for the eradication of *Helicobacter pylori.*

Pantoprazole (Protonix®)

__ 20 mg __ 40 mg PO __ qd __ other

Dosage: for erosive esophagitis associated with gastroesophageal reflux: age $\geq$ 5 years: weight $\geq$ 15 to < 40 kg, 20 mg daily; weight $\geq$ 40 kg, 40 mg daily

Maximum: usual single dose 40 mg

Formulations: tablets: 20 mg, 40 mg; oral pack: 40 mg

Comments: Used with the co-administration of antibiotics for the eradication of *Helicobacter pylori* (unlabeled use in the United States).

Histamine-2-Receptor Antagonist
Famotidine (Pepcid®)

___ mg __IV ___PO administered as __ suspension __ tablets ___ bid ___ qd

Dosage: usual PO dose: child 0.5 mg/kg/dose every 12–24 hours; IV dose 0.25 mg/kg/dose every 12–24 hours

Maximum: single dose 40 mg PO, single dose 20 mg IV

Formulations: oral suspension: 40 mg/5 mL, tablet: 10 mg, 20 mg, 40 mg

Laxatives
Polyethylene glycol – electrolyte solution (Miralax®)

__ mg PO __ qd

Dosage: usual initial PO dose for age $\geq$ 6 months 0.2 – 0.8 grams/kg

Maximum: dose 17 grams/day

Formulations: 17 grams powder dissolved in 8 ounces clear liquid

Comments: Do not use for more than 2 weeks

Radiology Studies for Patients with Contrast Allergy

Prestudy Orders

Prednisone __ mg __ 50 mg at 13, 7, 1 hour prior to study and diphenhydramine __ mg __ 50 mg at 1 hour prior to the study

Dosage: usual dose: prednisone 1 mg/kg up to 50 mg given 13 hours, 7 hours, and 1 hour prior to study and diphenhydramine 1 mg/kg up to 50 mg given 1 hour prior to the study

Other _____, _____, _____, _____

* This is not an all-inclusive list but gives some of the more commonly used medications with the dose, route, frequency, indications, and formulations. Commonly used brand names in the United States are listed. Dosing is primarily for the pediatric age group with adult doses also provided for pediatric patients eligible for adult dosing based on age and weight criteria. The dosing regimens listed do not take into account renal and/or hepatic impairment in which dosing adjustments may be necessary.

Inclusion of specific medications and medication regimens within these order sets and described throughout this textbook does not imply endorsement of any given medication, medication regimen, or product. The medication dosing regimens included are the usual suggested dosing ranges. However, patient-specific variables should always be taken into account as well as the most contemporary medical literature and standards of practice when determining the most appropriate therapeutic regimen for a given patient.

Generally, doses for only the first two days of therapy are provided since the observation unit is time limited, usually < 24 hours, so patients may be in the observation unit for part of one day and part of the next day only.

The formulations (e.g., oral, rectal, some subcutaneous) are listed because the health care provider may be initiating a medication in the observation unit and then subsequently writing a discharge prescription to continue the medication after observation unit discharge. However, the specific parenteral formulations of medications are not included within the order set due to significant variability secondary to manufacturing practices and institution-specific policies for preparation and administration.

Special considerations are needed for the use of medications in pediatric patients. Some medications commonly used in adults are not recommended in infants or young children. For example, tetracyclines (such as doxycycline and tetracycline) are not recommended in children < 8 years old due to effects related to permanent discoloration of the teeth, and fluoroquinolones (such as ciprofloxacin and levofloxacin) are not recommended as a first-line agent for pediatric patients due to reported adverse effects related to joints and/or surrounding tissues.

Because of concern for respiratory depression, opioids should be used with caution and patients receiving opioids, especially high doses, should probably be on continuous pulse oximetry and perhaps also capnography. Some institutions have used fentanyl for the treatment of sickle cell patients in observation units while others tend to use mainly morphine and hydromorphone, especially in pediatric patients.

Pediatric patients who may receive IV antibiotics for an infection, such as a non-immunocompromised patient with pharyngitis or cellulitis, may be appropriately managed in an observation unit; however, other patients requiring parenteral antibiotic therapy for indications such as osteomyelitis or endocarditis will likely require greater than 24 hours of inpatient hospital care and are therefore not appropriate candidates for pediatric observation. Similarly, some patients requiring opioid therapy for indications such as sickle cell disease may be appropriately treated in an ED observation unit; however, other patients requiring opioid therapy for indications such as pain associated with active malignancy will likely require inpatient care and would not be appropriate observation unit candidates.

Pediatric protocols with inclusion/exclusion criteria, diagnostic/treatment interventions, and disposition criteria can be developed for the pediatric observation unit similar to those for adults in observation status. These pediatric order sets are designed for use with pediatric protocols.

There are many advantages to utilizing order sets. Presenting preferred choices or options to a provider via an order set helps guide therapy decisions for patients. While providers have multiple options within an order set and can generate additional orders outside of order set recommendations, the order set provides specific guidance related to selected orders and related to management of specific disease states. Additionally, order sets can be utilized to restrict certain medication therapies to selected patients who meet pre-specified criteria to maximize patient safety and outcomes. Ultimately, the benefits of order sets include ease of use, increased provider efficiency, increased medication safety and patient safety, and promotion of "best practices."

IM = intramuscular
IV = intravenous
PO = per os = by or through the mouth
PR = per rectum
SQ = subcutaneous

Note: Weight based pediatric doses shouldn't exceed typical adult doses.

Chapter 96

Pediatric Order Sets
Generic or General Order Set

Sharon E. Mace, MD, FACEP, FAAP

Pediatric Generic (General) Order Set

Place in Emergency Department (ED)
Observation _____
Diagnosis _____, _____,
_____

ED Attending _____
Resident (if applicable) _____
Advanced Practice Provider (if applicable)
_____

Allergies: Yes _____ No _____

If yes, what _____, _____, _____, _____,
_____, _____

Vital Signs

Temperature __ Pulse __ Respiration __ BP__
Pulse oximetry ____
__ q 2 hours ___ q 4 hours ___ q 6 hours q ___
hours ___ q shift ___ qd ____ other
Cardiac monitoring (telemetry) _____
Orthostatic vital signs _____
Continuous pulse oximetry _____
Neurologic checks __ q 2 hours __ q 4 hours __
q 6 hours q __hours __ q shift __ qd __ other
Vascular checks __ q 2 hours __ q 4 hours __
q 6 hours q __hours __ q shift __ qd __ other
Other _____

Notify Physician if

Temperature (°C) > 38.0° ____ 38.5°____ 39° ____
40° ____ other _____
Systolic blood pressure (mmHg) ≤ 90 ___
≥ 160 __ ≥ 180 ___ ≥ 200 __ other _____
Diastolic blood pressure (mmHg) ≥ 120 ____
other _____
Heart rate ≤ 50 ___ ≥ 120 __ ≥ 150 ___
≥ 200 ___ other ____
Oxygen saturation < 90% _____ other _____
Any change in mental status _____

Any respiratory distress _____
Any new or worsening change in extremity (such
as color: pale or cyanotic, decreased capillary
fill, diminished or absent pulses, increased
pain, numbness or paresthesias) ____

Activity

Up ad lib _____
Assisted _____
Out of bed to chair _____
Bedrest with bathroom privileges _____
Bedrest with bedside commode _____
Bedrest _____
Other _____

Diet (Age Appropriate)

NPO _____
Regular _____
Advance diet as tolerated _____
Clear liquids ____
Dental, mechanical soft _____
Diabetic _____
Formula _____
Full liquids _____
Low added fat/No added salt _____
Low cholesterol ____
Pureed _____
Sodium: 1 gram ___ 2 gram ___
unrestricted____
Per feeding tube _____
Other _____

Nursing Interventions

Weight ___ on admission ___ qd ___ prior to
discharge ____ other
Height ____
I & Os _____ routine _____ strict _____
Fluid restriction ___ mL/hour ___ mL/shift
____ mL/24 hour ___ other
Fall precautions _____

Seizure precautions _____

Capillary blood glucose ___ × 1 q ___ hours ___ before meals and at bedtime

Foley catheter ___ Straight cath for urine _____

Elevation of extremity _____

Elevate head of bed at 30° _____

Wound Care

Dressing change q ___ hours ___ qd Wet to dry dressing q ___ hours ___ qd

Packing change in __ hours __ qd Packing removal in _____ hours

Respiratory Interventions

Oxygen __ liters nasal cannula __ venti mask at ___ liters per minute _____ other

Wean oxygen as tolerated without dyspnea, stridor or oxygen saturation < 90% ____

Peak flow __ on admission ___ prior to discharge ___ pre and post aerosols

Sleep apnea qhs __ CPAP BiPAP settings cm H_2O ___ inspiratory __ expiratory

Incentive spirometry __ q 2 hours __ q 4 hours __ q 6 hours q __ hours

Laboratory Tests

Amylase ___

Arterial blood gas ___ on room air ___ on other $FiO2$ ____

Basic metabolic panel _____

Blood alcohol level ____

Brain natriuretic peptide (BNP) _____

Calcium ____ total ___ ionized

Carbon monoxide _____

Cardiac enzymes __ × 1 __ with ECG ___ other

CBC _____ with differential

Complete metabolic panel _____

C-reactive protein (CRP) _____

Creatinine phosphokinase (total) (total CPK) __ × 1 __ repeat in a.m., repeat q __ hours × __

CK-MB (creatinine kinase – myocardial band) __ × 1 __ with ECG ___ other

D-dimer _____

Drug level _____, _____, _____

Erythrocyte sedimentation rate (ESR) _____

Fasting lipid panel ___

Glucose _____

Hemoglobin/hematocrit _____ Repeat hemoglobin/hematocrit ___ in a.m. ___ at ___ hours

Influenza studies (influenza A and B) (by nasal swab) _____

Lactate _____

Lipase ___

Liver function tests _____

Magnesium ____

Monospot ___

Phosphorus ___

Pregnancy test (qualitative urine) _____

Pregnancy test (quantitative blood) _____

Rapid Strept ___

Renal function tests (BUN, creatinine) _____

Respiratory antigen panel (by nasal swab) ___

Respiratory syncytial virus (RSV) swab (by nasal swab) ___

Toxicology: blood drug screen ____

Toxicology: urine drug screen ____

Troponin __ × 1 __ with ECG ___ other

TSH (thyroid stimulating hormone) ___

Thyroid function tests (T3, T4, TSH) ____

Type and cross for __ units packed red blood cells

Type and Screen _____

Urinalysis _____

Urine culture _____

Urine for amino acids ___

Urine 24 hour ___ for _____

Venous blood gas ____

Cultures:

Blood culture peripheral × ___ from central line × ___

Throat culture _____

Urine culture _____

Wound culture _____ site _____

Gonorrhea_____ site _____

Chlamydia _____ site _____

Trichomonas _____ site _____

Fungal (Candida, KOH) ___ site ____

Cerebrospinal Fluid (CSF) ___ culture ___ gram stain ___ CSF cell count ___ ___ CSF protein ___ CSF glucose ____ viral studies

CSF Other _____, _____, _____, _____, _____, _____, _____

Other _____

Radiology Studies

Plain X-rays

Acute abdominal series _____

Babygram _____

CXR portable_____

CXR (PA and lateral) _____

Extremity x-rays _____ right ___ left _____

KUB (Kidneys, ureters, bladder) x-ray

_____

Spine x-rays: Cervical ___ Thoracic ___
Lumbar _____

Soft tissue neck (PA and lateral) _____

Other _____, _____, _____

CT (Computed Tomography) Scans

CT abdomen/pelvis _____ without contrast _____
with contrast ___ IV ___ PO ___ PR

CT abdomen, renal stone protocol _____

CT brain _____ without contrast _____ with
contrast

CT chest _____ without contrast _____ with
contrast

CT face _____ without contrast _____ with
contrast

CT neck ___ without contrast _____ with
contrast

CT kidneys _____ without contrast _____ with
contrast

CT enterography _____

CTA (computed tomography angiography)
of brain without contrast ___ ___ with
contrast

Other _____, _____, _____

Ultrasound

Ultrasound abdomen (right upper quadrant)

_____

Ultrasound carotids: right ___ left ___
bilateral _____

Ultrasound extremity (rule out deep vein
thrombosis) ___ Upper ___ Lower ___ Right
___ Left

Ultrasound kidneys _____

Ultrasound pelvis _____

Ultrasound _____

MRI (Magnetic Resonance Imaging)

MRI (Magnetic resonance imaging) of brain
_____ without contrast _____ with contrast

MRA (Magnetic resonance angiography)
Circle of Willis and of Carotids ___
without contrast _____ with contrast

MRI chest ___ without contrast ___ with
contrast

MRI abdomen ___ without contrast ___ with
contrast

MRI extremity ___ without contrast ___ with
contrast

MRI spine: ___ cervical ___ thoracic ___
lumbar ___ without contrast ___ with
contrast

MRI _____

Other Radiology Studies

Cholescintigraphy (hepatic iminodiacetic acid
[HIDA] scan) _____

Transcranial doppler of brain vessels _____

Other _____, _____, _____

Interventional Radiology Procedures

Lumbar puncture under fluoroscopy

_____

Line placement _____

Feeding tube placement _____

Allergy Pretreatment for CT scans if contrast
given for contrast allergy

Administer 13 hours prior to the study:
prednisone 1–2 mg/kg (up to 50 mg) PO,
administer 7 hours prior to the study:
prednisone 1–2 mg/kg (up to 50 mg) PO,
and administer 1 hour prior to the study:
prednisone 1–2 mg/kg (up to 50 mg PO) and
diphenhydramine 1–2 mg/kg (up to 50 mg)
PO _____

Cardiac Studies

Serial ECGs ___ × 1 ___ q 4 hours × 3 ___ q
4 hours × 4 ___ other _____ with cardiac
enzymes

Echocardiogram (transthoracic) ___ with
agitated (bubble) study ___ without agitated
(bubble)

Neurologic Studies

Electroencephalogram (EEG) _____

Consultants

Pediatric cardiology _____ Notified:
Name _____ Time _____

Care coordinator (Case manager)_____
    Notified: Name _____ Time _____
Dentistry _____ Notified:
    Name _____ Time _____
Pediatric dermatology _____ Notified: Name
    _____ Time _____
Dietician _____ Notified:
    Name _____ Time _____
Pediatric endocrinology ____ Notified:
    Name _____ Time _____
Family practice _____ Notified:
    Name _____ Time _____
Pediatric gastroenterology ____Notified:
    Name _____ Time _____
Pediatric surgery _____Notified:
    Name _____ Time _____
Hand surgery _____ Notified:
    Name _____ Time _____
Pediatric nephrology _____Notified:
    Name _____ Time _____
Pediatric neurology _____Notified:
    Name _____ Time _____

Pediatric neurosurgery _____ Notified:
    Name _____ Time _____
Pediatric orthopedics _____ Notified:
    Name _____ Time _____
PICC line _____ Notified:
    Name _____ Time _____
Pediatric pulmonary_____ Notified:
    Name _____ Time _____
Pediatric radiology_____ Notified:
    Name _____ Time _____
Pediatric rheumatology_____ Notified:
    Name _____ Time _____
Social work _____ Notified:
    Name _____ Time _____
Pediatric Urology _____ Notified:
    Name _____ Time _____
Other _____ Notified:
    Name _____ Time _____

Education: patient _____ family _____
    Other _____

Prologue

Observation Medicine Is Not the Same as Observation Status

Sharon E. Mace, MD, FACEP, FAAP

Robert E. O'Connor, MD, MPH, FACEP

There has been a steady increase in the use of observation medicine in the emergency department (ED) in recent years. There has also been an unfortunate adoption of the use of "observation" to denote patients admitted to the hospital under observation status. Observation medicine is not the same as observation status, and we need to be clear when we use the terms, as they have very different meanings.

Approximately 2.1% of all ED visits in the United States result in observation care.[1] Observation medicine has shown tremendous benefit in terms of patient care and cost-effectiveness (see Table 1.3 in Chapter 1). Observation medicine has been applied to a host of clinical conditions, including chest pain, heart failure, and respiratory ailments (see Part IV for a more complete list). Considering the advantages of observation medicine, the question should be asked: If you are not doing observation, what's stopping you? (See evidence-based Chapters 80 and 81.)

On the other hand, the Centers for Medicare and Medicaid (CMS) has defined observation status as

> a well-defined set of specific, clinically appropriate services, which include ongoing short-term treatment, assessment, and reassessment before a decision can be made regarding whether patients will require further treatment as hospital inpatients or if they are able to be discharged from the hospital. Observation status is commonly assigned to patients who present to the emergency department and who then require a significant period of treatment or monitoring before a decision is made concerning their admission or discharge, (and) in the majority of cases, the decision can be made in less than 48 hours, usually in less than 24 hours. In only rare and exceptional cases do outpatient observation services span more than 48 hours.[2]

The caveat is that the benefits of observation medicine are best attained and may only be achievable in an observation unit (OU) that is "operationally and physically distinct"[3] or a type I unit.[4] (See Chapter 1.) Studies that fail to document the benefits of observation care generally are those in which patients in observation status differ markedly from the CMS definition of observation, and thus are not treated in a type I unit.[5] (See Chapter 1.)

Why then the controversy surrounding observation medicine? The issue does not pertain to the clinical utility and the financial benefits using of observation medicine practiced in a type I unit, but instead is associated with the occasional case where there is an unanticipated and high out-of-pocket cost to the patient.[6–8]

According to the Office of Inspector General's (OIG) report, of the 1.5 million observation stays in 2012, 78% began with the beneficiary being treated in the ED, 9% began with an operating room procedure, and 13% other. "The most common operating room procedure was coronary stent insertion … The remaining observation stays began in other ways, such as with scheduled clinic visits, minor procedures, or laboratory and imaging services."[8] Thus, we may be comparing apples and oranges. It seems obvious that ED patients are not the same as post–operating room patients or post–coronary stent patients.

Short inpatient stays are "inpatient stays that lasted less than 2 nights," per the CMS definition.[9] This time frame is similar to the CMS definition of observation as noted earlier.[2] The OIG report compared short inpatient stays with observation stays and found "on average, Medicare paid nearly three times more for a short inpatient stay than an observation stay and beneficiaries paid almost two times more." Medicare paid an average of $5,142 per stay for short inpatient stays and only $1,741 for observation stays.[9] Thus, there is a concern by CMS and others about beneficiaries spending long periods of time in observation status without being admitted as inpatients."[9, 10]

When the patient is considered, "Beneficiaries also paid more for short inpatient stays than for observation stays." Beneficiaries paid an average of $725 for a short inpatient stay, compared with only $401 on an average for the observation stay. "Beneficiaries typically paid more for short inpatient stays than for observation stays when they were treated for the same reason, although there were some exceptions."[9]

For all but two of the most common reasons, beneficiaries paid more for short inpatient stays, with these stays costing an average of $359 to $572 more than observation stays. For the two exceptions – coronary stent insertions and circulatory disorders – beneficiaries paid more on average for short inpatient stays. For these stays, the difference in average payments was $817 and $167, respectively. In 94% of all of the 1.5 million observation stays, beneficiaries did not pay more than the inpatient deductible, while in only 6% "of all observation stays, beneficiaries paid more than the inpatient deductible."[9]

Two issues are at the core of the controversy. Patients in observation status lack coverage for their chronic routine medications and do not qualify under Medicare for skilled nursing facility (SNF) services. Medicare coverage for SNF services requires a three-day inpatient stay. According to the OIG report, "for 4 percent of these stays, beneficiaries received SNF services for which they did not qualify"[9] and conversely the other 96% of beneficiaries did qualify for SNF services. Please note that the OIG defined patients as not qualifying for SNF services based on their placement in observation status and not on the nature of their medical condition or post-hospitalization needs. For example, a patient who has suffered a stroke and is placed in observation status would be defined by CMS as not qualifying for SNF services even if they required extensive rehabilitation following release from the hospital.

Why the problems or controversy with Medicare coverage? Inpatients are covered under Part A Medicare and outpatients are covered under Part B Medicare. Observation is considered outpatient care, and so an observation stay is covered by an outpatient insurance benefit. While patients are in observation status, any chronic routine medications that are administered during the observation stay are not covered. Beneficiaries who are not admitted as inpatients may not qualify for SNF services following discharge from the hospital and may end up paying out of pocket for their SNF services. Moreover, if a patient is in the ED or observation and then is admitted to the hospital, the time spent in the ED or observation is not counted toward the three-day SNF requirement.

What are the solutions? This "loophole in coverage has been previously identified as a policy failure, and advocacy groups and politicians are leading ongoing efforts to fix this."[12] Several Observation Status bills have been introduced in Congress.[5, 13] Even though there are efforts to provide temporary solutions to the financial implications of this loophole, we still need to continue the advocacy for patients in order to address these issues.[12]

This is one of the many reasons why we make the distinction throughout this textbook that the correct, appropriate use of observation is time limited, specifically less than 24 hours, and is best accomplished through a type I OU. In the authors' opinion, we agree with CMS that long, extended observation stays are inappropriate and should be discouraged.

Observation medicine holds great promise for your practice. By using an OU, emergency physicians are able to contain cost and provide for patient safety by reducing unnecessary hospital admissions and mitigating the risk of managing patients with potentially life-threatening chief complaints. This text provides information on how to start and manage an OU, including the proper identification of patients and the appropriate use of protocols. Everything you need to start an OU in your hospital is contained in this book. What are you waiting for?

Sharon E. Mace, M.D., FACEP, FAAP
Robert E. O'Connor, M.D., MPH, FACEP

References

1. Wiler JL, Ross MA, Ginde AA. National study of emergency department observation services. *Acad Emerg Med* 2011; 18(9):959–965.

2. Centers for Medicare and Medicaid Services (CMS). Medicare benefit policy manual, chapter 6, hospital services covered under Part B [Internet]. Baltimore, MD: CMS [revised Mar 1, 2013]. www.cms.gov/Regulations-and Guidance/Guidance/ Transmittals/downloads/ R42BP.pdf (last accessed December 5, 2014)

3. Macy ML, Hall M, and Shah SS, et al. Differences in designation of observation care in US freestanding Children's Hospitals: are they virtual or are they real? *J Hosp Med* 2012: 7(4): 287–293.

4. Ross MA, Hockenberry JM, Mutter R, et al. Protocol-driven emergency department observation units offer savings, shorter stays and reduced admissions. *Health Affairs* 2013: 32(12):2149–2156.

5. Sheehy AM, Graf B, Gangireddy S, et al. Hospitalized but not admitted characteristics of patients with "observation status" at an academic medical center. *JAMA Intern Med* 2013:173 (21):1991–1998.

6. Center for Medicare Advocacy. Observation status & Bagnall v. Sebelius. www.medicare advocacy.org/medicare-info/ observation-status (last accessed December 4, 2014)

7. Jaffe S. $18 for a baby aspirin? Hospitals hike costs for everyday drugs for some patients. *Kaiser Health News.* April 30, 2012.

8. Span, P. In the hospital, but not really a patient. *The New York Times,* New Old Age Blog, http://newoldage.blogs .nytimes.com/2012/06/22/in- the-hospital-but-not-really-a- patient/ (last accessed December 5, 2014)

9. Wright S. Memorandum report: hospitals' use of observation stays and short inpatient stays for Medicare beneficiaries, OEI-02-12-00040.

Department of Health and Human Services, Office of Inspector General. July 29, 2013, http://oig.hhs.gov/oei/ reports/oei-02-12-00040.pdf (last accessed December 21, 2015)

10. CMS, Listening Session: Hospital Observation Beds, Aug. 24, 2010. Transcript available: www.cms.gov/ hospitaloutpatientpps/ downloads/94244031Hospital ObservationBedsListening Session082410.pdf

11. Figel, C. Lawmakers try to eliminate Medicare coverage technicality. *American Medical News,* Nov. 7, 2011. www .amednews.com/article/ 20111107/government/ 311079953/7/ (last accessed December 5, 2014)

12. Natsui S, Baugh C. What's your policy on home meds for observation patients? *ACEP News,* November 2014, pp. 14.

13. United States Congress HR 1179 and S 569. Improving access to Medicare coverage act of 2013. 113th Congress, 1st Session.

Index